COTTRELL AND YOUNG'S NEUROANESTHESIA

COTTRELL AND YOUNG'S NEUROANESTHESIA

FIFTH EDITION

James E. Cottrell, MD, FRCA

Distinguished Service Professor and Chairman
Department of Anesthesiology
State University of New York Downstate College of Medicine
Brooklyn, New York

William L. Young, MD

James P. Livingston Professor and Vice-Chair
Department of Anesthesia and Perioperative Care
Professor of Neurological Surgery and Neurology
University of California, San Francisco School of Medicine
Director, UCSF Center for Cerebrovascular Research
San Francisco, California

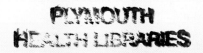
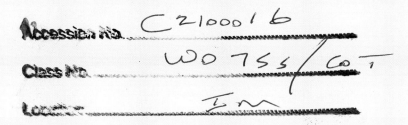
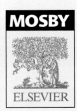

MOSBY

ELSEVIER

1600 John F. Kennedy Blvd.
Ste 1800
Philadelphia, PA 19103-2899

COTTRELL AND YOUNG'S NEUROANESTHESIA   ISBN: 978-0-323-05908-4

Copyright © 2010, 2001, 1994, 1986, 1980 by Mosby, Inc., an affiliate of Elsevier Inc.

Notice

Knowledge and best practice in this field are constantly changing. As new research and experience broaden
our knowledge, changes in practice, treatment, and drug therapy may become necessary or appropriate.
Readers are advised to check the most current information provided (i) on procedures featured or (ii) by
the manufacturer of each product to be administered to verify the recommended dose or formula, the
method and duration of administration, and contraindications. It is the responsibility of the practitioner,
relying on his or her own experience and knowledge of the patient, to make diagnoses, to determine dosages
and the best treatment for each individual patient, and to take all appropriate safety precautions. To the
fullest extent of the law, neither the Publisher nor the Authors assume any liability for any injury and/or
damage to persons or property arising out of or related to any use of the material contained in this book.

The Publisher

Library of Congress Cataloging-in-Publication Data

Cottrell's neuroanesthesia / [edited by] James E. Cottrell, William L.
Young. — 5th ed.
    p. ; cm.
  Rev. ed. of: Anesthesia and neurosurgery / [edited by] James E.
Cottrell, David S. Smith. 4th ed. c2001.
  Includes bibliographical references and index.
  ISBN 978-0-323-05908-4
  1. Nervous system—Surgery. 2. Anesthesia in neurology. I. Cottrell,
James E. II. Young, William L. III. Anesthesia and neurosurgery. IV.
Title: Neuroanesthesia.
  [DNLM: 1. Anesthesia. 2. Neurosurgical Procedures. WO 200 C851
2010]
  RD593.A5 2010
  617.9'6748—dc22   2009039629

Executive Publisher: Natasha Andjelkovic
Editorial Assistant: Bradley McIlwain
Publishing Services Manager: Hemamalini Rajendrababu
Project Manager: Srikumar Narayanan
Design Direction: Ellen Zanolle

Printed in the United States of America

Last digit is the print number: 9 8 7 6 5 4 3 2 1

CONTRIBUTORS

Alan A. Artru, MD
Professor, Associate Medical Director, and Chief of Anesthesia
Department of Anesthesiology
University of Washington School of Medicine
Seattle, Washington

Audrée A. Bendo, MD
Professor and Vice-Chair for Education
Department of Anesthesiology
SUNY Downstate Medical Center
Brooklyn, New York

Paolo A. Bolognese, MD
Department of Neurosurgery
The Chiari Institute, Harvey Cushing Institute of Neuroscience
North Shore-Long Island Jewish Health System
Manhasset, New York

Meredith R. Brooks, MD, MPH
Clinical Instructor, Department of Anesthesia
Lucile Salter Packard Children's Hospital
Stanford University Medical Center
Stanford, California

Nicolas Bruder, MD
Professor of Anesthesiology and Intensive Care
Medical Director
CHU Timone, Université de la Méditerranée
Marseille, France

Jean Charchaflieh, MD, MPH
Associate Professor of Anesthesiology and Critical Care
Director of Anesthesiology Critical Care Program
SUNY Downstate Medical Center
Brooklyn, New York

Daniel J. Cole, MD
Professor of Anesthesiology
College of Medicine, Mayo Clinic
Chairman, Department of Anesthesiology
Mayo Clinic Arizona
Phoenix, Arizona

James E. Cottrell, MD, FRCA
Distinguished Professor and Chairman
Department of Anesthesiology
SUNY Downstate Medical Center
Brooklyn, New York

Gregory Crosby, MD
Associate Professor of Anesthesia
Harvard Medical School
Brigham and Women's Hospital
Boston, Massachusetts

Deborah J. Culley, MD
Assistant Professor of Anesthesia
Harvard Medical School
Boston, Massachusetts

Marek Czosnyka, PhD
Reader in Brain Physics
Department of Clinical Neurosciences
Neurosurgical Unit, University of Cambridge
Addenbrooke's Hospital
Cambridge, United Kingdom

Karen B. Domino, MD, MPH
Professor of Anesthesiology and Pain Medicine
Vice Chair of Clinical Research
Adjunct Professor of Neurological Surgery
University of Washington School of Medicine
Seattle, Washington

Christopher F. Dowd, MD
Clinical Professor of Radiology and Biomedical Imaging,
Neurosurgery, Neurology, and Anesthesia and Perioperative Care
The Neurovascular Medical Group
Interventional Neuroradiology
University of California, San Francisco
San Francisco, California

Cassie L. Gabriel, MD
Chief Resident
Department of Anesthesiology
Loma Linda University
Loma Linda, California

Adrian W. Gelb, MBChB, FRCPC
Professor and Vice Chair for Faculty Affairs
Department of Anesthesia and Perioperative Care
University of California, San Francisco
San Francisco, California

Ian A. Herrick, MD, MPA, FRCPCA

Associate Professor of Anesthesia and Clinical Pharmacology
University of Western Ontario
Director, Department of Anesthesia and Perioperative Medicine
London Health Sciences Centre
London, Ontario, Canada

Randall T. Higashida, MD

Clinical Professor of Radiology, Neurological Surgery,
  Neurology and Anesthesia
Chief, Division of Neurointerventional Radiology
University of California, San Francisco Medical Center
San Francisco, California

Leslie Jameson, MD

Associate Professor and Vice Chair of Anesthesia
University of Colorado – Denver
Aurora, Colorado

Daniel Janik, MD

Associate Professor of Anesthesia
University of Colorado – Denver
Aurora, Colorado

Shailendra Joshi, MD

Assistant Professor
Department of Anesthesiology
College of Physicians and Surgeons of Columbia University
New York, New York

Ira Sanford Kass, PhD

Professor of Anesthesiology and Physiology and
  Pharmacology
State University of New York Downstate Medical Center
Brooklyn, New York

W. Andrew Kofke, MD, MBA, FCCM

Professor of Anesthesiology and Critical Care Medicine
Director of Neurosurgical Anesthesiology
Co-Director, Neurosurgical Critical Care
University of Pennsylvania
Philadelphia, Pennsylvania

Arthur M. Lam, MD, FRCPC

Professor of Anesthesiology and Neurological Surgery
University of Washington
Attending Anesthesiologist and Neurointensivist
Director of Cerebrovascular Laboratory
Harborview Medical Center
Seattle, Washington

Michael T. Lawton, MD

Professor of Neurological Surgery
Tong-Po Kan Endowed Chair
Chief, Cerebrovascular and Skull Base Surgery Programs
Director, Cerebrovascular Disorders Program
University of California, San Francisco
San Francisco, California

Carlos J. Ledezma, MD

Department of Radiology
Morristown Memorial Hospital
Morristown, New Jersey

Baiping Lei, MD, PhD

Research Assistant Professor
Anesthesiology Department
SUNY Downstate Medical Center
Brooklyn, New York

Alex John London, PhD

Associate Professor of Philosophy
Director, Center for the Advancement of Applied Ethics
  and Political Philosophy
Carnegie Mellon University
Pittsburgh, Pennsylvania

Michelle Lotto, MD

Oregon Anesthesiology Group
Portland, Oregon

Mishiya Matsumoto, MD

Professor of Anesthesiology
Yamaguchi University Graduate School of Medicine
Ube, Yamaguchi, Japan

Basil Matta, MD, FRCA

Divisional Director
Emergency and Perioperative Care
Associate Medical Director
Cambridge University Trust Hospitals
Cambridge, United Kingdom

Michael L. McManus, MD, MPH

Senior Associate in Medicine, Anesthesia and Critical Care
Children's Hospital Boston
Associate Professor
Harvard Medical School
Boston, Massachusetts

Thomas H. Milhorat, MD

Department of Neurosurgery
The Chiari Institute, Harvey Cushing Institute of Neuroscience
North Shore-Long Island Jewish Health System
Manhasset, New York

Jonathan D. Moreno, PhD

David and Lyn Silfen University Professor
Professor of Medical Ethics, History and Sociology of Science
University of Pennsylvania
Philadelphia, Pennsylvania

Eugene Ornstein, MD, PhD

Associate Professor
Department of Anesthesiology
College of Physicians and Surgeons of Columbia University
New York, New York

Ryan P. Pong, MD
Anesthesiology Faculty
Department of Anesthesiology
Virginia Mason Medical Center
Seattle, Washington

Patrick A. Ravussin, MD
Professor
Head of Department of Anesthesiology
CHCVs Sion Hospital
Sion, Switzerland

Angelique M. Reitsma, MD, MA
Program Manager
Scattergood Program for the Applied Ethics of Behavioral
    Health
University of Pennsylvania
Philadelphia, Pennsylvania

Irene Rozet, MD
Associate Professor of Anesthesiology
University of Washington
Seattle, Washington

Renata Rusa, MD
Associate Professor of Anesthesiology and Perioperative Medicine
Oregon Health and Science University
Portland, Oregon

Takefumi Sakabe, MD, PhD
Professor of Anesthesiology
Yamaguchi University Graduate School of Medicine
Ube, Yamaguchi, Japan

Armin Schubert, MD, MBA
Chair
Department of Anesthesiology
Ochsner Health System
New Orleans, Louisiana

Tod B. Sloan, MD, MBA, PhD
Professor of Anesthesia
University of Colorado Denver
Aurora, Colorado

David S. Smith, MD, PhD
Associate Professor of Anesthesiology and Critical Care
Department of Anesthesiology
University of Pennsylvania
Philadelphia, Pennsylvania

Sulpicio G. Soriano, MD, FAAP
Associate Professor of Anesthesia
Harvard Medical School
Children's Hospital Endowed Chair in Pediatric
    Neuroanesthesia
Senior Associate in Anesthesiology
Children's Hospital Boston
Boston, Massachusetts

Gary R. Stier, MD
Associate Professor and Program Director
Department of Anesthesiology and Critical Care
Loma Linda University School of Medicine
Loma Linda, California

Helen R. Stutz, DO
Assistant Professor
Department of Anesthesiology and Critical Care
Albany Medical Center
Albany, New York

Pekka Talke, MD
Professor
Department of Anesthesia and Perioperative Care
University of California, San Francisco
San Francisco, California

Lela Weems, MD
Clinical Assistant Professor of Anesthesiology
SUNY Downstate Medical Center
Brooklyn, New York

Max Wintermark, MD
Associate Professor of Radiology, Neurology and Neurosurgery
Director
Neuroradiology Division
University of Virginia
Charlottesville, Virginia

David J. Wlody, MD
Professor of Clinical Anesthesiology
Vice Chair for Clinical Affairs and Director of Obstetric
    Anesthesia
SUNY Downstate Medical Center
Chairman of Anesthesiology
Long Island College Hospital
Brooklyn, New York

William L. Young, MD
James P. Livingston Professor and Vice Chair
Department of Anesthesia and Perioperative Care
Professor of Neurological Surgery and Neurology
Director
Center for Cerebrovascular Research
University of California, San Francisco
San Francisco, California

Mark H. Zornow, MD
Professor of Anesthesiology and Perioperative Medicine
Oregon Health Science University
Portland, Oregon

Connie Zuckerman, JD
Attorney and Consultant
Health Law and Bioethics
White Plains, New York

FOREWORD

There have been many textbooks concerning the anesthetic care of neurosurgical patients. Most appeared in one or two versions and then disappeared. But this one has returned, edition after edition, since its inception in 1980, evolving and improving with each version. I have got all four previous editions lined up in my bookcase. For this fifth edition, Dr. Cottrell is joined as co-editor by Dr. William Young, Professor of Anesthesia at UCSF. Like Dr. Cottrell, Dr. Young has been involved in neurosurgical anesthesia for a very, very long time. In fact, on the basis of the dates of their initial publications, these two editors have 60 years of clinical and scientific experience with this specialty between them.

In my foreword to the previous edition, I made the comment, "This is not a book for educating technicians, it's a book for educating professionals." This remains true. There are some new chapters and authors, some old chapters have disappeared, others have been rearranged. But the focus on the underlying medicine and science of neuroanesthesia remains.

Why is this important? I realize that I'm repeating myself. There are lots of "handbooks" on the market that provide recipes for all sorts of clinical scenarios—along with lots of "board questions." If your only interest in neuroanesthesia is in passing your boards, or if neurosurgical patients are a rare part of your practice, these are OK. But if you think of yourself as a neuroanesthesiologist and deal with such patients daily, you must understand the underpinnings of your work. You need to know the surgical diseases (and what to expect of patients with such diseases), you need to understand the surgery itself, you need to know the anatomy and physiology of the brain and spinal cord, you need to know the science behind the practice. No "handbook" can cover every situation that you encounter. Doing anesthesia by recipe is an invitation to disaster—What happens when the recipe wasn't in your book? Nearly every time I'm in the operating room, I encounter a patient who "isn't in the book": the severely retarded and uncooperative adult with hydrocephalus who has undergone a previous occiput-C1 fusion; the pregnant woman with a subarachnoid hemorrhage; the patient with a swollen, bleeding AVM; the patient in whom the interventional radiologist has just perforated an aneurysm; the patient undergoing an awake temporal lobectomy who convulses; the patient undergoing endoscopic transsphenoidal hypophysectomy complicated by an inadvertent biopsy of the basilar artery—or in whom florid diabetes insipidus develops on the table; the postop aneurysm patient with severe vasospasm returning to the OR for an acute abdomen; the tumor patient who herniates in front of my eyes; the quadriparetic patient undergoing both an anterior cervical spine decompression *and* posterior fusion—or the C-spine patient who awakens with an unexpected major deficit.

To develop an intelligent plan of action, to avoid or manage these situations requires that you *understand* what you need to do—not just depend on experience and do what you've been told by your teachers. This is the definition of a medical professional.

This is a book for professionals. It is as up-to-date and as comprehensive as it can be, in terms of both its science and its practice. This is a book for anesthesiologists who truly see themselves as real doctors, not just technicians.

Michael Todd, MD
Professor and Chairman
Department of Anesthesia
University of Iowa
Iowa City, Iowa

PREFACE

With a new editor, William L. Young, and twenty-three new authors, seven new chapters, three chapters with all new authors, and eleven chapters with one or more new authors, the fifth edition of *Cottrell and Young's Neuroanesthesia* is both track-tested and up-to-date. There was, of course, no option. Ours is a fast-moving field. As the Red Queen said to Alice in Wonderland, "Now, *here,* you see, it takes all the running you can do, to keep in the same place." In this case, "*here*" is neurosurgical anesthesiology, and "the same place" is state-of-the-art knowledge.

Medicine advances through a sort of trickle-down process. Information flows from basic scientists to laboratory animal researchers to clinical investigators to scientific journals to clinical textbooks, and, finally, to clinicians. The closer the connections between the first four way stations and the textbook, the better clinicians are served. We have kept those connections tight by gathering authors who are, in various combinations, basic scientists, laboratory researchers, clinical investigators, journal authors, journal editors, and, of course, clinicians.

The emphasis of this book has always been clinical application, and that focus has only been sharpened in this fifth edition. We want this book to serve its readers by helping them serve their patients.

James E. Cottrell and William L. Young
Editors

ACKNOWLEDGMENTS

We thank our respective departments of anesthesiology, each of which has provided, despite recent economic adversity, the practical and intellectual background that makes it possible for colleagues like ourselves to write, assemble, and edit such books as *Cottrell and Young's Neuroanesthesia*. Special thanks are also due to Michael Todd for the new Foreword; Voltaire Gungab, John Hartung, Christine Waters, and Samrat Worah for editorial assistance; Anne Minaidis for coordinating the project; the publishing staff at Elsevier, Natasha Andjelkovic and Bradley McIlwain; and especially the contributing authors whose expertise has been particularly important in making this edition possible.

James E. Cottrell

William L. Young

CONTENTS

Chapter 1

BRAIN METABOLISM, THE PATHOPHYSIOLOGY OF BRAIN INJURY, AND POTENTIAL BENEFICIAL AGENTS AND TECHNIQUES

Ira S. Kass • James E. Cottrell • Baiping Lei

Brain metabolism involves both the production and the utilization of energy; catabolism is the breakdown and anabolism is the synthesis of components and molecules in the cells. For energy formation the main catabolic process is the breakdown of glucose with the ultimate formation of high-energy phosphate in the form of adenosine triphosphate (ATP). Other catabolic processes break down structural and enzymatic proteins, lipids, and carbohydrates; these processes are necessary to replace damaged and nonfunctional molecules. These molecules are resynthesized by anabolic processes that renew the cells and maintain optimal function. Cellular function also requires the maintenance of ionic homeostasis, which for neurons requires a large amount of energy. The pathophysiologic mechanisms of brain injury are incompletely understood but ultimately represent a failure of anabolic processes to maintain normal cell function. In this chapter we explore the putative mechanisms of brain injury. The causes of neuronal damage are multifaceted, and one pathway alone cannot explain how the injury occurs. Some pathophysiologic mechanisms are common to damage caused by ischemic, epileptogenic, and traumatic injury, whereas others are discrete for each of these processes. This review focuses on some common triggers of neuronal damage, such as altered ionic gradients, and explores how they in turn lead to long-term damage. We also discuss pharmacologic agents and clinical procedures that may lead to a reduction in long-term brain damage.

BRAIN METABOLISM

The main substance used for energy production in the brain is glucose. Because glucose is not freely permeable across the blood-brain barrier, it requires a transporter to enter the brain. This transporter does not require energy and can move glucose only down its concentration gradient, from a higher to a lower concentration. Normally the blood levels of glucose are well regulated so glucose concentrations in the brain are adequate; however, if blood levels of glucose fall, there can be net movement of glucose out of the brain. Thus adequate blood glucose levels are critical for normal brain activity. During insulin shock or other conditions that cause a reduction in blood glucose, unconsciousness can result from insufficient energy due to low brain glucose levels. When glucose and oxygen levels are sufficient, glucose is metabolized to pyruvate in the glycolytic pathway (Fig. 1-1). This biochemical process generates ATP from adenosine diphosphate (ADP) and inorganic phosphate and produces nicotinamide adenine dinucleotide reduced (NADH) from nicotinamide adenine dinucleotide (NAD). Pyruvate from this reaction then enters the citric acid cycle which, with regard to energy production, primarily generates NADH from NAD. The mitochondria use oxygen to couple the conversion of NADH back to NAD with the production of ATP from ADP and inorganic phosphate. This process, called *oxidative phosphorylation*, forms three ATP molecules for each NADH converted and yields a maximum of 38 ATP molecules for each glucose molecule metabolized.[1] Because numerous parts of this pathway supply other metabolic requirements, such as amino acid synthesis and the formation of reducing equivalents for other synthetic pathways, the normal yield of this energy pathway is approximately 30 to 35 ATP molecules for each glucose molecule.

This pathway requires oxygen; if oxygen is not present the mitochondria can neither make ATP nor regenerate NAD from NADH. The metabolism of glucose requires NAD as a cofactor and is blocked in its absence. Thus, in the absence of oxygen, glycolysis proceeds by a modified pathway termed "anaerobic glycolysis"; this modification involves the conversion of pyruvate to lactate, regenerating NAD. This process produces hydrogen ion, which may accentuate neuronal damage if the intracellular pH falls. A major problem with anaerobic glycolysis, in addition to lowering pH, is that only two molecules of ATP are formed for each molecule of glucose metabolized. This level of ATP production is insufficient to meet the brain's energy needs. In addition, ischemia cuts off the supply of glucose so even anaerobic glycolysis is blocked.

When the oxygen supply to a neuron is reduced, mechanisms that reduce and/or slow the fall in ATP levels include the following: (1) the utilization of phosphocreatine stores (a high-energy phosphate that can donate its energy to maintain ATP levels), (2) the production of ATP at low levels by anaerobic glycolysis, and (3) a rapid cessation of spontaneous electrophysiologic activity.

CELLULAR PROCESSES THAT REQUIRE ENERGY

Pumping ions across the cell membrane is the largest energy requirement in the brain. The sodium, potassium, and calcium concentrations of a neuron are maintained against large

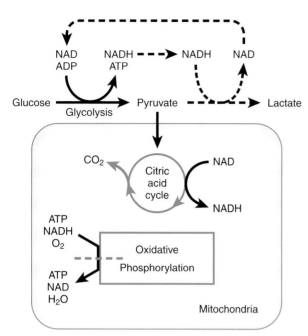

Figure 1–1 Energy metabolism in the brain. *Dotted lines* indicate reactions that occur during ischemia. Lines indicate metabolic pathways, dashed lines indicate anaerobic glycolysis. The *dotted line* across the oxidative phosphorylation reaction indicates this reaction is blocked during ischemia. ADP, adenosine diphosphate; ATP, adenosine triphosphate; NAD, nicotinamide adenine dinucleotide; NADH, nicotinamide adenine dinucleotide reduced. *(From Bendo AA, Kass IS, Hartung J, Cottrell JE: Anesthesia for Neurosurgery. In Barash PG, Cullen BF, Stoelting RK [eds]: Clinical Anesthesia, 5th ed. Philadelphia, Lippincott Williams & Wilkins, 2006.)*

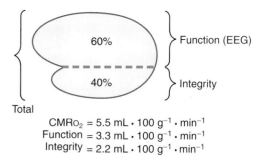

$$CMRO_2 = 5.5 \ mL \cdot 100 \ g^{-1} \cdot min^{-1}$$
$$Function = 3.3 \ mL \cdot 100 \ g^{-1} \cdot min^{-1}$$
$$Integrity = 2.2 \ mL \cdot 100 \ g^{-1} \cdot min^{-1}$$

Figure 1–2 Oxygen requirements of the normal brain. Values are those obtained in the canine. $CMRO_2$, cerebral metabolic rate for oxygen; EEG, electroencephalogram. *(From Michenfelder JD: The hypothermic brain. In Anesthesia and the Brain: Clinical, Functional, Metabolic, and Vascular Correlates. New York, Churchill Livingstone, 1988.)*

electrochemical gradients with respect to the outside of the cell. When sodium (Na), calcium (Ca) and potassium (K) are mentioned throughout the chapter we are referring to their ionic form (Na^+, Ca^{++} and K^+), this is the only form of these compounds that is present in living cells. When a neuron is not excited, there are slow leaks of potassium out of the cells and of sodium into the cells. The resting potential of a neuron depends mainly on the electrochemical equilibrium potential for potassium, which in most neurons is approximately −94 mV. There is some permeability to sodium and calcium so the resting potential for a neuron is usually −60 to −70 mV. Because the cell's membrane potential is not equal to the equilibrium potential for an ion, there is leakage of ions down their electrochemical gradients. If this leakage were not corrected by energy-dependent ion pumps, the membrane potential would fall to 0 mV and the cell would depolarize and die. The ion pumps fall into two major categories, (1) those that use ATP directly to pump ions and (2) those that use the energy of the Na gradient to cotransport another ion. The ultimate energy for the latter pumps comes from ATP via the Na/K ATPase, which transports Na ions and maintains the energy gradient of Na; examples of these are the Na/Ca and the Na/H transporters. Examples of the former category of pump are the Na/K ATPase, the major user of energy in neurons, and the Ca ATPase. Indeed, during ischemia these pumps do not have enough energy to operate, and this condition is a primary cause of neuronal depolarization and cell death. Neuronal activity markedly increases the flow of sodium, potassium, and calcium by opening Na, K, and Ca ion channels; this opening raises the rate of ion pumping required to maintain normal cellular ion concentrations. Because ion pumping uses ATP as an energy source, the ATP requirement of active neurons is greater than that of unexcited neurons. Approximately 60% of

the energy the brain uses is required for functional activity, and the remainder is used to maintain cellular integrity (Fig. 1-2). Anesthetics reduce neuronal activity and thereby ATP utilization by functional activity, but they do not reduce the energy required for the integrity of the brain. If energy production does not meet the demand of energy use in the brain, the neurons become first unexcitable and then irreversibly damaged.

Neurons require energy to maintain their structure and internal function. Each cell's membranes, internal organelles, and cytoplasm are made of carbohydrates, lipids, and proteins that require energy for their synthesis. Ion channels, enzymes, and cell structural components are important protein molecules that are continuously formed, modified, and broken down in the cell. If ATP is not available, protein synthesis cannot continue, and the neuron will die. Carbohydrates and lipids are also continuously synthesized and degraded in normally functioning neurons; their metabolism also requires energy. Most cellular synthesis takes place in the cell body, and energy is required for transport of components down the axon to the nerve terminals. Thus, energy is required to maintain the integrity of neurons even in the absence of electrophysiologic activity.

PATHOPHYSIOLOGY

Ischemia

When the blood supply to the brain is limited, ischemic damage to neurons can occur; the brain is the organ most sensitive to ischemic damage. The central event precipitating damage by hypoxia or ischemia is reduced energy production due to blockage of oxidative phosphorylation. This causes ATP production per molecule of glucose to be reduced by 95%. At this rate of production, ATP levels fall, leading to the loss of energy-dependent homeostatic mechanisms. Additionally, during ischemia the supply of glucose is interrupted, as is the washout of metabolites. The activity of ATP-dependent ion pumps is reduced and the intracellular levels of sodium and calcium increase, whereas intracellular potassium levels decrease (Fig. 1-3).[2] These ion changes cause the neurons to depolarize and release excitatory amino acids such as glutamate.[3,4] In addition glutamate is released from neurons owing to the reversal of the glutamate transporter, which pumps glutamate into the extracellular compartment when the cellular sodium and potassium ion gradients are disrupted.[5] High levels of glutamate further depolarize the neurons by activating AMPA (α-amino-3-hydroxyl-5-methyl-4-isoxazole-propionate) and

NMDA (*N*-methyl-D-aspartate) receptors, increasing sodium and potassium ion conductance.[6,7] The NMDA receptor also allows calcium to enter, triggering additional damaging pathways. Glutamate activates metabotropic receptors, which via second-messenger systems can increase the release of calcium from intracellular stores and activate other biochemical processes.[8,9] The damage due to excess glutamate has been termed *excitotoxicity* and is caused by activation of glutamate receptors and the accompanying ionic and biochemical changes.[10]

In addition to increased influx through membrane channels, cytosolic calcium is increased through reduced calcium pumping from the cell and the enhanced release of calcium from intracellular organelles such as the mitochondria and the endoplasmic reticulum (Fig. 1-4).[11,12] The high cytoplasmic calcium level is thought to trigger a number of events that lead to the ischemic damage. These include increasing the activity of proteases and phospholipases. Phospholipases raise the levels of free fatty acids, such as arachidonic acid, and free radicals. Free radicals are also generated by incomplete mitochondrial oxidation.[11] One of the most damaging free radicals is peroxynitrite, which is formed by the combination of nitric oxide and another free radical.[11] Free radicals are known to damage proteins and lipids, whereas free fatty acids interfere with membrane function. There is a buildup of lactate and hydrogen ions during ischemia, and this decrease in pH can lead to further formation of free radicals.[13] All of these processes, coupled with the reduced ability to synthesize proteins and lipids, contribute to the irreversible damage that occurs with ischemia (Box 1-1).

Additionally, phospholipase activation leads to the production of excess arachidonic acid, which upon reoxygenation can form eicosanoids, including thromboxane, prostaglandins, and leukotrienes. These substances can cause strong vasoconstriction, reduce blood flow in the postischemic period, alter the blood-brain barrier, and enhance free radical formation after reperfusion.[14,15]

Procedures that protect against ischemic damage should interfere with the cellular changes brought on by ischemia (Box 1-2). In addition to these direct triggering events, there is long-term damage that becomes apparent hours and days after the ischemic insult. Some of this delayed damage is necrotic; lysis of the cells causes microglial activation.[16] Lymphocytes,

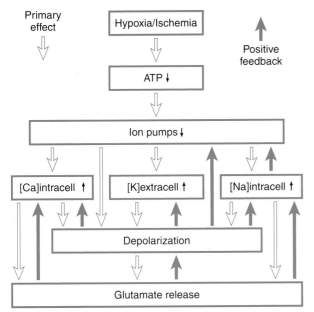

Figure 1–3 Line diagram of cellular ionic events occurring during anoxia or ischemia. The events indicated are the primary triggers of events leading to neuronal cell death. Positive feedback loops are unstable and rapidly worsen events. ATP, adenosine triphosphate; extracell, extracellular; intracell, intracellular; ↑, increase; ↓, decrease.

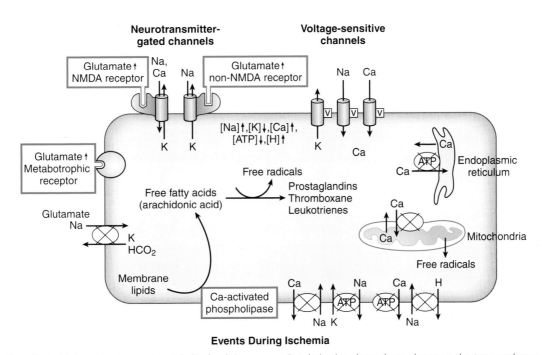

Events During Ischemia

Figure 1–4 The effect of ischemia on ion and metabolite levels in neurons. For clarity, ion channels are shown on the *top* membrane and ion pumps on the *bottom* membrane; their actual location can be on any membrane surface. *Circles* indicate energy-driven pumps; an *x* through a *circle* indicates that the pump is blocked or has reduced activity during ischemia. *V* indicates a voltage-dependent channel. ATP, adenosine triphosphate; NMDA, *N*-methyl-D-aspartate. *(Modified from Bendo AA, Kass IS, Hartung J, Cottrell JE: Anesthesia for neurosurgery. In Barash PG, Cullen BF, Stoelting RK [eds]: Clinical Anesthesia, 5th ed. Philadelphia, Lippincott Williams & Wilkins, 2006.)*

BOX 1–1 *Brain Metabolism and Cell Death: Triggers, Effectors, and Functional Changes*

Triggers

Adenosine triphosphate ↓
Extracellular potassium ↑
Intracellular sodium ↑
Intracellular calcium ↑
Free radical levels ↑
Depolarization ↑
Glutamate level ↑

Effectors

Protease activity ↑
Free radical action ↑
DNA damage ↑
Phospholipase activity ↑
Mitochondrial factors ↑ (cytochrome *c* → caspase activation)

Critical Functional Changes

Mitochondrial damage ↑
Apoptotic cascade activation ↑
Antiapoptotic factors ↓
Protein damage ↑
Protein synthesis ↓
Cytoskeletal damage ↑

End Stage

Apoptosis ↑ (programmed cell death)
Necrosis ↑ (cell disintegration)

↑, increases; ↓, decreases; →, leads to.
Adapted from Lipton P. Ischemic cell death in brain neutrons. Physiol Rev 1999;79:1431-1568.

BOX 1–2 *Consequences of Ischemia*

Vascular Changes

Vasospasm
Red cell sludging
Hypoperfusion

Neuronal Changes

Adenosine triphosphate reduction
Sodium influx
Potassium efflux
Intracellular acidosis
High cellular calcium concentrations
Calcium-activated proteases
Caspase activation
Phospholipase activation
Arachidonic acid formation and breakdown
Free radical production
Excitatory amino acid release
Disruption of ion and amino acid transporters

---

polymorphonuclear cells, and macrophages can invade the nervous system, leading to additional damage.[17,18] Although histamine receptor activation is generally associated with immune system activation, the histamine receptor involved with this is the H_1 receptor. In the central nervous system, the H_2 receptor is the one primarily activated, and it reduces immunologic processes and improves recovery from ischemia.[19-21] Indeed, blocking immune system activation can reduce damage.[19] It is clear there is also genetically programmed cell death as a result of the insult.[22] This programmed cell death, which is similar to apoptotic cell death during neuronal development, can occur days after the initial insult.

Necrosis versus Apoptosis

There are two major processes leading to neuronal death. The first, necrosis, is due to a more severe insult in which mitochondrial function is lost; it is characterized by a disintegration of the cell and an activation of microglia and the immune response.[16] The immune response and inflammation activate and recruit neutrophils and macrophages, which produce free radicals and damage adjacent neurons. This process expands the lesion in volume and time, allowing for continued and expanded neuronal damage.[16] In the second, apoptosis, the cell dies without breaking apart and there is no microglial or immune system involvement with the potential for excess damage to adjacent neurons. This process is frequently delayed and can lead to the activation of immediate early genes (IEGs) such as c-Jun and c-Fos; these genes are thought to affect gene expression and lead to the production of apop-

totic or antiapoptotic proteins, which determine whether the neurons will survive or die.[22,23] One set of proteins that lead to neuronal death are the cysteine proteinases, referred to as *caspases*. These enzymes are expressed as proenzymes, which undergo proteolytic processing to yield active enzymes that degrade important proteins in the cell (Fig. 1-5).[24,25] Blockade of caspases has been shown to block apoptosis.[26] Because these enzymes are now known to be present as proenzymes before ischemia, new protein synthesis is not needed to induce apoptosis.[27] However, proapoptotic proteins are synthesized under certain conditions, and their synthesis may lead to delayed neuronal cell death. Another set of proteins can be induced that block apoptosis and promote neuronal survival after ischemia; examples of these proteins are neuronal apoptosis inhibitory protein, heat shock proteins, and Bcl-2 family proteins.[28,29] Thus the fate of ischemic neurons rests in balance between apoptotic inhibitory and activating processes (Fig. 1-6).[29,30] The synthesis of certain trophic factors can improve neuronal survival by inhibiting apoptosis (see Fig. 1-5). The activation and release of certain cytokines, such as tumor necrosis factor and interleukin-1β, are thought to be damaging.[31,32]

Thus necrosis and apoptosis can be contrasted, with the former being a result of more severe ischemia and leading to damage of adjacent tissue (Fig. 1-7). Apoptosis is subject to modulation, so once started down the apoptotic pathway, cells have a chance of being rescued by trophic substances (see Fig. 1-6).

Global versus Focal Ischemia

Ischemia can be either global or focal in nature; an example of the former would be cardiac arrest, and of the latter, localized stroke. Although the mechanisms leading to neuronal damage are probably similar for the two types of ischemia, there are important distinctions between them. In focal ischemia there are three regions. The first region receives no blood flow and responds the same as globally ischemic tissue; the second region, called the *penumbra*, receives collateral flow and is partially ischemic; the third region is normally perfused. If the insult is maintained for a prolonged period, the neurons in the penumbra die. More neurons in the penumbra region survive if collateral blood flow is increased or if reperfusion is established in a timely manner by opening of the blocked vessel. With total global ischemia, the time until the circulation

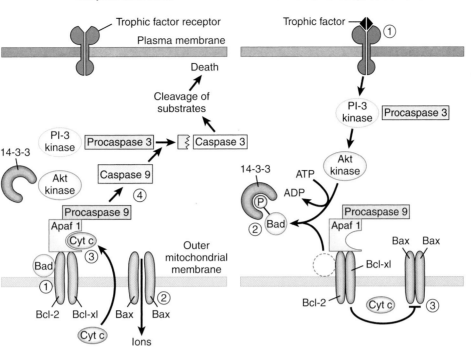

(a) Absence of trophic factor: Caspase activation

(b) Presence of trophic factor: Inhibition of caspase activation

Figure 1–5 Trophic factors and apoptosis. ADP, adenosine diphosphate; ATP, adenosine triphosphate; Cyt c, cytochrome c; PI, phosphoinositide; other abbreviations (Akt, Apaf, Bad, Bax, Bcl, 14-3-3) are names of proteins. The numbers on the diagram refer to the apoptotic pathway and its inhibition a) activated apoptotic pathway: 1) Bad protein inhibits Bcl-2, Bcl-xl proteins; 2) these proteins can no longer inhibit Bax and therefore Bax allows ion flow into the mitochondria; 3) this leads to cytochrome c release and the activation of Apaf 1 which finally 4) activates caspase 9 and apoptosis. b) apoptosis inhibited 1) trophic factor binds to a receptor and activates protein kinases; 2) this leads to the phophorylation of Bad and its inactivation; 3) Bad can no longer inhibit Bcl-2 and Bcl-xl and these 2 proteins can now inhibit Bax, blocking ion flow and apoptosis. *(From Lodish H, Berk A, Matsudaira P, et al [eds]: Molecular Cell Biology, 5th ed. New York, WH Freeman and Co, 2004: page 929, as adapted from Pettmann B, Henderson CE: Neuronal cell death. Neuron 1998;20:633-647.)*

is reestablished is critical, and only very short ischemic times (on the order of minutes) are survivable. The selective neurologic damage after survival subsequent to global ischemia is mainly due to the differential sensitivity of certain neurons and brain regions. The hippocampus, especially the cornus ammonis 1 (CA1) pyramidal cell region, is extremely vulnerable to ischemic damage; loss of learning and memory is common after global ischemia and hypoxia.[33,34]

Genetic Influences on Neuronal Damage

Genetic factors play an important role in an individual's susceptibility to ischemic brain injury. Both environmental (such as diet and stress) and genetic factors combine to determine the risk of stroke. A study of the Icelandic population found that polymorphisms (genetic changes) in genetic locus ALOX5AP, which encodes 5-lipoxygenase–activating protein, and PDE4D, which encodes phosphodiesterase 4D, increase the susceptibility to stroke.[35,36] In addition polymorphisms of both apolipoprotein B and apolipoprotein E have been found to enhance the susceptibility to stroke.[37,38] The genetic factors could target neuronal risk but more likely raise the vascular risk, which is associated with an increase in both stroke and cardiac disease. If a patient's genetic susceptibility to injury were known, it would be possible to choose therapeutic strategies individually for the patient, especially if those strategies carry their own morbidity or are costly.

In addition to neuronal dysfunction following stroke and global cerebral ischemia, postoperative cognitive deficit is frequently found after anesthesia and surgery even in the absence of ischemia. This deficit also shows genetic variation. The genetic alleles that reduced serum C-reactive protein and platelet activation were associated with a reduction in cognitive deficit after cardiac surgery. These studies indicate that the immune response may enhance postoperative cognitive deficits and that targeting the immune activation in certain patients may be beneficial.[39]

POTENTIAL TREATMENTS FOR CEREBRAL ISCHEMIA

Reperfusion Strategies

The most successful technique for improving recovery from embolic stroke is prompt restoration of spontaneous perfusion through the use of thrombolytic agents (such as tissue plasminogen activator [TPA]) or other anticlotting drugs in the period directly after the onset of a stroke (<3 hours); as one would predict, hemorrhagic strokes are made markedly worse by this treatment.[40,41] Thus detecting, classifying, and treating stroke rapidly after its onset is critical to a successful outcome.[42] Thrombolytics can not be used during or recently after surgery because of the risk of bleeding. The use of anticlotting agents such as warfarin is also thought to reduce the incidence and severity of subsequent strokes.[43]

The major side effect of this strategy is intracerebral hemorrhage, which can be devastating. It is essential that a noncontrast computed tomography scan be performed and analyzed shortly after patient presentation to the hospital in order to

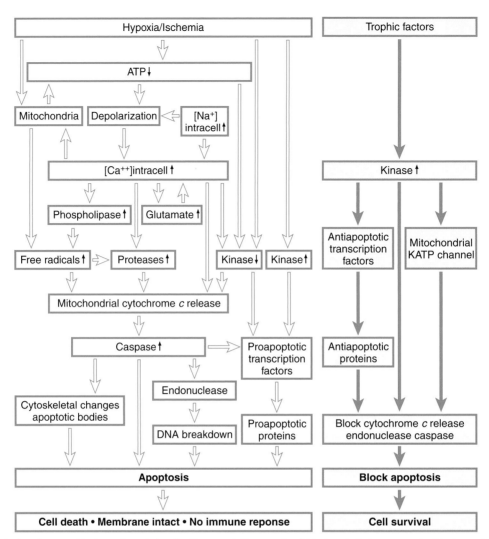

Figure 1–6 Apoptosis subsequent to hypoxia or ischemia: The apoptotic cascade of biochemical changes evoked by hypoxia or ischemia. Similar events may also be occurring during epileptic and trauma-induced damage; they lead to depolarization, reduced adenosine triphosphate (ATP), sodium influx, and high cytosolic calcium levels. There is no cellular membrane disruption during apoptosis, and inflammation is not triggered. The apoptotic biochemical cascade can be modulated and opposed by trophic factors. intracell, intracellular; KATP channel, ATP-sensitive potassium channel; ↑, increase; ↓, decrease; the large open arrows indicate damaging pathways, the large closed arrows indicate protective pathways.

rule out a hemorrhagic stroke, because TPA must be administered within 3 hours of an occlusive stroke onset to be effective. Other drugs are being evaluated for reperfusion strategy, such as desmoteplase, which is more fibrin specific and has a longer half-life, but only TPA has been approved by the U.S. Food and Drug Administration for this indication.

Although these strategies have shown benefit only when administered to patients within 3 hours of stroke onset, there are currently studies to identify patients who might benefit from these agents at later time points. The key is to identify patients in whom an area of reduced perfusion has not progressed to irreversible neuronal damage. These studies use advanced imaging to identify at-risk tissue that can still be salvaged if reperfusion can be established. Diffusion-weighted magnetic resonance imaging (DWI) identifies core ischemic areas where water has shifted into the intracellular compartment and has reduced diffusibility. Areas that have not yet converted to core ischemia can potentially be rescued from irreversible damage. Perfusion-weighted magnetic resonance imaging indicates regions with reduced perfusion that will ultimately proceed to irreversible damage if not reperfused. A region with reduced perfusion that

has not yet progressed to irreversible damage (as shown on diffusion-weighted imaging) would benefit from delayed reperfusion therapy.[44] It is likely that patients in this category would benefit from delayed TPA; the issue is under current investigation and some centers have extended the time for tPA to 4.5 hours. (ref 45) However it is clear that the sooner TPA is given the better the outcome is likely to be. Some studies are being done to examine intra-arterial application of TPA after unsuccessful intravenous TPA some studies have found no significance but a trend toward infarct reduction.[45] These results were encouraging but not enough to recommend a change in clinical practice. A study with a relatively small number of patients indicates that administration of desmoteplase 3 to 9 hours after the onset of an embolic stroke yields a high rate of reperfusion and better clinical outcome than administration of placebo in carefully selected patients with perfusion /diffusion mismatch.[46] However a larger well designed study was not able to confirm a benefit of desmoteplase under these same conditions, this indicates the difficulties and complications in finding agents that improve outcome.[47] It also indicates the importance of cautiously interpreting positive studies of

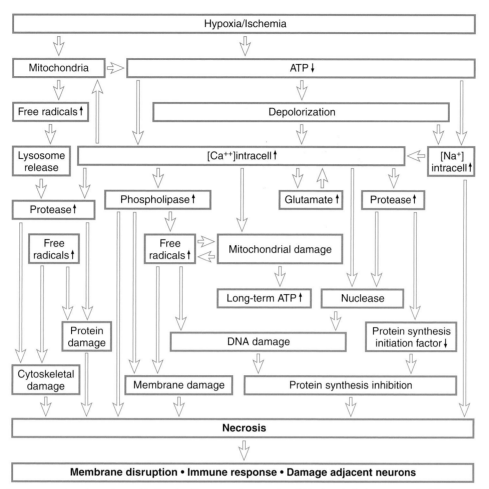

Figure 1–7 Necrosis subsequent to hypoxia and ischemia: The necrotic cascade of biochemical changes evoked by hypoxia or ischemia. Similar events may also be occurring during epileptic and trauma-induced damage; they lead to depolarization, reduced adenosine triphosphate (ATP), sodium influx, and high cytosolic calcium levels. These changes are more severe than those with apoptosis and lead to the disruption of the cells and activation of inflammation. The damage cannot be reversed, and surrounding intact neurons can be damaged by secondary processes. intracell, intracellular; ↑, increase; ↓, decrease; large arrows indicate damaging pathways.

clinical brain protection in which small groups of patients are examined.

In addition to chemical dissolution of the clot, mechanically assisted recanalization is possible. The Merci Retriever (Concentric Medical, Inc., Mountain View, CA) and the Penumbra System (Penumbra, Inc., Alameda, CA) are approved by the U.S. Food and Drug Administration for mechanical removal of clots. The Merci Retriever has been shown to provide a higher rate of good clinical outcome compared to historical controls, although the intracranial hemorrhage rate was 7.8%.[48] The Penumbra System successfully reopened 82% of the treated vessels, however the symptomatic intracerebral hemorrhage rate was 11%. The authors concluded that the Penumbra System allowed safe and effective revascularization up to 8 hours after symptom onset.[49]

Both intra-arterial thrombolysis and mechanical removal are confined to specialist centers and clinical trials. The only widely used treatment is administration TPA within 3 hours of stroke onset, however most recently it has been extended for up to 4.5 hours for certain patients.[50] This treatment is underutilized, in part because of the time restraints for imaging and the frequent delay in presentation of patients to the hospital after the onset of symptoms. The latter problem can and is being addressed by community education about the signs of stroke and the emergency nature of transport to an appropriate hospital with a stroke center. The guidelines for early management and treatment of stroke are frequently updated and should be consulted and examined for the latest recommendations.[45]

Hypothermia

Profound hypothermia has long been used in neonatal heart surgery to provide protection against irreversible brain injury when the heart is stopped. It has also been used during the repair of giant aneurysms. However there are numerous complications of profound hypothermia (Box 1-3). Profound hypothermia reduces cerebral metabolism to such an extent that the brain can survive relatively long periods without perfusion (Box 1-4). Experimental studies indicate that moderate hypothermia has a protective effect without many of the complications of profound hypothermia, although myocardial depression has been documented.[51-53] There are many in vitro and in vivo animal studies to support the use of moderate hypothermia to protect against ischemic damage, and a prospective clinical study is beginning. Indeed moderate hypothermia has come into common use even though it has not been unequivocally shown to improve recovery in a major clinical trial.[54,55] A European study published in

---

BOX 1–3 *Complications of Deep Hypothermia*

Cardiovascular Complications

Myocardial depression
Dysrhythmia including ventricular fibrillation
Hypotension
Inadequate tissue perfusion
Ischemia

Coagulation

Thrombocytopenia
Fibrinolysis
Platelet dysfunction
Increased bleeding

Metabolism

Slowed metabolism of anesthetic agents
Prolonged neuromuscular blockade
Increased protein catabolism

Shivering

Increased oxygen consumption
Increased carbon dioxide production
Increased cardiac output
Arterial oxygen desaturation
Hemodynamic instability

BOX 1–4 *Proposed Mechanisms of Protection by Hypothermia*

Decrease in cerebral metabolism
Delayed anoxic/ischemic depolarization
Preservation of ion homeostasis
Decrease excitatory neurotransmission
Prevention or reduction of damaging secondary biochemical changes

---

2002 indicates that mild hypothermia, target temperature 32° to 34° C, after hospital cardiac arrest improves neurologic outcome and survival 6 months after the arrest.[56] Even patients with out-of-hospital cardiac arrest benefit from mild hypothermia.[57]

It is clear that even minor amounts of hyperthermia worsen clinical outcome of ischemia and increase neuronal damage, and so must be carefully guarded against.[58,59]

Glucose

Glucose is the main source of energy for neurons in the brain, and some in vitro studies reported improved recovery with hyperglycemia. However, in vivo and clinical studies found a clear worsening of damage with hyperglycemia, which is thought to be due to enhanced cellular acidosis.[13,60] The precise mechanism by which hyperglycemia exacerbates damage is not known. Clinical recommendations are to maintain normal serum glucose levels and to treat hyperglycemia in order to reduce the glucose value to near normal range.[61] It is important for the patient not to be hypoglycemic, as hypoglycemia would also worsen outcome. The difficulty in doing this and the overall recommendations for glucose management are likely to be effected by a recent study on intensive glucose control which demonstrated a higher mortality in patients managed from 81-108 mg per deciliter compared to patients managed to a target of 180 mg or less per deciliter.[62]

Pharmacologic Agents

Many drugs have been proposed as potential agents to reduce permanent neuronal damage subsequent to ischemia, but very few have proved useful in clinical trials.[58,63] The theoretical basis for choosing drugs that block specific damaging pathways is sound. Blocking one pathway to damage may not be efficacious, however, owing to the many parallel paths that lead to permanent damage (see Fig. 1-6). For example, one can block voltage-sensitive calcium channels but cytoplasmic calcium can increase through influx via the NMDA receptor ion channel or release from intracellular organelles. Thus effective therapy might require multiple agents to block all of the parallel pathways simultaneously.

It must be recognized that no pharmacologic agent has been shown to improve neurologic recovery clinically after a stroke. Pharmacologic agents that have been studied in clinical trials have not been shown to be efficacious for the improvement of stroke outcome. This is an extremely controversial field, as evidenced by two 2008 editorials in the journal *Stroke*, entitled "Neuroprotection: Still achievable in humans"[64] and "Neuroprotection does not work!"[65] That said, some agents appear promising in animal studies and may prove efficacious clinically.[59,65,68]

One major problem with stroke treatments and a reason for the discrepancy between animal and human results is that most animal studies apply the protective agents either before or during the insult, whereas clinical stroke treatment is always delayed. In the perioperative environment, drugs and treatments can be applied before an insult, at the beginning of a high-risk surgery; thus, agents that fail to protect against stroke when used after the insult may be efficacious if given before surgery. Because only very few patients undergoing high-risk surgery will suffer an ischemic insult, the agents used must have a high safety factor and/or must be required for surgery (e.g., anesthetics). The deleterious effects will be shared among all patients, but the protective effects will benefit only ischemic patients.

Sodium Blockade

Blocking sodium influx during anoxia and ischemia has been shown to improve recovery both in vivo and in vitro.[67-69] The neuronal depolarization during anoxia and ischemia leads to massive flux of sodium and calcium into the neurons and of potassium out of the neurons.[70-73] Blocking sodium influx delays and attenuates the depolarization and delays the drop in ATP during anoxia and ischemia.[74-76] Lidocaine has improved recovery by delaying and attenuating the anoxic/ischemic depolarization and reducing anoxic sodium influx when given at concentrations that do not block sodium channels under normal conditions.[74,77] In one study, lidocaine reduced the infarct size and improved neurologic outcome following focal cerebral ischemia.[78] This agent appears to work, at least in part, by blocking apoptotic pathways in the penumbra.[79] When lidocaine application was delayed until 45 minutes after the onset of focal cerebral ischemia, there was improved neuronal survival in the core and penumbra, but the size of the infarct was not significantly reduced.[82] Studies in our laboratory have found that an antiarrhythmic dose of lidocaine administered

30 minutes before during and 60 minutes after ischemia improves the survival of CA1 pyramidal neurons after temporary global cerebral ischemia; there was enhanced neuronal survival at both 1 week and 4 weeks following the ischemia.[83] We also found that performance on a cognitive task that requires hippocampal involvement was improved with lidocaine treatment.[82] Two small clinical studies of lidocaine have indicated better cognitive outcome following cardiac surgery; a larger clinical study examining the effect of this agent on cerebral ischemia is required to demonstrate its efficacy for stroke.[83,84]

Calcium Blockade

Blockers of the voltage sensitive calcium channel such as nimodipine have been demonstrated to improve recovery from subarachnoid hemorrhage; they are recommended. Along with hypertension, hypervolemia and hemodilution to treat vasospasm.[85] A large clinical study of the effectiveness of nimodipine after stroke was discontinued due to higher mortality in the nimodipine group.[86] Clearly nimodipine can not be recommended subsequent to cerebral ischemia. Indeed during ischemia and anoxia calcium channels are already inhibited and direct protection of neurons with nimodipine was not observed in in vitro preparations.[87,88] Magnesium, an agent that blocks many voltage sensitive and transmitter activated channels which allow the influx of calcium and other ions, has recently been shown to be of benefit during focal cerebral ischemia, however a clinical trial did not show benefit from intravenous magnesium after stroke.[89-91] There was a subgroup of lacunar stroke that did show benefit with magnesium, but this would require a large new trial to confirm.[92] A study of magnesium in preterm birth to protect infant brains from damage did not yield significant improvement with magnesium treatment.[93] Clearly further studies are needed before it can be recommended. A major problem is its limited access to the central nervous system due to poor permeability across the blood-brain barrier. Blockade of secondary calcium activated pathways during and after ischemia appears promising in animal studies.[94]

Free Radical Scavenging

Free radicals have been implicated as causing cellular damage and leading to neuronal damage after ischemia. Both apoptotic damage and necrotic damage are thought to have a component of free radical damage. Use of free radical scavengers such as NXY-059, alpha-tocopherol and N-tert-alpha-phenyl-butyl nitrone (PBN) have shown to improve ischemia in animals.[95-98] However, an initial encouraging clinical result with NXY-059[99] was not confirmed in a later study.[100] Tirilazad has shown some promise in in vivo studies and with clinical trials for trauma and subarachnoid hemorrhage.[101] However, clinical studies have found that patients given methylprednisolone for 48 hours had a better outcome after spinal cord injury than patients given either methylprednisolone for 24 hours or tirilazad for 48 hours.[102] Neither methylprednisolone nor tirilazad has been demonstrated to improve recovery after cortical trauma or any ischemic lesion, and current practice is to use methylprednisolone only after spinal cord trauma.[103,104] Corticosteroids suppress the immune system, increase infection, and may actually enhance some free radical damage, so their use is not without consequences. Nitric oxide has been implicated as enhancing neuronal damage, and lubeluzole, an inhibitor of nitric oxide formation, has shown some promise in animals[105,106] but has not be found to benefit patients with ischemia.[107]

Excitotoxicity

Excitatory amino acids are implicated in the damaging cascade following ischemia, trauma, and epilepsy. Although blockers of NMDA and AMPA glutamate receptors have improved recovery in vitro and in vivo in a number of preparations, the results of clinical trials have been disappointing.[63,107] It appears that these agents are toxic and may themselves cause neuronal damage. Indeed, clinical trials with some of these agents have been terminated early owing to adverse outcome.[108,109] Magnesium, previously described as a potential protective agent for calcium blockade, is known to reduce NMDA receptor activation, perhaps one of its potential protective effects. As stated previously, magnesium has not been shown to improve clinical outcome if administered after a stroke.

Antiapoptotic Agents

Work with apoptosis indicates that specific blockers of caspases and modulators of apoptosis might improve recovery after ischemia, trauma, or epilepsy.[24,110,111,112] Although in vivo animal experiments are encouraging, these agents have not been shown to improve outcome clinically. A more useful technique might be to encourage neurons to synthesize antiapoptotic proteins, such as Bcl-2 and Bcl-xl, by inducing preconditioning with certain volatile anesthetics.

Cytokines and Trophic Factors

Cytokines such as tumor necrosis factor-alpha and interleukin-1β can activate the immune system and enhance damage; indeed, antibodies to these compounds have been shown to reduce cerebral ischemic damage in some animals.[63] However, tumor necrosis factor-alpha can also be beneficial, assisting neuronal survival in some circumstances, so targeting it can have mixed results.

Neurons have receptors for trophic factors such as nerve growth factor, neurotrophins, and brain-derived growth factor, which are required for neuronal survival even in the absence of any injury. These factors activate receptors that phosphorylate amino acids on certain proteins, thereby inhibiting apoptosis.[30,113] If these growth factors are not present, the receptors are not activated and the proteins are not phosphorylated; then the neurons do undergo apoptosis.[31] The loss of growth factors subsequent to neuronal degeneration after ischemia can exacerbate the delayed neuronal loss.

Erythropoietin is a trophic factor for blood cells that is also present in the nervous system. Animal studies indicate that it may protect neurons from apoptosis after ischemia by activating the trophic factor antiapoptotic pathway.[114] This is currently an area of active investigation for the protection against ischemic neuronal damage, and at least one small clinical trial has indicated that it is effective.[115]

Anesthetic Agents

Anesthetic agents have been examined for their ability to improve recovery from ischemia. The intuitive theory is that they reduce neuronal activity and metabolic rate and therefore should lower energy demand, enhance energy supply, and attenuate ischemic damage (Table 1-1).

However the different anesthetics also have specific actions, including effects on intracellular signalling pathways, ion conductances and neurotransmitters; these other actions may help explain their differential effects on neuronal damage (Table 1-2).

Barbiturates

Barbiturates are the only anesthetics that have been shown to have protective efficacy clinically, and in a highly specific context.[112] The mechanism of their protection has not been established and indeed may be multifaceted. Among its many actions, thiopental blocks Na, K, and calcium fluxes, scavenges free radicals, blocks seizures, improves regional blood flow, and decreases intracranial pressure (ICP).[117,118] Perhaps it is the multiple actions blocking parallel damaging pathways that allow this agent to protect against ischemic damage. It is important to note that very high barbiturate coma doses were needed to demonstrate clinical improvement after cardiac surgery.[116] In vitro studies also showed improved efficacy with very high doses.[117]

Etomidate and Propofol

Both etomidate and propofol, like thiopental, reduce the cerebral metabolic rate if given to burst suppression doses; however, they do not share many of thiopental's other actions. Etomidate has not been demonstrated to improve recovery from ischemic and anoxic damage under normal conditions.[54,118-121] Animal studies indicate that propofol may reduce ischemic damage, but it may not be as potent as thiopental.[122,123] It cannot be assumed that an anesthetic that reduces the cerebral metabolic rate to the same extent as thiopental will provide the same cerebral protection.

Nitrous Oxide

Nitrous oxide has been demonstrated to reduce recovery from ischemia and anoxia in comparison with other anesthetics, and its use should probably be avoided when perfusion of the brain might be compromised.[124,125]

Benzodiazepines

The most commonly used benzodiazepine in anesthesia practice is midazolam, and its effect on cerebral metabolism and ischemic damage has been examined. Benzodiazepines enhance neuronal inhibition in the nervous system and reduce brain metabolism by potentiating the effect of the neuronal transmitter gamma-aminobutyric acid (GABA) on the GABA$_A$ receptor. High doses of midazolam have been shown to reduce cerebral metabolism and cerebral blood flow, an effect that is reversed by the benzodiazepine antagonist flumazenil.[126,127] Midazolam improved neuronal recovery after anoxia and ischemia in animals, but there are no studies showing a better clinical outcome.[127-131] Flumazenil should be used cautiously, if at all, to reverse benzodiazepine effects in situations in which an increase in cerebral metabolic rate is undesirable, because this agent has been shown to increase the cerebral metabolic rate, cerebral blood flow, and ICP.[126]

Table 1-1 Effects of Anesthetics on Cerebral Blood Flow (CBF) and the Cerebral Metabolic Rate for Oxygen (CMRo$_2$)

Anesthetic	CBF	CMRo$_2$	Direct Cerebral Vasodilation
Halothane	↑↑↑	↓	Yes
Enflurane	↑↑	↓	Yes
Isoflurane	↑	↓↓	Yes
Desflurane	↑	↓↓	Yes
Sevoflurane	↑	↓↓	Yes
N$_2$O	↑	↑	—
N$_2$O with NO volatile anesthetics	↑↑	↑	—
N$_2$O with NO intravenous anesthetics	0	0	—
Thiopental	↓↓↓	↓↓↓	No
Etomidate	↓↓	↓↓	No
Propofol	↓↓	↓↓	No
Midazolam	↓	↓	No
Ketamine	↑↑	↑	No
Fentanyl	↓/0	↓/0	No

↑, increases; ↓, decreases (number of arrows indicates relative strength of effect); 0, no effect; —, not determined.
From Bendo AA, Kass IS, Hartung J, Cottrell JE: Anesthesia for Neurosurgery. In Barash PG, Cullen BF, Stoelting RK (eds): Clinical Anesthesia, 5th ed. Philadelphia, Lippincott Williams & Wilkins, 2006.

Table 1-2 Effect of Anesthetics on Recovery after and Biochemical Changes during Hypoxia*

Agent	Protects Physiologic Response	Delays Hypoxic Depolarization	Reduce Na$^+$ in	Improves Adenosine Triphosphate	Reduce Ca^{2+} in
Thiopental (600 µM)	Yes	Yes	Yes	Yes	Yes
Midazolam (100 µM)	Yes	—	—	Yes	Yes
Propofol (20 µg/mL)	No	No	Yes	Yes	Yes
Etomidate (3 µg/mL)	No	—	No	No	—
Lidocaine (10 µM)	Yes	Yes	Yes	Yes	No
Lidocaine (100 µM)	Yes	Yes	Yes	Yes	Yes
Nitrous oxide (50%)	No	—	No	No	No
Isoflurane (2%)	No	No	Yes	Yes	No
Sevoflurane (4%)	Yes	Yes	Yes	Yes	Yes
Desflurane (6%)	Yes	Yes	Yes	Yes	Yes

—, not determined, experiment not done; Na$^+$ in, cytosolic sodium; Ca^{2+} in, cytosolic calcium.
*Data from rat hippocampal slices at 37° C, in references 11,74,113,114,120,124,126.

Volatile Anesthetic Agents

Isoflurane is a volatile anesthetic whose protective efficacy is controversial. It does not cause greater damage and appears to have a better outcome than fentanyl–nitrous oxide anesthesia.[54,118,131,132] The advantage of volatile anesthetics are that they allow rapid awakening, for example, as might be required for an intraoperative wake-up test of neurologic function.

Sevoflurane and desflurane are two new volatile agents with metabolic and blood flow effects similar to those of isoflurane, and they have been reported to have neuroprotective effects (see Box 1-1).[133] There is an indication that isoflurane, but not sevoflurane, increases cytosolic Ca levels and can be cytotoxic to neurons in cell culture.[134] Sevoflurane was found to improve recovery in brain slices; it delayed and attenuated the hypoxic/ischemic depolarization and reduced the Ca and Na rises inside neurons. At equal minimal alveolar concentrations, sevoflurane was more effective than isoflurane.[135] It demonstrated sustained improvement after cerebral ischemia in comparison with nitrous oxide–fentanyl anesthesia.[136] Desflurane was also protective in brain slices and after cerebral ischemia in vivo.[137-141]

Preconditioning

In both heart and brain tissue, ischemic preconditioning—a short period of ischemia that allows recovery—can make tissue more resistant to a longer, normally damaging, period of ischemia. However ischemic preconditioning can lead to subtle damage.[136] Anesthetics, when given before ischemia, have been shown to induce preconditioning; these agents are most likely less damaging than ischemic preconditioning. There is much evidence indicating that isoflurane improves recovery from cerebral ischemia by preconditioning the neurons, but most of the studies have been done on male animals. A later study indicates that male, but not female mice, have better recovery from isoflurane-induced preconditioning administered 1 day before ischemia.[143] Thus it is important to remember there may be gender-specific aspects to protection from ischemic brain damage. This is a topic requiring further investigation.

Both anesthetic preconditioning and ischemic preconditioning have two time courses: Delayed preconditioning is demonstrated beginning a day after the preconditioning stimulus and lasts for several days; immediate preconditioning requires treatment only minutes to an hour before the ischemia.[144] Sevoflurane has been shown to induce preconditioning in vitro and in vivo if present only shortly before the ischemia.[34] The mechanism and extent of protection with sevoflurane in vitro was similar to that when sevoflurane was present before and during hypoxia; this finding suggests that a major portion of sevoflurane-induced protection is due to an alteration of biochemical pathways before the insult.[34] Sevoflurane preconditioning for 60 minutes, starting 90 minutes before the ischemia, with either 4% or 2% sevoflurane, increased the number of surviving CA1 pyramidal cells 6 weeks after temporary global cerebral ischemia in rats (Fig. 1-8).[34] Anesthetic preconditioning must be demonstrated clinically before it can be applied widely; however, if one is choosing an anesthetic in a patient at risk for ischemia, it might be prudent to use an agent that has been shown to be beneficial in animals.

Treatment

In summary, anesthetics have differential effects on neuronal metabolism, ionic fluxes, and membrane potentials. Anesthetics have multiple mechanisms of action; this feature complicates scientific studies but may enhance clinical protection. Hypothermia, lidocaine, thiopental, and sevoflurane have been shown to be protective against ischemia in animal studies.

Clinically, hypothermia and lidocaine show the most promise, but there is no conclusive evidence that they improve recovery from ischemia in patients. Thiopental requires very high barbiturate coma concentrations to exert its protection, whereas sevoflurane needs further study to see whether it will protect patients when given in clinically usable concentrations. Because anesthesia is required during surgery, it may prove prudent to choose an anesthetic that appears protective in animals even if it has not been demonstrated to be protective clinically; sevoflurane might be a good choice because it appears to be protective in the clinical dose range. Thiopental requires too high a dose to be used as an anesthetic in these cases, because awakening would be delayed; however, its use in the critical care setting, in which awakening is not an issue, might be beneficial. Limiting the ischemia by improving perfusion is the most effective mechanism of preventing neuronal damage from stroke. Thrombolysis and the prevention of clot formation are effective strategies.[42,145]

EPILEPTOGENIC DAMAGE

Epileptic activity is sudden, excessive, and synchronous discharges of large numbers of neurons.[146] Aside from those patients with established epilepsy, this massive increase in activity is seen in patients with ionic and electrolyte imbalances, disorders of brain metabolism, infection, brain tumor, brain trauma, and elevated body temperature. The electroencephalographic record shows spikes, which are rapid changes in voltage corresponding to excess activity in many neurons. During the epileptiform activity, sodium and calcium ions enter the cells, and potassium leaves. Thus the cells use more energy (ATP) for ion pumping. High extracellular potassium may be responsible for the large and progressive depolarization of the neurons that is commonly found. The mechanisms that lead to permanent neuronal damage with epilepsy may be similar to those that damage cells during ischemia. The enhanced excitability leads to glutamate release and excitotoxicity, which can exacerbate damage and contribute to enhanced activity due to NMDA receptor activation.[146] Activation of metabotropic glutamate receptors can contribute to the excess excitability and prolong seizures.[147] Intracellular calcium levels rise, possibly precipitating the damage. There is evidence that at least some of the permanent neuronal damage is apoptotic-like. It is clear that during epileptiform activity the energy demand and, therefore, the cerebral metabolic rate and blood flow increase greatly. Thus, in conditions in which blood flow to the brain may be compromised, it is imperative to avoid excess brain activity. Anticonvulsant medications increase neuronal inhibition or reduce excitatory processes in the brain.[148] Epileptic activity may be accompanied by systemic lactic acidosis, reduced arterial oxygenation, and increased carbon dioxide; therefore it is important to maintain ventilation, oxygenation, and blood pressure in a patient with such activity.[149] Prolonged or recurring epileptic activity can lead to profound brain damage.

Epileptic Treatment

For patients in status epilepticus, immediate treatment is necessary. Benzodiazepines such as midazolam and lorazepam are used to rapidly stop the seizure. If these agents do not stop the epileptiform activity, barbiturates (e.g., phenobarbital) are

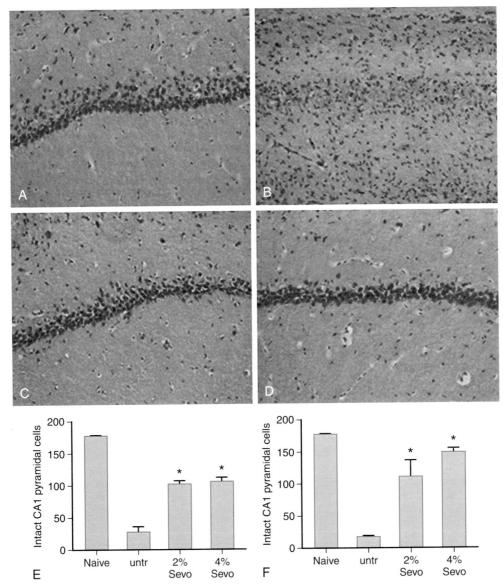

Figure 1–8 CA1 pyramidal neurons after global cerebral ischemia. **A** to **D,** Representative hematoxylin and eosin–stained cryostat sections (16 μm) from the CA1 pyramidal cell layer of the experimental groups 6 weeks after the global cerebral ischemia are shown at approximately ×250 magnification. **A,** Tissue from naïve rats not subjected to ischemia. **B,** Tissue from rats subjected to 10 minutes of global ischemia without preconditioning. **C,** Tissue from rats preconditioned with 2% sevoflurane for 1 hour before ischemia. **D,** Tissue from rats preconditioned with 4% sevoflurane for 1 hour before ischemia. **E** and **F,** The data were quantitated through counting the number of intact CA1 neurons per 475-μm length of stratum pyramidale in each hemisphere at the same level of coronal section under light microscopy (250× magnification); the observer was blind to the experimental treatment. The numbers were averaged across both hemispheres to yield a single value for each rat and expressed as number/mm (mean ± standard deviation). There were significantly more intact CA1 pyramidal cells in the rats with sevoflurane treatment (Sevo) than in the untreated ischemic group (untr) ($P < .01$) at both 1 week **(E)** and 6 weeks **(F)** after ischemia. From Wang J, Lei B, Popp S, Cottrell JE, Kass IS. Sevoflurane immediate preconditioning alters hypoxic membrane potential changes in rat hippocampal slices and improves recovery of CA1 pyramidal cells after hypoxia and global cerebral ischemia. Neuroscience 145: 1097-1107, 2007.

indicated. Loading with maintenance anticonvulsants, such as phenytoin and fosphenytoin, may proceed after acute control has been achieved.[149] In combination with ischemia, seizures can cause rapid and devastating neuronal damage and should be treated aggressively.

TRAUMA

Head trauma can lead directly to permanent physical neuronal damage. This primary damage can be caused by direct neuronal injury, brain herniation, or severing of blood vessels in the brain that results in hematoma or direct ischemia. Reversal of the primary damage is not possible; however, much of the brain injury in trauma patients is secondary, occurring after the initial insult.[150,151] Calcium influx resulting from the trauma has been implicated as a trigger for the damage. It is important to prevent the secondary ischemia that frequently follows brain trauma and is possibly due to the release of vasoconstrictive substances during reperfusion. Cerebral edema commonly follows head trauma and can lead to a marked increase in ICP. This leads to hypoperfusion of the brain even if blood pressure is maintained, as shown in the following equation:

Cerebral perfusion pressure = Mean arterial blood pressure
− Intracranial pressure

A cornerstone of treatment for cerebral edema and its subsequent high ICP is diuretic therapy with agents such as mannitol, hypertonic saline, and furosemide to remove excess fluid from the brain. In addition hemorrhage may increase intracranial blood volume and ICP, also reducing cerebral perfusion pressure. The intracranial blood can cause damage by directly promoting free radical formation using the iron in hemoglobin. Secondary damage may be reduced with proper monitoring and treatment. Hypotension has been associated with markedly worse outcome, so one of the most important interventions for improving outcome in trauma patients is maintaining normal blood pressure to prevent secondary cerebral ischemia, which is a common finding in histologic studies of terminal trauma cases.[152]

Trauma Treatment

Treatment involves lowering ICP, maintaining blood flow, reducing vasospasm, removing blood from the subarachnoid space, and, perhaps, using pharmacologic agents that interfere with the cascade of events leading to neuron damage.[151] High-dose corticosteroids, specifically methylprednisolone, have been shown to improve recovery after spinal cord trauma, although they have not been shown to be effective in treating cortical trauma.[102] These agents do increase the risk of infection and pneumonia, and some studies indicate that they may actually enhance free radical injury.[153,154] Magnesium sulfate may also improve recovery following trauma, but no large clinical studies have substantiated this observation.[155] Nimodipine has not been shown to improve recovery after head trauma but has been shown to be beneficial in patients with subarachnoid hemorrhage.[85] Although the prophylactic use of barbiturates to prevent high ICP is not justified, barbiturates did improve outcome in patients in whom high ICP was refractory to standard agents such as mannitol and furosemide.[156,157]

SUMMARY

For several pathophysiologic events in the brain, ionic imbalance (particularly, high intracellular calcium levels) and energy depletion have been implicated as possible triggers of the brain damage. In neurons subsequent to a pathophysiologic insult, molecular biological and biochemical changes are triggered, which can lead to either apoptotic-like or necrotic cell death. Thus common mechanisms of neuronal cell death for various pathophysiologic events may exist.

Thrombolysis is recommended for embolic stroke if it can be instituted within 4.5 hours of onset; this treatment worsens hemorrhagic stroke, so careful diagnosis is required. Very high-dose barbiturates and mild hypothermia have also been shown to improve ischemic outcome; other encouraging agents such as sodium channel blockers, free radical scavengers, and antiapoptosis agents have not yet been shown to have clear clinical benefits. Clinical trials with NMDA and calcium channel blockers have been disappointing; however, some encouraging results have been noted with magnesium, which blocks both NMDA and calcium channels. Methylprednisolone has been shown to improve recovery after spinal cord trauma, but not brain trauma; therefore it is only recommended after the former. Prevention of hypoperfusion and ischemia after trauma is important to reduce secondary injury. Anticonvulsant medications should be used to immediately arrest status epilepticus in surgical patients. Thus a number of treatments can be employed with some hope of reducing permanent brain damage.

References

1. Alberts B, Bray D, Johnson A, et al: How cells obtain energy from food. In *Essential Cell Biology: An Introduction to the Molecular Biology of the Cell*, New York, 1998, Garland, pp 107–124.
2. Hansen AJ: Effect of anoxia on ion distribution in the brain, *Physiol Rev* 65:101–148, 1985.
3. Rothman SM, Olney JW: Glutamate and the pathophysiology of hypoxic-ischemic brain damage, *Ann Neurol* 19:105–111, 1986.
4. Choi DW: Excitotoxic cell death, *J Neurobiol* 23:1261–1276, 1992.
5. Roettger V, Lipton P: Mechanism of glutamate release from rat hippocampal slices during in vitro ischemia, *Neuroscience* 75:677–685, 1996.
6. Watkins JC, Evans RH: Excitatory amino acid transmitters, *Annu Rev Pharmacol Toxicol* 21:165–204, 1981.
7. MacDermott AB, Dale N: Receptors, ion channels and synaptic potentials underlying the integrative actions of excitatory amino acids, *Trends Neurosci* 10:280–284, 1987.
8. Berridge MJ: Regulation of ion channels by inositol triphosphate and diacylglycerol, *J Exp Biol* 124:323, 1986.
9. Maiese K, Swiriduk M, TenBroeke M: Cellular mechanisms of protection by metabotropic glutamate receptors during anoxia and nitric acid toxicity, *J Neurochem* 66:2419–2428, 1996.
10. Olney JW: Inciting excitotoxic cytocide among central neurons, *Adv Exp Med Biol* 203:631–645, 1986.
11. Kristian T, Siesjo BK: Calcium in ischemic cell death, *Stroke* 29:705–718, 1998.
12. Tymianski M, Tator CH: Normal and abnormal calcium homeostasis in neurons: A basis for the pathophysiology of traumatic and ischemic central nervous system injury, *Neurosurgery* 38:1176–1195, 1996.
13. Siesjo BK, Katsura K, Kristian T: Acidosis-related damage, *Adv Neurol* 71:209–236, 1996.
14. Betz AL: Alterations in cerebral endothelial cell function in ischemia, *Adv Neurol* 71:301–314, 1996.
15. Chopp M, Zhang R-L, Jiang N: The role of adhesion molecules in reducing cerebral ischemic cell damage, *Adv Neurol* 71:315–328, 1996.
16. Minghetti L, Levi G: Microglia as effector cells in brain damage and repair: focus on prostanoids and nitric oxide, *Prog Neurobiol* 54:99–125, 1998.
17. Koroshetz WJ, Moskowitz MA: Emerging treatments for stroke in humans, *Trends Pharmacol Sci* 17:227–233, 1996.
18. Wang Q, Tang XN, Yenari MA: The inflammatory response in stroke, *J Neuroimmunol* 184:53–68, 2007.
19. Adachi N: Cerebral ischemia and brain histamine, *Brain Res Brain Res Rev* 50:275–286, 2005.
20. Hamami G, Adachi N, Liu K, Arai T: Alleviation of ischemic neuronal damage by histamine H2 receptor stimulation in the rat striatum, *Eur J Pharmacol* 484:167–173, 2004.
21. Hiraga N, Adachi N, Liu K, et al: Suppression of inflammatory cell recruitment by histamine receptor stimulation in ischemic rat brains, *Eur J Pharmacol* 557:236–244, 2007.
22. MacManus JP, Linnik MD: Gene expression induced by cerebral ischemia: an apoptotic perspective, *J Cereb Blood Flow Metab* 17:815–832, 1997.
23. Herdegen T, Claret FX, Kallunki T, et al: Lasting *N*-terminal phosphorylation of c-Jun and activation of c-Jun *N*-terminal kinases after neuronal injury, *J Neurosci* 18:5124–5135, 1998.
24. Namura S, Zhu J, Fink K, et al: Activation and cleavage of caspase-3 in apoptosis induced by experimental cerebral ischemia, *J Neurosci* 18:3659–3668, 1998.
25. Chen J, Nagayama T, Jin K, et al: Induction of caspase 3 like protease may mediate delayed neuronal death in the hippocampus after transient cerebral ischemia, *J Neurosci* 18:4914–4928, 1998.
26. Cheng Y, Deshmukh M, D'Costa A, et al: Caspase inhibitor affords neuroprotection with delayed administration in a rat model of neonatal hypoxic-ischemic brain injury, *J Clin Invest* 101:1992–1999, 1998.
27. Thornberry NA, Lazebnik Y: Caspases: Enemies within, *Science* 281:1312–1316, 1998.
28. Xu DG, Crocker SJ, Doucet J-P, et al: Elevation of neuronal expression of NIAP reduces ischemic damage in the rat hippocampus, *Nat Med* 3:997–1004, 1997.
29. Abe H, Nowak TS Jr: The stress response and its role in cellular defense mechanisms after ischemia, *Adv Neurol* 71:451–468, 1996.
30. Wieloch T, Hu B-R, Boris-Moller A, et al: Intracellular signal transduction in the postischemic brain: Implications for neurotransmission and neuronal survival, *Adv Neurol* 71:371–388, 1996.

31. Nikolics K, Hefti F, Thomas R, Gluckman PD: Trophic factors and their role in the post ischemic brain, *Adv Neurol* 71:389–404, 1996.

32. Lavine SD, Hofman FM, Zlokovic BV: Circulating antibody against tumor necrosis factor-alpha protects rat brain from reperfusion injury, *J Cereb Blood Flow Metab* 18:52–58, 1998.

33. Zola-Morgan S, Squire LR, Amaral DG: Human amnesia and the medial temporal region: Enduring memory impairment following a bilateral lesion limited to field CA1 of the hippocampus, *J Neurosci* 6:2950–2967, 1986.

34. Wang J, Lei B, Popp S, et al: Sevoflurane immediate preconditioning alters hypoxic membrane potential changes in rat hippocampal slices and improves recovery of CA1 pyramidal cells after hypoxia and global cerebral ischemia, *Neuroscience* 145:1097–1107, 2007.

35. Gretarsdottir S, Thorleifsson G, Reynisdottir ST, et al: The gene encoding phosphodiesterase 4D confers risk of ischemic stroke, *Nat Genet* 35:131–138, 2003.

36. Helgadottir A, Manolescu A, Thorleifsson G, et al: The gene encoding 5-lipoxygenase activating protein confers risk of myocardial infarction and stroke, *Nat Genet* 36:233–239, 2004.

37. Mustafina OE, Novikova LB, Nasibullin TR, et al: An analysis of association between the apolipoprotein B gene EcoR1 polymorphism and ischemic stroke [Russian]. Zh Nevrol Psikhiatr Im S S Korsakova, (Suppl 17):66–70, 2006.

38. Saidi S, Slamia LB, Ammou SB, et al: Association of apolipoprotein E gene polymorphism with ischemic stroke involving large-vessel disease and its relation to serum lipid levels, *J Stroke Cerebrovasc Dis* 16:160–166, 2007.

39. Mathew JP, Podgoreanu MV, Grocott HP, et al: Genetic variants in P-selectin and C-reactive protein influence susceptibility to cognitive decline after cardiac surgery, *J Am Coll Cardiol* 49:1934–1942, 2007.

40. Tissue plasminogen activator for acute ischemic stroke: The National Institute of Neurological Disorders and Stroke rt-PA Stroke Study Group, *N Engl J Med* 333:1581–1587, 1995.

41. Intracerebral hemorrhage after intravenous T-PA therapy for stroke: The NINDS t-PA Stroke Study Group, *Stroke* 28:2109–2118, 1997.

42. Charchaflieh J: Management of acute ischemic stroke, *Progress in Anesthesiology* 12:195–212, 1998.

43. Albers GW: Anticoagulant therapy for stroke prevention. In Sacco RL, editor: *Ischemic Brain Attack: Update on Management and Prevention*, New York, 1998, Health Science Communications, pp 46–50.

44. Suwanwela N, Koroshetz WJ: Acute ischemic stroke: Overview of recent therapeutic developments, *Annu Rev Med* 58:89–106, 2007.

45. Adams HP, Zoppo G del, Alberts MJ, et al: Guidelines for the Early Management of Adults with Ischemic Stroke, Stroke 38: 1655-1711, 2007.

46. Hacke W, Albers G, Al-Rawi Y, et al: The Desmoteplase in Acute Ischemic Stroke Trial (DIAS): A phase II MRI-based 9-hour window acute stroke thrombolysis trial with intravenous desmoteplase, *Stroke* 36:66–73, 2005.

47. Hacke W, Furlan AJ, Al-Rawi Y et al: Intravenous desmoteplase in patients with acute ischaemic stroke selected by MRI perfusion-diffusion weighted imaging or perfusion CT (DIAS-2): a prospective, randomised, double-blind, placebo-controlled study. Lancet Neurol. 8:141–50, 2009.

48. Smith WS, Sung G, Starkman S, et al: Safety and efficacy of mechanical embolectomy in acute ischemic stroke: results of the MERCI trial, *Stroke* 36:1432–1438, 2005.

49. Penumbra pivotal stroke trial investigators, The Penumbra Pivotal Stroke Trial. Stroke 40:2761-2768, 2009.

50. Hacke W, Kaste M, Bluhmki E, Thrombolysis with Alteplase 3 to 4.5 hours after acute ischemic stroke. New England Journal of Medicine 359:1317-29, 2008.

51. Busto R, Dietrich WD, Globus MY-T, et al: Small differences in intraischemic brain temperature critically determine the extent of ischemic neuronal injury, *J Cereb Blood Flow Metab* 7:729–738, 1987.

52. Ridenour TR, Warner DS, Todd MM, McAllister AC: Mild hypothermia reduces infarct size resulting from temporary but not permanent focal ischemia in rats, *Stroke* 23:733–738, 1992.

53. Frank SM, Beattie C, Christopherson R, et al: Unintentional hypothermia is associated with postoperative myocardial ischemia: The Perioperative Ischemia Randomized Anesthesia Trial Study Group, *Anesthesiology* 78:468–476, 1993.

54. Todd MM: Anesthesia for Intracranial Vascular Surgery. 1997 ASA Annual Refresher Course Lectures. Park Ridge, IL, American Society of Anesthesiologists, 1997, pp 151-1-151-7.

55. Cottrell JE: Brain protection in neurosurgery. 1997 Annual Refresher Course Lectures. Park Ridge, IL, American Society of Anesthesiologists, 1997, pp 153-1-153-7

56. Mild therapeutic hypothermia to improve the neurologic outcome after cardiac arrest: Hypothermia after Cardiac Arrest Study Group, *N Engl J Med* 346:549–556, 2002.

57. Bernard SA, Gray TW, Buist MD, et al: Treatment of comatose survivors of out-of-hospital cardiac arrest with induced hypothermia, *N Engl J Med* 346:557–563, 2002.

58. Fukuda S, Warner DS: Cerebral protection, *Br J Anaesth* 99:10–17, 2007.

59. Kammersgaard LP, Jorgensen HS, Rungby JA, et al: Admission body temperature predicts long-term mortality after acute stroke: The Copenhagen Stroke Study, *Stroke* 33:1759–1762, 2002.

60. Myers RE, Yamaguchi M: Effects of serum glucose concentration on brain response to circulatory arrest, *J Neuropathol Exp Neurol* 35:301, 1976.

61. Gentile NT, Seftchick MW, Huynh T, et al: Decreased mortality by normalizing blood glucose after acute ischemic stroke, *Acad Emerg Med* 13:174–180, 2006.

62. NICE-SUGAR study Investigators. Intensive versus conventional glucose control in critically ill patients. New England Journal of Medicine 360:1283-97, 2009.

63. Green AR: Pharmacological approaches to acute ischaemic stroke: reperfusion certainly, neuroprotection possibly, *Br J Pharmacol* 153(Suppl 1):S325–S338, 2008.

64. Donnan GA, Davis SM: Neuroprotection: Still achievable in humans, *Stroke* 39:525, 2008.

65. Rother J: Neuroprotection does not work!, *Stroke* 39:523–524, 2008.

66. Mehta SL, Manhas N, Raghubir R: Molecular targets in cerebral ischemia for developing novel therapeutics, *Brain Res Rev* 54:34–66, 2007.

67. Boening JA, Kass IS, Cottrell JE, Chambers G: The effect of blocking sodium influx on anoxia damage in the rat hippocampal slice, *Neuroscience* 33:263–268, 1989.

68. Taylor CP, Narasimhan LS: Sodium channels and therapy of central nervous system diseases, *Adv Pharmacol* 39:47–98, 1997.

69. Cao H, Kass IS, Cottrell JE, Bergold PJ: Pre- or postinsult administration of lidocaine or thiopental attenuates cell death in rat hippocampal slice cultures caused by oxygen-glucose deprivation, *Anesth Analg* 101:1163–1169, 2005.

70. Hansen AJ, Hounsgaard J, Jahnsen H: Anoxia increases potassium conductance in hippocampal nerve cells, *Acta Physiol Scand* 115:301–310, 1982.

71. Kass IS, Lipton P: Mechanisms involved in irreversible anoxic damage to the in vitro rat hippocampal slice, *J Physiol* 332:459–472, 1982.

72. Tanaka E, Yamamoto S, Kudo Y, et al: Mechanisms underlying the rapid depolarization produced by deprivation of oxygen and glucose in rat hippocampal CA1 neurons in vitro, *J Neurophysiol* 78:891–902, 1997.

73. Wang T, Raley-Susman KM, Wang J, et al: Thiopental attenuates hypoxic changes of electrophysiology, biochemistry, and morphology in rat hippocampal slice CA 1 pyramidal cells, *Stroke* 30:2400–2407, 1999.

74. Raley-Susman KM, Kass IS, Cottrell JE, et al: Sodium influx blockade and hypoxic damage to CA1 pyramidal neurons in rat hippocampal slices, *J Neurophysiol* 86:2715–2726, 2001.

75. Liu K, Adachi N, Yanase H, et al: Lidocaine suppresses the anoxic depolarization and reduces the increase in the intracellular Ca++ concentration in gerbil hippocampal neurons, *Anesthesiology* 87:1470–1478, 1997.

76. Seyfried FJ, Adachi N, Arai T: Suppression of energy requirement by lidocaine in the ischemic mouse brain, *J Neurosurg Anesthesiol* 17:75–81, 2005.

77. Fried E, Amorim P, Chambers G, et al: The importance of sodium for anoxic transmission damage in rat hippocampal slices: Mechanisms of protection by lidocaine, *J Physiol* 489:557–565, 1995.

78. Lei B, Cottrell JE, Kass IS: Neuroprotective effect of low-dose lidocaine in a rat model of transient focal cerebral ischemia, *Anesthesiology* 95:445–451, 2001.

79. Lei B, Popp S, Capuano-Waters C, et al: Lidocaine attenuates apoptosis in the ischemic penumbra and reduces infarct size after transient focal cerebral ischemia in rats, *Neuroscience* 125:691–701, 2004.

80. Lei B, Popp S, Capuano-Waters C, et al: Effects of delayed administration of low-dose lidocaine on transient focal cerebral ischemia in rats, *Anesthesiology* 97:1534–1540, 2002.

81. Popp S, Lei B, Cottrell JE, Kass IS: Effects of low-dose lidocaine administration on transient global cerebral ischemia in rats, *Anesthesiology* 032005:A115.

82. Popp SS, Kelemen E, Fenton A, et al: Effects of low-dose lidocaine administration on transient global cerebral ischemia in rats. Presented at American Society of Anesthesiologists Annual Meeting, San Francisco, Oct 13-17, 2007.

83. Mitchell SJ, Pellett O, Gorman DF: Cerebral protection by lidocaine during cardiac operations, *Ann Thorac Surg* 67:1117–1124, 1999.

84. Wang D, Wu X, Li J, et al: The effect of lidocaine on early postoperative cognitive dysfunction after coronary artery bypass surgery, *Anesth Analg* 95:1134–1141, 2002.

85. Mayberg MR, Batjer HH, Dacey R, et al: Guidelines for the management of aneurysmal subarachnoid hemorrhage, *Circulation* 90:2592–2605, 1994.

86. Legault SW, Furberg CD, Wagenknecht LE, et al: Nimodipine neuroprotection in cardiac valve replacement: Report of an early terminated trial, *Stroke* 27:593–598, 1996.

87. Kass IS, Abramowicz AE, Cottrell JE, et al: Anoxia reduces depolarization induced calcium uptake in the rat hippocampal slice, *Brain Res* 633:262–266, 1994.

88. Kass IS, Cottrell JE, Chambers G: Magnesium and cobalt, not nimodipine protect neurons against anoxic damage in the rat hippocampal slice, *Anesthesiology* 69:710–715, 1988.

89. Marinov MB, Harbaugh KS, Hoopes PJ, et al: Neuroprotective effects of preischemic intraarterial magnesium sulfate in reversible focal cerebral ischemia, *J Neurosurg* 85:117–124, 1996.

90. Muir KW: New experimental and clinical data on the efficacy of pharmacological magnesium infusions in cerebral infarcts, *Magnes Res* 11:43–56, 1998.

91. Muir KW, Lees KR, Ford I, Davis S: Magnesium for acute stroke (Intravenous Magnesium Efficacy in Stroke trial): randomised controlled trial, *Lancet* 363:439–445, 2004.

92. Aslanyan S, Weir CJ, Muir KW, Lees KR: Magnesium for treatment of acute lacunar stroke syndromes: Further analysis of the IMAGES trial, *Stroke* 38:1269–1273, 2007.

93. Marret S, Marpeau L, Zupan-Simunek V, et al: Magnesium sulphate given before very-preterm birth to protect infant brain: The randomised controlled PREMAG trial*, *BJOG* 114:310–318, 2007.

94. Saatman KE, Murai H, Bartus RT, et al: Calpain inhibitor AK295 attenuates motor and cognitive deficits following experimental brain injury in the rat, *Proc Natl Acad Sci U S A* 93:3428–3433, 1996.

95. van der Worp HB, Bar PR, Kappelle LL, Wildt DJ: Dietary vitamin E levels affect outcome of permanent focal cerebral ischemia in rats, *Stroke* 29:1002–1005, 1998.

96. Cao X, Phillis JW: alpha-Phenyl-tert-butyl-nitrone reduces cortical infarct and edema in rats subjected to focal ischemia, *Brain Res* 644: 267–272, 1994.

97. Kuroda S, Tsuchidate R, Smith ML, et al: Neuroprotective effects of a novel nitrone, NXY-059, after transient focal cerebral ischemia in the rat, *J Cereb Blood Flow Metab* 19:778–787, 1999.

98. Zhao Z, Cheng M, Maples KR, et al: NXY-059, a novel free radical trapping compound, reduces cortical infarction after permanent focal cerebral ischemia in the rat, *Brain Res* 909:46–50, 2001.

99. Lees KR, Zivin JA, Ashwood T, et al: NXY-059 for acute ischemic stroke, *N Engl J Med* 354:588–600, 2006.

100. Shuaib A, Lees KR, Lyden P, et al: NXY-059 for the treatment of acute ischemic stroke, *N Engl J Med* 357:562–571, 2007.

101. Hall ED: Lipid peroxidation, *Adv Neurol* 71:247–258, 1996.

102. Bracken MB, Shepard MJ, Holford TR, et al: Administration of methylprednisolone for 24 or 48 hours or tirilazad mesylate for 48 hours in the treatment of acute spinal cord injury: Results of the third national acute spinal cord injury randomized controlled trial, *JAMA* 277:1597–1604, 1997.

103. Haley EC Jr, Kassell NF, Apperson-Hansen CE, et al: A randomized, double blind, vehicle controlled trial of tirilazad mesylate in patients with aneurysmal subarachnoid hemorrhage: A cooperative study in North America, *J Neurosurg* 86:467–474, 1997.

104. Haley EC: Jr: High-dose tirilazad for acute stroke (RANTTAS II). RANTTAS II investigators [letter], *Stroke* 29:1256–1257, 1998.

105. Feuerstein GZ, Wang X, Barone FC: Inflammatory gene expression in cerebral ischemia and trauma: Potential new therapeutic targets, *Ann N Y Acad Sci* 825:179–193, 1997.

106. De Ryck M: Protection of neurological function in stroke models and neuroprotective properties of lubeluzole, *Cerebrovasc Dis* 7(Suppl 2):18–30, 1997.

107. Lyden P, Wahlgren NG: Mechanisms of action of neuroprotectants in stroke, *J Stroke Cerebrovasc Dis* 9:9–14, 2000.

108. Onal MZ, Fisher M: Acute ischemic stroke therapy: A clinical overview, *Eur Neurol* 38:141–154, 1997.

109. Pettigrew LC: Neuroprotection: Theory and practice. In Sacco RL, editor: *Ischemic Brain Attack: Update on management and Prevention*, New York, 1998, Health Science Communications, pp 25–32.

110. Barinaga M: Stroke-damaged neurons may commit cellular suicide, *Science* 218:1302–1303, 1998.

111. Green DG, Reed JC: Mitochondria and apoptosis, *Science* 281: 1309–1312, 1998.

112. Mehta SL, Manhas N, Raghubir R, Molecular targets in cerebral ischemia for developing novel therapeutics. Brain Research Reviews 54:34-66, 2007.

113. Lodish H, Berk A, Matsudaira P, et al: *Cell birth lineage and death, Molecular Cell Biology*. ed 5, New York, 2004, WH Freeman, 899–934.

114. Wang Y, Zhang ZG, Rhodes K, et al: Post-ischemic treatment with erythropoietin or carbamylated erythropoietin reduces infarction and improves neurological outcome in a rat model of focal cerebral ischemia, *Br J Pharmacol* 151:1377–1384, 2007.

115. Ehrenreich H, Hasselblatt M, Dembowski C, et al: Erythropoietin therapy for acute stroke is both safe and beneficial, *Mol Med* 8:495–505, 2002.

116. Nussmeier NA, Arlund C, Slogoff S: Neuropsychiatric complications after cardiopulmonary bypass: Cerebral protection by a barbiturate, *Anesthesiology* 64:165–170, 1986.

117. Kass IS, Abramowicz AE, Cottrell JE, Chambers G: The barbiturate thiopental reduces ATP levels during anoxia but improves electrophysiological recovery and ionic homeostasis in the rat hippocampal slice, *Neuroscience* 49:537–543, 1992.

118. Drummond JC, Shapiro HM: Cerebral physiology. In Miller RD, editor: *Anesthesia*, ed 4, New York, 1994, Churchill Livingstone, pp 689–730.

119. Amadeu ME, Abramowicz AE, et al: Etomidate does not alter recovery after anoxia of evoked population spikes recorded from the CA1 region of rat hippocampal slices, *Anesthesiology* 88:1274–1280, 1998.

120. Amorim P, Chambers G, Cottrell JE, Kass IS: Propofol reduces neuronal transmission damage and attenuates the changes in Ca, K and Na during hyperthermic anoxia in the rat hippocampal slice, *Anesthesiology* 83:1254–1265, 1995.

121. Zhu H, Cottrell JE, Kass IS: The effect of thiopental and propofol on NMDA- and AMPA-mediated glutamate excitotoxicity, *Anesthesiology* 87:944–951, 1997.

122. Engelhard K, Werner C, Eberspacher E, et al: Influence of propofol on neuronal damage and apoptotic factors after incomplete cerebral ischemia and reperfusion in rats: A long-term observation, *Anesthesiology* 101:912–917, 2004.

123. Kobayashi M, Takeda Y, Taninishi H, et al: Quantitative evaluation of the neuroprotective effects of thiopental sodium, propofol, and halothane on brain ischemia in the gerbil: Effects of the anesthetics on ischemic depolarization and extracellular glutamate concentration, *J Neurosurg Anesthesiol* 19:171–178, 2007.

124. Amorim P, Chambers G, Cottrell J, Kass IS: Nitrous oxide impairs electrophysiologic recovery after severe hypoxia in rat hippocampal slices, *Anesthesiology* 87:642–651, 1997.

125. Sugaya T, Kitani Y: Nitrous oxide attenuates the protective effect of isoflurane on microtubule-associated protein2 degradation during forebrain ischemia in the rat, *Brain Res Bull* 44:307–309, 1997.

126. Fleischer JE, Milde JH, Moyer TP, Michenfelder JD: Cerebral effects of high-dose midazolam and subsequent reversal with Ro 15-1788 in dogs, *Anesthesiology* 68:234–242, 1988.

127. Baughman VL, Hoffman WE, Miletich DJ, Albrecht RF: Cerebral metabolic depression and brain protection produced by midazolam and etomidate in the rat, *J Neurosurg Anesthesiol* 1:22–28, 1989.

128. Abramowicz AE, Kass IS, Chambers G, Cottrell JE: Midazolam improves electrophysiologic recovery after anoxia and reduces the changes in ATP levels and calcium influx during anoxia in the rat hippocampal slice, *Anesthesiology* 74:1121–1128, 1991.

129. Ito H, Watanabe Y, Isshiki A, Uchino H: Neuroprotective properties of propofol and midazolam, but not pentobarbital, on neuronal damage induced by forebrain ischemia, based on the GABAA receptors, *Acta Anaesth Scand* 43:153–162, 1999.

130. Lei B, Popp S, Cottrell JE, Kass IS. Effects of midazolam on brain injury after transient focal cerebral ischemia in rats. Jorunal of Neurosurgical Anesthesiology 21:131–9, 2009.

131. Kass IS, Amorim P, Chambers G, et al: The effect of isoflurane on biochemical changes during and electrophysiological recovery after anoxia in rat hippocampal slices, *J Neurosurg Anesthesiol* 9:280–286, 1997.

132. Patel PM, Drummond JC, Cole DJ, et al: Isoflurane and pentobarbital reduce the frequency of transient ischemic depolarizations during focal ischemia in rats, *Anesth Analg* 86:773–780, 1998.

133. Pasternak JJ, Lanier WL: Neuroanesthesiology review—2006, *J Neurosurg Anesthesiol* 19:70–92, 2007.

134. Wang QJ, Li KZ, Yao SL, et al: Different effects of isoflurane and sevoflurane on cytotoxicity, *Chin Med J (Engl)* 121:341–346, 2008.

135. Wang J, Meng F, Cottrell J, Kass I: The differential effects of volatile anesthetics on electrophysiological and biochemical changes during and recovery after hypoxia in rat hippocampal slice CA1 pyramidal cells, *Neuroscience* 140:957–967, 2006.

136. Pape M, Engelhard K, Eberspacher E, et al: The long-term effect of sevoflurane on neuronal cell damage and expression of apoptotic factors after cerebral ischemia and reperfusion in rats, *Anesth Analg* 103: 173–179, 2006.

137. Dimaculangan D, Bendo AA, Sims R, et al: Desflurane improves the recovery of evoked postsynaptic population spike from CA1 pyramidal cells after hypoxia in rat hippocampal slices, *J Neurosurg Anesthesiol* 18:78–82, 2006.

138. Haelewyn B, Yvon A, Hanouz JL, et al: Desflurane affords greater protection than halothane against focal cerebral ischemia in the rat, *Br J Anaesth* 91:390–396, 2003.

139. Tsai SK, Lin SM, Hung WC, et al: The effect of desflurane on ameliorating cerebral infarction in rats subjected to focal cerebral ischemia-reperfusion injury, *Life Sci* 74:2541–2549, 2004.

140. Wise-Faberowski L, Raizada MK, Sumners C: Desflurane and sevoflurane attenuate oxygen and glucose deprivation-induced neuronal cell death, *J Neurosurg Anesthesiol* 15:193–199, 2003.

141. Wang J, Cottrell JE, Kass IS. Effects of desflurane and propofol on electrophysiological parameters during and recovery after hypoxia in rat hippocampal slice CA1 pyramidal cells. Neuroscience 160:140–8, 2009.

142. Sommer C: Ischemic preconditioning: Postischemic structural changes in the brain, *J Neuropathol Exp Neurol* 67:85–92, 2008.

143. Kitano H, Young JM, Cheng J, et al: Gender-specific response to isoflurane preconditioning in focal cerebral ischemia, *J Cereb Blood Flow Metab* 27:1377–1386, 2007.

144. Clarkson AN: Anesthetic-mediated protection/preconditioning during cerebral ischemia, *Life Sci* 80:1157–1175, 2007.

145. Libman R: Thrombolysis in the first three hours. In Sacco RL, editor: *Ischemic Brain Attack: Update on Management and Prevention,* New York, 1998, Health Sciences Communications, pp 12–16.

146. Meldrum B: Epileptic seizures. In Siegel GJ, Agranoff BW, Albers RW, Molinoff PB, editors: *Basic Neurochemistry,* New York, 1994, Raven Press, pp 885–898.

147. Wong RKS, Merlin LR, Bianchi R, Taylor GW: Role of metabotropic glutamate receptors in epilepsy. In Delgado-Escueta AV, Wilson WA, Olsen RW, Porter RJ, editors: *Jasper's Basic Mechanisms of the Epilepsies,* ed 3, Philadelphia, 1998, Lippincott-Raven.

148. Dichter MA: Basic mechanisms of epilepsy: Targets for therapeutic intervention, *Epilepsia* 38(Suppl 9):S2–S6, 1997.

149. Lowenstein DH, Alldredge BK: Status epilepticus, *N Engl J Med* 338:970–976, 1998.

150. Chestnut RM: The management of severe traumatic brain injury, *Emerg Med Clin N Am* 15:581–604, 1997.

151. Prough DS: *Management of head trauma. 1997 Annual Refresher Course Lectures. Park Ridge IL, American Society of Anesthesiologists* 1997: 253-1–253-7.

152. Pietropaoli JA, Rogers FB, Shackford SR, et al: The deleterious effects of intraoperative hypotension on outcome in patients with severe head injuries, *J Trauma* 33:403–407, 1992.

153. Gerndt SJ, Rodriguez JL, Pawlik JW, et al: Consequences of high-dose steroid therapy for acute spinal cord injury, *J Trauma* 42:279–284, 1997.

154. McIntosh LJ, Sapolsky RM: Glucocorticoids may enhance oxygen radical-mediated neurotoxicity, *Neurotoxicology* 17:873–882, 1996.

155. Feldman Z, Gurevitch B, Artru AA, et al: Effect of magnesium given 1 hour after head trauma on brain edema and neurological outcome, *J Neurosurg* 85:131–137, 1996.

156. Ward JD, Becker DP, Miller JD: Failure of prophylactic barbiturate coma in the treatment of severe head injury, *J Neurosurg* 62:383–388, 1985.

157. Eisenberg HM, Frankowski RF, Contant CF, et al: High-dose barbiturate control of elevated intracranial pressure in patients with severe head injury, *J Neurosurg* 69:15–23, 1988.

Chapter 2

CEREBRAL AND SPINAL CORD BLOOD FLOW

Shailendra Joshi • Eugene Ornstein • William L. Young

Studies of cerebral circulation have improved the understanding of the function and pathophysiology of the central nervous system (CNS).[1] This chapter focuses on the regulation of cerebral circulation. It begins with a discussion on regulation of cerebral blood flow in health and the failure of regulation in disease states, and proceeds to discuss the methodology for measuring cerebral blood flow (CBF). A discussion of spinal cord blood flow follows; the chapter ends with a discussion of the applied aspects of manipulating cerebral blood flow and monitoring CBF in the clinical setting. The purpose of this chapter is to review the basic mechanisms of CNS circulatory behavior and the tools used to understand them.

PHYSIOLOGY OF THE CEREBRAL CIRCULATION

Cerebral Metabolism

Under most circumstances, neuronal function depends totally on oxidative metabolism of glucose to provide adenosine triphosphate (ATP), which ultimately fuels all cellular processes. Although the brain accounts for only 2% of body weight, it utilizes 20% of the oxygen needed by the body under resting conditions. Lack of substrate storage in the brain and its high metabolic rate account for the relative sensitivity of the brain to glucose and oxygen deprivation.

Brain metabolism can be split into two parts, the portion that drives the "work" of the brain—that is, synaptic transmission (*activation metabolism*)—and the portion necessary for cellular integrity (*basal metabolism*). A large part of the basal metabolism is devoted to the maintenance of the normal transmembrane ionic gradients (i.e., keeping potassium ions [K^+] inside and sodium and calcium ions [Na^+ and Ca^{2+}] outside the cell). The remainder of basal metabolism is concerned with protein and neurotransmitter synthesis and other basic cellular functions.

Regional Cerebral Blood Flow Requirements

The lack of a substrate reserve in the CNS and its inability to sustain anaerobic metabolism for more than a few minutes requires a constant blood flow that is finely tuned to the metabolic needs of the tissue. The CNS is a complex and structurally diverse organ that comprises multiple functional subdivisions. Neurons account for approximately half of the brain volume; the remainder consists of glial and vascular elements. In addition to mechanical support of neurons, the glia has important regulatory functions (e.g., neurotransmitter handling and maintenance of the metabolic milieu of the neuropile) that, at present, are imperfectly understood.

The metabolic rates differ considerably within the brain tissue; for instance, there is an approximately fourfold difference in cerebral metabolic rate for oxygen (CMR_{O_2}) and CBF between cortical gray matter and white matter. Flow and metabolism are said to be coupled, and under physiologic conditions, including sedation and general anesthesia, this coupling is generally preserved (Figs. 2-1 and 2-2).[2-4] Intravenous anesthetic agents such as propofol seem to preserve flow-metabolism coupling better than volatile agents.[5] In humans, this coupling is evident during anesthetic-induced burst suppression on the electroencephalogram (EEG), as demonstrated by transcranial Doppler ultrasonography (TCD) studies during normothermia[6,7] and during mild to moderate hypothermic cardiopulmonary bypass.[8]

Regulation of Cerebral Blood Flow

A rapid and precise regulatory system has evolved in the CNS whereby instantaneous increases in metabolic demand can be rapidly met by a local increase in CBF and substrate delivery. As known for a long time and demonstrated with multiple imaging modalities, the time course of this regulatory process is rapid.[9,10] Contralateral cortical areas "light up," demonstrating increased flow with hand movement, and a variety of motor and cognitive tasks can be mapped with CBF techniques.[11-13] Visual stimulation results in almost immediate increases in flow velocity through the posterior cerebral arteries. Positron emission tomography (PET), magnetic resonance imaging (MRI) and time-resolved near-infrared spectroscopy are beginning to unravel the interrelated functions and their temporal relationships in various cortical areas activated by complex phenomena such as language and visual processing.[14-16] As in most specialized vascular beds, this flow-metabolism coupling is critical during times of stress or extreme physiologic conditions, such as hypotension, hypoxia and hypothermia.[8] These pathologic processes engage regulatory mechanisms to keep flow at physiologic levels.

The term autoregulation is used by some to describe the hemodynamic response of flow to changes in perfusion pressure independent of flow-metabolism coupling. The problem with this approach is that the precise mechanisms responsible for maintenance of CBF are poorly understood.[17] We argue for the general case; that is, that *autoregulation* implies a general matching of flow to metabolism, irrespective of mechanism. For example, the ability of the cerebral vasculature to dilate in response to tissue hypoxia certainly qualifies as an autoregulatory phenomenon, and it may be an oxygen-sensitive mechanism that regulates vascular resistance in the normoxic or hyperoxic range.[18] Perhaps when the mediators of these "autoregulatory" events are more precisely known, better terminology can be devised. *Autoregulatory* responses

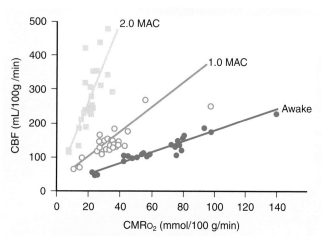

Figure 2–1 Cerebral blood flow (CBF) as a function of the cerebral metabolic rate for oxygen (CMRo₂) in different brain regions of the rat, as determined by autoradiography during isoflurane anesthesia. Three groups are shown: awake, 1.0 MAC, and 2.0 MAC. Note that the volatile anesthetic does not uncouple flow and metabolism; rather, flow-metabolism coupling is "reset" along a different line. *(Modified from Maekawa T, Tommasino C, Shapiro HM, et al: Local cerebral blood flow and glucose utilization during isoflurane anesthesia in the rat. Anesthesiology 1986;65:144-151. Figure courtesy Dr. David S. Warner, University of Iowa.)*

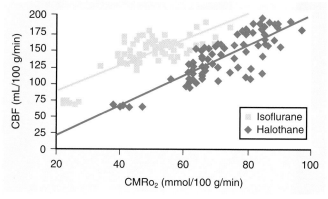

Figure 2–2 Cerebral blood flow (CBF) as a function of the cerebral metabolic rate for oxygen (CMRo₂) in different brain regions of the rat, as determined by autoradiography during halothane and isoflurane anesthesia. As in Figure 2-1, flow and metabolism remained coupled for both anesthetics. Note that for a given CMRo₂ value, flow is actually higher for isoflurane than for halothane. *(From Hansen TD, Warner DS, Todd MM, et al: The role of cerebral metabolism in determining the local cerebral blood flow effects of volatile anesthetics: Evidence for persistent flow-metabolism coupling. J Cereb Blood Flow Metab 1989;9:323-328.)*

are those that maintain the internal milieu of the CNS. Those that endanger CNS well-being are *dysregulatory*. Semantics aside, a clinical distinction can be made between two distinct processes that may or may not be mechanistically related—flow-metabolism coupling and active vasomotion in response to circulatory perturbation. There seems to be an elegant dichotomy of control in the cerebral vascular bed. The "distal vascular" bed can respond rapidly to the sudden changes in the metabolic needs of the tissue, whereas the "proximal vasculature" ensures adequate delivery of blood across a range of perfusion pressures. The two systems probably communicate with each other, in part through nonadrenergic, noncholinergic neurons that innervate the distal penetrating arterioles.[19,20]

Since Roy and Sherrington[21] put forth their hypothesis more than 100 years ago, the prevailing paradigm has been that local metabolic factors are involved in flow-metabolism coupling. However, pure changes in perfusion pressure undoubtedly involve a myogenic response in vascular smooth muscle as well (Bayliss effect).[22] This myogenic response may actually consist of two separate mechanisms, one responding to mean blood pressure changes and the other sensitive to pulsatile pressure.[23] Evidence shows that flow, irrespective of pressure, may affect vascular resistance.[24] An overwhelming number of metabolic mediators for CBF regulation have been proposed, including hydrogen ion, potassium, adenosine, glycolytic intermediates, and phospholipid metabolites.[17,22] Both neurons and astrocytes seem to participate in flow-metabolism coupling.[25] Endothelium-derived factors[26] such as nitric oxide (NO) enable the endothelium to function as a transducer that controls the tone of the vascular smooth muscles.[27] The interactions between the endothelium and the smooth muscle cells are complex and have built in redundancy. Cellular mechanisms within the endothelium and the vascular smooth muscles often converge on intracellular Ca²⁺ as their final common pathway. However, no single mechanism seems to be playing a preeminent role in regulating blood flow to the brain.[20,28]

Independent assessment of CBF and oxygen utilization by means of PET reveals that the increase in brain activity in response to sensory stimulation results in a minimal increase in O₂ consumption (CMRo₂, ~5%) but a considerably greater increase (~30% to 50%) in blood flow.[29] Such an increase in CBF is coupled to the increase in the cerebral metabolic rate for glucose. The disproportionate increases in CBF and cerebral metabolic rate for glucose in comparison with CMRo₂ raise the possibility of anaerobic metabolism in the brain.[30]

The issue of anaerobic metabolism in the brain has been debated ever since these observations were first made in the last decade, and conflicting evidence has been presented in this area. In support of anaerobic metabolism, evidence shows transient lactate production during photoptic stimulation.[31] On the other hand, evidence of an early rapid increase in tissue deoxyhemoglobin concentrations during cortical activity suggests a rise in oxygen use.[32] The emerging consensus is that cortical activity increases CMRo₂ but that there seems to be a much greater increase in CBF, which is coupled to an increased cerebral metabolic rate for glucose. The temporal relationship among neuronal activation, glucose utilization, and blood flow coupling is still being debated. It is now believed that neuronal activation prompts immediate anaerobic glucose metabolism to meet the energy demands for glutamate release. However, clearance of glutamate requires oxidation of glucose in amounts that are in excess of oxygen utilization, resulting in a net efflux of lactate.[33] Under physiologic conditions lactate is subsequently oxidized to generate additional energy.

Perivascular innervation in the brain has been recognized since Willis first described the cerebral circulation in 1664. Nevertheless, the precise function of this innervation remains obscure. The current paradigm holds that autonomic nerves are not necessary for regulatory responses but may modify them in several important ways.[34] Nonetheless, this view may change because growing attention is being paid to neural control mechanisms.[17,35] A major deficiency in the "local metabolic" theory is that the necessary temporal relationship between accumulation of vasoactive metabolites and flow increases has not been adequately demonstrated. In addition, in many situations, CBF and CMRo₂ change in the same direction but CBF increases out of proportion to metabolic rate, such as during seizure activity. Lou and associates[17] proposed that flow and metabolism level may be maintained after they have been set in place by a "rapid initiator" that involves a neurogenic mechanism.

Cellular Mechanisms of Cerebral Vasomotion

The remarkable ability of the cerebral vessels to respond to changes in cerebral metabolism, perfusion pressure, and milieu interior, such as $PaCO_2$, are mediated by a number of cellular mechanisms. These mechanisms involve nitric oxide, prostaglandins (PGE_2, PGI_2, and $PGF_{2\alpha}$), vasoactive peptides, potassium channels, and endothelin.[20,28,36]

Nitric Oxide

Although unlikely to be directly involved in pressure auto-regulation itself,[37] NO is the subject of intense scrutiny as a mediator of vascular tone[38] and as a neurotransmitter.[39,40] The interest in NO results from the identification of the multiple biologic roles it plays as a messenger molecule.[39] Although until recently no evidence had shown it to have any biologic function at all in vertebrates, NO now appears to have at least the following major roles: (1) as having bactericidal and tumoricidal effects in white blood cells, (2) as a neurotransmitter, and (3) as a moderator/mediator of vascular tone, functioning as an "endothelium-derived relaxing factor."[20]

NO is synthesized from L-arginine by nitric oxide synthase (NOS). There are at least three isoforms of NOS: endothelial (eNOS), neuronal (nNOS), and inducible (iNOS).[41] Of these, eNOS and neuronal NOS exist in the normal brain, whereas inducible NOS synthesis can be induced by endotoxins and cytokines. Endogenous inhibitors of NOS, such as asymmetric dimethyl-L-arginine (ADMA), are produced during protein catabolism and may reach concentrations sufficient to inhibit NOS activity in the brain.[36] NO action has been studied through the use of arginine analogues such as NG-nitro-L-arginine methyl ester (L-NAME), 7-nitroindazole, and aminoguanidine, which can nonselectively or selectively block NO synthesis. NO appears to influence basal tone,[42] including the endothelium-dependent response to acetylcholine in cerebral arteries[43] and vasogenic dilation from stimulation of nonadrenergic, noncholinergic nerves.[44] In general, topical, systemic, and intra-arterial application of NO donors increases CBF in several animal species.[45,46] In humans, intra-arterial injection of the NO donor nitroprusside into angiographically normal territories in patients with cerebral arteriovenous malformations failed to augment CBF.[47,48] In contrast, a study in human volunteers found that systemic and intra-arterial administration of NG-monomethyl-L-arginine (L-NMMA), a nonspecific inhibitor of eNOS, decreases CBF.[49,50] The latter findings suggest that NO may be involved in regulation of basal cerebrovascular tone. After synthesis, NO diffuses into the vascular myocyte and activates guanylate cyclase, forming cyclic guanosine monophosphate (cGMP). A protein kinase is stimulated by cyclic guanosine monophosphate, resulting in phosphorylation of the light chain of myosin and thus vascular relaxation.[39] NO may also act partly through calcitonin gene–related peptide (CGRP) and ATP-sensitive potassium (KATP) channels.[51] NO partly acts also by suppressing endothelial generation of vasoconstrictors such as thromboxane A_2. In pathologic settings, such as vasospasm and hypoxia, Rho kinase, a serine threonine kinase, is emerging as a potent mechanism of sustained vasoconstriction that in part acts through the NO pathway.[52] Inhibition of Rho kinase increases cerebral blood flow.[53] In middle cerebral artery occlusion models, Rho kinase inhibition improves neurologic outcome.[54,55] Rho kinase inhibition increases eNOS synthesis, and Rho kinase seems to negatively regulate eNOS activity.[56] Calcium is intimately involved in vascular relaxation by NO. NO appears to be formed on demand and is not stored in vesicles—the traditional fate of neurotransmitters.

The role of NO in the response to vasodilation due to changes in perfusion pressure or carbon dioxide (CO_2) remains to be coherently defined. For example, nonspecific inhibition of NOS in primates does not affect pressure auto-regulation but impairs response to carbon dioxide.[37] However, in humans, nonspecific inhibition of NOS results in a decrease in CBF that does not affect response to hypercapnia.[50] In rodents, nonspecific inhibition of NOS impairs autoregulatory response to hypotension in basilar artery irrigation,[57] but selective neuronal NOS inhibition by 7-nitroindazole has no effect on baseline blood flow, although 7-nitroindazole can prevent the increase in blood flow due to neural activation.[58] However, 7-nitroindazole decreases collateral blood flow during middle cerebral artery occlusion in dogs.[59]

Some investigators have reported that NO appears to play a role in dilation in response to CO_2[60-63]; in other experiments, however, its participation in hypocapnia-induced vasoconstriction could not be demonstrated.[43] Iadecola and Zhang[64] proposed that NO plays a "permissive" role in hypercapnic vasodilation. During cerebral vasodilation, NO may play either an "obligatory" or a "permissive" role. Obligatory implies that NO directly mediates vasodilation through that mechanism. For example, topical application of glutamate agonists results in vasodilation that can be markedly attenuated by inhibition of NOS. Therefore, NO seems to play an obligatory role in glutamate-mediated vasodilation. Permissive implies that NO facilitates relaxation but near-complete inhibition of NOS only partly attenuates the vasodilator response. Because hypercapnic response is only partly attenuated by NOS inhibition, NO's role is described as permissive, with other mechanisms also contributing to hypercapnic dilation. NO appears to play a much greater role in hypercapnic vasodilation in adults than in neonates.[51] The site of action for CO_2-induced NO production may be not in the endothelium but, rather, in the perivascular structures, such as astrocytes.[60]

The participation of NO in hypoxia-induced vasodilation does not appear to be physiologically important.[61,65,66] In regard to anesthetic effects on CBF, NO appears to interact with the cerebral vasodilatory effects of both halothane[67] and isoflurane.[68] The role of NO as a neurotransmitter undoubtedly will prove to be significant for care of the patient with neurologic disease through its interactions with anesthetic depth[69] and cerebral ischemic states,[66,70] in particular the pathogenesis of vasospasm after subarachnoid hemorrhage (SAH).[28] Inhibition of NO synthesis leads to vasoconstriction due to unopposed effects of endothelial prostanoids, such as thromboxane A_2 and prostaglandin $F_{2\alpha}$.[71] Vascular abnormalities in disease states that significantly predispose the brain to damage, such as diabetes mellitus, may also be related to an NO-mediated mechanism.[61]

Vasoactive Peptides

In the cerebral circulation, perivascular nerves contain several vasodilator peptides, including CGRP, substance P, and neurokinin A.[72-75] Vasodilation with CGRP, unlike with substance P and neurokinin A, is independent of endothelium. CGRP acts by increasing intracellular cyclic adenosine monophosphate (cAMP) concentrations and partly mediates cerebral vasodilation in response to hypotension, cortical spreading depression, and cerebral ischemia. Vasodilation by NO is in part mediated by CGRP.[74,75] CGRP probably does not play a role in vasodilator response to hypoxia or hypercapnia.[76] The physiologic roles of substance P and neurokinin A are not yet understood. Substance P may mediate vasodilation during pathologic derangements such as cerebral and meningeal inflammation and edema.[36]

Potassium Channels

Of the several potassium channels in the cerebral vessels,[77] two are of particular importance in the regulation of vascular tone: KATP channel and calcium-activated potassium (KCa) channel. A third potassium channel, pH-sensitive delayed rectifier potassium channel, may play a role in hypercapnia. Opening of potassium channels triggers potassium efflux from the vascular smooth muscle cell, hyperpolarizes the cell membrane, closes the voltage-dependent calcium channels, decreases calcium entry into the cells, and ultimately relaxes the muscles.[78] KATP channels are opened by a decrease in intracellular pH and are inhibited by an increase in intracellular ATP concentrations and by sulfonylureas.[79] Activation of KATP channels may partly mediate vasodilation by acetylcholine, CGRP, or noradrenaline.[80] KATP channels may play some role in vasodilation during hypotension, hypercapnia, acidosis, and hypoxia.[81-83] KCa channel–mediated vasodilation is due partly to astrocyte-derived carbon monoxide, which diffuses into the smooth muscle cells. Large-conductance KCa (BKCa) channels are the most important of the several KCa channels found in the cerebral circulation.[81] These channels can be selectively blocked by tetraethylammonium, charybdotoxin, and iberiotoxin.[84] Inhibition of BKCa channels results in cerebral vasoconstriction in the large arteries, suggesting that BKCa channels may be involved in the regulation of basal cerebrovascular tone in these vessels.[85] BKCa channels are activated by cyclic guanosine monophosphate, cyclic adenosine monophosphate, and NO and are partly responsible for hypoxia-induced vasodilation of cerebral arteries.[77,83,86,87]

Prostaglandins

Prostaglandins such as PGE_2 and PGI_2 are vasodilators but thromboxane A_2 and $PGF_{2\alpha}$ are vasoconstrictors in the cerebral circulation. Synthesis of prostaglandin H_2 from membrane phospholipids involves two critical enzymes, phospholipase and cyclooxygenase. Prostaglandin H_2 is converted into other prostaglandins by subsequent enzymatic steps. Although cyclooxygenase can be inhibited by aspirin, naproxen, and indomethacin,[88,89] only indomethacin impairs hypercapnic vasodilation in humans.[90,91]

Prostaglandins probably play a more significant role in the regulation of neonatal CBF than of adult CBF.[92] Inhibition of phospholipase by quinacrine hydrochloride abolishes the cerebrovascular response, hypercapnia, and hypoxia in newborn animals.[93] Endothelial damage and indomethacin also abolish hypercapnia-induced vasodilation and an increase in cerebrospinal fluid (CSF) PGI_2 concentrations.[94-96] However, indomethacin-impaired CO_2 reactivity can be restored by very low concentrations of PGE_2.[97] This suggests that prostaglandins may not be direct mediators of hypercapnic vasodilation but that small amounts of prostaglandins are necessary for permitting CO_2 response to hypercapnia and that prostaglandins thus play a so-called permissive role.[96]

Endothelin

Endothelin is a vasoactive peptide that is synthesized by the brain and the vascular endothelium. There are three isoforms of endothelin. The brain synthesizes endothelin-1 (ET-1) and endothelin-3 (ET-3) but not endothelin-2 (ET-2). The vascular endothelium synthesizes ET-1. The two receptors for endothelin are endothelin A (ETA) and endothelin B (ETB).[98] Activation of ETA receptors causes vasoconstriction, and activation of ETB receptors may cause vascular relaxation or constriction. Vascular relaxation is thought to be mediated by endothelin receptors on the endothelium, whereas constriction is probably mediated by endothelin receptors located on the smooth muscle cells.[36] ETA receptors are probably more sensitive to ET-1 and ET-2 than to ET-3. The ETB receptor is equally sensitive to all isoforms of endothelin.[98,99] Endothelin most likely acts through influx of extracellular calcium, which is probably mediated by protein kinases.[100] The vascular smooth muscle contraction caused by endothelin is sustained, suggesting that endothelin is not involved in rapid adjustment of cerebrovascular resistance (CVR).[101] Topical applications of endothelin receptor antagonists do not alter CVR.[102] Endothelin has been implicated in vascular spasm after SAH.[103,104] In experimental models of SAH, ETA and ETB receptor antagonists prevent evolution of vasospam.[105] Endothelin-induced vasospasm can also be reversed nonspecifically by calcium channel blockade and seems to be more responsive to intraarterial nicardipine than to verapamil.[106] Early results of clinical trials showed that intravenous infusion of an ETA receptor antagonist, clazosentan, resulted in a decrease in the incidence of vasospasm after SAH. Intravenous clazosentan infusion reduces the severity of the established cerebral vasospasm.[107]

Anatomic Considerations

The primary arterial supply to the brain consists of the anterior circulation, which comprises the two carotid arteries and their derivations, and the posterior circulation, consisting of the two vertebral arteries, which join to form the basilar artery. Collateral arterial inflow channels are a cornerstone of CBF compensation during ischemia. The principal pathways are embodied in the circle of Willis. This hexagonal ring of vessels lies in the subarachnoid space and circles the pituitary gland (Fig. 2-3; see Fig. 2-2). In many patients the circle of Willis is incomplete. The primary routes of collateral circulation are the Willisian channels (anterior communicating artery [ACA] and posterior communicating artery [PCA]) and the ophthalmic via the external carotid artery. In a normal individual, there is probably no net flow through these communicating vessels but rather a to-and-fro movement of blood that maintains patency by preventing thrombosis and atresia. These vessels allow flow when a pressure differential develops. The second main recourse for collateral flow in the hemispheres is the surface connections between pial arteries that bridge major arterial territories (ACA-PCA, ACA–middle cerebral artery [MCA], MCA-PCA). These connections are called by various names. "Pial-to-pial anastomoses" or "collaterals" seem to be the most logical terms, but they are also called "leptomeningeal pathways."[108] These pathways may protect the so-called border zones or watershed areas between vascular territories. A considerable amount of confusion in terminology is found in this domain.[109] Physiologically, a more precise term might be "equal pressure boundary,"[110] that is, where, under normal circumstances, pial flow does not

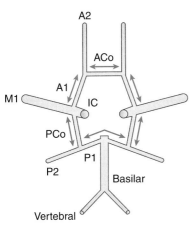

Figure 2–3 Circle of Willis with collateral pathways. Principal pathways for collateral flow are marked by *arrows*. Not shown are potential pathways from the extracranial circulation (e.g., retrograde flow through the ophthalmic artery). A1, proximal anterior cerebral arteries; A2, distal anterior cerebral arteries; ACo, anterior communicating artery; IC, internal carotid artery; Ma, middle cerebral artery; P1, proximal posterior cerebral arteries; P2, distal posterior cerebral arteries; PCo, posterior communicating artery. *(From Young W: Clinical Neuroscience Lectures. Munster, Cathenart, 1999.)*

cross collateral pathways into an adjacent territory because the pressures on either side of this distal territorial boundary are equal. Considerable variation exists in the anatomic location of these boundaries, and they may change during the course of treatment if the vascular architecture is altered, such as after multiple arteriovenous malformation (AVM) embolizations.

Collateral pathways are most efficacious during chronic ischemia, when they may gradually enlarge over time. In the acute stage, it is frequently necessary to augment blood pressure to effectively drive flow across them. Absence of adequate collateral pathways, especially in the circle of Willis, is a normal anatomic variant, so deliberate hypertension is not guaranteed to succeed. A complete circle of Willis with well-developed symmetrical components is present in only 18% to 20% of the population. Hypoplasia of the PCA, the proximal segment of the anterior cerebral artery, or the ACA is often encountered.[111] The size of the collateral vessels may influence the clinical course of acute vascular occlusion. Computer modeling suggests that any change in the ACA diameter, even in the normal range (0.6 to 1.4 mm), has a profound effect on collateral blood flow when an internal carotid artery is occluded.[112] Clinical observations suggest that a PCA diameter of less than 1 mm, measured by MR angiography, may be associated with an increased risk of watershed stroke.[113] The external and internal carotid arteries have the potential for communication, which most commonly manifests as flow from the external carotid artery, via facial pathways, to the ophthalmic artery. Thus retrograde flow is provided to the circle of Willis. Several other pathways may develop between the carotid and vertebrobasilar systems.[108] In rare situations, meningeal collaterals may develop into the intracranial circulation (e.g., AVMs and moyamoya disease).

In summary, an elegant microcirculatory arrangement is provided for recruiting accessory inflow channels to the endarterial perfusion territories of the brain. In normal circumstances these channels either lie dormant or are underused, becoming functional (critical) only when a pathologic stress is imposed on the circulation. In general, the circle of Willis and the leptomeningeal communications compensate for an acute interruption of the circulation; other pathways described previously are more likely to compensate for chronic cerebral insufficiency.

Regulation of CVR takes place primarily in the smaller arteries and arterioles (muscular or resistance vessels) and not the larger arteries that are visible on an angiogram (elastic or conductance vessels). However, the contribution of both venules and capillaries[114] and larger conductance arteries to regulatory activity is a subject of controversy.[115,116] There is probably a continuum of varying participation in autoregulatory function as one proceeds distally on the arterial tree.[116,117] In humans the venous drainage of the brain is complex and considerably more variable than drainage of the arterial tree. The typically thin-walled and valveless intracerebral conduits terminate into thicker-walled venous sinuses, which are rigid by virtue of bony attachments. Because of the confluence of the larger venous sinuses, a considerable admixture of venous blood draining the cerebral hemispheres takes place, and it is not uncommon to note, in the later venous phase of an angiogram, that one side of the venous drainage appears to be dominant. This finding may be of interest in the choice of internal jugular vein for cannulation.

Cerebral Microcirculation

The cerebral capillary vascular bed is a complex network of communicating vessels in which capillaries are supplied by several arterioles and drained by several venules. The precapillary vessels divide and reunite to form an anastomotic circle, the "circle of Duret." The capillary density is three times greater in gray matter than in white matter.[118] The capillaries arise from this anastomotic circle. These capillary beds are highly tortuous and irregular.

The velocity of red blood cell (RBC) flow in these capillary beds is higher than in other tissues. However, because of tortuosity and an increased path length, high RBC flow velocity in these capillaries does not decrease capillary transit time.[119] There is considerable variability in the blood flow velocities even in a given arterial distribution. In theory, changes in blood flow velocity can affect uptake of substrate and nutrients by the brain.[120] Blood flow velocity could provide an adaptive mechanism during cerebral hypoperfusion. It is believed that a small proportion of the brain capillaries that have high blood flow velocities are nonfunctional—that is, they do not participate in capillary fluid or substrate exchange. During cerebral hypoperfusion, whether through an increase in intracranial pressure (ICP) or a decrease in the mean arterial pressure (MAP), a greater decrease in blood flow velocity is observed in the faster capillaries than in the slower ones, resulting in an improvement of capillary function. Thus capillary dynamics provides a functional reserve to cope with hemodynamic stress.

It is still unclear whether the capillary bed of the brain is fully perfused at all times, that is, whether capillary recruitment takes place.[121-123] Mechanical influences on local flow through sphincter mechanisms at the microcirculatory level are likely.[114,124] At present, flow changes in the cerebral microcirculatory bed in response to hypoxia, hypercapnia, or reduced cerebral perfusion pressure are believed to be largely mediated by changes in blood flow velocity and not by recruitment of blood vessels.[119]

Efforts have been made to model human microcirculation on the basis of postmortem morphometric measurements. The models reveal differences in capillary density sizes and length based on their location. The capillaries are most densely distributed in the middle third of the cortex; the average length of capillaries, their surface area, and their volume in a given volume of brain tissue are 505 mm/mm^3, 11.8 mm^2/mm^3, and 2.7%, respectively. Accurate models of human cerebral microcirculation can provide insights into physical factors that affect blood flow, such as the distribution of pressure and shear stress, static and dynamic regulation of flow, substrate diffusion, and accurate interpretation of blood flow data on MRI.[125]

Hemodynamic Factors

Pressure Regulation

Conceptually, a convenient way to model the cerebral circulation is to envision a parallel system of rigid pipes in which Ohm's law would apply:

$$F = \frac{P_i - P_o}{R} \qquad (2\text{-}1)$$

where F is flow, P_i is input pressure, P_o is outflow pressure, and R is resistance.

The term $P_i - P_o$ is usually referred to as *cerebral perfusion pressure* (CPP) and is calculated as MAP minus the outflow pressure. The cerebral venous system is compressible and may act as a "Starling resistor." Therefore P_o is whichever pressure is higher, intracranial or venous pressure. True CPP often is overestimated because a small gradient exists between systemic and cerebral vessels,[126] which may be particularly important in patients with cerebral AVMs.[127] It is useful to conceptualize pressure and resistance as independent variables in the preceding equation and flow as the dependent variable (i.e., the pressure or resistance is affected by disease or treatment, and flow follows suit). For example, drugs exert effects on CBF by changing CPP and CVR (directly for vasodilators and indirectly by metabolic depressants).

Circulatory resistance can be modeled in terms of the Hagen-Poiseuille relationship (Equation 2-2), as follows:

$$R = \frac{8l\mu}{r^4} = \frac{P_i - P_o}{F} \qquad (2\text{-}2)$$

where l is length of conduit; μ is blood viscosity; and r is radius of vessel. Other symbol definitions were given previously. As is the case for Ohm's law, when this equation is applied to an intact vascular system, a number of critical assumptions are clearly not met. The equation applies to newtonian fluids during nonturbulent flow through rigid tubes; circulation, in contrast, is pulsatile with capacitance and the potential for turbulence. Also, a decrease in CPP can be a result of a decrease in systemic blood pressure or an increase in ICP or jugular venous pressure. Some groups have reported that the cerebral vascular bed responds in a similar way to either of the two changes in CPP, as a result of a decrease in the MAP or an increase in intracranial or jugular venous pressure.[128] However, other investigators have reported that the effect of changing CPP on vessel inner radius due to an increase in ICP may be quite different from that due to a decrease in MAP.[129]

From a purely practical standpoint, examination of the previous relationship leaves little question as to why vessel diameter evolved into the preeminent mode of vascular regulation. Although viscosity and vessel length influence resistance in a linear manner, the fact that flow is proportional to the fourth power of the conduit's radius makes this the most efficient means of controlling resistance.

In normal individuals, CBF is constant between a CPP of approximately 50 to 150 mm Hg (Fig. 2-4). As the ability of the cerebral vasculature to respond to changes in pressure is exhausted, CBF passively follows changes in CPP. At the

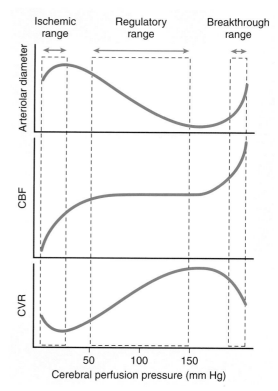

Figure 2–4   Idealized depiction of pressure autoregulation in terms of cerebral blood flow (CBF), cerebrovascular resistance (CVR), and arteriolar diameter. See text for further explanation. *(From Young W: Clinical Neuroscience Lectures. Munster, Cathenart, 1999.)*

extremes, resistance probably does not stay fixed. Vessel collapse and passive vascular dilation may actually potentiate the predicted decline or increase caused by CPP changes: Resistance does not remain linearly related to pressure. Although the general concept put forth in Figure 2-4 is important, it is only a statistical description of how the general population responds, and a value of 50 mm Hg, even in a nonhypertensive individual, does not guarantee that a particular patient's cerebral circulation remains within the "autoregulatory plateau." Individual responses vary widely.[130] Ideally, at the lower limit of cerebral autoregulation, a near maximal vasodilation is thought to take place. However, evidence shows that even below the lower limit of autoregulation, pharmacologic vasodilation may be possible.[131,132] The relevance of the idealized cerebral autoregulation curve, in particular the lower limit of autoregulation, has been questioned by some writers.[133]

In its simplest form, a cerebral autoregulation curve expressing CBF as a function of CPP is often represented by three straight lines. Two sloping lines intersect a horizontal line at points that represent the lower and upper limits of cerebral autoregulation. The horizontal segment represents the pressure-independent flow within the autoregulatory range, whereas the sloping lines represent pressure-dependent flow outside the range of autoregulation. In mathematical terms, an autoregulatory curve can be characterized by four principal autoregulatory parameters: lower limit of pressure autoregulation, upper limit of pressure autoregulation, slope below the lower limit of autoregulation, and slope above the lower limit of autoregulation. Using mathematical compartmental modeling, Gao and colleagues[125] observed that the three previously described autoregulatory curves did not accurately predict the experimentally observed principal autoregulatory parameters

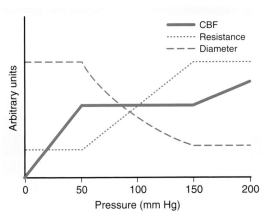

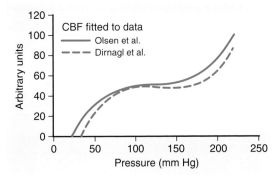

Figure 2–7 Cerebral blood flow (CBF) of autoregulation curves of type 3. CBF curve was obtained by curve-fitting to the third-order polynomial of data reported by Dirnagl and Pulsinelli[429] (*dashed line*) and Olsen et al.[478] (*solid line*). The prediction that blood flow ceases if pressure is below 30 or 20 mm Hg conflicts with experimental observations. *(From Gao E, Young WL, Pile-Spellman J, et al: Mathematical considerations for modeling cerebral blood flow autoregulation to systemic arterial pressure. Am J Physiol 1998;274:H1023-H1031.)*

Figure 2–5 Fixed maximal vasoreactivity type of autoregulation. Cerebral blood flow (CBF), cerebrovascular resistance, and arteriolar diameter are shown for the fixed maximal vasoreactivity type of autoregulation. Between the lower limit of autoregulation (LLA) and the upper lower limit of autoregulation (ULA), the CBF is autoregulated through a change of the vessel diameter. The vessel dilates as pressure decreases, and reaches its maximal size when pressure falls to less than LLA. Similarly, the vessel constricts as pressure increases, and maintains its minimal size when pressure exceeds ULA. Note that the two *sloped lines* are not parallel with each other (compare with variable maximal vasoreactivity type shown in Fig. 2-6). *(From Gao E, Young WL, Pile-Spellman J, et al: Mathematical considerations for modeling cerebral blood flow autoregulation to systemic arterial pressure. Am J Physiol 1998;274:H-1023-H1031.)*

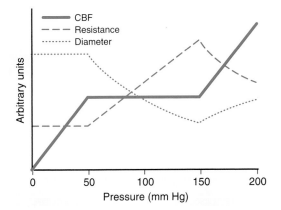

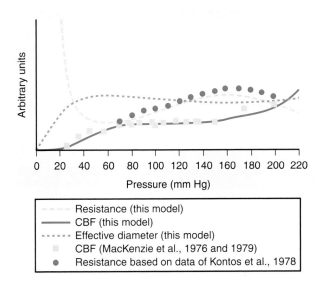

Figure 2–6 Variable maximal vasoreactivity type of autoregulation. Cerebral blood flow (CBF), cerebrovascular resistance, and arteriolar diameter are shown for the variable maximal vasoreactivity type of autoregulation. At the pressure below the upper lower limit of autoregulation (ULA), this type is the same as the fixed maximal vasoreactivity type. However, when pressure exceeds ULA, CBF increases at the same rate as it does when pressure is below LLA. This pattern implies that the arteriole dilates when pressure exceeds ULA. Note that the two *sloped lines* are parallel with each other (compare with Fig. 2-5). *(From Gao E, Young WL, Pile-Spellman J, et al: Mathematical considerations for modeling cerebral blood flow autoregulation to systemic arterial pressure. Am J Physiol 1998;274:H1023-H1031.)*

Figure 2–8 Regression results of cerebrovascular resistance, blood flow, and effective diameter of an autoregulation device (ARD) in the compartmental model. When the pressure decreases below the lower limit of autoregulation (LLA), the vessel continues to dilate until it finally reaches the maximum at a lower pressure of 40 mm Hg for three small vessels (diameter = 50, 150, and 200 μm) or 70 mm Hg for the large vessel (diameter = 300 μm). Some experimental data are also plotted in the figure. Resistance (*closed circles*) is calculated directly from experimental data of Kontos et al.,[116] The experimental data for CBF are readings of two head-fitted curves of the data reported by MacKenzie et al.[478,480] *(From Gao E, Young WL, Pile-Spellman J, et al: Mathematical considerations for modeling cerebral blood flow autoregulation to systemic arterial pressure. Am J Physiol 1998;274:H1023-H1031.)*

(Figs. 2-5 to 2-8). Computer modeling was most successful in predicting experimental results when the arterial resistive bed was compartmentalized into a series of four compartments on the basis of arterial/arteriolar diameter. These study findings suggest that there are multiple sites of autoregulation in the cerebral arterial resistive bed.[125,134]

A time constant is associated with autoregulatory changes. Figure 2-9A depicts the response of a simple tube (or a dysregulating vascular bed) to a step change in pressure. Because resistance does not change (assuming nonturbulent flow), flow passively follows the change in pressure. Figure 2-9B depicts the response that is typical of a normal circulatory bed. With the step change in pressure comes an instantaneous drop in flow, but as the bed actively autoregulates and resistance decreases, flow gradually increases and returns to baseline. When the pressure is returned to normal, there is a transient period of hyperemia while the resistance is reset.[135]

Venous Physiology

The influence of the cerebral venous system on overall autoregulation is unclear, primarily because of the difficulty of direct observation. The smooth muscle content and the

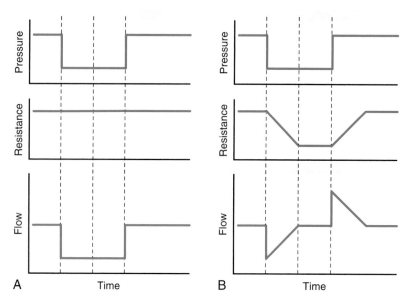

Figure 2–9 Flow, resistance, and pressure as a function of time. *Dotted vertical lines* represent a time scale of "minutes." **A,** In a rigid pipe (or a totally vasoparalyzed circulation), a step decrease in pressure leads to an instantaneous drop in flow, because resistance stays fixed. **B,** In a conduit with autoregulation, a step decrease in pressure is first met with an instantaneous drop in flow. As resistance falls, however, flow increases toward baseline. With the step restoration of pressure to control level, there is an instantaneous hyperemic response, and subsequently, flow decreases as resistance decreases toward control levels. *(From Young W: Clinical Neuroscience Lectures. Munster, Cathenart, 1999.)*

innervation of the venous system are less extensive than those of the arterial system, and many believe that the venous system is a passive recipient of the "regulated" arterial inflow. Asymptomatic occlusion of cortical veins in animals can impair the local autoregulatory response to systemic hypotension.[136] In addition, the venous system contains most of the cerebral blood volume (CBV); therefore slight changes in vessel diameter may have a profound effect on intracranial blood volume. Available evidence suggests that the venous system may be regulated more by neurogenic than by myogenic or metabolic factors.[137]

Pulsatile Perfusion

Both a fast component and a slow component to the myogenic response to changes in perfusion pressure have been proposed. This consideration is of particular interest in the patient undergoing cardiac surgery.[138] During cardiopulmonary bypass, the pulsatile variations in blood pressure transmitted to the cerebral vasculature appear to influence CBF, perhaps by interaction with endothelium-derived mediators of vascular tone.[139] Although the importance of these effects has not been completely determined, the loss of pulsatility may worsen the outcome of a cerebral ischemic event.[126] Sudden restoration of pulsatile perfusion to a previously dampened circulatory bed may be a mechanism to explain certain instances of cerebral hyperemia.[140]

Cardiac Output

A proposed theory is that cardiac output may be responsible for improved CBF and outcome after SAH. However, there is little evidence for increased cardiac output in the operative mechanism of improving cerebral perfusion. Improvement in perfusion by volume loading is indirectly accomplished by improving blood rheology and directly accomplished by increasing systemic blood pressure and preventing occult decreases in systemic pressure in a patient population that is already subject to volume depletion (i.e., decreased circulating blood volume).[141] Studies examining the possible relationship

between a change in cardiac output and a change in CBF have, for the most part, assessed the effect of drugs that increase cardiac output during either normotension or induced hypertension. Some investigators suggest, however, that during deliberate drug-induced hypotension, a decrease in cardiac output might be reflected by a decrease in CBF, even when blood pressure is kept above the lower autoregulatory threshold.[142] The effects of altering cardiac output on CBF are more likely to be indirect effects on central venous pressure and large cerebral vessel tone (i.e., sympathetic tone).

Rheologic Factors

Clinically, hematocrit is the main influence on blood viscosity,[143] and, as shown in Equation 2-2, blood viscosity is a major determinant of vascular resistance. Muizelaar and associates[144] have proposed that viscosity directly participates in hemodynamic autoregulation. As discussed later, viscosity may be the only determinant of CVR subject to manipulation in certain settings. An inverse relationship exists between hematocrit (Hct) and CBF. A continuing controversy concerns whether this relationship is, in fact, purely rheologic or a function of changes in oxygen delivery to the tissue.[145]

Todd and coworkers[146] demonstrated a significant CBF increase, from 30 ± 14 mL/100 g/min (baseline Hct = $42 \pm 2\%$, mean $\pm$ SD) to 100 ± 20 mL/100 g/min at Hct = $12 \pm 1\%$ in normal cerebral hemispheres of rabbits. The increase in regional CBF was markedly smaller after focal cryogenic cerebral injury, suggesting that a CBF increase produced by hemodilution is an active vasodilatory process rather than a passive response to changing blood viscosity. In another animal experiment, when blood was replaced by ultrapurified polymerized bovine hemoglobin, the viscosity of which does not depend on shear rate, a fourfold increase in viscosity did not significantly affect CBF. This finding suggests that blood viscosity alone may not significantly affect CBF.[147]

The Hagen-Poiseuille model does not accurately describe the behavior of flow at the microcirculatory level.[148,149] When RBCs flow near vessel walls, they create shear forces, which add resistance. (The *shear rate* is the change in velocity moving from the wall toward the center of the vessel.) Therefore in all vessels the RBC velocity is faster in the center of the vessel and slower at the periphery. In small vessels, cells move faster than the plasma (the Fahraeus effect), thereby reducing microvascular hematocrit. This reduction in hematocrit causes a reduction in viscosity (the Fahraeus-Lindqvist effect).[150] Another contribution of the smaller microvascular hematocrit is that as the vessels become progressively smaller, the relative size of the annular periphery (with reduced flow velocity) becomes larger.

Cerebral hematocrit in humans is approximately 75% of systemic values, but it is affected by $Paco_2$[151] and presumably by other vasoactive influences. Relative hypercapnia reduces cerebral hematocrit, and it is presumed that the other vasodilators do as well.

Metabolic and Chemical Influences

Carbon Dioxide

Carbon dioxide is a powerful modulator of CVR. At one time, CO_2 was thought to be the "coupler" between flow and metabolism, because an increase in metabolism generates CO_2 and therefore releases a cerebral vasodilator into the local environment. Rapid diffusion across the blood-brain barrier (BBB) allows CO_2 to modulate extracellular fluid pH and affect arteriolar resistance.[152] Metabolically induced changes in pH in the systemic circulation do not have the same effect in the presence of an intact BBB, but metabolic production of H^+ released into the CSF or extracellular space from ischemic lactic acidosis does. The mechanism of vasodilation by CO_2 may be different in adults and neonates (Fig. 2-10). Evidence shows that NO and cyclic guanosine monophosphate pathways are probably more important in adults, whereas prostaglandins and cyclic adenosine monophosphate are more important in neonates.[51] By active, though somewhat sluggish, exchange of HCO_3^-, the CSF eventually buffers itself against alterations in pH by CO_2 diffusion. Although CO_2-induced cerebral vasoconstriction wanes over a period of 6 to 10 hours,[153] this period can be variable in an individual patient. Also important in this regard are chronic states of either hypocapnia or hypercapnia because sudden normalization of $Paco_2$ can result in relative hypoperfusion or hyperperfusion.

At normotension, there is a nearly linear response of CBF at a $Paco_2$ between 20 and 80 mm Hg (CBF changes about 2% to 4% for each mm Hg change in $Paco_2$). The linearity of the response breaks down as $Paco_2$ approaches the extremes. The values quoted for either percentage change or absolute levels in CBF change per unit CO_2 are highly variable, depending on the methods employed and whether hemispheric or cortical flow is measured.[154,155]

In general, doubling $Paco_2$ from 40 to 80 mm Hg doubles CBF, and halving $Paco_2$ from 40 to 20 mm Hg halves CBF. This highly reproducible cerebrovascular CO_2 response is often used as a way of validating and comparing different CBF methods.[154]

In a fashion analogous to blood pressure autoregulation, the CO_2 response is limited by either maximal vasodilation at extreme hypercapnia or maximal vasoconstriction at extreme hypocapnia. Hypocapnia, however, may adversely affect cellular metabolism and shift the oxyhemoglobin dissociation curve to the left.[156] Severe hypocapnia (approximately 10 mm Hg) can result in anaerobic glucose metabolism and lactate production.[157,158] Although clinical experience clearly

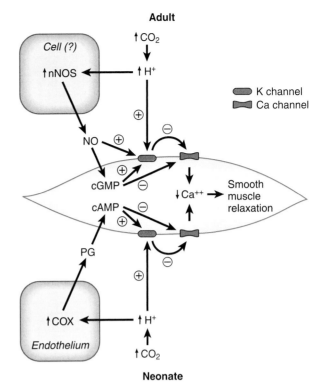

Adult

K channel
Ca channel

Smooth muscle relaxation

Neonate

Figure 2–10 The exact mechanism of hypercapnic vasodilation remains to be fully defined and may differ in adults and neonates. This figure illustrates one proposed sequence of events that results in hypercapnic vasodilation. In adults, hypercapnia decreases extracellular pH, activates the neuronal isoform of nitric oxide synthase (nNOS), and increases production of nitric oxide (NO) and cyclic guanosine monophosphate (cGMP). Subsequent activation of potassium channels by NO or cGMP results in hyperpolarization of the vascular smooth muscle (VSM) cell membrane. Extracellular acidosis may activate potassium channels directly. Hyperpolarization of VSM cell membrane inhibits voltage-gated calcium channels and decreases intracellular calcium concentrations. cGMP can also directly inhibit calcium channels, reducing intracellular calcium concentrations. A decrease in intracellular calcium results in vasorelaxation. In neonates, hypercapnia-induced extracellular acidosis increases prostaglandin (PG) synthesis by activating endothelial cyclooxygenase (COX). Prostaglandins play a "permissive role" in hypercapnic vasodilation (see text). Increased prostaglandin concentration activates adenylate cyclase and results in an increased intracellular cyclic adenosine monophosphate (cAMP) concentration in VSM. Increased cAMP concentrations in VSM activate potassium (K) channels and inhibit calcium (Ca) channels, resulting in a decrease in intracellular calcium (Ca^{++}) concentration and vascular relaxation. As in adults, extracellular acidosis may also directly activate potassium channels and hyperpolarize the VSM cell membrane. CO_2, carbon dioxide; H^+, hydrogen ion. *(Modified from Brian JE Jr: Carbon dioxide and the cerebral circulation. Anesthesiology 1998;88:1365-1386.)*

demonstrates impaired mentation with less severe degrees of hyperventilation, it is not clear whether this impairment represents impairment of tissue oxygenation or some effect of tissue alkalosis and transcellular ionic shifts. Clinically, inducing such extreme levels of hypocapnia is almost never necessary, and $Paco_2$ levels below 25 mm Hg are best avoided except in extraordinary circumstances. The routine use of profound hypocapnia in all neurosurgical settings should undergo reevaluation.[159,160]

Arteriolar tone, set by the systemic arterial blood pressure, modulates the effect of $Paco_2$ on CBF. Moderate hypotension blunts the ability of the cerebral circulation to respond to changes in $Paco_2$, and severe hypotension abolishes it altogether (Fig. 2-11).[161] Conversely, $Paco_2$ modifies pressure autoregulation, and from hypercapnia to hypocapnia there is a widening of the "autoregulatory plateau" (Fig. 2-12).[162]

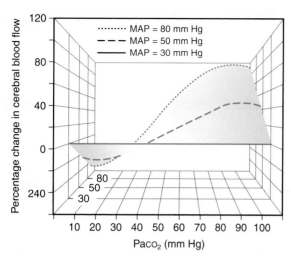

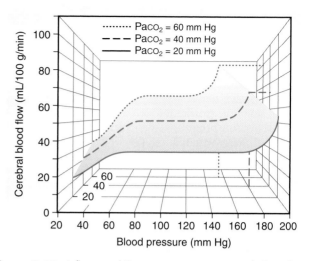

Figure 2–11 Influence of blood pressure on CBF response to Paco2. Effects of alteration in Paco2 on cortical blood flow in dogs with normotension (mean arterial pressure [MAP]: 80 mm Hg, *upper trace*), moderate hypotension (50 mm Hg, *middle trace*), and severe hypotension (30 mm Hg, *lower trace*).[161] *(From Harper AM: The inter-relationship between a Pco-2 and blood pressure in the regulation of blood flow through the cerebral cortex. Acta Neurol Scand Suppl 1965;41:94-103. Modified from McCulloch J. In Knezevic S, Maximilian VA, Mubrin Z, et al (eds): Handbook of Regional Cerebral Blood Flow. Hillsdale, Lawrence Erlbaum Associates,1988, p 1, using data from Harper AM: Autoregulation of cerebral blood flow: Influence of the arterial blood pressure on the blood flow through the cerebral cortex. J Neurol Neurosurg Psychiatry 1966;29:398-403.)*

Figure 2–12 Influence of Paco2 on pressure autoregulation of cerebral blood flow. *(Modified from Paulson OB, Strandgaard S, Edvinsson L: Cerebral autoregulation. Cerebrovasc Brain Metab Rev 1990;2:161-192.)*

There might be gender-based differences in CO_2 reactivity due to the underlying levels of prostaglandins. For example, suppression of prostaglandin synthesis by indomethacin treatment causes a greater attenuation of CO_2 reactivity in premenopausal women than in men.[163] Paco2 responsiveness also varies by region.[164] This difference may be due to the relative metabolic requirements present in each area, but this mechanism is not understood. Healthy female subjects demonstrated a greater increase in MCA flow velocity after 5% CO_2 inhalation than male subjects. This finding suggests a gender-dependent response to CO_2 in healthy subjects.[165] Decreased CO_2 reactivity can be a function of local decreases in CPP distal to a spastic or stenotic vessel. In addition, it may reflect deranged metabolism or structural damage in a number of disease states, including head injury,[166] SAH,[167,168] and ischemic cerebrovascular disease.[169] In comatose patients, impaired CO_2 reactivity suggests a poor prognostic outcome.[170]

Oxygen

Within physiologic ranges, Pao2 does not affect CBF. Hypoxemia, however, is a potent stimulus for arteriolar dilation,[171] as a result of tissue hypoxia and concomitant lactic acidosis, although the precise mechanism is unclear. Vasodilation in response to hypoxia probably involves adenosine and KATP channels.[172] CBF begins to increase at a Pao2 of about 50 mm Hg and roughly doubles at a Pao2 of 30 mm Hg. States that impair CO_2 reactivity are likely to interfere with O_2 reactivity as well. The response of CBF to changes in both Pao2 and the oxygen content of blood is shown in Figure 2-13. Hyperoxia decreases CBF, producing a modest 10% to 15% decrease at 1 atmosphere. Hyperbaric oxygenation in humans decreases CBF, but high atmospheric pressure alone probably does not affect CBF.[173]

Temperature

As is true for other organ systems, cerebral metabolism decreases with diminishing temperature. For each 1° C decrease in body temperature, $CMRo_2$ drops by approximately 7%. Alternatively, this relationship may be characterized by the metabolic temperature coefficient, *Q10*, which is defined as the ratio of $CMRo_2$ at temperature T, divided by the $CMRo_2$ at a temperature that is 10 degrees lower (T − 10). The value for cerebral Q10 in the physiologic range of 27° to 37° C is between 2.0 and 3.0.[174] Below 27° C, however, Q10 increases to near 4.5. This finding has been explained on the basis of the neuroelectrical effects, wherein the major suppression of neuronal function occurs between 17° and 27° C. Thus the lower Q10 between 27° and 37° C simply reflects the decrease in the rates of biochemical reaction (basal $CMRo_2$), and the higher Q10 between 17° and 27° C is due to the additive effect of the decrease in neuronal function.[153,174] Because moderate hypothermia, without major suppression of neuronal functions, provides better neuroprotection than isoelectric doses of barbiturates, identifying the biochemical mechanisms that contribute to basal $CMRo_2$ is important.[175]

Because the regulation of CBF is known to be closely coupled to cerebral metabolism, it is not surprising that this hypothermia-induced reduction in $CMRo_2$ is reflected by a parallel decrease in CBF. Some heterogeneity is found in this response, however; so CBF changes are most apparent in the cerebral and cerebellar cortex, less apparent in the thalamus, and not significant in the hypothalamus and brainstem.[176]

Intraoperative hypothermia is most often encountered during cardiopulmonary bypass. CBF in this setting has been shown to correlate with nasopharyngeal temperature, with a maximum 55% reduction in CBF occurring, in one study, at the lowest measured temperature, 26° C. This finding corresponds to a 56% calculated reduction in $CMRo_2$.[177] $CMRo_2$ continues to decrease with further lowering of temperature up to the point of EEG silence. In dogs, this level is reached at 18° C. CBF during cardiopulmonary bypass with profound hypothermia (18° to 20° C) is disproportionately maintained[178] and is determined by arterial blood pressure and not pump flow rate.[179,180] However, during rewarming, CBF velocity remains lower than the pre-bypass value, probably

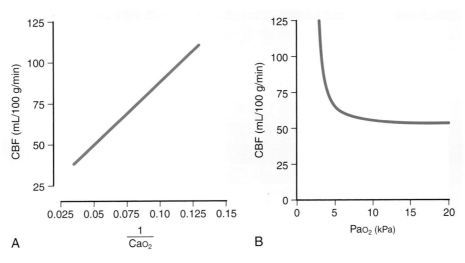

Figure 2–13 Influence of oxygen content (Ca_{O_2}) and Pa_{O_2} on cerebral flood flow (CBF). **A,** CBF is inversely proportional to Ca_{O_2}. **B,** Replotting the straight line in **A** by applying a sigmoid O_2 dissociation curve and taking the reciprocal produces the more familiar asymptotic curve of Pa_{O_2} versus CBF, which disguises the dependence of CBF on Ca_{O_2}. 5 kPa is approximately 40 mm Hg. *(Redrawn by Lesser PJA, Jones JG. In Scurr C, Feldman S, Soni N [eds]: Scientific Foundations of Anaesthesia: The Basis of Intensive Care, 2nd ed. St. Louis, Mosby, 1990, p 205; from original data reported by Brown MM, Wade JPH, Marshall J: Fundamental importance of arterial oxygen content in the regulation of cerebral blood flow in man. Brain 1985;108:81-93.)*

because of hypothermia-induced changes in the cerebral vasculature. A period of cold full-flow reperfusion may improve cerebral perfusion during rewarming.[181]

The effects of hypothermia and anesthetic drugs may be additive to the point at which EEG activity ceases. Thiopental administered during hypothermia in doses that enhance the hypothermia-induced suppression of EEG activity produces a further reduction in CMR_{O_2}, which is paralleled by an additional decrease in CBF. Although similar effects on CMR_{O_2} can be brought about by isoflurane, no additional drop in CBF appears to take place.[182]

Autoregulation, as well as CO_2 reactivity, is well preserved during cardiopulmonary bypass at moderate hypothermia.[177] Some investigators suggest, however, that autoregulation may become impaired if the CO_2 content of blood is allowed to rise. This effect can occur when exogenous CO_2 is administered to provide a "normal" Pa_{CO_2} corrected to the patient's actual temperature during "pH-stat" acid-base management.[183] Recalculating the Pa_{CO_2} at 37° C for "alpha-stat" acid-base management reveals patients so treated to be markedly hypercapnic, which explains the grossly elevated values of CBF reported in some cardiopulmonary bypass studies.[184,185]

Pharmacology

Dose-related anesthetic or drug effects (e.g., isoflurane, desflurane, and sevoflurane) can alter vasoactive responses just as blood pressure and CO_2 do (Fig. 2-14).[186,187] The vasodilatory effects of volatile anesthetic agents are apparent at minimum alveolar concentrations (MACs) exceeding 1.5. Beyond 1.5 MAC concentrations, volatile anesthetic agents can blunt the CO_2 response or render CBF pressure passive. Absolute CO_2 reactivity is preserved during intraoperative use of a narcotic, such as fentanyl or remifentanil.[188] CO_2 reactivity is also preserved with intravenous propofol anesthesia. Total intravenous anesthesia with propofol and remifentanil generally preserves response to CO_2 and protects pressure autoregulation better than that with volatile anesthetic agents. Because of preserved flow-metabolism coupling, progressively increasing depth of propofol anesthesia results in a decrease in CBF. In contrast, volatile anesthetic agents in concentrations

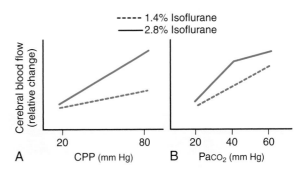

Figure 2–14 Influence of vasodilators on blood pressure autoregulation and CO_2 reactivity in the isoflurane-anesthetized dog. Comparing 1 and 2 MAC isoflurane: **A,** With changing cerebral perfusion pressure (CPP), autoregulation for blood pressure is not as efficient, and cerebral blood flow (CBF) appears to increase more between 20 and 40 mm Hg than between 40 and 60 mm Hg. **B,** However, CBF increases at each of the three levels of Pa_{CO_2} (at 1 MAC isoflurane). With 2 MAC isoflurane, CBF increases only between 20 and 40 mm Hg. Presumably the circulation is maximally vasodilated at 2 MAC isoflurane and a Pa_{CO_2} of 40 mm Hg, so that raising Pa_{CO_2} to 60 mm Hg has less of an effect on total cardiovascular resistance. *(Redrawn from data in McPherson RW, Brian JE, Traystman RJ: Cerebrovascular responsiveness to carbon dioxide in dogs with 1.4% and 2.8% isoflurane. Anesthesiology 1989;70: 843-850.)*

exceeding 1.5 MAC are associated with increasing CBF, suggesting an uncoupling of flow and metabolism. Although intravenous anesthetic agents such as propofol seem to preserve flow-metabolism coupling better than volatile agents,[189] the addition of nitrous oxide further impairs flow-metabolism coupling.[190] Interestingly, intracarotid injections of intravenous anesthetic drugs in doses sufficient to cause burst suppression do not decrease blood flow, suggesting an uncoupling of blood flow and metabolism with intra-arterial injections.[191] The apparent loss of flow-metabolism coupling with intra-arterial injections of anesthetic drugs may be due either to the biomechanical effects of the injection or to direct vascular effects.

Vasoactive drugs may affect different aspects of autoregulatory behavior, as illustrated by evidence that nitroprusside

27

impairs the ability of the circulation to maintain CBF when CPP is lowered but not when CPP is increased.[192] Apparently independent of autoregulatory impairment,[193] anesthesia with volatile drugs appears to result in a trend for CBF to decrease over time in animal models.[194-196] It does not, however, involve an effect on CSF pH. Not only do absolute flow levels decrease, but CO_2 changes responsiveness as well.[197] This time-dependent CBF decrease has been proposed to be operative during cardiopulmonary bypass in humans.[198]

The cause of these flow decreases (or, possibly, return to "normal") has not been adequately explained. Evidence that flow does not decrease in other carefully controlled studies raises the question that this time effect may be a methodologic artifact.[199,200] In conditions of temperature flux, declines in CBF during the initial period of cardiopulmonary bypass with the skull closed probably reflect temperature equilibration in the brain. Interestingly, however, with the skull open and direct monitoring of cortical temperature, there does not appear to be a time lag during cooling and rewarming during cardiopulmonary bypass.[201]

Neurogenic Influences

One of the most striking differences between the systemic and cerebral circulations is the relative lack of humoral and autonomic influences on normal cerebrovascular tone. The systemic circulation is regulated to a large extent by sympathetic nervous activity, but autonomic factors do not appear to control the cerebral circulation. Thus autonomic nerves are not necessary for regulatory responses, but they may modify these responses in several important ways.

The innervation of the cerebral vasculature is extensive,[202,203] involving serotonergic, adrenergic, and cholinergic systems of both intracranial and extracranial origin. The physiologic significance of this intricate and extensive system of innervation is not fully understood. One confounding factor in the interpretation of experimental studies is a marked interspecies difference in the CBF response to sympathetic stimulation.[115] Thus in monkeys, acute sympathetic denervation has no effect on CBF, but acute sympathetic stimulation reduces CBF during normotension and during hypertension. In cats and dogs, by contrast, sympathetic stimulation has no effect during normotension. However, when acute hypertension is induced in cats by aortic ligation, electrical stimulation of the cervical sympathetic chain attenuates the increase in CBF and decreases disruption of the BBB.[203]

Under normal circumstances, the presence of baseline sympathetic tone exerted on the cerebral vasculature in humans is controversial. The lack of baseline tone is supported by studies demonstrating that phentolamine-induced α-adrenergic receptor blockade does not affect CBF.[204] In contrast, Hernandez and colleagues[205] have demonstrated in monkeys that unilateral superior cervical ganglion excision leads to a 34% increase in CBF on the affected side, with no effect on autoregulation.

The effect of increased sympathetic tone on CBF in altered physiologic states, on the other hand, is well recognized. For example, using intense stimulation of the stellate ganglion in dogs, D'Alecy[206] could produce a decrease in CBF greater than 60%. Thus acute sympathetic stimulation can shift the autoregulatory curve to the right. Reflex increases in sympathetic tone have been shown to attenuate the transient increases in CBF that are observed during severe hypertensive episodes.[207] Sympathetic stimulation is also associated with

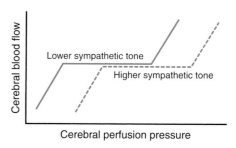

Figure 2–15 Autonomic effects on autoregulation. Higher sympathetic tone, through the addition of a "proximal resistor" to the arteriolar bed, shifts the upper and lower ends of autoregulation to the right.

a small decrease in the hyperemia seen during hypercapnia in normotensive rabbits.[208] The cerebrovascular effects are more pronounced during bilateral sympathetic nerve stimulation.[209] These effects are seen despite acidosis, which inhibits the release of noradrenaline.[210,211]

Sympathetic stimulation probably constricts the larger conductance and pial vessels, thereby interposing an additional "resistor" proximal to the arterioles. In those situations in which an increase in CBF occurs as a result of a rise in cerebral metabolic rate (i.e., seizures), even bilateral activation of sympathetic nerves has no effect on CBF. In such situations, metabolic factors are the overwhelming determinants of CBF, with only a minimal contribution from the sympathetic nervous system.[212]

At the lower limits of autoregulation, sympathetic activity modifies the autoregulatory response of CBF to a decrease in arterial blood pressure (Fig. 2-15). At equivalent blood pressures, CBF is lower during hemorrhagic hypotension than during pharmacologically induced hypotension.[213] Thus when reflex sympathetic constriction of larger cerebral arteries in response to hypotension is prevented by acute surgical sympathectomy or α-adrenergic receptor blockade, CBF is better maintained because autoregulation is preserved to a MAP that is 35% of control, in contrast to 65% of control pressure in untreated baboons. This observation explains why drug-induced hypotension during anesthesia is better tolerated than hypotension resulting from hemorrhagic shock. Although never studied, the sympathetic stimulation that occurs with severe pain may also shift the autoregulatory curve to the right.

Parasympathetic fibers surround the vessels of the circle of Willis and the cortical pial vessels. These fibers contain a wide variety of vasodilatory mediators, which include substance P, neurokinin A, and CGRP, whose mechanism of action was discussed earlier. Stimulation of parasympathetic fibers promotes a vasodilatory reaction to ischemia. Thus in rats rendered ischemic by branch occlusion of the MCA, sectioning of these nerves has been shown to lead to a greater cerebral infarction volume.[214] Any protective effect, however, may be overshadowed by an increase in postischemic hyperemia mediated by stimulation of these same fibers.[215] Parasympathetic fibers may also attenuate cerebral hyperemia after release of carotid arterial occlusion. Parasympathetic vasoconstrictor response is probably mediated by neuropeptide Y.[216] Because of species differences, these results cannot reasonably be extrapolated to humans. In summary, despite extensive innervation of the intracerebral vessels, the purpose of these pathways currently remains baffling.

Other Clinical Considerations

The Hypertensive Patient

Chronic hypertension is accompanied by a rightward shift of the autoregulation curve. Although this shift has some effect in protecting the brain against "breakthrough" caused by surpassing the upper limit of autoregulation, it occurs at the expense of the lower limit. In contrast to normotensive individuals, in whom CBF is preserved as long as MAP remains above 60 mm Hg, the lower limit of autoregulation in uncontrolled hypertensive patients may occur at a MAP as high as 120 mm Hg or more. Thus, although symptoms of cerebral hypoxia do not generally occur with a MAP above 35 to 40 mm Hg in the normotensive patient, these symptoms may occur at significantly higher blood pressures in the patient with chronic hypertension.[217] In one study, cerebral ischemia became apparent at an average MAP of 68 mm Hg.[218] Both the lower limit of autoregulation and the blood pressure at which cerebral hypoxia occurs appear to correlate with the extent to which the resting blood pressure is elevated. The significance of this rightward shift of the lower autoregulatory threshold is that, with decreases in blood pressure—whether caused by hemorrhage, shock, overly aggressive antihypertensive therapy, or deliberate hypotension—hypertensive patients may suffer cerebral ischemia at blood pressure levels well tolerated by normal patients. The mechanism responsible for the shift of the curve is not precisely known.

Vascular hypertrophy, accompanied by an increase in media thickness and a resulting decrease in the size of the intravascular lumen (thicker wall-to-lumen ratio), increases proximal conductance vessel resistance.[219] Neurogenic factors may also contribute.[220] Thus when cerebrovascular dilation in the resistance vessels is maximal, total vascular resistance is higher in the hypertensive subject, as it is with acute sympathetic stimulation. Despite the autoregulatory shift seen with chronic hypertension, CO_2 reactivity in this group is no different from that in the normotensive population.[221] This finding underscores the probable difference in mechanisms between CO_2-induced and blood pressure–induced cerebral vasomotion.

The significance of this rightward shift of the upper autoregulatory threshold is that the hypertensive patient is provided with a protective mechanism,[222] whereby increases in blood pressure—which in normal patients would increase CBF, possibly compromising the competence of the BBB or leading to hypertensive encephalopathy—have little effect. Cerebral vessel hypertrophy resists the tendency toward forced vasodilation, predominately in the smaller arterioles. Anesthetics that diminish cerebrovascular tone (e.g., halothane) have been shown to attenuate this protective effect during extreme elevations of blood pressure.[222]

The vascular changes and autoregulatory shift induced by chronic hypertension are modified by long-term antihypertensive therapy.[223,224] The extent of reversal appears to be related to the length of treatment and correlates with the resultant fall in blood pressure.[225] Treatment of blood pressure in spontaneously hypertensive rats restores the lower limit of autoregulation to the normal range.[226] With regard to acute antihypertensive therapy, the question whether the method of blood pressure reduction in the chronically hypertensive subject has an effect on the resultant CBF has been studied by several investigators.[227] The net effect of any antihypertensive drug can be attributed to some combination of the predicted fall in CBF that is due to autoregulatory failure and the direct pharmacologic effect of the drug on the cerebral vasculature.[228-231] Barry and colleagues[232] have proposed a system for categorizing the effects of antihypertensive agents on autoregulatory phenomena, as follows:

Group 1: Systemic direct vasodilators—without an action on cerebrovascular smooth muscle

Group 2: Systemic direct vasodilators—with an action on cerebrovascular smooth muscle

Group 3: α-adrenergic receptor and ganglion blocking agents

Group 4: Converting enzyme inhibitors

Their study and others suggest that agents in groups 1 and 3 should not have an effect on cerebrovascular autoregulation, in that they do not independently influence cerebrovascular tone. On the other hand, vasodilators that affect either the conductance or resistance vessels in the brain, such as hydralazine, sodium nitroprusside, nitroglycerin, and calcium channel blockers, may influence autoregulation. As discussed by Paulson and associates[22] and Michenfelder and coworkers,[233] determining the exact interaction and extent of pharmacologic and autoregulatory vasomotion is currently an imprecise science.

Captopril appears to foreshorten the autoregulatory plateau, but it shifts the autoregulatory curve to the left. This shift probably accounts for the fact that patients with captopril-treated congestive heart failure tolerate lower perfusion pressure without evidence of cerebral ischemia than untreated patients.[228,234,235] This tolerance may be due to direct involvement of the renin-angiotensin system in maintaining some influence on resting cerebrovascular tone or alleviation of sympathetically mediated conductance vessel constriction in low cardiac output states. Treatment of congestive heart failure may also improve cerebral perfusion by lowering central venous pressure, thus reducing cerebral venous outflow resistance and improving CPP.

The Elderly Patient

Normal resting hemispheric CBF in humans is known to diminish with increasing age[234-236]; however, the significance of this decreased perfusion is unclear. In the absence of brain electrical activity (i.e., high-dose barbiturates), CMR_{O_2} has been demonstrated to be decreased in elderly rats. Thus one reason proposed for a decrease in CBF with age may be a drop in metabolic demand for nonelectrical neuronal function.[237]

Accompanying this change in total CBF is a redistribution of regional CBF (rCBF): Relative frontal hyperemia in the young contrasts with a more uniformly distributed gray matter flow in the elderly. (This CBF pattern, called "hyperfrontality," is considered normal.) Thus the total CBF decrease with age is primarily a result of a rapid decrement of flow in the frontal regions, an intermediate decrement in the parietal regions, and a minor decrement in occipital rCBF.[235] This anterior circulation predominance of age-related changes correlates with previously demonstrated increases in regional CVR and a decrease in gray matter weight in the MCA territory.[234]

One may question whether the decreased resting CBF in the elderly represents a similar decrease in cerebrovascular reserve. In one study, CBF in newborn and juvenile pigs was 48 and 44 mL/100 g/min, respectively, compared with 27 mL/100 g/min in adults. CBF reserve was also shown to be lower in adult pigs, with EEG flattening occurring at significantly higher levels of CBF than in juveniles and newborns.[238]

Concerning cerebrovascular reactivity, the cerebral vasoconstrictive response to hypocapnia in humans diminishes with advancing age.[239] CO_2 reactivity at age 65 years is roughly half that at age 20 years. This change is seen whether CO_2 reactivity is expressed as an absolute value or as a percentage change in CBF. Some authorities postulate that this change in reactivity may be due to minor atherosclerosis or the loss of cerebral vascular elasticity. Alternatively, this finding may simply be due to the fact that at normocapnia, CBF in the elderly is significantly lower than it is in the young. Thus with hypocapnia, cerebrovascular constriction in the elderly is more likely to reduce CBF to the ischemic threshold. Below this CO_2 value, compensatory mechanisms may prevent the further reduction of CBF, yielding an artifactual impression of reduced CO_2 reactivity.[236]

The vasodilatory response to hypercapnia is also altered in the elderly. Yamamoto and colleagues[240] found that the decline in this response parallels the baseline decrease in CBF seen with advancing age. In normal healthy subjects, however, when CO_2 reactivity is expressed as percentage change in CBF rather than absolute change, the age-related differences found in response to hypercapnia are minimal. Regional impairment of vasodilatory responsiveness to hypercapnia becomes increasingly more significant as one moves across the spectrum from normal patients to patients with risk factors for cerebrovascular disease and, finally, to patients with symptomatic cerebral ischemia. Both resting CBF and the hyperemic response to hypercapnia may, however, be well preserved in patients with angiographically documented cerebrovascular occlusion.[237]

In animals, with advancing age comes an increase in the lower limit of pressure autoregulation and an impaired vasodilator response in brainstem blood vessels during systemic hypotension.[241] The increase in the lower limit of pressure autoregulation with progressive aging can be prevented by treatment with angiotensin-converting enzyme inhibitors.[242] The underlying cellular mechanisms of impaired cerebrovascular reactivity with aging remain to be fully understood. In the peripheral arteries, a progressive decline to NO-mediated vasodilation occurs with increasing age,[243] whereas vasoconstrictor response to serotonin is augmented in cerebral vessels of aged rats.[244]

Although, as mentioned previously, most studies have shown a decrease in CBF as well as deterioration in CBF regulation with advancing age, this premise is not universally accepted because isolating age as an independent factor is often difficult. Thus one study demonstrated no change in CBF between the ages of 50 and 85 years despite the presence of an age-related increase in brain atrophy. Of significance, in this combined stable xenon (sXE) computed tomography (CT) and PET study, is the fact that patients were carefully screened to exclude those with any brain lesions or mental deterioration as determined by psychological examination. These older patients may thus be characterized as the fittest of the fit.[245] Earlier studies, however, have shown that although risk factors for stroke enhance the age-related reduction in CBF, a reduction in CBF in the elderly is demonstrable even without the presence of these confounding factors.[234]

AUTOREGULATORY FAILURE

Cerebral autoregulation is disturbed in a number of disease states. Most diseases that affect the CNS will, in one way or another, affect the ability of the circulation to regulate itself. Examples are acute ischemia, mass lesions, trauma, inflammation, prematurity, neonatal asphyxia, and diabetes mellitus.

Despite a wide range of causes, the final common pathway of dysfunction, in its most extreme state, may be termed *vasomotor paralysis*.

What causes autoregulation to fail? The simplistic approach is to invoke tissue acidosis or local accumulation of "noxious metabolites," but it does not account for all cases. Localized damage that results in loss of autoregulation at sites distant from the injury is more difficult to explain.[246] Furthermore, Paulson and associates[22] coined the term "dissociated vasoparalysis" to describe retained CO_2 responsiveness with loss of autoregulatory capacity to changes in blood pressure.[162] This response can be observed in regions contralateral to tumor or infarction or during hyperperfusion after AVM resection.[247] Such a dissociation between two preeminent vasomotive stimuli emphasizes that pressure regulation is much more vulnerable than is loss of CO_2 reactivity or, possibly, other metabolic influences on regulatory mechanisms. Total loss of CO_2 responsiveness is probably a preterminal event. A related phenomenon is *diaschisis*, the occurrence of hypoperfusion and hypometabolism remote from a damaged area.[248,249]

"False autoregulation" is an additional phenomenon that has been described in the setting of head injury.[250] In a paralyzed circulatory bed, pressure-passive increases in CBF may result in local pressure gradients in the most damaged areas. Local swelling may then keep CBF constant despite rising systemic pressures.

Autoregulatory failure (Fig. 2-16) can be divided into "right-sided" (hyperperfusion) and "left-sided" (hypoperfusion) autoregulatory failure. Although the following sections discuss the parenchymal consequences of dysregulation in a homogeneous light, there are differing regional susceptibilities to ischemia and circulatory "breakthrough." Portions of the hippocampus, for example, are exquisitely sensitive to ischemia. Previously this feature was thought to be simply a function of the basal metabolic state of the tissue—that is, the higher the metabolic rate, the more susceptible the tissue is to ischemia. However, this sensitivity undoubtedly involves other mechanisms.[251]

Hypoperfusion and Ischemia

Hypoperfusion leads to cerebral ischemia. However, there is no reason to believe that the fundamental metabolic consequences of reduced CBF to the neurons are any different for any of the various modes of flow reduction. The distinction of complete versus incomplete ischemia, however, may have metabolic consequences and, most importantly, regional or focal ischemia carries with it the possibility of collateral supply of CBF.

Figure 2-16 is an idealized expansion of the left side of the autoregulatory curve shown in Figure 2-4. As CPP decreases toward the lower limit of autoregulation (approximately 50 mm Hg), arteriolar resistance vessels dilate and CBV increases. At the lower limit of autoregulation, however, the capacity for vasodilation is exhausted, the circulation cannot decrease resistance further to maintain flow, and CBF begins to decline passively as CPP decreases further. At first, an increase in oxygen extraction compensates for the passive decline in CBF. When oxygen extraction is maximum, CMR_{O_2} begins to diminish. Accordingly, synaptic transmission becomes impaired and eventually fails completely, as manifested by an isoelectric EEG. At this point, sufficient energy is available to keep the neurons alive, but neuronal "work" is abolished. Proceeding to even lower flow levels results in "membrane failure" (Na^+, Ca^{2+}, and water enter, and K^+ exits the cell; i.e.,

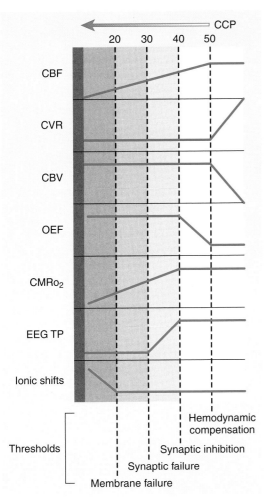

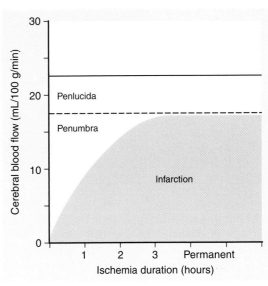

Figure 2–17 Interaction of extent and duration of flow reductions on neurologic function. Tissue receiving flow between approximately 18 and 23 mL/100 g/min is functionally inactive, but function can be restored at any time with re-institution of increased perfusion (*penlucida*). For tissue perfused at lower blood flows, the development of infarction is a function of time. If tissue is restored to adequate perfusion before the time limit for infarction, it will recover function (*penumbra*). *(From Young W: Clinical Neuroscience Lectures. Munster, Cathenart, 1999; modified from data in Jones TH, Morawetz RB, Crowell RM, et al: Thresholds of focal cerebral ischemia in awake monkeys. J Neurosurg 1981;54:773-782.)*

Figure 2–16 Autoregulatory failure is expanded here to show idealized changes in various physiologic functions (some of the pathophysiologic events indicated overlap). The values for cerebral perfusion pressure (CPP) are only approximate, and many of the changes in the various covariates may overlap. They are stylized here for the sake of clarity. Cerebral blood flow (CBF), cerebrovascular resistance (CVR), cerebral blood volume (CBV), oxygen extraction fraction (OEF), cerebral metabolic rate for oxygen (CMRo2), total power of the cortical EEG signal (EEG TP), and ionic shifts (e.g., water and Na+ into the cells and K+ out of the cells) are shown along the *left* of the figure. The various CBF thresholds are indicated by the *broken lines* and labeled at the bottom of the figure. The functional state between thresholds is shown along the *bottom*. In this figure the loss of EEG power is still above the line for membrane failure. Clinically, any event that results in EEG signs of ischemia should be assumed to represent the potential for irreversible damage and should be treated accordingly. *(From Young W: Clinical Neuroscience Lectures. Munster, Cathenart, 1999.)*

cytotoxic edema). Such reductions in CBF are in the lethal range and result in infarction if not corrected.

The development of cerebral infarction depends both on the degree to which flow is reduced to ischemic levels and on its duration (Fig. 2-17). Neuronal tissue can receive flow at a level that prevents normal function but does not result in permanent damage. If flow is returned to adequate levels, function returns. As shown in Figure 2-17, two such states may exist, the penlucida, from which tissue recovers function irrespective of the ischemic time, and the penumbra, from which tissue is salvageable only if flow is restored within a certain time. The term penumbra, which means "almost shadow," was introduced by Branston and associates.[252] They originally used the term to denote all such tissue that was nonfunctional

but that had the capacity to regain function. To make the distinction between tissue that survives without intervention and tissue that succumbs if left untended, Drummond and colleagues[253] designated the former as ischemic penlucida ("almost light").

Although any clinical event that results in EEG changes suggesting ischemia should be assumed to represent a threat for irreversible damage and should be treated accordingly, many such events probably reflect flow reduction to the penumbral range (see Fig. 2-16). An example of this phenomenon is the patient undergoing carotid endarterectomy in whom EEG changes suggesting ischemia develop after carotid clamping. With shunt placement, the EEG normalizes, and the patient awakens without sequelae.

Hyperperfusion and Circulatory Breakthrough

If CPP exceeds the upper limit of autoregulation, flow initially increases with a fixed maximal arteriolar resistance. At some point, the arteriolar bed dilates under the increasing pressure, and the resistance falls as well. Clinically, one may observe brain swelling from this intravascular engorgement, vasogenic edema from opening of the BBB, and intracerebral hemorrhage from vessel rupture.[22,247,254] The different types of brain swelling and their primary fluid compartment alterations are shown in Table 2-1.

To explain the occurrence of postoperative brain swelling and intracerebral hemorrhage after AVM resection, the concept "normal pressure perfusion breakthrough" (NPPB)[255] or "circulatory breakthrough"[256] has been proposed. This theory holds that the low-resistance AVM shunt system results in arterial hypotension and venous hypertension in the relatively normal circulatory beds irrigated by vessels in continuity with feeding arteries and draining veins adjacent to the lesion. Regional CBF in these neighboring areas is kept in a normal

Table 2–1   Types of Brain Swelling

Type of Swelling	Primary Fluid Compartment Alteration
Cytotoxic	Shift of fluid from extracellular to intracellular space
Vasogenic	Shift of fluid from intravascular to extracellular space
Interstitial	Shift of cerebrospinal fluid into extracellular space
Hyperemic	Increase in intravascular volume

range by appropriate autoregulatory vasodilation. This long-standing state of maximal dilation may result in vasomotor paralysis; the resistance vessels may no longer be capable of autoregulation should perfusion pressure increase. When the AVM fistula is interrupted, the pressure "normalizes" in the neighboring circulation. However, the presence of a vasomotor paralysis in newly normotensive circulatory beds prevents the appropriate increase in CVR necessary to maintain flow at a constant level, and cerebral hyperemia occurs. This hyperperfusion and abrupt increase in perfusion pressure may result in swelling and hemorrhage, although the precise mechanism is speculative. Postoperative swelling and hemorrhage after carotid endarterectomy[254] and after obliteration of a jugular-carotid fistula[257] are probably mechanistically related to normal pressure perfusion breakthrough.

Many of the aspects of "perfusion breakthrough" are controversial and supported by anecdotal evidence only. As observed in rats, 12 weeks after creation of carotid-jugular fistulas that result in chronic cerebral hypoperfusion, perfusion breakthrough occurs at a much lower systemic pressure than in normal animals (130 vs. 180 mm Hg). This finding suggests that chronic cerebral hypoperfusion decreases the upper limit of autoregulation and could account for the pressure breakthrough phenomena when CPP is restored in hypoperfused vascular beds.[258] The syndromes of pressure breakthrough that result in postoperative catastrophes are clearly a clinical problem, but the precise mechanisms and relative importance of the contributing circulatory physiology remain to be elucidated.[259] Young and colleagues[260] reported that after AVM resection, cerebral hyperemia—not feeding artery pressure—was the predictor of "breakthrough" complications.[260] This finding argues against a simple hydraulic explanation of the breakthrough complications and points toward other possible causes.[261] There is growing interest in the notion that neuroeffector mechanisms[19,43] may participate in the pathogenesis of pressure breakthrough phenomena.

Reperfusion Injury

Many of the pathophysiologic events leading to irreversible neuronal damage are probably due to injury sustained during reperfusion of the ischemic tissue, perhaps as a result of reoxygenation.[262] Specifically in regard to CBF, the syndrome of delayed hypoperfusion is evident.[263]

The significance of the hypoperfusion in relation to neuronal damage is not clear. Most likely, CBF is grossly and appropriately coupled to a decreased metabolic rate after ischemia[264]; however, certain areas of the brain may be left with a mismatched CBF-metabolism ratio.[263] Adhesion of neutrophils to the vascular endothelium may also prevent restoration of tissue perfusion after cerebral ischemia. Mice deficient in intercellular adhesion molecules are relatively resistant to stroke following transient cerebral ischemia.[265] Reperfusion injury can also be mitigated by aminoguanidine, a selective inhibitor of inducible NOS, and ifenprodil, a polyamine site N-methyl-D-aspartate (NMDA) receptor antagonist.[266,267]

Hemodynamic Considerations during Autoregulatory Failure

Cerebrovascular Reserve

If cerebral vessels are stenotic, specific areas may have reduced inflow pressure. These regions often follow the distribution of a main arterial supply, such as the anterior, middle, or posterior cerebral arteries, or may be limited to a smaller distribution. Distal to an area of stenosis, a drop in perfusion pressure occurs, and, thus, even at normal systemic blood pressure, the arterial bed distal to the stenosis is relatively hypotensive and may operate near or on the pressure-passive area of the autoregulatory curve (see Figs. 2-4 and 2-16). The resting flow to a tissue bed may be normal, but there is no further potential for vasodilation if a drop in perfusion pressure occurs. Therefore these areas have an exhausted "cerebrovascular reserve,"[268] that is, the capacity for further vasodilation and maintenance of flow at appropriate levels. A way to assess cerebrovascular reserve is by challenging the circulation with a vasodilator.

Clinically, both acetazolamide and carbon dioxide are used.[269] In structurally normal regions (i.e., on routine MRI or CT scans) that have decreased vasodilatory response to such challenges, one may infer that the perfusion pressure is decreased. Application of this sort of testing has been proposed, for example, to determine which patients might benefit from extracranial-to-intracranial revascularization procedures or to assess the effects of an acute arterial occlusion. Use of such methods, however, is still in its infancy in clinical practice. PET[270] and single-photon emission computed tomography (SPECT)[271] may ultimately provide more sensitive measures by simultaneously determining the ratio of CBF to CBV as an index of cerebrovascular reserve.

CBF is lower in patients with cerebrovascular disease than control levels. In fact, patients with risk factors only for cerebrovascular disease have reductions in CBF and CO_2 reactivity.[240] These reductions do not necessarily depend on the presence of angiographically demonstrable vessel occlusions. The mechanism of these flow reductions and impaired vasomotion remains to be elucidated.

Newer theories on the pathogenesis of stroke in sickle cell disease combine elements of the concepts discussed in this and previous sections concerning hemodynamic regulation. Pavlakis and colleagues[271] and Prohovnik and associates[272] have proposed that the pathogenesis of infarcts in patients with sickle cell disease is due to large proximal vessel occlusion with resultant drop in distal perfusion pressure; the distal irrigation of major vascular territories (e.g., MCA) is rendered hypotensive. These patients, however, have already exhausted their arteriolar vasodilatory capacity to compensate for decreased oxygen delivery resulting from the anemia. Watershed infarcts are the clinical result.

Cerebral Steal

A concept related to reserve is cerebral "steal." Steal is a colorful but physiologically misleading term.[273] It refers to the decreased flow to ischemic areas caused by blood vessel dilation in nonischemic areas, such as can be induced by hypercapnia.[274] Blood is "stolen" from one area and given to another only if a pressure gradient exists between the two circulatory beds. Cerebral steal is also said to occur in patients with cerebral AVMs in whom significant blood flow occurs through the lesion and results in progressive focal neurologic symptoms. However, in a large sample of patients with AVM, no pressure gradient between feeding and nonfeeding vessels to the lesion could be demonstrated, raising debate about whether steal is responsible for neurologic symptoms in such patients.[275]

If an ischemic area is maximally vasodilated, addition of CO_2 causes vasodilation of normal adjacent brain regions and may result in a net decrease in flow, presumably by lowering local input pressure, to the ischemic focus. Conversely, vasoconstriction in the normal brain may result in redistribution of blood to ischemic regions, a condition referred to as *inverse steal* or the Robin Hood effect. This mechanism may also be operative for other cerebral vasodilators, such as volatile anesthetics, and systemic vasodilators, such as nitroprusside, hydralazine, and nitroglycerin, although data are lacking on the clinical importance of all such interactions.

Vessel Length and Viscosity

After exhaustion of vasodilatory capacity, flow is both pressure passive and highly dependent on vessel length and blood viscosity (primarily determined by hematocrit).[143] Thus with maximal distal vasodilation, the areas with the lowest pressure are those farthest from the arterial input. These regions therefore have the highest resistance and the lowest flow. This concept is important clinically because brain regions that are farthest from their arterial input, watershed areas (such as the border between the arterial distributions of the MCA and ACA), are the regions most likely to become ischemic during systemic hypotension.

Viscosity reduction is also pertinent to the prevention or treatment of cerebral vasospasm in patients with aneurysmal SAH.[276] Although the conductance vessels (as visualized angiographically) are seen to be in spasm (with a large pressure drop across constricted segments), the distal resistive bed may be maximally vasodilated.[277] In Equation 2-2, therefore, the resistance term can no longer be influenced by changing vessel caliber. Because the vessel length term stays fixed, only blood viscosity can potentially affect CVR, provided that oxygen-carrying capacity is not adversely affected.[143] In the clinical setting, however, the relative influence of hemodilution on the improved outcome with volume loading remains to be determined.

Excessive hemoglobin concentration may produce a hyperviscous state. Although polycythemia decreases CBF and is a risk factor for thromboembolic stroke, uniform guidelines for phlebotomy are lacking in clinical practice. Certainly patients with hematocrit values in excess of 60% should be anesthetized only in urgent circumstances.

Collateral Failure

After carotid occlusion in a patient with a normal cerebral circulation, the vessels in the ipsilateral hemisphere experience a fall in input pressure; accordingly, the resistance network of arteriolar vessels undergoes vasodilation. This response allows collateral blood flow from a patent circle of Willis or other channels to compensate and restore perfusion. However, if these channels do not exist or the affected resistance vessels are already maximally vasodilated, no compensation occurs, and a condition of cerebral ischemia ensues.

THERAPY FOR ENHANCING PERFUSION

Induced Hypertension

Rationale

Maintenance of a high perfusion pressure, in concert with optimal viscosity and oxygen delivery, may reduce cell death in a threatened vascular territory. As reviewed by Young and Cole,[140] ample experimental evidence is given for this strategy in the form of improvements in cerebral perfusion, electrophysiologic evoked responses, and histopathologic and neurologic outcomes. By augmenting systemic perfusion pressure, one can mitigate the pressure drop across a stenotic vessel or collateral pathway to an ischemic area (Fig. 2-18).[278] Even small increases in CBF may shift a region from the penumbra (destined for infarction) to the penlucida and perhaps to a level of perfusion enabling normal function. However, the hazards of induced hypertension include worsening ischemic (vasogenic) edema and transformation of a pale infarct into a hemorrhagic one. If blood pressure is used to increase CPP during brief periods of carotid or intracranial artery occlusion,[274,279] these concerns are less important. However, pharmacologically induced hypertension and any attendant tachycardia would raise the risk of cardiac ischemia; hence, α-adrenergic agonists may be preferable in these settings.[280]

Applications

Application of induced hypertension during acute thromboembolic stroke is controversial[140] but has relevance to anesthetic practice. Elevation of blood pressure during carotid endarterectomy has been discussed for some time; many writers have recommended keeping blood pressure elevated during the period of temporary occlusion of the carotid artery.[274,281,282] Both anastomotic CPP,[281,282] as measured in the distal stump of the carotid artery after clamping, and CBF[274] are increased by elevation of systemic pressure. Fortunately, phenylephrine only minimally increases venous sinus pressure; therefore during induced hypertension, the drug is unlikely to adversely affect CPP.[282] Despite claims that distal stump pressures do not correlate with CBF changes during carotid endarterectomy,[283] the technique is a simple, low-risk, and cost-effective method to assess the adequacy of CPP.[284] False-negative results may occur (i.e., normal stump pressure with inadequate CBF); however, if the angiogram demonstrates normal intracranial vessels, a severe stump pressure reduction (i.e., 20 mm Hg) is potentially useful information.

An evolving practice during neurovascular surgery is the use of temporary vascular occlusion to secure cerebral aneurysms.[285] Temporary occlusion techniques require some modification of the traditional anesthetic management of cerebral aneurysm clipping.[279,286] During temporary vascular occlusion of a major intracranial artery, not only must systemic hypotension be avoided but also blood pressure augmentation may be necessary.[140,278,287]

Induced hypertension has been used in the management of aneurysmal SAH.[288-290] In this setting, hypertension is employed in conjunction with hypervolemic hemodilution; thus the relative contribution made by raising perfusion pressure is not well defined.[291]

Inverse Steal

Undoubtedly, inverse steal can redistribute CBF to ischemic areas, with unequivocal studies documenting its clinical relevance.[292] Ideally, treatment should be tailored to individual

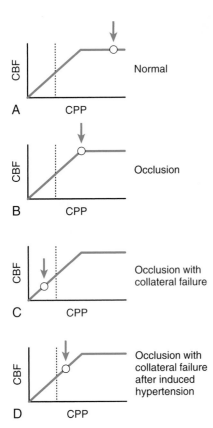

Figure 2–18 Induced hypertension model. **A,** Normal. *Arrow* indicates operating point on the autoregulatory curve; in this case, the circulatory bed is in mid-position in the full range of autoregulation. Lower limit of autoregulation is the knee of the curve. *Dotted vertical line* represents the ischemic flow threshold. **B,** Inflow occlusion. If a major inflow channel to this vascular territory is interrupted, input pressure drops in the resistive bed. Autoregulatory function now adjusts for this decrease in input pressure by vasodilation of the bed. How much the input pressure falls after the major inflow occlusion is determined by the number and caliber of available collateral vascular pathways. In the example shown, there is sufficient collateral perfusion pressure (CPP) to keep the operating point above the threshold for ischemia, although the operating point has entered the pressure-passive range (i.e., this bed is maximally vasodilated). **C,** Inflow occlusion with collateral failure. If one assumes atresia or stenosis of collateral pathways (high collateral resistance), then, with occlusion of the major inflow channel, input pressure drops to a much lower level distal to the occlusion. Cerebral blood flow (CBF) is lower because the drop in pressure has exhausted the ability of the resistive bed to compensate by further vasodilation. Now the operating point is below the ischemic threshold. This situation demands treatment. **D,** Augmentation of CPP. At this point, systemic mean arterial pressure is increased. Pressure transmitted across the collateral pathways, although not sufficient to restore normal pressure in the ischemic bed, is sufficient to raise input pressure, allowing CBF to rise to just above the ischemic threshold (albeit still on the pressure-passive point on the curve). This small shift above the ischemic threshold may be crucial in determining the final extent of the infarct and the ultimate functional outcome after an ischemic event. *(From Young W: Clinical Neuroscience Lectures. Munster, Cathenart, 1999.)*

patients' responses, which are probably variable. A practical problem is the lack of bedside methods to assess regional cerebral perfusion.

Hypocapnia

The concept that hypocapnia can favorably influence CBF during ischemia is not new,[293,294] but not all investigators have been able to demonstrate favorable flow redistribution.[295]

Many of the early studies did not support a beneficial effect of hypocapnia (see Artru and Merriman[296]).

Early animal models used prolonged ischemia.[297] Furthermore, human studies showing trends of improved outcome with hypocapnia lacked sufficient statistical power.[298,299] As in the case of induced hypertension in the setting of carotid endarterectomy, collateral perfusion pressure appears to improve in the presence of hypocapnia.[282,300-302] Therefore it is reasonable to consider a modest induced hypocapnia as an adjunct to induced hypertension.

Pharmacologic Manipulation

Vasoactive drugs that cause constriction of the normal vasculature may produce a favorable intracerebral redistribution of CBF to an ischemic focus, and vasodilators would be expected to work in a fashion analogous to hypercapnia. However, no good evidence supports improvement in outcome from such an effect.

One of the mechanisms proposed for the salutary effects of barbiturates on focal ischemia has been the redistribution of CBF from normal to ischemic areas.[252,303] Despite this idea, the clinical role of barbiturates remains a controversial topic. Except in cardiopulmonary bypass, outcome studies are lacking, if not impractical.[147] Nevertheless, most authorities would agree that in the intraoperative setting, barbiturates are to be recommended in the setting of acute temporary focal ischemia. Whether steal or inverse steal has any bearing on clinical anesthetic management is open to debate.[304] At present, other than agents such as propofol and etomidate (which have not been convincingly demonstrated to be cerebroprotective), no other pharmacologic agents can accomplish inverse steal.

Augmenting CBF is often necessary in the settings of cerebral vasospasm. Both proximal and distal vasospasms are initially treated with hypertensive, hypervolemic hemodilution therapy. Endovascular interventions are usually reserved for drug-resistant vasospasm. There is emerging evidence that vasospasm in the proximal and distal cerebral arteries may require different interventions.[305] Proximal vasospasm is often better treated with mechanical stenting that has a sustained benefit, whereas distal vasospasm is best treated with intra-arterial vasodilator therapy. Intra-arterial papaverine has been the mainstay of such treatment.[306] Owing to transient neurologic complications, calcium channel blocking drugs, such as verapamil and nicardipine, are emerging as alternatives to papaverine.[307-310] Because of the risk of increased ICP with intra-arterial vasodilator therapy, optimum treatment of cerebrovascular insufficiency during vasospasm requires monitoring of ICP.[311]

Intra-Arterial Drug Delivery

Advances in endovascular surgery now permit highly targeted intra-arterial delivery of drugs for the treatment of a variety of brain diseases.[307,308,312] However the keys to effective drug delivery to the brain are the careful adjustment of bolus characteristics (volume and concentration) and, if possible, the careful transient reduction of blood flows.[313-316] Although computer simulations and experimental evidence suggest that the increase in regional blood flow will raise the local concentrations of intra-arterial drug, there is no clinical consensus yet as to the role of blood flow manipulations in augmenting drug deposition in brain tissue.[315,317-320] In the treatment of brain tumors, doses of intra-arterial drugs are often increased with greater regional blood flows so as to increase the maximum dose that can be safely delivered.[320] In other centers, cardiac output, and thereby CBF, is increased during intra-arterial chemotherapy to enhance local delivery.[321] One of the fundamental challenges in the understanding of drug kinetics is the inability to determine tissue drug concentrations within the short time it takes for the drug to transit the cerebral circulation.[322] Modern optical technology promises to overcome this limitation with tissue-noninvasive, high-speed drug concentration measurements.[323-325] Another major hurdle to intra-arterial delivery of drugs is the precise control of BBB disruption.[326] Intra-arterial mannitol is often used to disrupt the BBB.[327] Reducing CBF seems to augment dose response to intra-arterial mannitol.[328] Monitoring CBF therefore is likely to play a critical role in the understanding of the kinetics of intra-arterial drugs and improvement of drug delivery. Intra-arterial drug delivery is likely to be used for delivery of "smart" neuropharmaceuticals and stem cells.

MEASUREMENT OF CEREBRAL BLOOD FLOW

The choice of CBF measurement method depends on many considerations: local availability of equipment and expertise, cost, subject (human vs. animal), desired anatomic resolution, and so on. The method used is important because it determines the range of normal and pathologic values, the anatomic specificity or resolution, and the set of assumptions necessary for interpreting the data. A particularly important consideration is the ability to perform repeated measures in a given patient or subject. (For a general review of CBF methods, including historical aspects, see Bell.[1]) A summary of CBF methods is presented in Table 2-2.

Kety-Schmidt (Arteriovenous Difference) Method

Although attempts had been made earlier, measurement of brain tissue perfusion was perfected by the pioneering work of Kety and Schmidt.[329] All CBF techniques in use today are either conceptually derived from their method or have been validated by some variation of it. Their work was based on the principle, first described by Fick, that the amount of tracer taken up by an organ per unit time (Q_b) must equal the amount of tracer delivered to the organ via the arterial blood ($F \cdot C_a$) less that recovered by the venous effluent ($F \cdot C_v$) in the same amount of time; thus:

$$Q_b = F \cdot (C_a - C_v) \qquad (2-3)$$

After the administration of a tracer but before the attainment of steady state, for any small time epoch, Δt, the quantity of tracer within the organ increases by an amount that can be expressed as follows:

$$\Delta Q_b = [C_a(t) - C_v(t)] \, (F) \, (\Delta t) \qquad (2-4)$$

Similarly, the total quantity of tracer present in the organ at steady state is determined by the following integral:

$$Q_b = \int F[C_a(t) - C_v(t)] dt \qquad (2-5)$$

This integration encompasses the period beginning with the commencement of tracer input and ends with the attainment of steady state.

Manipulation of Equation 2-5 yields the following:

$$F \, (mL/min) = \frac{Q_b(mg)}{\int [C_a(t) - C_v(t)] dt \, (mg/mL/min)} \qquad (2-6)$$

Therefore CBF is equal to the equilibrium brain tracer content divided by the integral of the arteriovenous concentration differences.

The amount of tracer in the brain is equal to its concentration (C_b) times brain weight (W_b). Substituting in the previous equation yields the following:

$$Q_b = C_b \cdot W_b \qquad (2-7)$$

$$F = \frac{C_b \cdot W_b}{\int [C_a(t) - C_v(t)] dt} \qquad (2-8)$$

However, this equation requires determination of absolute cerebral concentration and weight, which is not feasible in humans. At equilibrium (*eq*), however, the venous and brain concentrations are no longer changing, and the brain and venous concentrations are thus related by the partition coefficient, λ, where:

$$\lambda = \frac{C_{beq}}{C_{veq}} \qquad (2-9)$$

Substituting for λ yields the following equation:

$$F = \frac{C_{veq} \cdot \lambda \cdot W_b}{\int [C_a(t) - C_v(t)] \, dt} \qquad (2-10)$$

where *F* is the flow to the entire organ.

If one divides each side of the equation by the weight of the brain, the blood flow per gram of brain tissue can be determined. Multiplying both sides of the equation by 100 introduces the well-known units for CBF of milliliters per 100 g per minute, and this "flow" is usually written with a lower-case *f* to distinguish it from the upper case *F* denoting total brain blood flow in milliliters per minute, as follows:

$$f \, (mL/100 \, g/min) = \frac{100 \, \lambda \cdot C_{veq}}{\int [C_a(t) - C_v(t)] dt} \qquad (2-11)$$

Kety and Schmidt initially used nitrous oxide as the best available approximation of an inert, freely diffusible tracer. Subjects breathed a gas mixture containing 15% N_2O for 10 to 15 minutes. Blood samples were taken intermittently from a peripheral artery and the jugular bulb for determination of tracer concentration (Fig. 2-19). This measurement is a reasonable approximation of hemispheric CBF, and because of the confluence of sinuses, it is really a global measure of CBF. There is "contamination" from the contralateral hemisphere, as each jugular bulb represents roughly one third of the contralateral hemispheric drainage. There is a small (<5%) extracerebral component as well. Because nitrous oxide is not truly an inert tracer, later modifications of this CBF technique used radioactive tracers such as krypton Kr 85 and xenon Xe 133, which are truly inert in the quantities used. One may measure arterial and venous desaturation rather than saturation curves; this may be easier to apply in certain clinical settings.

The Kety-Schmidt method has the disadvantage of being cumbersome and invasive; it requires puncture or retrograde catheterization of the jugular bulb and direct sampling of the

Table 2-2 A Comparison of Cerebral Blood Flow Measurement Methodologies

Methodology	Human (H) or Animal (A)	Relative Cost†	Resolution	Time Scale	Repeated Measurement Possible?	Invasiveness	Tracer(s)	Radiation?	Relative Flow Values‡ (mL/100 g/min unless noted)
Hemispheric									
Kety-Schmidt	H	+	Hemispheric	15 min	Yes	Jugular puncture	N_2 / ^{133}Xe / ^{83}Kr	No / Yes / Yes	50
AVDo$_2$	H	+	Hemispheric	<1 min	Yes	Jugular puncture	Not applicable (NA)	No	Relative change
Two-Dimensional Clearance									
Intracarotid ^{133}Xe	H	+	3-4 cm cortical§	<1 min for gray matter 3-11 min for white matter	Yes	Carotid puncture or transfemoral catheter	^{133}Xe	Yes	80 gray matter 20 white matter 50 initial slope index (mean hemispheric flow)
Intravenous ^{133}Xe	H	+	3-4 cm cortical	3-11 min	Yes	IV	^{133}Xe	Yes	As intracarotid ^{133}Xe
Inhaled ^{133}Xe	H	+	3-4 cortical	3-11 min	Yes	No	^{133}Xe	Yes	As intracarotid ^{133}Xe
Thermal clearance	H	+	<1-2 cm cortical	<1 min	Yes	Exposed cortex	Heat	No	Relative change
Hydrogen clearance	A	+	<5 mm cortical	<1 min	Yes	Exposed cortex, electrode placement	H_2	No	150-220
Cold xenon	H	+++	<1 cm, three dimensional	Several minutes	Limited	No	sXe	Yes¶¶	
Perfusion-computed tomography	H	++	2-3 cm sections	Several minutes	Limited	IV	Iodinated contrast	Yes¶¶	
Positron emission tomography	H	++++++	<1 cm, three-dimensional	Several minutes per section level	Limited	IV	Short t$_{1/2}$, lighter-weight positron emitters; see text	Yes	50-70 gray matter 20 white matter
Single-photon emission computed tomography	H	+++	<1 cm, three-dimensional	Several minutes per section level	Limited	IV	(1)Longer t$_{1/2}$, heaver-weight γ emitters or (2)^{127}Xe or ^{133}Xe; see text	Yes	Relative change for γ emitters; quantitive change for Xe

Table 2–2 A Comparison of Cerebral Blood Flow Measurement Methodologies—cont'd

Methodology	Human (H) or Animal (A)	Relative Cost[†]	Resolution	Time Scale	Repeated Measurement Possible?	Invasiveness	Tracer(s)	Radiation?	Relative Flow Values[‡] (mL/100 g/min unless noted)
Perfusion-weighted magnetic resonance imaging, with contrast Gd-DTPA	H[¶]	+++	<1 cm, three dimensional	Several minutes	Limited	IV	Gadopentate dimeglumine (Gd-DTPA)	Magnetic[¶¶]	
Perfusion-weighted magnetic resonance imaging Spin-labeling	H	++++	<1 cm, three dimensional	Several minutes	Limited	None	None	Magnetic[¶¶]	
Autoradiography	A	++	<5 mm, three-dimensional	<1 min	No	Sacrifice	^{3}H, ^{14}C, ^{18}F	Yes	90-150 gray matter 20-30 white matter
Other Methodology									
Microspheres	A	+++	<1 cm	<1 min	Yes	Sacrifice	^{153}Gd, ^{57}Co, ^{141}Ce, ^{51}Cr, ^{113}Sn, ^{103}Rd, ^{46}Sc, ^{85}Sr, ^{95}Nb	Yes	50-70 gray matter 20 white matter
Doppler Methods									
Laser Doppler flowmetry	H	+	<5 mm	<1 min	Yes	Exposed cortex	NA	Light	Relative changes
Transcranial Doppler ultrasonography	H	+	Hemispheric	<1 min	Yes	No	NA	Ultrasound	40-80 cm/s
Mixed Methodologies									
Sagittal sinus outflow	A	+	Hemispheric	<1 min	Yes	Sagittal sinus cannulation	NA	No	50

†Does not separate equipment investment from individual study cost.
‡Values are approximate normal values for rough comparison between methods; for precise details, refer to reference citations in text.
§Depends on detector size and collimator angle.
¶¶No radiation from the tracer, only from the scan itself.
¶No clinically approved tracers for tissue perfusion; current paramagnetic tracers are for transit time with rapid-sampling magnetic resonance imaging.

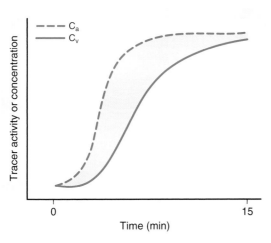

Figure 2–19 Graphic depiction of the Kety-Schmidt cerebral blood flow (CBF) technique. A freely diffusible tracer is given until (theoretically) equilibrium exists between the arterial (C_a) and venous (C_v) concentrations. The area between the two curves is proportional to CBF.

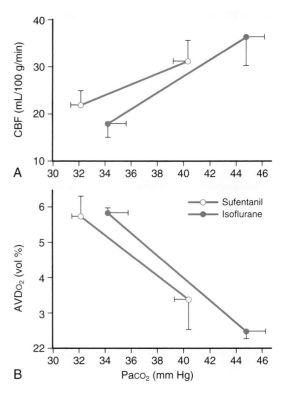

Figure 2–20 **A** and **B,** Simultaneous cerebral blood flow (CBF) and arteriovenous difference in oxygen content (AVDo$_2$) measurements. Comparison of CBF and AVDo$_2$ values for sufentanil (*open circles*) and isoflurane (*closed circles*) anesthesia. The abscissa is Paco$_2$ for both **A** and **B**. There was a significant effect of Paco$_2$ concentration on the increase in CBF ($P < .0001$) and the decrease in AVDo$_2$ ($P < .001$); the product of CBF and AVDo$_2$, which reflects cerebral metabolic oxygen consumption, remained constant ($P = .364$). There was no significant difference in effect between anesthetics. (*From Young WL, Prohovnik I, Correll JW, et al: A comparison of the cerebral hemodynamic effects of sufentanil and isoflurane in humans undergoing carotid endarterectomy. Anesthesiology 1989;71:863-869.*)

arterial blood. CBF may be overestimated in the case of low perfusion states, in which brain and venous blood may not equilibrate during the measurement interval.

After CBF is known, the arteriovenous difference of glucose and oxygen content across the brain can be calculated. The cerebral metabolic rate for a given substrate (oxygen or glucose) is calculated as CBF multiplied by the arteriovenous difference for substrate (milligrams per 100 mL), as follows:

$$CMR = CBF\ (C_a - C_v) \qquad (2\text{-}12)$$

Arteriovenous Difference in Oxygen Content

If cerebral metabolic activity remains constant, the relative changes in the arteriovenous difference in oxygen content (AVDo$_2$) must reflect global CBF (Fig. 2-20), and a "CBF equivalent" can be calculated as follows:

$$CBF = \alpha\ (C_a - C_v) \qquad (2\text{-}13)$$

where α is the proportionality constant.

This is a great leap of faith in most circumstances and should always be interpreted cautiously. However, it is a practical way of assessing CBF changes when metabolism is expected to stay constant (e.g., examination of CO$_2$ reactivity) if a "calibration" has been done with another method (see Madsen et al.[330]). The AVDo$_2$ can be used to monitor changes in patients through placement of an oximetric catheter in the jugular bulb, but this is a case in which the assumption of an unchanged underlying metabolic rate is tenuous. Nonetheless, AVDo$_2$ monitoring can be useful as an "early warning system" for disturbances in flow-metabolism coupling.[331]

Monitoring AVDo$_2$ has particular relevance to care of the head-injured patient in the intensive care unit, in which minute ventilation is adjusted to reduce brain volume because inducing hypocapnia after head injury[332] without regard to CBF may adversely affect outcome.[159,333] A thermodilution method for measurement of jugular blood flow, similar to the technique used for measuring coronary sinus flow, has been described and validated by comparison with measurements made by the Kety-Schmidt technique. The measurement technique involves placement of a thermodilution catheter in the jugular venous bulb. It uses on-line computer analysis of the indicator (cold fluid) washout curve 25 mm downstream of the infusion site and provides a continuous assessment of cerebral blood flow.[333]

Radioactive Xenon

Intra-Arterial Xenon Xe 133 Methods

On the basis of Kety's work, the method of CBF determination described by Lassen and Ingvar[334] allowed progression from "one-dimensional" (i.e., global measurements) to two-dimensional maps of cortical CBF patterns. The technique involves injecting a radioactive tracer ([85]Kr or ^{133}Xe) as a bolus directly into the cerebral arterial supply and following the cerebral washout with external scintillation counters placed over the skull, thus making it possible to perform regional determination of CBF. The higher energy of ^{133}Xe makes it preferable to [85]Kr, the lower-energy beta emissions of which do not effectively penetrate the skull.

Conceptually, the rate at which the tracer washes out of the brain is proportional to CBF. An important assumption here is that the bolus delivers all molecules of tracer to the tissue at the same time before washout begins. In its simplest form (i.e., a single-compartment system), the radioactive count rate decays from a maximum value, C(0), as a single exponential whose rate constant is proportional to the flow rate:

$$C(t) = C(0)e^{-kt} = C(0)e^{-ft/\lambda} \qquad (2\text{-}14)$$

where k is f/λ, or flow/partition coefficient.

Absolute tissue weight, absolute tracer amounts, and blood volume are not needed for calculation of CBF. Because under many circumstances the washout of tracer from the brain is bicompartmental, reflecting gray (fast-clearing) and white (slow-clearing) compartments, the previous equation may be expanded. Compartmental analysis is described elsewhere,[335] but conceptually it is illustrated in Figure 2-21.

How to extract a usable number from these equations depends on the time scale of the measurement (rapid vs. slow) and the inclination of the user. Possible variations include the initial slope technique (suggested by Olesen[11]), which uses the logarithm of the previous equation and differentiating as follows:

$$\frac{f}{\lambda} = \frac{d\ln C(t)}{dt} \qquad (2\text{-}15)$$

This method is useful for 1 to 2 minutes of tracer washout. Because of the mathematical instability of compartmental analysis, stochastic methods (i.e., height-over-area) have also been developed (see Appendix I at the end of this chapter for a discussion of transit time and its relation to CBF).

Problems with intra-arterial ^{133}Xe include the necessity for carotid artery injection, which currently in humans is feasible only during carotid surgery or cerebral angiography. The technique also requires the use of a volatile radionuclide.

Any method that uses isotope clearance techniques has an inherent weakness, in that areas that are not perfused remain invisible—the "look-through phenomenon." "Look-through" results when a region in the field of view for a detector is not perfused but adjacent or underlying regions are normally irrigated. This means that although the isotope is not delivered to the ischemic area, it does reach adjacent regions. The ischemic region is "invisible" to the detector because no (or little) washout is recorded from it, and the detector registers only normal washout from adjacent regions. Obrist and Wilkinson[335] have discussed some mathematical approaches to minimizing this problem of invisibility, but it remains of practical significance in the application of washout techniques to regional mapping of focal cerebral ischemia. How can one measure hemispheric CBF after the carotid occlusion? One method would be to inject the tracer bolus into the carotid artery, allow a few seconds for it to wash into the hemisphere, and then occlude the artery.[336] The washout then is determined by the availability, if any, of collateral perfusion.

Scattered radiation is a problem for all CBF techniques using external counting of radioactive decay. *Compton scattering* describes the situation in which relatively low-energy photons emitted from the isotope pass through the tissue and collide with molecules, producing a change in direction and some loss of energy. Because the detection device is set to measure photons at a specific energy (81 keV in the case of ^{133}Xe), true activity is underestimated.

Finally, the partition coefficient for xenon changes with both physiologic and pathologic conditions. The most important determinants are temperature and hematocrit.[337] The assumption, however, is made often that λ does not change with pathologic states, and this assumption must be considered a potential source of error.

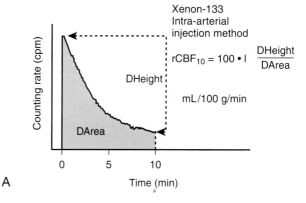

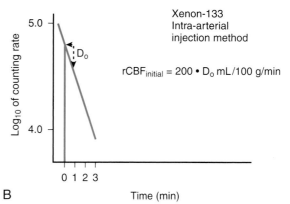

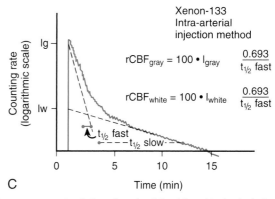

Figure 2–21 Depiction of cerebral blood flow (CBF) calculations for the intracarotid radioactive (^{133}Xe) method. CBF indices used by the intracarotid method. **A,** Height-over-area determination of mean flow, based on integration of the area under the curve to 10 minutes. **B,** Initial slope estimate of gray matter flow obtained from the first minute of clearance on a semilog plot. The constant, 200, represents 100 times the product of λ (assumed to be 0.87) and the factor for converting base 10 to natural logarithms. **C,** Compartmental analysis, in which the curve is resolved into fast-clearing (gray matter) and slow-clearing (white matter) components, calculated from the half-times ($t_{1/2}$) on a semilog plot. cpm, counts per minute; D₀, determinants; I, xx; rCBF, regional CBF *(From Obrist WD, Wilkinson WE: Regional cerebral blood flow measurement in humans by xenon-133 clearance. Cerebrovasc Brain Metab Rev 1990;2:283-327.)*

Intravenous and Inhaled Xenon Methods

Intravenous and inhaled ^{133}Xe methods are often lumped together under the rubric "noninvasive techniques" because carotid artery puncture is not necessary. These methods use mathematical models developed primarily by Obrist and colleagues[338] and later modified by Risberg and coworkers.[339]

The inhalation method employs a 1-minute ^{133}Xe inhalation period followed by a 10-minute washout period.[338]

External scintillation detection is performed as for intracarotid injection techniques. The kinetics of tracer washout from the brain is similar to that obtained with intra-arterial injection, with one important difference: Instead of an instantaneous input of tracer to the brain, there is a "smeared" input, owing to mixing of the tracer in the heart and lungs. With use of the tracer concentration in end-tidal expired gas as an estimate of arterial concentration, the "history" of the arterial input function is obtained and transformed into a series of weighted impulses. By the theory of superposition, the total time-activity response of a linear system to such a series of weighted impulse inputs equals the sum of all responses to the component inputs, and a mathematical technique known as *deconvolution* can be used to determine the input function. A "virtual" intracarotid washout curve is then obtained, and thereafter, the slow and fast components of flow are determined in a manner conceptually similar to that with direct intracarotid injection.

Data analysis for intravenous injection of ^{133}Xe in saline is handled in exactly the same manner. The primary differences between systemic administration and intracarotid administration of ^{133}Xe are summarized in Figure 2-22. Strictly speaking, the algorithms used for noninvasive methods render them compartmental, in that they are based on slope analysis. Because the slow compartment (corresponding to white matter flow for the intracarotid method) is contaminated by extracranial clearance (primarily muscle, skin, and connective tissue), the noninvasive methods are most suited for either gray matter flow or gray matter–weighted indices such as the initial slope index (ISI).[340]

In the inhaled method, an artifact is introduced because of high radioactivity in the air passages. This artifact is present to a much lesser extent with the intravenous method, which involves only exhaled activity. With endotracheal intubation, the contribution becomes even more negligible. The Obrist method for bicompartmental curve-fitting process involved a "start-fit time,"[338] which was introduced to exclude data obtained during the first 60 to 90 seconds of data collection. This model delays curve-fitting until the peak activity of the end-tidal air curve has decreased to 20% of its maximal value. The model calculates the tissue transfer function by solving for four unknowns (two rate constants and two weight coefficients). To achieve solution of even the earliest parts of the clearance curve and eliminate the statistical variability associated with the start-fit time, Prohovnik and coworkers[272] expanded the model to include two additional linear unknowns representing tracer concentrations in air and blood compartments. The curve-fitting procedure with this model, termed M2, is performed on the entire head curve.

With these common rate constants and weight coefficients, a value for CBF may be generated. Unfortunately, a bewildering number of different indices have been proposed for reporting CBF data.[338,341] Strictly compartmental indices, such as the slope of the fast compartment (*fg*), are prone to inaccuracy because of a mathematical instability of compartmental analysis, sometimes referred to as "slippage," in which too much relative weight is assigned to one or another compartment (see Prohovnik[341]). Although *fg* is the most sensitive flow index and conceptually the easiest to understand, it is the least stable of the indices.

The ISI (not the initial slope as described in the discussion of the intra-arterial method) was originally proposed by Risberg and colleagues[339]; it is the mono-exponential slope of the deconvoluted clearance curve between minutes 2 and 3 of tracer washout. Prohovnik and coworkes[272] modified the ISI calculation to use the curve between 0.5 and 1.5 minutes to reduce noise and increase sensitivity. The ISI reflects clearance from both fast and slow compartments but is dominated by the fast compartment. Because of its use of both compartments, it is inherently more stable, although less sensitive, than *fg*.[339] Strictly speaking, the ISI is a rate constant, but it can be expressed in milliliters per 100 g per minute, assuming a xenon λ of 1 for the perfused tissue, a mixture of gray matter ($\lambda = 0.82$) and white matter ($\lambda = 1.5$).

Another useful model, proposed by Wyper and associates[342] uses only the first 3 minutes of tracer washout. This method has application when physiologic conditions are not likely to remain in a steady state for 11 minutes.[343] However, even 3 minutes' analysis of washout curve may not be possible after intracarotid injection of drugs, such as adenosine, that have a very transient effect on CBF. In one study, initial slope analysis was abbreviated to 5 and 25 seconds after intracarotid ^{133}Xe injection to provide a semiquantitative measure of CBF change, *early initial slope*. Early initial slope and standard initial slope analyses yielded similar results after intracarotid nicardipine, but bolus adenosine increased only early initial slope.[340] Early slope analysis has not yet been validated as a quantitative measure of CBF, but under certain conditions, it seems possible to undertake rapid analysis of the washout curve within 30 seconds of intracarotid ^{133}Xe injection.

The noninvasive ^{133}Xe methods have many advantages. Like the intracarotid method, they provide reproducible information primarily about cortical perfusion. Repeat studies are easily performed and are limited only by cumulative radiation exposure, which, in comparison with that for routine radiologic procedures, is minimal. CBF may be measured over both hemispheres and in the posterior fossa with a fair degree of spatial (two-dimensional) resolution because the isotope is delivered to all perfused areas of the brain. The inhalation and

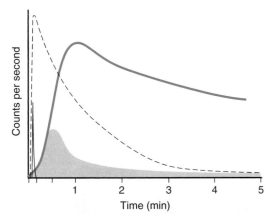

Figure 2–22 Idealized input functions and washout curves recorded at the scalp after intracarotid and intravenous injections of radioactive xenon (^{133}Xe). Intracarotid head curve (*dotted line*) is shown with its input function (*shaded spike*), which is considered to be instantaneous and purely cerebral. Intravenous head curve (*solid line*) is accompanied by its input function (as recorded from continuous end-tidal sampling of expired ^{133}Xe), which is shared by extracerebral compartments. Note that the input function (*shaded curve* underneath) is delayed (and smeared). This results in a slower rise and decay of head curve activity after intravenous injection. Solutions for calculating cerebral blood flow rely on deconvolution of the head curve by the delayed input function. (*From Young WL, Prohovnik I, Schroeder TT, et al: Intraoperative ^{133}Xe cerebral blood flow measurements by intravenous versus intracarotid methods. Anesthesiology 1990;73:637-643.*)

intravenous methods may be less reliable in the presence of pulmonary disease because end-tidal concentration of tracer may not reflect arterial concentration.[344] Although contamination of the head clearance by the extracranial tissue compartment may result in underestimation of CBF results, this is rarely a significant problem. Errors caused by isotope recirculation (which are small) are handled by quantitation of the arterial input function.

During most circumstances the noninvasive techniques yield information similar to that obtained by the intracarotid method.[345] An important caveat is that under extremely low-flow states, especially at ischemic levels, the noninvasive methods have not been validated and may not give equivalent quantitative information. This knowledge is important because many studies examining the flow thresholds for ischemia have used direct carotid injection.[346]

Hydrogen Clearance

The hydrogen clearance method, confined primarily to animal experimentation, is conceptually similar to the methods previously described in that it depends on "wash-in" and wash-out of a tracer, in this case molecular hydrogen.[347] It is a polarographic method, whereby, typically, a platinum electrode is inserted into the brain. A current is used to polarize the electrode, positive with respect to a reference electrode, which is usually made of silver/silver chloride (Ag/AgCl). Molecular hydrogen (H_2) is administered and then is allowed to wash out (be cleared from the blood). The H_2 in the vicinity of the platinum electrode is oxidized into two protons and two electrons, the latter being accepted by the electrode, thus generating current flow that is proportional to the relative concentration of H_2 in the vicinity of the electrode. As with the isotope techniques, measurement of absolute concentration is not required. The algorithms for CBF calculation are conceptually identical. Hydrogen clearance has been used to validate other methods of CBF, such as laser Doppler flow measurements.[348] The hydrogen clearance method suggests that CBF in the range of 15 to 20 mL/100 g/min is associated with energy failure, as demonstrated by magnetic resonance spectroscopy.[349]

The advantages of the hydrogen clearance method include the possibility of multiple repeated measures in a single subject, simple data analysis, low cost, and the ability to measure other physiologic events, such as pH or K^+ in proximity of the electrode. The tissue partition coefficient for H_2 is relatively stable in comparison with xenon. Disadvantages include the requirement for an exposed cortex, measurement of an unknown tissue volume, and tissue damage by the probe.[350]

Autoradiography

Autoradiographic determination of experimental animal CBF is based on Kety and Schmidt's original work and was developed in Kety's laboratory.[351] Modern techniques use an inert, freely diffusible nonmetabolized tracer that is trapped in the tissue.[352] The most common tracer is radioactive carbon (^{14}C)–labeled iodoantipyrine, although others, such as radioactive hydrogen–labeled nicotine,[350] have been used. The tracer is infused intravenously (usually over 45 seconds), and the arterial "history" of the tracer is recorded through sampling of arterial blood. Thin sections of brain are placed against photographic film along with standards of known radioactivity. The tracer trapped in tissue exposes the film

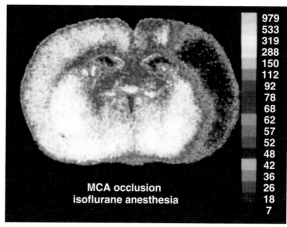

Figure 2–23 Example of cerebral autoradiography. This coronal section of brain is from a rat that was subjected to middle cerebral artery (MCA) occlusion during isoflurane anesthesia. The lookup table, shown on the *right* side of the illustration, corresponds to flow units of mL/100 g/min. Note that the low-flow cortical infarct area is sharply delineated from the remainder of the section. *(Courtesy of Dr. David S. Warner, University of Iowa.)*

(thus autoradiography). By calculating the optical density of brain against known standards, one can deduce tissue activity. Knowing the tissue activity and arterial input function, one can solve for CBF. Data are commonly presented by constructing a color lookup table (Fig. 2-23).

A variation of this method, "indicator fractionation," assumes the tracer enters the tissue, and the brain is removed after all tracer has arrived but before any of it leaves.[353] The calculation of CBF is similar to that used for microspheres, described later. Indicator fractionation is best avoided during high-flow states.

The primary advantage of autoradiography is outstanding anatomic resolution, even in small laboratory animals. Disadvantages are expense, radiation exposure concerns (although usually β emitters, as opposed to higher-energy γ emitters, are used for many of these techniques), and the need to sacrifice the animal. The long turnaround time for cutting the brains, developing the film, and conducting computerized optical density analysis is a relative disadvantage. Repeat studies currently are not practical. Double labeling can provide for simultaneous measurement of CBF and another physiologic variable, such as cerebral glucose metabolism.

A hybrid of autoradiography and microspheres (see following discussion) might be termed the "chunk" method. The experiment is done exactly the same as for autoradiography, except that instead of using optical density to infer tissue activity, one uses direct radioactivity counting of cerebral tissue samples.[354] In this instance, one may use tracers that are cheaper but not suited for autoradiography because of volatility, such as ^{14}C-butanol. Butanol is more freely diffusible than iodoantipyrine at high flow rates.[355]

Microspheres

The radioactive microsphere technique is a widely used method for determining not only CBF but also flow in other organs. It is an embolic technique that relies on delivery of particles into capillary beds, where they are trapped. Typically, 15-μm latex spheres are used. The tissue being investigated is removed and its radioactivity counted in a gamma counter. Although a number of different approaches can be used, the usual design and calculation involve setting up an "artificial organ," usually by withdrawing blood with a pump from a femoral artery at a known rate. Knowing the reference "artificial organ" flow and activity in the sample, C(reference), and the activity C(brain), in the region of interest, one then can solve for CBF, F(brain), as follows:

$$\frac{F_{(brain)}}{F_{(reference)}} = \frac{C_{(brain)}}{C_{(reference)}} \quad (2\text{-}16)$$

Critical assumptions for the method include complete mixing of the microspheres in the circulation, complete trapping in the tissues, and an adequate number of particles in the counted tissue. Repeated measurements are limited by the number of isotope labels. The radionuclides currently used include gadolinium (^{153}Gd), cobalt (^{57}Co), cerium (^{141}Ce), chromium (^{51}Cr), tin (^{113}Sn), ruthenium (^{103}Ru), scandium (^{46}Sc), strontium (^{85}Sr), and niobium (^{95}Nb). They can be discriminated from one another because each isotope has a unique emission "signature"; that is, the emitted photons' energy peaks in different energy ranges. Depending on the size of the brain involved, regional measures of perfusion are possible. Disadvantages of this method include high cost, the need to sacrifice the animal, which precludes outcome studies, and the use of radioisotopes.

Xenon-Enhanced Computed Tomography

Nonradioactive or stable xenon (sXe) in sufficiently high concentrations is radiodense. Therefore it may also be used in conjunction with rapid sequential CT scanning to quantitate CBF.[356] In contrast to radionuclide studies, which use emission CBF tracers, sXe is used as a transmission tracer.

The advantages of this technique include relative availability, because CT scanners are widely available, and the fact that this technique is fully quantitative. Regions of interest for the quantitative determination of rCBF are easily selected visually from the anatomic delineation of known structures on the CT scans. Besides the ability to quantitate rCBF, the CT scans enable one to qualitatively visualize changes in CBF. In addition, visualization of delayed scans permits the qualitative evaluation of BBB disruption. The disadvantages are an unfavorable signal/noise ratio (possibly degrading the inherently superior spatial resolution), difficulty in determining absolute flow values, possible anesthetic effects from the dose of xenon used, significant radiation exposure, the current limitation of analysis to only three CT slices at a time, and the requirement that the patient remain still for 7 to 9 minutes.

Mathematically, stable xenon–enhanced CT (sXe-CT) is based on the Kety algorithm and as such differs little from the previously mentioned radioisotope techniques. Instead of quantitation of the washout of radioactivity, the estimated concentration of cold xenon is quantitated in terms of CT enhancement ($\Delta Ct[t]$). Unlike radionuclide techniques that use standardized λ values, this method computes tissue-specific partition coefficients, a process that may help minimize errors and may have some diagnostic implications.[357] Major sources of error result from CT noise, tissue heterogeneity, and inaccuracies in the estimation of arterial xenon concentration. The degree of inaccuracy or error appears to be inversely related to the size of the area of interest.[358] Thus there is a tradeoff between resolution and accuracy.

The validity of sXe-CT would be questionable if it could be shown that sXe itself modifies CBF. In addition, any sXe-induced increase in ICP would severely limit the usefulness of the technique. Thus for some time, sXe-CT was controversial. Several reports have implied that the concentration of xenon used (approximately 33%) might raise ICP by augmenting CBF.[359] This possibility now appears, in fact, not to be a matter of concern. A study in monkeys with cortical freeze injury has shown that when the conditions under which CBF is measured are well controlled, ICP is not affected by 33% xenon, despite a small drop in MAP attributed to the anesthetic effect of xenon.[360]

sXe-CT suffers from many of the shortcomings of previously mentioned CBF techniques. Great variation is evident in the relative contribution of gray matter and white matter to the flows obtained in different regions of interest. Even so, the technique has been shown to be useful in delineating rCBF changes within a given patient after pharmacologic intervention and has been validated for the determination of rCBF during low-flow states.[361] Because the technique was somewhat controversial, no standardized technique had been established for the conduct of sXe-CT analysis, so the delineation of normal reference values is still to be completed.[362]

sXe-CT has also been used to determine CBV. The technique is based on consecutive determination of CBF by sXe-CT and tissue mean transit time (MTT) by dynamic CT after rapid bolus injection of an iodinated contrast agent. CBV maps are produced by multiplication of CBF and MTT in accordance with the central volume principle. The *central volume principle* holds that blood flow (CBF) through a system is the ratio of the vascular volume (CBV) of the system and the MTT of the contrast agent through the system; that is, CBF = CBV/MTT. The method is rapid and is easily implemented on CT scanners with sXe-CT capability. It yields CBV values expressed in milliliters of blood per 100 grams of tissue.[363] Although this approach is theoretically appealing, limited experimental validation has been provided.

Another related technology that is being developed to determine CBF and CBV is slip-ring (helical or spiral) CT. The technique uses third- or fourth-generation CT scanners that use slip-ring technology to transmit power to the x-ray tube, permitting its continuous unidirectional rotation and data acquisition. As the table is steadily moved forward, the rotating x-ray tube describes a spiral path along the body. Tracking a bolus of radio opaque contrast makes it possible to determine the CBV. The MTT through brain tissue can be determined by measuring the difference in MTTs observed in the common carotid artery and the sagittal sinus. CBF can then be determined by application of the central volume principle.[364]

Positron Emission Tomography

Current PET technology allows precise imaging of glucose and oxygen use, CBV, CBF, pH, numerous presynaptic and postsynaptic receptor and transmitter events, and protein synthesis.[270,365] For example, critical reduction in CBF after SAH can be assessed by studies using ^{15}O-labeled water ($H_2{}^{15}O$),[366,367] and ^{11}C-labeled flumazenil may be able to demonstrate irreversible cell damage after ischemic brain injury.[368] This technique's great disadvantages, compared with all other techniques, are cost and complexity. Few anesthesiologists have used it.[369-372]

Certain unstable radioisotopes decay by producing positrons, which are equal in mass to an electron but have the opposite charge. After a few millimeters' travel through the tissue, the positron encounters an electron, and mutual annihilation takes place. This collision results in the formation of two γ energy photons, which are emitted in exactly opposite directions. By recording the simultaneous arrival of these photons on each side of the head with electronically linked coincidence detectors, one can reconstruct tomographic, three-dimensional images of tracer activity. An advantage of this method is that it controls for tissue scattering because random deflections result in the loss of coincidence.

The resolution of PET is excellent (≤1 cm), but limitations of current instruments include the fact that point sources of tracer activity cannot be perfectly separated. Reconstruction of the image results in partial volume averaging; that is, the radioactivity is smeared somewhat, and any activity in a region of interest is partially contaminated by adjacent regions. The ability to discern point sources in brain imaging is referred to as full-width, half-maximum (FWHM), which denotes the separation between two point sources required for the instrument to discern them.

Isotopes currently used are those that can be incorporated into naturally occurring organic molecules (e.g., ^{11}C, ^{13}N, and ^{15}O) or isotopes that can be used to label biologically occurring molecules, such as ^{18}F. The positron-emitters are all short lived and, except for ^{18}F, require on-site production with a cyclotron. The short half-life allows repeat studies and enables large doses to be used without excessive radiation exposure for the patient.

Measurement of CBF with the use of several tracers and techniques has been described. The earliest method developed used inhaled ^{15}O-labeled CO_2. The ^{15}O (half-life 123 seconds) is rapidly transferred to H_2^{15}O by carbonic anhydrase in the RBCs. After 10 minutes, tracer entry into brain is in equilibrium, with venous outflow and radioactivity decay. The arterial input function is assessed from peripheral blood. With use of the model described previously for tissue autoradiography, CBF can be calculated. A variation of this approach is to use an intravenous infusion, thus avoiding air passage artifact. Several variations using bolus injections have also been proposed. Alternative tracers include ^{18}F-fluoromethane and ^{15}O-butanol.[30] Albumin microspheres have also been used.[373] The many methodologic issues are beyond the scope of this chapter, but partition coefficient and the flow limitations of H_2^{15}O as a tracer are some of the drawbacks of current PET CBF studies.

Single-Photon Emission Computed Tomography

SPECT is the image produced by gamma scintillation counting (like two-dimensional ^{133}Xe methods) that is reconstructed in three dimensions by some form of rotating or moving camera (Fig. 2-24).[374] It is a general term, and any camera that views an organ from more than one angle and uses a computer to achieve tomographic reconstruction may be considered a SPECT instrument. Most nuclear medicine departments have rotating gamma cameras that fulfill this definition. However, dedicated brain scanners that are specifically optimized for the intracranial cavity have become increasingly available. SPECT technology offers slightly less resolution than PET yet has formidable anatomic specificity. Although it requires expensive hardware and software, it is significantly cheaper than PET. The full-width, half-maximum value with newer generation devices (7 to 9 mm) approaches that of PET scanners. Scattered radiation problems and partial volume effects produce inherent problems with data analysis.

For perfusion imaging, the only tracers that currently can be reliably quantitated are Xe isotopes. Although ^{133}Xe can be used, it provides poor resolution, and ^{127}Xe is preferable

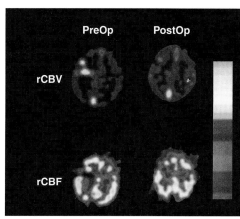

Figure 2–24 Example of single-photon emission computed tomography (SPECT). Double-label methodology is used to simultaneously image both regional cerebral blood flow (rCBF) (SPECTamine; ^{131}I-iodoamphetamine) and cerebral blood volume (rCBV) (technetium Tc99m–labeled red blood cells [RBCs]). The lookup table is relative, and the *lighter shades* reflect increasing flow or volume. Flow and volume imaging currently cannot be quantitated (unlike as positron emission tomography techniques). This patient had a temporal cerebral arteriovenous malformation (AVM), and these scans were obtained before (PreOp) and after (PostOp) surgery. The CBF was normal except for a flow defect that corresponded to the AVM location demonstrated on magnetic resonance imaging. The CBF tracer does not image the fistula because there are no capillaries. In the rCBV image, a hot spot can be seen on the posterior midline that represents the sagittal sinus. The larger temporal enhancement is the AVM nidus; the smaller one is a large draining vein. *(Courtesy Isak Prohovnik, PhD, and W.L. Young, MD, Columbia University.)*

because of its higher energy. Unfortunately, however, ^{127}Xe has a significantly longer half-life. Administration and CBF calculations are roughly similar to those for the two-dimensional ^{133}Xe methods.

One may also use lipophilic tracers that are taken up by the tissue in proportion to flow and then trapped or bound. These include, at present, SPECTamine (N-isopropyl-^{123}I-p-iodoamphetamine) and Ceretec (^{99m}Tc-HMPAO, a propylene-amine oxime).[375] SPECT tracers are generally heavier metallic elements with longer half-lives (hours) that decay by single-photon γ emission, as opposed to PET tracers, which are low–atomic number organic elements with short half-lives (minutes) decaying by positron emission. A problem with repeat SPECT studies in patients with subacute ischemic strokes is hyperfixation of ^{99m}Tc-HMPAO, which may lead to spuriously high subsequent estimates of CBF.[376] Technetium-99m-L,L-ethyl cysteinate dimer (ECD) has been proposed as a chemical microsphere for SPECT studies. It has been shown that the ECD count density correlates with the regional CBF measurements with 133Xe SPECT.[377]

SPECT is increasingly being used for the diagnosis and management of cerebrovascular diseases, provides an early assessment of the hemodynamic effects of cerebral thromboembolism, and can be used with CO_2 or acetazolamide to assess cerebrovascular reserve.[378,379] It is being used with increasing frequency to assess the adequacy of collateral circulation before surgical procedures in which the internal carotid artery must be sacrificed, such as skull base tumor resection.

In addition to CBF, CBV can be assessed with plasma or RBC labeling.[151] Some units can image ^{18}F, offering the possibility of studying receptor systems and cerebral metabolism of glucose. Several single-photon–emitting receptor ligands are now becoming available for SPECT (for instance, dopaminergic [d_2], cholinergic, muscarinic, and some types of benzodiazepine and opiate receptors). [18]F has a longer half-life than most positron emitters, making it an appealing choice for use in centers with no on-site cyclotron.

Magnetic Resonance Imaging

MRI is becoming increasingly important to the study of vascular anatomy as MR angiography begins to supplant standard contrast x-ray techniques. Two approaches have evolved in determining blood flow with MRI. The first technique uses paramagnetic tracers that can be excited in a magnetic field, so that one may directly examine cerebral perfusion.[380] Capillary transit time can be assessed with currently available intravascular tracers, such as gadolinium-labeled agents, thus providing an indirect index of CBF and CBV.[249,381] CBF values are similar when CBF is determined by MRI after injection of gadodiamide injection and $H_2^{15}O$ PET imaging. However, it is possible that MRI values are more weighted toward the more numerous smaller (30- to 4-μm) blood vessels and hence are more suitable for investigating flow changes in small blood vessels, such as those in tumors.[382] More importantly, with development of freely diffusible paramagnetic drugs, wash-in and wash-out can be determined in ways similar to those with current radioisotope methods.[383]

The second technique, known as *spin labeling*, uses radiofrequency to magnetically label arterial water content. The basic concept is that water, being freely diffusible, transfers its magnetic properties to the brain tissue. By comparing perfusion images with and without spin contrast, one can determine the blood flow. Other things being equal, the rate of transfer of magnetic properties is a function of blood flow. The spin labeling could be continuous or pulsed. In continuous spin labeling, radiofrequency pulses are continuously applied to the feeding artery and magnetic transfer is assessed downstream at the imaging plane. Continuous spin labeling therefore has to correct for the decay of the spin from the magnetization plane to the imaging plane and magnetization transfer characteristic of the tissue.[384] The alternative approach, known as *pulsed spin labeling*, is to apply a short pulse of radiofrequency close to the imaging plane so that there is a minimal delay in contrast transfer. Several techniques use pulsed spin labeling to measure blood flow, as discussed in the reviews by Calamante and associates.[385-387]

MRI resolution and the ability to correlate CBF information with structural information could potentially make this the "gold standard".[383] MRI also can image other cerebral physiologic functions, such as hemoglobin saturation, intracellular energy stores, sodium, and pH.[387-389] The noninvasive nature of MRI permits longitudinal follow-up of physiologic and anatomical parameters, thus providing valuable insights into brain diseases.[390]

Thermal Clearance

Thermal clearance is a well-known technique for quantitating cardiac output. Bolus thermal techniques applied to the brain, however, introduce artifact because of the effects of temperature on physiologic function (e.g., CO_2 reactivity).[391] However, thermal conductivity of cortical tissue varies proportionally with CBF, and measurement of thermal gradients (diffusion) at the cortical surface can be used for quantitative CBF determination.[392] The probe is placed directly on the cortical surface but away from large surface vessels or areas of direct brain retraction. There are several measurement variations. In one system, a large gold disk at the tip of the probe is equipped with an active temperature sensor and a heater, and a smaller disk with a neutral thermistor temperature sensor. When power is applied to the heater, the temperature of the gold disk increases while the temperature of the smaller disk remains at brain temperature. The difference in temperature between the two disks is inversely proportional to the thermal conductivity of the brain tissue.

The resulting thermal gradient would be maximal when there is no flow through the opposing cerebral cortex. As CBF increases, the temperature difference (recorded in millivolts) decreases in proportion to CBF, so that the following equation would apply:

$$1CoCBF = \emptyset \left(\frac{1}{\Delta V} - \frac{1}{\Delta V_0} \right) \qquad (2-17)$$

where *1CoCBF* is local cortical CBF; $\emptyset$ is a constant value used as a scale factor; ΔV_0 is maximum temperature difference at zero blood flow; and ΔV is the actual temperature difference.

The thermal diffusion CBF technique has been used to describe autoregulatory dysfunction in a number of surgical settings, including cerebral aneurysm and AVM surgery. The greatest strength of thermal diffusion is the ability to obtain continuous quantitative assessment of cortical perfusion.[393,394] The time resolution is 1 to 2 seconds.[395] Currently, no commercial units are sufficiently reliable for routine use. If CBF changes take place in an entire vascular supply territory (e.g., MCA), the focal flow changes in the probe's area should reflect the regional changes.

Extraneous thermal influences, such as operating room lights, electrocautery interference, and irrigation of the surgical field, may result in erroneous CBF measurements. Another problem is frequent separation of the probe from the cortical surface. Therefore any detected CBF change must be carefully related to activity in the operative field. The use of the probe is sometimes also limited in febrile patients so as to avoid local thermal injury.[396]

Several assumptions are made in the derivation of the CBF values. First, the thermal conductivity of tissue from patient to patient is assumed to be constant. Thermal conductivity depends on the chemical composition of normal cortical tissue and appears to be constant within many different species, including humans. Proper calibration depends on knowledge of the ΔV_0 term in Equation 2-17, which represents no flow. Although this term has been experimentally determined in animals, it cannot be done in the clinical setting. Therefore the nature of the CBF information is probably better viewed as a reflection of relative changes in perfusion rather than as the frequently reported absolute values. Because the method does not require sophisticated equipment, does not use ionizing radiation, and is theoretically easy to use, it deserves further development for use during neurosurgery.[397]

Doppler Techniques

Transcranial Doppler Ultrasonography

TCD was introduced by Aaslid and colleagues[398,399] in 1982. Doppler-based devices are in wide use for clinical imaging, and the general method is similar for all applications. TCD uses a 2-MHz probe and is range gated; therefore the ultrasonic beam can be focused on a target volume at a specific depth. No actual image of the vessel is obtained, as with "duplex" devices. The probe is placed over low-density bone regions of the skull, and the beam is focused on the desired vessel. The Doppler shift of the ultrasonic beam after its reflection on the moving blood column within the vessel is proportional to blood flow velocity.

This technique can provide continuous assessment of the systolic, diastolic, and mean flow velocities in the target vessel. Evidence has shown that the downstream vascular resistance is proportional to the difference between systolic and diastolic velocities. Several resistance indices have been proposed; a currently popular one is the "pulsatility index" (*PI*), defined as follows[400]:

$$PI = \frac{\text{Systolic velocity} - \text{Diastolic velocity}}{\text{Mean velocity}} \quad (2\text{-}18)$$

Although a correlation may be found between PI and CVR, it was not evident in an experimental study. During hypercapnia, PI correlated with the change in CVR, but there was no correlation with CVR during hemorrhagic hypotension, trimetaphan-induced systemic hypotension, or increased ICP.[401]

Flow velocity in large vessels in the circle of Willis and its major branches can be determined. The signals obtained document the direction and velocity of the vessel flow insonated by the beam. In addition, spectrum analysis of the signal allows estimation of the severity of stenosis much as extracranial duplex Doppler ultrasonography does. To insonate the distal internal carotid, anterior cerebral, middle cerebral, and posterior cerebral arteries, the probe is positioned above the zygomatic arch from 1 to 5 cm in front of the ear, the so-called temporal bone window. The basilar artery is insonated by directing the probe through the foramen magnum suboccipitally over the first cervical vertebra. For intraoperative application, a probe can be affixed to the temporal bone window with a strap. During craniotomy, adhesive can be used to directly mount a small probe against the skin.

TCD does not measure CBF; rather, it determines velocity and direction of the moving column of blood in a major artery (Fig. 2-25). The bulk flow (*F* [mL/min], not *f* [mL/100 g/min]), is the product of the diameter of the vessel (*d*) and the velocity (*v*), as follows:

$$F = dv \quad (2\text{-}19)$$

Ample criticisms of the technique have been made.[402] TCD indirectly estimates flow from the peak flow velocity in a given blood vessel. Hence, to equate TCD measurements over a given vessel with "CBF velocity" is inappropriate, because doing so implies measurement of hemispheric CBF. If flow in the MCA is being described, "MCA velocity" is preferable.

Although tissue perfusion is relatively constant among similar patient populations, there is a much greater between-subject variation with TCD velocities because of varying proportions of hemispheric flow carried by the different vessels and the natural variability in arterial diameters. When TCD is used to monitor clinical changes with repeated measurement, the key assumption is that the diameter of the insonated vessel remains the same. This is probably true in the majority of cases.[403,404] Yet, evidence has shown that vasoactive drugs such as L-NMMA may lead to constriction of the MCA such that a decrease in CBF with this agent may not be evident by flow velocity measurements over the artery.[50] Dynamic change in vessel diameter may also be observed during cerebral vasospasm, which limits the applicability of flow measurements by TCD in such settings.[405] Furthermore, the traditional Doppler measurements are based on laminar flows through rigid tubes

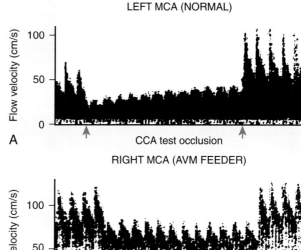

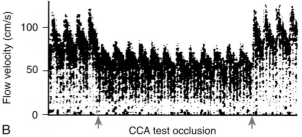

Figure 2–25 Transcranial Doppler ultrasonography studies in a patient with an arteriovenous malformation (AVM). **A,** Carotid compression of the ipsilateral normal carotid artery yields a drop in the left middle cerebral artery (MCA) velocity. Gradually, over the course of the compression, flow is recruited from collateral pathways. With release of compression, there is a brief period of hyperemia. **B,** The right MCA also feeds a large AVM. The low-resistance fistula of the AVM results in much higher flow velocities through the MCA stem. Ratio of systolic to diastolic velocities is different, with the diastolic velocity being much higher in relation to systolic velocity, indicating decreased pulsatility. There is no apparent autoregulatory recruitment of collateral flow and no reperfusion increase in flow velocity, in comparison with the ipsilateral, normal side. (*From Aaslid R: Transcranial Doppler Sonography. New York, Springer-Verlag, 1986.*)

in which the maximal Doppler shift is proportional to the axial flow velocity. In clinical settings, these assumptions may not be valid. One approach to overcome the problem of nonlaminar flow is to measure the so-called intensity-weighted mean velocity. This approach differs from the traditional Doppler measurements, because it takes into consideration the entire spectrum and not merely the maximal frequency of Doppler shift. The intensity-weighted velocity indices yield blood flow velocities with nonlaminar flows and can also be used to estimate the diameter of the blood vessels.[404,406,407]

Other problems with TCD are related to the inherent error in the natural variability of the exact angle of insonation. The error is proportional to the cosine of the angle of insonation, and with less than 20-degree angles, this error is negligible in normal patients. Nonetheless, in certain neurosurgical patients with distorted intracranial anatomy, this error can become significant.[408] Another problem is difficulty in finding the vessel. With experience, this difficulty should occur less than 5% to 10% of the time, but its incidence depends on the patient population.[409]

TCD's greatest advantages are that it is relatively inexpensive, noninvasive, and nonradioactive and that it furnishes beat-to-beat (i.e., continuous) information about the cerebral circulation. It has proved valuable to the neurologist in the diagnosis of intracranial stenoses and abnormal collateral blood flow patterns.[300,410] It might have potential as a powerful monitoring method during anesthesia and critical care. Also, it can be used to study functional[411] and pressure[412] autoregulatory phenomena noninvasively on a beat-to-beat basis. Spontaneous fluctuations in MCA flow velocity (MCAFV) can be detected and quantified by frequency domain analysis and can provide a useful tool to investigate the nature and dynamic regulation of cerebral circulation. For example, MCAFV, much like the arterial blood pressure (ABP), can be diffracted into three specific frequency ranges: high, low, and very low. High-frequency and low-frequency components of MCAFV are coherent with ABP, indicating a similarity of MCAFV and ABP in these frequency ranges.[413] TCD may also provide information about the venous circulation.[13]

Some writers have proposed absolute values for TCD that correspond to EEG ischemic thresholds during carotid endarterectomy.[414] In a comparison of TCD, near infrared spectroscopy (NIRS), stump pressure, and somatosensory evoked responses during carotid artery surgery, the percentage changes in TCD velocity and in NIRS and stump pressure values had similar accuracy in detecting ischemia. However TCD measurements were not possible in 21% of the patients.[415] Thus, technical difficulties in insonating cerebral arteries often limit applications of TCD. As with many other methods, however, TCD information is best considered in relative terms. Flow information is most reproducible when coupled with a physiologic challenge, such as CO_2.[416] Relative CO_2 reactivity of TCD velocities is roughly similar to those reported for CBF.[417,418] Possible routes of development for TCD, in addition to monitoring of hemispheric perfusion, include noninvasive ICP monitoring,[419] determining the adequacy of pulsatile perfusion during cardiopulmonary bypass,[420] and detection of intracranial arterial air emboli.[421] In general, volatile anesthetic agents such as sevoflurane, desflurane, isoflurane, and nitrous oxide increase blood flow velocity through a decrease in cerebral vascular resistance. Intravenous anesthetic agents such as propofol and sodium thiopental, but not ketamine, decrease the velocity of blood flow. Narcotics, on the other hand, have variable effect; remifentanil does not alter blood flow velocity, fentanyl increases it, and sufentanil decreases it.[422]

Other Ultrasound Methods

With a 20-MHz probe, direct interrogation of surface vessels exposed during neurosurgical procedures is possible.[422,423] This method has potential application during neurovascular surgery, including revascularization, aneurysm clipping, and AVM resection.

Intravascular Doppler ultrasonography is used primarily for cardiac purposes and has been adapted to neuroradiologic purposes with the introduction of a 0.018-inch flexible, steerable guidewire that has an integrated 12-MHz piezoelectric transducer. This system allows continuous determination of blood flow velocity in intracranial vessels.[424-426]

Experiments suggest that the injection of albumin "microspheres" during Doppler interrogation give the technique greater sensitivity than existing techniques and offer the possibility of quantitatively measuring intravascular transit time. Furthermore, it is possible to simulate "autoradiography" of the exposed brain by interrogating a field of view during passage of the tracer.[427]

Laser Doppler Ultrasonography

Laser Doppler ultrasonography is another CBF technique that can register CBF from the surface of exposed cortex during surgery. It detects the Doppler shift of laser light

reflected off RBCs moving in a small volume of cortical tissue. The cortical area interrogated by the probe is probably only several cubic millimeters in diameter. The laser light is dispersed in a small hemispherical area, and the depth of CBF measurements is approximately 100 to 400 μm.[348] The technique is similar to thermal diffusion, is relatively inexpensive and nonradioactive, and furnishes continuous information. In addition, one can adjust the time resolution to examine events with a very short time constant, such as the effects of pulsatile pressure on local flow.[428] It is noninvasive in the sense that it may be used during an open skull operation with no additional preparation. It is well suited to animal studies,[429-431] and small-diameter implantable fiberoptic probes, have been used in human subjects.[432-434] Although current instruments claim to be calibrated in terms of absolute flow (mL/100 g/min), relative changes are probably the most meaningful. An interesting application of laser Doppler imaging is its ability to scan large areas of brain tissue when exposed during surgery. Intraoperative laser Doppler scans have been used to map out ischemic injury and CO_2 reactivity.[434] However, the brain surface shows heterogeneous response to physiologic and pathologic challenges that limits applications of such scans.[435] Development of better algorithms that correct for the spatial variability in laser Doppler imaging, such as those using cluster analysis, could improve the accuracy of the technique.[436]

Other Cerebral Blood Flow Quantitation Methods

Isolation of the sagittal sinus outflow and quantitation by either timed collection or flowmeters is a widely used experimental method.[437] Conceptually, the global outflow method is easy to understand (what exits must equal what enters), permits rapid repeated or continuous measurements, and allows simultaneous blood sampling for metabolic calculations. However, it involves a fair degree of physiologic trespass because obliteration of accessory outflow tracts is required. Physiologic or pharmacologic manipulations may recruit additional accessory outflow pathways and thus confound interpretation of results.[438] A variation on this technique involves determining regional venous efflux, particularly for phenomena with a short time constant,[439] but this approach has largely been replaced by newer methods, such as laser Doppler ultrasonography.

Umbelliferone, a hydroxycoumarin, is a pH-sensitive tracer that can be used to investigate highly focal areas of perfusion in the exposed cortex of the brain.[154] Various plethysmographic techniques have also been proposed for the indirect evaluation of cerebral perfusion (e.g., ocular plethysmography in adult patients and head plethysmography in neonates)[440,441] or CBV.[442] Two forms of near infrared spectroscopy (NIRS) technology are currently available: transmission spectroscopy and reflectance spectroscopy. The former uses transillumination through the skull of neonates, whereas the latter measures light reflected from brain tissue in adults. NIRS technology makes several critical assumptions in characterizing the optical path lengths, the relative paths through the extracranial versus deeper tissues, and the proportions of arterial and venous blood. These assumptions may not always remain constant during NIRS measurements and therefore limit the application of the technology.[443] However, NIRS technology may provide a bedside tool for measuring CBF in the future. NIRS probes placed over the intact skull can quantify clearance of indocyanine green after an intravenous bolus injection. Preliminary results suggest that NIRS assessment of indocyanine green clearance may provide a measure of CBF.[444] Through the use of multiple optodes, the NIRS technique has been used to map out brain functions. Simultaneous NIRS- and MRI-based measurements have been investigated for flow-metabolism coupling.[445] NIRS has been used to monitor blood flow in a variety of situations, such as during carotid surgery and cardiopulmonary bypass, in critical units for detection of cerebral vasospasm, in the emergency room to guide resuscitation, However, despite a 30-year history, the technology is still evolving, and many fundamental concerns discussed previously remain unresolved.[446,447]

Synthesis and Comment

An often confusing aspect of the medical literature in general and CBF techniques in particular is that different methods often appear to be in competition. However, the various methods examine different aspects of the same or related biologic phenomena, and different techniques may be required to completely elucidate a process. Examples of complementary methods are shown in Figures 2-24 to 2-26.

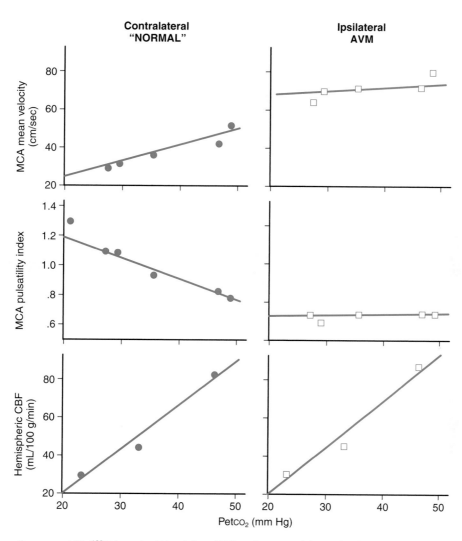

Figure 2–26 Intraoperative xenon 133 (^{133}Xe) cerebral blood flow (CBF) and transcranial Doppler ultrasonography (TCD) studies in a patient with an arteriovenous malformation (AVM) fed by the middle cerebral artery (MCA). CBF was measured 5 to 6 cm away from the AVM nidus and in an equivalent homologous site over the contralateral hemisphere. TCD mean velocity was recorded from the proximal MCA via the temporal bone window. These data illustrate the different natures of the information obtained from these two complementary imaging techniques. As shown by the ^{133}Xe CBF study, $Paco_2$ reactivity was preserved in both hemispheres. Values for ^{133}Xe washout, which measures tissue perfusion in the cortex underlying the detectors, were similar in the two hemispheres. The TCD responses to increased $Paco_2$ are similar on the contralateral hemisphere, in that mean velocity increases and the pulsatility index decreases, reflecting vasodilation of the resistance vessels with increasing end-tidal CO_2 pressure ($Petco_2$). TCD examination of the ipsilateral hemisphere reveals a different response. Because there is a large shunt in parallel with the normal resistance bed, its effect overshadows that of the normal adjacent circulation. The law of parallel resistances states that normal resistance (R_{normal}) decreases with increasing $Paco_2$, as follows:

$$\frac{1}{R_{total}} = \frac{1}{R_{AVM}} + \frac{1}{R_{normal}}$$

where R_{total} is total resistance and R_{AVM} is resistance of the AVM shunt. The extremely low resistance of the AVM shunt (R_{AVM}), however, completely masks resistance changes in the adjacent circulation. Although a high baseline mean velocity and a low pulsatility are present, these parameters remain relatively constant with increased $Paco_2$ because R_{total} changes so little. (*From Young W: Clinical Neuroscience Lectures. Munster, Cathenart, 1999.*)

SPINAL CORD BLOOD FLOW

Compared with the voluminous literature about regulation of CBF, there has been limited experience in delineating the determinants of spinal cord blood flow (SCBF). Technology readily applicable to measurement of CBF has not yet had a major effect on the study of SCBF. Some of the difficulties encountered are (1) the lack of a suitable site for venous sampling, in light of the complexity and small size of the spinal cord venous drainage system, (2) the difficulty in cannulation and the tendency for vasospasm with radicular artery injection, and (3) the difficulty in isolating spinal cord tissue and the resultant low count rates with external scintillation detectors.[448] An often-asked question is whether the spinal cord is a vascular microcosm of the brain.[449]

Measurement Techniques

The first measurements of SCBF historically were obtained with autoradiography. Because this method requires the sacrifice of the animal for the generation of flow values, repeated measurements in the same subject over a prolonged period are not possible. Thus this technique offers little in the ability to detect changes caused by drug administration or other provocative challenges. SCBF values obtained with this technique have varied from 10 to 20 mL/100 g/min for white matter and from 41 to 63 mL/100 g/min for gray matter.[450]

A variation of the ^{133}Xe clearance technique was used by Smith and colleagues[448] to study SCBF in goats. An isotope was injected directly into the spinal cord, and tissue washout was measured with external scintillation detectors. With this technique, the response to manipulation of $Paco_2$ could be demonstrated as an increase in SCBF with hypercapnia and as a decrease with hypocapnia.

The same technique was used to systematically study the effect of changes in $Paco_2$, Pao_2, and blood pressure on SCBF in dogs.[451-453] White matter flow values during anesthesia were relatively independent of the spinal cord segment at which the isotope was injected and varied from 10 to 30 mL/100 g/min. Under halothane anesthesia, an increase in $Paco_2$ from 43 to 80 mm Hg led to a 57% rise in SCBF. In a fashion analogous to CBF, SCBF does not change with decreased O_2 tension unless Pao_2 drops below 60 mm Hg, at which point there is a rise in SCBF. The response of SCBF during hemorrhagic hypotension was also investigated. In normocapnic, normoxic dogs, SCBF was well maintained to an MAP of 60 mm Hg. Below this level, blood flow decreased with further reduction of pressure. With concurrent hypoxia, autoregulation was usually, but not invariably, impaired. The lower limit of autoregulation shifted to 110 mm Hg in some cases. With hypercapnia to a $Paco_2$ of 80 mm Hg, autoregulation was either markedly impaired or absent, with SCBF becoming blood pressure passive. This series of studies, however, did not examine the response to increases in blood pressure, so the upper limit of SCBF autoregulation could not be determined.

Intraspinal injection of xenon has been criticized, for several reasons. It is often difficult to determine the anatomic location of the injection or to characterize the variable contributions of gray matter and white matter. Spinal cord damage may result from intramedullary injection and may affect the flow measurements. In addition, this method is limited to flow measurement in one small cord area at a time.

The application of the noninvasive radioisotope technology (intravenous or inhalational) for the measurement of SCBF is limited primarily by the necessity of a reasonable count rate, which can be ensured only by the use of large doses of isotope. Were large doses practical, separation of the region of interest from surrounding tissue and background would still be difficult.

Attempts made to circumvent these problems in the early 1970s involved the placement of detectors close to the spinal cord. These include small vacuum mass spectrometer probes for the aspiration of cold argon tracer and miniature platinum electrodes for the detection of clearance of hydrogen gas that had been added to the inspired gas mixture. Neither of these techniques has had widespread acceptance.[450] To improve the technique, attempts have been made to measure hydrogen delivery by intra-arterial injections and by measuring clearance with catheters placed in the epidural space.[454]

There seems to be no consensus yet as regarding the best techniques to measure SCBF noninvasively, and different techniques seem to yield different perfusion parameters. Clearance of the contrast agent iohexol during CT yields the following values: SCBF 8.9 mL/100 g/min, blood volume approximately 1.2 mL/100 g, and contrast transit time 1.9 seconds. These measurements differ from data obtained by MRI; however CT measurements are consistent among observers and with different methods of data analysis.[455] In rodents, SCBF has been measured with arterial spin labeling technique during MRI. The spinal gray matter blood flow value (330 ± 90 mL/100/min) is similar to the brain gray matter value (295 ± 22 mL/min).[456] Pre- and post-contrast administration image analysis during MRI yields a spinal blood volume in humans of approximately 4.3 ± 0.7 mL per 100 mL of tissue volume.[457] During surgery the exposure of the spinal cord offers the possibility of measuring blood flow directly. Doppler ultrasound techniques have been used to measure distal arterial blood flow during aortic clamping.[458] SCBF changes can be investigated with laser Doppler flow measurements in experimental animals and in clinical settings.[459-461] Although the method is invasive, it can provide continuous data. Laser Doppler blood flow measurements during scoliosis surgery suggest that unilateral occlusion of the segmental spinal artery is usually well tolerated but bilateral occlusion critically decreases the blood flow.[462]

Comparison of Cerebral Blood Flow and Spinal Cord Blood Flow

Sato and colleagues[164] obtained simultaneous recordings of blood flow from different parts of the cat central nervous system by using hydrogen clearance during ketamine–nitrous oxide anesthesia. The SCBF of 46 mL/100 g/min during normocapnia and normotension was significantly lower than the 86 mL/100 g/min recorded in the cerebrum. In the spinal cord, gray matter blood flow is approximately five times greater than white matter blood flow.

Regional differences in blood flow exist for the spinal cord in much the same way as they do in the brain. Thus mean blood flow is approximately 40% higher in the cervical and lumbar segments than in the thoracic segments. This difference is most likely related to the relative paucity of gray matter in the thoracic cord.[463] SCBF is metabolically linked to the local level of electrical activity. Thus unilateral stimulation of the sciatic and femoral nerves is reflected by a 50% increase in flow in the ipsilateral lumbosacral gray matter.[464]

Blood Pressure

Autoregulation of SCBF has been demonstrated in many species. In rats, SCBF seems to be autoregulated in the range of 50 to 140 mm Hg and is not affected by propofol anesthesia.[465] Using hydrogen clearance in the monkey, Kobrine and associates[466] determined that, as a result of compensatory vasoconstriction, there was no change in SCBF with MAP values between 50 and 135 mm Hg. At MAP below 50 mm Hg, the vasculature became maximally dilated, leading to a passive drop in SCBF with decreasing blood pressure. After the upper autoregulatory limit of 135 mm Hg was exceeded, vascular resistance actually decreased, presumably because of physical dilation resulting from high intraluminal pressure. This finding was accompanied by a marked increase in SCBF. Hickey and coworkers[449] demonstrated that during thiopental anesthesia, autoregulation in several regions of the rat spinal cord roughly mirrors regional autoregulation in the brain.

Comparing autoregulation in the spinal cord with that in the cerebrum, Sato and colleagues[164] found that the upper and lower limits of the autoregulatory plateau were strikingly similar for the two regions in cats. Despite this finding, simultaneously evoked potential data obtained during reduction of blood pressure below the autoregulatory minimum suggest that the spinal cord is less susceptible than the brain to ischemic damage due to reductions in regional blood flow.

Carbon Dioxide and Oxygen Tension

As mentioned previously, SCBF increases with hypercapnia and decreases with hypocapnia.[453] Inasmuch as baseline blood flow levels are lower in the spinal cord than in the cerebrum, the absolute change in CBF per unit change in carbon dioxide tension (between 20 and 80 mm Hg) is greater than the corresponding change in SCBF. Blood flow changes expressed as percentage change are, however, the same for the two regions.[164] Nitric oxide plays a major role in CO_2 responsiveness in the spinal cord. Inhibition of NOS by NG-nitro-L-arginine normally decreases SCBF; however, after spinal cord injury it may cause a regional increase in blood flow.[459] The manipulation of SCBF by regulation of arterial CO_2 tension seems to have no beneficial effect on the outcome of spinal cord injury. Therefore it has been proposed that the complex phenomena steal and inverse steal known to occur in the brain probably exist in the spinal cord as well.[467]

Temperature

Studies have confirmed that SCBF decreases with hypothermia.[468] Local spinal cord hypothermia within 4 hours of injury has been advocated for limiting the progression of spinal cord injury.[469] However, in both experimental and clinical settings, the effects of spinal hypothermia remain unproven, in part because of a concomitant reduction in blood flow.[470-472]

Neurogenic Control

Data is limited regarding the autonomic control of SCBF. Neither chemoreceptor nor baroreceptor stimulation seems to affect SCBF in dogs, despite the fact that spinal cord blood vessels are richly innervated.[462]

Anesthetics

SCBF is affected by anesthetics in much the same way as CBF. Thus thiopental administered to dogs in a dose sufficient to induce EEG burst suppression reduced SCBF by 50%, prompting the investigators to suggest that barbiturate coma may provide spinal cord protection.[473] Pentobarbital–nitrous oxide anesthesia in sheep resulted in a decrease in SCBF, which became more apparent with longer exposure times (up to 3 hours).[474] SCBF was better preserved with isoflurane anesthesia than with ketamine anesthesia during experimental intraoperative cardiac tamponade. In assessment of the effects of anesthetic drugs on SCBF, due attention must be paid to their hemodynamic effects.[475] Low doses of midazolam preserved SCBF, but higher doses result in a decrease owing to the reduction in perfusion pressure.[476]

Although not as completely studied as CBF, SCBF measurement suggests that SCBF in many ways mimics CBF. The spinal cord gray matter–white matter flow ratio, 5:1, is similar to that seen in the CNS. Autoregulation keeps both CBF and SCBF relatively constant, despite wide blood pressure fluctuations. Regional differences in both rCBF and regional SCBF can be elicited as responses to variations in local metabolic activity. Carbon dioxide tension is the single most significant physiologic variable affecting both CBF and SCBF.

SUMMARY

CBF monitoring has elucidated mechanisms in a number of specific disease states and has offered a means to both instigate treatment and monitor its effects for SAH, AVM, head injury, and thromboembolic stroke. CBF monitoring has also been used as an adjunct in the determination of brain death. Nevertheless, the method must realistically be viewed as remaining in its infancy in regard to the clinical care of patients.[477] In the care of the anesthetized or critically ill patient, the clinician must either make an educated guess about what is happening to the cerebral circulation or resort to logistically improbable imaging modalities (transport to the radiology department for angiography or SPECT). However, with the development of bedside methods, discussed previously, physicians will be able to more rationally care for the patient with actual or impending brain injury.

One particular bias in the anesthesia community that has held back the development of such methods is the somewhat unreasonable expectation that CNS monitoring must have absolute prognostic meaning rather than simple descriptive use. With the development of reasonably priced methods to assess cerebral perfusion at the bedside, physicians will no longer be faced with a plethora of questions regarding patient management, particularly those about blood pressure and ventilation.

Acknowledgments

The authors would like to thank Mei Wang, MPH, for assistance in preparation of the manuscript. The writing was supported in part by National Institutes of Health (NIH) grant NCI R01 127500 grant (SJ).

REFERENCES

1. Bell BA: A history of the study of the cerebral circulation and the measurement of cerebral blood flow [review article], *Neurosurgery* 14:238–246, 1984.

2. Veselis R, Reinsel R, Feshchenko V, et al: Midazolam sedation decreases rCBF in brain regions important in memory: A PET study [abstract]. Association of University Anesthesiologists, 43rd Annual Meeting, Boston, May 16-19 1996, p 33.

3. Alkire MT: Quantitative EEG correlations with brain glucose metabolic rate during anesthesia in volunteers, *Anesthesiology* 89:323–333, 1998.

4. Sturzenegger M, Newell DW, Aaslid R: Visually evoked blood flow response assessed by simultaneous two-channel transcranial Doppler using flow velocity averaging, *Stroke* 27:2256–2261, 1996.

5. Oshima T, Karasawa F, Satoh T: Effects of propofol on cerebral blood flow and the metabolic rate of oxygen in humans, *Acta Anaesthesiol Scand* 46:831–835, 2002.

6. Lam AM, Matta BF, Mayberg TS, Strebel S: Change in cerebral blood flow velocity with onset of EEG silence during inhalation anesthesia in humans: Evidence of flow-metabolism coupling? *J Cereb Blood Flow Metab* 15:714–717, 1995.

7. Doyle PW, Matta BF: Burst suppression or isoelectric encephalogram for cerebral protection: Evidence from metabolic suppression studies, *Br J Anaesth* 83:580–584, 1999.

8. Arrica M, Bissonnette B: Therapeutic hypothermia, *Semin Cardiothorac Vasc Anesth* 11:6–15, 2007.

9. Feng CM, Liu HL, Fox PT, Gao JH: Dynamic changes in the cerebral metabolic rate of O_2 and oxygen extraction ratio in event-related functional MRI, *Neuroimage* 18:257–262, 2003.

10. Mackert BM, Leistner S, Sander T, et al: Dynamics of cortical neurovascular coupling analyzed by simultaneous DC-magnetoencephalography and time-resolved near-infrared spectroscopy, *Neuroimage* 39:979–986, 2008.

11. Olesen J: Contralateral focal increase of cerebral blood flow in man during arm work, *Brain* 94:635–646, 1971.

12. Lassen NA, Ingvar DH, Skinhoj E: Brain function and blood flow: Changes in the amount of blood flowing in areas of the human cerebral cortex, reflecting changes in the activity of those areas, are graphically revealed with the aid of a radioactive isotope, *Sci Am* 239:62–71, 1978.

13. Aaslid R, Newell DW, Stooss R, Sorteberg W, Lindegaard K-F: Assessment of cerebral autoregulation dynamics from simultaneous arterial and venous transcranial Doppler recordings in humans, *Stroke* 22:1148–1154, 1991.

14. Hammeke TA, Yetkin FZ, Mueller WM, et al: Functional magnetic resonance imaging of somatosensory stimulation, *Neurosurgery* 35:677–681, 1994.

15. Petersen SE, Fox PT, Snyder AZ, Raichle ME: Activation of extrastriate and frontal cortical areas by visual words and word-like stimuli, *Science* 249:1041–1044, 1990.

16. Martin C, Martindale J, Berwick J, Mayhew J: Investigating neural-hemodynamic coupling and the hemodynamic response function in the awake rat, *Neuroimage* 32:33–48, 2006.

17. Lou HC, Edvinsson L, MacKenzie ET: The concept of coupling blood flow to brain function: Revision required? *Ann Neurol* 22:289–297, 1987.

18. Wei EP, Kontos HA: Increased venous pressure causes myogenic constriction of cerebral arterioles during local hyperoxia, *Circ Res* 55:249–252, 1984.

19. Faraci FM, Heistad DD: Regulation of large cerebral arteries and cerebral microvascular pressure, *Circ Res* 66:8–17, 1990.

20. Iadecola C: The role of nitric oxide in cerebrovascular regulation and stroke. In Mathie RT, Griffith TM, editors: *The Hemodynamic Effects of Nitric Oxide*, London, 1999, Imperial College Press, pp 207–253.

21. Roy CS, Sherrington CS: On the regulation of the blood-supply of the brain, *J Physiol* 11:85–108, 1890.

22. Paulson OB, Strandgaard S, Edvinsson L: Cerebral autoregulation, *Cerebrovasc Brain Metab Rev* 2:161–192, 1990.

23. Symon L: Physiological studies of blood flow in the middle cerebral arterial territory, *Stroke* IX:5–8, 1974.

24. Garcia-Roldan J-L, Bevan JA: Flow-induced constrictions and dilation of cerebral resistance arteries, *Circ Res* 66:1445–1448, 1990.

25. Koehler RC, Gebremedhin D, Harder DR: Role of astrocytes in cerebrovascular regulation, *J Appl Physiol* 100:307–317, 2006.

26. Harder DR, Kauser K, Lombard JH, et al: Pressure-induced activation of renal and cerebral arteries depends upon an intact endothelium. In Rubanyi GM, Vanhoutte PM, editors: *Endothelium-Derived Contracting Factors:1st International Symposium on Endothelium-Derived Vasoactive Factors*, Philadelphia, 1990, Basel S Karger AG, May 1-3, 1989, pp 8–13.

27. Faraci FM: Endothelium-derived vasoactive factors and regulation of the cerebral circulation, *Neurosurgery* 33:648–659, 1993.

28. Dietrich HH, Dacey RG Jr: Molecular keys to the problems of cerebral vasospasm, *Neurosurgery* 46:517–530, 2000.

29. Fox PT, Mintun MA, Raichle ME, et al: Mapping human visual cortex with positron emission tomography, *Nature* 323:806–809, 1986.

30. Fox PT, Raichle ME, Mintun MA, Dence C: Nonoxidative glucose consumption during focal physiologic neural activity, *Science* 241:462–464, 1988.

31. Prichard J, Rothman D, Novotny E, et al: Lactate rise detected by ¹H NMR in human visual cortex during physiologic stimulation, *Proc Natl Acad Sci U S A* 88:5829–5831, 1991.

32. Malonek D, Grinvald A: Interactions between electrical activity and cortical microcirculation revealed by imaging spectroscopy: Implications for functional brain mapping, *Science* 272:551–554, 1996.

33. Shulman RG, Hyder F, Rothman DL: Lactate efflux and the neuroenergetic basis of brain function, *NMR Biomed* 14:389–396, 2001.

34. Hamel E: Perivascular nerves and the regulation of cerebrovascular tone, *J Appl Physiol* 100:1059–1064, 2006.

35. Macfarlane R, Moskowitz MA, Sakas DE, et al: The role of neuroeffector mechanisms in cerebral hyperperfusion syndromes, *J Neurosurg* 75:845–855, 1991.

36. Brian JE Jr, Faraci FM, Heistad DD: Recent insights into the regulation of cerebral circulation, *Clin Exp Pharmacol Physiol* 23:449–457, 1996.

37. Thompson BG, Pluta RM, Girton ME, Oldfield EH: Nitric oxide mediation of chemoregulation but not autoregulation of cerebral blood flow in primates, *J Neurosurg* 84:71–78, 1996.

38. Long CJ, Berkowitz BA: What is the relationship between the endothelium derived relaxant factor and nitric oxide? *Life Sci* 45:1–14, 1989.

39. Bredt DS, Snyder SH: Nitric oxide, a novel neuronal messenger, *Neuron* 8:3–11, 1992.

40. Johns RA: EDRF/nitric oxide: The endogenous nitrovasodilator and a new cellular messenger, *Anesthesiology* 75:927–931, 1991.

41. Pelligrino DA: Saying NO to cerebral ischemia, *J Neurosurg Anesth* 5:221–231, 1993.

42. Tanaka K, Gotoh F, Gomi S, et al: Inhibition of nitric oxide synthesis induces a significant reduction in local cerebral blood flow in the rat, *Neurosci Lett* 127:129–132, 1991.

43. Faraci FM: Role of endothelium-derived relaxing factor in cerebral circulation: Large arteries vs. microcirculation, *Am J Physiol* 261:H1038–H1042, 1991.

44. Gonzalez C, Estrada C: Nitric oxide mediates the neurogenic vasodilation of bovine cerebral arteries, *J Cereb Blood Flow Metab* 11:366–370, 1991.

45. Fernandez N, Garcia JL, Garcia-Villalon AL, et al: Cerebral blood flow and cerebrovascular reactivity after inhibition of nitric oxide synthesis in conscious goats, *Br J Pharmacol* 110:428–434, 1993.

46. Auer L: The action of sodium nitroprusside on the pial vessels, *Acta Neurochir (Wien)* 43:297–306, 1978.

47. Joshi S, Young WL, Pile-Spellman J, et al: Intra-arterial nitrovasodilators do not increase cerebral blood flow in angiographically normal territories of arteriovenous malformation patients, *Stroke* 28:1115–1122, 1997.

48. Joshi S, Young WL, Duong H, et al: Intracarotid nitroprusside does not augment cerebral blood flow in human subjects, *Anesthesiology* 96:60–66, 2002.

49. Joshi S, Young WL, Duong DH, et al: Intracarotid infusion of the nitric oxide synthase inhibitor, L-NMMA, modestly decreases cerebral blood flow in human subjects, *Anesthesiology* 93:699–707, 2000.

50. White RP, Deane C, Vallance P, Markus HS: Nitric oxide synthase inhibition in humans reduces cerebral blood flow but not the hyperemic response to hypercapnia, *Stroke* 29:467–472, 1998.

51. Brian JE: Jr: Carbon dioxide and the cerebral circulation, *Anesthesiology* 88:1365–1386, 1998.

52. Janjua N, Mayer SA: Cerebral vasospasm after subarachnoid hemorrhage, *Curr Opin Crit Care* 9:113–119, 2003.

53. Shin HK, Salomone S, Potts EM, et al: Rho-kinase inhibition acutely augments blood flow in focal cerebral ischemia via endothelial mechanisms, *J Cereb Blood Flow Metab* 27:998–1009, 2007.

54. Riley RH, Lincoln CA: Intra-arterial injection of propofol, *Anaesth Intensive Care* 18:269–270, 1990.

55. Yamashita K, Kotani Y, Nakajima Y, et al: Fasudil, a Rho kinase (ROCK) inhibitor, protects against ischemic neuronal damage in vitro and in vivo by acting directly on neurons, *Brain Res* 1154:215–224, 2007.

56. Jin HG, Yamashita H, Nagano Y, et al: Hypoxia-induced upregulation of endothelial small G protein RhoA and Rho-kinasc/ROCK2 inhibits eNOS expression, *Neurosci Lett* 408:62–67, 2006.

57. Toyoda K, Fujii K, Ibayashi S, et al: Role of nitric oxide in regulation of brain stem circulation during hypotension, *J Cereb Blood Flow Metab* 17:1089–1096, 1997.

58. Stefanovic B, Schwindt W, Hoehn M, Silva AC: Functional uncoupling of hemodynamic from neuronal response by inhibition of neuronal nitric oxide synthase, *J Cereb Blood Flow Metab* 27:741–754, 2007.

59. Robertson SC, Loftus CM: Effect of *N*-methyl-D-aspartate and inhibition of neuronal nitric oxide on collateral cerebral blood flow after middle cerebral artery occlusion, *Neurosurgery* 42:123–124, 1998.

60. Iadecola C: Does nitric oxide mediate the increases in cerebral blood flow elicited by hypercapnia? *Proc Natl Acad Sci U S A* 89:3913–3916, 1992.

61. Pelligrino DA, Miletich DJ, Albrecht RF: Diminished muscarinic receptor-mediated cerebral blood flow response in streptozotocin-treated rats, *Am J Physiol* 262:E447–E454, 1992.

62. Iadecola C, Yang G, Xu S: 7-Nitroindazole attenuates vasodilation from cerebellar parallel fiber stimulation but not acetylcholine, *Am J Physiol* 270:R914–R919, 1996.

63. Wang Q, Paulson OB, Lassen NA: Effect of nitric oxide blockade by N^G-nitro-L-arginine on cerebral blood flow response to changes in carbon dioxide tension, *J Cereb Blood Flow Metab* 12:947–953, 1992.

64. Iadecola C, Zhang F: Permissive and obligatory roles of NO in cerebrovascular responses to hypercapnia and acetylcholine, *Am J Physiol* 271:R990–R1001, 1996.

65. Kozniewska E, Oseka M, Stys T: Effects of endothelium-derived nitric oxide on cerebral circulation during normoxia and hypoxia in the rat, *J Cereb Blood Flow Metab* 12:311–317, 1992.

66. Iadecola C: Bright and dark sides of nitric oxide in ischemic brain injury, *Trends Neurosci* 20:132–139, 1997.

67. Koenig HM, Pelligrino DA, Albrecht RF: Halothane vasodilation and nitric oxide in rat pial vessels [abstract], *J Neurosurg Anesth* 4:301, 1992.

68. Moore L, Kirsch J, Helfaer M, et al: Isoflurane induced cerebral hyperemia: Role of prostanoids and nitric oxide in pigs [abstract], *J Neurosurg Anesth* 4:304, 1992.

69. Johns RA, Moscicki JC, DiFazio CA: Nitric oxide synthase inhibitor dose-dependently and reversibly reduces the threshold for halothane anesthesia, *Anesthesiology* 77:779–784, 1992.

70. Siesjo BK: Pathophysiology and treatment of focal cerebral ischemia, *Part I: Pathophysiology. J Neurosurg* 77:169–184, 1992.

71. Roman RJ, Renic M, Dunn KM, et al: Evidence that 20-HETE contributes to the development of acute and delayed cerebral vasospasm, *Neurol Res* 28:738–749, 2006.

72. McCulloch J, Uddman R, Kingman TA, Edvinsson L: Calcitonin gene-related peptide: Functional role in cerebrovascular regulation, *Proc Natl Acad Sci U S A* 83:5731–5735, 1986.

73. Edvinsson L, Hamel E: Perivascular nerves in brain vessels. In Edvinsson L, Krause DN, editors: *Cerebral Blood Flow and Metabolism*, ed 2, Philadelphia, 2002, Lippincott Williams & Wilkins, pp 43–67.

74. Hong KW, Pyo KM, Lee WS, et al: Pharmacological evidence that calcitonin gene-related peptide is implicated in cerebral autoregulation, *Am J Physiol* 266:H11–H16, 1994.

75. Wei EP, Moskowitz MA, Boccalini P, Kontos HA: Calcitonin gene-related peptide mediates nitroglycerin and sodium nitroprusside-induced vasodilation in feline cerebral arterioles, *Circ Res* 70:1313–1319, 1992.

76. Moskowitz MA: Trigeminovascular system, *Cephalalgia* 12:127, 1992.

77. Nishimura M, Takahashi H, Nanbu A, et al: Cerebral ATP-sensitive potassium channels during acute reduction of carotid blood flow, *Hypertension* 25:1069–1074, 1995.

78. Kitazono T, Faraci FM, Taguchi H, Heistad DD: Role of potassium channels in cerebral blood vessels, *Stroke* 26:1713–1723, 1995.

79. Faraci FM, Brian JE Jr: Nitric oxide and the cerebral circulation, *Stroke* 25:692–703, 1994.

80. Kitazono T, Heistad DD, Faraci FM: Role of ATP-sensitive K^+ channels in CGRP-induced dilatation of basilar artery in vivo, *Am J Physiol* 265:H581–H585, 1993.

81. Nelson MT, Quayle JM: Physiological roles and properties of potassium channels in arterial smooth muscle, *Am J Physiol* 268:C799–C822, 1995.

82. Faraci FM, Sobey CG: Role of potassium channels in regulation of cerebral vascular tone, *J Cereb Blood Flow Metab* 18:1047–1063, 1998.

83. Taguchi H, Heistad DD, Kitazono T, Faraci FM: ATP-sensitive K+ channels mediate dilatation of cerebral arterioles during hypoxia, *Circ Res* 74:1005–1008, 1994.

84. Nelson M, Bonsor G, Lamb JT: Cost implications of different policies for the treatment of arteriovenous malformations of the brain, *Neuroradiology* 33(Suppl):203–205, 1991.

85. Brayden JE, Nelson MT: Regulation of arterial tone by activation of calcium-dependent potassium channels, *Science* 256:532–535, 1992.

86. Robertson BE, Schubert R, Hescheler J, Nelson MT: cGMP-dependent protein kinase activates Ca-activated K channels in cerebral artery smooth muscle cells, *Am J Physiol* 265:C299–C303, 1993.

87. Paterno R, Faraci FM, Heistad DD: Role of Ca^{2+}-dependent K^+ channels in cerebral vasodilatation induced by increases in cyclic GMP and cyclic AMP in the rat, *Stroke* 27:1603–1608, 1996.

88. Eriksson S, Hagenfeldt L, Law D, et al: Effect of prostaglandin synthesis inhibitors on basal and carbon dioxide stimulated cerebral blood flow in man, *Acta Physiol Scand* 117:203–211, 1983.

89. Onoue H, Katusic ZS: Role of potassium channels in relaxations of canine middle cerebral arteries induced by nitric oxide donors, *Stroke* 28:1264–1271, 1997.

90. Wang Q, Paulson OB, Lassen NA: Indomethacin abolishes cerebral blood flow increase in response to acetazolamide-induced extracellular acidosis: A mechanism for its effect on hypercapnia?, *J Cereb Blood Flow Metab* 13:724–727, 1993.

91. Markus HS, Vallance P, Brown MM: Differential effect of three cyclooxygenase inhibitors on human cerebral blood flow velocity and carbon dioxide reactivity, *Stroke* 25:1760–1764, 1994.

92. Brian JE Jr, Heistad DD, Faraci FM: Effect of carbon monoxide on rabbit cerebral arteries, *Stroke* 25:639–643, 1994.

93. Wagerle LC, Mishra OP: Mechanism of CO_2 response in cerebral arteries of the newborn pig: Role of phospholipase, cyclooxygenase, and lipoxygenase pathways, *Circ Res* 62:1019–1026, 1988.

94. Leffler CW, Busija DW: Prostanoids in cortical subarachnoid cerebrospinal fluid and pial arterial diameter in newborn pigs, *Circ Res* 57:689–694, 1985.

95. Leffler CW, Mirro R, Shanklin DR, et al: Light/dye microvascular injury selectively eliminates hypercapnia-induced pial arteriolar dilation in newborn pigs, *Am J Physiol* 266:H623–H630, 1994.

96. Leffler CW, Mirro R, Pharris LJ, Shibata M: Permissive role of prostacyclin in cerebral vasodilation to hypercapnia in newborn pigs, *Am J Physiol* 267:H285–H291, 1994.

97. Wagerle LC, DeGiulio PA: Indomethacin-sensitive CO_2 reactivity of cerebral arterioles is restored by vasodilator prostaglandin, *Am J Physiol* 266:H1332–H1338, 1994.

98. Sakurai T, Yanagisawa M, Takuwa Y, et al: Cloning of a cDNA encoding a non-isopeptide-selective subtype of the endothelin receptor, *Nature* 348:732–735, 1990.

99. Arai H, Hori S, Aramori I, et al: Cloning and expression of a cDNA encoding an endothelin receptor, *Nature* 348:730–732, 1990.

100. Murray MA, Faraci FM, Heistad DD: Effect of protein kinase C inhibitors on endothelin- and vasopressin-induced constriction of the rat basilar artery, *Am J Physiol* 263:H1643–H1649, 1992.

101. Durieu-Trautmann O, Federici C, Creminon C, et al: Nitric oxide and endothelin secretion by brain microvessel endothelial cells: regulation by cyclic nucleotides, *J Cell Physiol* 155:104–111, 1993.

102. Kitazono T, Heistad DD, Faraci FM: Enhanced responses of the basilar artery to activation of endothelin-B receptors in stroke-prone spontaneously hypertensive rats, *Hypertension* 25:490–494, 1995.

103. Foley PL, Caner HH, Kassell NF, Lee KS: Reversal of subarachnoid hemorrhage-induced vasoconstriction with an endothelin receptor antagonist, *Neurosurgery* 34:108–112, 1994.

104. Zuccarello M: Endothelin: the "prime suspect" in cerebral vasospasm, *Acta Neurochir Suppl* 77:61–65, 2001.

105. Zuccarello M, Boccaletti R, Romano A, Rapoport RM: Endothelin B receptor antagonists attenuate subarachnoid hemorrhage-induced cerebral vasospasm, *Stroke* 29:1924–1929, 1998.

106. Lavine SD, Wang M, Etu JJ, et al: Augmentation of cerebral blood flow and reversal of endothelin-1-induced vasospasm: A comparison of intracarotid nicardipine and verapamil, *Neurosurgery* 60:742–748, 2007.

107. Vajkoczy P, Meyer B, Weidauer S, et al: Clazosentan (AXV-034343), a selective endothelin A receptor antagonist, in the prevention of cerebral vasospasm following severe aneurysmal subarachnoid hemorrhage: Results of a randomized, double-blind, placebo-controlled, multicenter phase IIa study, *J Neurosurg* 103:9–17, 2005.

108. Day AL: Arterial distributions and variants. In Wood JH, editor: *Cerebral Blood Flow Physiologic and Clinical Aspects*, New York, 1987, McGraw-Hill, pp 19–36.

109. Bladin CF, Alexandrov AV, Norris JW: Carotid endarterectomy and the measurement of stenosis, *Stroke* 25:709–712, 1994.

110. Van der Zwan A, Hillen B, Tulleken CAF, et al: Variability of the territories of the major cerebral arteries, *J Neurosurg* 77:927–940, 1992.

111. Riggs HE, Rupp C: Variations in form of circle of Willis, *Arch Neurol* 8:24–30, 1963.

112. Cassot F, Vergeur V, Bossuet P, et al: Effects of anterior communicating artery diameter on cerebral hemodynamics in internal carotid artery disease: A model study, *Circulation* 92:3122–3131, 1995.

113. Schomer DF, Marks MP, Steinberg GK, et al: The anatomy of the posterior communicating artery as a risk factor for ischemic cerebral infarction, *N Engl J Med* 330:1565–1570, 1994.

114. Nakai K, Imai H, Kamei I, et al: Microangioarchitecture of rat parietal cortex with special reference to vascular "sphincters": Scanning electron microscopic and dark field microscopic study, *Stroke* 12:653–659, 1981.

115. Heistad DD, Marcus ML, Abboud FM: Role of large arteries in regulation of cerebral blood flow in dogs, *J Clin Invest* 62:761–768, 1978.

116. Kontos HA, Wei EP, Navari RM, et al: Responses of cerebral arteries and arterioles to acute hypotension and hypertension, *Am J Physiol* 234:H371–H383, 1978.

117. Shapiro HM, Stromberg DD, Lee DR, Wiederhielm CA: Dynamic pressures in the pial arterial microcirculation, *Am J Physiol* 221:279–283, 1971.

118. Hudetz AG: The cerebral microcirculation in ischemia and hypoxemia. The Arisztid G.B. Kovach Memorial Lecture, *Adv Exp Med Biol* 530:347–357, 2003.

119. Hudetz AG: Cerebral microcirculation. In Welch KMA, Caplan LR, Reis DJ, et al: *Primer on Cerebrovascular Diseases*, San Diego, CA, 1997, Academic Press, pp 45–51.

120. Gobel U, Theilen H, Schrock H, Kuschinsky W: Dynamics of capillary perfusion in the brain, *Blood Vessels* 28:190–196, 1991.

121. Francois-Dainville E, Buchweitz E, Weiss HR: Effect of hypoxia on percent of arteriolar and capillary beds perfused in the rat brain, *J Appl Physiol* 60:280–288, 1986.

122. Frankel H, Dribben J, Kissen I, et al: Effect of carbon dioxide on the utilization of brain capillary reserve and flow, *Microcirc Endoth Lymphatics* 5:391–415, 1989.

123. Gobel U, Theilen H, Kuschinsky W: Congruence of total and perfused capillary network in rat brains, *Circ Res* 56:271–281, 1990.

124. Halsey JH Jr, McFarland S: Oxygen cycles and metabolic autoregulation, *Stroke* 5:219–225, 1974.

125. Gao E, Young WL, Pile-Spellman J, et al: Mathematical considerations for modeling cerebral blood flow autoregulation to systemic arterial pressure, *Am J Physiol* 274:H1023–H1031, 1998.

126. Fein JM, Lipow K, Marmarou A: Cortical artery pressure in normotensive and hypertensive aneurysm patients, *J Neurosurg* 59:51–56, 1983.

127. Kader A, Young WL: The effects of intracranial arteriovenous malformations on cerebral hemodynamics, *Neurosurg Clin N Am* 7:767–781, 1996.

128. Wagner EM, Traystman RJ: Hydrostatic determinants of cerebral perfusion, *Crit Care Med* 14:484–490, 1986.

129. Auer LM, Ishiyama N, Pucher R: Cerebrovascular response to intracranial hypertension, *Acta Neurochir (Wien)* 84:124–128, 1987.

130. Strandgaard S: The lower and upper limits for autoregulation of cerebral blood flow [abstract], *Stroke* 4:323, 1973.

131. Joshi S, Young WL, Pile-Spellman J, et al: Manipulation of cerebrovascular resistance during internal carotid artery occlusion by intraarterial verapamil, *Anesth Analg* 85:753–759, 1997.

132. Joshi S, Hashimoto T, Ostapkovich N, et al: Effect of intracarotid papaverine on human cerebral blood flow and vascular resistance during acute hemispheric arterial hypotension, *J Neurosurg Anesthesiol* 13:146–151, 2001.

133. Drummond JC: The lower limit of autoregulation: Time to revise our thinking, *Anesthesiology* 86:1431–1433, 1997.

134. Gao E, Young WL, Hademenos GJ, et al: Theoretical modelling of arteriovenous malformation rupture risk: a feasibility and validation study, *Med Eng Phys* 20:489–501, 1998.

135. Florence G, Seylaz J: Rapid autoregulation of cerebral blood flow: A laser-Doppler flowmetry study, *J Cereb Blood Flow Metab* 12:674–680, 1992.

136. Nakase H, Nagata K, Otsuka H, et al: Local cerebral blood flow autoregulation following "asymptomatic" cerebral venous occlusion in the rat, *J Neurosurg* 89:118–124, 1998.

137. Capra NF, Kapp JP: Anatomic and physiologic aspects of venous system. In Wood JH, editor: *Cerebral Blood Flow Physiologic and Clinical Aspects*, New York, 1987, McGraw-Hill, pp 37–58.

138. Hickey PR, Buckley MJ, Philbin DM: Pulsatile and nonpulsatile cardiopulmonary bypass: Review of a counterproductive controversy, *Ann Thorac Surg* 36:720–737, 1983.

139. Murkin JM, Martzke JS, Buchan AM, et al: A randomized study of the influence of perfusion technique and pH management strategy in 316 patients undergoing coronary artery bypass surgery. II: Neurologic and cognitive outcomes, *J Thorac Cardiovasc Surg* 110:349–362, 1995.

140. Young WL, Cole DJ: Deliberate hypertension: Rationale and application for augmenting cerebral blood flow, *Probl Anesth* 7:140–153, 1993.

141. Solomon RA, Post KD, McMurtry JG III: Depression of circulating blood volume in patients after subarachnoid hemorrhage: Implications for the management of symptomatic vasospasm, *Neurosurgery* 15:354–361, 1984.

142. Ornstein E, Young WL, Prohovnik I, et al: Effect of cardiac output on CBF during deliberate hypotension [abstract], *Anesthesiology* 73:A169, 1990.

143. Gaehtgens P, Marx P: Hemorheological aspects of the pathophysiology of cerebral ischemia, *J Cereb Blood Flow Metab* 7:259–265, 1987.

144. Muizelaar JP, Wei EP, Kontos HA, Becker DP: Cerebral blood flow is regulated by changes in blood pressure and in blood viscosity alike, *Stroke* 17:44–48, 1986.

145. Todd MM, Weeks JB, Warner DS: Cerebral blood flow, blood volume, and brain tissue hematocrit during isovolemic hemodilution with hetastarch in rats, *Am J Physiol* 263:H75–H82, 1992.

146. Todd MM, Wu B, Warner DS: The hemispheric cerebrovascular response to hemodilution is attenuated by a focal cryogenic brain injury, *J Neurotrauma* 11:149–160, 1994.

147. Todd MM, Hindman BJ, Warner DS: Barbiturate protection and cardiac surgery: A different result, *Anesthesiology* 74:402–405, 1991.

148. Chien S, Usami S, Skalak R: Blood flow in small tubes. In Renkin EM, Michel CC, Geiger SR, editors: *Handbook of Physiology A Critical Comprehensive Presentation. Section 2: The Cardiovascular System Volume 4 Microcirculation Part 1*, Bethesda, MD, 1984, American Physiological Society, pp 217–249.

149. Zweifach BW, Lipowsky HH: Pressure-flow relations in blood and lymph microcirculation. In Renkin EM, Michel CC, Geiger SR, editors: *Handbook of Physiology A Critical Comprehensive Presentation. Section 2: The Cardiovascular System Volume 4 Microcirculation Part 1*, Bethesda, MD, 1984, American Physiological Society, Handbook of Physiology-Microcirculation, pp 251–307.

150. Hudetz AG: Blood flow in the cerebral capillary network: A review emphasizing observations with intravital microscopy, *Microcirculation* 4:233–252, 1997.

151. Sakai F, Nakazawa K, Tazaki Y, et al: Regional cerebral blood volume and hematocrit measured in normal human volunteers by single-photon emission computed tomography, *J Cereb Blood Flow Metab* 5:207–213, 1985.

152. Koehler RC, Traystman RJ: Bicarbonate ion modulation of cerebral blood flow during hypoxia and hypercapnia, *Am J Physiol* 243:H33–H40, 1982.

153. Raichle ME, Posner JB, Plum F: Cerebral blood flow during and after hyperventilation, *Arch Neurol* 23:394–403, 1970.

154. Anderson RE, Sundt TM Jr, Yaksh TL: Regional cerebral blood flow and focal cortical perfusion: A comparative study of ^{133}Xe, ^{85}Kr, and umbelliferone as diffusible indicators, *J Cereb Blood Flow Metab* 7:207–213, 1987.

155. Kety SS, Schmidt CF: The effects of altered arterial tensions of carbon dioxide and oxygen on cerebral blood flow and cerebral oxygen consumption of normal young men, *J Clin Invest* 27:484–492, 1948.

156. Siesjo BK: *Brain Energy Metabolism*, New York, 1978, John Wiley & Sons, pp 297-300.

157. Alexander SC, Smith TC, Strobel G, et al: Cerebral carbohydrate metabolism of a man during respiratory and metabolic alkalosis, *J Applied Physiol* 24:66–72, 1968.

158. Wollman H, Smith TC, Stephen GW, et al: Effects of extremes of respiratory and metabolic alkalosis on cerebral blood flow in man, *J Appl Physiol* 24:60–65, 1968.

159. Muizelaar JP, Marmarou A, Ward JD, et al: Adverse effects of prolonged hyperventilation in patients with severe head injury: A randomized clinical trial, *J Neurosurg* 75:731–739, 1991.

160. Young WL, Fremond D, Ravussin PA: Is there still a place for routine deep hypocapnia for intracranial surgery? *Ann Fr Anesth Reanim* 14:70–76, 1995.

161. Harper AM: Autoregulation of cerebral blood flow: Influence of the arterial blood pressure on the blood flow through the cerebral cortex, *J Neurol Neurosurg Psychiatry* 29:398–403, 1966.

162. Paulson OB, Olesen J, Christensen MS: Restoration of autoregulation of cerebral blood flow by hypocapnia, *Neurology* 22:286–293, 1972.

163. Kastrup A, Happe V, Hartmann C, Schabet M: Gender-related effects of indomethacin on cerebrovascular CO_2 reactivity, *J Neurol Sci* 162:127–132, 1999.

164. Sato M, Pawlik G, Heiss W-D: Comparative studies of regional CNS blood flow autoregulation and responses to CO_2 in the cat: Effects of altering arterial blood pressure and $PaCO_2$ on rCBF of cerebrum, cerebellum, and spinal cord, *Stroke* 15:91–97, 1984.

165. Kastrup A, Thomas C, Hartmann C, Schabet M: Sex dependency of cerebrovascular CO_2 reactivity in normal subjects, *Stroke* 28:2353–2356, 1997.

166. Enevoldsen EM, Jensen FT: Autoregulation and CO_2 responses of cerebral blood flow in patients with acute severe head injury, *J Neurosurg* 48:689–703, 1978.

167. Ishii R: Regional cerebral blood flow in patients with ruptured intracranial aneurysms, *J Neurosurg* 50:587–594, 1979.

168. Shinoda J, Kimura T, Funakoshi T, et al: Acetazolamide reactivity on cerebral blood flow in patients with subarachnoid haemorrhage, *Acta Neurochir (Wien)* 109:102–108, 1991.

169. Bullock R, Mendelow AD, Bone I, et al: Cerebral blood flow and CO_2 responsiveness as an indicator of collateral reserve capacity in patients with carotid arterial disease, *Br J Surg* 72:348–351, 1985.

170. Berre J, Moraine J-J, Melot C: Cerebral CO_2 vasoreactivity evaluation with and without changes in intrathoracic pressure in comatose patients, *J Neurosurg Anesth* 10:70–79, 1998.

171. Brown MM, Wade JPH, Marshall J: Fundamental importance of arterial oxygen content in the regulation of cerebral blood flow in man, *Brain* 108:81–93, 1985.

172. Armstead WM: Role of nitric oxide, cyclic nucleotides, and the activation of ATP-sensitive K^+ channels in the contribution of adenosine to hypoxia-induced pial artery dilation, *J Cereb Blood Flow Metab* 17:100–108, 1997.

173. Omae T, Ibayashi S, Kusuda K, et al: Effects of high atmospheric pressure and oxygen on middle cerebral blood flow velocity in humans measured by transcranial Doppler, *Stroke* 29:94–97, 1998.

174. Steen PA, Newberg L, Milde JH, Michenfelder JD: Hypothermia and barbiturates: Individual and combined effects on canine cerebral oxygen consumption, *Anesthesiology* 58:527–532, 1983.

175. Klementavicius R, Nemoto EM, Yonas H: The Q_{10} ratio for basal cerebral metabolic rate for oxygen in rats, *J Neurosurg* 85:482–487, 1996.

176. Hoffman WE, Albrecht RF, Miletich DJ: Regional cerebral blood flow changes during hypothermia, *Cryobiology* 19:640–645, 1982.

177. Govier AV, Reves JG, McKay RD, et al: Factors and their influence on regional cerebral blood flow during nonpulsatile cardiopulmonary bypass, *Ann Thorac Surg* 38:592–600, 1984.

178. Schwartz AE, Michler RE, Young WL: Cerebral blood flow during low-flow hypothermic cardiopulmonary bypass in baboons [abstract], *Anesth Analg* 74:S267, 1992.

179. Schwartz AE, Kaplon RJ, Young WL, et al: Cerebral blood flow during low-flow hypothermic cardiopulmonary bypass in baboons, *Anesthesiology* 81:959–964, 1994.

180. Schwartz AE, Minanov O, Stone JG, et al: Phenylephrine increases cerebral blood flow during low-flow hypothermic cardiopulmonary bypass in baboons, *Anesthesiology* 85:380–384, 1996.

181. Jonassen AE, Quaegebeur JM, Young WL: Cerebral blood flow velocity in pediatric patients is reduced after cardiopulmonary bypass with profound hypothermia, *J Thorac Cardiovasc Surg* 110:934–943, 1995.

182. Woodcock TE, Murkin JM, Farrar JK, et al: Pharmacologic EEG suppression during cardiopulmonary bypass: Cerebral hemodynamic and metabolic effects of thiopental or isoflurane during hypothermia and normothermia, *Anesthesiology* 67:218–224, 1987.

183. Hindman BJ, Funatsu N, Harrington J, et al: Differences in cerebral blood flow between alpha-stat and pH-stat management are eliminated during period of decreased systemic flow and pressure: A study during cardiopulmonary bypass in rabbits, *Anesthesiology* 74:1096–1102, 1991.

184. Henriksen L, Hjelms E, Lindeburgh T: Brain hyperperfusion during cardiac operations: Cerebral blood flow measured in man by intra-arterial injection of xenon 133. Evidence suggestive of intraoperative microembolism, *J Thorac Cardiovasc Surg* 86:202–208, 1983.

185. Stephan H, Sonntag H, Lange H, Rieke H: Cerebral effects of anaesthesia and hypothermia, *Anaesthesia* 44:310–316, 1989.

186. Hoffman WE, Edelman G, Kochs E, et al: Cerebral autoregulation in awake versus isoflurane-anesthetized rats, *Anesth Analg* 73:753–757, 1991.

187. McPherson RW, Brian JE, Traystman RJ: Cerebrovascular responsiveness to carbon dioxide in dogs with 1.4% and 2.8% isoflurane, *Anesthesiology* 70:843–850, 1989.

188. Ostapkovich ND, Baker KZ, Fogarty-Mack P, et al: Cerebral blood flow and CO_2 reactivity is similar during remifentanil/N_2O and fentanyl N_2O anesthesia, *Anesthesiology* 89:358–363, 1998.

189. Koenig HM, Pelligrino DA, Albrecht RF: Halothane vasodilation and nitric oxide in rat pial vessels, *J Neurosurg Anesth* 5:264–271, 1993.

190. Kaisti KK, Langsjo JW, Aalto S, et al: Effects of sevoflurane, propofol, and adjunct nitrous oxide on regional cerebral blood flow, oxygen consumption, and blood volume in humans, *Anesthesiology* 99:603–613, 2003.

191. Wang M, Joshi S, Emerson RG: Comparison of intracarotid and intravenous propofol for electrocerebral silence in rabbits, *Anesthesiology* 99:904–910, 2003.

192. Stange K, Lagerkranser M, Sollevi A: Nitroprusside-induced hypotension and cerebrovascular autoregulation in the anesthetized pig, *Anesth Analg* 73:745–752, 1991.

193. Albrecht RF, Miletich DJ, Madala LR: Normalization of cerebral blood flow during prolonged halothane anesthesia, *Anesthesiology* 58:26–31, 1983.

194. Brian JE Jr, Traystman RJ, McPherson RW: Changes in cerebral blood flow over time during isoflurane anesthesia in dogs, *J Neurosurg Anesth* 2:122–130, 1990.

195. Turner DM, Kassell NF, Sasaki T, et al: Time-dependent changes in cerebral and cardiovascular parameters in isoflurane-nitrous oxide-anesthetized dogs, *Neurosurgery* 14:135–141, 1984.

196. Warner DS, Turner DM, Kassell NF: Time-dependent effects of prolonged hypercapnia on cerebrovascular parameters in dogs: Acid-base chemistry, *Stroke* 18:142–149, 1987.

197. McPherson R, Levitt R: Effect of time and dose on scalp-recorded somatosensory evoked potentials wave augmentation by etomidate, *J Neurosurg Anesthesiol* 1:142–149, 1989.

198. Rogers AT, Stump DA, Gravlee GP, et al: Response of cerebral blood flow to phenylephrine infusion during hypothermic cardiopulmonary bypass: Influence of $PaCO_2$ management, *Anesthesiology* 69:547–551, 1988.

199. Bissonnette B, Leon JE: Cerebrovascular stability during isoflurane anaesthesia in children, *Can J Anaesthesia* 39:128–134, 1992.

200. Roald OK, Forsman M, Steen PA: The effects of prolonged isoflurane anaesthesia on cerebral blood flow and metabolism in the dog, *Acta Anaesthesiol Scand* 33:210–213, 1989.

201. Stone JG, Young WL, Smith CR, et al: Do temperatures recorded at standard monitoring sites reflect actual brain temperature during deep hypothermia [abstract]? *Anesthesiology* 75:A483, 1991.

202. Edvinsson L, Owman C, Siesjo B: Physiological role of cerebrovascular sympathetic nerves in the autoregulation of cerebral blood flow, *Brain Res* 117:519–523, 1976.

203. Beausang-Linder M, Bill A: Cerebral circulation in acute arterial hypertension: Protective effects of sympathetic nervous activity, *Acta Physiol Scand* 111:193–199, 1981.

204. Skinhoj E: The sympathetic nervous system and the regulation of cerebral blood flow, *Eur Neurol* 6:190–192, 1971/72.

205. Hernandez MJ, Raichle ME, Stone HL: The role of the sympathetic nervous system in cerebral blood flow autoregulation, *Eur Neurol* 6:175–179, 1971/72.

206. D'Alecy LG: Relation between sympathetic cerebral vasoconstriction and CSF pressure, *Eur Neurol* 6:180–184, 1971/72.

207. Heistad DD: Summary of symposium on cerebral blood flow: Effect of nerves and neurotransmitters: Cardiovascular Center, University of Iowa, Iowa City, Iowa, June 16-18, 1981. *J Cereb Blood Flow Metab* 1981;1:447–450

208. Beausang-Linder M: Effects of sympathetic stimulation on cerebral and ocular blood flow, *Acta Physiol Scand* 114:217–224, 1982.

209. Busija DW, Heistad DD: Effects of activation of sympathetic nerves on cerebral blood flow during hypercapnia in cats and rabbits, *J Physiol* 347:195, 1974.

210. Puig M, Kirpekar SM: Inhibitory effect of low pH on norepinephrine release, *J Pharmacol Exp Ther* 176:134–138, 1967.

211. Verhaeghe RH, Lorenz RR, McGrath MA, et al: Metabolic modulation of neurotransmitter release—adenosine, adenine nucleotides, potassium, hyperosmolarity, and hydrogen ion, *Fed Proc* 37:208–211, 1978.

212. Faraci FM, Mayhan WG, Werber AH, Heistad DD: Cerebral circulation: Effects of sympathetic nerves and protective mechanisms during hypertension, *Circ Res* 61:II-102–II-106, 1987.

213. Fitch W, Ferguson GG, Sengupta D, et al: Autoregulation of cerebral blood flow during controlled hypotension in baboons, *J Neurol Neurosurg Psychiatry* 39:1014–1022, 1976.

214. Kano M, Moskowitz MA, Yokota M: Parasympathetic denervation of rat pial vessels significantly increases infarction volume following middle cerebral artery occlusion, *J Cereb Blood Flow Metab* 11:628–637, 1991.

215. Moskowitz MA, Sakas DE, Wei EP, et al: Postocclusive cerebral hyperemia is markedly attenuated by chronic trigeminal ganglionectomy, *Am J Physiol* 257:H1736–H1739, 1989.

216. Branston NM, Umemura A, Koshy A: Contribution of cerebrovascular parasympathetic and sensory innervation to the short-term control of blood flow in rat cerebral cortex, *J Cereb Blood Flow Metab* 15:525–531, 1995.

217. Lassen NA: Cerebral blood flow and oxygen consumption in man, *Physiol Rev* 39:183–238, 1959.

218. Strandgaard S, Olesen J, Skinhoj E, Lassen NA: Autoregulation of brain circulation in severe arterial hypertension, *Br Med J* 1:507–510, 1973.

219. Nordborg C, Johansson BB: Morphometric study on cerebral vessels in spontaneously hypertensive rats, *Stroke* 11:266–270, 1980.

220. Sadoshima S, Fujii K, Yao H, et al: Regional cerebral blood flow auto-regulation in normotensive and spontaneously hypertensive rats: Effects of sympathetic denervation, *Stroke* 17:981–984, 1986.

221. Tominaga S, Strandgaard S, Uemura K, et al: Cerebrovascular CO_2 reactivity in normotensive and hypertensive man, *Stroke* 7:507–510, 1976.

222. Forster A, Van Horn K, Marshall LF, Shapiro HM: Anesthetic effects on blood-brain barrier function during acute arterial hypertension, *Anesthesiology* 49:26–30, 1978.

223. Hoffman WE, Miletich DJ, Albrecht RF, et al: Cerebrovascular response to hypotension in hypertensive rats: Effect of antihypertensive therapy, *Anesthesiology* 58:326–332, 1983.

224. Vorstrup S, Barry DI, Jarden JO, et al: Chronic antihypertensive treatment in the rat reverses hypertension-induced changes in cerebral blood flow autoregulation, *Stroke* 15:312–318, 1984.

225. Fujishima M, Ibayashi S, Fujii K, et al: Effects of long-term antihypertensive treatment on cerebral, thalamic and cerebellar blood flow in spontaneously hypertensive rats (SHR), *Stroke* 17:985–988, 1986.

226. Toyoda K, Fujii K, Ibayashi S, et al: Attenuation and recovery of brain stem autoregulation in spontaneously hypertensive rats, *J Cereb Blood Flow Metab* 18:305–310, 1998.

227. Ooboshi H, Sadoshima S, Fujii K, et al: Acute effects of antihypertensive agents on cerebral blood flow in hypertensive rats, *Eur J Pharmacol* 179:253–261, 1990.

228. Hoffman WE, Albrecht RF, Miletich DJ: The influence of aging and hypertension on cerebral autoregulation, *Brain Res* 214:196–199, 1981.

229. Barry DI, Paulson OB, Jarden JO, et al: Effects of captopril on cerebral blood flow in normotensive and hypertensive rats, *Am J Med* 76:79–85, 1984.

230. Hoffman WE, Albrecht RF, Miletich DJ: Nitroglycerin induced hypotension will maintain CBF in hypertensive rats, *Stroke* 13:225–228, 1982.

231. Pearson RM, Griffith DN, Woollard M, et al: Comparison of effects on cerebral blood flow of rapid reduction in systemic arterial pressure by diazoxide and labetalol in hypertensive patients: Preliminary findings, *Br J Clin Pharmacol* 8(Suppl):195S–198S, 1979.

232. Barry DI, Jarden JO, Paulson OB, et al: Cerebrovascular aspects of converting-enzyme inhibition. I: Effects of intravenous captopril in spontaneously hypertensive and normotensive rats, *J Hypertens* 2: 589–597, 1984.

233. Michenfelder JD, Sundt TM, Fode N, Sharbrough FW: Isoflurane when compared to enflurane and halothane decreases the frequency of cerebral ischemia during carotid endarterectomy, *Anesthesiology* 67:336–340, 1987.

234. Naritomi H, Meyer JS, Sakai F, et al: Effects of advancing age on regional cerebral blood flow: Studies in normal subjects and subjects with risk factors for atherothrombotic stroke, *Arch Neurol* 36:410–416, 1979.

235. Sullivan HG, Kingsbury TB 4th, Morgan ME, et al: The rCBF response to Diamox in normal subjects and cerebrovascular disease patients, *J Neurosurg* 67:525–534, 1987.

236. Yamaguchi F, Meyer JS, Sakai F, Yamamoto M: Normal human aging and cerebral vasoconstrictive responses to hypocapnia, *J Neurol Sci* 44:87–94, 1979.

237. Baughman VL, Hoffman WE, Miletich DJ, Albrecht RF: Effects of phenobarbital on cerebral blood flow and metabolism in young and aged rats, *Anesthesiology* 65:500–505, 1986.

238. Harada J, Takaku A, Endo S, et al: Differences in critical cerebral blood flow with age in swine, *J Neurosurg* 75:103–107, 1991.

239. Nishiyama T, Sugai N, Hanaoka K: Cerebrovascular CO_2 reactivity in elderly and younger adult patients during sevoflurane anaesthesia, *Can J Anaesth* 44:160–164, 1997.

240. Yamamoto M, Meyer JS, Sakai F, Yamaguchi F: Aging and cerebral vasodilator responses to hypercarbia: Responses in normal aging and in persons with risk factors for stroke, *Arch Neurol* 37:489–496, 1980.

241. Toyoda K, Fujii K, Takata Y, et al: Effect of aging on regulation of brain stem circulation during hypotension, *J Cereb Blood Flow Metab* 17:680–685, 1997.

242. Lartaud I, Makki T, Bray-des-Boscs L, et al: Effect of chronic ANG I-converting enzyme inhibition on aging processes. IV: Cerebral blood flow regulation, *Am J Physiol* 267:R687–R694, 1994.

243. Gerhard M, Roddy MA, Creager SJ, Creager MA: Aging progressively impairs endothelium-dependent vasodilation in forearm resistance vessels of humans, *Hypertension* 27:849–853, 1996.

244. Hajdu MA, McElmurry RT, Heistad DD, Baumbach GL: Effects of aging on cerebral vascular responses to serotonin in rats, *Am J Physiol* 264:H2136–H2140, 1993.

245. Itoh M, Hatazawa J, Miyazawa H, et al: Stability of cerebral blood flow and oxygen metabolism during normal aging, *Gerontology* 36:43–48, 1990.

246. Shiokawa O, Sadoshima S, Kusuda K, et al: Cerebral and cerebellar blood flow autoregulations in acutely induced cerebral ischemia in spontaneously hypertensive rats: Transtentorial remote effect, *Stroke* 17:1309–1313, 1986.

247. Young WL, Prohovnik I, Ornstein E, et al: The effect of arteriovenous malformation resection on cerebrovascular reactivity to carbon dioxide, *Neurosurgery* 27:257–267, 1990.

248. Andrews RJ: Transhemispheric diaschisis: A review and comment, *Stroke* 22:943–949, 1991.

249. Edelman RR, Mattle HP, Atkinson DJ, et al: Cerebral blood flow: Assessment with dynamic contrast-enhanced T2*-weighted MR imaging at 1.5 T., *Radiology* 176:211–220, 1990.

250. Cold G, Christensen M, Schmidt K: Effect of two levels of induced hypocapnia on cerebral autoregulation in the acute phase of head injury coma, *Acta Anaesth Scand* 25:397–401, 1981.

251. Choi DW: Cerebral hypoxia: Some new approaches and unanswered questions, *J Neurosci* 10:2493–2501, 1990.

252. Branston NM, Hope DT, Symon L: Barbiturates in focal ischemia of primate cortex: Effects on blood flow distribution, evoked potential and extracellular potassium, *Stroke* 10:647–653, 1979.

253. Drummond JC, Oh Y-S, Cole DJ, Shapiro HM: Phenylephrine-induced hypertension reduces ischemia following middle cerebral artery occlusion in rats, *Stroke* 20:1538–1544, 1989.

254. Schroeder T, Sillesen H, Engell HC: Hemodynamic effect of carotid endarterectomy, *Stroke* 18:204–209, 1987.

255. Spetzler RF, Wilson CB, Weinstein P, et al: Normal perfusion pressure breakthrough theory, *Clin Neurosurg* 25:651–672, 1978.

256. Nornes H, Wikeby P: Cerebral arterial blood flow and aneurysm surgery. Part 1: Local arterial flow dynamics, *J Neurosurg* 47:810–818, 1977.

257. Halbach V, Higashida RT, Hieshima G, Norman D: Normal perfusion pressure breakthrough occurring during treatment of carotid and vertebral fistulas, *Am J Neuroradiol* 8:751–756, 1987.

258. Irikura K, Morii S, Miyasaka Y, et al: Impaired autoregulation in an experimental model of chronic cerebral hypoperfusion in rats, *Stroke* 27:1399–1404, 1996.

259. Young WL, Kader A, Prohovnik I, et al: Pressure autoregulation is intact after arteriovenous malformation resection, *Neurosurgery* 32:491–497, 1993.

260. Young WL, Kader A, Ornstein E, et al: The Columbia University Arteriovenous Malformation Study Project Cerebral hyperemia after arteriovenous malformation resection is related to "breakthrough" complications but not to feeding artery pressure, *Neurosurgery* 38:1085–1093, 1996.

261. Joshi S, Young WL: Arteriovenous malformation. In Atlee JL, editor: *Complications in Anesthesia*, Philadelphia, 1999, WB Saunders, pp 744–747.

262. Halsey JH Jr, Conger KA, Garcia JH, Sarvary E: The contribution of reoxygenation to ischemic brain damage, *J Cereb Blood Flow Metab* 11:994–1000, 1991.

263. Pulsinelli WA, Levy DE, Duffy TE: Regional cerebral blood flow and glucose metabolism following transient forebrain ischemia, *Ann Neurol* 11:499–509, 1982.

264. Michenfelder JD, Milde JH, Katusic ZS: Postischemic canine cerebral blood flow is coupled to cerebral metabolic rate, *J Cereb Blood Flow Metab* 11:611–616, 1991.

265. Connolly E Jr, Winfree CJ, Springer TA, et al: Cerebral protection in homozygous null ICAM-1 mice after middle cerebral artery occlusion: Role of neutrophil adhesion in the pathogenesis of stroke, *J Clin Invest* 97:209–216, 1996.

266. Cockroft KM, Meistrell M 3rd, Zimmerman GA, et al: Cerebroprotective effects of aminoguanidine in a rodent model of stroke, *Stroke* 27:1393–1398, 1996.

267. Dogan A, Rao AM, Baskaya MK, et al: Effects of ifenprodil, a polyamine site NMDA receptor antagonist, on reperfusion injury after transient focal cerebral ischemia, *J Neurosurg* 87:921–926, 1997.

268. Prohovnik I, Knudsen E, Risberg J: Accuracy of models and algorithms for determination of fast-compartment flow by noninvasive ^{133}Xe clearance. In Magistretti PL, editor: *Functional Radionuclide Imaging of the Brain*, New York, 1983, Raven Press, pp 87–115.

269. Kazumata K, Tanaka N, Ishikawa T, et al: Dissociation of vasoreactivity to acetazolamide and hypercapnia: Comparative study in patients with chronic occlusive major cerebral artery disease, *Stroke* 27:2052–2058, 1996.

270. Powers WJ, Raichle ME: Positron emission tomography and its application to the study of cerebrovascular disease in man, *Stroke* 16:361–376, 1985.

271. Pavlakis S, Bello J, Prohovnik I, et al: Brain infarction in sickle cell anemia: Magnetic resonance imaging correlates, *Ann Neurol* 23:125–130, 1988.

272. Prohovnik I, Knudsen E, Risberg J: Theoretical evaluation and simulation test of the initial slope index for noninvasive rCBF. In Hartmann A, Hoyer S, editors: *Cerebral Blood Flow and Metabolism Measurement*, Berlin, 1985, Springer-Verlag, pp 56–60.

273. Wade JPH, Hachinski VC: Cerebral steal: Robbery or maldistribution? In Wood JH, editor: *Cerebral Blood Flow Physiologic and Clinical Aspects*, New York, 1987, McGraw-Hill, pp 467–480.

274. Boysen G, Engell HC, Henriksen H: The effect of induced hypertension on internal carotid artery pressure and regional cerebral blood flow during temporary carotid clamping for endarterectomy, *Neurology* 22:1133–1144, 1972.

275. Mast H, Mohr JP, Osipov A, et al: "Steal" is an unestablished mechanism for the clinical presentation of cerebral arteriovenous malformations, *Stroke* 26:1215–1220, 1995.

276. Solomon RA, Fink ME, Lennihan L: Prophylactic volume expansion therapy for the prevention of delayed cerebral ischemia after early aneurysm surgery, *Arch Neurol* 45:325–332, 1988.

277. Grubb RL, Raichle ME, Eichling JO, Gado MH: Effects of subarachnoid hemorrhage on cerebral blood volume, blood flow, and oxygen utilization in humans, *J Neurosurg* 46:446–453, 1977.

278. Duong H, Hacein-Bey L, Vang MC, et al: Management of cerebral arterial occlusion during endovascular treatment of cerebrovascular disease, *Problems in Anesthesia: Controversies in Neuroanesthesia* 9:99–111, 1997.

279. Young WL, Solomon RA, Pedley TA, et al: Direct cortical EEG monitoring during temporary vascular occlusion for cerebral aneurysm surgery, *Anesthesiology* 71:794–799, 1989.

280. Miller JA, Dacey RG Jr, Diringer MN: Safety of hypertensive hypervolemic therapy with phenylephrine in the treatment of delayed ischemic deficits after subarachnoid hemorrhage, *Stroke* 26:2260–2266, 1995.

281. Ehrenfeld WK, Hamilton FN, Larson CP Jr, et al: Effect of CO$_2$ and systemic hypertension on downstream cerebral arterial pressure during carotid endarterectomy, *Surgery* 67:87–96, 1970.

282. Fourcade HE, Larson CP Jr, Ehrenfield WK, et al: The effects of CO$_2$ and systemic hypertension on cerebral perfusion pressure during carotid endarterectomy, *Anesthesiology* 33:383–390, 1970.

283. McKay RD, Sundt TM, Michenfelder JD, et al: Internal carotid artery stump pressure and cerebral blood flow during carotid endarterectomy: Modification by halothane, enflurane, and Innovar, *Anesthesiology* 45:390–399, 1976.

284. Archie JP: Jr: Technique and clinical results of carotid stump backpressure to determine selective shunting during carotid endarterectomy, *J Vasc Surg* 13:319–327, 1991.

285. Batjer HH, Frankfurt AI, Purdy PD, et al: Use of etomidate, temporary arterial occlusion, and intraoperative angiography in surgical treatment of large and giant cerebral aneurysms, *J Neurosurg* 68:234–240, 1988.

286. Buckland MR, Batjer HH, Giesecke AH: Anesthesia for cerebral aneurysm surgery: Use of induced hypertension in patients with symptomatic vasospasm, *Anesthesiology* 69:116–119, 1988.

287. Drummond JC: Deliberate hypotension for intracranial aneurysm surgery: Changing practices, *Can J Anaesth* 38, 1991, pp 935–936.

288. Kassell NF, Peerless SJ, Durward QJ, et al: Treatment of ischemic deficits from vasospasm with intravascular volume expansion and induced arterial hypertension, *Neurosurgery* 11:337–343, 1982.

289. Awad IA, Carter LP, Spetzler RF, et al: Clinical vasospasm after subarachnoid hemorrhage: Response to hypervolemic hemodilution and arterial hypertension, *Stroke* 18:365–372, 1987.

290. Muizelaar JP, Becker D: Induced hypertension for the treatment of cerebral ischemia after subarachnoid hemorrhage, *Surg Neurol* 25:317–325, 1986.

291. Joshi S, Ornstein E, Young WL: Augmenting cerebral perfusion pressure: When is enough too much? *J Neurosurg Anesthesiol* 8:249–253, 1996.

292. Warner DS, Hansen TD, Vust L, Todd MM: Distribution of cerebral blood flow during deep halothane vs pentobarbital anesthesia in rats with middle cerebral artery occlusion, *J Neurosurg Anesth* 1:219–226, 1989.

293. Soloway M, Moriarty G, Fraser JG, White RJ: Effect of delayed hyperventilation on experimental cerebral infarction, *Neurology* 21:479–485, 1971.

294. Soloway M, Nadel W, Albin MS, White RJ: The effect of hyperventilation on subsequent cerebral infarction, *Anesthesiology* 29:975–980, 1968.

295. Drummond JC, Ruta TS, Cole DJ, et al: The effect of hypocapnia on cerebral blood flow distribution during middle cerebral artery occlusion in the rat, *J Neurosurg Anesth* 1:163–164, 1989.

296. Artru AA, Merriman HG: Hypocapnia added to hypertension to reverse EEG changes during carotid endarterectomy, *Anesthesiology* 70:1016–1018, 1989.

297. Michenfelder JD, Sundt TM Jr: The effect of Paco$_2$ on the metabolism of ischemic brain in squirrel monkeys, *Anesthesiology* 38:445–453, 1973.

298. Baker WH, Rodman JA, Barnes RW, Hoyt JL: An evaluation of hypocarbia and hypercarbia during carotid endarterectomy, *Stroke* 7:451–454, 1976.

299. Christensen MS, Brodersen P, Olesen J, Paulson OB: Cerebral apoplexy (stroke) treated with or without prolonged artificial hyperventilation. 2: Cerebrospinal fluid acid-base balance and intracranial pressure, *Stroke* 4:620–631, 1973.

300. Mohr JP, Petty GW, Sacco RL: Recent advances in cerebrovascular disease, *Curr Neurol* 9:77–108, 1989.

301. Pistolese GR, Faraglia V, Agnoli A, et al: Cerebral hemispheric "countersteal" phenomenon during hyperventilation in cerebrovascular diseases, *Stroke* 3:456–461, 1972.

302. Boysen G, Ladegaard-Pedersen HJ, Henriksen H, et al: The effects of PaCO$_2$ on regional cerebral blood flow and internal carotid arterial pressure during carotid clamping, *Anesthesiology* 35:286–300, 1971.

303. Ochiai C, Asano T, Takakura K, et al: Mechanisms of cerebral protection by pentobarbital and nizofenone correlated with the course of local cerebral blood flow changes, *Stroke* 13:788–795, 1982.

304. Young WL, Prohovnik I, Correll JW, et al: Cerebral blood flow and metabolism in patients undergoing anesthesia for carotid endarterectomy: A comparison of isoflurane, halothane, and fentanyl, *Anesth Analg* 68:712–717, 1989.

305. Oskouian RJ Jr, Martin NA, Lee JH, et al: Multimodal quantitation of the effects of endovascular therapy for vasospasm on cerebral blood flow, transcranial Doppler ultrasonographic velocities, and cerebral artery diameters, *Neurosurgery* 51:41–43, 2002.

306. Kassell NF, Helm G, Simmons N, et al: Treatment of cerebral vasospasm with intra-arterial papaverine, *J Neurosurg* 77:848–852, 1992.

307. Joshi S, Emala CW, Pile-Spellman J: Intra-arterial drug delivery: A concise review, *J Neurosurg Anesthesiol* 19:111–119, 2007.

308. Joshi S, Meyers PM, Ornstein E: Intracarotid delivery of drugs: The potential and the pitfalls, *Anesthesiology* 109:543–564, 2008.

309. Feng L, Fitzsimmons BF, Young WL, et al: Intraarterially administered verapamil as adjunct therapy for cerebral vasospasm: Safety and 2-year experience, *AJNR Am J Neuroradiol* 23:1284–1290, 2002.

310. Badjatia N, Topcuoglu MA, Pryor JC, Rabinov JD, et al: Preliminary experience with intra-arterial nicardipine as a treatment for cerebral vasospasm, *AJNR Am J Neuroradiol* 25:819–826, 2004.

311. Cross DT III, Moran CJ, Angtuaco EE, et al: Intracranial pressure monitoring during intraarterial papaverine infusion for cerebral vasospasm, *AJNR Am J Neuroradiol* 19:1319–1323, 1998.

312. Joshi S, Ornstein E, Bruce JN: Targeting the brain: Rationalizing the novel methods of drug delivery to the central nervous system *J Neurocrit Care* 6:200–212, 2007.

313. Joshi S, Wang M, Etu JJ, et al: Cerebral blood flow affects dose requirements of intracarotid propofol for electrocerebral silence, *Anesthesiology* 104:290–298, 2006.

314. Joshi S, Wang M, Etu JJ, Pile-Spellman J: Bolus configuration affects dose requirements of intracarotid propofol for electroencephalographic silence, *Anesth Analg* 102:1816–1822, 2006.

315. Joshi S, Wang M, Etu JJ, et al: Transient cerebral hypoperfusion enhances intraarterial carmustine deposition into brain tissue, *J Neurooncol* 86:123–132, 2008.

316. Joshi S, Wang M, Etu JJ, Pile-Spellman J: Reducing cerebral blood flow increases the duration of electroencephalographic silence by intracarotid thiopental, *Anesth Analg* 101:851–858, 2005.

317. Dedrick RL: Arterial drug infusion: Pharmacokinetic problems and pitfalls, *J Natl Cancer Inst* 80:84–89, 1988.

318. Dedrick RL: Interspecies scaling of regional drug delivery, *J Pharm Sci* 75:1047–1052, 1986.

319. Cloughesy TF, Gobin YP, Black KL, et al: Intra-arterial carboplatin chemotherapy for brain tumors: A dose escalation study based on cerebral blood flow, *J Neurooncol* 35:121–131, 1997.

320. Gobin YP, Cloughesy TF, Chow KL, et al: Intraarterial chemotherapy for brain tumors by using a spatial dose fractionation algorithm and pulsatile delivery, *Radiology* 218:724–732, 2001.

321. Elkassabany NM, Bhatia J, Deogaonkar A, et al: Perioperative complications of blood brain barrier disruption under general anesthesia: A retrospective review, *J Neurosurg Anesthesiol* 20:45–48, 2008.

322. Jones DR, Hall SD, Jackson EK, et al: Brain uptake of benzodiazepines: Effects of lipophilicity and plasma protein binding, *J Pharmacol Exp Ther* 245:816–822, 1988.

323. Mourant JR, Johnson TM, Los G, Bigio IJ: Non-invasive measurement of chemotherapy drug concentrations in tissue: preliminary demonstrations of in vivo measurements, *Physics Med Biol* 44:1397–1417, 1999.

324. Kanick SC, Eiseman JL, Joseph E, et al: Noninvasive and nondestructive optical spectroscopic measurement of motexafin gadolinium in mouse tissues: Comparison to high-performance liquid chromatography, *J Photochem Photobiol B* 88:90–104, 2007.

325. Reif R, Wang M, Joshi S, et al: Optical method for real-time monitoring of drug concentrations facilitates the development of novel methods for drug delivery to brain tissue, *J Biomed Opt* :12, 2007:034036.

326. Neuwelt E, Abbott NJ, Abrey L, et al: Strategies to advance translational research into brain barriers, *Lancet Neurol* 7:84–96, 2008.

327. Bellavance MA, Blanchette M, Fortin D: Recent advances in blood-brain barrier disruption as a CNS delivery strategy, *AAPS J* 10:166–177, 2008.

328. Wang M, Etu J, Joshi S: Enhanced disruption of the blood brain barrier by intracarotid mannitol injection during transient cerebral hypoperfusion in rabbits, *J Neurosurg Anesthesiol* 19:249–256, 2007.

329. Kety SS, Schmidt CF: The determination of cerebral blood flow in man by the use of nitrous oxide in low concentrations, *Am J Physiol* 14:353–366, 1945.

330. Madsen JB, Cold GE, Hansen ES, Bardrum B: The effect of isoflurane on cerebral blood flow and metabolism in humans during craniotomy for small supratentorial cerebral tumors, *Anesthesiology* 66:332–336, 1987.

331. Sutton LN, McLaughlin AC, Dante S, et al: Cerebral venous oxygen content as a measure of brain energy metabolism with increased intracranial pressure and hyperventilation, *J Neurosurg* 73:927–932, 1990.

332. Cruz J, Miner ME, Allen SJ, et al: Continuous monitoring of cerebral oxygenation in acute brain injury: Assessment of cerebral hemodynamic reserve, *Neurosurgery* 29:743–749, 1990.

333. Melot C, Berre J, Moraine J-J, Kahn RJ: Estimation of cerebral blood flow at bedside by continuous jugular thermodilution, *J Cereb Blood Flow Metab* 16:1263–1270, 1996.

334. Lassen NA, Ingvar DH: The blood flow of the cerebral cortex determined by radioactive krypton85, *Experientia* 17:42–43, 1961.

335. Obrist WD, Wilkinson WE: Regional cerebral blood flow measurement in humans by xenon-133 clearance, *Cerebrovasc Brain Metab Rev* 2:283–327, 1990.

336. Sundt TM, Sharbrough FW, Piepgras DG, et al: Correlation of cerebral flood flow and electroencephalographic changes during carotid endarterectomy, *Mayo Clinic Proc* 56:533–543, 1981.

337. Chen RYZ, Fan F-C, Kim S, et al: Tissue-blood partition coefficient for xenon: Temperature and hematocrit dependence, *J Appl Physiol* 49:178–183, 1980.

338. Obrist WD, Thompson HK Jr, Wang HS, Wilkinson WE: Regional cerebral blood flow estimated by 133xenon inhalation, *Stroke* 6:245–256, 1975.

339. Risberg J, Ali Z, Wilson EM, et al: Regional cerebral blood flow by 133xenon inhalation, *Stroke* 6:142–147, 1975.

340. Joshi S, Young WL, Pile-Spellman J, et al: The feasibility of intracarotid adenosine for the manipulation of human cerebrovascular resistance, *Anesth Analg* 87:1291–1298, 1998.

341. Prohovnik I: Data quality, integrity and interpretation. In Knezevic S, Maximilian VA, Mubrin Z, et al: *Handbook of Regional Cerebral Blood Flow*, Hillsdale, NJ, 1988, Lawrence Erlbaum Associates, pp 51–78.

342. Wyper DJ, Lennox GA, Rowan JO: Two minute slope inhalation technique for cerebral blood flow measurement in man. 2: Clinical appraisal, *J Neurol Neurosurg Psych* 39:147–151, 1976.

343. Young WL, Prohovnik I, Ornstein E, et al: Rapid monitoring of intraoperative cerebral blood flow using 133Xe, *J Cereb Blood Flow Metab* 8:691–696, 1988.

344. Hansen M, Jakobsen M, Enevoldsen E, Egede F: Problems in cerebral blood flow calculation using xenon-133 in patients with pulmonary diseases, *Stroke* 21:745–750, 1990.

345. Young WL, Prohovnik I, Schroeder T, et al: Intraoperative 133Xe cerebral blood flow measurements by intravenous *versus* intracarotid methods, *Anesthesiology* 73:637–643, 1990.

346. Branston NM, Strong AJ, Symon L: Extracellular potassium activity, evoked potential and tissue blood flow: Relationships during progressive ischaemia in baboon cerebral cortex, *J Neurol Sci* 32:305–321, 1977.

347. Young W: H2 clearance measurement of blood flow: A review of technique and polarographic principles, *Stroke* 11:552–564, 1980.

348. Fukuda O, Endo S, Kuwayama N, et al: The characteristics of laser-Doppler flowmetry for the measurement of regional cerebral blood flow, *Neurosurgery* 36:358–364, 1995.

349. Gadian DG, Allen K, van Bruggen N, et al: Applications of NMR spectroscopy to the study of experimental stroke in vivo, *Stroke* 24(Suppl I): I-57–I-59, 1993.

350. Tomida S, Wagner HG, Klatzo I, Nowak TS Jr: Effect of acute electrode placement on regional CBF in the gerbil: A comparison of blood flow measured by hydrogen clearance, [3H]nicotine, and [14C]iodoantipyrine techniques, *J Cereb Blood Flow Metab* 9:79–86, 1989.

351. Kety SS: The measurement of cerebral blood flow by means of inert diffusible tracers, *Keio J Med* 43:9–14, 1994.

352. Sakurada O, Kennedy C, Jehle J, et al: Measurement of local cerebral blood flow with iodo[14C]antipyrine, *Am J Physiol* 234:H59–H66, 1978.

353. Patlak CS, Blasberg RG, Fenstermacher JD: An evaluation of errors in the determination of blood flow by the indicator fractionation and tissue equilibration (Kety) methods, *J Cereb Blood Flow Metab* 4:47–60, 1984.

354. Young WL, Josovitz K, Morales O, Chien S: The effect of nimodipine on post-ischemic cerebral glucose utilization and blood flow in the rat, *Anesthesiology* 67:54–59, 1987.

355. Van Uitert RL, Sage JI, Levy DE, Duffy TE: Comparison of radio-labeled butanol and iodoantipyrine as cerebral blood flow markers, *Brain Res* 222:365–372, 1981.

356. Gur D, Yonas H, Good WF: Local cerebral blood flow by xenon-enhanced CT: Current status, potential improvements, and future directions, *Cerebrovasc Brain Metab Rev* 1:68–86, 1989.

357. Moossy J, Martinez J, Hanin I, et al: Thalamic and subcortical gliosis with dementia, *Arch Neurol* 44:510–513, 1987.

358. Good WF, Gur D, Yonas H, Herron JM: Errors in cerebral blood flow determinations by xenon-enhanced computed tomography due to estimation of arterial xenon concentrations, *Med Phys* 14:377–381, 1987.

359. Gur D, Yonas H, Jackson DL, et al: Measurements of cerebral blood flow during xenon inhalation as measured by the microspheres method, *Stroke* 16:871–874, 1985.

360. Darby JM, Nemoto EM, Yonas H, John M: Stable xenon does not increase intracranial pressure in primates with freeze-injury-induced intracranial hypertension, *J Cereb Blood Flow Metab* 11:522–526, 1991.

361. Tarr RW, Johnson DW, Rutigliano M, et al: Use of acetazolamide-challenge xenon CT in the assessment of cerebral blood flow dynamics in patients with arteriovenous malformations, *Am J Neuroradiol* 11:441–448, 1990.

362. Yonas H, Darby JM, Marks EC, et al: CBF measured by Xe-CT: Approach to analysis and normal values, *J Cereb Blood Flow Metab* 11:716–725, 1991.

363. Muizelaar JP, Fatouros PP, Schroder ML: A new method for quantitative regional cerebral blood volume measurements using computed tomography, *Stroke* 28:1998–2005, 1997.

364. Hamberg LM, Hunter GJ, Halpern EF, et al: Quantitative high-resolution measurement of cerebrovascular physiology with slip-ring CT, *Am J Neuroradiol* 17:639–650, 1996.

365. Frost JJ, Wagner HN Jr: *Quantitative Imaging: Neuroreceptors, Neurotransmitters, and Enzymes*, New York, 1990, Raven Press.

366. Enblad P, Valtysson J, Andersson J, et al: Simultaneous intracerebral microdialysis and positron emission tomography in the detection of ischemia in patients with subarachnoid hemorrhage, *J Cereb Blood Flow Metab* 16:637–644, 1996.

367. Ingvar M, Eriksson L, Greitz T, et al: Methodological aspects of brain activation studies: Cerebral blood flow determined with [15O] butanol and positron emission tomography, *J Cereb Blood Flow Metab* 14: 628–638, 1994.

368. Heiss W-D, Graf R, Fujita T, et al: Early detection of irreversibly damaged ischemic tissue by flumazenil positron emission tomography in cats, *Stroke* 28:2045–2052, 1997.

369. Alkire MT, Haier RJ, Shah NK, Anderson CT: Positron emission tomography study of regional cerebral metabolism in humans during isoflurane anesthesia, *Anesthesiology* 86:549–557, 1997.

370. Archer DP, Labrecque P, Tyler JL, et al: Measurement of cerebral blood flow and volume with positron emission tomography during isoflurane administration in the hypocapnic baboon, *Anesthesiology* 72:1031–1037, 1990.

371. Firestone LL, Gyulai F, Mintun M, et al: Human brain activity response to fentanyl imaged by positron emission tomography, *Anesth Analg* 82:1247–1251, 1996.

372. Alkire M, Haier RJ, Barker SJ, et al: Cerebral metabolism during propofol anesthesia in humans studied with positron emission tomography, *Anesthesiology* 82:393–403, 1995.

373. Brooks DJ, Frackowiak RSJ, Lammertsma AA: A comparison between regional cerebral blood flow measurements obtained in human subjects using 11C-methylalbumin microspheres, the C15O2 steady-state method, and positron emission tomography, *Acta Neurol Scand* 73:415–422, 1986.

374. Van Heertum RL, Tikofsky RS: *Advances in Cerebral SPECT Imaging: An Atlas and Guideline for Practitioners*, Philadelphia, Lea & Febiger, 1989.

375. Lassen NA, Blasberg RG: Technetium-99m-*d, l*-HM-PAO, The development of a new class of ^{99m}Tc-labeled tracers: An overview, *J Cereb Blood Flow Metab* 8:S1–S3, 1988.

376. Sperling B, Lassen NA: Hyperfixation of HMPAO in subacute ischemic stroke leading to spuriously high estimates of cerebral blood flow by SPECT, *Stroke* 24:193–194, 1993.

377. Devous Sr MD, Payne JK, Lowe JL, Leroy RF: Comparison of technetium-99m-ECD to xenon-133 SPECT in normal controls and in patients with mild to moderate regional cerebral blood flow abnormalities, *J Nucl Med* 34:754–761, 1993.

378. Yudd AP, Van Heertum RL, Masdeu JC: Interventions and functional brain imaging, *Semin Nucl Med* 21:153–158, 1991.

379. Hirano T, Minematsu K, Hasegawa Y, et al: Correlation with positron emission tomography parameters Acetazolamide reactivity on ^{123}I-IMP single photon emission computed tomography in patients with major cerebral artery occlusive disease, *J Cereb Blood Flow Metab* 14:763–770, 1994.

380. Roussel SA, van Bruggen N, King MD, Gadian DG: Identification of collaterally perfused areas following focal cerebral ischemia in the rat by comparison of gradient echo and diffusion-weighted MRI, *J Cereb Blood Flow Metab* 15:578–586, 1995.

381. Belliveau JW, Cohen MS, Weisskoff RM, et al: Functional studies of the human brain using high-speed magnetic resonance imaging, *J Neuroimag* 1:36–41, 1991.

382. Branch CA, Helpern JA, Ewing JR: Welch KMA ^{19}F NMR imaging of cerebral blood flow, *Magn Reson Med* 20:151–157, 1991.

383. Larson KB, Perman WH, Perlmutter JS, et al: Tracer-kinetic analysis for measuring regional cerebral blood flow by dynamic nuclear magnetic resonance imaging, *J Theor Biol* 170:1–14, 1994.

384. Calamante F, Gadian DG, Connelly A: Quantification of perfusion using bolus tracking magnetic resonance imaging in stroke: Assumptions, limitations, and potential implications for clinical use, *Stroke* 33:1146–1151, 2002.

385. Calamante F, Thomas DL, Pell GS, et al: Measuring cerebral blood flow using magnetic resonance imaging techniques, *J Cereb Blood Flow Metab* 19:701–735, 1999.

386. Thomas DL, Lythgoe MF, Calamante F, et al: Simultaneous noninvasive measurement of CBF and CBV using double-echo FAIR (DEFAIR), *Magn Reson Med* 45:853–863, 2001.

387. Posse S, Olthoff U, Weckesser M, et al: Regional dynamic signal changes during controlled hyperventilation assessed with blood oxygen level-dependent functional MR imaging, *Am J Neuroradiol* 18:1763–1770, 1997.

388. Litt L, Gonzalez-Mendez R, Severinghaus JW, et al: Cerebral intracellular changes during supercarbia: An in vivo ^{31}P nuclear magnetic resonance study in rats, *J Cereb Blood Flow Metab* 5:537–544, 1985.

389. Ra JB, Hilal SK, Oh CH, Mun IK: In vivo magnetic resonance imaging of sodium in the human body, *Magn Reson Med* 7:11–22, 1988.

390. Calamante F, Vonken EJ, van Osch MJ: Contrast agent concentration measurements affecting quantification of bolus-tracking perfusion MRI, *Magn Reson Med* 58:544–553, 2007.

391. Hoehner PJ, Dean JM, Rogers MC, Traystman RJ: Comparison of thermal clearance measurement of regional cerebral blood flow with radiolabelled microspheres, *Stroke* 18:606–611, 1987.

392. Carter LP: Surface monitoring of cerebral cortical blood flow, *Cerebrovasc Brain Metab Rev* 3:246–261, 1991.

393. Mazzeo AT, Bullock R: Effect of bacterial meningitis complicating severe head trauma upon brain microdialysis and cerebral perfusion, *Neurocrit Care* 2:282–287, 2005.

394. Vajkoczy P, Roth H, Horn P, et al: Continuous monitoring of regional cerebral blood flow: Experimental and clinical validation of a novel thermal diffusion microprobe, *J Neurosurg* 93:265–274, 2000.

395. Joshi S, Hartl R, Wang M, et al: The acute cerebrovascular effects of intracarotid adenosine in nonhuman primates, *Anesth Analg* 97:231–237, 2003.

396. Jaeger M, Soehle M, Schuhmann MU, et al: Correlation of continuously monitored regional cerebral blood flow and brain tissue oxygen, *Acta Neurochir (Wien)* 147:51–56, 2005.

397. Vajkoczy P, Roth H, Horn P, et al: Continuous monitoring of regional cerebral blood flow: Experimental and clinical validation of a novel thermal diffusion microprobe, *J Neurosurg* 93:265–274, 2000.

398. Aaslid R, Markwalder T-M, Nornes H: Noninvasive transcranial Doppler ultrasound recording of flow velocity in basal cerebral arteries, *J Neurosurg* 57:764–769, 1982.

399. Aaslid R: *Transcranial Doppler Sonography*, New York, 1986, Springer-Verlag.

400. Gosling RG, King DH: Arterial assessment by Doppler-shift ultrasound, *Proc Roy Soc Med* 67:447–449, 1974.

401. Czosnyka M, Richards HK, Whitehouse HE, Pickard JD: Relationship between transcranial Doppler-determined pulsatility index and cerebrovascular resistance: an experimental study, *J Neurosurg* 84:79–84, 1996.

402. Kontos HA: Validity of cerebral arterial blood flow calculations from velocity measurements, *Stroke* 20:1–3, 1989.

403. Huber P, Handa J: Effect of contrast material, hypercapnia, hyperventilation, hypertonic glucose and papaverine on the diameter of the cerebral arteries: Angiographic determination in man, *Invest Radiol* 2:17–32, 1967.

404. Poulin MJ, Robbins PA: Indexes of flow and cross-sectional area of the middle cerebral artery using Doppler ultrasound during hypoxia and hypercapnia in humans, *Stroke* 27:2244–2250, 1996.

405. Laumer R, Steinmeier R, Gonner F, et al: Cerebral hemodynamics in subarachnoid hemorrhage evaluated by transcranial Doppler sonography. Part 1: Reliability of flow velocities in clinical management, *Neurosurgery* 33:1–9, 1993.

406. Romner B, Bellner J, Kongstad P, Sjoholm H: Elevated transcranial Doppler flow velocities after severe head injury: Cerebral vasospasm or hyperemia? *J Neurosurg* 85:90–97, 1996.

407. Giller CA, Hatab MR, Giller AM: Estimation of vessel flow and diameter during cerebral vasospasm using transcranial Doppler indices, *Neurosurgery* 42:1076–1082, 1998.

408. Finn JP, Quinn MW, Hall-Craggs MA, Kendall BE: Impact of vessel distortion on transcranial Doppler velocity measurements: Correlation with magnetic resonance imaging, *J Neurosurg* 73:572–575, 1990.

409. Halsey JH: Effect of emitted power on waveform intensity in transcranial Doppler, *Stroke* 21:1573–1578, 1990.

410. Lindegaard K-F, Grolimund P, Aaslid R, Nornes H: Evaluation of cerebral AVM's using transcranial Doppler ultrasound, *J Neurosurg* 65:335–344, 1986.

411. Aaslid R: Visually evoked dynamic blood flow response of the human cerebral circulation, *Stroke* 18:771–775, 1987.

412. Aaslid R, Lindegaard K-F, Sorteberg W, Nornes H: Cerebral autoregulation dynamics in humans, *Stroke* 20:45–52, 1989.

413. Kuo TB-J, Chern C-M, Sheng W-Y, et al: Frequency domain analysis of cerebral blood flow velocity and its correlation with arterial blood pressure, *J Cereb Blood Flow Metab* 18:311–318, 1998.

414. Halsey JH, McDowell HA, Gelmon S, Morawetz RB: Blood velocity in the middle cerebral artery and regional cerebral blood flow during carotid endarterectomy, *Stroke* 20:53–58, 1989.

415. Moritz S, Kasprzak P, Arlt M, et al: Accuracy of cerebral monitoring in detecting cerebral ischemia during carotid endarterectomy: A comparison of transcranial Doppler sonography, near-infrared spectroscopy, stump pressure, and somatosensory evoked potentials, *Anesthesiology* 107:563–569, 2007.

416. Bishop CCR, Powell S, Rutt D, Browse NL: Transcranial Doppler measurement of middle cerebral artery blood flow velocity: A validation study, *Stroke* 17:913–915, 1986.

417. Markwalder T-M, Grolimund P, Seiler RW, et al: Dependency of blood flow velocity in the middle cerebral artery on end-tidal carbon dioxide partial pressure: A transcranial ultrasound Doppler study, *J Cereb Blood Flow Metab* 4:368–372, 1984.

418. Pilato MA, Bissonnette B, Lerman J: Transcranial Doppler: Response of cerebral blood-flow velocity to carbon dioxide in anaesthetized children, *Can J Anaesth* 38:37–42, 1991.

419. Lam AM, Manninen PH, Ferguson GG, Nantau W: Monitoring electrophysiologic function during carotid endarterectomy: A comparison of somatosensory evoked potentials and conventional electroencephalogram, *Anesthesiology* 75:15–21, 1991.

420. Murkin JM, Lee DH: Transcranial Doppler verification of pulsatile cerebral blood flow during cardiopulmonary bypass [abstract], *Anesth Analg* 72:S194, 1991.

421. Bunegin L, Wahl D, Albin MS: Detection and volume estimation of embolic air in the middle cerebral artery using transcranial Doppler sonography, *Stroke* 25:593–600, 1994.

422. Gilsbach J, Hassler W: Intraoperative Doppler and real time sonography in neurosurgery, *Neurosurg Rev* 7:199–208, 1984.

423. Hassler W: *Hemodynamic Aspects of Cerebral Angiomas*, Vienna, Springer-Verlag, 1986.

424. Chaloupka JC, Vinuela F, Malanum RP, et al: Technical feasibility and performance studies of a Doppler guide wire for potential neuroendovascular applications, *Am J Neuroradiol* 15:503–507, 1994.

425. Chaloupka JC, Vinuela F, Kimme-Smith C, et al: Use of a Doppler guide wire for intravascular blood flow measurements: A validation study for potential neurologic endovascular applications, *AJNR Am J Neuroradiol* 15:509–517, 1994.

426. Henkes H, Nahser HC, Klotzsch C, et al: Endovascular Doppler sonography of intracranial blood vessels. Technical indications and potential applications, *Radiologe* 33:645–649, 1993.

427. Rampil IJ: Cerebral perfusion mapping with ultrasound contrast, *Anesthesiology* 751991:A1006.

428. Meyerson BA, Gunasekera L, Linderoth B, Gazelius B: Bedside monitoring of regional cortical blood flow in comatose patients using laser Doppler flowmetry, *Neurosurgery* 29:750–755, 1991.

429. Dirnagl U, Pulsinelli W: Autoregulation of cerebral blood flow in experimental focal brain ischemia, *J Cereb Blood Flow Metab* 10:327–336, 1990.

430. Kramer MS, Vinall PE, Katolik LI, Simeone FA: Comparison of cerebral blood flow measured by laser-Doppler flowmetry and hydrogen clearance in cats after cerebral insult and hypervolemic hemodilution, *Neurosurgery* 38:355–361, 1996.

431. Fabricius M, Lauritzen M: Laser-Doppler evaluation of rat brain microcirculation: Comparison with the [^{14}C]-iodoantipyrine method suggests discordance during cerebral flow increases, *J Cereb Blood Flow Metab* 16:156–161, 1996.

432. Steinmeier R, Fahlbusch R, Powers AD, et al: Pituitary microcirculation: Physiological aspects and clinical implications. A laser-Doppler flow study during transsphenoidal adenomectomy, *Neurosurgery* 29:47–54, 1991.

433. Johnson WD, Bolognese P, Miller JI, et al: Continuous postoperative ICBF monitoring in aneurysmal SAH patients using a combined ICP-laser Doppler fiberoptic probe, *J Neurosurg Anesthesiol* 8:199–207, 1996.

434. Nakase H, Kaido T, Okuno S, et al: Novel intraoperative cerebral blood flow monitoring by laser-Doppler scanner, *Neurol Med Chir (Tokyo)* 42:1–4, 2002.

435. Steinmeier R, Bondar I, Bauhuf C, Fahlbusch R: Laser Doppler flowmetry mapping of cerebrocortical microflow: Characteristics and limitations, *Neuroimage* 15:107–119, 2002.

436. Friedrich DH, Baethmann A, Plesnila N: Cluster analysis: A useful tool for the analysis of cerebral laser-Doppler scanning data, *J Neurosci Methods* 146:91–97, 2005.

437. Artru AA, Michenfelder JD: Effects of hypercarbia on canine cerebral metabolism and blood flow with simultaneous direct and indirect measurement of blood flow, *Anesthesiology* 52:466–469, 1980.

438. Wagner EM, Traystman RJ: Cerebral venous outflow and arterial microsphere flow with elevated venous pressure, *Am J Physiol* 244:H505–H512, 1983.

439. Symon L, Held K, Dorsch NWC: A study of regional autoregulation in the cerebral circulation to increased perfusion pressure in normocapnia and hypercapnia, *Stroke* 4:139–147, 1973.

440. Hayes AC, Baker WH, Reichman OH: Non-invasive evaluation of patients with extracranial to intracranial bypass, *Stroke* 13:365–368, 1982.

441. Nioka S, Chance B, Smith DS, et al: Cerebral energy metabolism and oxygen state during hypoxia in neonate and adult dogs, *Pediatr Res* 28:54–62, 1990.

442. Gupta AK, Menon DK, Czosnyka M, et al: Non-invasive measurement of cerebral blood volume in volunteers, *Br J Anaesth* 78:39–43, 1997.

443. Pollard V, Prough DS: Cerebral near-infrared spectroscopy: A plea for modest expectations, *Anesth Analg* 83:673–674, 1996.

444. Terborg C, Bramer S, Harscher S, et al: Bedside assessment of cerebral perfusion reductions in patients with acute ischaemic stroke by near-infrared spectroscopy and indocyanine green, *J Neurol Neurosurg Psychiatry* 75:38–42, 2004.

445. Huppert TJ, Hoge RD, Diamond SG, et al: A temporal comparison of BOLD, ASL, and NIRS hemodynamic responses to motor stimuli in adult humans, *Neuroimage* 29:368–382, 2006.

446. Wolf M, Ferrari M, Quaresima V: Progress of near-infrared spectroscopy and topography for brain and muscle clinical applications, *J Biomed Opt* :12, 2007:062104.

447. Nicklin SE, Hassan IA, Wickramasinghe YA, Spencer SA: The light still shines, but not that brightly? The current status of perinatal near infrared spectroscopy, *Arch Dis Child Fetal Neonatal Ed* 88:F263–F268, 2003.

448. Smith A, Pernder J, Alexander S: Effects of PCO_2 in spinal cord blood flow, *Am J Physiol* 216:1158–1163, 1969.

449. Hickey R, Albin MS, Bunegin L, Gelineau J: Autoregulation of spinal cord blood flow: Is the cord a microcosm of the brain? *Stroke* 17:1183–1189, 1986.

450. Sandler AN, Tator CH: Review of the measurement of normal spinal cord blood flow, *Brain Res* 118:181–198, 1976.

451. Griffiths IR: Spinal cord blood flow in dogs: The effect of blood pressure, *J Neurol Neurosurg Psychiatry* 36:914–920, 1973.

452. Griffiths IR: Spinal cord blood flow in dogs. 1: The 'normal' flow, *J Neurol Neurosurg Psychiatry* 36:34–41, 1973.

453. Griffiths IR: Spinal cord blood flow in dogs: 2. The effects of the blood gases, *J Neurol Neurosurg Psychiatry* 36:42–49, 1973.

454. Harakawa I, Yano T, Sakurai T, et al: Measurement of spinal cord blood flow by an inhalation method and intraarterial injection of hydrogen gas, *J Vasc Surg* 26:623–628, 1997.

455. Bisdas S, Rumboldt Z, Surlan K, et al: Perfusion CT measurements in healthy cervical spinal cord: Feasibility and repeatability of the study as well as interchangeability of the perfusion estimates using two commercially available software packages, *Eur Radiol* 18:2321–2328, 2008.

456. Duhamel G, Callot V, Cozzone PJ, Kober F: Spinal cord blood flow measurement by arterial spin labeling, *Magn Reson Med* 59:846–854, 2008.

457. Lu H, Law M, Ge Y, et al: Quantitative measurement of spinal cord blood volume in humans using vascular-space-occupancy MRI, *NMR Biomed* 21:226–232, 2008.

458. Shibata K, Takamoto S, Kotsuka Y, et al: Doppler ultrasonographic identification of the critical segmental artery for spinal cord protection, *Eur J Cardiothorac Surg* 20:527–532, 2001.

459. Hitchon PW, Mouw LJ, Rogge TN, et al: Response of spinal cord blood flow to the nitric oxide inhibitor nitroarginine, *Neurosurgery* 39:795–803, 1996.

460. Milhorat TH, Kotzen RM, Capocelli AL Jr, et al: Intraoperative improvement of somatosensory evoked potentials and local spinal cord blood flow in patients with syringomyelia, *J Neurosurg Anesth* 8:208–215, 1996.

461. Schneider SJ, Rosenthal AD, Greenberg BM, Danto J: A preliminary report on the use of laser-Doppler flowmetry during tethered spinal cord release, *Neurosurgery* 32:214–218, 1993.

462. Hempfing A, Dreimann M, Krebs S, et al: Reduction of vertebral blood flow by segmental vessel occlusion: an intraoperative study using laser Doppler flowmetry, *Spine (Phila Pa 1976)* 30:2701–2705, 2005.

463. Marcus ML, Heistad DD, Ehrhardt JC, Abboud FM: Regulation of total and regional spinal cord blood flow, *Circ Res* 41:128–134, 1977.

464. Marcoux FW, Goodrich JE, Dominick MA: Ketamine prevents ischemic neuronal injury, *Brain Res* 452:329–335, 1988.

465. Werner C, Hoffman WE, Kochs E, et al: The effects of propofol on cerebral and spinal cord blood flow in rats, *Anesth Analg* 76:971–975, 1993.

466. Kobrine A, Doyle T, Rizzoli H: Spinal cord blood flow as affected by changes in systemic arterial blood pressure, *J Neurosurg* 44:12–15, 1976.

467. Ford RWJ, Malm DN: Therapeutic trial of hypercarbia and hypocarbia in acute experimental spinal cord injury, *J Neurosurg* 61:925–930, 1984.

468. Sakamoto T, Monafo WW: Regional blood flow in the brain and spinal cord of hypothermic rats, *Am J Physiol* 257:H785–H790, 1989.

469. Albin MS: Resuscitation of the spinal cord, *Crit Care Med* 6:270–276, 1978.

470. Westergren H, Farooque M, Olsson Y, Holtz A: Spinal cord blood flow changes following systemic hypothermia and spinal cord compression injury: An experimental study in the rat using Laser-Doppler flowmetry, *Spinal Cord* 39:74–84, 2001.

471. Halstead JC, Wurm M, Etz C, et al: Preservation of spinal cord function after extensive segmental artery sacrifice: Regional variations in perfusion, *Ann Thorac Surg* 84:789–794, 2007.

472. Bernhard M, Gries A, Kremer P, Bottiger BW: Spinal cord injury (SCI): Prehospital management, *Resuscitation* 66:127–139, 2005.

473. Hitchon P, Kassell N, Hill T, et al: The response of spinal cord blood flow to high-dose barbiturates, *Spine* 7:41–45, 1982.

474. Hitchon P, Lobosky J, Yamada T, Torner J: Effect of laminectomy and anesthesia upon spinal cord blood flow, *J Neurosurg* 61:545–549, 1984.

475. Crystal GJ, Metwally AA, Salem MR: Isoflurane preserves central nervous system blood flow during intraoperative cardiac tamponade in dogs, *Can J Anaesth* 51:1011–1017, 2004.

476. Nishiyama T: Spinal cord blood flow change by intravenous midazolam during isoflurane anesthesia, *Anesth Analg* 101:5–242, 2005.

477. Young WL: Neuroanesthesia: A look into the future, *Anesthesiol Clin N Am* 10:727–746, 1992.

478. Olsen KS, Svendsen LB, Larsen FS, Paulson OB: Effect of labetalol on cerebral blood flow, oxygen metabolism and autoregulation in healthy humans. *Br J Anaesth* 75:51–54, 1995.

479. MacKenzie ET, Farrar JK, Fitch W, et al: Effects of hemorrhagic hypotension on the cerebral circulation: I. Cerebral blood flow and pial arteriolar caliber. *Stroke* 10:711–718, 1979.

480. MacKenzie ET, Strandgaard S, Graham DI, et al: Effects of acutely induced hypertension in cats on pial arteriolar caliber, local cerebral blood flow, and the blood-brain barrier. *Circ Res* 39:33–41, 1976.

Appendix I   TRANSIT TIME

A more simplistic approach can be taken if one assumes that at any given time, the concentration of isotope, $c(t)$, within the region of interest is homogeneous. In this case, the amount of blood that leaves (or enters) this region in a small increment of time, dt, is defined by the product of the flow rate and time, Fdt. The amount of isotope carried away from the region by this departing blood is described as $c(t)Fdt$. Again, by conservation of mass, the dose of isotope injected into the region of interest, q, must be the same as the amount leaving during all subsequent periods, as follows:

$$q = \int c(t)Fdt \qquad (2\text{-}20)$$

Rearranging this equation, one finds that flow can be described as the initially injected tracer dose within the region of interest divided by the area under the curve of the concentration vs. time relationship:

$$F = \frac{q}{\int c(t)dt} \qquad (2\text{-}21)$$

If one takes the relationship derived in Equation 2-21 a step further, the rate at which tracer leaves the region of interest is the product of the flow rate and the concentration of isotope in the departing blood at that given time, $F = c(t)$. At this point, it is useful to define the frequency function as follows:

$$h(t) = \frac{F\,c(t)}{q} \qquad (2\text{-}22)$$

The frequency function, simply stated, describes the fractional rate at which tracer leaves the region of interest. Because all tracer must ultimately leave, as expressed by the following equation:

$$\int h(t)dt = 1 \qquad (2\text{-}23)$$

For any small time interval between t and $t + dt$, the fraction of the original tracer leaving the system is thus $h(t) \cdot dt$. The quantity of tracer leaving is thus $q = h(t) \cdot dt$. By virtue of the fact that the tracer is assumed to follow the same kinetics as the trace, a similar analysis can be made regarding the volume of blood (tracee) entering into the region of interest per unit time, F. The fraction of this blood leaving between t and $t + dt$ is, again, $h(t) \cdot dt$. Thus the blood that is present in the region of interest leaves at a rate of $F \cdot h(t) \cdot dt$ until the time when all such particles have left. With transformation from rates to volumes, the volume of blood that departs from the region of interest between t and $t = dt$, denoted as dV, is the product of the egress rate and the time required for this blood to leave, $t \cdot F \cdot (t) h(dt)$. Integrating over all time intervals, one obtains the following equation:

$$\int dv = \int tFh(T)dt = F \int th(t)dt \qquad (2\text{-}24)$$

Because $h(t)$ is the frequency function of the transit times of the tracer, the integral expression $\int th(t)dt$ is simply the mean transit time, t, which statistically defines the average time that any particle of tracer, or for that matter tracee (blood), remains within the system. Substituting Equation 2-22 and then Equation 2-20 into the expression for t yields the following:

$$\bar{t} = \infty \int_{t=0} th(t)dt = \frac{\infty \int_{t=0} tFc(t)dt}{q} = \frac{\infty \int_{t=0} t\,c(t)\,dt}{\infty \int_{t=0} c(t)dt} \qquad (2\text{-}25)$$

Mean transit time thus can easily be calculated from the concentration versus time curve. Once again, invoking conservation of mass, it is clear that for any time interval, the volumes of blood entering and leaving a region of interest are equal. For the inert gas system being discussed, the mean transit time of the inert gas particles (the tracer) is equal to the mean transit time of the blood particles (the tracee). Thus the blood volume contained in the region of interest is equal to the product of the blood flow into (or out of) this region and the mean transit time through the region of interest, expressed as follows:

$$rCBV = rCBF \times I \text{ or (Flow) } \bar{t} \qquad (2\text{-}26)$$

Chapter 3

CEREBROSPINAL FLUID

Alan A. Artru

The first section of this chapter reviews cerebrospinal fluid (CSF) with respect to anatomy of the CSF-containing spaces, physiology, and the effects of anesthetics and other influences. The second section reviews the relationship between CSF dynamics and intracranial pressure (ICP), anesthetics and drug-induced changes in CSF dynamics that increase or decrease ICP, and clinical situations wherein therapy to alter CSF dynamics may affect neurologic outcome.

ANATOMY OF CSF SPACES AND PROPERTIES OF CSF

The CSF is formed in the brain and circulates through macroscopic and extracellular fluid (ECF) spaces that are in continuity. The total volume of these spaces ranges from 50 mL in infants to 140 to 150 mL in adults (Table 3-1). Ventricular volume accounts for about 16% to 17% of macroscopic CSF volume in adults. Studies to determine the volumes of portions of the macroscopic CSF space using noninvasive imaging technology are ongoing.[1] The ECF space surrounds the neuronal and glial elements of the central nervous system. Brain ECF volume is about 300 to 350 mL in adults.

Macroscopic Spaces

The choroid plexuses (CPs) of the lateral ventricles extend from the inferior horn to the central part of the ventricle. The CPs in the body of the lateral and third ventricles receive their blood supply from the posterior and anterior choroidal arteries, respectively. The CPs in the temporal horns and the fourth ventricle are supplied by the superior and posterior inferior cerebellar arteries, respectively.[2] The nervous supply to the CPs includes branches of the vagus, glossopharyngeal, and sympathetic nerves.

Table 3–1 Cerebrospinal Fluid (CSF) Pressure and Volume in Humans

	Range*
CSF pressure (mm Hg):	
Children	3.0-7.5
Adults	4.5-13.5
CSF volume (mL):	
Infants	40-60
Young children	60-100
Older children	80-120
Adults	100-160

*Values based on references 97-99.

Extracellular Fluid Spaces

The ECF spaces of the brain and spinal cord, unlike those of other organs in the body, are small in diameter (180 Å). Exchange between cerebral capillaries and the ECF is limited because the capillary membrane is highly impermeable. This blood-brain barrier (BBB) consists of two elements. First, the cells of the cerebral capillary endothelium are joined by tight junctions (zonula occludens) that restrict the intercellular movement of molecules having a diameter of 20 Å or more. Second, astrocyte foot processes surround the capillaries. Evidence shows that the ECF spaces communicate with lymphatic channels.

COMPOSITION OF CSF

CSF is a clear aqueous solution that, compared with plasma, contains higher concentrations of sodium, chloride, and magnesium and lower concentrations of glucose, proteins, amino acids, uric acid, potassium, bicarbonate, calcium, and phosphate (Table 3-2). Differences between the composition of CSF and an ultrafiltrate of plasma indicate that active secretion occurs during CSF formation. The concentrations of

Table 3–2 Composition of Cerebrospinal Fluid (CSF) and Plasma in Humans

Feature or Component	Mean CSF Value or Concentration*	Mean Plasma Value or Concentration*
Specific gravity	1.007	1.025
Osmolality (mOsm/kg H_2O)	289	289
pH	7.31	7.41
P_{CO_2} (mm Hg)	50.5	41.1
Sodium (mEq/L)	141	140
Potassium (mEq/L)	2.9	4.6
Calcium (mEq/L)	2.5	5.0
Magnesium (mEq/L)	2.4	1.7
Chloride (mEq/L)	124	101
Bicarbonate (mEq/L)	21	23
Glucose (mg/100 mL)	61	92
Protein (mg/100 mL):	28	7000
Albumin	23	4430
Globulin	5	2270
Fibrinogen	0	300

*Average values based on references 108-110.

these and other substances in the macroscopic spaces vary according to the sampling site because diffusion between CSF and ECF occurs as CSF passes through the ventricles and subarachnoid spaces. Concentrations of CSF constituents are significantly altered during neuroendoscopy.[3]

CSF FORMATION

The rate of CSF formation ($\dot{V}_f$) is about 0.35 to 0.40 mL/min, or 500 to 600 mL/day in humans. Approximately 0.25% of total adult CSF volume is replaced by freshly formed CSF each minute. The turnover time for total CSF volume is 5 to 7 hours, yielding a turnover rate of about four times per day. About 40% to 70% of CSF enters the macroscopic spaces via the CP, and 30% to 60% enters across the ependyma and pia.

CSF Formation at the Choroid Plexus

Unlike the capillary endothelium of other cerebral vessels, the capillary endothelium of the CP does not possess tight junctions between its cells. Instead, the capillary endothelium of the CP is fenestrated. Blood entering CP capillaries is filtered across this endothelium and forms a protein-rich fluid within the CP stroma that is similar in composition to interstitial fluid in other tissues of the body. Selected constituents of the stromal fluid are transported across the relatively impermeable CP epithelium by the combined processes of ultrafiltration and secretion. Stroma fluid enters clefts between the CP epithelial cells as a result of hydrostatic pressure and bulk flow (Fig. 3-1).

Extrachoroidal CSF Formation

Sixty percent of extrachoroidal CSF formation results from oxidation of glucose by the brain, and 40% from ultrafiltration from cerebral capillaries.[4] In most of the cerebral vasculature, passage of large and polar molecules across the "blood-ECF" interface is restricted by capillary tight junctions and specialized heterolytic vesicles within endothelial cells. Water, electrolytes, glucose, amino acids, urea, lipid-soluble materials, and a number of small nonelectrolytes pass more freely across this interface. Some of these substances may be actively transported by the astrocyte layer that envelops the capillary endothelium, whereas others may diffuse into the brain ECF. This glucose-rich and protein-poor "lymph" diffuses through the ECF space toward the macroscopic CSF spaces (Fig. 3-2).

Movement of Glucose

The concentration of glucose in CSF at the CP or in mixed samples is approximately 60% of that in blood. This ratio remains constant unless blood glucose rises to more than 15 to 20 mM (270 to 360 mg/dL). Glucose in blood enters CSF by facilitated transport, so that glucose crosses the blood-CSF barrier more quickly than would be predicted on the basis of its lipid solubility.[5] Transport follows saturable kinetics, with the rate being directly related to serum glucose concentration and independent of the serum-to-CSF glucose concentration gradient.[6] Movement of glucose in the opposite direction, from the cerebral ventricles into the surrounding brain and blood, occurs via ouabain-sensitive and ouabain-insensitive fluxes and diffusion.

Movement of Protein

Protein entry into CSF from blood at the CP and extrachoroidal sites is limited, so CSF protein concentrations are normally 0.5% or less of the respective plasma or serum concentrations. The permeability of the blood-CSF "barrier" to albumin increases with age and does not differ between genders.[7] If a structural barrier between the brain ECF and the macroscopic CSF space is absent, proteins entering the brain

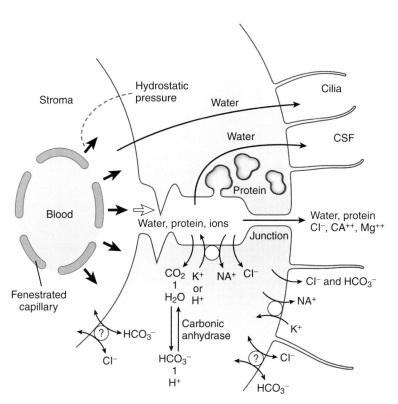

Figure 3-1 Some of the processes involved in cerebrospinal fluid (CSF) formation at the choroid plexus are shown in schematic form. Adenosine triphosphate–dependent membrane "pumps" transport Na^+ across the abluminal surface to within the choroid plexus cell and across the secretory surface, into the macroscopic CSF space, in exchange for K^+ and H^+. Water moves from the stroma into CSF as it follows the concentration gradient produced by the ionic "pumps." *(From Cucchiara RF, Michenfelder JD [eds]: Clinical Neuroanesthesia. New York, Churchill Livingstone, 1990.)*

ECF drain into the macroscopic CSF space by bulk flow. Once in CSF, proteins are transported along with CSF through the macroscopic pathways and are cleared from the CSF space into dural venous sinuses. This "sink effect" of flowing CSF keeps the CSF and brain protein concentration low and far from equilibrium with blood.[4] In normal infants and adults, CSF protein concentrations are lowest in the ventricles (about 26 mg/100 mL), intermediate in the cisterna magna (about 32 mg/100 mL), and highest in the lumbar sac (42 mg/100 mL).[8] Under normal conditions, 60% of protein entry into CSF occurs at the CP, and 40% at extrachoroidal sites.

Effects of Increased Intracranial Pressure on CSF Formation

The negative correlation between $\dot{V}_f$ and increased ICP is weak; the relationship between $\dot{V}_f$ and cerebral perfusion pressure (CPP) is somewhat stronger.[9] Increase of ICP to 20 mm Hg produces no change in $\dot{V}_f$ as long as CPP remains above ~70 mm Hg.[10] When CPP falls below ~70 mm Hg, whether from arterial hypotension or because of the combination of arterial hypotension with increased ICP, $\dot{V}_f$ diminishes. These $\dot{V}_f$ results are consistent with reported effects of changes in CPP on cerebral blood flow (CBF), lateral ventricle CP blood flow (CPBF), and fourth ventricle CPBF.[9] A decrease of CPP to 70 mm Hg by arterial hypotension, combined with increased ICP, reduces CBF and CPBF. A drop of CPP to 50 mm Hg causes a further decline in CPBF when CPP is reduced by an even greater increase in ICP, but not when CPP is reduced solely by arterial hypotension.

CIRCULATION OF CSF

The hydrostatic pressure of CSF formation, 15 cm H_2O, produces CSF flow where it is freshly formed. Cilia on ependymal cells generate currents that propel CSF toward the fourth ventricle and its foramina into the subarachnoid spaces. Respiratory variations and vascular pulsations of the cerebral arteries and CP cause ventricular excursions, supplying additional momentum for CSF movement. The pressure difference between mean CSF pressure, 15 cm H_2O, and superior sagittal sinus pressure, 9 cm H_2O, provides a 6 cm H_2O pressure gradient for passage of CSF across the arachnoid villi. The high velocity of blood flow through the fixed diameter of the sinuses and the low intraluminal pressure that develops at the circumference of the sinus wall where the arachnoid villi enter cause a "suction-pump" action that may explain how the circulation of the CSF continues through a wide range of postural pressures.

Radioisotope studies show that labeled CSF moves from the ventricles to the basal cisterns within a few minutes and collects along the superior sagittal sinus area at 12 to 24 hours. The labeled fluid enters the low cervical–high thoracic region at 10 to 20 minutes, the thoracolumbar area at 30 to 40 minutes, the lumbosacral cul de sac at 60 to 90 minutes, and the basal cisterns at 2 to 2.5 hours.[11] About 20% to 33% of the labeled CSF reaches the intracranial cavity within 12 hours. CSF circulation concludes with reabsorption across arachnoid villi into the superior sagittal sinus and spinal dural sinusoids located on dorsal nerve roots (Fig. 3-3).

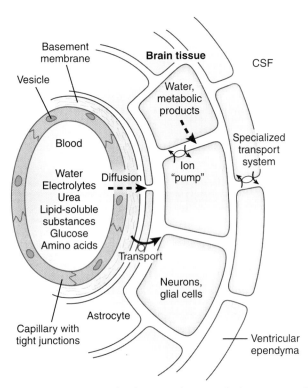

Figure 3–2 Water and other constituents of plasma cross the blood-brain barrier (capillary endothelial cells, basement membrane, and astrocyte foot processes) into the brain extracellular fluid (ECF) space by diffusion or transport. This fluid diffuses toward the macroscopic cerebrospinal fluid (CSF) space and subarachnoid space. Water and other cellular metabolites are added to the ECF from neurons and glial cells.

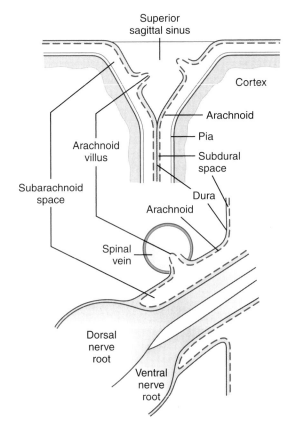

Figure 3–3 Cerebrospinal fluid is reabsorbed via arachnoid villi at the sagittal sinus and at spinal veins on dorsal nerve roots. (*From Cucchiara RF, Michenfelder JD [eds]: Clinical Neuroanesthesia. New York, Churchill Livingstone, 1990.*)

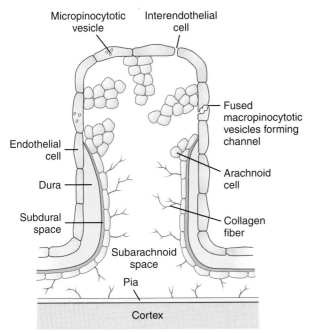

Figure 3–4 Schematic drawing of the microscopic anatomy of an arachnoid villus. *(From Cucchiara RF, Michenfelder JD, editors: Clinical Neuroanesthesia. New York, Churchill Livingstone, 1990.)*

Labels on figure: Micropinocytotic vesicle; Interendothelial cell; Fused macropinocytotic vesicles forming channel; Arachnoid cell; Collagen fiber; Endothelial cell; Dura; Subdural space; Subarachnoid space; Pia; Cortex

REABSORPTION OF CSF

CSF passes from the subarachnoid space into venous blood through microscopic arachnoid villi and macroscopic arachnoid granulations. Intracranial arachnoid villi are located within the dural wall bordering the superior sagittal sinus and venous lacunae, and spinal arachnoid villi are located within the dural wall bordering dural sinusoids on dorsal nerve roots. Under usual conditions, 85% to 90% of CSF is reabsorbed at intracranial sites, and 10% to 15% at spinal sites. The arachnoid villus or granulation is composed of arachnoid cells protruding from the subarachnoid space into and through the wall of an adjacent venous sinus[12] (Fig. 3-4). Under normal conditions, an endothelium composed of arachnoid cells joined by tight junctions covers the villus. In adults, this endothelial covering may be multilayered.

Normal Intracranial Pressure

The endothelium covering the villus acts as a CSF-blood barrier that limits the rate of passage of CSF and solute into venous blood. The rate at which CSF passes through the subarachnoid space and arachnoid villi and across the endothelium is determined by (1) the transvillous hydrostatic pressure gradient (CSF pressure − venous sinus pressure) and (2) a pressure-sensitive resistance to CSF outflow at the arachnoid villus. Because the endothelium is highly permeable, transvillous osmotic differences probably do not play a major role in determining CSF movement through arachnoid villi. CSF may exit the villus by passing between or through endothelial cells. CSF may pass through endothelial cells via pinocytotic vesicles and transcellular openings formed by chains of fused vesicles extending from one surface of the epithelium to the other.[13] These vesicles transport macromolecular tracers, as well as fluid, from CSF to blood. Although micropinocytotic vesicles appear to be the primary route of CSF transport at resting CSF

pressure, both pathways contribute to the total resistance to CSF outflow.

Increased Intracranial Pressure

The rate of reabsorption of CSF ($\dot{V}_a$) increases as the pressure gradient across the villus (CSF pressure − venous sinus pressure) increases. Resistance to reabsorption of CSF (R_a) remains close to "normal" as CSF pressure increases to more than 30 cm H_2O. Thereafter, with further increases in CSF pressure, R_a declines.[14-17] An increase in the size and number of endothelial vesicles was reported when CSF pressure was increased from 9 to 30 cm H_2O.[18] At CSF pressures greater than 30 cm H_2O, growing numbers of transcellular channels were present concurrent with progressive increases in steady-state pressures and decreases in R_a.

Clearance of Brain Interstitial Fluid

Normal Intracranial Pressure

Under normal conditions, there is relatively little bulk flow across cerebral capillaries and through the parenchyma of the brain.[19] Molecules in the brain ECF move through that space primarily by diffusion. The rate at which molecules exit the brain ECF relates to their molecular size, tissue concentration gradients, and the ability of the molecules to cross the BBB and reenter the vascular system.

Cerebral Edema

Vasogenic brain edema results from damage to cerebral vessels. Vasogenic edema resolves in part through passage of edema fluid into ventricular CSF. One factor favoring fluid movement out of brain ECF is the pressure gradient between edematous brain tissue and CSF. A second factor is the "sink" action of CSF.[20] Clearance of edema fluid was reported to increase when ICP was decreased, presumably because of a rise in the pressure gradient between edematous brain tissue and CSF.[21] Clearance of brain ECF proteins occurs by intraglial uptake, and this step is believed to play an important role in the resolution of vasogenic brain edema.[22]

FUNCTION OF CSF

The varied and complex functions of CSF include protection, support, and chemical regulation of the brain. The low specific gravity of CSF (1.007) relative to that of the brain (1.040) reduces the effective mass of a 1400-g brain to only 47 g. In continuity with the brain ECF, CSF provides a stable supply of substrates, primarily glucose, even though concentrations of substrates in plasma are continuously changing. CSF maintains the chemically precise environment required for neurotransmission and removes metabolic products, unwanted drugs, and harmful substances resulting from CNS injury.

Nutrition

Certain nutritive and other substrates for the brain are actively transported by systems in the capillary-glial complex. Simple sugars, certain vitamins, eicosanoids, monosaccharides, neutral and basic amino acids (brain tissue does not appear to contain an acidic amino acid transport system), and monocarboxylic acids are transported by specialized pump mechanisms (equilibrating carriers) between blood and brain ECF.[23-25] Also, CSF may mediate uptake of certain vitamins, such as ascorbic acid.

Control of the Chemical Environment

Exchange between CSF and neural tissue ECF occurs readily because the maximum distance for diffusion between CSF and any brain area in humans is 15 mm and the interstitial space of the brain and spinal cord is continuous with the macroscopic CSF spaces. The acid-base characteristics of CSF influence respiration, CBF, autoregulation of CBF, and cerebral metabolism.[26] CSF calcium, potassium, and magnesium levels influence heart rate, blood pressure, vasomotor and other autonomic reflexes, respiration, muscle tone, and emotional states. Calcium, potassium, magnesium, and bicarbonate ions are actively transported by "primary pumps," whereas hydrogen and chloride ions are passively transferred by "secondary pumps." Within limits, CSF composition of larger molecules is regulated by the BBB with the almost total exclusion of toxic or potentially toxic large, polar, and lipid-insoluble drugs, humoral agents, and metabolites.

Excretion

Accumulation of metabolites and substances in brain ECF is prevented by their passage into CSF, cerebral veins, or cervical lymphatics. Although passage into CSF may occur by two mechanisms, net diffusion and bulk flow of ECF, bulk flow accounts for most passages of many substrates of different molecular weights.[27]

Intracerebral Transport

Because CSF circulates to regions of the brain known to participate in neuroendocrine activity, it serves as a convenient vehicle for intracerebral transport of neurotransmitters. Neurohormone-releasing factors are synthesized in the hypothalamus and released into the brain ECF and CSF by means of axonal contact between neurons with specialized cells of the ependyma. These factors are carried by the CSF to the median eminence, where they stimulate the dendrites of receptor neurons. Opioid effects—such as analgesia and respiratory depression—may be mediated by third-ventricle cellular elements in contact with CSF, because electrical stimulation of the medial thalamus or periaqueductal gray matter increases the level of β-endorphins in ventricular CSF.[28-30]

EFFECTS OF ANESTHETICS AND OTHER INFLUENCES ON FORMATION AND REABSORPTION OF CSF

Methods of Determining CSF Formation Rate and Resistance to CSF Reabsorption

Experimental Animals

Three currently used methods for determining $\dot{V}_f$, R_a, and other CSF dynamics in animals are ventriculocisternal perfusion, manometric infusion, and volume injection or withdrawal. Ventriculocisternal perfusion was first described by Heisey and colleagues[31] and Pappenheimer and associates[32]

in the early 1960s. The method requires placement of cannulas in one or both lateral ventricles and in the cisterna magna. Labeled, mock CSF is infused into the ventricles, and a mixed sample composed of labeled, mock CSF and native CSF is collected from the cisterna magna. A portion of the continuous outflow of mock-native CSF from the cisternal cannula is collected, and the volume of the sample is determined. The concentration of the label in the outflow sample is measured, and the time over which the sample was obtained is noted. $\dot{V}_f$ is calculated according to the following formula:

$$\dot{V}_f = \dot{V}_i \left(\frac{C_i - C_o}{C_o} \right) \tag{3-1}$$

where $\dot{V}_i$ is mock CSF inflow rate, C_i is concentration of the label in mock CSF, and C_o is concentration of the label in the mixed outflow solution.

$\dot{V}_a$ is calculated by either of two formulas; the first is as follows:

$$\dot{V}_a = \frac{\dot{V}_i C_i - \dot{V}_o C_o}{C_o} \tag{3-2}$$

where $\dot{V}_o$ is the outflow rate of CSF from the cisternal cannula. The second formula for calculation of $\dot{V}_a$ is as follows:

$$\dot{V}_a = \dot{V}_i + \dot{V}_f - \dot{V}_o \tag{3-3}$$

R_a is a reciprocal measure of the slope relating $\dot{V}_a$ to CSF pressure. For calculation of R_a, $\dot{V}_a$ must be determined at several CSF pressures. If the slope relating $\dot{V}_a$ to CSF pressure is linear, a single R_a value adequately describes the data. If the $\dot{V}_a$/CSF pressure slope is not linear, multiple R_a values must be calculated. For any CSF pressure, the corresponding R_a value is the inverse of tangent to the $\dot{V}_a$/CSF pressure slope.

Manometric infusion, as it is currently used, was described by Maffeo and colleagues[33] and Mann and associates[16] in the late 1970s. For this technique, a manometric infusion device is inserted into the spinal or supracortical subarachnoid space. Mock CSF is infused into the subarachnoid space, and CSF pressure is measured at the same site as the infusion. Each steady-state CSF pressure (P_S) is paired with its associated $\dot{V}_i$. Next, each pair of $\dot{V}_i$:P_S values is plotted on a semilog plot of $\dot{V}_i$ versus P_S. A linear slope is then fit through the three to six data points. For determination of $\dot{V}_f$, the linear slope is extrapolated toward the origin (to the left). The $\dot{V}_i$ value at resting CSF pressure (P_o)—that is, the $\dot{V}_i$ value corresponding to the intersection of a perpendicular from P_o and the extrapolated semilog plot—is considered to be $\dot{V}_f$. R_a is determined with the use of observed values and two calculated, species-dependent parameters: M (transport capacity) and P_R (pressure at maximum resistance). These species-dependent parameters are calculated on the basis of the following formula:

$$\dot{V}_i = \frac{1}{M} e^{P_S/P_R} \tag{3-4}$$

Simultaneously solving this equation for the three to six pairs of $\dot{V}_i$:P_S values used to calculate $\dot{V}_f$ yields one unique pair of M and P_R values. R_a is then calculated according to the following formula:

$$R_a = MP_e - P_S/P_R \tag{3-5}$$

In addition, the compliance (C) of the CSF compartment can be calculated according to the following formula:

$$C = \frac{\dot{V}_i}{\Delta P / \Delta t} \quad (3\text{-}6)$$

where P is CSF pressure, t is time, and $\Delta P / \Delta t$ is the slope of the linear rise in CSF pressure during infusion of mock CSF.

Volume injection or withdrawal was described by Marmarou and colleagues[34] and Miller[35] in the mid-1970s. A ventricular or spinal subarachnoid catheter is inserted to permit injection or withdrawal of CSF and measurement of the CSF pressure change that accompanies injection or withdrawal. P_o is determined, and then a known volume of CSF (ΔV) is injected into (or withdrawn from) the catheter while a timed recording of CSF pressure is made. $\dot{V}_f$ and R_a are determined first through a calculation of the pressure volume index (PVI) as follows:

$$PVI = \Delta V / [\log P_P / P_o] \quad (3\text{-}7)$$

where P_P is peak CSF pressure (increase after volume injection and decrease after volume withdrawal).

R_a is then calculated on the basis of the following formula:

$$R_a = \frac{t \cdot P_o}{PVI \cdot \log_{10}\left(\frac{P_2(P_P - P_o)}{P_P(P_2 - P_o)}\right)} \quad (3\text{-}8)$$

where P_2 is CSF pressure measured some time between P_P and the return of CSF pressure to P_o and t is time from volume injection or withdrawal to P_2.

$\dot{V}_f$ is calculated on the basis of the following formula:

$$P_o = P_v - (R_a \cdot \dot{V}_f) \quad (3\text{-}9)$$

which can be rewritten as follows:

$$\dot{V}_f = \frac{P_v - P_o}{R_a} \quad (3\text{-}10)$$

where P_v is the venous blood pressure of the sagittal sinus.

C is calculated on the basis of the following formula:

$$C = \frac{0.4343 \cdot PVI}{P_o} \quad (3\text{-}11)$$

Humans

Ventriculocisternal perfusion, manometric infusion, and volume injection or withdrawal have also been used to calculate $\dot{V}_f$, R_a, and C in patients.[16] For ventriculocisternal perfusion, the outflow catheter is placed in the lumbar subarachnoid space, and ventricular and spinal CSF pressures are closely monitored to ensure that CSF pressure does not increase to potentially hazardous levels as a result of obstructed perfusion. For manometric infusion, the number of infusions is reduced, and infusion rates are limited to 1.5 to 15 times the $\dot{V}_f$ —that is, 0.01 to 0.1 mL/sec. Infusions are restricted to 20 to 60 seconds, being discontinued at CSF pressures of 60 to 70 cm H_2O or if a rapid rise in CSF pressure with no apparent tendency toward stabilization is observed. The procedures and formulas for calculation of $\dot{V}_f$, R_a, and C in humans are the same as those in experimental animals.

Because of the hazards associated with prolonged infusion of mock CSF, ventriculocisternal perfusion and manometric infusion are less commonly used in patients than volume injection or withdrawal. An obvious advantage of this last method is that when ICP is of concern, CSF withdrawal is therapeutic—as well as useful for calculating $\dot{V}_f$, R_a, and C. The risk of infection is minimized because the system can remain completely closed. For repeated testing, CSF can be alternately withdrawn and then injected, with the net change of CSF volume being made according to the patient's ICP responses. Calculation of CSF dynamics requires only a single change of CSF volume and pressure lasting for several minutes. In contrast, with ventriculocisternal perfusion, more than 1 hour of infusion of mock CSF may be needed for tracer equilibration, and the manometric technique requires multiple infusions.

Anesthetic- and Drug-Induced Changes in CSF Formation Rate and Resistance to CSF Reabsorption and Transport of Various Molecules into CSF and the Central Nervous System

Anesthetics

Anesthetics influence many aspects of CSF dynamics (Table 3-3). Early studies with enflurane reported that 1 minimum alveolar concentration (MAC) increased $\dot{V}_f$ by 50% to 80% on initial exposure in rats and dogs.[36,37] $\dot{V}_f$ gradually returned to normal over several hours. Enflurane also increased R_a, but R_a did not return to normal when administration of enflurane was continued for several hours.[37,38] Enflurane produced these alterations of CSF dynamics when administered with either nitrogen (60% to 70%) or nitrous oxide (60% to 70%) in oxygen. Later studies with enflurane reported that its effects on $\dot{V}_f$ and R_a are dose related. High concentrations of enflurane (2.6% and 3.5% end-expired) increased $\dot{V}_f$ (by about 40% when corrected for the effects of time), whereas low concentrations (0.9% and 1.8%) did not.[39] Conversely, low concentrations increased R_a, but high concentrations did

Table 3–3 Effects of Inhaled Anesthetics on Cerebrospinal Fluid (CSF) Dynamics

Inhaled Anesthetic	$\dot{V}_f$	R_a	Predicted Effect on Intracranial Pressure
Desflurane	0,+,a	0	0,+,a
Enflurane:			
Low concentration	0	+	+
High concentration	+	0	+
Halothane	−	+	+
Isoflurane:			
Low concentration	0	0,+,b	0,+,b
High concentration	0	−	−
Nitrous oxide	0	0	0
Sevoflurane	−	+	?

R_a, Resistance to reabsorption of CSF; $\dot{V}_f$, rate of CSF formation; +, increase; 0, no change; −, decrease; a, effect occurs only during hypocapnia combined with increased CSF pressure, and under such conditions treatment with furosemide (but not mannitol, dexamethasone, or fentanyl) decreases $\dot{V}_f$; b, effect depends on dose; ?, uncertain.

not. Halothane (1 MAC) generally is reported to decrease $\dot{V}_f$[40] and increase R_a.[41] In addition, halothane enhances transport of glucose into brain[42] as well as movement of albumin and immunoglobulin (Ig) G[43,44] and of sodium, chloride, and water[45,46] into CSF. Nitrous oxide (66%) is reported to produce no change in R_a or $\dot{V}_f$[36,40] and to decrease brain glucose influx and efflux.[47]

Early studies with isoflurane reported that 1 MAC of that anesthetic decreased R_a and caused no change in $\dot{V}_f$.[38,48] Later studies with isoflurane reported that its effects on R_a are dose related. R_a was normal at 0.6% (end-expired) isoflurane, increased at 1.1%, and decreased at 1.7% and 2.2%.[39] At 2% (inspired) isoflurane, the BBB transfer coefficient for small hydrophilic molecules was decreased.[49] The concentration of glutamate in CSF was higher during isoflurane anesthesia than during propofol anesthesia.[50] Sevoflurane (1 MAC) is reported to decrease $\dot{V}_f$ by about 40% and to increase R_a in comparison with 50% nitrous oxide in oxygen.[51] Studies with desflurane reported that its effects on $\dot{V}_f$ are related to CSF pressure and Pa_{CO_2}. At normocapnia and normal CSF pressure, normocapnia and increased CSF pressure, and hypocapnia and normal CSF pressure, both 0.5 and 1 MAC desflurane caused no change in $\dot{V}_f$ or R_a.[52] However, at hypocapnia and increased CSF pressure, both concentrations of desflurane increased R_a. During the combination of desflurane, hypocapnia, and increased CSF pressure, furosemide (2 mg/kg)—but not dexamethasone (0.2 mg/kg), mannitol (2 g/kg), nor fentanyl (48 μg/kg followed by 0.6 μg/kg/min)—decreased $\dot{V}_f$, whereas none of the treatments significantly altered R_a.[53]

Ketamine (40 mg/kg/hr) increases R_a but does not alter $\dot{V}_f$ (Table 3-4).[37] In addition, ketamine (150 mg/kg) decreases the transport of small hydrophilic molecules across the BBB.[54] Low doses of etomidate (0.86 mg/kg, followed by 0.86 or 1.72 mg/kg/hr) do not alter R_a or $\dot{V}_f$, whereas high doses (2.58 or 3.44 mg/kg/hr) decrease both R_a and $\dot{V}_f$.[55] Low doses of thiopental (6 mg/kg, followed by 6 or 12 mg/kg/hr) increase or do not alter R_a and do not alter $\dot{V}_f$, whereas high doses (18 or 24 mg/kg/hr) decrease both R_a and $\dot{V}_f$.[55] Thiopental (100 μg/mL but not 25 or 50 μg/mL) but not methohexital (10 to 50 μg/mL) increases the permeability of brain microvascular endothelial cells to α-aminoisobutyric acid but not to sucrose nor Evans blue albumin.[56] Propofol (6 mg/kg, followed by 12, 24, and 48 mg/kg/hr) and pentobarbital (40 mg/kg) produce no change in R_a or $\dot{V}_f$.[37,57] In addition, pentobarbital decreases transport of glucose,[58] amino acids,[59] and small hydrophilic molecules[54] into the brain.

Among the sedative-hypnotic drugs, the effects of midazolam appear to be the most variable. Low doses of midazolam (1.6 mg/kg, followed by 0.5 mg/kg/hr) increase R_a and do not alter $\dot{V}_f$, intermediate doses (1 to 1.5 mg/kg/hr) cause no change, and high doses (2 mg/kg/hr) increase R_a and decrease $\dot{V}_f$.[55] The benzodiazepine antagonist, flumazenil, caused no change in $\dot{V}_f$ when given to dogs receiving midazolam (1.6 mg/kg, followed by 1.25 mg/kg/hr) nor dogs not receiving midazolam.[60] Low-dose flumazenil (0.0025 mg/kg) caused no change in R_a, and high-dose flumazenil (0.16 mg/kg) decreased R_a. In dogs receiving midazolam, low-dose flumazenil increased R_a (perhaps because of partial reversal of midazolam so that CSF dynamics approximated those of low-dose midazolam), whereas after high-dose flumazenil, R_a returned to normal (that is, to values characteristic of dogs not receiving midazolam).

Early studies with fentanyl reported that 60 μg/kg, followed by 0.2 μg/kg/min decreased R_a[41] and did not alter $\dot{V}_f$.[40]

Table 3–4 Effects of Sedative-Hypnotics and Antagonist Drugs on Cerebrospinal Fluid (CSF) Dynamics

Sedative-Hypnotic	$\dot{V}_f$	R_a	Predicted Effect on Intracranial Pressure
Etomidate:			
Low dose	0	0	0
High dose	−	0, −, a	−
Midazolam*:			
Low dose	0	+, 0, a	+, 0, a
High dose	−	0, +, a	−, ?, a
Pentobarbital	0	0	0
Propofol	0	0	0
Thiopental:			
Low dose	0	+, 0, a	+, 0, a
High dose	−	0, −, a	−
Antagonists			
Flumazenil:			
Low dose	0	0	0
High dose	0	−	−

R_a, Resistance to reabsorption of CSF; $\dot{V}_f$, rate of CSF formation; +, increase; 0, no change; −, decrease; a, effect depends on dose; ?, uncertain.
*Partial reversal with flumazenil causes CSF dynamics similar to that with lowest dose of midazolam, and complete reversal with flumazenil causes CSF dynamics similar to that with pre-midazolam (control) values.

More recent studies reported that its effects on $\dot{V}_f$ and R_a are dose related (Table 3-5). High doses of fentanyl decreased $\dot{V}_f$, whereas low doses did not.[61] R_a was decreased at the two low doses, normal at one high dose, and increased at the highest dose. Fentanyl (25 to 100 μg/mL) causes no change in the permeability of brain microvascular endothelial cells to α-aminoisobutyric acid, sucrose, or Evans blue albumin.[56] All doses of sufentanil studied caused no change in $\dot{V}_f$.[61] R_a was decreased at the two low doses, increased at one high dose, and normal at the highest dose. In addition, sufentanil (0.5 μg/kg, followed by 0.1 μg/kg/hr) combined with thiopental (2 to 5 mg/kg, followed by 1 to 4 mg/kg/hr) caused no greater movement of albumin or IgG into CSF.[44] None of the doses of alfentanil studied caused a change in $\dot{V}_f$.[61] R_a was decreased at the two low doses and normal at the two high doses. Lidocaine (0.5 mg/kg followed by 1 μg/kg/min, 1.5 mg/kg followed by 3 μg/kg/min, and 4.5 mg/kg followed by 9 μg/kg/min) produced a dose/time-related decrease of $\dot{V}_f$ with no change in R_a.[62] Cocaine, in the same doses as lidocaine, caused no significant change of $\dot{V}_f$ or R_a.[62]

The mechanism(s) by which inhalational and intravenous anesthetics alter CSF dynamics is uncertain. The increase in $\dot{V}_f$ with enflurane may result from an enflurane-induced increase in CP metabolism.[63] The decrease of $\dot{V}_f$ with halothane may result from halothane-induced stimulation of vasopressin receptors.[64]

Anesthetics and analgesics move from blood into CSF at varying rates. The free concentration of propofol in CSF was about 30% of the total concentration in CSF and about 60%

Table 3–5 Effects of Opioids and Other Anesthetics on Cerebrospinal (CSF) Dynamics			
	$\dot{V}_f$	R_a	Predicted Effect on Intracranial Pressure
Opioids			
Alfentanil:			
Low dose	0	−	−
High dose	0	0	0
Fentanyl:			
Low dose	0	−	−
High dose	−	0, +	−, ?
Sufentanil:			
Low dose	0	−	−
High dose	0	+, 0	+, 0
Other Anesthetics			
Cocaine	0	0	0
Ketamine	0	+	+
Lidocaine	0, −, a	0	0, −, a

R_a, Resistance to reabsorption of CSF; $\dot{V}_f$, rate of CSF formation; +, increase; 0, no change; −, decrease; a, effect depends on dose; ?, uncertain.

of the free plasma concentration when propofol was infused intravenously as a component of total intravenous anesthesia.[65-68] Entry of intravenous ketoprofen, indomethacin, and ketorolac into CSF is limited.[69-71] Intravenous acetaminophen and ibuprofen permeate readily into CSF.[72,73] CSF concentrations frequently exceed free plasma concentrations. Acetaminophen reaches peak concentrations in CSF at about 1 hour, and concentrations are sufficient to enable rapid central analgesic and antipyretic effects. Ibuprofen peak CSF concentrations occur at about 30 to 40 minutes.

Diuretics

Although diuretics differ in their mechanisms of action, most are reported to decrease $\dot{V}_f$. Acetazolamide reduces $\dot{V}_f$ by up to 50%. Acetazolamide inhibits carbonic anhydrase, the enzyme that catalyzes the hydration of intracellular carbon dioxide, which decreases the amount of hydrogen ions available for exchange with sodium on the abluminal border of the epithelial cell. Acetazolamide may also decrease $\dot{V}_f$ through an indirect action on ion transport mediated by an effect on bicarbonate. Another view is that acetazolamide constricts CP arterioles, reducing CPBF. Methazolamide, another carbonic anhydrase inhibitor, also is reported to reduce $\dot{V}_f$ by up to 50%. The effects of carbonic anhydrase inhibitors are additive with those produced by drugs that work by other mechanisms. For example, the combination of acetazolamide and ouabain decreases $\dot{V}_f$ by 95%.

Ethacrynic acid decreases $\dot{V}_f$, presumably by inhibiting the exchange of sodium ions for potassium or hydrogen at the abluminal border of the cell. Spironolactone and amiloride decrease $\dot{V}_f$, probably by minimizing the entry of sodium into cells at the abluminal transport site. Furosemide decreases $\dot{V}_f$, by reducing either sodium or chloride transport, which is linked to sodium transport on the abluminal surface but follows an electrochemical gradient on the luminal surface. Mannitol decreases $\dot{V}_f$ because of reductions in both CP

output and ECF flow from cerebral tissue to the macroscopic CSF compartment.[74-76]

Steroids

Numerous steroids are reported to alter R_a and $\dot{V}_f$. With increased R_a secondary to pneumococcal meningitis, methylprednisolone reduced R_a to a value that was intermediate between control and untreated animals.[77] It was speculated that methylprednisolone improved CSF flow in the supracortical subarachnoid space or arachnoid villi. When R_a was increased as a result of pseudotumor cerebri, prednisone decreased R_a to a value that was intermediate between pretreatment and normal values for patients.[78] CSF reabsorption may have risen because impaired transport across arachnoid epithelial cells was improved or because metabolically induced changes in the structure of the villi were reversed. Cortisone was reported to decrease $\dot{V}_f$. Rapid uptake of radioactively labeled hydrocortisone into the CP suggests that cortisone exerts its action at the CP rather than at extrachoroidal sites. Dexamethasone decreases $\dot{V}_f$ by up to 50%, probably because it inhibits sodium-potassium adenosine triphosphatase, thereby reducing the activity of the sodium-potassium pump at the CP epithelial membrane.

Other Drugs

Many other drugs are reported to alter $\dot{V}_f$ and R_a. Theophylline increases $\dot{V}_f$, presumably because inhibition of phosphodiesterase elevates CP cyclic adenosine monophosphate levels, stimulating the CP epithelial sodium-potassium pump.[79] Cholera toxin is also reported to increase $\dot{V}_f$.[80] Vasopressin decreases $\dot{V}_f$, perhaps by constricting CP blood vessels. Others contend that physiologic doses of vasopressin provide insufficient CP vascular effect to explain the observed decrease of $\dot{V}_f$.[79,80] Vasopressin also decreases R_a.[80] Hypertonic saline (3%) decreases $\dot{V}_f$, presumably by reducing the osmolality gradient for movement of fluid out of plasma and into the CP stroma or across brain tissue and into CSF.[81] Hypertonic saline increases R_a at some doses but not others. Dinitrophenol decreases $\dot{V}_f$, probably as a result of its ability to uncouple oxidative phosphorylation, thereby reducing the energy available for active secretory and transport processes, such as the membrane pumps. Atrial natriuretic peptides decrease $\dot{V}_f$ by stimulating production of cyclic guanine monophosphate.[80] Digoxin and ouabain decrease $\dot{V}_f$ by inhibition of the sodium-potassium adenosine triphosphatase of the CP epithelial sodium-potassium pump.

In contrast to the aforementioned drugs, both succinylcholine (continuous infusion) and vecuronium (continuous infusion) produce no change in $\dot{V}_f$ or R_a.[82] Prostaglandin E$_1$, when used to induce deliberate, controlled hypotension, caused no change in $\dot{V}_f$.[83]

Neurogenic Regulation of CSF Formation and Resistance to its Reabsorption

Structural Aspects

Adrenergic nerves form networks around the small arteries and veins of the CP, and their nerve terminals are located between the CP endothelium and the underlying fenestrated capillaries.[84] For the most part, these adrenergic nerves originate in the superior cervical ganglia, although some fibers in the CP of the fourth ventricle derive from lower ganglia.[85] Innervation of the lateral ventricles is unilateral, whereas innervation of the midline ventricles is bilateral.

Cholinergic nerves also form networks around the small arteries and veins of the CP, with terminals located between the endothelium and adjacent capillaries.[86] The CP of the third ventricle is richly supplied by cholinergic nerves, but the fourth ventricle is almost devoid of cholinergic innervation. Adrenergic and cholinergic terminals have been identified at the bases of choroid epithelial cells, in the clefts between cells, and near the smooth muscle cells of the choroid arterioles.

Peptidergic nerves are also found in the CP, but their density is less than that of adrenergic and cholinergic nerves.[87] As in the adrenergic and cholinergic networks, peptidergic nerves are located between the small blood vessels of the CP and the overlying CP epithelium.[88] Peptidergic nerves contain vasoactive intestinal peptide or substance P, both of which are potent dilators of cerebral vessels.

Functional Aspects

Studies of the effects of adrenergic stimulation on isolated anterior CP arteries suggest that the adrenergic system plays a role in regulating CPBF.[89] Constriction occurs via α-adrenergic receptors, and relaxation occurs via β-adrenergic receptors. The adrenergic system also appears to exert a functional influence on CP epithelial cells. Carbonic anhydrase activity increased by 125% to 150% in CP homogenate after sympathectomy achieved by surgical removal of the superior cervical ganglion or injection of reserpine. In another study, sympathetic denervation was found to alter epithelial cell transport of organic acids and bases in isolated CP.[90]

In addition, the adrenergic system is reported to alter $\dot{V}_f$. Cervical sympathetic stimulation decreased $\dot{V}_f$ by 32%,[85,91,92] and bilateral excision of the superior cervical ganglia increased $\dot{V}_f$ by 33%. Low norepinephrine concentrations decreased $\dot{V}_f$ by a β-adrenoreceptor–mediated effect on the secretory epithelium, whereas the reduction at high concentrations represents α-adrenoreceptor–mediated CP vasoconstriction. The β-adrenoceptor–induced decrease in $\dot{V}_f$ appears to derive from a direct, inhibitory action on the CP epithelium via β_1-adrenoreceptors.

The cholinergic system is also reported to alter $\dot{V}_f$. Intraventricular perfusion with carbocholine or with acetylcholine in the presence of the cholinesterase inhibitor neostigmine reduced $\dot{V}_f$ by 25% to 55%.[93] Cholinergic receptors presumably are muscarinic because the effect of carbachol is blocked by atropine but is not altered by hexamethonium. The site of action of cholinergic agonists or antagonists is uncertain. They are believed to act on the CP epithelium, rather than on the CP vasculature, because carbocholine has no vasomotor effect on isolated anterior choroidal arteries.

Metabolic Regulation of CSF Formation and Resistance to its Reabsorption

Alterations in metabolism or physiologic status affect $\dot{V}_f$ and $\dot{V}_a$. Hypothermia decreases $\dot{V}_f$, probably by reducing the activity of active secretory and transport processes and by decreasing CBF.[2] Each 1° C reduction in temperature between 41° and 31° C decreases $\dot{V}_f$ by 11%. In one study, hypercapnia raised $\dot{V}_f$ to normal values if $\dot{V}_f$ was decreased at normocapnia but did not change $\dot{V}_f$ if it was normal at normocapnia.[94] Normalization of $\dot{V}_f$ by hypercapnia may have occurred because CPBF improved. In contrast, hypocapnia acutely decreases $\dot{V}_f$, because of reductions of either CPBF or the availability of hydrogen ion for exchange with sodium at the abluminal surface of the CP epithelial cells. After several

hours of hypocapnia, $\dot{V}_f$ returns to normal values.[95,96] Prolonged hypercapnia or hypocapnia does not significantly change $\dot{V}_f$.[94,95] Metabolic acidosis does not change $\dot{V}_f$, but metabolic alkalosis decreases $\dot{V}_f$, presumably as a result of a pH effect unrelated to ion or substrate availability.

Wald and associates[97] found that reduced osmolarity of ventricular CSF or increased osmolarity of serum decreased $\dot{V}_f$; similarly, increased osmolarity of ventricular CSF or reduced osmolarity of serum increased $\dot{V}_f$. The increase or decrease of $\dot{V}_f$ caused by the change in serum osmolarity was four times greater than that caused by a comparable change in ventricular fluid osmolarity. Presumably the changes in $\dot{V}_f$ resulting from altered ventricular fluid osmolarity occurred at the CP, whereas the changes resulting from altered serum osmolarity occurred at extrachoroidal sites.

CSF DYNAMICS AND INTRACRANIAL PRESSURE

Equilibrium Between CSF Formation and Reabsorption

Within limits, $\dot{V}_f$ is not affected by an increase or decrease of ICP. Thus $\dot{V}_f$ remains "normal" whether ICP is 2 cm H_2O or 22 cm H_2O (Fig. 3-5). Only when ICP rises sufficiently to reduce CPP below ~70 mm Hg will $\dot{V}_f$ decrease. In contrast, $\dot{V}_a$ is quite sensitive to change of ICP. At ICPs below ~7 cm H_2O, minimal reabsorption occurs.[98] At ICPs greater than 17 cm H_2O, $\dot{V}_a$ increases directly as ICP increases. The relationship between $\dot{V}_a$ and ICP is linear for ICPs up to ~30 cm H_2O. The equilibrium pressure occurs at the intersection of the plots of $\dot{V}_f$/ICP and $\dot{V}_a$/ICP. At that ICP, $\dot{V}_f$ equals $\dot{V}_a$, and no net change in CSF volume occurs.

Anesthetic- and Drug-Induced Changes in Intracranial Pressure

Treatments that alter $\dot{V}_f$ or $\dot{V}_a$ alter ICP. For example, theophylline is reported to increase $\dot{V}_f$.[79] Assuming no change in $\dot{V}_a$, the plots of $\dot{V}_f$/ICP and $\dot{V}_a$/ICP after administration of

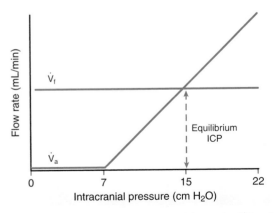

Figure 3–5 Rates of cerebrospinal fluid (CSF) formation ($\dot{V}_f$) and reabsorption ($\dot{V}_a$) are plotted as functions of intracranial pressure (ICP). As long as choroid plexus pressure (CPP) remains above ≈70 mm Hg, $\dot{V}_f$ is unaffected by ICP. At ICP < 7 cm H_2O, $\dot{V}_a$ is minimal. At ICP values between 7 and 25 to 30 cm H_2O, the resistance to CSF reabsorption (R_a) is relatively constant, and $\dot{V}_a$ is linearly related to ICP. ICP stabilizes at a value where $\dot{V}_f$ equals $\dot{V}_a$. *(From Cucchiara RF, Michenfelder JD [eds]: Clinical Neuroanesthesia. New York, Churchill Livingstone, 1990.)*

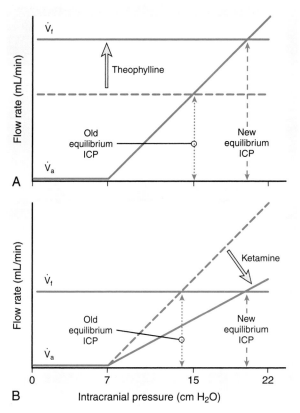

Figure 3–6 **A,** Theophylline increases the rate of cerebrospinal fluid (CSF) formation ($\dot{V}_f$) ("elevating" the slope of $\dot{V}_f$ plotted against intracranial pressure [ICP]). **B,** Ketamine increases the resistance to CSF resorption (R_a) ("flattening" the $\dot{V}_f$/ICP slope). With both treatments, $\dot{V}_f$ equals rate of CSF absorption $\dot{V}_a$ at increased ICP. *(From Cucchiara RF, Michenfelder JD [eds]: Clinical Neuroanesthesia. New York, Churchill Livingstone, 1990.)*

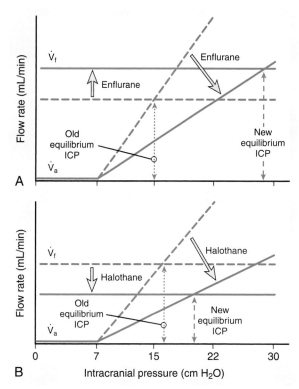

Figure 3–7 **A,** Enflurane at intermediate concentrations increases both the rate of cerebrospinal fluid (CSF) formation $\dot{V}_f$ ("elevating" the slope of $\dot{V}_f$ plotted against intracranial pressure [ICP]) and resistance to CSF reabsorption (R_a) ("flattening" the $\dot{V}_f$/ICP slope). **B,** Halothane decreases $\dot{V}_f$ ("lowering" the $\dot{V}_f$/ICP slope) and increases R_a. With both anesthetics, $\dot{V}_f$ equals $\dot{V}_a$ at increased ICP. *(From Cucchiara RF, Michenfelder JD [eds]: Clinical Neuroanesthesia. New York, Churchill Livingstone, 1990.)*

theophylline intersect at an ICP value that is higher than "normal" (Fig. 3-6A). Stated another way, theophylline increases $\dot{V}_f$ so that the volume of CSF formed each minute exceeds the volume reabsorbed each minute. As a result, CSF volume expands, causing ICP to increase. ICP continues to rise as CSF volume expands, and as ICP rises it provides an increasingly greater "driving force" for reabsorption of CSF. $\dot{V}_a$ increases as ICP increases until $\dot{V}_a$ equals $\dot{V}_f$. A new equilibrium state is achieved when formation and reabsorption are equal and no net change in CSF volume or further change in ICP occurs. The net effect of these changes is that by increasing $\dot{V}_f$, theophylline should cause a rise in ICP, provided that other CSF dynamics are not altered.

Ketamine is reported to increase R_a.[37] By definition, R_a is the inverse of the slope of the relationship between $\dot{V}_a$ and ICP. Increased R_a produces a "flattening" of the $\dot{V}_a$/ICP regression line. Assuming no change in $\dot{V}_f$, the plots of $\dot{V}_f$/ICP and $\dot{V}_a$/ICP after administration of ketamine intersect at an ICP that is higher than normal (Fig. 3-6B). Stated another way, ketamine reduces $\dot{V}_a$ because "normal" ICP does not provide sufficient driving force to cause the usual amounts of CSF to be reabsorbed now that R_a has increased. As a result, the volume of CSF formed each minute exceeds the volume reabsorbed each minute. CSF volume expands, causing ICP to increase. ICP continues to increase as CSF volume expands, and as ICP increases it provides a progressively greater driving force for reabsorption of CSF. $\dot{V}_a$ increases as ICP increases until $\dot{V}_a$ equals $\dot{V}_a$. A new equilibrium is achieved, at which formation and reabsorption are equal and no net change in

CSF volume or further change of ICP occurs. The net effect of these changes is that by increasing R_a, ketamine should cause a rise in ICP, provided that other CSF dynamics are not altered.

Enflurane alters ICP because it increases both $\dot{V}_f$ and R_a (Fig. 3-7A).[36,38,39] Halothane also has combined effects on $\dot{V}_f$ and R_a.[40,41] However, unlike those of enflurane, its effects are opposing rather than additive (Fig. 3-7B).[99] Fentanyl is an example of a drug that decreases ICP. Fentanyl decreases R_a, so the $\dot{V}_a$/ICP regression line becomes "steeper" (Fig. 3-8).[61] Consequently, "normal" ICP, the driving force for reabsorption of CSF, is in excess of what is needed for "normal" $\dot{V}_a$. $\dot{V}_a$ is greater than $\dot{V}_f$, causing a contraction of CSF volume and a reduction of ICP. ICP gradually diminishes, resulting in a lesser driving force for reabsorption of CSF. $\dot{V}_a$, initially greater than $\dot{V}_f$, gradually decreases until, at some reduced ICP, $\dot{V}_a$ is lowered to a value that matches $\dot{V}_f$. A new equilibrium between formation and reabsorption is achieved, and ICP drops no farther.

Furosemide is another example of a drug that decreases ICP. Furosemide decreases $\dot{V}_f$, "lowering" the $\dot{V}_f$/ICP regression line (Fig. 3-9A). As a result, at "normal" ICP, $\dot{V}_a$ exceeds $\dot{V}_f$, causing a contraction of CSF volume and a reduction in ICP. ICP continues to decrease, providing a lesser driving force for reabsorption of CSF. At some reduced ICP, $\dot{V}_a$ is decreased enough to match the reduced $\dot{V}_f$. Formation and reabsorption are in equilibrium at that reduced ICP, and no further decrease of ICP occurs. High doses of etomidate reduce ICP through combined effects on $\dot{V}_f$ and R_a (Fig. 3-9B).[55]

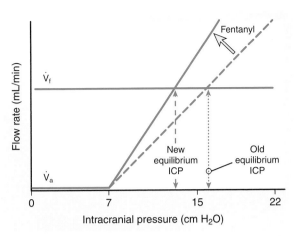

Figure 3–8 Fentanyl in low doses decreases resistance to cerebrospinal fluid (CSF) reabsorption (R_a) ("steepening" the slope of the plot of CSF absorption [$\dot{V}_a$] against intracranial pressure [ICP]). As a result, the rate of CSF formation ($\dot{V}_f$) equals $\dot{V}_a$ at decreased ICP.

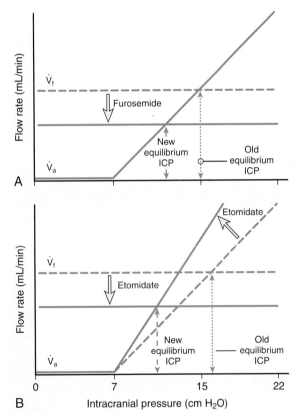

Figure 3–9 **A,** Furosemide decreases the rate of cerebrospinal fluid (CSF) formation ($\dot{V}_f$) ("lowering" the slope of $\dot{V}_f$ plotted against intracranial pressure [ICP]). **B,** Etomidate in high doses decreases $\dot{V}_f$ and the resistance to CSF reabsorption (R_a) ("steepening" the slope of CSF fluid reabsorption [$\dot{V}_a$] plotted against ICP). With both treatments, $\dot{V}_f$ equals $\dot{V}_a$ at decreased ICP. *(From Cucchiara RF, Michenfelder JD [eds]: Clinical Neuroanesthesia. New York, Churchill Livingstone, 1990.)*

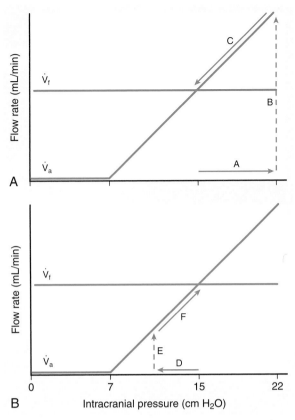

Figure 3–10 Plots of cerebrospinal fluid (CSF) formation ($\dot{V}_f$) versus intracranial pressure (ICP) and rate of CSF reabsorption $\dot{V}_a$ versus ICP show how CSF volume changes to offset changes in intracranial volume, thereby minimizing ICP changes. **A,** Increase in intracranial volume raises ICP. (A) At higher ICP, $\dot{V}_a$ exceeds $\dot{V}_f$, (B) so CSF volume decreases. As CSF volume decreases, ICP decreases (C) until $\dot{V}_f$ equals $\dot{V}_a$. If $\dot{V}_f$ and the resistance to CSF reabsorption (R_a) are not altered, ICP returns to "normal." **B,** Decrease in intracranial volume decreases ICP (D). At decreased ICP, $\dot{V}_a$ (E) is less than $\dot{V}_f$, so CSF volume increases. As CSF volume increases, ICP increases (F) until $\dot{V}_f$ equals $\dot{V}_a$. If $\dot{V}_f$ and R_a are not altered, ICP returns to "normal." *(From Cucchiara RF, Michenfelder JD [eds]: Clinical Neuroanesthesia. New York, Churchill Livingstone, 1990.)*

CSF Volume Change to Compensate for Intracranial Volume Change

When the volume of intracranial blood, brain tissue, gas, or other material increases, CSF volume contracts through translocation of intracranial CSF to the spinal subarachnoid space and through reabsorption of CSF. Conversely, the volume of intracranial blood, brain tissue, gas, or other material decreases, CSF volume expands by means of cephalad translocation and a temporary decrease in $\dot{V}_a$. CSF volume and ICP responses to increases or decreases in intracranial volume are easily illustrated by use of the $\dot{V}_f$/ICP and $\dot{V}_a$/ICP relationships discussed previously. For example, subdural hematoma adds volume to the intracranial contents, thereby raising ICP, as shown in Figure 3-10A: Increased ICP *(A)* provides a driving force for reabsorption of CSF, so $\dot{V}_a$ increases *(B)* to a value greater than $\dot{V}_f$ (which does not change). Consequently, the volume of CSF reabsorbed each minute exceeds the volume of CSF formed each minute. Gradually, CSF volume contracts, and as it does, total intracranial volume decreases, causing ICP to fall *(C)* from its increased level. As ICP approaches "normal," $\dot{V}_a$ falls toward "normal," and the mismatch between $\dot{V}_a$ and $\dot{V}_f$ becomes progressively reduced. When ICP returns to pre-hematoma values, $\dot{V}_f$ and $\dot{V}_a$ once again are in equilibrium, and no further change of CSF volume or ICP occurs. At the new equilibrium state, ICP and total intracranial volume are much the same as before the subdural hematoma, but cerebral blood volume (CBV) (part of it in the form of the hematoma) is increased, and CSF volume is decreased.

Conversely, surgical removal of brain tissue reduces intracranial volume, thereby decreasing ICP, as shown in Figure 3-10B: Reduced ICP (*D*) provides only a weak driving force for reabsorption of CSF, so $\dot{V}_a$ (*E*) is less than $\dot{V}_f$ (which does not change). Thus over the ensuing minutes, the volume of CSF reabsorbed is less than the volume formed. Gradually, CSF volume expands, and as it does, total intracranial volume increases, causing ICP to rise (*F*) from its reduced level. Rising ICP stimulates $\dot{V}_a$. When ICP reaches presurgical values, $\dot{V}_f$ and $\dot{V}_a$ once again are in equilibrium, and no further change of CSF volume or ICP occurs. At the new equilibrium state, ICP and total intracranial volume are much the same as before surgical removal of brain tissue, but brain tissue volume is decreased and CSF volume is increased.

CONDITIONS IN WHICH ALTERED CSF DYNAMICS CHANGE INTRACRANIAL PRESSURE

Responses to Increased Intracranial Pressure

Work in animal models and in clinical studies has demonstrated how $\dot{V}_f$ and R_a affect CSF volume and contribute to ICP change in clinically relevant ways.

Intracranial Mass

Rapid expansion of an intracranial mass causes an increase in ICP followed by compensatory decreases in CBV, CSF volume, and brain tissue volume. For delineation of these changes and the contribution of $\dot{V}_f$ and R_a, three groups of dogs were studied.[100] As reported, hypocapnia initially reduced CBV, and during 4 hours of hypocapnia, CBV reexpanded and CSF volume changed reciprocally (group 1). In group 2, an increase in ICP with an intracranial balloon caused a decrease in CBV and an increase in R_a that were stable for 4 hours. In group 3, balloon inflation reduced CBV, hypocapnia caused a further decrease of CBV, and, during 4 hours of hypocapnia, CBV reexpanded and CSF volume changed reciprocally. Brain tissue composition was not different among the groups.

Effects of Anesthetics

Anesthetics may affect the initial increase in ICP and subsequent compensatory decreases in CBV, CSF volume, and brain tissue volume caused by rapid expansion of an intracranial mass. For examination of these changes and the contribution of $\dot{V}_f$ and R_a, five groups of dogs were anesthetized with inhalational or intravenous agents while an intracranial mass was present, and hypocapnia was used to reduce ICP.[45] With enflurane- and halothane-induced anesthesia, $\dot{V}_f$, R_a, or both were high, and ICP progressively rose because CSF volume did not contract to the same extent that CBV reexpanded. With isoflurane-, fentanyl-, or thiopental-induced anesthesia, $\dot{V}_f$ and R_a were normal, and ICP did not progressively increase because reexpansion of CBV was minimal (fentanyl) or because CSF volume contracted to the same extent that CBV reexpanded (isoflurane and thiopental).

Causes of Increased Intracranial Pressure

Many clinical conditions are accompanied by an increase in ICP. Laboratory and clinical studies have demonstrated the role of altered $\dot{V}_f$ or R_a in clinical conditions in which ICP is increased.

Acute Subarachnoid Hemorrhage

Acute subarachnoid hemorrhage often results in increased ICP. In studies examining the effect of blood components on $\dot{V}_f$ and $\dot{V}_a$ and determining the effects of $\dot{V}_f$ and $\dot{V}_a$ on ICP, animals were intrathecally given (1) heparinized whole blood, (2) plasma, (3) dialysate of plasma, (4) serum (fibrinogen free), and (5) saline.[15,16,101,102] $\dot{V}_a$ values were determined by manometric infusion. Whole blood and plasma raised ICP and produced a threefold to tenfold rise in R_a, respectively. Electron microscopic examination of the arachnoid villi revealed decreased numbers of transendothelial channels and fibrin deposits within the villi.

Chronic Changes after Subarachnoid Hemorrhage

Hydrocephalus often follows subarachnoid hemorrhage. In both animals and patients examined at various intervals after subarachnoid hemorrhage, scanning electron microscopic studies of the CSF pathways and arachnoid villi revealed extensive fibrosis resulting from blood within these spaces.[103] The researchers concluded that after subarachnoid hemorrhage, as well as after other clinical conditions in which leptomeningeal scarring exists, chronic obstruction to CSF outflow results from functional narrowing or blockage of CSF outflow pathways. By this mechanism, R_a is increased within both the subarachnoid space and the arachnoid villi.

Bacterial Meningitis

Bacterial meningitis is often accompanied by increased ICP. In a study examining the effect of meningitis on $\dot{V}_f$ and $\dot{V}_a$ and determining the effects of $\dot{V}_f$ and $\dot{V}_a$ on ICP, animals were intrathecally given (1) *Streptococcus pneumoniae* or (2) *Escherichia coli*.[77] $\dot{V}_f$ and $\dot{V}_a$ were determined before inoculation, 16 to 24 hours after inoculation, and after therapy. ICP rose in both groups. R_a was increased 25-fold with *S. pneumoniae* and 36-fold with *E. coli*, and although antibiotic therapy sterilized the CSF and prevented mortality, R_a remained elevated at 2 weeks after treatment. Methylprednisolone reduced R_a to a value that was intermediate between those in control and infected animals.

Pseudotumor Cerebri

The increased ICP seen in pseudotumor cerebri is thought to result from either (1) increased R_a, (2) increased $\dot{V}_f$, (3) greater water movement into brain across cerebral capillaries, (4) increased CBF and CBV, or (5) glial or neuronal cellular edema.[78] Currently, most evidence favors altered CSF dynamics as the principal cause of increased ICP.[104] In a study to determine the role of CSF dynamics, $\dot{V}_f$ and R_a were measured in both control patients and patients with pseudotumor cerebri.[105] Resting ICP was 33 cm H_2O in patients with pseudotumor cerebri and 14 cm H_2O in controls. Maximal R_a was 10 times greater, and R_a at resting ICP was 6 times greater in the pseudotumor patients than in controls. $\dot{V}_f$ was decreased 39% in the pseudotumor patients, as compared with controls. These results are comparable with results previously reported by others and support the view that in pseudotumor patients, impaired CSF reabsorption is a principal mechanism leading to increased ICP.[106] Prednisone decreased R_a to a value that was intermediate between controls and untreated pseudotumor patients.

Head Injury

Head injury often results in increased ICP. In one study, the PVI was used to determine $\dot{V}_f$, R_a, and the contribution of altered $\dot{V}_f$ and R_a to increased ICP in head-injured patients.[107]

Results showed that R_a was increased but $\dot{V}_f$ was within normal limits for 75% of the patients studied. As calculated, about 20% of the ICP rise in this population derived from $\dot{V}_f$ and R_a.

SUMMARY

CSF plays a key role in brain well-being. It cushions the brain, provides pathways for nutrients and other substrates, regulates the concentrations of ions and other chemicals, provides routes of clearance for unwanted substances, and transports neurohormones and neurotransmitters. Alteration of $\dot{V}_f$ causes a change in ICP, with an increase (or decrease) in $\dot{V}_f$ causing an increase (or decrease) in CSF volume. Alteration of R_a not only causes a change in ICP but also determines the pressure-buffering capacity of the CSF "compartment," with an increase in R_a reducing the ability of CSF volume to contract in response to greater intracranial volume, and vice versa. Studies in animal models of increased ICP report that anesthetic-induced changes in $\dot{V}_f$ and R_a significantly alter the effectiveness of treatments employed to lower ICP. Studies in patients with increased ICP report that $\dot{V}_f$ and R_a may be significant (though not the major) factors altering the effectiveness of treatments to lower ICP.

REFERENCES

1. Sullivan JT, Grouper S, Walker MT, et al: Lumbosacral cerebrospinal fluid volume in humans using three-dimensional magnetic resonance imaging, *Anesth Analg* 103:1306–1310, 2006.
2. Milhorat TH: Pediatric neurosurgery. In Plum F, McDowell FH, editors: *Contemporary Neurology Series*, vol 16, Philadelphia, 1978, FA Davis, pp 91–135.
3. Salvador L, Valero R, Carrero E, et al: Cerebrospinal fluid composition modifications after neuroendoscopic procedures, *Minim Invasive Neurosurg* 50:51–5, 2007.
4. Rapoport SI: *The Blood-Brain Barrier in Physiology and Medicine*, New York, 1976, Raven Press, pp 43–86.
5. Hochwald GM, Gandhi M, Goldman S: Transport of glucose from blood to cerebrospinal fluid in the cat, *Neuroscience* 10:1035–1040, 1983.
6. Hochwald GM, Magee J, Ferguson V: Cerebrospinal fluid glucose: Turnover and metabolism, *J Neurochem* 44:1832–1837, 1985.
7. Pakulski C, Drobnik L, Millo B: Age and sex as factors modifying the function of the blood-cerebrospinal fluid barrier, *Med Sci Monit* 6:314–318, 2000.
8. Weisner B, Bernhardt W: Protein fractions of lumbar, cisternal and ventricular cerebrospinal fluid, *J Neurol Sci* 37:205–214, 1978.
9. Pollay M, Stevens FA, Roberts PA: Alteration in choroid-plexus blood flow and cerebrospinal fluid formation by increased ventricular pressure. In Wood JH, editor: *Neurobiology of Cerebrospinal Fluid*, vol 2, New York, 1983, Plenum Press, pp 687–695.
10. Weiss MH, Wertman N: Modulation of CSF production by alterations in cerebral perfusion pressure, *Arch Neurol* 35:527–529, 1978.
11. DiChiro G, Hammock MK, Bleyer WA: Spinal descent of cerebrospinal fluid in man, *Neurology* 26:1–8, 1976.
12. Upton ML, Weller RO: The morphology of cerebrospinal fluid drainage pathways in human arachnoid granulations, *J Neurosurg* 63:867–875, 1985.
13. Simionescu N, Simionescu M, Palade GE: Structural basis of permeability in sequential segments of the microvasculature of the diaphragm. II: Pathways followed by microperoxidase across the endothelium, *Microvasc Res* 15:17–36, 1978.
14. Johnson RN, Maffeo CJ, Butler AB, et al: Intracranial hypertension in experimental animals and man: Quantitative approach to system dynamics of circulatory cerebrospinal fluid. In Wood JH, editor: *Neurobiology of Cerebrospinal Fluid*, vol 2, New York, 1983, Plenum Press, pp 697–706.
15. Johnson RN, Maffeo CJ, Mann JD, et al: Intracranial pressure regulation: A comparative model of cerebrospinal fluid systems, *TIT J Life Sci* 8:79–92, 1978.
16. Mann JD, Butler AB, Rosenthal JE, et al: Regulation of intracranial pressure in rat, dog, and man, *Ann Neurol* 3:156–165, 1978.
17. Mann JD, Butler AB, Johnson RN, et al: Clearance of macromolecular and particulate substances from the cerebrospinal fluid system of the rat, *J Neurosurg* 50:343–348, 1979.
18. Butler AB, Mann JD, Maffeo CJ, et al: Mechanisms of cerebrospinal fluid absorption in normal and pathologically altered arachnoid villi. In Wood JH, editor: *Neurobiology of Cerebrospinal Fluid*, vol 2, New York, 1983, Plenum Press, pp 707–726.
19. Fenstermacher JD, Patlak CS: The movement of water and solutes in the brain of mammals. In Pappius HM, Feindel W, editors: *Dynamics of Brain Edema*, New York, 1976, Springer-Verlag, p 87.
20. Reulen HJ, Graham R, Spatz M, et al: Role of pressure gradients and bulk flow in dynamics of vasogenic brain edema, *J Neurosurg* 46:24–35, 1977.
21. Reulen HJ, Prioleau GR, Tsuyumu M, et al: Clearance of edema fluid into cerebrospinal fluid: Mechanisms for resolution of vasogenic brain edema. In Wood JH, editor: *Neurobiology of Cerebrospinal Fluid*, vol 2, New York, 1983, Plenum Press, pp 777–787.
22. Klatzo I, Chui E, Fujiwara K, et al: Resolution of vasogenic brain edema (VBE), *Adv Neurol* 28:359–373, 1980.
23. Bito LZ: Absorptive transport of prostaglandins and other eicosanoids across the blood-brain barrier system and its physiological significance. In Suckling AJ, Rumsby MG, Bradbury MWB, editors: *The Blood-Brain Barrier in Health and Disease*, Chichester, UK, 1986, Ellis Horwood Ltd, pp 109–121.
24. Pratt OE, Greenwood J: Movement of vitamins across the blood-brain barrier. In Suckling AJ, Rumsby MG, Bradbury MWB, editors: *The Blood-Brain Barrier in Health and Disease*, Chichester, UK, 1986, Ellis Harwood Ltd, pp 87–97.
25. Rosenberg GA: Glucose, amino acids, and lipids. In Rosenberg GA, editor: *Brain Fluids and Metabolism*, New York, 1990, Oxford University Press, pp 119–144.
26. Leusen IR, Weyne JJ, Demeester GM: Regulation of acid-base equilibrium of cerebrospinal fluid. In Wood JH, editor: *Neurobiology of Cerebrospinal Fluid*, vol 2, New York, 1983, Plenum Press, pp 25–42.
27. Cserr HF, Cooper DM, Milhort TJ: Flow of cerebral interstitial fluid as indicated by the removal of extracellular markers from rat caudate nucleus, *Exp Eye Res* (Suppl) 25:461–473, 1977.
28. Akil H, Richardson DE, Borchas JD, et al: Appearance of beta-endorphin-like immunoreactivity in human ventricular cerebrospinal fluid upon analgesic electrical stimulation, *Proc Natl Acad Sci U S A* 75:5170–5172, 1978.
29. Hosobuchi Y, Rossier J, Bloom FE, et al: Stimulation of human periaqueductal gray for pain relief increases immunoreactive beta-endorphin in ventricular fluid, *Science* 203:279–281, 1979.
30. Jeffcoate WJ, Rees LH, McLoughlin L, et al: β-Endorphin in human cerebrospinal fluid, *Lancet* 2(8081):119–121, 1978.
31. Heisey SR, Held D, Pappenheimer JR: Bulk flow and diffusion in the cerebrospinal fluid system of the goat, *Am J Physiol* 203:775–781, 1962.
32. Pappenheimer JR, Heisey SR, Jordan EF, et al: Perfusion of the cerebral ventricular system in unanesthetized goats, *Am J Physiol* 203:763–774, 1962.
33. Maffeo CJ, Mann JD, Butler AB, et al: Constant flow perfusion of the cerebrospinal fluid system of rat, dog, and man: A mathematical model. In Saha S, editor: *Proceedings of the Fourth New England Bioengineering Conference*, New York, 1976, Pergamon Press, p 447.
34. Marmarou A, Shapiro K, Shulman K: Isolating factors leading to sustained elevations of the ICP. In Beks JWF, Bosch DA, Brock M, editors: *Intracranial Pressure III*, New York, 1976, Springer-Verlag, pp 33–35.
35. Miller JD: Intracranial pressure-volume relationships in pathological conditions, *J Neurosurg Sci* 20:203–209, 1976.
36. Artru AA, Nugent M, Michenfelder JD: Enflurane causes a prolonged and reversible increase in the rate of CSF production in the dog, *Anesthesiology* 57:255–260, 1982.
37. Mann JD, Mann ES, Cookson SL: Differential effect of pentobarbital, ketamine hydrochloride, and enflurane anesthesia on CSF formation rate and outflow resistance in the rat. In Miller JD, Becker DP, Hochwald G, et al, editors: *Intracranial Pressure IV*, New York, 1980, Springer-Verlag, pp 466–471.
38. Artru AA: Effects of enflurane and isoflurane on resistance to reabsorption of cerebrospinal fluid in dogs, *Anesthesiology* 61:529–533, 1984.
39. Artru AA: Concentration-related changes in the rate of CSF formation and resistance to reabsorption of CSF during enflurane and isoflurane anesthesia in dogs receiving nitrous oxide, *J Neurosurg Anesthesiol* 1:256–262, 1989.
40. Artru AA: Effects of halothane and fentanyl on the rate of CSF production in dogs, *Anesth Analg* 62:581–585, 1983.
41. Artru AA: Effects of halothane and fentanyl anesthesia on resistance to reabsorption of CSF, *J Neurosurg* 60:252–256, 1984.

42. Nemoto EM, Stezoski SW, MacMurdo D: Glucose transport across the rat blood-brain barrier during anesthesia, *Anesthesiology* 49:170–176, 1978.

43. Hannan CJ Jr, Kettler TM, Artru AA, et al: Blood-brain barrier permeability during hypocapnia in halothane-anesthetized monkeys, *Ann N Y Acad Sci* 528:172–174, 1988.

44. Pashayan AG, Mickle JP, Vetter TR, et al: Blood-CSF barrier function during general anesthesia in children undergoing ventriculoperitoneal shunt placement [abstract], *Anesth Rev* 15:30–31, 1988.

45. Artru AA: Reduction of cerebrospinal fluid pressure by hypocapnia: Changes in cerebral blood volume, cerebrospinal fluid volume and brain tissue water and electrolytes. II: Effects of anesthetics, *J Cereb Blood Flow Metab* 8:750–756, 1988.

46. Schettini A, Furniss WW: Brain water and electrolyte distribution during the inhalation of halothane, *Br J Anaesth* 51:1117–1124, 1979.

47. Alexander SC, Helmer PH, Ramirez O, et al: Effects of general anesthesia on canine blood-brain barrier glucose transport. In Harper M, Jennett B, Miller O, et al, editors: *Blood Flow and Metabolism in the Brain,* Edinburgh, 1975, Churchill Livingstone, pp 9-37–9-41.

48. Artru AA: Isoflurane does not increase the rate of CSF production in the dog, *Anesthesiology* 60:193–197, 1984.

49. Chi OZ, Anwar M, Sinha AK, et al: Effects of isoflurane anesthesia on the blood-brain barrier transport, *Anesthesiology* 73:A682, 1990.

50. Stover JF, Kempski OS: Anesthesia increases circulating glutamate in neurosurgical patients, *Acta Neurochir (Wien)* 147:847–853, 2005.

51. Sugioka S: Effects of sevoflurane on intracranial pressure and formation and absorption of cerebrospinal fluid in cats, *Masui (Jap J Anesth)* 41:1434–1442, 1992.

52. Artru AA: Rate of cerebrospinal fluid formation, resistance to reabsorption of cerebrospinal fluid, brain tissue water content, and electroencephalogram during desflurane anesthesia in dogs, *J Neurosurg Anesth* 5:178–186, 1993.

53. Artru AA, Powers KM: Furosemide decreases cerebrospinal fluid formation during desflurane anesthesia in rabbits, *J Neurosurg Anesth* 9:166–174, 1997.

54. Saija A, Princi P, Pasquale R, et al: Modifications of the permeability of the blood-brain barrier and local cerebral metabolism in pentobarbital- and ketamine-anaesthetized rats, *Neuropharmacology* 28:997–1002, 1989.

55. Artru AA: Dose-related changes in rate of cerebrospinal fluid formation and resistance to reabsorption of cerebrospinal fluid following administration of thiopental, midazolam, and etomidate in dogs, *Anesthesiology* 69:541–546, 1988.

56. Fischer S, Renz D, Schaper W, et al: In vivo effects of fentanyl, methohexital, and thiopental on brain endothelial permeability, *Anesthesiology* 82:451–458, 1995.

57. Artru AA: Propofol combined with halothane or with fentanyl/halothane does not alter the rate of CSF formation or resistance to reabsorption of CSF in rabbits, *J Neurosurg Anesthesiol* 5:250–257, 1993.

58. Gjedde A, Rasmussen M: Pentobarbital anesthesia reduces blood-brain glucose transfer in the rat, *J Neurochem* 35:1382–1387, 1980.

59. Sage JI, Duffy TE: Pentobarbital anesthesia: Influence on amino acid transport across the blood-brain barrier, *J Neurochem* 33:963–965, 1979.

60. Artru AA: The rate of CSF formation, resistance to reabsorption of CSF, and aperiodic analysis of the EEG following administration of flumazenil to dogs, *Anesthesiology* 72:111–117, 1990.

61. Artru AA: Dose-related changes in the rate of CSF formation and resistance to reabsorption of CSF during administration of fentanyl, sufentanil, or alfentanil in dogs, *J Neurosurg Anesthesiol* 3:283–290, 1991.

62. Artru AA, Bernards CM, Mautz DS, et al: Intravenous lidocaine decreases but cocaine does not alter the rate of cerebrospinal fluid formation in anesthetized rabbits, *J Neurosurg Anesthesiol* 9:31–43, 1997.

63. The 1978 ASA Annual Meeting was held in Chicago, Oct. 21—25, 1978. It was held at the Conrad Hilton & Chicago Marriott.

64. Maktabi MA, El Bokl FF, Todd MM: Effect of halothane anesthesia on production of cerebrospinal fluid: Possible role of vasopressin V1 receptors [abstract], *J Cereb Blood Flow Metab* 11:S268, 1991.

65. Dawidowicz AL, Kalitynski R, Fijalkowska A: Free and bound propofol concentrations in human cerebrospinal fluid, *Br J Clin Pharmacol* 56:545–550, 2003.

66. Dawidowicz AL, Kalitynski R, Fijalkowska A: Relationships between total and unbound propofol in plasma and CSF during continuous drug infusion, *Clin Neuropharmacol* 27:129–132, 2004.

67. Luo W, Li YH, Yang JJ, et al: Cerebrospinal fluid and plasma propofol concentration during total intravenous anaesthesia of patients undergoing elective intracranial tumor removal, *J Zhejian Univ Sci B* 6:865–868, 2005.

68. Dawidowicz AL, Kalitynski R, Mardarowicz M: The changes of propofol concentration in human cerebrospinal fluid after drug infusion, *Clin Neuropharmacol* 29:3–5l, 2006.

69. Mannila A, Hokki H, Heikkinen M, et al: Cerebrospinal fluid distribution of ketoprofen after intravenous administration in young children, *Clin Pharmacokinet* 45:737–743, 2006.

70. Mannila A, Kumpulainen E, Lehtonen M, et al: Plasma and cerebrospinal fluid concentrations of indomethacin in children after intravenous administration, *J Clin Pharmacol* 47:94–100, 2007.

71. Kumpulainen E, Kokki H, Laisalmi M, et al: How readily does ketorolac penetrate cerebrospinal fluid in children? *J Clin Pharmacol* 48:495–501, 2008.

72. Kumpulainen E, Kokki H, Halonen T, et al: Paracetamol (acetaminophen) penetrates readily into the cerebrospinal fluid of children after intravenous administration, *Pediatrics* 119:766–771, 2007.

73. Kokki H, Kumpulainen E, Lehtonen M, et al: Cerebrospinal fluid distribution of ibuprofen after intravenous administration in children, *Pediatrics* 120:e1002–e1008, 2007.

74. Rosenberg GA, Kyner WT: Effect of mannitol-induced hyperosmolarity on transport between brain interstitial fluid and cerebrospinal fluid. In Wood JH, editor: *Neurobiology of Cerebrospinal Fluid,* vol 2, New York, 1983, Plenum Press, pp 765–775.

75. Rosenberg GA, Kyner WT, Estrada E: Bulk flow of brain interstitial fluid under normal and hyperosmolar conditions, *Am J Physiol* 238:F42–F49, 1980.

76. Sahar A, Tsipstein E: Effects of mannitol and furosemide on the rate of formation of cerebrospinal fluid, *Exp Neurol* 60:584–591, 1978.

77. Dacey RGJ, Scheld WM, Winn HR: Bacterial meningitis: Selected aspects of cerebrospinal fluid pathophysiology. In Wood JH, editor: *Neurobiology of Cerebrospinal Fluid,* vol 2, New York, 1983, Plenum Press, pp 727–738.

78. Mann JD, Johnson RN, Butler AB, et al: Cerebrospinal fluid circulatory dynamics in pseudotumor cerebri and response to steroid therapy. In Wood JH, editor: *Neurobiology of Cerebrospinal Fluid,* vol 2, New York, 1983, Plenum Press, pp 739–751.

79. Wright EM: Transport processes in the formation of cerebrospinal fluid, *Rev Physiol Biochem Pharmacol* 83:1–34, 1978.

80. Rosenberg GA: Physiology of cerebrospinal and interstitial fluids. In Rosenberg GA, editor: *Brain Fluids and Metabolism,* New York, 1990, Oxford University Press, pp 36–57.

81. Foxworthy JCI, Artru AA: Cerebrospinal fluid dynamics and brain tissue composition following intravenous infusion of hypertonic saline in anesthetized rabbits, *J Neurosurg Anesthesiol* 2:256–265, 1990.

82. Artru AA: Muscle relaxation with succinylcholine or vecuronium does not alter the rate of CSF production or resistance to reabsorption of CSF in dogs, *Anesthesiology* 68:392–396, 1988.

83. Fujita N: Prostaglandin E1-induced hypotension: Its effect on rate of cerebrospinal fluid formation in anesthetized cats, *J Osaka Dent Univ* 27:67–76, 1993.

84. Lindvall M: Fluorescence histochemical study on regional differences in the sympathetic nerve supply of the choroid plexus from various laboratory animals, *Cell Tissue Res* 198:261–267, 1979.

85. Lindvall M, Edvinsson L, Owman C: Sympathetic nervous control of cerebrospinal fluid production from the choroid plexus, *Science* 201:176–207, 1978.

86. Lindvall M, Edvinsson L, Owman C: Histochemical study on regional differences in the cholinergic nerve supply of the choroid plexus from various laboratory animals, *Exp Neurol* 55:152–159, 1977.

87. Larsson LI, Edvinsson L, Fohrenkrug J, et al: Immunohistochemical localization of a vasodilatory peptide (VIP) in cerebrovascular nerves, *Brain Res* 113:400–404, 1976.

88. Lindvall M, Alumets J, Edvinsson L, et al: Peptidergic (VIP) nerves in the mammalian choroid plexus, *Neurosci Lett* 9:77–82, 1978.

89. Edvinsson L, Lindvall M: Autonomic vascular innervation and vasomotor reactivity in the choroid plexus, *Exp Neurol* 62:394–404, 1978.

90. Winbladh B, Edvinsson L, Lindvall M: Effect of sympathectomy on active transport mechanisms in choroid plexus in vitro, *Acta Physiol Scand* 102:85A, 1978.

91. Haywood JR, Vogh BP: Some measurements of autonomic nervous system influence on production of cerebrospinal fluid in the cat, *J Pharmacol Exp Ther* 208:341–346, 1979.

92. Lindvall M, Edvinsson L, Owman C: Effect of sympathomimetic drugs and corresponding receptor antagonists on the rate of cerebrospinal fluid production, *Exp Neurol* 64:132–148, 1979.

93. Lindvall M, Edvinsson L, Owman C: Reduced cerebrospinal fluid formation through cholinergic mechanisms, *Neurosci Lett* 10:311–316, 1978.

94. Heisey SR, Adams T, Fisher MJ, et al: Effect of hypercapnia and cerebral perfusion pressure on cerebrospinal fluid production in the cat, *Am J Physiol* 244:R224–R227, 1983.

95. Artru AA, Hornbein TF: Prolonged hypocapnia does not alter the rate of CSF production in dogs during halothane anesthesia or sedation with nitrous oxide, *Anesthesiology* 67:66–71, 1987.

96. Martins AN, Doyle TF, Newby N: PCO2 and rate of formation of cerebrospinal fluid in the monkey, *Am J Physiol* 231:127–131, 1976.

97. Wald A, Hochwald GM, Gandhi M: Evidence for the movement of fluid, macromolecules and ions from the brain extracellular space to the CSF, *Brain Res* 151:283–290, 1978.

98. Brumback RA: Anatomic and physiologic aspects of the cerebrospinal fluid space. In Herndon RM, Brumback RA, editors: *The Cerebrospinal Fluid*, Boston, 1989, Kluwer Academic, pp 15–43.

99. Artru AA: Relationship between cerebral blood volume and CSF pressure during anesthesia with halothane or enflurane in dogs, *Anesthesiology* 58:533–539, 1983.

100. Artru AA: Reduction of cerebrospinal fluid pressure by hypocapnia: Changes in cerebral blood volume, cerebrospinal fluid volume, brain tissue water and electrolytes, *J Cereb Blood Flow Metab* 7:471–479, 1987.

101. Butler AB, Maffeo CJ, Johnson RN, et al: Impaired absorption of CSF during experimental subarachnoid hemorrhage: Effects of blood components on vesicular transport in arachnoid villi. In Shulman K, Marmarou A, Miller JD, et al, editors: *Intracranial Pressure IV*, New York, 1980, Springer-Verlag, pp 245–248.

102. Johnson RN, Maffeo CJ, Dacey RG, et al: Mechanism for intracranial hypertension during experimental subarachnoid hemorrhage: Acute malfunction of arachnoid villi by components of plasma, *Trans Am Neurol Assoc* 103:138–142, 1978.

103. Suzuki S, Ishii M, Iwabuchi T: Posthaemorrhagic subarachnoid fibrosis in dogs: Scanning electron microscopic observation and dye perfusion study, *Acta Neurochir* 46:105–117, 1979.

104. Johnston I: The definition of a reduced CSF absorption syndrome: A reappraisal of benign intracranial hypertension and related syndromes, *Med Hypotheses* 1:10–14, 1975.

105. Mann JD, Johnson RN, Butler AB, et al: Impairment of cerebrospinal fluid circulatory dynamics in pseudotumor cerebri and response to steroid treatment [abstract], *Neurology* 29:550, 1979.

106. Johnston I, Paterson A: Benign intracranial hypertension. II: CSF pressure and circulation, *Brain* 97:301–312, 1974.

107. Becker DP: *Isolation of factors leading to raised ICP in head-injured patients*, Atlanta, 1985, A preliminary report [abstract]. Presented at 53rd Annual Meeting of the American Association of Neurological Surgeons.

108. Cerebrospinal fluid. In Diem K, Lentner C, editors: *Scientific Tables*, ed 7, Basel, 1970, JR Geigy, pp 635–640.

109. Hochwald GM: Cerebrospinal fluid mechanisms. In Cottrell JRE, Turndorf H, editors: *Anesthesia and Neurosurgery*, St Louis, 1986, Mosby, pp 33–53.

110. Wood JH: Physiology, pharmacology, and dynamics of cerebrospinal fluid. In Wood JH, editor: *Neurobiology of Cerebrospinal Fluid*, vol 1, New York, 1980, Plenum Press, pp 1–16.

Chapter 4

INTRACRANIAL PRESSURE MONITORING

Paolo A. Bolognese • Thomas H. Milhorat

The intracranial pressure (ICP) is the final result of a complex interaction of hemodynamic, metabolic, and anatomic factors. The purpose of this chapter is to provide the reader with an array of basic concepts with which to tackle the needs of daily clinical practice.

NORMAL AND PATHOLOGIC DETERMINANTS OF INTRACRANIAL PRESSURE

Simplifying to the extreme, the skull is a rigid box with three contents: brain, blood, and cerebrospinal fluid (CSF).[1] The box is lightly stuffed by its contents, resulting in a mildly positive baseline pressure. Metabolic requirements, as well as cardiac and respiratory variations, modulate the cerebral blood flow (CBF), with repercussions for the cerebral blood volume. Small amounts of CSF are periodically shifted on demand from the intracranial to the intraspinal compartment to buffer the effects of the cerebral blood volume variations on the ICP. The normal brain volume is on average around 1400 mL, whereas the intracranial CSF volume averages 75 to 100 mL, and the cerebral blood volume is about 150 mL. The fine mechanisms that are the suprastructure of this basic scenario are quite complicated.

The skull is not a single-chambered box; it is divided in compartments by semirigid dural structures (falx and tentorium). In early life it is a somewhat pliable encasement, and even later in life the rigidity of the skull is not an absolute concept.

At a macroscopic level, the brain is not a uniform structure (cerebral and cerebellar hemispheres, the brainstem, etc.). Instead, it has a biphasic composition (white and gray matter). At a microscopic level, there is an intracellular compartment as well as an extracellular compartment.

The brain's metabolism is also not uniform and constant but instead has regional surges connected to the electrical activity. The regional metabolism is the major determinant of the regional CBF, via the intervention of vasoactive agents that change the regional cerebrovascular resistance (CVR) by constricting or dilating microvascular networks. Carbon dioxide (CO_2), pH, and adenosine are among the strongest vasoactive agents.

A further level of safety is autoregulation, a buffer system that (in the face of changing metabolic requirements) provides a constant CBF corresponding to the physiologic and pathologic swings of the arterial blood pressure. This mechanism is achieved through a direct control on the CVR (vasodilation and vasoconstriction) and is active between an upper level and a lower level of arterial blood pressure. The autoregulatory function is modulated by a number of physiologic and pathologic factors, including age, hormones, and hypertension.

The pressure differential between the arterial side and the venous side is the driving force of the blood navigating through the vascular network. This pressure differential is called *cerebral perfusion pressure* (CPP) when applied to the brain circulation.[2] The arterial pressure in the major arteries of the circle of Willis is mildly lower than the aortic blood pressure. The bridging veins to the dural sinuses are the electrical equivalent of a resistor and are easily compressible by steady surges of intraparenchymal or CSF pressure; the pressure within these veins is considered almost equivalent to the CSF pressure and the ICP.[3] The pressure in the dural sinuses is subatmospheric in the standing position. The dural sinuses are poorly compressible and are not affected by moderate elevations in ICP. The "zero reference hemodynamic level" for the cerebral circulation is set at the jugular foramen; this fact should be remembered when accurate CPP estimates need to be obtained in an intensive care unit setting, with the patient in a semi-Fowler's position.

According to Ohm's law, perfusion pressure and blood flow are linked by a third entity that expresses the resistance to flow. In cerebral hemodynamic terms, the CPP is equal to the product of CBF and CVR.[4]

The CSF is an extracellular fluid that has a number of functions, including waste removal and mechanical protection. Part of it is contained inside the brain and spinal cord, and part outside. It has a passive circulation, like the lymphatic fluid outside the central nervous system. Part of it is produced by the choroid plexuses, but its bulk is "sweated" by the central nervous system. Its volume is modulated by a number of factors, including the general level of hydration of the body, the renal function, as well as hormonal agents like progesterone.

In physiologic conditions, the ICP has a mean value, with superimposed cardiac, respiratory, and vasomotor variations. Sudden and short-lasting elevations in intra-abdominal and intrathoracic pressures (such as during coughing or straining) result in parallel and significant elevations of the ICP, with minimal or no interference with the brain metabolism and function. In certain pathologic conditions, the compliance of the intracranial system is compromised and the same intra-abdominal and intra-thoracic elevations can result in prolonged ICP surges, which will interfere with the cerebral metabolism and function; this breakdown is linked to the activation of a number of complex vicious circles. For example, the elevated ICP compresses the cerebral bridging veins, causing venous stasis, which slows down the microcirculatory flow, causing hypoxia and the consequent release of vasoactive agents, which further increase the CBV, and promotes cerebral edema (in both its cytotoxic and vasogenic components), which increases the distance between the capillaries and the target neural cells, further promoting hypoxia and ischemia.

The ICP and the overall intracranial volume (the sum of the volumes of blood, brain, and CSF) tend to display a linear relationship under physiologic and paraphysiologic conditions, until a critical point, defined as the "breakpoint," at which the destabilizing positive feedback of the pathologic vicious cycles kick in. Above the breakpoint, the relationship between ICP and intracranial volume is no longer linear but becomes exponential, meaning that small changes in volume dictate far larger changes in pressure. The pitch of the pressure-volume plot, in both its physiologic and pathologic segments, is influenced by any factor affecting the compliance of the system, such as age, hormones, and hematocrit value.

Elevations of the ICP can be diffuse, as in the case of pseudotumor cerebri (PTC), or focal, as in the case of a frontal glioblastoma. In the first case, the overall brain function is affected, whereas in the second, the pressures are not homogeneous and can be represented in the same fashion as atmospheric pressures on a weather map, with isobars (contour lines of equal pressure). The orientation of the isobars is affected by poorly compressible mechanical obstacles, such as bone and dural septations, with the formation of pressure cones that can acutely distort nearby neural and vascular structures along anatomic "choke points" like the subfalcine and transtentorial regions.[5,6] The previously mentioned distortions can generate secondary foci of brain damage and cerebral ischemia, with overall destabilizing effects on the ICP.[7]

Under pathologic conditions, the suppression of the autoregulatory mechanisms of negative feedback brings about a destabilization of the ICP equilibrium, with the formation of periodic variations, defined as the *Lundberg's waves*. Lundberg's A waves (also called "plateau waves") are characterized by a sudden steep ICP increase to 80 to 100 mm Hg that is sustained over several minutes and then rapidly extinguished.[8] Lundberg's B and C waves are respectively related to the effects of vasomotor variations and Traube-Hering respiratory variations on the ICP; their magnitude and duration are less than those of the A waves.[9,10]

As explained previously, changes in the CVR (via vasodilatation and vasoconstriction) can be affected by Pco_2 levels (the CO_2 vasoreactivity) and take part in the mechanisms of pressure-flow autoregulation. The autoregulation is more fragile than the CO_2 vasoreactivity. When only the first mechanism is compromised by pathologic events, the scenario is defined as *dissociated vasoparalysis*. When both mechanisms are disrupted by more severe pathologic events, we face *total vasoparalysis*. The difference between dissociated vasoparalysis and total vasoparalysis is of key importance to the ICU care of neurosurgical patients, because hyperventilation can be effective in the first condition but not in the second. Disruption of the pressure-flow autoregulation through the use of vasopressor drugs can be used to the patient's advantage. If total vasoparalysis is present in one area of the brain, but dissociated vasoparalysis is present in an adjacent region, therapeutic hyperventilation can trigger the so-called Robin Hood effect. This effect, in essence, occurs when the vessels in the less damaged area vasoconstrict and the blood flow is shifted toward the vasoparalyzed circulation of the more compromised area, leading to greater vasoactive edema and hemorrhagic infarction.[11]

TECHNIQUES OF INTRACRANIAL PRESSURE MONITORING

ICP monitoring is an important component of neurointensive care. A number of technical modalities have been available over the years, though none of them is perfect from a pure engineering point of view. All of them violate in different amounts the principle requiring the monitor not to interfere with the observed parameter.

Some of them, like epidural ICP monitoring, are now obsolete. Others, such as subdural ICP monitoring, have limited applications, being used primarily in postoperative situations. Lumbar CSF pressure monitoring, which should not be used in the presence of intracranial disorders because of the risk of downward herniation, is affected by inaccuracies caused by the small caliber and the long length of the indwelling catheter.

Two modalities of ICP monitoring are currently favored, the intraparenchymal and intraventricular techniques.

The intraventricular technique is accurate but requires cannulation of one of the ventricular frontal horns in situations in which the ventricles are very small and subject to midline shifting.[12] The ventriculostomy tubing requires some maintenance, because brain tissue or clots can plug the lumen. CSF infection, overshunting, and intraparenchymal and intraventricular hemorrhages are among the most common complications associated with this technique. The ventricular catheter requires antibiotic prophylaxis. Antibiotic-coated indwelling tubing has been introduced on the market, with claims of reduced infection rates. In our experience, the best-protecting factors against ventriculostomy infections are a combination of maintenance, antibiotic prophylaxis, and careful occlusive sterile dressing. For accurate readings, the system should be zeroed on a daily basis, with the jugular foramen (projected at the tragus) as the zero reference level.

Intraparenchymal techniques rely on technical variations of the strain gauge method. Zeroing is performed once, prior to intraparenchymal insertion of the sensor, and the catheter is held in place by a variety of devices, the most popular being the bolt screw. This method is user friendly, requires minimal maintenance, and is easily movable during patient transport. A technical drawback is represented by the zero drift, with the zero reference line drifting upward at rates of 1 to 2 mm Hg per day.[13]

During the last decades, efforts have been made to combine ICP information with the monitoring of other parameters. CPP can be now calculated and plotted in real time by modern overhead digital intensive care unit monitors, once ICP and arterial blood pressure are fed to such systems.

CBF can be now monitored in real time by thermal diffusion and laser Doppler flowmetry. Thermal diffusion provides regional CBF values, whereas laser Doppler flowmetry measures local CBF because of its smaller sample volume. Commercially available systems allow simultaneous CBF and ICP monitoring through combined probes. The simultaneous availability of ICP, CPP, and CBF values allows the calculation of CVR. Limitations of these CBF monitoring techniques include intensive maintenance, small sample volume, and invasiveness.

Intraparenchymal Po_2, Pco_2, and pH can be monitored through small indwelling intraparenchymal probes. The readings are accurate, but the technique is labor intensive.[14,15]

ICP monitoring can also be coupled with other noninvasive techniques, such as near-infrared spectroscopy (NIRS) for the measurement of CBF, and somatosensory evoked potentials (SSEPs).

A number of noninvasive techniques have been developed to provide approximate estimates of ICP. Optical coherence tomography (OCT) explores the fundus and quantifies elevation of the papilla, whereas another method relies on the measurement of the cochlear impedance.

CLINICAL INDICATIONS FOR INTRACRANIAL PRESSURE MONITORING

Trauma and subarachnoid hemorrhage are the two prime indications for ICP monitoring.[16,17] The classic indication is in the patient in a coma with a Glasgow Coma Scale score of 7 or less.[18] Control of the mean ICP values, prompt treatment of A waves, and optimization of the CPP are the mainstay of applied monitoring.

ICP monitoring is sometimes used in non-comatose patients in selected cases of hydrocephalus and pseudotumor cerebri.[19] The ICP information is used to choose the most suitable shunting strategy in difficult cases.[20]

ICP monitoring is occasionally used in the postoperative or postembolic management of arteriovenous malformations, when swelling and perfusion breakthrough are at their peaks.

Autoregulation can be easily tested in patients with combined ICP/CBF monitoring, with repercussions on the management of systemic blood pressure.

CO_2 vasoreactivity, once a mainstay of critical care in patients with head trauma, is now subject to a revisionist view because of its tendency to cause rebound hyperemia and Robin Hood effect, as well as loss of efficacy when used over prolonged periods.

THE FUTURE OF INTRACRANIAL PRESSURE MONITORING

ICP monitoring is and will remain an important tool in the management of the patient with critical neurologic status.[21] In the future, current efforts will deliver monitoring techniques that are more reliable, less invasive, and more accurate. Another impetus will reside in more sophisticated mathematical analyses of the ICP information, to derive a better insight into the mechanisms of pathology and to allow prediction of catastrophic events, as in the case of applied fractal analysis, which has been applied to the analysis of heart rate dynamics to predict myocardial ischemia and related mortality.

REFERENCES

1. Monro A: *Observations on the Structure and the Function of the Nervous System*, Edinburgh, 1783, Creech & Johnson.
2. Rosner MJ, Rosner SD, Johnson AH: Cerebral perfusion pressure: Management protocol and clinical results [see comments], *J Neurosurg* 83:949–962, 1995.
3. Ryder HW, Espey FF, Kimbell FD, et al: Effect of changes in systemic venous pressure on cerebrospinal fluid pressure, *Arch Neurol Psychiatry* 68:175–179, 1952.
4. Czosnyka M, Smielewski P, Kirkpatrick P, et al: Continuous assessment of the cerebral vasomotor reactivity in head injury, *Neurosurgery* 41:11–17, 1997:discussion, 17-19.
5. Jefferson G: The tentorial pressure cone, *Arch Neurol Psychiatry* 40: 857–875, 1938.
6. Meyer A: Herniation of the brain, *Arch Neurol Psychiatry* 4:387, 1920.
7. Ropper AH: A preliminary study of the geometry of brain displacement and level of consciousness in patients with acute intracranial masses, *Neurology* 39:622–627, 1989.
8. Risberg J, Lundberg N, Ingrav DH: Regional cerebral blood volume during acute rises of the intracranial pressure (plateau waves), *J Neurosurg* 31:303–310, 1969.
9. Newell DW, Aaslid R, Stooss R, et al: The relationship of blood flow velocity fluctuations to intracranial pressure B waves, *J Neurosurg* 75:415–421, 1992.
10. Kjallgvist A, Lundberg N, Ponten U: Respiratory and cardiovascular changes during spontaneous variations of ventricular fluid pressure in patients with intracranial hypertension, *Acta Neurol Scand* 40:291–317, 1964.
11. The use of hyperventilation in the acute management of severe traumatic brain injury. Brain Trauma Foundation, *J Neurotrauma* 13:699–703, 1996.
12. Lundberg N: Continuous recording and monitoring of ventricular fluid pressure in neurosurgical practice, *Acta Psychiatr Neurol Scand* 36(Suppl 149):1–193, 1960.
13. Bavetta S, Norris JS, Wyatt M, et al: Prospective study of zero drift in fiberoptic pressure monitors used in clinical practice, *J Neurosurg* 86:927–930, 1997.
14. Kiening KL, Unterberg AW, Bardt TF, et al: Monitoring of cerebral oxygenation in patients with severe head injuries: Brain tissue PO_2 versus jugular vein oxygen saturation, *J Neurosurg* 85:751–757, 1996.
15. Persson L, Hillered L: Chemical monitoring of neurosurgical intensive care patients using intracerebral microdialysis, *J Neurosurg* 76:72–80, 1992.
16. Obrist WD, Langfitt TW, Jaggi JL, et al: Cerebral blood flow and metabolism in comatose patients with acute head injury: Relationship to intracranial hypertension, *J Neurosurg* 61:241–253, 1984.
17. Lundberg N, Troupp H, Lorin H: Continuous recording of ventricular fluid pressure in patients with severe acute traumatic brain injury: A preliminary report, *J Neurosurg* 22:581–590, 1965.
18. Indications for intracranial pressure monitoring: Brain Trauma Foundation, *J Neurotrauma* 13:667–679, 1996.
19. Shulman K, Ransohoff J: Sagittal sinus venous pressure in hydrocephalus, *J Neurosurg* 23:169–173, 1965.
20. Chapman PH, Cosman ER, Arnold MA: The relationship between ventricular fluid pressure and body position in normal subjects and subjects with shunts: a telemetric study, *Neurosurgery* 26:181–189, 1990.
21. Marshall LF, Smith RW, Shapiro HM: The outcome with aggressive treatment in severe head injuries. I: The significance of intracranial pressure monitoring, *J Neurosurg* 50:20–25, 1979.

Chapter 5

EFFECTS OF ANESTHETIC AGENTS AND OTHER DRUGS ON CEREBRAL BLOOD FLOW, METABOLISM, AND INTRACRANIAL PRESSURE

Takefumi Sakabe • Mishiya Matsumoto

Major goals in neurosurgical anesthesia are to provide adequate tissue perfusion to the brain (and spinal cord) so that the regional metabolic demand is met and to provide adequate surgical conditions (a "relaxed brain"). If anesthetic drugs or anesthetic techniques are improperly used, they can worsen the existing intracranial pathologic condition and may produce new damage. Some anesthetics or anesthetic techniques may help protect the brain subjected to metabolic stress or even ameliorate damage from such an insult. Thus knowledge of the effects of anesthetics and anesthetic techniques on cerebral circulation, metabolism, and intracranial pressure (ICP) both in normal and pathologic conditions is important. In addition, special attention must be paid to these effects during functional neurosurgery or minimally invasive surgery such as awake surgery, stereotaxic surgery, identification of epileptic foci, and neuroradiologic interventional procedures, in which anesthesiologists should consider using anesthetics and adjuvant drugs that allow control of asleep-awake-asleep status or sedation with analgesia and with no or minimal interference with brain electrophysiologic monitoring or neurologic findings. While providing such a state, the anesthesiologist should assure patency of the airway with well-maintained ventilation and circulatory stability.

In this chapter, physiologic and pharmacologic considerations in relation to neurosurgical anesthesia are summarized, followed by a review of the effects of anesthetics and other drugs on cerebral blood flow (CBF), cerebral metabolism, and ICP. The clinical relevance of these issues to the practice of neurosurgical anesthesia is discussed.

PHYSIOLOGIC AND PHARMACOLOGIC CONSIDERATIONS IN RELATION TO NEUROSURGICAL ANESTHESIA

Blood Flow and Metabolism Changes in Relation to Functional Changes

Under physiologic conditions, the brain vessel diameter changes within seconds in response to the changes in neuronal activity that immediately influence metabolic demand. Although the cellular mechanisms underlying the coupling of neuronal activation to cerebral blood vessel responses are not yet fully determined, there may be two types of local cerebral blood flow (lCBF) modulation, the phasic response mediated by transient neuronal activity and the tonic activation by local astrocytes—the latter mechanism being supported by evidence that astrocytes control vascular tone and supply energy metabolites to neurons on demand.[1] Phasic (fast and transient) vasomodulation is regulated by various substances released from neurons, including nitric oxide (NO), vasoactive intestinal peptide, and potassium ion (K^+), whereas tonic (slow and long-lasting) vasomodulation is regulated by metabolites of the arachidonic acid from astrocytes, including 20-hydroxyeicosatetraenoic acid, prostaglandin E_2, and epoxy icosatrienoic acid. The cerebral vessel is constricted by 20-hydroxyeicosatetraenoic acid but dilated by prostaglandin E_2 and epoxye (epoxyeicosatrienoic) icosatrienoic acid.[1] These metabolites are generated as a result of astrocytic calcium ion (Ca^{2+}) surges triggered by glutamate released from neurons. However, what determines whether the vessel constricts or dilates in relation to astrocytic function in a given condition remains unknown.

Cerebral activation can result in a much greater increase in glucose consumption than in oxygen consumption. This phenomenon can be explained by "the astrocyte-neuron lactate shuttle hypothesis," in which astrocytic activation by glutamate released from neurons stimulates glucose uptake into astrocytes; glucose is processed glycolytically, resulting in a release of lactate as an energy substrate for neurons.[2] How metabolic changes from this shuttle system influence cerebral vascular tone remains to be clarified.

Anesthetics cause functional alterations in the central nervous system and produce metabolic changes. In general, intravenous anesthetics decrease cerebral metabolic rate (CMR) and CBF in parallel fashion, whereas most inhalational anesthetics decrease CMR with an increase in CBF. At first sight, the coupling of CMR and CBF is maintained with intravenous anesthetics, whereas it is lost with inhalational anesthetics. However, a strong correlation exists between CMR and CBF within individual brain structures during anesthesia. Indeed, during burst and suppression phases of the electroencephalogram (EEG) with isoflurane anesthesia, cerebral blood flow velocity of middle cerebral artery (Vmca) appears to increase and decrease, respectively.[3,4] In addition, seizure activity or noxious stimuli during anesthesia produce parallel increases in CBF and CMR. Because the net effect of anesthetics on CBF is a balance between their direct effects on cerebral vessels and indirect effects caused by CMR changes, it is probable that the coupling of CMR and CBF is maintained with anesthetics but is modified by direct effects of anesthetics on vascular tone.

Blood Flow Changes in Relation to Cerebral Perfusion Pressure and Carbon Dioxide

Cerebral perfusion pressure (CPP) and carbon dioxide tension in the arterial blood (Paco2) are the important variables that influence CBF. Autoregulation is the physiologic maintenance of constant CBF over a wide range of CPP values. Traditionally, CPP is determined as the difference between mean arterial blood pressure (MABP) and the greater of ICP or CVP. In the patient with intracranial hypertension, effective downstream pressure is determined by ICP. Advances in flow measurement techniques have demonstrated beat-to-beat flow changes and the concept of apparent zero flow pressure, at which flow ceases. Apparent zero flow pressure has been proposed as an estimate of critical closing pressure that may better estimate CPP.[5] In conditions of increased cerebrovascular tone, such as hypocapnia or pharmacologically induced vasoconstriction, ICP does not uniquely determine effective downstream pressure. Impairment of CBF induced by hypocapnia may be related to the reduction in CPP associated with the increase in effective downstream pressure.

CO2 can produce marked changes in Cerebrovascular resistance (CVR) and CBF. Over a range of Paco2 values of 20 to 80 mm Hg, for each 1–mm Hg increase or decrease in Paco2 there is a 2% to 4% increase or decrease in CBF. Changes in the extracellular hydrogen ion (H+) concentration, NO, prostanoids, cyclic nucleotides, intracellular calcium, and potassium channel activity have been regarded as regulatory factors for cerebrovascular reactivity to CO2.[6] Compared with adults, children have less cerebral reactivity to CO2 changes. Whether this difference is related to possible domination of prostaglandin and cyclic guanosine monophosphate in regulating vascular tone in children remains to be determined.

Changes in Cerebral Blood Flow and Intracranial Pressure Regulation in Pathologic Conditions

Patients who undergo neurosurgery may have various types of intracranial pathologic as well as systemic diseases, and their responses to anesthetics may be different from those of normal subjects. Brain tissue hypoxia, acidosis, and edema are the main pathologic consequences of most brain disorders. Cerebral vasoparalysis occurs, and coupling between blood flow and metabolism is impaired. Under these circumstances, autoregulation and CO2 reactivity are also disturbed. Strict blood pressure control and respiratory management are required.

In the event of focal cerebral ischemia, hypercapnia can dilate the vessels in the normal area but not in the damaged area, and consequently, blood flow may be shunted from the ischemic to the normal area (intracerebral steal). Conversely, hypocapnia can divert blood from the normal area to the ischemic area (inverse intracerebral steal, or the "Robin Hood effect"). Because of a lack of evidence indicating the possible deleterious effects of hyperventilation or its beneficial effect on outcome, hyperventilation cannot be recommended in patients who have experienced stroke.[7]

Although the effect is not confirmed for every anesthetic, experimental data in animals suggest that intracerebral steal or inverse intracerebral steal may also be induced pharmacologically. However, it is not easy to predict the efficacy of inverse intracerebral steal by anesthetics because the cerebral vessel constriction by anesthetics is affected by both their direct vasoconstrictive property and indirect effects caused by CMR changes, as well as any additional intrinsic neuroprotective effects.

Anesthesia alters ICP through changes in cerebral blood volume (CBV). Although correlation between CBV and CBF does not always exist, the changes in CBV, in general, appear to be proportional to the changes in CBF. Therefore an increase in CBF causes an increase in CBV and, thus, in ICP. Increases in blood pressure, especially when autoregulation is impaired, also produce an increase in CBV. Mechanical effects, such as the patient's position and respiratory pattern (by influencing intrathoracic pressure) also may affect ICP.[8,9] Muscle activity during patient movement may raise central venous pressure (CVP) and ICP. Anesthetic agents also affect ICP by changing the rate of production and reabsorption of cerebrospinal fluid (CSF) (see Chapter 3). CBV control is the most important measure to be rapidly performed by anesthesiologists to prevent ICP elevation. Practically, hyperventilation can rapidly control intracranial hypertension. However, prolonged and extreme hypocapnia has been demonstrated to result in a marked decrease in CBF in patients with head trauma.[10] Only short duration of mild to moderate hyperventilation (hypocapnia) should be instituted for emergencies, and other pharmacologic or surgical intervention should be undertaken subsequently for controlling critical intracranial hypertension. Intracranial physiology and pathophysiology in relation to the use of anesthetics and adjuvant drugs are summarized in Figure 5-1.

EFFECTS OF SPECIFIC ANESTHETIC DRUGS AND OTHER DRUGS

Inhalational Anesthetics

In general, all inhalational anesthetics are cerebral vasodilators and possess the capability of increasing ICP. Inhalational anesthetics, with the possible exception of nitrous oxide (N2O), usually depress metabolism. Despite the disassociation of CBF and CMRo2, changes in the magnitude of cerebral vasodilation appear to be related to the level of tissue metabolism. Table 5-1 summarizes the effects of inhalational anesthetics on CBF, CMR, and ICP.

Nitrous Oxide

N2O continues to generate debate in neurosurgical anesthesia because it is not inert as has classically been thought, in terms of its effect on CBF, CMR and ICP. Classic studies in humans demonstrated that N2O did not significantly affect CBF, although it decreased the Cerebral metabolic rate for oxygen (CMRo2). However, results might have been affected by premedication, anesthetic induction drugs, or body temperature. It is now generally agreed that N2O increases CBF, CMRo2, and ICP, although the magnitude varies substantially. The cause of this variation may be a species specific as to the values of minimum alveolar concentration (MAC) and its use in combination with other drugs that may modify its original effect. The most dramatic increases in CBF and ICP occurred when N2O was administered alone or with other minimal background anesthetics. The increases in CBF and CMRo2 with N2O do not appear to be related solely to sympathetic hyperactivity. N2O appears to have no direct vasodilating effect.[11]

Marked heterogeneity in regional cerebral blood flow (rCBF), regional CBV, and regional CMR (rCMR) during administration of N2O has been revealed with positron emission tomography (PET) and magnetic resonance imaging (MRI). Subanesthetic concentrations of N2O (20%) increase rCBF and rCMR in the anterior cingulate cortex,

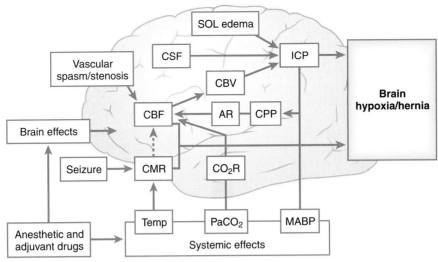

Figure 5–1 Intracranial physiology and pathophysiology in relation to the use of anesthetics and adjuvant drugs. The interaction of brain effects with the systemic effects of anesthetics and adjuvant drugs must be considered. Improvement of oxygen (substrate) supply/demand balance and prevention of intracranial hypertension are key points to prevent brain tissue hypoxia or ischemia and brain herniation and to obtain a better outcome. AR, autoregulation; CBF, cerebral blood flow; CBV, cerebral blood volume; CMR, CO$_2$R, cerebrovascular reactivity to CO$_2$; ICP, intracranial pressure; MABP, mean arterial blood pressure; SOL, space-occupying lesion; Temp, temperature.

Table 5–1 Summary of the effects of inhalational anesthetics on CBF, CMR, and ICP

	CBF	CMR	ICP
N$_2$O	↑↑	↑ or →	↑↑
Xenon	↓ (Gray) ↑ (White)	↓	↑ or →
Isoflurane	↑ or →	↓↓	→ or ↗ or ↑
Sevoflurane	↓ or → or ↗	↓ or ↓↓	→ or ↗ or ↑
Desflurane	↓ or ↑	↓↓	↑ or →

Arrows indicate semi-quantitative changes.
↗:slight increase, ↑:increase, ↑↑:marked increase, →:unchanged
↓:decrease, ↓↓:marked decrease

with opposite effects in the posterior cingulate, hippocampus, parahippocampal gyrus, and visual cortices.[12] At N$_2$O 50%, rCBF and regional CBV increased in all gray matter regions, although the increase in rCBF was less pronounced in basal ganglia.[13] Global cerebral metabolic rates for glucose (CMRGL) was unchanged with N$_2$O 50%, but metabolism was changed; regional CMRGL increased in the basal ganglia and thalamus, and this effect was present 1 hour after discontinuation of N$_2$O.[14]

N$_2$O, when added to volatile anesthetics, raises both CBF and CMR.[15-17] Indirect evidence—measurements of Vmca—has shown that N$_2$O raises CBF.[18,19] In patients with brain tumors, N$_2$O increased Vmca, but the increase was completely reversed by hyperventilation.[20,21]

Intravenous anesthetics, thiamylal, fentanyl plus pentobarbital, and midazolam have been shown to attenuate N$_2$O-induced increases in CBF or CMRO$_2$. Regional metabolic studies in rats demonstrated that N$_2$O raised local cerebral metabolic rates for glucose (lCMRGL) in subcortical structures and in the spinal cord. A higher lCMRGL was observed when subjects were lightly anesthetized with pentobarbital after the addition of N$_2$O but not when anesthetized with doses of pentobarbital that produced a flat (isoelectric) EEG.[22] In contrast, the addition of N$_2$O 70% to anesthesia with propofol (EEG

isoelectric) in nonneurosurgical patients produced a 20% increase in Vmca with greater oxygen and glucose use in association with EEG activation.[23] A PET study in humans showed that N$_2$O 70% counteracted almost all rCBF reductions and some of the regional CMRO$_2$ reductions produced by propofol at a dose of clinical anesthesia (EEG activity remained). No data are available for high doses of propofol and an isoelectric EEG.[17] Whether the differences in modification of N$_2$O-induced increases in CBF or CMR by other anesthetics are due to the differences in species, methods, or dose ranges of the anesthetics examined is not clear.

An increase in ICP caused by N$_2$O has been repeatedly demonstrated. The rise in ICP can be attenuated by prior administration of thiopental, diazepam, or morphine or by induction of hypocapnia. It is advisable to use hypocapnia, cerebral vasoconstricting drugs, or both when N$_2$O is administered, especially in patients with reduced intracranial compliance.

Some authorities have proposed that N$_2$O has neurotoxic properties. It has been reported that N-methyl-D-aspartate (NMDA) receptor blockade during synaptogenesis in the immature brain can induce neuronal degeneration. This effect occurs not only with anesthetics with an NMDA receptor–blocking property (N$_2$O, xenon, and ketamine) but also with those acting as gamma-aminobutyric acid (GABA) receptor modulators (propofol, midazolam, barbiturates, and isoflurane).[24] However, it has been demonstrated that NMDA receptor antagonists protect against ischemic brain injuries. N$_2$O may therefore have both neuroprotective[25] and neurotoxic[26] properties.

N$_2$O enlarges the volume of potential air space, and thus its use is restricted in the patient with an intracranial or intravascular air compartment. Further, the incidence of nausea and vomiting appears to be high after N$_2$O anesthesia, which may also restrict its use in neurosurgical patients.[27]

Xenon

During steady state xenon 70% inhalation in rats, with stable cardiovascular conditions was achieved, mean values of CBF and CMRg1 did not change from conscious control values, but, during short inhalation of xenon 70%, CBF increased by 40-50%.[28] In pigs, xenon 79% increased rCBF approximately 40% more than total intravenous anesthesia control.[29]

In humans, PET showed that xenon 1 MAC decreases absolute rCBF by 11% in the gray matter and increases it by 22% in the white matter,[30] with greater reductions in the cerebellum (by 35%), thalamus (by 23%), and cortical areas (by 9%). The decreased rCBF in the gray matter may be a result of reduced metabolism, as evidenced by the comparable reductions in CMRGL in the corresponding brain areas.[31] Though the reduction in CMR is less pronounced than those reported with volatile anesthetics, the metabolic pattern produced with xenon resembles those produced with volatile anesthetics rather than with N_2O.[14,32,33]

In animals either with normal ICP[34] or with elevated ICP,[35,36] xenon did not change ICP. This agent's effects in patients with head injury are variable; ICP has been found to either increase by 7 mm Hg[37] or not to change.[38] It should be noted that MAC of xenon varies among species (71% in humans, 119% in pigs, 85% in rabbits, 161% in rats), and this variation may explain the different results among the species. At present, in humans, xenon appears to be a mild cerebral metabolic depressant and its effect on CBF and ICP is mild.

Because xenon is an antagonist of the NMDA receptor, it may have neuroprotective effects. Indeed, neuroprotection by inhalation of xenon before injury was demonstrated both in vitro[41] and in vivo models,[39-41] the effect being observed even with post-treatment after hypoxic-ischemic insult in neonatal rats.[42] In combination with either hypothermia (35° C)[43] or the α_2-adrenergic agonist dexmedetomidine,[44] xenon exhibited neuroprotection in the same model. Also, it was reported that preconditioning by xenon 70% reduced brain damage from hypoxia-ischemia in neonatal rats.[45] A later study has demonstrated that xenon 50% provides long-term neuroprotection in a neonatal hypoxia-ischemia model and that this protection is augmented by concomitant application of moderate hypothermia (32° C).[46]

With its low blood/gas partition coefficient of 0.115, xenon may offer advantages for neuroanesthesia use, because early neurologic examination after the emergence period is possible and may be desirable. However, this agent's effects when combined with other anesthetics should be further determined.

Halothane

In most animal experiments, halothane produces an increase in CBF in association with a decrease in CVR. The varying magnitude of the increase in CBF reported may be due not only to species differences but also to the level of CPP. If the blood pressure decrease is not corrected, the increase in CBF is less. At low concentrations, CBF changes are not consistent, and some subjects have shown a decrease.[47] It is possible that at low concentrations, the cerebral vasodilatory effect of halothane is weak, and flow may be determined by the metabolic depressive effect. At higher concentrations, the vasodilating effect overcomes this metabolism-dependent vasoconstrictive action, resulting in a net increase in CBF. Regional flow measurement in the rat demonstrated that vasodilation with halothane is more prominent in the cerebral cortex, but isoflurane dilates vessels in the subcortical structures.

In humans, most studies demonstrated that halothane induces cerebral vasodilation and increases CBF, provided that the systemic blood pressure is maintained. The increase in cortical CBF appears greater with halothane than with enflurane or isoflurane at equi-MAC concentrations. It is probably true that the potency of the overall vasodilating property of halothane appears to be most prominent among available volatile anesthetics.

The mechanism of the cerebral vasodilation produced by halothane (and other volatile anesthetics) has not been thoroughly understood. A direct effect on vascular smooth muscle or an increase in cyclic adenosine monophosphate (cAMP) in the brain has been postulated, but the evidence is inconclusive. Nitric oxide (NO) might be an important mediator of cerebral vasodilation produced by volatile agents[48-50] as evidenced by an attenuation of either pial vasodilation or CBF increase with N-nitro-L-arginine methyl ester (L-NAME), an inhibitor of NO synthase. However, because further attenuation was observed when treatment with indomethacin was given, NO does not seem to be an obligatory mediator in halothane-induced cerebral vasodilation.[51]

A dose-related cerebral metabolic depressive effect of halothane has been demonstrated repeatedly both in animals and humans. Metabolic changes show regional variations, as evidenced by a more marked decrease in lCMRGL in the occipital lobe, brainstem, cerebellar cortex, and anterior commissure than in other parts of the brain. At clinical levels of anesthesia in humans, the decrease in global $CMRO_2$ ranges from 10% to 30%. A study using PET demonstrated that halothane anesthesia titrated to a point just beyond the loss of consciousness is associated with 40% reduction of whole-brain glucose metabolism,[33] the magnitude of reduction being similar to that with isoflurane. Although halothane was reported to reduce the global $CMRO_2$ less than isoflurane in an animal experiment at 0.5 to 1.5 MAC,[52] the percentage of absolute reduction of whole-brain glucose metabolism caused by anesthesia at the point just beyond the loss of consciousness in humans may be almost the same.[33]

In both animals and humans, halothane raises ICP in a dose-related fashion, and the rise in ICP is parallel to that in CBF. The elevation of ICP with halothane appears to be most prominent among the commonly used volatile anesthetics. However, at 0.5 MAC or less, the effect on ICP is minimal. The increased ICP that, with halothane, often occurs in association with systemic hypotension results in reduced CPP. This response may augment the risk of cerebral ischemia. The increase in ICP may be attenuated either by hyperventilation or by barbiturates. However, the beneficial effects of hypocapnia may not be obtained when the initial ICP is very high or reactivity to CO_2 is lost globally.

An increase in CBF with halothane in association with a decrease in $CMRO_2$ does not necessarily mean that halothane may provide a neuroprotective effect against cerebral ischemia. Worse neurologic outcome and greater infarct volume have been reported after experimental focal ischemia in animals. High concentrations of halothane can be toxic. At inspired concentrations of halothane above 2.3% (more obviously at those above 4%), brain tissue hypoxia seems to occur even when CBF is maintained by extracorporeal circulation.

In summary, considerable discussion has taken place concerning the use of halothane during surgery for intracranial space-occupying lesions, and some authorities are against its use. Although halothane in low concentrations (less than 1%) can be safely used in clinical neuroanesthesia practice when $PaCO_2$ is reduced and barbiturates (and probably propofol) also are given, the margin of safety is probably wider with isoflurane, desflurane, or sevoflurane than with halothane.

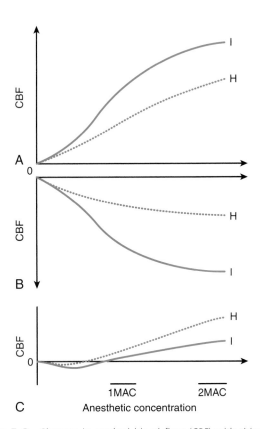

Figure 5–2 Changes in cerebral blood flow (CBF) with rising anesthetic concentrations. The graph is drawn on the basis of the hypothesis that CBF changes exhibit a net result of the direct effect and the metabolism-coupled effect of anesthetics. Also, the graph is based on the assumption that isoflurane (I) possesses greater direct vasodilating effect and metabolic-depressing effect than halothane (H). **A,** CBF changes caused by the direct vasodilating effect of anesthetics. **B,** CBF changes caused by the metabolic depressive effects of anesthetics (metabolism-coupled changes). **C,** Net CBF changes caused by both direct and metabolism-coupled effects. In normal subjects, halothane produces greater increase in CBF than isoflurane **(C).** In contrast, in patients whose baseline metabolism is maximally depressed either with other drugs or from an intracranial pathologic condition, metabolism-coupled flow changes may not occur, and CBF changes are simply determined by direct vasodilating effects of anesthetics, provided that the mechanisms for direct vasodilating effects are intact. If this is the case, isoflurane produces a greater increase in CBF than halothane, with rising anesthetic concentration **(A).** MAC, minimum alveolar concentration.

Isoflurane

Most animal studies show that isoflurane produces an increase in CBF that is accompanied by a decrease in CVR and CMRo$_2$, except at low concentration. In general, the increase in global CBF is smaller with isoflurane than with halothane. However, at a given level of metabolic rate, isoflurane possesses greater cerebral vasodilating capabilities than halothane. It has been demonstrated that halothane, isoflurane, and desflurane at 0.5 MAC produce similar increases in Vmca in humans during propofol-induced isoelectric EEG, whereas at 1.5 MAC, isoflurane and desflurane have greater vasodilating effects than halothane.[53] The net effect of inhalational anesthetics on CBF is a balance between a reduction in CBF due to CMR suppression and augmentation of CBF due to direct cerebral vasodilation; the reported smaller increases in CBF with isoflurane than with halothane may occur from a more potent cerebral metabolic depressive effect of isoflurane. The hypothetical illustrations of changes in CBF with

rising concentrations of halothane and isoflurane are shown in Figure 5-2.

In a PET study in humans, isoflurane (0.2-1.0 MAC) was reported to produce no change in global CBF[54] but to cause regional increases (anterior cingulate and insula regions) and decreases (cerebellum, thalamus, and lingual gyrus) in relative CBF.

It is unlikely that any single mechanism is entirely responsible for vasodilative property of isoflurane. Some investigators speculate that the vasodilative properties of isoflurane may be related to NO. It was also reported that approximately one third of the cortical hyperemic response to isoflurane measured by laser Doppler flowmetry is mediated by NO, prostaglandins, and epoxyeicosatrienoic acid and that the remaining part of the response appears to be mediated by a direct action on smooth muscle.[55] A study using a closed cranial window model demonstrated that an adenosine triphosphate (ATP)–sensitive K$^+$ channel blocker, glibenclamide, attenuates isoflurane (and sevoflurane)–induced cerebral vasodilation, suggesting that vasodilation with these anesthetics is mediated, at least in part, via activation of ATP-sensitive K$^+$ channels.[56]

In animal studies, isoflurane, decreased CMRo$_2$ in a dose-related manner until the EEG became flat (2 MAC); thereafter, no further decrease in CMRo$_2$ was observed despite an increase in isoflurane to 4 MAC. Also, isoflurane in humans produces a decrease in CMRo$_2$. Isoflurane (0.5%), as examined with PET, was reported to reduce whole-brain metabolism almost by half, and the reduction was fairly uniform throughout the brain.[32]

Animal studies show that isoflurane raises ICP minimally in normal subjects and in patients with intracranial hypertension, with the exception of a substantial increase in ICP when isoflurane and N$_2$O are used in combination. In humans, gray matter regional CBV is increased with isoflurane (0.45%),[57] and thus ICP can rise. However, clinical data have been inconsistent; lumbar cerebrospinal fluid pressure (CSFP) increased in one study[58] but did not change in another.[59] However, because ICP was reported to be lower in the patients anesthetized with propofol-fentanyl than those anesthetized with isoflurane-fentanyl, propofol may be preferable in the setting of unstable ICP.[60]

Because of its potent cerebral metabolic depressive effect, isoflurane was predicted to have cerebral protective effects, which may be produced by a variety of mechanisms, including inhibition of excitatory neurotransmission, potentiation of GABA$_A$ receptors, regulation of intracellular calcium responses, and activation of TWIK (tandem of P domains in a weak inwardly rectifying K$^+$ channel)–related K$^+$ (TREK)-1 two-pore-domain K$^+$ channels.[61] Indeed, many animal studies have demonstrated the neuroprotective properties of isoflurane within clinically relevant concentrations. However, the protection with isoflurane is applicable only to mild insults, being inferior to and less durable than mild hypothermia in its neuroprotective effect.[62] Also, it is important to note that isoflurane has preconditioning effects.[63,64]

In the clinical setting, there is no good evidence that isoflurane uniquely protects against ischemic central nervous system injury. Suggestive observations include those in a large retrospective review of changing anesthetic management practices during carotid endarterectomy in humans.[65] The critical CBF below which ischemic EEG changes occur was greater in patients anesthetized with halothane than in patients anesthetized with isoflurane. At a comparable level of rCBF, the incidence of EEG ischemic changes with isoflurane has been reported to be significantly lower than that seen with halothane.

In summary, isoflurane appears to produce a mild increase in CBF and a pronounced decrease in cerebral metabolism. The accumulated evidence in basic research strongly suggests that isoflurane may have a cerebral protective effect, although this effect is not proven clinically. However, isoflurane may be a desirable anesthetic for many neurosurgical procedures, including carotid endarterectomy. The increase in ICP caused by isoflurane, if it occurs, may be mild and can be prevented by hypocapnia. However, when ICP elevation should definitely be avoided, propofol in combination with a synthetic opioid may be preferable.

The effects of enflurane, a stereoisomer of isoflurane, are intermediate between those of isoflurane and halothane. Because of enflurane's potential effects on ICP and possible epileptogenic properties, high concentrations of the agent should be avoided in patients at risk. Low doses of enflurane can be safely used, but this agent does not seem to be useful in neurosurgical anesthesia.

Sevoflurane

Earlier studies in pigs demonstrated that sevoflurane decreased CBF. Several reports in other animals showed no change in CBF.[66-68] Increases in CBF have been reported only in spontaneously ventilated rats.[69] Sevoflurane also was found to decrease CMR_{O_2} in a dose-dependent manner.[68]

The results obtained with the use of the transcranial Doppler ultrasonography technique in humans vary also. Vmca has been reported to be either decreased,[18,59] unchanged,[3] or increased with sevoflurane (at less magnitude than with isoflurane).[70] Low CBF (and CMR_{O_2}) was reported in patients with known cerebrovascular disease who were anesthetized with sevoflurane and N_2O 33%.[71] CBF equivalent (an index of flow-metabolism relationship) was shown to be slightly higher than normal but was comparable to or slightly lower than that for equi-MAC isoflurane.[72]

Studies using PET demonstrated similar results, that either a decrease[73] or no change[74] in global CBF occurred with use of sevoflurane. No increase or even a decrease in CBF with sevoflurane can be a result of a reduction in CBF caused by CMR suppression.[17] Regarding rCBF, one study showed heterogeneity of response—an increase of relative rCBF in the anterior cingulate and a decrease in the cerebellum[74]—whereas the other showed unanimous decrease.[17] Taken together, studies show that sevoflurane decreases CMR but its effect on CBF seems weaker than that of isoflurane.

Sevoflurane, either with or without N_2O, produced no or small increases in ICP in animals and in humans. The increase in ICP, if any, can be blocked by hyperventilation.[75] When sevoflurane is compared with isoflurane and desflurane, the extent of the increase in ICP is in the following order in animals: desflurane > isoflurane > sevoflurane.[76] In patients undergoing transsphenoidal pituitary surgery (no mass effect),[77] lumbar CSFP was increased with sevoflurane, but the mean increase was small and comparable to those reported with isoflurane and desflurane.[58] In patients with cerebral tumors (midline shift less than 10 mm) anesthetized with either propofol-fentanyl, isoflurane-fentanyl, or sevoflurane-fentanyl, the values of ICP was in the order of propofol-fentanyl < isoflurane-fentanyl = sevoflurane-fentanyl anesthesia. The effect of propofol-fentanyl was less than those of isoflurane-fentanyl and sevoflurane-fentanyl

anaesthesia.[60] The ICP-raising properties of a clinical dose of sevoflurane appear to be mild, but propofol would be preferable in a patient for whom ICP mut be rigidly controlled.

The neuroprotective effect of sevoflurane reported earlier in the middle cerebral artery occlusion model in rats may be assumed to be due to temperature reduction with anesthetics.[78] However, several other studies demonstrated neuroprotective effects,[79] and the agent's favorable effect appears to be similar to that of isoflurane.[80] In addition, sevoflurane-induced early or late ischemic tolerance has been shown in rats.[81]

In the clinical setting, there is no unequivocal evidence for a neuroprotective effect of sevoflurane. Indirect evidence includes the observation that critical rCBF, below which ischemic EEG changes occur during carotid cross-clamping, was found to be similar to that previously determined in patients anesthetized with isoflurane.[82] At present, the neuroprotective effects of sevoflurane, though inconclusive, appear to be similar, if they occur, to those of isoflurane.

The disadvantages of sevoflurane are that this drug is biodegradable and that its metabolites may be toxic in high concentrations. Although the major degradation product, compound A, has renal toxicity, such toxicity has not yet been reported in humans with clinical use of sevoflurane. Nevertheless, prolonged anesthesia, which is often necessary for neurosurgical procedures, may increase the possibility of toxicity, especially in patients with preexisting renal disease. It is not recommended to use this drug in a low-flow circuit.

Desflurane

In animals, desflurane has been reported to produce a dose-dependent increase in CBF and a decrease in CMR_{O_2} or CMR_{GL}.[83] These effects appear comparable to those of isoflurane.[84] Cerebrovascular reactivity to changes in Pa_{CO_2} is preserved.[85]

In humans, during propofol-induced isoelectric EEG, desflurane at 0.5 MAC produced increases in Vmca that were similar to those seen with isoflurane. At 1.5 MAC, the increase produced by desflurane was also similar to that with isoflurane.[53] This finding may suggest that desflurane, used when cerebral metabolism is maximally suppressed, increases CBF in a dose-dependent, cerebral vasodilatory effect. During hypocapnia (Pa_{CO_2} 25 mm Hg) in patients receiving desflurane, the CBF at 1 MAC was lower, but the CBF at 1.5 MAC was similar to those measured during an equi-MAC isoflurane anesthesia.[86] Desflurane 1 MAC decreased CMR_{O_2} by half, CMR_{GL} by 35%, and CBF by 22%, and preserved cerebrovascular CO_2 reactivity.[87]

In animals, at normocapnia, desflurane causes progressive and greater increases of ICP than isoflurane; at hypocapnia, however, desflurane and isoflurane have similar and small effects.[88] When the animals were subjected to intracranial hypertension, desflurane increased ICP more than sevoflurane but less than isoflurane, whereas during hypocapnia, no significant differences in ICP were observed among the three agents.[76]

In patients with supratentorial mass lesions with a midline shift, desflurane 1 MAC (7%) was reported to produce an increase in CSFP despite prior establishment of hypocapnia,[89] but not to raise ICP in patients without a midline shift,[90] whereas isoflurane 1 MAC was reported not to change CSFP or ICP in either case.[89,90]

Many studies have demonstrated neuroprotective effects of desflurane in vivo[91-93] and in vitro[94] models in experimental animals. At present, the degree of protection afforded by desflurane appears to be comparable to that with isoflurane.[91-92] In the clinical setting, brain tissue oxygen pressure measured in patients undergoing craniotomy was elevated when desflurane concentration was increased from 3% to 9%, and the blood pressure was maintained with intravenous phenylephrine.[95]

In summary, because of a low blood/gas partition coefficient (0.42) relative to other clinically used volatile inhalational anesthetics, desflurane can provide rapid onset and offset of anesthesia, which facilitates early neurologic evaluation. In general, desflurane decreases CMR, but CBF may either be increased or decreased, depending on the doses used. Desflurane's neuroprotective effects appear to be comparable to those of isoflurane. However, because desflurane may have slightly greater ICP-elevating effects than isoflurane or sevoflurane, desflurane should be used cautiously in patients with unstable ICP.

Intravenous Anesthetics

In general, intravenous anesthetics cause a decrease in CBF and $CMRo_2$. However, these anesthetics might not be vasoconstrictors in a strict sense, because in vitro barbiturates, for example, dilate isolated cerebral vessels. The decrease in CBF induced by most intravenous anesthetics appears to be the result of reduced cerebral metabolism secondary to cerebral functional depression. Among the intravenous anesthetics, ketamine may be unique because it produces an increase in both CBF and $CMRo_2$. Table 5-2 summarizes the effects of intravenous anesthetics on CBF, CMR, and ICP.

Barbiturates

Thiopental produces a dose-dependent reduction in CBF and $CMRo_2$. Other barbiturates, such as phenobarbital and pentobarbital, essentially have similar effects. A dose-dependent reduction in CBF and $CMRo_2$ occurs until the EEG becomes flat. At the point of EEG isoelectricity, no further $CMRo_2$ reduction occurs despite a further increase in barbiturate dose. A burst-suppression dose of thiopental decreases both CBF and $CMRo_2$ to about 40% (near maximal reduction) of the awake value in humans. Thus, with barbiturates, functional depression appears to be coupled with the reduction in CBF and $CMRo_2$. If CMR is maximally depressed as a result of an intracranial pathologic condition, thiopental can increase CBF, possibly because of its direct effect, provided that blood pressure is maintained.

ICP is reduced by barbiturates, possibly through the reduction in CBF and CBV. Barbiturates have been shown to result in lower CBV values than those resulting from use of volatile anesthetics. This effect is exploited during the treatment of raised ICP in head-injured patients (although such use is controversial) as well as in the induction of anesthesia in patients with decreased intracranial compliance. Barbiturates attenuate the cerebral vasodilation produced by N_2O and ketamine and thus are useful as supplemental anesthetics.

The neuroprotective effect of barbiturates has been repeatedly demonstrated in focal ischemia. Significant reductions in infarct volume have been demonstrated in rats anesthetized with moderate doses of pentobarbital.[96] Increasing the doses sufficient to produce burst suppression on EEG did not further decrease infarct volume. It has been suggested that burst suppression of EEG is not necessary to provide neuroprotection and that mechanisms other than metabolic depression may be involved for protection.[96]

ICP-reducing effects and possible neuroprotective effects make the barbiturates favorable drugs for neurosurgical anesthesia, provided that cardiovascular stability is maintained. It should be noted, however, that prolonged use of barbiturate produces accumulated effects because of its slow metabolism. Because of similar cerebral hemodynamic effects and a shorter context-sensitive half-life, other intravenous agents, especially propofol, may be more appropriate for this application (see later).

Etomidate

Etomidate does not have cardiovascular side effects. Etomidate, like barbiturates, decreases $CMRo_2$ progressively until an isoelectric EEG appears. CBF decreases precipitously with the start of etomidate infusion. A maximal decrease in CBF was achieved before the maximal decrease in $CMRo_2$.[97] This finding may suggest that etomidate causes vasoconstriction through a different mechanism (possibly by direct action) than that of the barbiturates. Parallel decreases in ICP and CBF were observed. In humans, almost parallel reductions in CBF and $CMRo_2$ are induced with etomidate. With clinical doses, CBF and $CMRo_2$ are decreased by approximately 30% to 50%. Reactivity to CO_2 is preserved during etomidate anesthesia.

Etomidate effectively decreases ICP without diminishing CPP. In severely head-injured patients, etomidate reduced ICP while electrocortical activity was present but was not effective when cortical electrical activity was already maximally suppressed.[98] This finding indicates that the decrease in ICP may be caused by the reduction of CBF (and CBV) induced by the functional (metabolic) depressant effects of etomidate.

The reported results on neuroprotective effects of etomidate in animal experiments vary depending on the model used. In a forebrain ischemia model (bilateral carotid artery occlusion with hypotension) in rats, etomidate has been reported to have a small brain protective effect.[99] In contrast, poor outcome or larger infarct volume was reported after incomplete cerebral ischemia or middle cerebral artery occlusion, respectively.[100-102] The injury-enhancing effect of etomidate in middle cerebral artery occlusion has been attributed to its ability to reduce NO levels in the ischemic brain tissue.[103] In addition, in some patients who underwent cerebral aneurysm surgery, etomidate led to cerebral deoxygenation, which was exaggerated with temporal cerebral artery occlusion.[104] Further study may be necessary before one can conclude that etomidate is a neuroprotectant.

Table 5–2 Summary of the effects of intravenous anesthetics on CBF, CMR, and ICP

	CBF	CMR	ICP
Barbiturates	⇓	⇓	⇓
Etomidate	⇓	⇓	⇓
Propofol	⇓	⇓	⇓
Ketamine	⇑	↑ or →	↑ or ⇑
Benzodiazepines	↓	↓	↓ or →
Synthetic Opioids	→ or ↗	→ or ↓	→ or ↗
Dexmedetomidine	↓	→ or ↓	→

Arrows indicate semi-quantitative changes.
↗:slight increase, ↑:increase, ⇑:marked increase, →:unchanged
↘:slight decrease, ↓:decrease, ⇓:marked decrease

Adverse effects of this drug include adrenocortical suppression and frequent occurrence of involuntary muscle activity and seizure activity. Etomidate should be used with caution in patients with a history of seizures. Etomidate dissolved in propylene glycol can have various adverse effects, including pain on injection, thrombophlebitis, and histamine release, whereas the preparation in lipid emulsion (Lipofundin) is devoid of those side effects.[105]

Propofol

Propofol produces dose-related decreases in both CBF and $CMRO_2$, with minimum $CMRO_2$ values being 40% to 60% of control values. In PET studies, variation of rCBF reductions has been demonstrated; large decreases occurred preferentially in the brain regions implicated in the regulation of arousal, performance of associative functions, and autonomic control.[106] As with barbiturates, the CBF decrease with propofol is attributable to its metabolic depressant effect. However, several studies demonstrated that the reduction of CBF was larger than the reduction of $CMRO_2$, suggesting that propofol may have direct cerebral vasoconstrictive activity. The vasoconstrictive activity of propofol may be suitable for carotid endarterectomy[107] and revascularization surgery for moyamoya disease,[108] because the cerebral steal phenomenon can be avoided with propofol.

As with the regional variation in CBF decrease, propofol was reported not only to depress CMR but to do so differentially according to region.[109] Overall metabolism in the cortex was depressed more than overall metabolism in the subcortical brain areas; in the cortical lobes, rCMR was significantly lower in the frontal, parietal, and occipital lobes.

In patients with cerebral tumors with midline shift less than 10 mm, ICP was reported to be lower and CPP higher in patients anesthetized with propofol than in those anesthetized with isoflurane or sevoflurane.[60] Nevertheless, in most circumstances, MABP is reduced with propofol. Therefore, if propofol, like any other drug, is given to treat intracranial hypertension, attention should be paid to maintaining MABP (CPP). CO_2 reactivity is preserved with propofol. Thus, hyperventilation can decrease ICP during propofol anesthesia. However, because the incidence of a decrease in jugular bulb venous Hemoglobin (Hb) ($SjvO_2$) of less than 50% is higher (suggesting cerebral hypoperfusion) during hyperventilation, hyperventilation should be cautiously applied in patients anesthetized with propofol.[110] However, the significance of these low values in relatively intact hemispheres remains to be demonstrated.

Regarding the neuroprotective effects of propofol, many studies in animals,[111,112] but not all,[113,114] demonstrated favorable effects of burst-suppression doses of propofol. The possible neuroprotective mechanisms include CMR reduction, antioxidant activity, activation of GABA receptors, attenuation of glutamate-mediated excitotoxicity, prevention of mitochondrial swelling, and interaction of the endocannabinoid system.[115] Interestingly, protection was observed even in a light depth of propofol anesthesia (not a burst-suppression dose) and even when propofol was administered after ischemic insults.[116] Though there is yet no clinical evidence showing improvement of neurologic outcome after its use in acute cerebral injury in patients, propofol has a rapid onset and offset of action with minimal interference with electrophysiologic monitoring, including motor evoked potentials, and thus propofol seems to be a favorable anesthetic for various types of neurosurgery.

A number of case reports suggest that prolonged use of propofol caused systemic acidosis and progressive cardiac failure and even death in children.[117,118] Until this phenomenon is better understood, use of prolonged propofol infusions in children is unjustified.

In summary, propofol seems to have cerebral hemodynamic and metabolic effects similar to those of barbiturates. This drug may be useful in patients with intracranial pathologic conditions, provided that hypotension is prevented.

Ketamine

Increases in CBF and $CMRO_2$ with ketamine have been reported both in animals and in humans, with some inconsistency for global $CMRO_2$. The rCBF increases in frontal and parietooccipital areas are remarkable and might be related to the dreams or hallucinations peculiar to ketamine. In animals, lCMRGL is increased in the hippocampus and extrapyramidal structures.[119] In humans, PET studies showed that subanesthetic doses of ketamine increased rCBF and regional CMRGL without a global change in regional $CMRO_2$ [120,121]; the greatest rCBF increases were seen in the anterior cingulate, thalamus, putamen, and frontal cortex, and the greatest regional CMRGL increases were detected in the thalamus and the frontal and parietal cortices.[120]

These data have been obtained with the use of commercially available formulations of ketamine containing both S(+)- and R(−)-ketamine enantiomers. S(+)-ketamine is more effective as an analgesic and anesthetic than a racemic mixture of two enantiomers (racemic ketamine) or R(−)-ketamine. The changes in CBF and CMR with S(+)-ketamine appear essentially similar with minor quantitative difference; subanesthetic doses increased global CBF by 14% without a change in global $CMRO_2$, with greatest increase in CBF detected in the anterior cingulate. The anesthetic dose increased global CBF by 36% without changes in global $CMRO_2$ or CMRGL,[122] with the greatest increase in CBF detected in the insula, whereas $CMRO_2$ rose only in the frontal cortex, and CMRGL only in the thalamus. Vasodilation by ketamine has been attributed, in part, to its metabolic stimulating effect, a direct dilating effect, and a cholinergic mechanism. Pretreatment with thiopental completely blocks these CBF and $CMRO_2$ effects of ketamine. Diazepam pretreatment attenuates the increase in lCMRGL in the hippocampus.

Ketamine markedly raises ICP. An increase in ICP can be blocked or attenuated by induced hypocapnia or by administration of thiopental or benzodiazepine. During propofol sedation in patients with traumatic brain injury, ketamine decreases ICP.[123] In patients with supratentorial tumor who are anesthetized with isoflurane (0.3% to 0.4%)/N_2O 50%, ketamine 1 mg/kg did not significantly raise ICP.[124] However, some reports demonstrate failure to block ketamine-induced ICP elevation by secobarbital, droperidol, diazepam, or midazolam. A later study has shown that S(+)-ketamine does not increase ICP in comparison with fentanyl in patients with either severe traumatic brain injury or aneurysmal subarachnoid hemorrhage.[125] However, the study did find a persistent trend for S(+) ketamine–treated patients to have higher ICP values. Thus ketamine may not be a first choice in neuroanesthesia, especially in patients with elevated ICP or decreased intracranial compliance.

Some animal experiments,[126] but not all,[127] demonstrated neuroprotective effects of ketamine in various intracranial pathologic conditions, including ischemia and head injury, which could be related to NMDA receptor antagonism.

However, improved outcomes in animal experiments were reported only in the studies with brief recovery observation intervals.[128] In addition, clinical studies comparing ketamine sedation with fentanyl or sufentanil after traumatic brain injury failed to find any favorable effects on functional outcome after 6 months.[129,130] A definite neuroprotective effect of ketamine remains to be demonstrated in the clinical setting.

Benzodiazepines

Diazepam reduces CBF in animals. CMR_{O_2} is also decreased with this agent, except in rats, in which CMR_{O_2} decreases only when diazepam is combined with N_2O 70%. In dogs the decrease in CMR_{O_2} with diazepam is not influenced by the addition of N_2O. In normal humans, diazepam in combination with fentanyl and N_2O produces parallel decreases in CBF and CMR_{O_2}. In the head-injured patient, diazepam produces proportional 25% decreases in CBF and CMR_{O_2}. Contrary to the assumption that ICP would be reduced because of a lower CBF, diazepam (0.25 mg/kg) did not change ICP.[131]

Midazolam, like diazepam, produces parallel reductions in CBF and CMR_{O_2}. With rising doses, the effects appear to reach a plateau, possibly reflecting saturation of the benzodiazepine receptors. The effect of midazolam is completely blocked by the specific benzodiazepine antagonist flumazenil. The PET study in humans demonstrated that the decrease in rCBF with midazolam occurred in the areas associated with the functioning of arousal, attention, and memory, such as the insula, the cingulate gyrus, the prefrontal cortex, the thalamus, and parietal and temporal association areas.[132]

Midazolam produces either a decrease or no change in ICP. May be due to normal ICP before drug administration. Midazolam has been shown to maintain hemodynamic stability better than thiopental. However, caution must be used because of the possibility of CPP reduction in patients with critical conditions.

Midazolam may have protective effects against hypoxia or cerebral ischemia; the effects appear to be comparable with or slightly less than those of barbiturates. Lorazepam, triazolam, and flurazepam seem to have effects similar to those of diazepam and midazolam.

Because a specific receptor antagonist is now available, benzodiazepine derivatives are useful as induction or supplemental drugs during neuroanesthesia. However, flumazenil, a competitive benzodiazepine receptor antagonist, also antagonizes the effects of midazolam on CBF, CMR_{O_2}, and ICP. Thus one must use this drug cautiously when reversing benzodiazepine-induced sedation in patients with impaired intracranial compliance.

Synthetic Opioids

The reported effects of synthetic opioids on CBF, CMR_{O_2}, and ICP are variable. The variability appears to be due to the background anesthetic. When vasodilating drugs are used as the background anesthetic, the effect of the opioid is consistently that of a cerebral vasoconstrictor. Conversely, when a vasoconstrictor is used as the background anesthetic or when no anesthetic is given, opioids either have no effect or even increase CBF. When N_2O is also used, most opioids decrease CMR_{O_2}. Variable ICP effects also depend on the background anesthetic and on the systemic blood pressure autoregulation status.

Fentanyl and Sufentanil

When fentanyl and sufentanil are given to animals along with a background anesthetic—N_2O or volatile agents—they decrease CBF and CMR_{O_2}.[133] In an acute cryogenic brain injury model, fentanyl and sufentanil produced no change in CBF, even though animals were anesthetized with N_2O or volatile agents.[134] With no background anesthesia, sufentanil produced an increase in CBF in the absence of seizure activity in dogs.[135] When seizures were induced with high doses, rises in both CBF and CMR occurred. Whether cerebral metabolism is compromised during seizures and causes ischemic brain damage is not yet determined. High-dose fentanyl has been reported to reduce global CMR_{O_2} in rats but does not prevent a reduction in ATP and phosphocreatine (PCr) or an increase in lactate during hypoxemia.[136] In humans, the clinical significance of seizure activity observed with fentanyl in rats is not clear.

The combined use of fentanyl (5 µg/kg) and droperidol (0.25 mg/kg) had no significant effect on CBF and CMR_{O_2} in humans. Increases in Vmca were observed when fentanyl or sufentanil was used in unpremedicated humans,[137,138] but not in premedicated patients.[139] This difference also suggests that the CBF response depends on background state. Sufentanil decreased Vmca in patients with elevated ICP, and the decrease can be explained by low CPP.[140] A PET study in awake humans showed that fentanyl (1.5 µg/kg) increased rCBF in the cerebral region associated with a range of pain-related behaviors.[141]

Earlier studies show that ICP is either not elevated or may be slightly decreased with fentanyl used alone or in combination with droperidol. Reported ICP increases in patients with space-occupying lesions have been attributed to hypercapnia, and many authorities favor the use of these opioids during normocapnia or hypocapnia for neurosurgical anesthesia. Herrick and colleagues[142] reported that fentanyl, sufentanil, and alfentanil did not affect brain retractor pressure in hyperventilated neurosurgical patients anesthetized with isoflurane, suggesting that these opioids appear safe for intraoperative administration after the cranium is open. Better cerebral relaxation has been noted when fentanyl or sufentanil was used in patients anesthetized with N_2O and isoflurane during craniotomy, suggesting that both fentanyl and sufentanil probably have cerebrovasoconstrictive activity.[143]

However, some reports showed that fentanyl and sufentanil increased ICP (or CSFP) in patients with severe head trauma.[144,145] Werner and colleagues[146] reported that when MABP was controlled and remained unchanged, sufentanil (3 µg/mg) had significant effects on ICP in patients with brain injury, whereas the same dose of sufentanil caused a transient increase in ICP and a decrease in MABP. From these results, an increase in ICP appears to be attributable to the autoregulatory response.[140,147,148] However, in one study, there were no differences in the ICP-elevating effect of fentanyl between patients with head trauma who had preserved autoregulation and those who had impaired autoregulation.[149] Thus, the cerebrovascular autoregulation may not be the only probable mechanism responsible for fentanyl-induced increases in ICP in patients with head trauma. Although an ICP rise may be only transient after bolus administration of fentanyl and sufentanil, attention should be paid to this effect in patients with unstable ICP.

Alfentanil and Remifentanil

Alfentanil and remifentanil produce little changes or slight decreases in CBF[148,150] and Vmca[151,152] and essentially have a minimal effect on ICP.[153] These drugs have been used in neurosurgical anesthesia with satisfactory results.[142,154,155] No ICP elevation with alfentanil was observed in pediatric patients with hydrocephalus who were anesthetized with isoflurane and N_2O.[147] However, as with sufentanil, some reports showed a rise in lumbar CSFP associated with reduced MABP and CPP in patients with supratentorial tumors. In an experimental brain injury model, Souter and colleagues[148] reported that rapid infusion of alfentanil raised ICP concomitant with reduction in MABP but with no CBF changes.

In a PET study in human volunteers, either increases or decreases in relative rCBF were observed with an infusion of low doses of remifentanil (0.05 µg/kg/min), depending on the structures, the increases being observed within structures involved in pain processing.[156] With moderate doses (0.15 µg/kg/min), changes in relative rCBF were observed in structures involved in modulating vigilance and alertness.[156] The increases in relative rCBF with painful heat stimulation detected in various structures, including the thalamus, were suppressed with rising remifentanil dosage (0.05 to 0.15 µg/kg/min), whereas relative rCBF rose in the cingulofrontal cortex and periaqueductal gray, where descending antinociceptive pathways exist.[157] When higher doses (2-4 µg/kg/min) were administered in one study, CBF (stable xenon–enhanced computed tomography) and Vmca were decreased.[158]

In summary, clinically used doses of most opioids have minimal to modest depressive effects on CBF and CMR_{O_2}. During opioid-induced seizures in animals, there are substantial increases in CBF and CMR_{O_2} (CMR_{GL}), although they were not seen in humans. If adequate alveolar ventilation is instituted to maintain Pa_{CO_2} (and Pa_{O_2}) within the normal range and rigidity is prevented, clinical doses of opioids have minimal or negligible effects on ICP. However, the possibility of an increase in ICP with synthetic opioids cannot be completely excluded. Whenever these opioids are used, slow administration and care to maintain MABP are recommended.[159] It seems probable that remifentanil with either propofol or dexmedetomidine may be a useful regimen for various neurosurgical procedures, including minimally invasive surgery.

Muscle Relaxants

Succinylcholine

Many studies have demonstrated that succinylcholine elevates ICP in animals and humans, irrespective of the presence or absence of space-occupying intracranial lesions. The rise in ICP with succinylcholine was accompanied by muscle fasciculation, an increase in muscle spindle afferent activity, EEG arousal, and an elevation of CBF.[160] Fasciculation in the muscles of the neck, causing stasis in the jugular veins, might also be a factor contributing to increased ICP with succinylcholine. The rise in ICP was prevented or diminished by pretreatment with a nondepolarizing muscle relaxant,[161] the results contrasting with the animal study in which pretreatment with pancuronium did not attenuate the succinylcholine-induced increase in afferent muscle activity and CBF.[162]

Succinylcholine-induced increases in serum K^+ in a patient with subarachnoid hemorrhage is another concern but may not be significant at a relatively early stage (within 4 days).

Nevertheless, the use of succinylcholine has been diminishing in clinical neuroanesthesia practice, with the exception of emergency situations, such as the patient with a full stomach in whom a rapid-sequence induction of anesthesia is recommended. In this situation, prior administration of small doses of nondepolarizing muscle relaxant or lidocaine is recommended.

Nondepolarizing Muscle Relaxants

Some nondepolarizing muscle relaxants or their metabolites may affect the cerebral circulation through a histamine-releasing property that has pharmacologic activity. The clinical dose of atracurium appears to have no significant effect on CBF, CMR_{O_2}, or ICP. However, high doses of atracurium have the potential to release histamine, though the potential is considerably less than that of D-tubocurarine. Histamine can reduce CPP because of the increase in ICP caused by cerebral vasodilation and the decrease in MAP. The metabolite of atracurium, laudanosine, has been reported to cross the blood-brain barrier readily and cause seizures. However, the blood level of laudanosine after clinical doses of atracurium should not have undesirable consequences. No significant differences in seizure threshold for lidocaine have been reported in cats paralyzed with atracurium, pancuronium, and vecuronium.

Cisatracurium, an intermediate-acting muscle relaxant, produces and releases less laudanosine and histamine than atracurium. The cerebral effects of cisatracurium are essentially similar to or weaker than those of atracurium.[163]

Pancuronium, vecuronium, rocuronium, and pipecuronium have little or minimal effect on CBF, CMR_{O_2}, or ICP. Pancuronium raises blood pressure and heart rate, which could be disadvantageous for certain patients, such as those with hypertension, especially if they have disturbed autoregulation. In these patients, a substantial elevation of ICP could occur. Vecuronium does not induce histamine release, nor does it change blood pressure or heart rate, and thus may be preferable. Rocuronium, because of its rapid onset of action in comparison with other nondepolarizing muscle relaxants and its lack of adverse activity such as histamine release, may be preferable to succinylcholine during rapid induction of anesthesia.

In summary, if succinylcholine is used, prior administration of small doses of a nondepolarizing muscle relaxant or lidocaine is recommended, as well as maintenance of an adequate depth of anesthesia. With respect to the use of nondepolarizing muscle relaxants, in most clinical situations the changes in CBF and ICP are minimal if respiration is well controlled and an increase in Pa_{CO_2} is avoided.

Other Drugs

Lidocaine

Lidocaine has unique central nervous system effects that depend on the blood concentration; at low concentration, sedation occurs, but at higher concentration, seizures may occur. Non–seizure-inducing doses of lidocaine produce a dose-related reduction of CMR_{O_2} and CBF. Large doses of lidocaine reduce CMR_{O_2} by a maximum of 30% in dogs. If seizures are induced by lidocaine, CMR_{O_2} increases, as does CBF. Brain oxygenation seems to be adequate. However, regional flow–metabolism imbalance may not be excluded entirely.

Intravenous lidocaine 1.5 mg/kg has been reported to be effective in preventing circulatory changes and an elevation

ICP during tracheal intubation, endotracheal suctioning, or after application of a pin-type skull clamp or skin incision in patients undergoing craniotomy.

Several sodium channel blockers have been investigated and suggested as possible neuroprotectants.[164] Although the protective effect of lidocaine was not demonstrated in severe forebrain ischemia,[165] it was demonstrated in transient focal cerebral ischemia.[166] The dosage regimen was clinically relevant. The mechanism for protection appears to be related to preservation of mitochondrial function and inhibition of apoptosis.[167,168] A small clinical trial demonstrated a benefit of a clinically relevant dose of lidocaine infusion during cardiac surgery on long-term (6 months) neuropsychological condition.[169] A large-scale trial has not yet been performed.

α₂-Adrenergic Agonists

α_2-Adrenergic agonists appear to be potent cerebral vasoconstrictors.[170] In most animal studies, α_2 agonists decreased CBF with little if any influence on $CMRo_2$.[170] The cerebrovascular effects may depend on background anesthesia. The decrease in CBF caused by dexmedetomidine was observed in dogs anesthetized with isoflurane[170] but not during pentobarbital anesthesia.[171] α_2-Adrenergic agonists, topically applied through a cranial window, constricted pial arteries and veins. This effect was blocked by pretreatment of yohimbine, an α_2 antagonist.[172] The pretreatment with glibenclamide, a blocker of the ATP-sensitive potassium channel, potentiated the vasoconstriction of pial arteries, indicating that α_2-agonist–induced activation of ATP-sensitive potassium channels as a counterbalancing vasodilatory effect.[172] Neither inhibition of NO synthase nor a blockade of β-adrenoreceptor affects the cerebral vasoconstriction induced by dexmedetomidine.[173]

In humans, dexmedetomidine decreased Vmca in a dose-dependent manner, with the maximum reduction being approximately 25% at the hypnotic doses.[174] Dexmedetomidine was also reported to decrease both rCBF and global CBF.[175] As to the metabolic effect, contrary to the data derived from the animal investigations, dexmedetomidine reduced CMR equivalent (CMRe; this value is calculated by multiplying Vmca by the difference between arterial and cerebral jugular venous oxygen contents) in healthy volunteers in a dose-dependent manner.[176] The decreases in the CBF/CMR ratio that were anticipated from animal studies were not observed. A PET study in humans demonstrated a significant negative linear correlation between clonidine concentration and rCBF in the thalamus, prefrontal, orbital, and parietal association cortex, posterior cingulate cortex, and precuneus, suggesting that the pattern of regional deactivation during the sedation induced by clonidine is very close to the pattern of the physiologic early stage of non–rapid eye movement (REM) sleep.[177] Because the metabolic effects of clonidine were not examined in this study, the CBF/CMR ratio is not known.

Dexmedetomidine in a small dose decreased both MABP and ICP, and in higher doses it did not influence ICP, despite a significant increase in MABP in halothane-anesthetized rabbits.[178] In healthy human volunteers, oral administration of clonidine 5 µg/kg decreased Vmca by approximately 20% with slight attenuation of CO_2 reactivity.[179] In severely head-injured patients, a single dose of clonidine (2.5 µg/kg IV) did not significantly affect ICP but significantly reduced MABP and CPP.[180] Some patients displayed a transient increase (>10 mm Hg) in ICP concomitant with a decrease in MABP, which may have resulted from a cerebral autoregulatory vasodilation mechanism.[180]

A variety of in vivo and in vitro models demonstrated the neuroprotective effects of α_2 agonists, especially dexmedetomidine.[181] However the neuroprotective mechanism of dexmedetomidine remains unclear. No clinical evidence of neuroprotective effects of dexmedetomidine is available as yet. Nevertheless, because of the rapid onset and offset of effective sedation without respiratory depression, dexmedetomidine may be advantageous for awake craniotomy.

ANESTHETIC INTERACTIONS

Modification of autoregulation and CO_2 responses with anesthetics is important because these changes lead to unsatisfactory operative conditions and a potentially poor clinical outcome. Other important aspects are the interaction of anesthetics with surgical stimulation and with time (duration of anesthesia).

Autoregulation during Anesthesia

Autoregulation is preserved with intravenous anesthetics, barbiturates, propofol, and fentanyl, either alone or in combination even at high doses. Autoregulation appears to be impaired with volatile anesthetics, especially at high concentrations.[182] Impairment of autoregulation has lasted even after the depth of anesthesia was decreased. Such findings suggest that rapid normalization of blood pressure after induced hypotension might increase CBF profoundly and thus should be avoided. Reports have shown that autoregulation is partly preserved with isoflurane at 1 to 2 MAC.[183] Sevoflurane 1.5%, with or without N_2O, preserves autoregulation in patients with chronic cerebrovascular disease.[71] N_2O alone or in combination with morphine was reported not to disturb autoregulation.[184] Xenon appears to preserve autoregulation.[185,186] However, a study in humans demonstrated that N_2O has potential to impair "dynamic" autoregulation.[187]

Autoregulation is influenced not only by the anesthetic itself but also by the level of $Paco_2$. In general, autoregulation is impaired more easily when vasodilatory anesthetics are used or patients are kept hypercapnic than when vasoconstricting agents, including intravenous anesthetics, are in use and during hypocapnia.

Autoregulation is usually impaired in patients with intracranial space-occupying lesions. When autoregulation is lost or disturbed, sudden blood pressure changes can produce ischemia or brain edema. Therefore deep inhalational anesthesia and hypercapnia should definitely be avoided in such patients. During surgical incision and after extubation, suggestive increases in CBF in association with an increase in MABP were observed.[188] Thus careful management of blood pressure is critical in patients with intracranial pathologic conditions.

Cerebrovascular Reactivity to Carbon Dioxide

Cerebrovascular reactivity to CO_2 has been considered to be regulated by the change in extracellular H^+ concentration. The pH effect appears to be mediated by NO, prostanoids, cyclic nucleotides, and intracellular calcium as well as by potassium channel activity.[6] The extent of involvement of these mediating factors appears somewhat different in adults and neonates. Anesthetics may affect these parameters and influence the cerebrovascular reactivity to CO_2, although this process has not been well understood.

Nevertheless, at clinical levels of anesthesia, cerebrovascular responses to alterations in $Paco_2$ are preserved when both inhalational and intravenous agents are used, although the magnitude of response may vary according to agent and anesthetic depth. CO_2 reactivity is maintained to barbiturate concentrations that produce burst suppression in humans. In general, CO_2 reactivity appears to be greater when vasodilatory anesthetics are used than when vasoconstrictor drugs are used. In the rabbit, halothane increased CBF at all $Paco_2$ levels examined (20, 40, and 50 mm Hg).[189] In contrast, with isoflurane, CBF decreased during hypocapnia; it was unchanged during normocapnia and increased during hypercapnia. In another report, CO_2 reactivity has been shown to be greater with isoflurane than with halothane.[190] At a $Paco_2$ of 18 to 20 mm Hg, CBF was significantly less with isoflurane than with halothane. The explanation could be that the cerebral metabolic depression is greater than the ability to dilate cerebral vessels. The different CO_2 reactivity with different anesthetics may be related to the agents' potency of metabolic depression.

CO_2 reactivity has been reported to be impaired or lost when blood pressure diminishes during high concentrations of inhalational anesthetics. Whether the loss of reactivity to CO_2 is due to the anesthetic or to hypotension is unclear. However, it was reported that cerebrovascular reactivity to hypocapnia was better preserved during hypotension with isoflurane than with sodium nitroprusside.[191] Cerebrovascular reactivity to hypercapnia, in contrast, was blunted with high concentration of isoflurane. This may be the result of the maximally dilated vasculature with high concentrations of isoflurane.

Reactivity to CO_2 has been shown to be present in anesthetized patients with intracranial space-occupying lesions. For this reason, hyperventilation is recommended in patients with increased ICP or decreased intracranial compliance. However, hyperventilation may cause ischemia, both in patients with head injury and in patients with ischemic cerebrovascular disease, and thus, prolonged extreme hyperventilation should be avoided.[192] In moyamoya disease, both hypocapnia and hypercapnia appear to decrease CBF. CO_2 reactivity also varies by region. It also may be attenuated during anesthesia by associated diseases such as diabetes mellitus and peripheral vascular disease.[193]

Many neurosurgical procedures have been performed with the patient under mild to moderate hypothermia because decreases in temperature provide neuroprotective effects, although the multicenter Intraoperative Hypothermia for Aneurysm Surgery Trial (IHAST) did not demonstrate a significant protective effect for intraoperative mild hypothermia (33° C) during surgery for intracranial aneurysm.[194] CO_2 reactivity at a corresponding level of moderate hypothermia appears to be maintained.

Surgical Stimulation

The changes in CBF, $CMRo_2$, and ICP that occur during surgical stimulation are important to note. Sciatic nerve stimulation has been shown to produce coupled increases in CBF and $CMRo_2$, accompanied by EEG desynchronization, during 0.5% and 1.0% halothane in dogs. During 1.4% halothane, stimulation produced an increase in CBF without a change in $CMRo_2$ or EEG or an increase in arterial blood pressure. During morphine anesthesia (0.5 mg/kg and 1.5 mg/kg with or without N_2O), nerve stimulation produced almost parallel increases in CBF and $CMRo_2$ and was accompanied by EEG desynchronization. During deep thiopental anesthesia, stimulation-induced increases in CBF and $CMRo_2$ were abolished but were seen during light thiopental anesthesia. Therefore, irrespective of anesthetic depth, a tight relationship exists among changes in CBF, $CMRo_2$, and EEG with stimulation during thiopental anesthesia. These results suggest that anesthetics possessing cerebral vasodilator effects attenuate the coupling between flow and metabolism with stimulation and may disturb it at higher concentration, whereas cerebral vasoconstrictor drugs tend to maintain it.

Through autoradiographic techniques, cerebral vasodilation elicited by focal stimulation within the medullary reticular formation in rats anesthetized with α-chloralose has been reported.[195] Local glucose use in the brain (the hindlimb projection area) and in the dorsal horn of the lumbar spinal cord was increased by unilateral sciatic nerve stimulation in rats anesthetized with 0.5% and 2% enflurane. At 4% enflurane, stimulation induced an increase in glucose use in the spinal cord but not in the brain.[196] The results show that a threshold exists at which enflurane suppresses the metabolic responses to peripheral stimulation in the somatosensory cortex but not in the spinal cord. If electrical stimulation is regarded as analogous to surgical stimulation, a considerable increase in spinal cord metabolism may occur during surgery, even in a deeply anesthetized subject, even though the cerebral cortical responses are blocked with high anesthetic concentrations.

In humans anesthetized with 3.5% enflurane, no apparent increases in global CBF or $CMRo_2$ were observed with surgical stimulation, despite changes in EEG.[197] However, in that study, CBF and $CMRo_2$ were measured by the Kety-Schmidt method, and the regional changes in CBF and $CMRo_2$ with stimulation may not have been detected. Another study showed that cerebral Vmca increased with surgical stimulation at 1 and 2 MAC isoflurane anesthesia. The increase was not a function of changes in blood pressure. These data suggest that surgical stimulation raises CBF, possibly because of the changes in cerebral functional activity.[198] CBF changes evoked by surgical stimulation were reported to be dependent on the $Paco_2$ level. In patients anesthetized with sevoflurane 1.7% and N_2O 60%, the increase in Vmca was attenuated by hypocapnia and augmented by hypercapnia, even within clinically relevant ranges of $Paco_2$.[199]

Comparing these reported data in animals and humans, one must consider the possibility that, during light anesthesia, surgical stimulation provokes a CBF increase in association with metabolic activation and may cause an increase in ICP. Blocking the noxious stimuli by other drugs would be recommended. This recommendation is supported by a study in which Vmca remained stable during surgery at 1 MAC isoflurane anesthesia with concomitant use of epidural local anesthetic.[200]

Interactions with Time

Many studies in animals revealed that cerebral hyperemia induced by volatile anesthetics decreases during prolonged anesthesia. Similar reductions in CBF have been reported for N_2O. The mechanism for this gradual return of CBF to preanesthetic level is not clear. However, this phenomenon could not be modified by prior administration of α- and β-receptor blocking drugs. In addition, it is not related to time-dependent changes in autoregulation or CSF pH. Immobilization or mechanical ventilation has been postulated as the cause, but the data are inconclusive.

In some reports there was no gradual decrease in CBF over time in animals.[201] Because a volatile anesthetic–induced cerebral hyperemia is partially attributed to an increased production of NO,[49] sustained production of NO during prolonged anesthesia might have prevented the gradual decrease in CBF.[201] Further studies are necessary to determine the contribution of NO to CBF during prolonged exposure to volatile anesthetics.

Human studies of this time effect are rather limited because repeated measurements of CBF at short intervals for a prolonged period are hard to obtain owing to technical difficulties during surgical anesthesia in the operating room. In patients with intracranial mass lesions, no significant differences of CBF between two times of measurement during isoflurane or desflurane anesthesia appeared.[86] Although the measurements were made only twice, at the beginning and at the end of the study, the results suggest that CBF does not change over time during anesthesia in humans. Kuroda and associates[72] found that the elevated CBF equivalent was preserved during prolonged anesthesia (1.5 MAC) over 3 hours with halothane, isoflurane, and sevoflurane. However, CBF equivalent provides only the global ratio of CBF to CMR_{O_2} for a certain period. There are two possible explanations for these results: CBF remains stable or CBF changes in a parallel fashion to functional-metabolic changes during the observation period. As judged from relatively unchanged EEG patterns during 3 hours of anesthesia, it is unlikely the CMR_{O_2} exhibits consistent change over time. Thus the increase in CBF produced by volatile anesthetics is maintained during prolonged anesthesia without decay. The subsequent study using the transcranial Doppler ultrasonography technique showed no decay in Vmca over time during 3 hours of inhalation of volatile anesthetics at 1.5 MAC in humans.[3] No decay in Vmca over time is seen in children during isoflurane (1 MAC) exposure.[200] It seems likely that a time effect for gradual decrease in CBF does not take place in humans during prolonged administration of volatile anesthetics.

SUMMARY

Anesthetic drugs and techniques influence cerebral circulation, metabolism, and ICP. Some anesthetic drugs may have a potential for neuroprotective effects. The issues discussed in this chapter are important for the anesthetic management of both patients undergoing neurosurgery and patients with brain disorders. The severely damaged brain cannot be restored. Anesthetic management thus should focus on preventing the extension of damage, preventing new damage, and providing appropriate surgical conditions. If a potent cerebral vasodilatory anesthetic is used in patients with intracranial space-occupying lesions or decreased intracranial compliance, a marked rise in ICP may occur. Induction of cerebral hyperemia in a patient with a space-occupying intracranial lesion therefore should always be avoided. Induction of vasoconstriction, by either hyperventilation or concomitant use of vasoconstricting anesthetics such as barbiturates and propofol, decreases and stabilizes the ICP. During carotid endarterectomy and bypass surgery, normocapnia may be recommended because the rCBF response of an ischemic area to altered $Paco_2$ cannot be accurately predicted in individual patients. Autoregulation may be impaired by pathologic conditions as well as by deep volatile inhalational anesthesia.

Furthermore, the CPP necessary to maintain adequate cerebral perfusion cannot be easily determined in an individual patient. Thus, during surgery for ischemic cerebrovascular decreases, arterial blood pressure should be kept at a value no lower than the lowest preoperative pressure. The metabolic depressive effect of barbiturates and propofol may also be beneficial in such situations. Isoflurane and sevoflurane have been suggested as drugs of choice if an inhalational anesthetic is deemed desirable. However, other volatile anesthetics, when used at low concentration, would not cause harm. Noxious stimuli in a patient under inadequate anesthesia or with seizure activity can produce undesirable events, such as increases in metabolism, CBV, and ICP. Synthetic opioids and supplemental local anesthetics are recommended. Special attention must be paid, in the case of functional neurosurgery, to obtain rapid control of asleep-awake-asleep state or sedation with analgesia through the use of anesthetics and adjuvant drugs with easy controllability.

REFERENCES

1. Hirase H: A multi-photon window onto neuronal-glial-vascular communication, *Trends Neurosci* 28:217–219, 2005.
2. Pellerin L, Bouzier-Sore AK, Aubert A, et al: Activity-dependent regulation of energy metabolism by astrocytes: an update, *Glia* 55:1251–1262, 2007.
3. Kuroda Y, Murakami M, Tsuruta J, et al: Blood flow velocity of middle cerebral artery during prolonged anesthesia with halothane, isoflurane, and sevoflurane in humans, *Anesthesiology* 87:527–532, 1997.
4. Lam AM, Matta BF, Mayberg TS, et al: Change in cerebral blood flow velocity with onset of EEG electroencephalogram silence during inhalation anesthesia in humans: Evidence of flow-metabolism coupling?, *J Cereb Blood Flow Metab* 15:714–717, 1995.
5. Weyland A, Buhre W, Grund S, et al: Cerebrovascular tone rather than intracranial pressure determines the effective downstream pressure of the cerebral circulation in the absence of intracranial hypertension, *J Neurosurg Anesthesiol* 12:210–216, 2000.
6. Brian JE Jr: Carbon Dioxide and the cerebral circulation, *Anesthesiology* 88:1365–1386, 1998.
7. Bardutzky J, Schwab S: Antiedema therapy in ischemic stroke, *Stroke* 38:3084–3094, 2007.
8. Lanier WL, Iaizzo PA, Milde JH, et al: The cerebral and systemic effects of movement in response to a noxious stimulus in lightly anesthetized dogs: Possible modulation of cerebral function by muscle afferents, *Anesthesiology* 80:392–401, 1994.
9. Lanier WL, Albrecht RF 2nd, Laizzo PA: Divergence of intracranial and central venous pressures in lightly anesthetized, tracheally intubated dogs that move in response to a noxious stimulus, *Anesthesiology* 84:605–613, 1996.
10. Stocchetti N, Maas AI, Chieregato A, et al: Hyperventilation in head injury: A review, *Chest* 127:1812–1827, 2005.
11. Reinstrup P, Ryding E, Algotsson L, et al: Effects of nitrous oxide on human regional cerebral blood flow and isolated pial arteries, *Anesthesiology* 81:396–402, 1994.
12. Gyulai FE, Firestone LL, Mintun MA, et al: In vivo imaging of human limbic responses to nitrous oxide inhalation, *Anesth Analg* 83:291–298, 1996.
13. Lorenz IH, Kolbitsch C, Hormann C, et al: The influence of nitrous oxide and remifentanil on cerebral hemodynamics in conscious human volunteers, *Neuroimage* 17:1056–1064, 2002.
14. Reinstrup P, Ryding E, Ohlsson T, et al: Regional cerebral metabolic rate (positron emission tomography) during inhalation of nitrous oxide 50% in humans, *Br J Anaesth* 100:66–71, 2008.
15. Algotsson L, Messeter K, Rosen I, et al: Effects of nitrous oxide on cerebral haemodynamics and metabolism during isoflurane anaesthesia in man, *Acta Anaesthesiol Scand* 36:46–52, 1992.
16. Hoffman WE, Charbel FT, Edelman G, et al: Nitrous oxide added to isoflurane increases brain artery blood flow and low frequency brain electrical activity, *J Neurosurg Anesthesiol* 7:82–88, 1995.
17. Kaisti KK, Langsjo JW, Aalto S, et al: Effects of sevoflurane, propofol, and adjunct nitrous oxide on regional cerebral blood flow, oxygen consumption, and blood volume in humans, *Anesthesiology* 99:603–613, 2003.

18. Cho S, Fujigaki T, Uchiyama Y, et al: Effects of sevoflurane with and without nitrous oxide on human cerebral circulation: Transcranial Doppler study, *Anesthesiology* 85:755–760, 1996.

19. Strebel S, Kaufmann M, Anselmi L, et al: Nitrous oxide is a potent cerebrovasodilator in humans when added to isoflurane: A transcranial Doppler study, *Acta Anaesthesiol Scand* 39:653–658, 1995.

20. Hormann C, Schmidauer C, Haring HP, et al: Hyperventilation reverses the nitrous oxide-induced increase in cerebral blood flow velocity in human volunteers, *Br J Anaesth* 74:616–618, 1995.

21. Hormann C, Schmidauer C, Kolbitsch C, et al: Effects of normo- and hypocapnic nitrous-oxide-inhalation on cerebral blood flow velocity in patients with brain tumors, *J Neurosurg Anesthiol* 9:141–145, 1997.

22. Sakabe T, Tsutsui T, Maekawa T, et al: Local cerebral glucose utilization during nitrous oxide and pentobarbital anesthesia in rats, *Anesthesiology* 63:262–266, 1985.

23. Matta BF, Lam AM: Nitrous oxide increases cerebral blood flow velocity during pharmacologically induced EEG electroencephalogram silence in humans, *J Neurosurg Anesthiol* 7:89–93, 1995.

24. Culley DJ, Xie Z, Crosby G: General anesthetic-induced neurotoxicity: An emerging problem for the young and old?, *Curr Opin Anaesthesiol* 20:408–413, 2007.

25. David HN, Leveille F, Chazalviel L, et al: Reduction of ischemic brain damage by nitrous oxide and xenon, *J Cereb Blood Flow Metab* 23:1168–1173, 2003.

26. Jevtovic-Todorovic V, Beals J, Benshoff N, et al: Prolonged exposure to inhalational anesthetic nitrous oxide kills neurons in adult rat brain, *Neuroscience* 122:609–616, 2003.

27. Myles PS, Leslie K, Chan MT, et al: Avoidance of nitrous oxide for patients undergoing major surgery: A randomized controlled trial, *Anesthesiology* 107:221–231, 2007.

28. Frietsch T, Bogdanski R, Blobner M, et al: Effects of xenon on cerebral blood flow and cerebral glucose utilization in rats, *Anesthesiology* 94:290–297, 2001.

29. Schmidt M, Marx T, Kotzerke J, et al: Cerebral and regional organ perfusion in pigs during xenon anaesthesia, *Anaesthesia* 56:1154–1159, 2001.

30. Laitio RM, Kaisti KK, Laangsjo JW, et al: Effects of xenon anesthesia on cerebral blood flow in humans: A positron emission tomography study, *Anesthesiology* 106:1128–1133, 2007.

31. Rex S, Schaefer W, Meyer PH, et al: Positron emission tomography study of regional cerebral metabolism during general anesthesia with xenon in humans, *Anesthesiology* 105:936–943, 2006.

32. Alkire MT, Haier RJ, Shah NK, et al: Positron emission tomography study of regional cerebral metabolism in humans during isoflurane anesthesia, *Anesthesiology* 86:549–557, 1997.

33. Alkire MT, Pomfrett CJ, Haier RJ, et al: Functional brain imaging during anesthesia in humans: Effects of halothane on global and regional cerebral glucose metabolism, *Anesthesiology* 90:701–709, 1999.

34. Fukuda T, Nakayama H, Yanagi K, et al: The effects of 30% and 60% xenon inhalation on pial vessel diameter and intracranial pressure in rabbits, *Anesth Analg* 92:1245–1250, 2001.

35. Darby JM, Nemoto EM, Yonas H, et al: Stable xenon does not increase intracranial pressure in primates with freeze-injury-induced intracranial hypertension, *J Cereb Blood Flow Metab* 11:522–526, 1991.

36. Schmidt M, Marx T, Armbruster S, et al: Effect of xenon on elevated intracranial pressure as compared with nitrous oxide and total intravenous anesthesia in pigs, *Acta Anaesthesiol Scand* 49:494–501, 2005.

37. Plougmann J, Astrup J, Pedersen J, et al: Effect of stable xenon inhalation on intracranial pressure during measurement of cerebral blood flow in head injury, *J Neurosurg* 81:822–828, 1994.

38. Marion DW, Crosby K: The effect of stable xenon on ICP, *J Cereb Blood Flow Metab* 11:347–350, 1991.

39. Homi HM, Yokoo N, Ma D, et al: The neuroprotective effect of xenon administration during transient middle cerebral artery occlusion in mice, *Anesthesiology* 99:876–881, 2003.

40. Schmidt M, Marx T, Gloggl E, et al: Xenon attenuates cerebral damage after ischemia in pigs, *Anesthesiology* 102:929–936, 2005.

41. Wilhelm S, Ma D, Maze M, et al: Effects of xenon on in vitro and in vivo models of neuronal injury, *Anesthesiology* 96:1485–1491, 2002.

42. Dingley J, Tooley J, Porter H, et al: Xenon provides short-term neuroprotection in neonatal rats when administered after hypoxia-ischemia, *Stroke* 37:501–506, 2006.

43. Ma D, Hossain M, Chow A, et al: Xenon and hypothermia combine to provide neuroprotection from neonatal asphyxia, *Ann Neurol* 58:182–193, 2005.

44. Rajakumaraswamy N, Ma D, Hossain M, et al: Neuroprotective interaction produced by xenon and dexmedetomidine on in vitro and in vivo neuronal injury models, *Neurosci Lett* 409:128–133, 2006.

45. Ma D, Hossain M, Pettet GK, et al: Xenon preconditioning reduces brain damage from neonatal asphyxia in rats, *J Cereb Blood Flow Metab* 26:199–208, 2006.

46. Hobbs C, Thoresen M, Tucker A, et al: Xenon and hypothermia combine additively, offering long-term functional and histopathologic neuroprotection after neonatal hypoxia/ischemia, *Stroke* 39:1307–1313, 2008.

47. Brussel T, Fitch W, Brodner G, et al: Effects of halothane in low concentrations on cerebral blood flow, cerebral metabolism, and cerebrovascular autoregulation in the baboon, *Anesth Analg* 73:758–764, 1991.

48. Koenig HM, Pelligrino DA, Albrecht RF: Halothane vasodilation and nitric oxide in rat pial vessels, *J Neurosurg Anesthiol* 5:264–271, 1993.

49. MacPherson RW, Kirsch JR, Moore LE, et al: N omega-nitro-L-arginine-nitro-arginine methyl ester prevents cerebral hyperemia by inhaled anesthetics in dogs, *Anesth Analg* 77:891–897, 1993.

50. Moore LE, Kirsch JR, Helfaer MA, et al: Nitric oxide and prostanoids contribute to isoflurane-induced cerebral hyperemia in pigs, *Anesthesiology* 80:1328–1337, 1994.

51. Toda N, Toda H, Hatano Y: Nitric oxide: Involvement in the effects of anesthetic agents, *Anesthesiology* 107:822–842, 2007.

52. Todd MM, Drummond JC: A comparison of the cerebrovascular and metabolic effects of halothane and isoflurane in the cat, *Anesthesiology* 60:276–282, 1984.

53. Matta BF, Mayberg TS, Lam AM: Direct cerebrovasodilatory effects of halothane, isoflurane, and desflurane during propofol-induced isoelectric electroencephalogram in humans, *Anesthesiology* 83:980–985, 1995.

54. Schlünzen L, Cold GE, Rasmussen M, et al: Effects of dose-dependent levels of isoflurane on cerebral blood flow in healthy subjects studied using positron emission tomography, *Acta Anaesthesiol Scand* 50:306–312, 2006.

55. Kehl F, Shen H, Moreno C, et al: Isoflurane-induced cerebral hyperemia is partially mediated by nitric oxide and epoxyeicosatrienoic acids in mice in vivo, *Anesthesiology* 97:1528–1533, 2002.

56. Iida H, Ohata H, Iida M, et al: Isoflurane and sevoflurane induce vasodilation of cerebral vessels via ATP-sensitive K+ channel activation, *Anesthesiology* 89:954–960, 1998.

57. Lorenz IH, Kolbitsch C, Hormann C, et al: Influence of equianaesthetic concentrations of nitrous oxide and isoflurane on regional cerebral blood flow, regional cerebral blood volume, and regional mean transit time in human volunteers, *Br J Anaesth* 87:691–698, 2001.

58. Talke P, Caldwell J, Dodsont B, et al: Desflurane and isoflurane increase lumbar cerebrospinal fluid pressure in normocapnic patients undergoing transsphenoidal hypophysectomy, *Anesthesiology* 85:999–1004, 1996.

59. Artru AA, Lam AM, Johnson JO, et al: Intracranial pressure, middle cerebral artery flow velocity, and plasma inorganic fluoride concentrations in neurosurgical patients receiving sevoflurane or isoflurane, *Anesth Analg* 85:587–592, 1997.

60. Petersen KD, Landsfeldt U, Cold GE, et al: Intracranial pressure and cerebral hemodynamic in patients with cerebral tumors: A randomized prospective study of patients subjected to craniotomy in propofol-fentanyl, isoflurane-fentanyl, or sevoflurane-fentanyl anesthesia, *Anesthesiology* 98:329–336, 2003.

61. Fukuda S, Warner DS: Cerebral protection, *Br J Anaesth* 99:10–17, 2007.

62. Sano T, Drummond JC, Patel PM, et al: A comparison of the cerebral protective effects of isoflurane and mild hypothermia in a model of incomplete forebrain ischemia in the rat, *Anesthesiology* 76:221–228, 1992.

63. Kapinya KJ, Lowl D, Futterer C, et al: Tolerance against ischemic neuronal injury can be induced by volatile anesthetics and is inducible NO synthase dependent, *Stroke* 33:1889–1898, 2002.

64. Xiong L, Zheng Y, Wu M, et al: Preconditioning with isoflurane produces dose-dependent neuroprotection via activation of adenosine triphosphate-regulated potassium channels after focal cerebral ischemia in rats, *Anesth Analg* 96:233–237, 2003.

65. Messick JM, Casement B, Sharbrough FW, et al: Correlation of regional cerebral blood flow (rCBF) with EEG changes during isoflurane anesthesia for carotid endarterectomy: critical rCBF, *Anesthesiology* 66:344–349, 1987.

66. Conzen PF, Vollmar B, Habazettl H, et al: Systemic and regional hemodynamics of isoflurane and sevoflurane in rats, *Anesth Analg* 74:79–88, 1992.

67. Fujibayashi T, Sugiura Y, Yanagimoto M, et al: Brain energy metabolism and blood flow during sevoflurane and halothane anesthesia: Effects of hypocapnia and blood pressure fluctuations, *Acta Anaesthesiol Scand* 38:413–418, 1994.

68. Scheller MS, Nakakimura K, Fleischer JE, et al: Cerebral effects of sevoflurane in the dog: Comparison with isoflurane and enflurane, *Br J Anaesth* 65:388–392, 1990.

69. Crawford MW, Lerman J, Saldivia V, et al: Hemodynamic and organ blood flow responses to halothane and sevoflurane anesthesia during spontaneous ventilation, *Anesth Analg* 75:1000–1006, 1992.

70. Matta BF, Heath KJ, Tipping K, et al: Direct cerebral vasodilatory effects of sevoflurane and isoflurane, *Anesthesiology* 91:677–680, 1999.

71. Kitaguchi K, Ohsumi H, Kuro M, et al: Effects of sevoflurane on cerebral circulation and metabolism in patients with ischemic cerebrovascular disease, *Anesthesiology* 79:704–709, 1993.

72. Kuroda Y, Murakami M, Tsuruta J, et al: Preservation of the ration of cerebral blood flow/metabolic rate for oxygen during prolonged anesthesia with isoflurane, sevoflurane, and halothane in humans, *Anesthesiology* 84:555–561, 1996.

73. Kaisti KK, Metsahonkala L, Teras M, et al: Effects of surgical levels of propofol and sevoflurane anesthesia on cerebral blood flow in healthy subjects studied with positron emission tomography, *Anesthesiology* 96:1358–1370, 2002.

74. Schlünzen L, Vafaee MS, Cold GE, et al: Effects of subanaesthetic and anaesthetic doses of sevoflurane on regional cerebral blood flow in healthy volunteers: A positron emission tomographic study, *Acta Anaesthesiol Scand* 48:1268–1276, 2004.

75. Takahashi H, Murata K, Ikeda K: Sevoflurane does not increase intracranial pressure in hyperventilated dogs, *Br J Anaesth* 71:551–555, 1993.

76. Hölmstrom A, Åkeson J: Desflurane increases intracranial pressure more and sevoflurane less than isoflurane in pigs subjected to intracranial hypertension, *J Neurosurg Anesthesiol* 16:136–143, 2004.

77. Talke P, Caldwell JE, Richardson CA: Sevoflurane increases lumbar cerebrospinal fluid pressure in normocapnic patients undergoing transsphenoidal hypophysectomy, *Anesthesiology* 91:127–130, 1999.

78. Warner DS, McFarlane C, Todd MM, et al: Sevoflurane and halothane reduce focal ischemic brain damage in the rat, *Anesthesiology* 79:985–992, 1993.

79. Werner C, Mollenberg O, Kochs E, et al: Sevoflurane improves neurological outcome after incomplete cerebral ischaemia in rats, *Br J Anaesth* 75:756–760, 1995.

80. Nakajima Y, Moriwaki G, Ikeda K, et al: The effects of sevoflurane on recovery of brain energy metabolism after cerebral ischemia in the rat: a comparison with isoflurane and halothane, *Anesth Analg* 85:593–599, 1997.

81. Payne RS, Akca O, Roewer N, et al: Sevoflurane-induced preconditioning protects against cerebral ischemic neuronal damage in rats, *Brain Res* 1034:147–152, 2005.

82. Grady RE, Weglinski MR, Sharbrough FW, et al: Correlation of regional cerebral blood flow with ischemic electroencephalographic changes during sevoflurane-nitrous oxide anesthesia for carotid endarterectomy, *Anesthesiology* 88:892–897, 1998.

83. Lutz LJ, Milde JH, Milde LN: The cerebral functional, metabolic, and hemodynamic effects of desflurane in dogs, *Anesthesiology* 73:125–131, 1990.

84. Lenz C, Frietsch T, Futterer C, et al: Local coupling of cerebral blood flow to cerebral glucose metabolism during inhalational anesthesia in rats: desflurane versus isoflurane, *Anesthesiology* 91:1720–1723, 1999.

85. Lutz LJ, Milde JH, Milde LN: The response of the canine cerebral circulation to hyperventilation during anesthesia with desflurane, *Anesthesiology* 74:504–507, 1991.

86. Ornstein E, Young WL, Fleischer LH, et al: Desflurane and isoflurane have similar effects on cerebral blood flow in patients with intracranial mass lesions, *Anesthesiology* 79:498–502, 1993.

87. Mielck F, Stephan H, Buhre W, et al: Effects of 1 MAC desflurane on cerebral metabolism, blood flow and carbon dioxide reactivity in humans, *Br J Anaesth* 81:155–160, 1998.

88. Artru AA: Intracranial volume/pressure relationship during desflurane anesthesia in dogs: Comparison with isoflurane and thiopental/halothane, *Anesth Analg* 79:751–760, 1994.

89. Muzzi DA, Losasso TJ, Dietz NM, et al: The effect of desflurane and isoflurane on cerebrospinal fluid pressure in humans with supratentorial mass lesions, *Anesthesiology* 76:720–724, 1992.

90. Fraga M, Rama-Maceiras P, Rodino S, et al: The effects of isoflurane and desflurane on intracranial pressure, cerebral perfusion pressure, and cerebral arteriovenous oxygen content difference in normocapnic patients with supratentorial brain tumors, *Anesthesiology* 98:1085–1090, 2003.

91. Engelhard K, Werner C, Reeker W, et al: Desflurane and isoflurane improve neurological outcome after incomplete cerebral ischaemia in rats, *Br J Anaesth* 83:415–421, 1999.

92. Haelewyn B, Yvon A, Hanouz JL, et al: Desflurane affords greater protection than halothane against focal cerebral ischaemia in the rat, *Br J Anaesth* 91:390–396, 2003.

93. Tsai SK, Lin SM, Hung WC, et al: The effect of desflurane on ameliorating cerebral infarction in rats subjected to focal cerebral ischemia-reperfusion injury, *Life Sci* 74:2541–2549, 2004.

94. Dimaculangan D, Bendo AA, Sims R, et al: Desflurane improves the recovery of the evoked postsynaptic population spike from CA1 pyramidal cells after hypoxia in rat hippocampal slices, *J Neurosurg Anesthesiol* 18:78–82, 2006.

95. Hoffman WE, Charbel FT, Edelman G: Desflurane increases brain tissue oxygenation and pH, *Acta Anaesthesiol Scand* 41:1162–1166, 1997.

96. Warner DS, Takaoka S, Wu B, et al: Electroencephalographic burst suppression is not required to elicit maximal neuroprotection from pentobarbital in a model of focal cerebral ischemia, *Anesthesiology* 84:1475–1484, 1996.

97. Milde LN, Milde JH, Michenfelder JD: Cerebral functional, metabolic, and hemodynamic effects of etomidate in dogs, *Anesthesiology* 63:371–377, 1985.

98. Bingham RM, Procaccio F, Prior PF, et al: Cerebral electrical activity influences the effects of etomidate on cerebral perfusion pressure in traumatic coma, *Br J Anaesth* 57:843–848, 1985.

99. Sano T, Patel PM, Drummond JC, et al: A comparison of the cerebral protective effects of etomidate, thiopental, and isoflurane in a model of forebrain ischemia in the rat, *Anesth Analg* 76:990–997, 1993.

100. Drummond JC, Cole DJ, Patel PM, et al: Focal cerebral ischemia during anesthesia with etomidate, isoflurane, or thiopental: A comparison of the extent of cerebral injury, *Neurosurgery* 37:742–748, 1995.

101. Guo J, White JA, Batjer HH: Limited protective effects of etomidate during brainstem ischemia in dogs, *J Neurosurg* 82:278–283, 1995.

102. Hoffman WE, Charbel FT, Edelman G, et al: Comparison of the effect of etomidate and desflurane on brain tissue gases and pH during prolonged middle cerebral artery occlusion, *Anesthesiology* 88:1188–1194, 1998.

103. Drummond JC, McKay LD, Cole DJ, et al: The role of nitric oxide synthase inhibition in the adverse effects of etomidate in the setting of focal cerebral ischemia in rats, *Anesth Analg* 100:841–846, 2005.

104. Edelman GJ, Hoffman WE, Charbel FT: Cerebral hypoxia after etomidate administration and temporary cerebral artery occlusion, *Anesth Analg* 85:821–825, 1997.

105. Ostwald P, Doenicke AW: Etomidate revisited, *Curr Opin Anaesthesiol* 11:391–398, 1998.

106. Fiset P, Paus T, Daloze T, et al: Brain mechanisms of propofol-induced loss of consciousness in humans: A positron emission tomographic study, *J Neurosci* 19:5506–5513, 1999.

107. McCulloch TJ, Thompson CL, Turner MJ: A randomized crossover comparison of the effects of propofol and sevoflurane on cerebral hemodynamics during carotid endarterectomy, *Anesthesiology* 106:56–64, 2007.

108. Kikuta K, Takagi Y, Nozaki K, et al: Effects of intravenous anesthesia with propofol on regional cortical blood flow and intracranial pressure in surgery for moyamoya disease, *Surg Neurol* 68:421–424, 2007.

109. Alkire MT, Haier RJ, Barker SJ, et al: Cerebral metabolism during propofol anesthesia in humans studied with positron emission tomography, *Anesthesiology* 82:393–403, 1995.

110. Jansen GF, van Praagh BH, Kedaria MB, et al: Jugular bulb oxygen saturation during propofol and isoflurane/nitrous oxide anesthesia in patients undergoing brain tumor surgery, *Anesth Analg* 89:358–363, 1999.

111. Cervantes M, Ruelas R, Chavez-Carrillo I, et al: Effects of propofol on alterations of multineuronal activity of limbic and mesencephalic structures and neurological deficit elicited by acute global cerebral ischemia, *Arch Med Res* 26:385–395, 1995.

112. Kochs E, Hoffman WE, Werner C, et al: The effects of propofol on brain electrical activity, neurologic outcome, and neuronal damage following incomplete ischemia in rats, *Anesthesiology* 76:245–252, 1992.

113. Pittman JE, Sheng H, Pearlstein R, et al: Comparison of the effects of propofol and pentobarbital on neurologic outcome and cerebral infarct size after temporary focal ischemia in the rat, *Anesthesiology* 87:1139–1144, 1997.

114. Ridenour TR, Warner DS, Todd MM, et al: Comparative effects of propofol and halothane on outcome from temporary middle cerebral artery occlusion in the rat, *Anesthesiology* 76:807–812, 1992.

115. Adembri C, Venturi L, Pellegrini-Giampietro DE: Neuroprotective effects of propofol in acute cerebral injury, *CNS Drug Rev* 13:333–351, 2007.

116. Bayona NA, Gelb AW, Jiang Z, et al: Propofol neuroprotection in cerebral ischemia and its effects on low-molecular-weight antioxidants and skilled motor tasks, *Anesthesiology* 100:1151–1159, 2004.

117. Parke TJ, Stevens JE, Rice AS, et al: Metabolic acidosis and fatal myocardial failure after propofol infusion in children: Five case reports, *BMJ* 305:613–616, 1992.

118. Strickland RA, Murray MJ: Fatal metabolic acidosis in a pediatric patient receiving an infusion of propofol in the intensive care unit: Is there a relationship? *Crit Care Med* 23:405–409, 1995.

119. Cavazzuti M, Porro CA, Biral GP, et al: Ketamine effects on local cerebral blood flow and metabolism in the rat, *J Cereb Blood Flow Metab* 7:806–811, 1987.

120. Långsjö JW, Kaisti KK, Aalto S, et al: Effects of subanesthetic doses of ketamine on regional cerebral blood flow, oxygen consumption, and blood volume in humans, *Anesthesiology* 99:614–623, 2003.

121. Långsjö JW, Salmi E, Kaisti KK, et al: Effects of subanesthetic ketamine on regional cerebral glucose metabolism in humans, *Anesthesiology* 100:1065–1071, 2004.

122. Långsjö JW, Maksimow A, Salmi E, et al: S-ketamine anesthesia increases cerebral blood flow in excess of the metabolic needs in humans, *Anesthesiology* 103:258–268, 2005.

123. Albanese J, Arnaud S, Rey M, et al: Ketamine decreases intracranial pressure and electroencephalographic activity in traumatic brain injury patients during propofol sedation. Anesthesiology 87:1328-1334, 1997.

124. Mayberg TS, Lam AM, Matta BF, et al: Ketamine does not increase cerebral blood flow velocity or intracranial pressure during isoflurane/nitrous oxide anesthesia in patients undergoing craniotomy, *Anesth Analg* 81:84–89, 1995.

125. Schmittner MD, Vajkoczy SL, Horn P, et al: Effects of fentanyl and S(+)-ketamine on cerebral hemodynamics, gastrointestinal motility, and need of vasopressors in patients with intracranial pathologies: A pilot study, *J Neurosurg Anesthesiol* 19:257–262, 2007.

126. Shapira Y, Lam AM, Eng CC, et al: Therapeutic time window and dose response of the beneficial effects of ketamine in experimental head injury, *Stroke* 25:1637–1643, 1994.

127. Ridenour TR, Warner DS, Todd MM, et al: Effects of ketamine on outcome from temporary middle cerebral artery occlusion in the spontaneously hypertensive rat, *Brain Res* 565:116–122, 1991.

128. Himmelseher S, Durieux ME: Revising a dogma: Ketamine for patients with neurological injury?, *Anesth Analg* 101:524–534, 2005.

129. Bourgoin A, Albanese J, Wereszczynski N, et al: Safety of sedation with ketamine in severe head injury patients: Comparison with sufentanil, *Crit Care Med* 31:711–717, 2003.

130. Kolenda H, Gremmelt A, Rading S, et al: Ketamine for analgosedative therapy in intensive care treatment of head-injured patients, *Acta Neurochir (Wien)* 138:1193–1199, 1996.

131. Tateishi A, Maekawa T, Takeshita H, et al: Diazepam and intracranial pressure, *Anesthesiology* 54:335–337, 1981.

132. Veselis RA, Reinsel RA, Beattie BJ, et al: Midazolam changes cerebral blood flow in discrete brain regions: An $H_2^{15}O$ positron emission tomography study, *Anesthesiology* 87:1106–1117, 1997.

133. Werner C, Hoffman WE, Baughman VL, et al: Effects of sufentanil on cerebral blood flow, cerebral blood flow velocity, and metabolism in dogs, *Anesth Analg* 72:177–181, 1991.

134. Sheehan PB, Zornow MH, Scheller MS, et al: The effects of fentanyl and sufentanil on intracranial pressure and cerebral blood flow in rabbits with an acute cryogenic brain injury, *J Neurosurg Anesthesiol* 4:261–267, 1992.

135. Milde LN, Milde JH, Gallagher WJ: Effects of sufentanil on cerebral circulation and metabolism in dogs, *Anesth Analg* 70:138–146, 1990.

136. Keykhah MM, Smith DS, O'Neill JJ, et al: The influence of fentanyl upon cerebral high-energy metabolites, lactate, and glucose during severe hypoxia in the rat, *Anesthesiology* 69:566–570, 1988.

137. Kolbitsch C, Hormann C, Schmidauer C, et al: Hypocapnia reverses the fentanyl-induced increase in cerebral blood flow velocity in awake humans, *J Neurosurg Anesthesiol* 9:313–315, 1997.

138. Trindle MR, Dodson BA, Rampil IJ: Effects of fentanyl versus sufentanil in equianesthetic doses on middle cerebral artery blood flow velocity, *Anesthesiology* 78:454–460, 1993.

139. Hanel F, Werner C, von Knobelsdorff G, et al: The effects of fentanyl and sufentanil on cerebral hemodynamics, *J Neurosurg Anesthesiol* 9:223–227, 1997.

140. Weinstabl C, Mayer N, Spiss CK: Sufentanil decreases cerebral blood flow velocity in patients with elevated intracranial pressure, *Eur J Anaesthesiol* 9:481–484, 1992.

141. Firestone LL, Gyulai F, Mintun M, et al: Human brain activity response to fentanyl imaged by positron emission tomography, *Anesth Analg* 82:1247–1251, 1996.

142. Herrick IA, Gelb AW, Manninen PH, et al: Effects of fentanyl, sufentanil, and alfentanil on brain retractor pressure, *Anesth Analg* 72:359–363, 1991.

143. Bristow A, Shalev D, Rice B, et al: Low-dose synthetic narcotic infusions for cerebral relaxation during craniotomies, *Anesh Analg* 66:413–416, 1987.

144. Albanese J, Durbec O, Viviand X, et al: Sufentanil increases intracranial pressure in patients with head trauma, *Anesthesiology* 79:493–497, 1993.

145. Sperry RJ, Bailey PL, Reichman MV, et al: Fentanyl and sufentanil increase intracranial pressure in head trauma patients, *Anesthesiology* 77:416–420, 1992.

146. Werner C, Kochs E, Bause H, et al: Effects of sufentanil on cerebral hemodynamics and intracranial pressure in patients with brain injury, *Anesthesiology* 83:721–726, 1995.

147. Markovitz BP, Duhaime AC, Sutton L, et al: Effects of alfentanil on intracranial pressure in children undergoing ventriculoperitoneal shunt revision, *Anesthesiology* 76:71–76, 1992.

148. Souter MJ, Andrews PJ, Piper IR, et al: Effects of alfentanil on cerebral haemodynamics in an experimental model of traumatic brain injury, *Br J Anaesth* 79:97–102, 1997.

149. de Nadal M, Munar F, Poca MA, et al: Cerebral hemodynamic effects of morphine and fentanyl in patients with severe head injury: Absence of correlation to cerebral autoregulation, *Anesthesiology* 92:11–19, 2000.

150. Hoffman WE, Cunningham F, James MK, et al: Effects of remifentanil, a new short-acting opioid, on cerebral blood flow, brain electrical activity, and intracranial pressure in dogs anesthetized with isoflurane and nitrous oxide, *Anesthesiology* 79:107–113, 1993.

151. Mayberg TS, Lam AM, Eng CC, et al: The effect of alfentanil on cerebral blood flow velocity and intracranial pressure during isoflurane-nitrous oxide anesthesia in humans, *Anesthesiology* 78:288–294, 1993.

152. Paris A, Scholz J, von Knobelsdorff G, et al: The effect of remifentanil on cerebral blood flow velocity, *Anesth Analg* 87:569–573, 1998.

153. Warner DS, Hindman BJ, Todd MM, et al: Intracranial pressure and hemodynamic effects of remifentanil versus alfentanil in patients undergoing supratentorial craniotomy, *Anesth Analg* 83:348–353, 1996.

154. From RP, Warner DS, Todd MM, et al: Anesthesia for craniotomy: A double-blind comparison of alfentanil, fentanyl, and sufentanil, *Anesthesiology* 73:896–904, 1990.

155. Ostapkovich ND, Baker KZ, Fogarty-Mack P, et al: Cerebral blood flow and CO_2 reactivity is similar during remifentanil/N_2O and fentanyl/N_2O anesthesia, *Anesthesiology* 89:358–363, 1998.

156. Wagner KJ, Willoch F, Kochs EF, et al: Dose-dependent regional cerebral blood flow changes during remifentanil infusion in humans: A positron emission tomography study, *Anesthesiology* 94:732–739, 2001.

157. Wagner KJ, Sprenger T, Kochs EF, et al: Imaging human cerebral pain modulation by dose-dependent opioid analgesia: A positron emission tomography activation study using remifentanil, *Anesthesiology* 106:548–556, 2007.

158. Klimscha W, Ullrich R, Nasel C, et al: High-dose remifentanil does not impair cerebrovascular carbon dioxide reactivity in healthy male volunteers, *Anesthesiology* 99:834–840, 2003.

159. Lauer KK, Connolly LA, Schmeling WT: Opioid sedation does not alter intracranial pressure in head injured patients, *Can J Anaesth* 44:929–933, 1997.

160. Lanier WL, Iaizzo PA, Milde JH: Cerebral blood flow and afferent muscle activity following IV succinylcholine in dogs, *Anesthesiol Rev* 14:60–66, 1987.

161. Minton MD, Grosslight K, Stirt JA, et al: Increases in intracranial pressure from succinylcholine: prevention by prior nondepolarizing blockade, *Anesthesiology* 65:165–169, 1986.

162. Lanier WL, Iaizzo PA, Milde JH: Cerebral function and muscle afferent activity following intravenous succinylcholine in dogs anesthetized with halothane: the effects of pretreatment with a dafasciculating dose of pancuronium, *Anesthesiology* 71:87–95, 1989.

163. Schramm WM, Papousek A, Michalek-Sauberer A, et al: The cerebral and cardiovascular effects of cisatracurium and atracurium in neurosurgical patients, *Anesth Analg* 86:123–127, 1998.

164. Bacher A, Zornow MH: Lamotrigine inhibits extracellular glutamate accumulation during transient global cerebral ischemia in rabbits, *Anesthesiology* 86:459–463, 1997.

165. Warner DS, Godersky JC, Smith ML: Failure of pre-ischemic lidocaine administration to ameliorate global ischemic brain damage in the rat, *Anesthesiology* 68:73–78, 1988.

166. Lei B, Cottrell JE, Kass IS: Neuroprotective effect of low-dose lidocaine in a rat model of transient focal cerebral ischemia, *Anesthesiology* 95:445–451, 2001.

167. Lei B, Popp S, Capuano-Waters C, et al: Lidocaine attenuates apoptosis in the ischemic penumbra and reduces infarct size after transient focal cerebral ischemia in rats, *Neuroscience* 125:691–701, 2004.

168. Niiyama S, Tanaka E, Tsuji S, et al: Neuroprotective mechanisms of lidocaine against in vitro ischemic insult of the rat hippocampal CA1 pyramidal neurons, *Neurosci Res* 53:271–278, 2005.

169. Mitchell SJ, Pellett O, Gorman DF: Cerebral protection by lidocaine during cardiac operations, *Ann Thorac Surg* 67:1117–1124, 1999.

170. Zornow MH, Fleischer JE, Scheller MS, et al: Dexmedetomidine, an alpha2 adrenergic agonist, decreases cerebral blood flow in the isoflurane-anesthetized dog, *Anesth Analg* 70:624–630, 1990.

171. Fale A, Kirsch JR, McPherson RW: alpha2 adrenergic agonist effects on normocapnic and hypercapnic cerebral blood flow in the dog are anesthetic dependent, *Anesth Analg* 79:892–898, 1994.

172. Ishiyama T, Dohi S, Iida H: The vascular effects of topical and intravenous alpha2-adrenoceptor agonist clonidine on canine pial microcirculation, *Anesth Analg* 86:766–772, 1998.

173. McPherson RW, Kirsch JR, Traystman RJ: Inhibition of nitric oxide synthase does not affect alpha2-adrenergic-mediated cerebral vasoconstriction, *Anesth Analg* 78:67–72, 1994.

174. Zornow MH, Maze M, Dyck JB, et al: Dexmedetomidine decreases cerebral blood flow velocity in humans, *J Cereb Blood Flow Metab* 13: 350–353, 1993.

175. Prielipp RC, Wall MH, Tobin JR, et al: Dexmedetomidine-induced sedation in volunteers decreases regional and global cerebral blood flow, *Anesth Analg* 95:1052–1059, 2002.

176. Drummond JC, Dao AV, Roth DM, et al: Effect of dexmedetomidine on cerebral blood flow velocity, cerebral metabolic rate, and carbon dioxide response in normal humans, *Anesthesiology* 108:225–232, 2008.

177. Bonhomme V, Maquet P, Phillips C, et al: The effect of clonidine infusion on distribution of regional cerebral blood flow in volunteers, *Anesth Analg* 106:899–909, 2008.

178. Zornow MH, Scheller MS, Sheehan PB, et al: Intracranial pressure effects of dexmedetomidine in rabbits, *Anesth Analg* 75:232–237, 1992.

179. Lee HW, Caldwell JE, Dodson B, et al: The effect of clonidine on cerebral blood flow velocity, carbon dioxide cerebral vasoreactivity, and response to increased arterial pressure in human volunteers, *Anesthesiology* 87:553–558, 1997.

180. ter Minassian A, Beydon L, Decq P, et al: Changes in cerebral hemodynamics after a single dose of clonidine in severely head-injured patients, *Anesth Analg* 84:127–132, 1997.

181. Ma D, Hossain M, Rajakumaraswamy N, et al: Dexmedetomidine produces its neuroprotective effect via the α_{2A}-adrenoceptor subtype, *Eur J Pharmacol* 502:87–97, 2004.

182. Strebel S, Lam AM, Matta B, et al: Dynamic and static cerebral autoregulation during isoflurane, desflurane, and propofol anesthesia, *Anesthesiology* 83:66–76, 1995.

183. Todd MM, Drummond JC: A comparison of the cerebrovascular and metabolic effects of halothane and isoflurane in the cat, *Anesthesiology* 60:276–282, 1984.

184. Jobes DR, Kennell E, Bitner R, et al: Effects of morphine-nitrous oxide anesthesia on cerebral autoregulation, *Anesthesiology* 42:30–34, 1975.

185. Fink H, Blobner M, Bogdanski R, et al: Effects of xenon on cerebral blood flow and autoregulation: An experimental study in pigs, *Br J Anaesth* 84:221–225, 2000.

186. Schmidt M, Marx T, Papp-Jambor C, et al: Effect of xenon on cerebral autoregulation in pigs, *Anaesthesia* 57:960–966, 2002.

187. Girling KJ, Cavill G, Mahajan RP: The effects of nitrous oxide and oxygen on transient hyperemic response in human volunteers, *Anesth Analg* 89:175–180, 1999.

188. Engberg M, Øberg B, Christensen KS, et al: The cerebral arterio-venous oxygen content differences ($AVDO_2$) during halothane and neurolept anesthesia in patients subjected to craniotoy, *Acta Anaesthesiol Scand* 33:642–646, 1989.

189. Scheller MS, Todd MM, Drummond JC, et al: Isoflurane, halothane, and regional cerebral blood flow at various levels of $Paco_2$ in rabbits, *Anesthesiology* 64:598–604, 1986.

190. Drummond JC, Todd MM: The response of the feline cerebral circulation to $Paco_2$ during anethesia with isoflurane and halothane and during sedation with nitrous oxide, *Anesthesiology* 62:268–273, 1985.

191. Matta BF, Lam AM, Mayberg TS, et al: Cerebrovascular response to carbon dioxide during sodium nitroprusside- and isoflurane-induced hypotension, *Br J Anaesth* 74:296–300, 1995.

192. Muizelaar JP, Marmarou A, Ward JD, et al: Adverse effects of prolonged hyperventilation in patients with severe head injury: A randomized clinical trial, *J Neurosurg* 75:731–739, 1991.

193. Kawata R, Nakakimura K, Matsumoto M, et al: Cerebrovascular CO2 reactivity during anesthesia in patients with diabetes mellitus and peripheral vascular disease, *Anesthesiology* 89:887–893, 1998.

194. Todd M, Hindman B, Clarke W, et al: Intraoperative Hypothermia for Aneurysm Surgery Trial (IHAST) Investigators.: Mild intraoperative hypothermia during surgery for intracranial aneurysm, *New Engl J Med* 352:135–145, 2005.

195. Iadecola C, Nakai M, Arbit E, et al: Global cerebral vasodilatation elicited by focal electrical stimulation within the dorsal medullary reticular formation in anesthetized rat, *J Cereb Blood Flow Metab* 3:270–279, 1983.

196. Nakakimura K, Sakabe T, Takeshita H: Modulation of cerebrospinal metabolic responses to peripheral stimulation by enflurane anesthesia in rats, *J Neurosurg Anesthesiol* 1:333–338, 1989.

197. Sakabe T, Maekawa T, Fujii S, et al: Cerebral circulation and metabolism during enflurane anesthesia in humans, *Anesthesiology* 59:532–536, 1983.

198. von Knobelsdorff G, Kusagaya H, Werner C, et al: The effects of surgical stimulation on intracranial hemodynamics, *J Neurosurg Anesthesiol* 8:9–14, 1996.

199. Kawata R, Matsumoto M, Haranishi Y, et al: Changes in cerebral blood flow velocity elicited by surgical stimulation are dependent on the PaCO2 level, *Can J Anaesth* 48:1029–1033, 2001.

200. Bisonnette B, Leon JE: Cerebrovascular stability during isoflurane anaesthesia in children, *Can J Anaesth* 39:128–134, 1992.

201. MacPherson RW, Kirsch JR, Tobin JR, et al: Cerebral blood flow in primates is increased by isoflurane over time and is decreased by nitric oxide synthase inhibition, *Anesthesiology* 80:1320–1327, 1994.

Chapter 6

MODERN NEURORADIOLOGY RELEVANT TO ANESTHETIC AND PERIOPERATIVE MANAGEMENT

Carlos J. Ledezma • Max Wintermark

Imaging provides important diagnostic, prognostic, and pathophysiologic information integral in the evaluation and management of patients with neurologic disorders. Anatomical (structural) imaging modalities, such as computed tomography (CT) and magnetic resonance imaging (MRI), provide information about the structure of the skull, the meninges, the brain parenchyma, the vascular supply of the nervous system, and the cerebrospinal fluid (CSF) spaces and thus can help assess intracranial hemorrhage (ICH), fractures, and other structural lesions. Functional (or physiologic) imaging techniques, such as perfusion CT, perfusion-weighted MRI (PWI), diffusion-weighted MRI (DWI), and MR spectroscopy (MRS), can play a complementary role to anatomical imaging by providing invaluable molecular, physiologic and metabolic information to fully characterize a lesion. In this chapter, we provide an overview of the imaging modalities that are essential in the evaluation of central nervous system (CNS) lesions. Subsequently, we discuss representative neurologic disorders and describe how advancements in imaging technology have influenced the evaluation of these disorders.

IMAGING MODALITIES

Structural Imaging Modalities

Plain Radiographs

Although plain radiographs are a rapid, inexpensive, and accurate modality for evaluating osseous integrity and alignment, the advent of CT-based technology has diminished the clinical utility of plain radiographs in the evaluation of CNS disorders. Furthermore, although skull or spine radiographs can accurately detect skull or spine fractures, they are not as sensitive for evaluating associated intracranial or intraspinal injury.[1-3]

Computed Tomography

With its widespread availability, short scan time, noninvasiveness, and safety, CT has become the preferred imaging modality for the initial evaluation of many intracranial lesions. Owing to the short scan time and ease of acquisition, acute CT is of considerable benefit in the agitated or unstable patient, who might require prompt identification of potential surgical lesions such as acute hemorrhage with resultant mass effect and acute hydrocephalus. The ease of access and speed of data acquisition with this modality facilitates prompt early surgical intervention, which has been shown to improve outcome.[4] Modern CT scanners are able to acquire isotropic data, improving the capability to evaluate intracranial and spinal structures in reconstructed three-dimensional (3D) views. The principal disadvantages of CT are its ionizing radiation exposure (although technologic CT advancements such as dose modulation have effectively reduced the amount of radiation exposure) and its inability to assess lesions in areas that have a propensity to create "beam-hardening" artifacts (e.g., posterior fossa and floor of middle fossa lesions).

Magnetic Resonance Imaging

MRI is based on the relaxation properties of excited hydrogen nuclei in water. By varying the way in which images are obtained, one can alter the soft tissue contrast of the visualized anatomic structures. On T1-weighted images, fat appears bright and water-filled structures such as CSF appear black. On T2-weighted images, fat exhibits intermediate signal and appears gray, whereas water and CSF appear bright. Cortical bone, composed of relatively fixed protons, does not produce a signal. Flowing blood produces no signal (i.e., resulting in a so-called signal void). In general, pathologic processes usually contain excess amounts of free water and therefore are dark on T1-weighted images and bright on T2-weighted images. The use of a paramagnetic MRI contrast agent (e.g., gadolinium [Gd]–DTPA [diethylenetraminepenta-acetic acid]) permits greater conspicuity of vessels and of both intracranial and intraspinal pathologic lesions, which manifest as areas of increased enhancement or T1 signal.[5]

Employing a variety of different MRI sequences better characterizes CNS lesions. Fluid-attenuated inversion recovery (FLAIR) and gradient recalled echo (GRE) are particularly commonly used MRI sequences that assist in the evaluation of CNS pathology. FLAIR imaging increases the conspicuity of focal hyperintense T2 signal abnormalities by eliminating (or "nulling") the hyperintense CSF signal. Thus, focal bright gray matter abnormalities (e.g., contusions) and white matter abnormalities (e.g., shear injuries) are more easily appreciated against the adjacent "nulled" dark CSF spaces. Furthermore, sagittal and coronal FLAIR images are particularly helpful in the evaluation of diffuse axonal injury (DAI) involving the fornix and corpus callosum, two areas that are difficult to distinguish from adjacent CSF on routine T2-weighted imaging.[6] FLAIR also has increased sensitivity for the presence of acute or subacute subarachnoid hemorrhage (SAH), which appears as hyperintense signal within the sulci and cisterns.[7] GRE T2*-weighted MR images have been shown to be very sensitive for the detection of intracranial blood.[8-11]

With the growing number of biomedical implants, materials, and devices present in the general population, MRI safety protocols and extensive preprocedural screening are important for the safety of any patient prior to a MRI examination.[12,13] Contraindications to MRI include cardiac pacemakers, intraocular metallic fragments, mechanical device implants (e.g., cochlear implants, drug infusion pumps, neurostimulators for deep brain stimulation), and ferromagnetic aneurysm clips (non-ferromagnetic or weakly ferromagnetic clips, such as Elgiloy, Phynox, titanium alloy, and commercially pure titanium, have been shown to be MRI compatible and safe).[14] These and similar ferromagnetic objects may pose a risk of adverse effects such as magnetically induced movement, current, and heating.[14] Of secondary concern, ferromagnetic materials can produce image artifacts, thereby degrading MRI image quality.

Conventional Angiography

Conventional angiography entails the introduction of a flexible catheter via the right femoral artery. Alternative sites include the left femoral artery, and the axillary or brachial arteries. Mild intravenous sedation is often helpful as it improves patient comfort and cooperation and lessens patient anxiety. The clinical question and disease process usually dictate which vessel is examined, but a four-vessel (bilateral carotid and bilateral vertebral arteries) cerebral angiogram is routinely performed. Visualization of the cerebral vasculature is accomplished via the injection of iodinated contrast agent with subsequent digital subtraction angiography (DSA), which removes (subtracts) bony details.[15] Serial fluoroscopic spot images are obtained throughout the procedure, and standard angiographic views (i.e., anteroposterior and lateral) are obtained of the vessel of interest. The advent of endovascular surgery has led to the ability of cerebral angiographic techniques not only to be of diagnostic value but also to provide a conduit for definitive therapy.[16,17]

Although cerebral angiography is considered the gold standard for the evaluation of cerebrovascular disease, conventional cerebral angiography is an invasive procedure with associated procedural risk. The rate of neurologic complications is 0.3% to 1.3%, and 0.07% to 0.5% of these complications are permanent.[18-20] The majority of the complications are minor and transient (e.g., groin hematomas, femoral artery injury, and minor allergic reactions). However, more severe complications occasionally occur (e.g., cerebral infarction, seizure, and death). Spinal angiography imposes the same risks as cerebral angiography, with the added danger of cord infarction secondary to spinal artery embolus. For this reason, spinal angiography should be performed only when a vascular malformation is demonstrated by another imaging modality or when the patient has SAH with normal pancerebral angiographic findings and a spinal source is strongly suspected.

With improvements in the detection rates of cerebrovascular disease by newer noninvasive modalities such as CT angiography (CTA) and MR angiography (MRA), conventional catheter-based DSA has been replaced by CTA or MRA in some centers as the screening and diagnostic tools for intracranial vascular disease.

Magnetic Resonance Angiography and Computed Tomographic Angiography

MRA is noninvasive and offers the ability to accurately depict the intracranial vasculature from different angles through the use of a collection of related methods of obtaining angiographic data. Three different MRA techniques are routinely available: time-of-flight (TOF MRA), phase-contrast, and contrast-enhanced. The simplest and most widely used approach, time-of-flight MRA, relies on in-flow enhancement. Essentially, static tissue within a two-dimensional or 3D slice gives a low signal owing to the saturating effect of the long train of closely spaced excitation pulses used in forming the image. On flowing into the imaging volume, unsaturated blood appears hyperintense relative to the static surround.[21,22] Two-dimensional time-of-flight MRA is recommended for venous evaluation, and 3D time-of-flight MRA for arterial evaluation. Disadvantages of MRA include limited visualization of very small distal cortical or deep branches and dependence on flow or the patient's cooperation.[22] For better visualization of the veins and small arterial branches, intravenous contrast enhancement can be used, although it carries the disadvantages of increased cost and superimposition of veins and of enhanced soft tissues.

Similarly, advances in multidetector row CT (MDCT) have facilitated the quick and accurate examination of the cerebral vasculature. CTA is widely available, with fast, thin-section, volumetric spiral CT images acquired during the injection of a time-optimized bolus of contrast material for vessel opacification.[23] With modern multisection CT scanners, the entire region from the aortic arch up to the circle of Willis can be covered in a single data acquisition, with excellent, 3D spatial resolution, the required acquisition time being less than 10 seconds. Multiplanar reformatted images, maximum intensity projection images (MIP), and 3D reconstructions of axial CTA source images provide images comparable, or even superior, to those obtained with conventional angiography (Fig. 6-1).[24-26]

Myelography and Computed Tomography–Myelography

Routine myelography involves the injection of iodinated, water-soluble contrast material into the spinal subarachnoid space via a lumbar or lateral C1-C2 puncture. Plain radiographs are obtained in multiple projections while the contrast material is moved cranially or caudally for evaluation of multiple levels. Newer contrast agents and smaller-gauge spinal needles now permit myelography to be performed on an outpatient basis. After the study, the contrast agent is left in the subarachnoid space, from which it is absorbed and then excreted in the urine. Myelography is typically followed by immediate or delayed CT examination (CT-myelography). The newer, nonionic contrast agents have dramatically reduced the side effects and complications associated with myelography.[27] The most common postprocedural complication is mild-to-severe headache with nausea and/or vomiting. Because contrast material lowers the seizure threshold, patients with a history of seizures should be studied cautiously and patients taking a medication known to lower the seizure threshold (i.e., tricyclic antidepressants) are commonly instructed to stop taking the drug 3 days before the myelography procedure, to allow adequate drug clearance.

CT-myelography has all the features of routine CT with the added benefit of radiopaque contrast material outlining the spinal cord and nerve roots. Pathologic lesions appear as abnormal filling defects within the contrast column, and any cord enlargement or deviation from anatomic position is easily appreciated.

In the last decade, MRI has become the imaging spine modality of choice, superseding both myelography and CT-myelography. The capability for multiplanar imaging, the use of nonionizing radiation, and the ability to obtain a

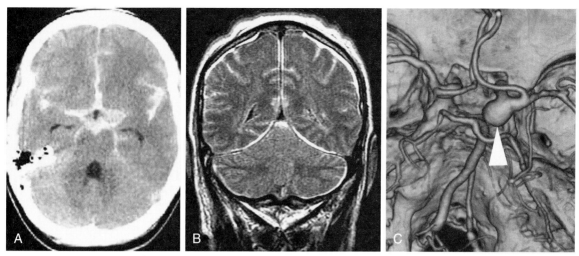

Figure 6–1 35-year-old woman who presented with thunderclap headaches. **A,** Noncontrast computed tomography (CT) scan of the brain shows diffuse subarachnoid hemorrhage. **B,** Confirmation of subarachnoid hemorrhage with fluid-attenuated inversion recovery magnetic resonance image. **C,** 3D reconstruction from a CT angiogram, viewed from above, depicts a ruptured aneurysm in the right posterior communicating artery (*arrowhead*), which is responsible for the subarachnoid hemorrhage.

myelography-like image without intrathecal contrast injection all give MRI distinct advantages.

Functional Imaging Modalities

Functional (or physiologic) imaging provides complementary information to structural imaging and thus facilitates a better characterization of CNS pathology. Indeed, imaging of cerebral function can possibly define the early pathophysiologic processes responsible for neuronal injury, assess the efficacy of therapeutic interventions, and potentially direct the design and implementation of future therapeutic interventions aimed at reversing or preventing neuronal injury.

Perfusion Computed Tomography

On the basis of the multicompartmental tracer kinetic model, dynamic perfusion CT (PCT) is performed by monitoring the first pass of an iodinated contrast agent bolus through the cerebral circulation (Fig. 6-2). Because the change in CT enhancement (in Hounsfield units [HU]) is proportional to the concentration of contrast agent, perfusion parameters are calculated by deconvolution from the changes in the density-time curve for each pixel with the use of mathematical algorithms based on the central volume principle as follows[28,29]:

1. Mean transit time (MTT) indicates the time difference between the arterial inflow and venous outflow.
2. Time to bolus peak (TTP) indicates the time from the beginning of contrast material injection to the maximum (peak) concentration of contrast material within a region of interest.
3. Cerebral blood volume (CBV) indicates the volume of blood per unit of brain mass (normal range in gray matter, 4-6 mL/100 g).
4. Cerebral blood flow (CBF) indicates the volume of blood flow per unit of brain mass per minute (normal range in gray matter, 50-60 mL/100 g/min).

The relationship between CBF and CBV is expressed by the following equation:

$$CBF = \frac{CBV}{MTT}$$

The main advantage of PCT is its wide availability and quantitative accuracy.[30] Its main limitation is its inability to

image the whole brain, because it is limited to a 2- to 3-cm section of brain tissue per bolus. The introduction of 256- and 320-slice CT scanners offering whole brain coverage is likely to overcome this limitation in the near future.

Diffusion-Weighted Magnetic Resonance Imaging and Diffusion Tensor Imaging

DWI is based on the measure of the random (brownian) motion of water molecules and detects the level of mobility (or diffusibility) of water molecules within tissues. Introducing spatial magnetic field gradients makes it possible to obtain MRI sequences that are sensitive to the diffusivity of water along a chosen direction, obtaining so-called diffusion-weighted images. From the ratio of diffusion-weighted images acquired at different levels of diffusion sensitization (known as b-value), it is possible to compute a quantitative measure of mean diffusivity, known as the *apparent diffusion coefficient* (ADC). The ADC measures water diffusion and, therefore, often mirrors changes in DWI signal. In areas of increased diffusion (e.g., vasogenic edema), DWI signal intensity is low, and there is an increase in ADC. In regions of restricted diffusion (e.g., cytotoxic edema), DWI signal intensity is increased, and the ADC signal decreases.

This technique is widely used in acute ischemic stroke, in which reduced DWI signal is seen before the onset of visible abnormalities on conventional MRI.[31,32] In the affected region, there is a temporal evolution from restricted diffusion (i.e., cytotoxic edema in the acute stroke setting) to unrestricted diffusion (i.e., vasogenic edema and encephalomalacia in the chronic setting). DWI has also been used to evaluate other CNS processes, such as cerebral and spinal abscesses, epidermoid cysts, and traumatic brain injury (TBI),[33,34] and to study brain maturation and development, especially the myelination process.

Water diffusion properties also play a role in related imaging technique called diffusion tensor imaging (DTI). Whereas gray matter is microstructurally arranged uniformly along directions, white matter bundles are arranged in a highly directional manner. For this reason, water usually diffuses in all directions (i.e., diffusion is isotropic), but in the brain, water diffuses preferentially along white matter tracts rather than across them (i.e., white matter is anisotropic).

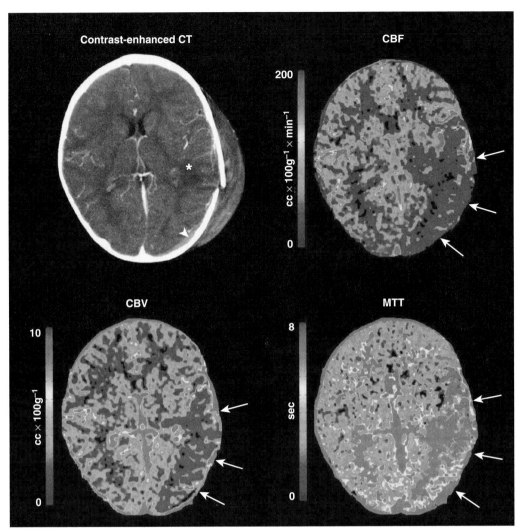

Figure 6–2 This patient had fallen from a 6-m height and was admitted with a Glasgow Coma Scale score of 9. Neurologic examination in the emergency department revealed an asymmetry of tone and deep tendon reflex involving both right upper and lower limbs. The admission contrast-enhanced cerebral computed tomography (CT) scan (*upper left*) demonstrated a displaced left parietal skull fracture associated with a large cephalhematoma. A small left parieto-occipital epidural hematoma (*arrowhead*) and a small contusion area (*star*) could also be identified on the conventional CT images. Perfusion CT scanning (*upper right* and *lower*) demonstrated a much wider area of brain perfusion compromise (white arrows), with involvement of the whole left temporal and parietal lobes, the latter showing increased mean transit time (MTT) and decreased cerebral blood flow (CBF) and volume (CBV). Thus, perfusion CT afforded a better understanding of the neurologic findings on admission than conventional CT.

A mathematical algorithm known as *diffusion tensor* is commonly used to model anisotropic diffusion in white matter. Fractional anisotropy (FA) maps can be created—the fractional anisotropy index varies between 0 (representing a symmetrical anisotropic medium in which there is no directionality of the diffusion, for instance in water) and 1 (representing maximum anisotropy). Also, directionally encoded color maps and 3D tractography can be performed to visually display white matter tracts (Fig. 6-3).[35]

Perfusion-Weighted Magnetic Resonance Imaging

Whereas DWI is most useful for detecting irreversibly infarcted tissue, PWI may be used to identify areas of reversible ischemia as well. PWI techniques rely either on an exogenous method of achieving perfusion contrast (i.e., the administration of an MRI contrast agent, typically gadopentetate dimeglumine [Gd-DTPA, Magnevist]) or on an endogenous method (i.e., use of an endogenous diffusible tracer to measure CBF by applying magnetic resonance pulses to tag inflowing water protons).[36,37] PWI is most commonly applied

as bolus tracking after the intravenous administration of a bolus of gadolinium contrast agent. The passage of the contrast agent through the brain capillaries causes a transient loss of signal because of the susceptibility (T2*) effects of the contrast agent. A hemodynamic time-signal intensity curve is produced, with subsequent calculation of MTT, time-to-peak, CBF, and CBV perfusion maps by means of the same principles as those underlying PCT (Fig. 6-4).[28,38]

PWI can also be performed with the use of T1-weighted imaging, also after an injection of a gadolinium contrast agent. This technique requires a longer acquisition but can measure the permeability of the blood-brain permeability.[39]

Finally, brain perfusion can be assessed using a third MRI technique called arterial spin labeling (ASL) (Fig. 6-5). This method uses not an exogenous contrast agent but, rather, an endogenous diffusible tracer to measure perfusion parameters by applying MR pulses to magnetically label inflowing water protons. However, because of the heavy processing involved, this method has largely remained a research tool rather than gaining widespread clinical applicability.

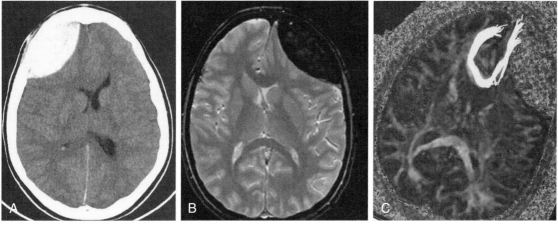

Figure 6–3 **A,** Noncontrast CT scan from a 20-year-old man involved in a motor vehicle accident demonstrates a right frontal epidural hematoma, with its typical biconvex shape and the absence of crossing of sutures. This epidural hematoma resulted from arterial bleeding caused by a right frontal calvarial fracture. **B** and **C,** Epidural hematoma displacing and compressing white matter tracts of the left frontal lobe, demonstrated by 3 Tesla magnetic resonance imaging (3T MRI) and diffusion tensor imaging (DTI) with fiber tractography. The patient is a 22-year-old woman who was imaged 6 days after mild traumatic brain injury and a Glasgow Coma Scale score of 15. **B,** The T2*-weighted gradient echo sequence from 3T MRI shows the large lentiform epidural hematoma as a dark-signal, space-occupying, extra-axial mass in the left frontal lobe. There is medial displacement and compression of white matter in the left frontal lobe as well as midline shift to the right, signifying subfalcine herniation. **C,** A directionally encoded color fractional anisotropy (FA) map from 3T DTI displays white matter tracts with left-to-right fiber orientation shown in red, anteroposterior orientation in green, and craniocaudal orientation in blue. Three-dimensional fiber tractography of the commissural tracts of the genu of the corpus callosum has been performed and is displayed in bright yellow. Medial deviation of the commissural fibers of the left frontal lobe is evident. *(Courtesy Drs. Pratik Mukherjee and Geoff Manley, San Francisco, California.)*

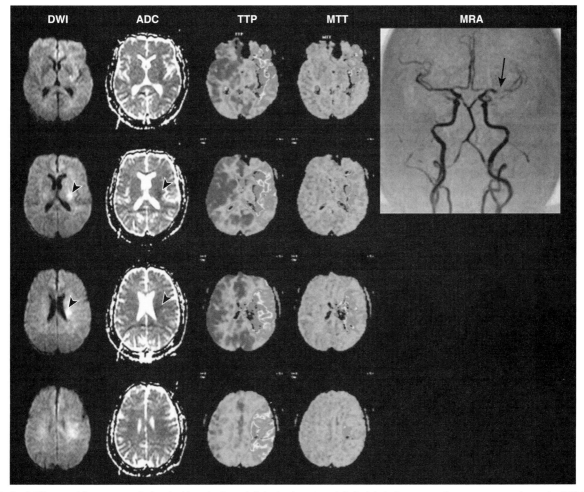

Figure 6–4 A 64-year-old man was admitted with aphasia and right-body motor deficit. Admission magnetic resonance angiography (MRA) shows a proximal stenosis of the left middle cerebral artery (MCA) (*arrow*). Diffusion-weighted MR imaging (DWI) and apparent diffusion coefficient (ADC) maps feature a focus of restricted diffusion in the deep territory of the MCA (*arrowheads*) consistent with acute stroke. Time-to-peak (TTP) and mean transit time (MTT) maps from perfusion-weighted MR imaging (PWI) demonstrate an extensive alteration of brain hemodynamics. The DWI-PWI mismatch is classically regarded as a hallmark of tissue at risk or penumbra. *(Courtesy Dr. Salvador Pedraza, Girona, Spain.)*

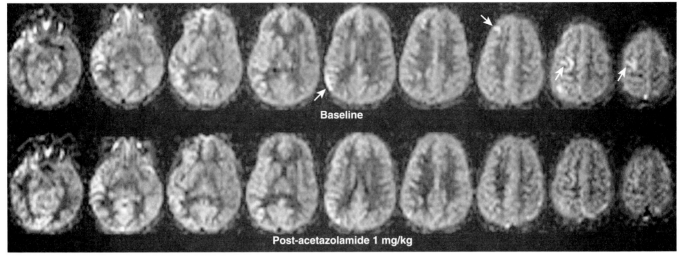

Figure 6–5 Arterial spin-labeled cerebral blood flow (CBF) magnetic resonance imaging obtained before (Baseline) and after arterial administration of acetazolamide in a 9-year-old girl with vasculitis, high-grade right proximal internal carotid artery stenosis, and multiple subacute strokes (*arrows*). Significant decrease in CBF is shown in the entire right hemisphere after administration of acetazolamide, indicative of cerebrovascular steal. The effect is particularly marked in the regions of the subacute strokes. *(Courtesy Dr. Greg Zaharchuk, Stanford, California.)*

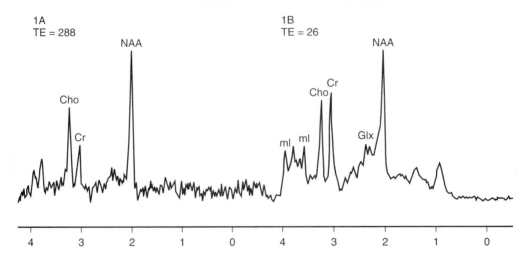

Figure 6–6 **A,** Normal long-echo (TE = 288 msec), single-voxel white matter spectrum from magnetic resonance spectroscopy (MRS) demonstrating the resonances of *N*-acetyl aspartate (NAA, 2.02 parts per million [ppm]), creatine (Cr; 3.02 ppm), and choline (Cho; 3.22 ppm). There is no evidence of lactate or lipid contributions at 0.9 to 1.3 ppm. **B,** Normal short-echo (TE = 26 msec) single-voxel white matter spectrum (MRS) demonstrating the resonances for NAA, Cr, and Cho at the same concentrations as in **A**. Contributions from glutamine and glutamate (Glx) are seen as a complex set of peaks at 2.2 to2.5 ppm. Primary resonance peaks of myo-inositol (mI) are present at 3.56 and 4.06 ppm.

Magnetic Resonance Spectroscopy

MRS allows noninvasive, in vivo assessment of brain metabolism. The physical basis of MRS is the chemical shift effect, that is, the fact that nuclei located in different molecular environments sense slightly different magnitudes of magnetic field, causing them to process at different rates. MRS provides plots or spectra of signal intensity, which is proportional to concentration, against precession rate shift with respect to a reference, expressed in parts per million (ppm). Various biologically relevant metabolites can be identified on the basis of subtly different resonant frequencies, which are a reflection of their specific chemical environment. These metabolites reflect aspects of neuronal integrity, energy metabolism, and cell membrane proliferation or degradation. In clinical practice, the following five major metabolites

containing hydrogen nuclei (1H-MRS) are typically evaluated (Fig. 6-6)[40,41]:

Creatine/Phosphocreatine (Cr/PCr), 3.04 ppm: Creatine and phosphocreatine are involved in cellular energy metabolism and adenosine triphosphate production. Because creatine and phosphocreatine levels tend to be relatively constant in the normal brain, they are used as a reference metabolite, with the concentrations of other metabolites expressed as the ratio of the peak areas compared with the creatine peak.

N-*acetyl aspartate (NAA), 2.02 ppm:* NAA, a cellular amino acid, is a neuronal marker as well as a measure of neuronal density and integrity.[42] Reduced NAA levels have been reported in a wide spectrum of conditions involving neuronal death or dysfunction, decreased neural metabolism, axonal/dendritic loss, and reduced myelination.[42] Because most brain tumors are of nonneuronal origin, NAA is absent or greatly reduced in patients with such lesions, as it is with other insults to the brain, such as infarction and demyelination, that produce neuronal dysfunction or loss. A decrease in NAA has also been observed after head injury.[43]

Choline (Cho), 3.24 ppm: Choline is a composite signal of choline compounds (glycerophosphocholine [GPC], phosphocholine [PC], and a small amount of free choline) and thus reflects total brain choline stores. Choline is a constituent of the phospholipid metabolism of cell membranes and reflects membrane turnover. A choline increase is characteristic of brain tumors due to accelerated membrane turnover in rapidly dividing cancer cells.

Lactate (Lac), 1.33 ppm: Under normal conditions, lactate is barely detectable by MRS in the normal healthy brain. Increased lactate production occurs in disorders of energy metabolism, suggests altered energy metabolism, and is consistent with cerebral ischemia.

Glutamate and glutamine (Glx), composite peak between 2.1 and 2.5 ppm: Glutamate is an excitatory neurotransmitter that plays a role in mitochondrial metabolism. Gamma-amino butyric acid (GABA) is an important product of glutamate. Glutamine plays a role in detoxification and regulation of neurotransmitter activities. Elevations of glutamate lead to excitotoxic cell damage. Greater glutamine synthesis occurs as a result of increased blood ammonia levels.

INTRACRANIAL DISORDERS

Imaging Patterns of Intracranial Disorders

Edema

By definition, cerebral edema or swelling results from an increase in one brain parenchymal compartment at the expense of another. Typically, brain edema can be vasogenic, cytotoxic, or interstitial.[44]

Vasogenic edema, which is predominantly associated with brain metastases, abscesses, trauma, and hemorrhage, develops as a result of a physical disruption of the vascular endothelium or functional alterations in endothelial tight junctions; subsequently, the migration of fluid occurs via bulk flow mechanisms, with transmural pressure gradients causing fluid extravasation from cerebral vessels to the extracellular fluid brain spaces. Vasogenic edema primarily involves the white matter (most commonly the deep white matter of the cerebral hemispheres).

Cytotoxic (intracellular) edema is defined as fluid accumulating within cells as a result of injury, usually from toxicity, ischemia, or hypoxia. The mechanism of injury leads to energy failure due to failure of the sodium-potassium, adenosine triphosphatase-dependent pumps. Cytotoxic edema involves both gray matter and white matter (in contrast to vasogenic edema). Hypo-osmolar states (e.g., dilutional hyponatremia, acute sodium depletion, inappropriate antidiuretic hormone [ADH] syndrome) and osmotic dysequilibrium syndromes (e.g., hemodialysis, diabetic ketoacidosis) can also cause cytotoxic edema. In the early stages of cytotoxic edema, fluid moves from the extracellular compartment to the intracellular compartment, with no net change in brain volume, but eventually the extracellular compartment equilibrates with the intravascular compartment.

Interstitial edema results from CSF migration into the periventricular white matter, which is commonly due to conditions that impede CSF circulation, absorption, or both.

Except for location and DWI (diffusion is reduced in cytotoxic edema and increased in vasogenic edema), the imaging appearance of edema is essentially similar for all pathologic processes. On CT, any increase in water is visualized as a dark, hypodense area. On MRI, an increase in water is visualized as an area of hypointensity (black) on T1-weighted images and as an area of hyperintensity (white) on T2-weighted images. Contrast enhancement may help define areas of edema and might suggest an etiology. As contrast agent accumulates in regions of blood-brain barrier breakdown, areas of vasogenic edema enhance, whereas areas of cytotoxic edema usually do not (or only at later stages).

Hemorrhage

ICH may be traumatic or nontraumatic in origin. When blood is seen in the extra-axial space (epidural, subdural, subarachnoid), trauma is the most likely cause. SAH may be traumatic or may be associated with ruptured berry (saccular) or fusiform aneurysms. Arterial dissection, often though not always associated with trauma, may also manifest as SAH. Parenchymal hemorrhage is more likely to be nontraumatic in origin, secondary to an underlying disease such as hypertension, neoplasm, or vascular anomaly. Regardless of location, acute hemorrhage is seen on a CT scan as a hyperdense area. Blood products evolve with time, progressively decreasing in density and subsequently becoming first isodense to brain parenchyma and then eventually hypodense. A negative CT scan result does not completely exclude hemorrhage. Severely anemic patients (hematocrit < 30%) may present with isodense extra-axial or intraparenchymal blood collections, and only the presence of mass effect suggests hemorrhage.

The appearance of hemorrhage on MRI is complicated because of varying paramagnetic properties of blood breakdown products. One should consider the age of hemorrhage in relation to these breakdown products.[8,45,46] During the first hours after parenchymal hemorrhage, intact red blood cells containing oxyhemoglobin accumulate. Being diamagnetic, oxyhemoglobin is slightly hypointense to isointense on T1-weighted images and hyperintense on T2-weighted images, mainly because of the concomitant presence of globin proteins. Over the next hours to days, hemoglobin becomes deoxygenated. Because deoxyhemoglobin is paramagnetic, the T2 intensity values fall (so that the hemorrhage becomes hypointense), whereas the T1 values essentially remain the same. With respect to brain parenchyma, the acute hematoma appears dark on T2-weighted images and slightly dark to isointense on T1-weighted images. Between 3 and 7 days after hemorrhage, intracellular methemoglobin begins to accumulate, beginning peripherally and advancing toward the center of the clot. During this stage, T2 signal intensity remains stable but T1 values begin to increase, with the periphery of the clot becoming hyperintense. The hematoma is dark on T2-weighted images and bright on T1-weighted images. Between 7 days and 2 to 3 months, intracellular methemoglobin is released from erythrocytes (extracellular methemoglobin). During this stage, the lesion's signal intensities on both T1 and T2 images increase (appearing hyperintense on both T1- and T2-weighted images). During the final stage, which may begin within the first 2 weeks and last for years, phagocytic degradation of methemoglobin to hemosiderin occurs. This process, which also begins peripherally and extends toward the center, effectively removes iron from the hematoma and deposits it at the periphery. The lesion's signal intensities again decrease, and hemosiderin appears black on

T2-weighted images, beginning at the periphery as a ring and eventually replacing the entire hemorrhage. This progression represents a continuum of changing intensity values and is not an all-or-nothing phenomenon.

In the acute/subacute phase, most hematomas produce a surrounding area of edema that should not be misinterpreted as an additional area of hemorrhage. Edema, dark on T1-weighted images and bright on T2-weighted images, gradually decreases over time.

Mass Effect, Shift, and Herniation

An enlarging mass (e.g., tumor or abscess), hemorrhage, or edema can cause mass effect and lead to brain herniation, which can directly compress vascular structures, resulting in ischemia and infarct, and directly impinge upon cranial nerves and vital structures, ultimately causing death. Because hemorrhages frequently progress and large contusions often develop delayed hemorrhage or edema, repeated serial imaging is usually indicated, especially if changes in neurologic status occur, as the severity of mass effect correlates with the level of consciousness.[47] Imaging features of intracranial mass effect include sulcal effacement, midline shift, basal cistern effacement, obstructive hydrocephalus, and herniation.

Different types of brain herniation are subfalcine, transtentorial, and tonsillar.

Subfalcine herniation occurs when a hemispheric mass pushes the cingulate or supracingulate gyri beneath the falx. It is easily recognized on CT or MRI from deviation of the falx and extension of hemispheric structures across the midline.

Transtentorial herniation occurs when a mass on either side of the tentorium causes brain herniation through the tentorial incisura, either descending (downward) or ascending (upward). Descending herniation is usually more commonly caused by a supratentorial mass displacing the medial temporal lobe through the tentorial incisura. It may be anterior (involving the uncus), posterior (involving the parahippocampal or lingual gyri), or complete. On CT or MRI, the herniated uncus or parahippocampal gyrus produces widening of the ipsilateral subarachnoid cistern and obliteration of the contralateral subarachnoid cistern as the brainstem is rotated and displaced to the opposite side.[48,49] Ascending transtentorial herniation is caused by an infratentorial mass that pushes the pons, vermis, and adjacent portions of the cerebellar hemispheres upward through the incisura. On CT or MRI, the subarachnoid cisterns are effaced symmetrically as the cerebellar vermis bulges up through the incisura. The upper pons is pushed forward against the clivus, and often acute hydrocephalus is caused by compression of the sylvian aqueduct. Occipital lobe infarction (ipsilateral or contralateral) may also occur if the posterior cerebral artery is compressed between the temporal lobe and the crus cerebri.[50]

Tonsillar herniation features inferior displacement of the cerebellar tonsils through the foramen magnum into the cervical spinal canal. It results in compression of the medulla, producing dysfunction of the vital respiratory and cardiac rhythm centers. MRI, with its sagittal imaging abilities, is the primary imaging modality for demonstrating the presence of tonsillar herniation and its secondary effects on the brainstem. On CT, the cerebellar tonsils can be seen below the level of the foramen magnum.[49,51]

Efforts have been made to correlate quantitative measures of herniation on imaging (i.e., the extent of shift of structures)

with clinical outcomes. For example, in subfalcine herniation (midline shift or cingulated herniation), the extent of displacement of the septum pellucidum from the midline is predictive of patient prognosis. In studies of descending transtentorial herniation, however, the extent of vertical descent does not always correlate well with neurologic signs. Prior studies have shown a correlation between extent of midline shift and level of consciousness.[47]

Hydrocephalus

Hydrocephalus is classified as either obstructive or communicating.

Communicating hydrocephalus results from excessive CSF production by choroid plexus tumors or from obstruction to CSF absorption by arachnoid villi, which may be caused by SAH, meningitis, or leptomeningeal carcinomatosis.[52] CT and MRI show symmetrical enlargement of the lateral, third, and fourth ventricles with effacement of cerebral sulci. With elevated pressure, CSF may leak from the ventricles into the brain (interstitial edema).

Obstructive hydrocephalus results secondary to obstruction along the CSF pathway between the lateral ventricles and the fourth ventricular outlet. The CT and MRI appearances are identical to those of communicating hydrocephalus, with the exception that in obstructive hydrocephalus not all ventricles are enlarged. The ventricles are dilated proximal but not distal to the obstruction. For example, in aqueduct obstruction, the fourth ventricle remains normal as the third and lateral ventricles enlarge. The cause of obstructive hydrocephalus can often be identified on CT or MRI. MRI is the preferred modality for evaluation of NCH for the following reasons:

1. MRI can provide multiplanar images, which are invaluable in demonstrating obstruction at the foramen of Monro, the aqueduct, or the level of the fourth ventricle.[53]
2. Tumors are readily seen, and webs or atresia of the aqueduct occasionally can be identified.
3. Newer techniques with CSF flow phenomena are helpful in classifying types of obstruction.[54]

Review of the Major Surgical Intracranial Disorders

Traumatic Brain Injury (TBI)

TBI represents the leading cause of morbidity and mortality among individuals younger than 45 years.[55] It is estimated that nearly 1.6 million head injuries occur in the United States each year, resulting in more than 50,000 deaths and more than 70,000 patients with permanent neurologic deficits.[56]

TBI has classically been subdivided into two simplified categories, (1) primary injury (e.g., cortical contusion, skull fracture, and white matter shearing injury), which is the result of the initial, mechanical insult, and (2) secondary (delayed) brain injury (e.g., edema, hypoxia, intracranial hypertension, vasospasm), which is a sequela of the initial trauma. This classification is clinically important because early medical intervention might possibly ameliorate the deleterious effects associated with secondary injury that ultimately can lead to brain compromise and permanent brain injury.[57] In addition, TBI may also be classified according to lesion location (i.e., intra-axial vs. extra-axial), clinical severity (minor, mild, moderate, severe) and mechanism of injury (penetrating vs. blunt/closed). The majority of TBIs are mild, and around 10% are moderate or severe.[58]

INDICATIONS FOR IMAGING IN PATIENTS WITH TRAUMATIC BRAIN INJURY

As CT is readily available, cost-effective, and fast and accurately detects injuries (i.e., hemorrhages and fractures) that might require surgical intervention, it is the preferred imaging modality for the initial assessment of acute TBI.[59-61] It has excellent ability to detect acute hemorrhage and to demonstrate resulting mass effect, basal cistern effacement, and presence of acute hydrocephalus. Excellent bone resolution facilitates assessment of skull base, calvarium, and facial bone fractures. Indications for head CT in acute trauma include: A Glasgow Coma Scale score less than 8 or a decrease of more than 3 in the score, headache, vomiting, worsening level of consciousness, loss of consciousness for more than 5 minutes, focal neurologic findings, seizure, penetrating skull injuries, signs of a basal or depressed skull fracture, and physical evidence of trauma above the clavicle.[62-64]

Although CT is best for acute injuries such as hemorrhages, a number of intracranial lesions (e.g., diffuse axonal injury, brainstem and deep gray matter injury) are difficult to appreciate on CT scans. MRI therefore shows greater sensitivity than CT for the detection of these subtle lesions and also is better suited for the evaluation of subacute and chronic TBI. In particular, MRI is ideal for the evaluation of a patient with unexplained neurologic deficits that cannot be explained by the CT findings.[65-67] MRI is superior to CT in detecting axonal injury, small areas of contusion, and subtle lesions in the brainstem, basal ganglia, and thalami.[68] It is estimated that CT "misses" approximately 10% to 20% of abnormalities subsequently seen on MRI.[69,70]

SPECIFIC TRAUMATIC BRAIN INJURIES

Primary traumatic brain injuries are divided into extra-axial and intra-axial lesions.

Extra-Axial Lesions. Extra-axial lesions include skull fractures, and epidural, subdural, subarachnoid, and intraventricular hemorrhages. CT is the preferred modality to assess skull fractures, because it facilitates identification of associated brain injuries (e.g., intra-axial or extra-axial hemorrhage, CSF leak) that are not always obvious on plain radiographs.[71,72] Basal skull fractures may be associated with cranial nerve (e.g., longitudinal and transverse temporal bone fractures are associated with facial paresis and sensorineural hearing loss, respectively) and vascular injury (vessels near skull base) (Fig. 6-7).[73,74] Diagnosis of these fractures require thin CT slice protocols and 3D multiplanar CT reformats.[75-78] Skull fractures can lead to CSF leaks. Radionuclide cisternography, contrast-enhanced CT cisternography, and high-definition CT have been used for posttraumatic CSF leak detection.[79-81]

Damage to the meninges may lead to hemorrhage into the subdural, epidural, or CSF space (SAH and intraventricular hemorrhage).

Epidural hematomas (see Fig. 6-3) are relatively uncommon (1%-4% of patients with head trauma). They have an overall mortality of 5%. An epidural hematoma, an extra-axial blood collection that accumulates in the potential space between the dura mater and the inner table of the skull, occurs in 85% to 95% of cases secondary to a laceration of the middle meningeal artery (90%) or a dural venous sinus (10%) by an associated skull fracture.[82] The classic clinical presentation of an epidural hematoma is a so-called lucid, conscious interval that is soon followed by neurologic deterioration; this "lucid interval" has been attributed to the absence of underlying brain injury with subsequent epidural hematoma enlargement that causes progressive neurologic deterioration. However, this classic presentation occurs in only 20% of patients.[83] Epidural hematomas exhibit a lent form or biconvex hyperdense appearance, and the majority occur in the temporoparietal area.[72] Less commonly, they may develop at the frontal pole, in the parieto-occipital region, between the occipital

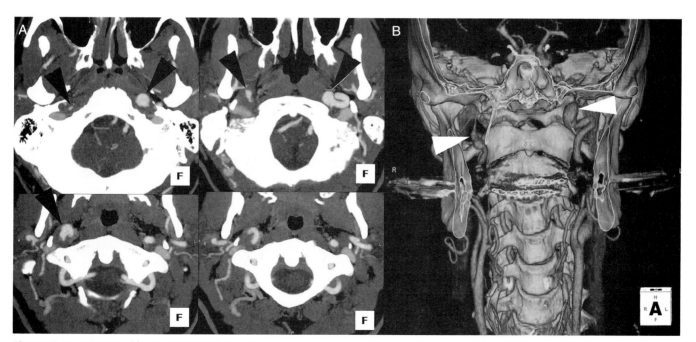

Figure 6-7 A 50-year-old man experienced several falls while snowboarding. Because of symptoms of transient ischemic attacks, the patient underwent computed tomographic angiography (CTA). **A.** Axial CT slices, and **B.** 3D reformation demonstrate bilateral internal carotid artery pseudoaneurysms (associated with a dissection on the right side) (arrowheads) just below the skull base. This segment of the internal carotid arteries is particularly vulnerable to shear trauma forces, because it is a mobile segment adjacent to an immobile segment in the petrous portion of the carotid canal.

lobes, or in the posterior fossa. These are most often venous in origin and occur from fractures of the overlying major dural sinuses (parasagittal region from a tear from the superior sagittal sinus; middle cranial fossa from injury to the sphenoparietal sinus or middle meningeal veins; posterior fossa/occipital region from rupture of the transverse or sigmoid sinus). Epidural hematomas usually do not cross the midline and suture lines (an exception being the sagittal suture). They can extend from the supratentorial to the infratentorial space, whereas the subdural hematoma (SDH) is limited by the tentorium. The presence of hypodense regions within an otherwise hyperdense epidural hematoma (the "swirl sign") may represent areas of active hemorrhage.[84]

SDHs are common (occurring in 10%-20% of patients with head trauma) and have a high mortality (50%-85%).[8] Typically, whereas epidural hematomas are located at the coup site, an acute SDH is a contrecoup lesion, which most commonly occurs from a deceleration mechanism that causes traumatic bridging vein rupture. SDHs exhibit certain specific traits. They are crescent-shaped, usually holohemispheric; they can cross suture lines and extend along the tentorium and the falx cerebri; and they usually do not extend from the supratentorial space into the infratentorial space. Common locations for SDHs include along the cerebral convexities, the falx cerebri, and the tentorium cerebelli. Although the common etiology for acute subdural hematomas is trauma, other etiologies are child abuse, rapid ventricular decompression, and spontaneous SDH (which usually occurs in the patient who is taking anticoagulants, is elderly, or has an existing coagulopathy).[85-87]

Subarachnoid hemorrhage is defined as bleeding into the subarachnoid space surrounding the brain (i.e., between the arachnoid and pia mater), and it may occur from trauma or spontaneously (spontaneous or primary SAH usually results from ruptured aneurysm).[88] The interpeduncular cistern and sylvian fissures are two common locations for the accumulation of subarachnoid blood.[89] CT and MRI with FLAIR are equally sensitive at detecting SAH.[90] Subarachnoid blood is toxic to the arteries coursing through the subarachnoid spaces, causing vasospasm. It can also interfere with normal CSF resorption at the level of the pacchionian (arachnoidal) granulations, thus leading to communicating hydrocephalus.

Traumatic intraventricular hemorrhage can occur by one of three methods—contiguous extension from a parenchymal hematoma, shearing of subependymal veins that line the ventricular cavities, and retrograde reflux of SAH through the foramina of the fourth ventricle.[91] It may be isolated but it is usually associated with superficial contusions and SAH. Subtle intraventricular hemorrhage can be detected from the appearance of a fluid-fluid level layering dependently within the occipital horns of the lateral ventricles (so-called hematocrit effect), which occurs because fibrinolytic activators within the CSF inhibit clotting. In some cases, the choroid plexus may act as a nidus for the blood to clot and form a ventricular cast or tumefactive blood clot. Large amounts of intraventricular blood may impede CSF flow and result in noncommunicating hydrocephalus.

Intra-Axial Lesions. Intra-axial lesions include hemorrhagic and nonhemorrhagic contusions, parenchymal hematomas, and diffuse axonal injuries (DAIs).

Cortical brain contusions are relatively common, occurring in up to 40% of patients with blunt trauma.[91] They are peripheral lesions, involving the gyral crests, particularly those in contact with irregular skull bony prominences (e.g., the orbital roof, sphenoid ridge, and petrous ridge). The terms coup and

contrecoup are often used to describe the cortical contusion lesions that are a result of the brain parenchyma's striking the inner table at the site of impact (*coup*) or at the opposite side of impact (*contrecoup*). On non–contrast-enhanced CT, contusions appear as low-attenuation foci if hemorrhage is absent and high-attenuation foci if hemorrhage is present. Nonhemorrhagic contusions are often difficult to detect initially on CT but become more conspicuous with time as they evolve and exhibit increased hypodensity owing to edema within the contused tissue. Moreover, delayed hemorrhage can develop within previously nonhemorrhagic lesions. For these reasons, repeat or serial CT is recommended.

If CT is optimal for the acute evaluation of contusions, subacute and chronic cortical contusions are better evaluated with MRI.[8] On MRI, contusions that appear nonhemorrhagic on CT are often demonstrated to have hemorrhagic components and consequently follow the time evolution of the MRI signal of blood products. Contusions are particularly conspicuous on GRE images. With time, contusions shrink into gliotic scars. An old contusion is seen as a wedge-shaped area of peripheral encephalomalacia with the apex of the wedge pointing centrally and the broad base facing the irregular surface of the skull. In the chronic stage, this triangular shape can resemble a remote ischemic infarct. The products of hemorrhage can be detected on MRI for years (rather than a few weeks, as on CT).

Diffuse axonal injury (DAI), or shear injury, typically occurs secondary to sudden acceleration and deceleration forces that cause microscopic axonal brain injury, preferentially to deep white matter or the gray/white matter interface. Pathologically, it is characterized by microscopic axonal lesions that most frequently involve the subcortical white matter, the corpus callosum (particularly the splenium), and the dorsolateral brain stem.[92-94] Early and exact identification of the extent of axonal injury is a major diagnostic challenge, because these injuries are seldom visible on CT or conventional MRI sequences. With the advent of advanced MRI modalities, such as GRE, DWI, and DTI, the ability to detect these shear injuries has improved dramatically.[94] Hemorrhagic DAI can sometimes be diagnosed on CT or conventional T1- or T2-weighted images but usually require GRE sequences.[95,96] Nonhemorrhagic DAI can usually be seen only on DWI or DTI.[97-99]

Brain Neoplasms

Neuroimaging plays a crucial role in diagnosing brain neoplasms, planning their treatment, and monitoring the effects of the therapies.

The radiologic appearances of brain tumors include some features that are common to most tumors: mass lesion, causing mass effect and sometimes hydrocephalus; abnormal CT hypodensity or MRI T2 signal, reflecting either edema or tumor infiltration; abnormal enhancement in most cases; and hemorrhagic complication, cystic necrosis, or both in some instances. Differential diagnosis can usually be narrowed on the basis of the patient's age and through determining whether the lesion is solitary or multiple and intra-axial or extra-axial. Primary brain gliomas are intra-axial. Extra-axial tumors include meningiomas and schwannomas. Metastases are typically multiple and can be both intra-axial and extra-axial.

In terms of imaging of brain tumors, CT is usually used to assess for tumor complications such as hemorrhage and mass effect, including hydrocephalus, whereas MRI is used for tumor diagnosis and classification, treatment planning, and post-treatment follow-up. Modern MRI techniques such

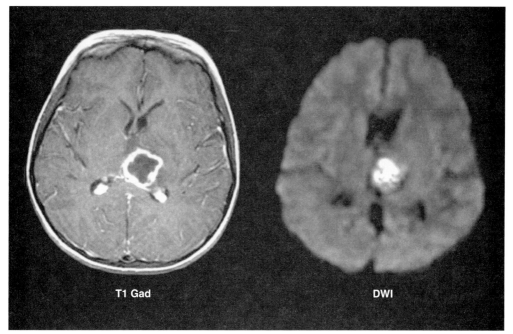

Figure 6–8 *Left,* T1-weighted magnetic resonance image with gadolinium enhancement from a 47-year-old man shows a rim-enhancing lesion in the left thalamus. *Right,* Diffusion-weighted imaging shows reduced diffusion within the rim-enhancing lesion, which is a typical feature of an abscess and distinguishes it from a necrotic tumor.

as PWI, DWI DTI, MRS, and functional MRI have allowed significant progress in accurate delineation of tumor margins, determination of tumor grade, distinction of treatment effects from residual or recurrent tumor, and differentiation of eloquent cortex or white matter tracts from tumor. DWI is also used to differentiate between necrotic tumors (increased ADC values) and abscesses (decreased ADC values) (Fig. 6-8).

IMAGING DETECTION OF TUMOR MARGINS

Gliomas have a propensity for infiltration of the adjacent brain parenchyma and tend to migrate along white matter tracts. Gliomas have been found to extend beyond the gross tumor margins as depicted by conventional MRI.[100,101] MRS has the ability to detect increased choline levels and reduced NAA peaks beyond the tumor margins, within the normal-appearing parenchyma infiltrated by the tumor.[102,103] Similarly, DTI detects tumoral infiltration as a decrease in fractional anisotropy.[101,104-106] However, although both DTI and MRS were shown to be better than conventional MRI at defining the tumor margins, further studies have shown mixed results in comparison with those of DTI in noninvasive tumors (e.g., meningiomas and metastases) MRS in normal brain and mild tumor infiltration.[107]

GRADING OF BRAIN TUMORS ON BASIS OF IMAGING

Although histology is the "gold standard" in determining tumor grade, MRI has sensitivity and specificity of 65% and 95%, respectively, for the characterization of high-grade tumors.[108] The presence or absence of abnormal contrast enhancement does not correlate with tumor histology.[109] Newer MRI techniques are needed for noninvasive elucidation of tumor biology—tumor cellularity (DWI), tumor metabolism (MRS), and tumor vascularity (PWI).

ADC and fractional anisotropy values correlate inversely with the level of tumor cellularity and the proliferation index of the glioma.[110-113] ADC values have been found to be significantly lower in higher-grade gliomas than in less

cellular low-grade gliomas.[113,114] Similarly, the choline peak, lactate/lipid peak, and the Cho/NAA ratio have been correlated with cell density, proliferation markers, and tumor grade (Fig. 6-9).[103,115-120] Lastly, because greater angiogenesis and microvascular proliferation are markers of a more malignant process, certain perfusion parameters such as CBV have been used to provide a noninvasive method of grading gliomas.[121-123] However, this approach has pitfalls. For instance, oligodendrogliomas have higher CBV values than astrocytic tumors.[124] As a result, a low-grade oligodendroglioma might possibly be falsely graded as a higher-grade tumor (Fig. 6-10).

IMAGING OF BRAIN TUMOR TREATMENT EFFECTS

Conventional MRI is limited to differentiate post-treatment effects from tumor residual or recurrence. Also, current MRI methods, all based on structural imaging, rely on changes in tumor size to determine treatment response; however, evaluation of tumor physiology could provide an earlier assessment of treatment response and could potentially serve as a surrogate marker of treatment success.

ADC changes have been shown to correspond to changes in tumor volume and cellularity.[113] ADC changes are usually noticeable prior to their appearance on conventional MRI.

PWI allows one to distinguish between glial tumor (preserved blood-brain barrier) and metastases (abnormally permeable blood-brain barrier), and between tumor recurrence (increased CBV) and treatment necrosis (decreased CBV) (Fig. 6-11).[125] PWI has been utilized to study the response for antiangiogenic or antivascular drugs and to radiotherapy.[126]

MRS has also been used to distinguish between tumor recurrence (increased choline, decreased NAA levels) and treatment necrosis (decreased choline, decreased NAA levels).[127] MRS has also been reported to predict the response to therapy. In a cohort of patients with high-grade gliomas receiving radical radiotherapy (i.e., 60 Gy in 30 fractions), the lactate/NAA ratio was the strongest predictor of response to radiotherapy and overall survival.[128]

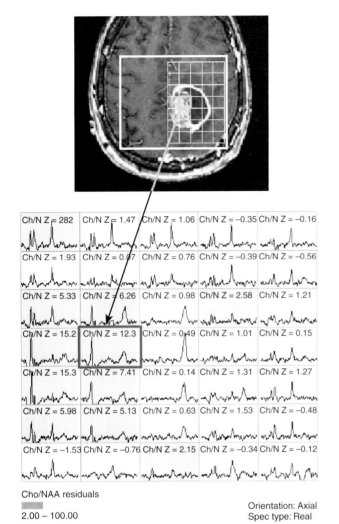

Ch/N Z = 282	Ch/N Z = 1.47	Ch/N Z = 1.06	Ch/N Z = −0.35	Ch/N Z = −0.16
Ch/N Z = 1.93	Ch/N Z = 0.07	Ch/N Z = 0.76	Ch/N Z = −0.39	Ch/N Z = −0.56
Ch/N Z = 5.33	Ch/N Z = 6.26	Ch/N Z = 0.98	Ch/N Z = 2.58	Ch/N Z = 1.21
Ch/N Z = 15.2	Ch/N Z = 12.3	Ch/N Z = 0.49	Ch/N Z = 1.01	Ch/N Z = 0.15
Ch/N Z = 15.3	Ch/N Z = 7.41	Ch/N Z = 0.14	Ch/N Z = 1.31	Ch/N Z = 1.27
Ch/N Z = 5.98	Ch/N Z = 5.13	Ch/N Z = 0.63	Ch/N Z = 1.53	Ch/N Z = −0.48
Ch/N Z = −1.53	Ch/N Z = −0.76	Ch/N Z = 2.15	Ch/N Z = −0.34	Ch/N Z = −0.12

Cho/NAA residuals

2.00 – 100.00

Orientation: Axial
Spec type: Real

Figure 6–9 *Top,* Long-echo (TE = 288 msec) point-resolved, three-dimensional magnetic resonance spectroscopy in a patient with glioblastoma multiforme. *Bottom,* The highlighted voxel corresponds to an area of abnormal enhancement on the diagnostic image at the margin of a cavitary lesion. An abnormal elevation of choline (Cho) (the dominant peak in the spectrum) with a notable absence of *N*-acetyl aspartate (NAA) is seen. Additionally, the second largest peak in the spectrum (at the far right of the voxel) represents lipid contributions from tumor necrosis. The three-dimensional acquisition facilitates comparison of normal and abnormal tissues in a single acquisition. Z-values represent abnormal primary peak ratios (NAA, creatinine [Cr], Cho) that are more than two standard deviations greater than the expected ratios. Voxels with abnormal Z-values are shaded *gray* for identification.

ELOQUENT CORTEX

DTI and functional MRI have the ability to "map" functional areas, whereby disruption would lead to focal neurologic deficits and to identify both areas of cortical activation and white matter tracts. This information may be important for the neurosurgeon in deciding which surgical approach is best to minimize a patient's deficit from tumor or AVM resection (Fig. 6-12).

Intracranial Aneurysms and Other Intracranial Vascular Malformations

Approximately 10% of patients presenting with ICH have a vascular malformation. SAH is the most highly morbid type of ICH; vascular malformations are the most common cause of nontraumatic SAH in patients younger than 40 years. The five types of vascular malformations of the brain are intracranial

aneurysms, AVMs and arteriovenous fistulas, capillary telangiectasias, developmental venous abnormalities, and cavernomas (cavernous malformations). An older term for cavernoma is "cryptic AVM." About 10% of cavernomas are associated with a heritable mutation and are associated with multiple lesions; single lesions tend to be sporadic and to have a higher rate of association with a developmental venous anomaly.

INTRACRANIAL ANEURYSMS

The four types of intracranial aneurysms are berry/saccular, fusiform/atherosclerotic, septic/mycotic, and pedicular aneurysms on the feeding arteries of AVMs. Berry (saccular) aneurysms are the most common, accounting for up to 90% of all aneurysms, and represent the leading cause of spontaneous SAH. The extent to which berry aneurysms are congenital is speculative; they can form during adult life, especially in patients with multiple aneurysms. Pathologically, there is thinning or absence of the arterial media with dilation of the lumen, usually at a bifurcation and almost always in the proximal circle of Willis. Common locations are the origin of the posterior communicating artery from the internal carotid artery, the anterior communicating artery, and the middle cerebral artery bifurcation. The probability of rupture strongly correlates with the size of the aneurysm and becomes significant when aneurysm diameter is more than 7 mm.

Noncontrast CT is usually used as a primary screening tool in patients in whom SAH is suspected. Moreover, the pattern of the SAH can offer clues to the possible location of the underlying cerebral aneurysm. The sensitivity of CT for SAH is more than 95% in the first 12 hours. Beyond 12 hours, normal CT findings do not rule out the diagnosis of acute SAH, and a lumbar puncture is needed.[129]

DSA is considered the gold standard for the detection of intracranial aneurysms and of aneurysm complications. It also represents a treatment modality because it permits coiling of ruptured and unruptured aneurysms and endovascular treatment of vasospasm (angioplasty and/or intra-arterial verapamil).[113]

CTA and MRA have been proposed as feasible alternatives for conventional angiography. CTA has been shown to exhibit 83% to 96% sensitivity and 97% to 100% specificity[130-134] for aneurysm detection (see Fig. 6-1), although the sensitivity decreases for smaller aneurysms, with a 40% to 91% sensitivity for aneurysms smaller 3 mm.[131,133,135] Similarly, MRA has shown to be highly sensitive and specific for the detection of intracranial aneurysms but, like CTA, decreases in sensitivity for smaller aneurysm (i.e., <3 mm in diameter).[134,135] PCT and CTA have also been reported as accurate noninvasive imaging techniques to assess for vasospasm (Fig. 6-13).[136,137]

ARTERIOVENOUS MALFORMATIONS

Arteriovenous malformation is a vascular anomaly characterized by a network of abnormal vessels with an abnormal connection, or shunt, between a feeding artery and a draining vein bypassing an intervening capillary bed.[138] Cortical arteriovenous fistulas, which are composed of one or a few arteriovenous shunts, are probably extreme cases of the more common angioarchitecture of an AVM, which is made up of a number of shunts within the AVM nidus.

As a result, arteriovenous shunting occurs with rapid flow, most probably accounting for the enlarged, flow-remodeled afferent and efferent vessels. AVMs are often presumed to be congenital lesions resulting from embryonic maldevelopment during the fourth to eighth week, but there is remarkably little

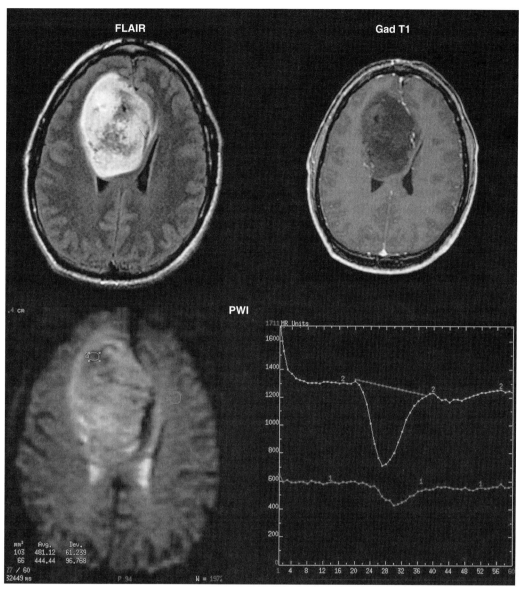

Figure 6–10 Magnetic resonance imaging (MRI) in a 28-year-old man with prior history of seizures. Conventional fluid-attenuated inversion recovery (FLAIR) and post–gadolinium administration, T1-wieghted images (Gad T1) demonstrated a right mesiofrontal, heterogenous, but well-delineated, mass. Perfusion-weighted dynamic susceptibility imaging (PWI) demonstrated an increased area over the curve in a (*green*) region of interest placed within the mass compared with a region of interest (*purple*) placed within the normal contralateral frontal white matter. This increased area over the curve, corresponding to higher cerebral blood volume, in combination with the low-grade appearance of the lesion on conventional imaging sequences, raised the suspicion for an oligodendroglioma, which is a low-grade tumor with a very rich blood supply. This diagnosis was confirmed histologically.

evidence for this assertion. Further, there have been multiple reports of AVMs that grow or regress. In addition, there are reported cases of de novo AVM formation.[139] AVMS have substantial hemodynamic effects, as reviewed elsewhere.[140]

DSA is the gold standard for the imaging evaluation of cerebral AVMs. Using DSA, one can obtain information about the angioarchitecture of brain AVMs, including vascular composition of the nidus, types of feeding arteries, and types and patterns of venous drainage. Ancillary findings include flow-related aneurysms, extranidal and intranidal aneurysms, venous strictures, and venous varices. The timing of imaging after hemorrhage is critical because nidus compression by the hematoma may lead to falsely negative DSA results if the procedure is performed soon after the initial hemorrhage.[141] CT and MRI play minor roles in the diagnosis and management of cerebral AVMs. CT is the first-line imaging technique for patients presenting with a suspicion of acute ICH. The

unruptured AVM may not be seen on noncontrast CT or may appear as a subtle, hyperdense region. After administration of a contrast agent, large, tortuous, high-density structures representing the serpentine vessels can be easily identified. MRI is used for AVM follow-up during and after treatment. On MRI, AVM features include enlarged cerebral arteries feeding the AVM, a cluster of signal voids representing the nidus, and enlarged draining veins. Secondary findings include gliosis or encephalomalacia from prior hemorrhage and areas of hypointensity caused by hemosiderin from prior hemorrhage.

Ischemic Strokes

Acute ischemic stroke is defined as abrupt onset of a focal neurologic deficit due to a disturbance in the blood supply to a vascular territory in the brain. Rapid and accurate assessment is crucial for treatment, because acute intracerebral hemorrhage must be ruled out prior to the administration of known

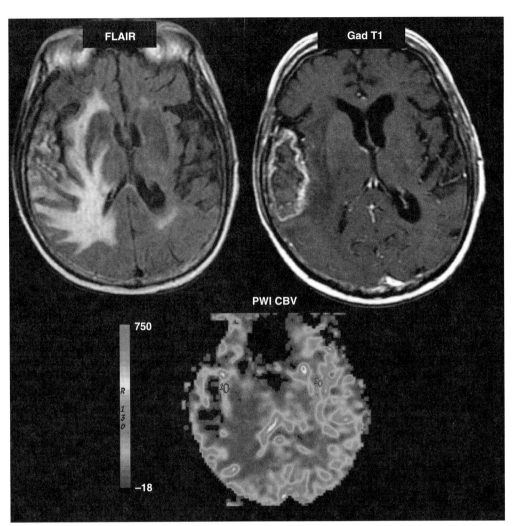

Figure 6–11 Magnetic resonance imaging (MRI) study of an 82-year-old man who had undergone radiation therapy for external ear cancer. Gadolinium-enhanced, T1-weighted (Gad T1) and fluid-attenuated inversion recovery (FLAIR) images showed an abnormally enhancing lesion in the right temporal lobe without significant mass effect. Perfusion-weighted dynamic susceptibility imaging (PWI) demonstrated no increased cerebral blood volume (CBV) (i.e., no red) within this lesion, confirming the clinical suspicion of radiation necrosis.

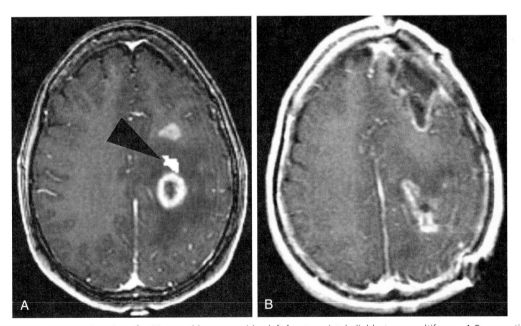

Figure 6–12 Magnetic resonance imaging of a 66-year-old woman with a left frontoparietal glioblastoma multiforme. A Preoperative Diffusion tensor imaging (DTI) demonstrated the corticospinal tract (*arrowhead*) to be located between two nodules of abnormal enhancement. The neurosurgeon took this information into consideration when planning surgery. He used two approaches and performed two resection cavities, one anterior and one posterior, in order to spare the corticospinal tract, as demonstrated on the postoperative images (B).

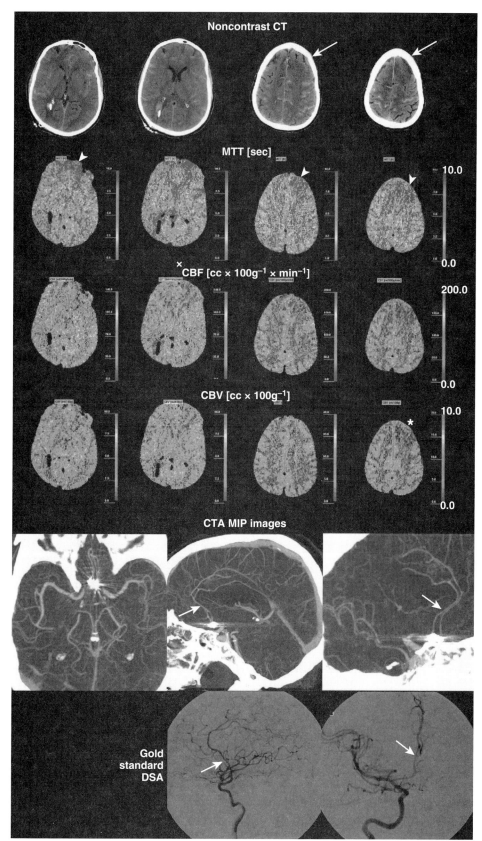

Figure 6–13 Patient who underwent coiling of a ruptured anterior communicating artery aneurysm at another institution was transferred on day 8 to our neurovascular intensive care unit (ICU). *Top row,* Noncontrast brain computed tomography (CT) scans obtained upon admission to the neurovascular ICU demonstrated extensive residual subarachnoid hemorrhage and suspicious loss of gray matter–white matter contrast in the left superior frontal gyrus (*white arrows*). The tip of a right ventricular drain catheter is also visible. *Second through fourth rows,* On perfusion CT, significantly abnormal brain perfusion in the distribution of the anterior and inferior branches of the left (and also, to a lesser extent, right) anterior cerebral arteries (ACAs) (*arrowheads*) and of the right posterior middle cerebral artery (MCA) branches is seen primarily on mean transit time (MTT) maps. The cerebral blood flow (CBF) was also slightly decreased in the same territories, whereas cerebral blood volume (CBV) was mainly preserved (it is lowered only in the left superior frontal gyrus [*]). *Fifth row,* CT angiography (CTA) confirmed the suspicion of moderate vasospasm of both A2 and A3 segments of the ACA (*arrows*), which was ultimately verified by "gold standard" digital subtraction angiography (DSA; *bottom row*). No abnormality of the right posterior MCA branches was identified. Of note, the artifacts created by the coils on the CTA MIP (maximum intensity projection) images obscure the A1 segments bilaterally and interfere with their evaluation. Endovascular therapy (intra-arterial verapamil) was performed in the ACA territories during the DSA.

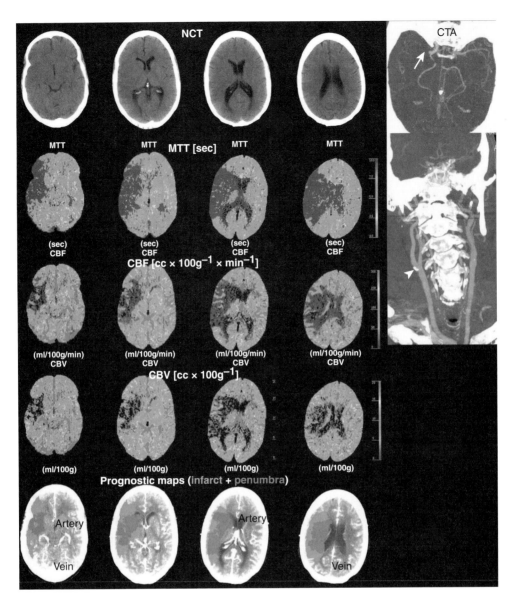

Figure 6–14 A modern computed tomography (CT) survey in a 57-year-old man admitted to our emergency department with a left hemisyndrome; unenhanced CT scans (*top row*), perfusion CT (PCT) scans (*second through fifth rows*), and CT angiography (CTA) (*right column*). The unenhanced CT scans ruled out a cerebral hemorrhage. From the PCT raw data, three parametric maps were extracted, relating to mean transit time (MTT; *second row*), cerebral blood flow (CBF; *third row*), and cerebral blood volume (CBV; *fourth raw*). Application of the concept of cerebral vascular autoregulation led to prognostic maps (*fifth row*) describing the infarct in *red* and the penumbra in *green*, the latter being the target of acute reperfusion therapies. CTA identified an occlusion at the right M1-M2 junction (*arrow*) as the origin of the hemodynamic disturbance demonstrated by PCT. CTA also revealed a calcified atheromatous plaque at the right carotid bifurcation (*arrowhead*). (*sec*, second).

effective therapies, such as intravenous thrombolytic drug therapy.[142] Moreover, imaging in patients with acute stroke should be targeted toward the assessment of the four Ps (parenchyma, pipes, perfusion, and penumbra).[143] In other words, one must establish a diagnosis as early as possible, rule out ICH, and obtain accurate information about the intracranial vasculature (i.e., identification of intravascular thrombi) and brain perfusion (differentiation of infarcted tissue from tissue at risk). Tissue at risk, or *penumbra*, is defined as an area of markedly reduced perfusion with compromised function yet still viable neurons that might benefit from timely reperfusion, which thus might prevent irreversible damage.[144,145]

COMPUTED TOMOGRAPHY AND ACUTE STROKE

Noncontrast CT of the brain has traditionally been the first-line imaging study in acute stroke because it can detect "early signs" of stroke and accurately rule out hemorrhage,

a contraindication to thrombolytic stroke therapies.[146-148] Early CT findings in brain ischemia include loss of contrast between white matter and gray matter (cortical ribbon and/or basal ganglia), early mass effect, and the presence of a hyperdense artery.[149-156] However, noncontrast CT has limited sensitivity for the hyperacute stage of ischemic stroke (55%-82%).[157,158] Also, noncontrast CT cannot reliably differentiate between irreversibly damaged brain tissue and penumbra.

Emerging CT-based techniques have facilitated a more comprehensive multimodal evaluation of acute stroke. Noncontrast CT enables the ruling out of hemorrhage, CTA identifies intracranial thrombus, and PCT evaluates the functional state of ischemic brain tissue by differentiating between "at-risk" brain tissue (the so-called penumbra) and irreversibly damaged brain tissue (Fig. 6-14).[157]

CTA allows a quick and detailed evaluation of the intracranial and extracranial vasculature with thin-section multiplanar views.[25,159] Its utility in acute stroke lies not only in its ability to detect large vessel thrombi within intracranial vessels and to evaluate the carotid and vertebral arteries in the neck[160-162] but also in its potential to guide therapy. In particular, the exact location (i.e., proximal vs. peripheral) and the extent of vascular occlusion have been shown to have prognostic value as to the response to thrombolytic agents, the determination of collateral circulation, and the possible risk of subsequent recanalization.[163] For example, patients with "top of carotid" occlusions, proximal middle cerebral artery branch occlusions, or significant thrombus burden might be poor candidates for intravenous thrombolytics and possibly may be better candidates for intra-arterial or mechanical thrombolysis.[164]

Within the last few years, PCT has become the third component in the multimodal CT assessment of acute ischemic stroke.[165] Compared with MRI imaging, xenon-enhanced CT, positron emission tomography, and single-photon emission CT, PCT is more widely available and can be performed quickly on any standard helical CT scanner immediately after noncontrast CT.[166] PCT maps can then be generated in a short time at a workstation equipped with a dedicated postprocessing software.[166] PCT has been shown to be more accurate than noncontrast CT for stroke detection[158] and for assessing the extent of the stroke.[167] MTT maps have been found to be more sensitive, and CBF and CBV maps to be more specific, for distinguishing ischemia from infarction.[167,168] PCT distinction of the infarct core from the penumbra is based on the concept of cerebral vascular autoregulation. In the penumbra, autoregulation is preserved, MTT is prolonged, but CBV is preserved because of vasodilatation and collateral recruitment as part of the autoregulation process. In the infarct core, autoregulation is lost, MTT is prolonged, and CBV is diminished.[169] Thus, with the use of appropriate MTT and CBV thresholds, infract core and penumbra can be distinguished on PCT maps (see Fig. 6-14).[170]

MAGNETIC RESONANCE IMAGING AND ACUTE STROKE

Multimodal MRI including DWI, PWI, and MRA affords results similar to those of the CT-based multimodal techniques already described. DWI shows the infarct core, the DWI-PWI mismatch represents the penumbra, and MRA allows assessment of vascular patency across the whole brain with high-resolution structural imaging (see Fig. 6-4).[171,172]

Although acute infarcts may be seen early on conventional MRI, DWI is more sensitive for detection of hyperacute ischemia. DWI hyperintensity and ADC hypointensity occur shortly after acute ischemia as a result of a failure of the adenosine triphosphatase pump, subsequent loss of ion homeostasis, and the movement of water into the intracellular compartment, where it is relatively restricted (cytotoxic edema).[28] These radiographic findings identify severely ischemic tissue within minutes of stroke onset, whereas conventional MRI and noncontrast CT findings might be normal.

PWI changes precede the development of DWI lesions, and in the absence of reperfusion, the area of restricted diffusion spontaneously progresses within the region of perfusion abnormality. Conversely, spontaneous or therapeutic recanalization tends to prevent progression of this process. By combing the DWI and PWI image information, one can generate a composite so-called diffusion-perfusion mismatch,[173] which is theorized to represent the tissue at risk, or penumbra. Penumbra as defined by the DWI-PWI mismatch is very similar to the penumbra characterized by PCT.[174] In as many as 70% of acute strokes caused by middle cerebral artery occlusion imaged within 6 hours of onset, a DWI-PWI mismatch is present, the PWI lesion (hypoperfusion) being larger than the DWI core.[173] The two other patterns that can be observed are (1) the DWI lesion size is equal to the PWI lesion size (i.e., tissue is irreversibly infarcted and no penumbra is present) and (2) the DWI lesion is larger than PWI lesion or there is a DWI lesion with no perfusion defect, a finding that usually indicates early reperfusion of ischemic tissue (the DWI lesion size does not change over time).[175]

However, there are some aspects of the mismatch concept that still need to be addressed. The initial DWI lesion abnormality can be reversible and thus includes areas of penumbral as well as infarcted tissue.[176,177] In addition, the PWI parameter most representative of hypoperfusion has not been clearly defined (e.g., prolonged MTT or TTP). Nevertheless, the importance of the DWI-PWI mismatch hypothesis is the ability to potentially appropriately identify patients in whom there is evidence of potentially salvageable tissue for therapeutic intervention. In the small Desmoteplase In Acute Ischemic Stroke (DIAS) trial,[178] intravenous thrombolytic treatment given to patients selected on the basis of a mismatch improved clinical and radiologic outcomes even though treatment began between 3 and 9 hours after stroke.

REFERENCES

1. Hofman PA, Nelemans P, et al: Value of radiological diagnosis of skull fracture in the management of mild head injury: Meta-analysis, *J Neurol Neurosurg Psychiatry* 68:416–422, 2000.
2. Lloyd DA, Carty H, Patterson M, et al: Predictive value of skull radiography for intracranial injury in children with blunt head injury, *Lancet* 349:821–824, 1997.
3. Masters S, McClean P, Arcarese JS, et al: Skull x-ray examinations after head trauma. Recommendations by a multidisciplinary panel and validation study, *N Engl J Med* 316:84–91, 1987.
4. Seelig JM, Becker DP, Miller JD, et al: Traumatic acute subdural hematoma: Major mortality reduction in comatose patients treated within four hours, *N Engl J Med* 304:1511–1518, 1981.
5. Bronen RA, Sze G: Magnetic resonance imaging contrast agents: Theory and application to the central nervous system, *J Neurosurg* 73:820–839, 1990.
6. Ashikaga R, Araki Y, Ishida O: MRI of head injury using FLAIR, *Neuroradiology* 39:239–242, 1997.
7. Singer MB, Atlas SW, Drayer BP: Subarachnoid space disease: Diagnosis with fluid-attenuated inversion-recovery MR imaging and comparison with gadolinium-enhanced spin-echo MR imaging—blinded reader study, *Radiology* 208:417–422, 1998.
8. Bradley WG: Jr: MR appearance of hemorrhage in the brain, *Radiology* 189:15–26, 1993.
9. Bradley WG Jr: Hemorrhage and hemorrhagic infections in the brain, *Neuroimaging Clin N Am* 4:707–732, 1994.
10. Edelman R, Johnson K, et al: MR of hemorrhage: A new approach, *AJNR Am J Neuroradiol* 7:751–756, 1986.
11. Tsushima Y, Aoki J, Endo K: Brain microhemorrhages detected on T2*-weighted gradient-echo MR images, *AJNR Am J Neuroradiol* 24:88–96, 2003.
12. Sawyer-Glover AM, Shellock FG: Pre-MRI procedure screening: Recommendations and safety considerations for biomedical implants and devices, *J Magn Reson Imaging* 12:92–106, 2000.
13. Woods TO: Standards for medical devices in MRI: Present and future, *J Magn Reson Imaging* 26:1186–1189, 2007.
14. Shellock FG, Crues JV: MR procedures: Biologic effects, safety, and patient care, *Radiology* 232:635–652, 2004.
15. Brant-Zawadzki M, Gould R, Mentzer W: Digital subtraction cerebral angiography by intraarterial injection: Comparison with conventional angiography, *Am J Roentgenol* 140:347–353, 1983.
16. Prestigiacomo CJ: Surgical endovascular neuroradiology in the 21st century: What lies ahead?, *Neurosurgery* 59:S48–S55, 2006:discussion S43-S13.
17. Wang H, Fraser K, Wang D, Lanzino G: The evolution of endovascular therapy for neurosurgical disease, *Neurosurg Clin N Am* 16:223–229, 2005:vii.

18. Cloft HJ, Joseph GJ, Dion JE: Risk of cerebral angiography in patients with subarachnoid hemorrhage, cerebral aneurysm, and arteriovenous malformation: A meta-analysis, *Stroke* 30:317–320, 1999.

19. Heiserman JE, Dean BL, Hodak JA, et al: Neurologic complications of cerebral angiography, *AJNR Am J Neuroradiol* 15:1408–1411, 1994:1401-1407; discussion.

20. Willinsky RA, Taylor SM, et al: Neurologic complications of cerebral angiography: Prospective analysis of 2,899 procedures and review of the literature, *Radiology* 227:522–528, 2003.

21. Ozsarlak O, Van Goethem JW, Maes M, Parizel PM: MR angiography of the intracranial vessels: Technical aspects and clinical applications, *Neuroradiology* 46:955–972, 2004.

22. Wilms G, Bosmans H, Demaerel P, Marchal G: Magnetic resonance angiography of the intracranial vessels, *Eur J Radiol* 38:10–18, 2001.

23. Vieco PT: CT angiography of the intracranial circulation, *Neuroimaging Clin N Am* 8:577–592, 1998.

24. Prokop M, Shin HO, Schanz A, Schaefer-Prokop CM: Use of maximum intensity projections in CT angiography: A basic review, *Radiographics* 17:433–451, 1997.

25. Prokop M: Multislice CT angiography, *Eur J Radiol* 36:86–96, 2000.

26. Lell MM, Anders K, Uder M, et al: New techniques in CT angiography, *Radiographics* 26(Suppl 1):S45–S62, 2006.

27. Katayama H, Heneine N, van Gessel R, et al: Clinical experience with iomeprol in myelography and myelo-CT: Clinical pharmacology and double-blind comparisons with iopamidol, iohexol, and iotrolan, *Invest Radiol* 36:22–32, 2001.

28. Latchaw RE, Yonas H, Hunter GJ, et al: Council on Cardiovascular Radiology of the American Heart Association. Guidelines and recommendations for perfusion imaging in cerebral ischemia: A scientific statement for healthcare professionals by the writing group on perfusion imaging, from the Council on Cardiovascular Radiology of the American Heart Association, *Stroke* 34:1084–1104, 2003.

29. Wintermark M, Maeder P, Thiran JP, et al: Quantitative assessment of regional cerebral blood flows by perfusion CT studies at low injection rates: A critical review of the underlying theoretical models, *Eur Radiol* 11:1220–1230, 2001.

30. Wintermark M, Thiran JP, Maeder P, et al: Simultaneous measurement of regional cerebral blood flow by perfusion CT and stable xenon CT: A validation study, *AJNR Am J Neuroradiol* 22:905–914, 2001.

31. Schaefer PW, Grant PE, Gonzalez RG: Diffusion-weighted MR imaging of the brain, *Radiology* 217:331–345, 2000.

32. Schaefer PW, Copen WA, Lev MH, Gonzalez RG: Diffusion-weighted imaging in acute stroke, *Neuroimaging Clin N Am* 15:503–530, 2005:ix-x.

33. Huisman TA, Sorensen AG, Hergan K, et al: Diffusion-weighted imaging for the evaluation of diffuse axonal injury in closed head injury, *J Comput Assist Tomogr* 27:5–11, 2003.

34. Rugg-Gunn FJ, Symms MR, Barker GJ, et al: Diffusion imaging shows abnormalities after blunt head trauma when conventional magnetic resonance imaging is normal, *J Neurol Neurosurg Psychiatry* 70:530–533, 2001.

35. Sorensen AG, Wu O, Copen WA, et al: Human acute cerebral ischemia: Detection of changes in water diffusion anisotropy by using MR imaging, *Radiology* 212:785–792, 1999.

36. Calamante F, Thomas DL, Pell GS, et al: Measuring cerebral blood flow using magnetic resonance imaging techniques, *J Cereb Blood Flow Metab* 19:701–735, 1999.

37. Petrella JR, Provenzale JM: MR perfusion imaging of the brain: Techniques and applications, *AJR Am J Roentgenol* 175:207–219, 2000.

38. Ostergaard L: Principles of cerebral perfusion imaging by bolus tracking, *J Magn Reson Imaging* 22:710–717, 2005.

39. Tofts PS, Brix G, Buckley DL, et al: Estimating kinetic parameters from dynamic contrast-enhanced T(1)-weighted MRI of a diffusable tracer: Standardized quantities and symbols, *J Magn Reson Imaging* 10:223–232, 1999.

40. Castillo M, Kwock L, Mukherji SK: Clinical applications of proton MR spectroscopy, *AJNR Am J Neuroradiol* 17:1–15, 1996.

41. Maheshwari SR, Fatterpekar GM, Castillo M, Mukherji SK: Proton MR spectroscopy of the brain, *Semin Ultrasound CT MR* 21:434–451, 2000.

42. Birken DL, Oldendorf WH: N-acetyl-L-aspartic acid: A literature review of a compound prominent in 1h-NMR spectroscopic studies of brain, *Neurosci Biobehav Rev* 13:23–31, 1989.

43. Garnett MR, Blamire AM, Corkill RG, et al: Early proton magnetic resonance spectroscopy in normal-appearing brain correlates with outcome in patients following traumatic brain injury, *Brain* 123:2046–2054, 2000.

44. Marmarou A: A review of progress in understanding the pathophysiology and treatment of brain edema, *Neurosurg Focus*, 22:E1, 2007.

45. Cohen ZR, Ram Z, Knoller N, et al: Management and outcome of nontraumatic cerebellar haemorrhage, *Cerebrovasc Dis* 14:207–213, 2002.

46. Gomori J, Grossman R: Mechanisms responsible for the MR appearance and evolution of intracranial hemorrhage, *Radiographics* 8:427–440, 1988.

47. Ropper A: Lateral displacement of the brain and level of consciousness in patients with an acute hemispheral mass, *N Engl J Med* 314:953–958, 1986.

48. Feldmann E, Gandy SE, Becker R, et al: MRI demonstrates descending transtentorial herniation, *Neurology* 38:697–701, 1988.

49. Johnson PL, Eckard DA, Chason DP, et al: Imaging of acquired cerebral herniations, *Neuroimaging Clin N Am* 12:217–228, 2002.

50. Wernick S, Wells RG: Sequelae of temporal lobe herniation: MR imaging, *J Comput Assist Tomogr* 13:323–325, 1989.

51. Hahn FJ, Gurney J: CT signs of central descending transtentorial herniation, *AJNR Am J Neuroradiol* 6:844–845, 1985.

52. Sze G: Diseases of the intracranial meninges: MR imaging features, *AJR Am J Roentgenol* 160:727–733, 1993.

53. Sherman JL, Citrin CM, Bowen BJ, Gangarosa RE: MR demonstration of altered cerebrospinal fluid flow by obstructive lesions, *AJNR Am J Neuroradiol* 7:571–579, 1986.

54. Levy LM: MR imaging of cerebrospinal fluid flow and spinal cord motion in neurologic disorders of the spine, *Magn Reson Imaging Clin N Am* 7:573–587, 1999.

55. Jennett B: Epidemiology of head injury, *J Neurol Neurosurg Psychiatry* 60:362–369, 1996.

56. Sosin DM, Sniezek JE, Waxweiler RJ: Trends in death associated with traumatic brain injury, 1979 through 1992. Success and failure, *JAMA* 273:1778–1780, 1995.

57. Werner C, Engelhard K: Pathophysiology of traumatic brain injury, *Br J Anaesth* 99:4–9, 2007.

58. Yates PJ, Williams WH, Harris A, et al: An epidemiological study of head injuries in a UK population attending an emergency department, *J Neurol Neurosurg Psychiatry* 77:699–701, 2006.

59. Ahmadi J, Destian S: Head trauma, *Top Magn Reson Imaging* 2:17–24, 1989.

60. Kelly AB, Zimmerman RD, Snow RB, et al: Head trauma: Comparison of MR and CT—experience in 100 patients, *AJNR Am J Neuroradiol* 9:699–708, 1988.

61. Quencer RM: Neuroimaging and head injuries: Where we've been—where we're going, *AJR Am J Roentgenol* 150:13–18, 1988.

62. Haydel MJ, Preston CA, Mills TJ, et al: Indications for computed tomography in patients with minor head injury, *N Engl J Med* 343:100–105, 2000.

63. Jeret JS, Mandell M, Anziska B, et al: Clinical predictors of abnormality disclosed by computed tomography after mild head trauma, *Neurosurgery* 32:15–16, 1993:9-15; discussion.

64. Moran SG, McCarthy MC, Uddin DE, Poelstra RJ: Predictors of positive CT scans in the trauma patient with minor head injury, *Am Surg* 60:535–536, 1994:533-535; discussion.

65. Cecil KM, Hills EC, Smith DH, et al: Proton magnetic resonance spectroscopy for detection of axonal injury in the splenium of the corpus callosum of brain-injured patients, *J Neurosurg* 88:795–801, 1998.

66. Gentry LR, Godersky JC, Thompson B, Dunn VD: Prospective comparative study of intermediate-field MR and CT in the evaluation of closed head trauma, *AJR Am J Roentgenol* 150:673–682, 1988.

67. Sinson G, Bagley LJ, Cecil KM, et al: Magnetization transfer imaging and proton MR spectroscopy in the evaluation of axonal injury: Correlation with clinical outcome after traumatic brain injury, *AJNR Am J Neuroradiol* 22:143–151, 2001.

68. Ogawa T, Sekino H, Uzura M, et al: Comparative study of magnetic resonance and CT scan imaging in cases of severe head injury, *Acta Neurochir Suppl (Wien)* 55:8–10, 1992.

69. Doezema D, King JN, Tandberg D, et al: Magnetic resonance imaging in minor head injury, *Ann Emerg Med* 20:1281–1285, 1991.

70. Mittl RL, Grossman RI, Hiehle JF, et al: Prevalence of MR evidence of diffuse axonal injury in patients with mild head injury and normal head CT findings, *AJNR Am J Neuroradiol* 15:1583–1589, 1994.

71. Thornbury JR, Campbell JA, Masters SJ, Fryback DG: Skull fracture and the low risk of intracranial sequelae in minor head trauma, *AJR Am J Roentgenol* 143:661–664, 1984.

72. Zee CS, Hovanessian A, Go JL, Kim PE: Imaging of sequelae of head trauma, *Neuroimaging Clin N Am* 12:325–338, 2002:ix.

73. Alvi A, Bereliani AT: Trauma to the temporal bone: Diagnosis and management of complications, *J Craniomaxillofac Trauma* 2:36–48, 1996.

74. Kruse JJ, Awasthi D: Skull-base trauma: Neurosurgical perspective, *J Craniomaxillofac Trauma* 4:8–14, 1998:discussion 17.

75. Alder ME, Deahl ST, Matteson SR: Clinical usefulness of two-dimensional reformatted and three-dimensionally rendered computerized tomographic images: Literature review and a survey of surgeons' opinions, *J Oral Maxillofac Surg* 53:375–386, 1995.

76. Fatterpekar GM, Doshi AH, Dugar M, et al: Role of 3d CT in the evaluation of the temporal bone, *Radiographics* 26(Suppl 1):S117–S132, 2006.

77. Holland BA, Brant-Zawadzki M: High-resolution CT of temporal bone trauma, *AJR Am J Roentgenol* 143:391–395, 1984.

78. Schuknecht B, Graetz K: Radiologic assessment of maxillofacial, mandibular, and skull base trauma, *Eur Radiol* 15:560–568, 2005.

79. Lloyd MN, Kimber PM, Burrows EH: Post-traumatic cerebrospinal fluid rhinorrhoea: Modern high-definition computed tomography is all that is required for the effective demonstration of the site of leakage, *Clin Radiol* 49:100–103, 1994.

80. Lund VJ, Savy L, Lloyd G, Howard D: Optimum imaging and diagnosis of cerebrospinal fluid rhinorrhoea, *J Laryngol Otol* 114:988–992, 2000.

81. Stone JA, Castillo M, Neelon B, Mukherji SK: Evaluation of CSF leaks: High-resolution CT compared with contrast-enhanced CT and radionuclide cisternography, *AJNR Am J Neuroradiol* 20:706–712, 1999.

82. Zimmerman R, Bilaniuk L: Computed tomographic staging of traumatic epidural bleeding, *Radiology* 144:809–812, 1982.

83. Bricolo AP, Pasut LM: Extradural hematoma: Toward zero mortality. A prospective study, *Neurosurgery* 14:8–12, 1984.

84. Al-Nakshabandi NA: The swirl sign, *Radiology* 218:433, 2001.

85. Lee KS, Bae WK, Bae HG, et al: The computed tomographic attenuation and the age of subdural hematomas, *J Korean Med Sci* 12:353–359, 1997.

86. Provenzale J: CT and MR imaging of acute cranial trauma, *Emerg Radiol* 14:1–12, 2007.

87. Smith WP Jr, Batnitzky S, Rengachary SS: Acute isodense subdural hematomas: A problem in anemic patients, *AJR Am J Roentgenol* 136:543–546, 1981.

88. van Gijn J, Kerr RS, Rinkel GJ: Subarachnoid haemorrhage, *Lancet* 369:306–318, 2007.

89. Yeakley JW, Patchall LL, Lee KF: Interpeduncular fossa sign: CT criterion of subarachnoid hemorrhage, *Radiology* 158:699–700, 1986.

90. Schellinger PD, Jansen O, Fiebach JB, et al: A standardized MRI stroke protocol: Comparison with CT in hyperacute intracerebral hemorrhage, *Stroke* 30:765–768, 1999.

91. Young RJ, Destian S: Imaging of traumatic intracranial hemorrhage, *Neuroimaging Clin N Am* 12:189–204, 2002.

92. Adams JH, Doyle D, Ford I, et al: Diffuse axonal injury in head injury: Definition, diagnosis and grading, *Histopathology* 15:49–59, 1989.

93. Adams JH, Graham DI, Gennarelli TA, Maxwell WL: Diffuse axonal injury in non-missile head injury, *J Neurol Neurosurg Psychiatry* 54:481–483, 1991.

94. Hammoud DA, Wasserman BA: Diffuse axonal injuries: Pathophysiology and imaging, *Neuroimaging Clin N Am* 12:205–216, 2002.

95. Scheid R, Preul C, Gruber O, et al: Diffuse axonal injury associated with chronic traumatic brain injury: Evidence from T2*-weighted gradient-echo imaging at 3 t, *AJNR Am J Neuroradiol* 24:1049–1056, 2003.

96. Tong KA, Ashwal S, Holshouser BA, et al: Diffuse axonal injury in children: Clinical correlation with hemorrhagic lesions, *Ann Neurol* 56:36–50, 2004.

97. Kinoshita T, Moritani T, Hiwatashi A, et al: Conspicuity of diffuse axonal injury lesions on diffusion-weighted MR imaging, *Eur J Radiol* 56:5–11, 2005.

98. Parizel PM, Ozsarlak O, Van Goethem JW, et al: Imaging findings in diffuse axonal injury after closed head trauma, *Eur Radiol* 8:960–965, 1998.

99. Pierallini A, Pantano P, Fantozzi LM, et al: Correlation between MRI findings and long-term outcome in patients with severe brain trauma, *Neuroradiology* 42:860–867, 2000.

100. Lunsford LD, Martinez AJ, Latchaw RE: Magnetic resonance imaging does not define tumor boundaries, *Acta Radiol Suppl* 369:154–156, 1986.

101. Price SJ, Jena R, Burnet NG, et al: Improved delineation of glioma margins and regions of infiltration with the use of diffusion tensor imaging: An image-guided biopsy study, *AJNR Am J Neuroradiol* 27:1969–1974, 2006.

102. Croteau D, Scarpace L, Hearshen D, et al: Correlation between magnetic resonance spectroscopy imaging and image-guided biopsies: Semiquantitative and qualitative histopathological analyses of patients with untreated glioma, *Neurosurgery* 49:823–829, 2001.

103. McKnight TR, von dem Bussche MH, Vigneron DB, et al: Histopathological validation of a three-dimensional magnetic resonance spectroscopy index as a predictor of tumor presence, *J Neurosurg* 97:794–802, 2002.

104. Price SJ, Jena R, Burnet NG, et al: Predicting patterns of glioma recurrence using diffusion tensor imaging, *Eur Radiol* 17:1675–1684, 2007.

105. Provenzale JM, McGraw P, Mhatre P, et al: Peritumoral brain regions in gliomas and meningiomas: Investigation with isotropic diffusion-weighted MR imaging and diffusion-tensor MR imaging, *Radiology* 232:451–460, 2004.

106. Tropine A, Vucurevic G, Delani P, et al: Contribution of diffusion tensor imaging to delineation of gliomas and glioblastomas, *J Magn Reson Imaging* 20:905–912, 2004.

107. van Westen D, Latt J, Englund E, et al: Tumor extension in high-grade gliomas assessed with diffusion magnetic resonance imaging: Values and lesion-to-brain ratios of apparent diffusion coefficient and fractional anisotropy, *Acta Radiol* 47:311–319, 2006.

108. Julia-Sapé M, Acosta D, Majós C, et al: Comparison between neuroimaging classifications and histopathological diagnoses using an international multicenter brain tumor magnetic resonance imaging database, *J Neurosurg* 105:6–14, 2006.

109. Ginsberg LE, Fuller GN, Hashmi M, et al: The significance of lack of MR contrast enhancement of supratentorial brain tumors in adults: Histopathological evaluation of a series, *Surg Neurol* 49:436–440, 1998.

110. Beppu T, Inoue T, Shibata Y, et al: Fractional anisotropy value by diffusion tensor magnetic resonance imaging as a predictor of cell density and proliferation activity of glioblastomas, *Surg Neurol* 63:56–61, 2005:discussion 61.

111. Provenzale JM, McGraw P, Mhatre P, et al: Peritumoral brain regions in gliomas and meningiomas: Investigation with isotropic diffusion-weighted MR imaging and diffusion-tensor MR imaging, *Radiology* 232:451–460, 2004.

112. Stadlbauer A, Ganslandt O, Buslei R, et al: Gliomas: Histopathologic evaluation of changes in directionality and magnitude of water diffusion at diffusion-tensor MR imaging, *Radiology* 240:803–810, 2006.

113. Sugahara T, Korogi Y, Kochi M, et al: Usefulness of diffusion-weighted MRI with echo-planar technique in the evaluation of cellularity in gliomas, *J Magn Reson Imaging* 9:53–60, 1999.

114. Kono K, Inoue Y, Nakayama K, et al: The role of diffusion-weighted imaging in patients with brain tumors, *AJNR Am J Neuroradiol* 22:1081–1088, 2001.

115. Fountas KN, Kapsalaki EZ, Gotsis SD, et al: In vivo proton magnetic resonance spectroscopy of brain tumors, *Stereotact Funct Neurosurg* 74:83–94, 2000.

116. Law M, Yang S, Wang H, et al: Glioma grading: Sensitivity, specificity, and predictive values of perfusion MR imaging and proton MR spectroscopic imaging compared with conventional MR imaging, *AJNR Am J Neuroradiol* 24:1989–1998, 2003.

117. Law M: MR spectroscopy of brain tumors, *Top Magn Reson Imaging* 15:291–313, 2004.

118. McKnight TR, Lamborn KR, Love TD, et al: Correlation of magnetic resonance spectroscopic and growth characteristics within grades II and III gliomas, *J Neurosurg* 106:660–666, 2007.

119. Murphy M, Loosemore A, Clifton AG, et al: The contribution of proton magnetic resonance spectroscopy (1HMRS) to clinical brain tumour diagnosis, *Br J Neurosurg* 16:329–334, 2002.

120. Nafe R, Herminghaus S, Raab P, et al: Preoperative proton-MR spectroscopy of gliomas—correlation with quantitative nuclear morphology in surgical specimen, *J Neurooncol* 63:233–245, 2003.

121. Hakyemez B, Erdogan C, Ercan I, et al: High-grade and low-grade gliomas: Differentiation by using perfusion MR imaging, *Clin Radiol* 60:493–502, 2005.

122. Shin JH, Lee HK, Kwun BD, et al: Using relative cerebral blood flow and volume to evaluate the histopathologic grade of cerebral gliomas: Preliminary results, *AJR Am J Roentgenol* 179:783–789, 2002.

123. Sugahara T, Korogi Y, Kochi M, et al: Correlation of MR imaging-determined cerebral blood volume maps with histologic and angiographic determination of vascularity of gliomas, *AJR Am J Roentgenol* 171:1479–1486, 1998.

124. Lev MH, Ozsunar Y, Lev MH, et al: Glial tumor grading and outcome prediction using dynamic spin-echo MR susceptibility mapping compared with conventional contrast-enhanced MR: Confounding effect of elevated RCBV of oligodendrogliomas [corrected], *AJNR Am J Neuroradiol* 25:214–221, 2004.

125. Sugahara T, Korogi Y, Tomiguchi S, et al: Posttherapeutic intraaxial brain tumor: The value of perfusion-sensitive contrast-enhanced MR imaging for differentiating tumor recurrence from nonneoplastic contrast-enhancing tissue, *AJNR Am J Neuroradiol* 21:901–909, 2000.

126. Barrett T, Brechbiel M, Bernardo M, Choyke PL: MRI of tumor angiogenesis, *J Magn Reson Imaging* 26:235–249, 2007.

127. Chernov MF, Hayashi M, Izawa M, et al: Multivoxel proton MRS for differentiation of radiation-induced necrosis and tumor recurrence after gamma knife radiosurgery for brain metastases, *Brain Tumor Pathol* 23:19–27, 2006.

128. Tomoi M, Kimura H, Yoshida M, et al: Alterations of lactate (+ lipid) concentration in brain tumors with in vivo hydrogen magnetic resonance spectroscopy during radiotherapy, *Invest Radiol* 32:288–296, 1997.

129. van der Wee N, Rinkel G, Hasan D, van Gijn J: Detection of subarachnoid haemorrhage on early CT: Is lumbar puncture still needed after a negative scan? *J Neurol Neurosurg Psychiatry* 58:357–359, 1995.

130. Chappell ET, Moure FC, Good MC: Comparison of computed tomographic angiography with digital subtraction angiography in the diagnosis of cerebral aneurysms: A meta-analysis, *Neurosurgery* 52:624–631, 2003:discussion 630-621.

131. Dammert S, Krings T, Moller-Hartmann W, et al: Detection of intracranial aneurysms with multislice CT: Comparison with conventional angiography, *Neuroradiology* 46:427–434, 2004.

132. Kangasniemi M, Mäkelä T, Koskinen S, et al: Detection of intracranial aneurysms with two-dimensional and three-dimensional multislice helical computed tomographic angiography, *Neurosurgery* 54:336–340, 2004:discussion 340-331.

133. Tipper G, U-King-Im JM, Price SJ, et al: Detection and evaluation of intracranial aneurysms with 16-row multislice CT angiography, *Clin Radiol* 60:565–572, 2005.

134. White PM, Teasdale EM, Wardlaw JM, Easton V: Intracranial aneurysms: CT angiography and MR angiography for detection prospective blinded comparison in a large patient cohort, *Radiology* 219:739–749, 2001.

135. White PM, Wardlaw JM, Easton V: Can noninvasive imaging accurately depict intracranial aneurysms? A systematic review, *Radiology* 217:361–370, 2000.

136. Chaudhary SR, Ko N, Dillon WP, et al: Prospective evaluation of multidetector-row CT angiography for the diagnosis of vasospasm following subarachnoid hemorrhage: A comparison with digital subtraction angiography, *Cerebrovasc Dis* 25:144–150, 2008.

137. Wintermark M, Ko NU, Smith WS, et al: Vasospasm after subarachnoid hemorrhage: Utility of perfusion CT and CT angiography on diagnosis and management, *AJNR Am J Neuroradiol* 27:26–34, 2006.

138. Hofmeister C, Stapf C, Hartmann A, et al: Demographic, morphological, and clinical characteristics of 1289 patients with brain arteriovenous malformation, *Stroke* 31:1307–1310, 2000.

139. Du R, Hashimoto T, Tihan T, et al: Growth and regression of arteriovenous malformations in a patient with hereditary hemorrhagic telangiectasia: Case report, *J Neurosurg* 106:470–477, 2007.

140. Young WL: Intracranial arteriovenous malformations: Pathophysiology and hemodynamics. In Jafar JJ RH, Rosenwasser AI, editors: *Vascular Malformations of the Central Nervous System*, New York, 1999, Lippincott Williams & Wilkins.

141. Hino A, Fujimoto M, Yamaki T, et al: Value of repeat angiography in patients with spontaneous subcortical hemorrhage, *Stroke* 29:2517–2521, 1998.

142. Tissue plasminogen activator for acute ischemic stroke: The National Institute of Neurological Disorders and Stroke rt-PA Stroke Study Group, *N Engl J Med* 333:1581–1587, 1995.

143. Rowley HA: The four Ps of acute stroke imaging: Parenchyma, pipes, perfusion, and penumbra, *AJNR Am J Neuroradiol* 22:599–601, 2001.

144. Astrup J, Siesjo BK, Symon L: Thresholds in cerebral ischemia—the ischemic penumbra, *Stroke* 12:723–725, 1981.

145. Heiss WD: Ischemic penumbra: Evidence from functional imaging in man, *J Cereb Blood Flow Metab* 20:1276–1293, 2000.

146. Manno EM, Nichols DA, Fulgham JR, Wijdicks EF: Computed tomographic determinants of neurologic deterioration in patients with large middle cerebral artery infarctions, *Mayo Clin Proc* 78:156–160, 2003.

147. Moulin T, Cattin F, Crépin-Leblond T, et al: Early CT signs in acute middle cerebral artery infarction: Predictive value for subsequent infarct locations and outcome, *Neurology* 47:366–375, 1996.

148. von Kummer R, Bourquain H, Bastianello S, et al: Early prediction of irreversible brain damage after ischemic stroke at CT, *Radiology* 219:95–100, 2001.

149. Barber PA, Demchuk AM, Hudon ME, et al: Hyperdense sylvian fissure MCA " dot" sign: A CT marker of acute ischemia, *Stroke* 32:84–88, 2001.

150. Leys D, Pruvo JP, Godefroy O, et al: Prevalence and significance of hyperdense middle cerebral artery in acute stroke, *Stroke* 23:317–324, 1992.

151. Rauch RA, Bazan C 3rd, Larsson EM, Jinkins JR: Hyperdense middle cerebral arteries identified on CT as a false sign of vascular occlusion, *AJNR Am J Neuroradiol* 14:669–673, 1993.

152. Schuierer G, Huk W: The unilateral hyperdense middle cerebral artery: An early CT-sign of embolism or thrombosis, *Neuroradiology* 30:120–122, 1988.

153. Tomsick T, Brott T, Barsan W, et al: Prognostic value of the hyperdense middle cerebral artery sign and stroke scale score before ultraearly thrombolytic therapy, *AJNR Am J Neuroradiol* 17:79–85, 1996.

154. Tomura N, Uemura K, Inugami A, et al: Early CT finding in cerebral infarction: Obscuration of the lentiform nucleus, *Radiology* 168:463–467, 1988.

155. Truwit CL, Barkovich AJ, Gean-Marton A, et al: Loss of the insular ribbon: Another early CT sign of acute middle cerebral artery infarction, *Radiology* 176:801–806, 1990.

156. von Kummer R, Meyding-Lamadé U, Forsting M, et al: Sensitivity and prognostic value of early CT in occlusion of the middle cerebral artery trunk, *AJNR Am J Neuroradiol* 15:16–18, 1994:9-15; discussion.

157. Kloska SP, Nabavi DG, Gaus C, et al: Acute stroke assessment with CT: Do we need multimodal evaluation?, *Radiology* 233:79–86, 2004.

158. von Kummer R, Nolte PN, Schnittger H, et al: Detectability of cerebral hemisphere ischaemic infarcts by CT within 6 h of stroke, *Neuroradiology* 38:31–33, 1996.

159. Lev MH, Farkas J, Rodriguez VR, et al: CT angiography in the rapid triage of patients with hyperacute stroke to intraarterial thrombolysis: Accuracy in the detection of large vessel thrombus, *J Comput Assist Tomogr* 25:520–528, 2001.

160. Cumming M, Morrow I: Carotid artery stenosis: A prospective comparison of CT angiography and conventional angiography, *Am J Roentgenol* 163:517–523, 1994.

161. Katz DA, Marks MP, Napel SA, et al: Circle of Willis: Evaluation with spiral CT angiography, MR angiography, and conventional angiography, *Radiology* 195:445–449, 1995.

162. Shrier DA, Tanaka H, Numaguchi Y, et al: CT angiography in the evaluation of acute stroke, *AJNR Am J Neuroradiol* 18:1011–1020, 1997.

163. Tan JC, Dillon WP, Liu S, et al: Systematic comparison of perfusion-CT and CT-angiography in acute stroke patients, *Ann Neurol* 61:533–543, 2007.

164. Zaidat OO, Suarez JI, Santillan C, et al: Response to intra-arterial and combined intravenous and intra-arterial thrombolytic therapy in patients with distal internal carotid artery occlusion, *Stroke* 33:1821–1826, 2002.

165. Miles KA: Brain perfusion: Computed tomography applications, *Neuroradiology* 46(Suppl 2):S194–S200, 2004.

166. Wintermark M, Sesay M, Barbier E, et al: Comparative overview of brain perfusion imaging techniques, *J Neuroradiol* 32:294–314, 2005.

167. Wintermark M, Fischbein NJ, Smith WS, et al: Accuracy of dynamic perfusion CT with deconvolution in detecting acute hemispheric stroke, *AJNR Am J Neuroradiol* 26:104–112, 2005.

168. Sparacia G, Iaia A, Assadi B, Lagalla R: Perfusion CT in acute stroke: Predictive value of perfusion parameters in assessing tissue viability versus infarction, *Radiol Med (Torino)* 112:113–122, 2007.

169. Wintermark M, Reichhart M, Thiran JP, et al: Prognostic accuracy of cerebral blood flow measurement by perfusion computed tomography, at the time of emergency room admission, in acute stroke patients, *Ann Neurol* 51:417–432, 2002.

170. Wintermark M, Flanders AE, Velthuis B, et al: Perfusion-CT assessment of infarct core and penumbra: Receiver operating characteristic curve analysis in 130 patients suspected of acute hemispheric stroke, *Stroke* 37:979–985, 2006.

171. Beauchamp NJ Jr, Ulug A, Passe TJ, van Zijl PC: MR diffusion imaging in stroke: Review and controversies, *Radiographics* 18:1269–1283, 1998.

172. Grandin CB, Duprez TP, Smith AM, et al: Which MR-derived perfusion parameters are the best predictors of infarct growth in hyperacute stroke? Comparative study between relative and quantitative measurements, *Radiology* 223:361–370, 2002.

173. Schlaug G, Benfield A, Baird AE, et al: The ischemic penumbra: Operationally defined by diffusion and perfusion MRI, *Neurology* 53:1528–1537, 1999.

174. Wintermark M, Reichhart M, Cuisenaire O, et al: Comparison of admission perfusion computed tomography and qualitative diffusion- and perfusion-weighted magnetic resonance imaging in acute stroke patients, *Stroke* 33:2025–2031, 2002.

175. Srinivasan A, Goyal M: Al Azri F, Lum C: State-of-the-art imaging of acute stroke, *Radiographics* 26(Suppl 1):S75–S95, 2006.

176. Fiehler J, Foth M, Knab R, et al: Severe ADC decreases do not predict irreversible tissue damage in humans, *Stroke* 33:79–86, 2002.

177. Kidwell CS, Saver JL, Mattiello J, et al: Thrombolytic reversal of acute human cerebral ischemic injury shown by diffusion/perfusion magnetic resonance imaging, *Ann Neurol* 47:462–469, 2000.

178. Hacke W, Albers G, Al-Rawi Y, et al: The Desmoteplase In Acute Ischemic Stroke Trial (DIAS): A phase II MRI-based 9-hour window acute stroke thrombolysis trial with intravenous desmoteplase, *Stroke* 36:66–73, 2005.

Chapter 7

EVOKED POTENTIALS

Tod B. Sloan • Leslie Jameson • Daniel Janik

The nervous system has the unique property of exchanging information through the chemical generation of electrical activity. Monitoring this activity allows assessment of the functional status of the nervous system during altered states of consciousness (e.g., coma, anesthesia), whereas traditional physiologic monitors (e.g., blood pressure and oxygenation) measure only parameters that are supportive of function. Although not a replacement for the awake neurologic examination, intraoperative neurophysiologic monitoring can detect an unfavorable surgical or physiologic environment that changes neuronal functions to allow maneuvers that improve intraoperative decision-making and therefore reduce operative morbidity.

It has been nearly 50 years since the first somatosensory evoked potentials (SSEPs) were recorded in humans, and more than 20 years since their use was reported in the operating room. In some cases monitoring has become indispensable (e.g., neuroma in situ), and in others, a standard of care (e.g., facial nerve monitoring in acoustic neuroma and spinal monitoring during scoliosis correction). The efficacy of SSEP monitoring has been demonstrated in many surgical procedures because it has become a valuable tool for assessing the consequences of surgical actions.

BASICS OF EVOKED POTENTIALS

Evoked potentials are simple in concept, despite the sophistication of the equipment that is used. Just as the electroencephalogram (EEG) records the spontaneous electrical activity of the brain (cerebral cortex), evoked potentials record the electrical potentials produced after stimulation of specific neural tracts. The most commonly utilized evoked potentials are those produced by stimulation of the sensory system, *sensory evoked potentials*. Stimulation of the sensory tract initiates an electrical volley that travels to the cerebral cortex and can be measured at several locations along the neural tracts involved.

The recorded plot of voltage versus time has an initial artifact representing the stimulation of the tract followed by the neuronal response, which is recorded as a series of peaks and valleys (Fig. 7-1). Peaks may be positive or negative (with respect to the active electrode) and may be plotted downward or upward, depending on convention. The peaks (and valleys) are thought to arise from specific neural generators (often more than one neural structure) in a fashion similar to the peaks on an electrocardiogram that follow a pacemaker-initiated response. The information recorded is usually the amplitude (peak to adjacent trough) and the time from the stimulation to the peak (called *latency*) (see Fig. 7-1). In addition, the time between peaks (interpeak latency or *conduction time*) may be measured. Peaks are usually named

by convention—I through V, P_a, P_b—or by polarity and latency—P (positive) or N (negative) followed by the latency in milliseconds (msec) (e.g., N_{20}).

When the response is large in comparison with background noise, one single measurement or response may be sufficient. However, for most sensory responses, the evoked response is very small (1-2 microvolts) compared with the much larger EEG (50-100 microvolts) and electrocardiogram (1000-2000 microvolts). Because the signals are often small, an amplifier reduces the electrical noise by subtracting the signal at a reference electrode from the recording electrode. Filtering of this signal and by further reducing noise in a third, ground electrode helps focus on the evoked response of interest. Because the evoked response always occurs at a set time after stimulation, averaging responses increases the time-locked response, whereas the background activity acts as a random signal and averages out to zero. The number of responses that are averaged varies from one to several thousand, depending on the ratio of evoked response to background noise.

The time required for this signal averaging may be sufficient to delay rapid feedback to the surgeon. To solve this problem, some novel monitoring techniques are employed. In some instances, new responses are averaged with previously recorded averages (e.g., moving average). More commonly, stimuli are staggered so that the second response does not overlap the first (e.g., left then right posterior tibial nerve SSEPs).

Effective intraoperative monitoring requires recording of responses to infer the functional health of the neural tracts involved. The monitoring goal is to identify impending neural compromise quickly, to allow intervention so that permanent injury is averted. This goal requires preoperative identification of the type and location of neural tissue at risk for vascular and mechanical injury during surgery. On the basis of this information, the monitoring team chooses the most appropriate evoked potentials to monitor for these insults. The potentials are then monitored during surgery to identify the onset of an insult, which is signaled by decreases in amplitude and increases in latency. In addition to monitoring for operative insult, evoked responses can be used for diagnostic testing during surgery, allowing educated operative decision-making (e.g., edge of tumor and functional neural tissue) as well as identification of nonsurgical problems that may need correction (e.g., positioning-related brachial plexus injury).

When an evoked response changes, the physiologic, anesthetic, and surgical environment must be assessed to determine its contribution to the change. Ischemia generally produces a loss of response, particularly if synaptic components are involved. In general, tolerance to ischemia (e.g., time to irreversible injury) is related directly to the residual blood flow and inversely to the metabolic demand of the tissue. Fortunately the evoked response is altered at a level of blood flow well above the level that produces irreversible injury. Hence, unless the permanent ischemic injury is very severe, time is usually available for intervention before permanent injury results. Studies suggest that a slow loss of response amplitude (and increase in latency) may be due to diffuse ischemia. Fast losses (with minimal latency change) may be due to mechanical injury or localized ischemia, especially in gray matter.[1,2] As a general principle, an amplitude reduction of 50% or latency increase of 10% of an evoked potential is considered significant, although smaller changes may indicate impending compromise. The experience of the monitoring team is critical to effective monitoring and to judging when to intervene. Anesthetic management often plays a critical role in the intervention.

SOMATOSENSORY EVOKED POTENTIALS

The most commonly monitored sensory evoked potential remains the SSEP, which is used in spinal cord and axial skeletal surgery.[3-12] The SSEP is a sensory evoked response in which

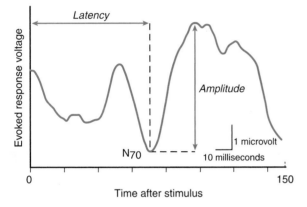

Figure 7–1 Visual evoked response tracing of amplitude versus time after stimulus. The measurement of latency and amplitude for the negative peak at 70 msec (N_{70}) is shown.

peripheral sensory nerves are stimulated electrically and the response is measured along the sensory pathway. The large, mixed motor and sensory nerves (and their component spinal roots) usually used are median (C6-T1), ulnar (C8-T1), common peroneal (L4-S1), and posterior tibial (L4-S2) nerves. Stimulation activates predominantly the large-diameter, fast-conducting Ia muscle afferent and group II cutaneous nerve fibers.[3] Anatomically, peripheral nerve stimulation produces both orthodromic (propagating in the normal direction) and antidromic (propagating in the reverse direction) neural transmission. The orthodromic motor stimulation elicits a muscle response, which is seen as a foot or hand twitch (verifying stimulation), and the orthodromic sensory stimulation produces the SSEP.

It is currently thought that the incoming volley of neural activity from stimulation represents primarily activity in the pathway of proprioception and vibration that ascends the ipsilateral dorsal column. It makes its first synapse near the nucleus cuneatus and nucleus gracilis and then decussates near the cervicomedullary junction, ascending via the contralateral medial lemniscus. A second synapse occurs in the ventroposterolateral nucleus of the thalamus, from which it projects to the contralateral sensory cortex. For the upper extremity, the evoked responses can be measured from electrodes placed over the antecubital fossa, supraclavicular fossa (brachial plexus), cervical spine, and cortex; for the lower extremity, they can be recorded over the popliteal fossa, along the spinal cord (surface or epidural electrodes), and at cervical and cortical locations (Fig. 7-2). Response recordings are usually conducted at multiple recording sites to verify that the nervous system is stimulated and to identify the location of neural compromise if the response is lost.

The cortical response is best recorded over the primary somatosensory cortex appropriate for the nerve stimulated. However, some response components are widely distributed over the cortex.[3] The major cortical peaks recorded after median nerve and posterior tibial nerve stimulation (N_{20} and P_{38}, respectively) are likely the result of the thalamocortical projections to the primary sensory cortex.[3] Responses recorded posteriorly over the cervical spine

Figure 7–2 Example of the somatosensory evoked potential peaks and the corresponding anatomy as recorded from the sensory cortex (C_4 in the international 10-20 system referenced to the knee). Positive peaks are labeled as "P" followed by the approximate time in milliseconds from median nerve stimulation. *(From Wiederholt WC, Meyer-Hardting E, Budnick B, et al: Stimulating and recording methods used in obtaining short-latency somatosensory evoked potentials [SEPs] in patients with central and peripheral neurologic disorders. Ann N Y Acad Sci 1982;388:349.)*

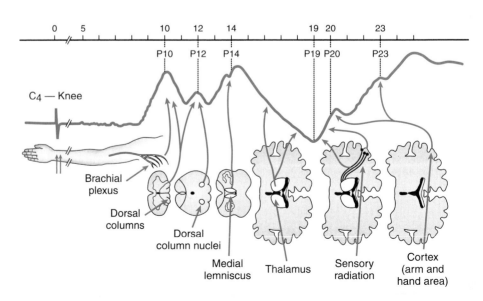

probably represent responses of the tracts in the spinal cord or brainstem.[3]

Cortical Monitoring Using Somatosensory Evoked Potentials

The cortical SSEP has been used to detect ischemia in and to localize specific areas of cortical tissue. Numerous studies have demonstrated a threshold relationship between regional cerebral blood flow and cortical evoked responses.[13] Although clinical functional neurologic findings become abnormal at a cortical blood flow of about 25 mL/min/100 g, the SSEP remains normal until cortical blood flow is reduced to about 20 mL/min/100 g. SSEP responses are lost at a local blood flow of between 15 and 18 mL/min/100 g. Subcortical regions, brainstem, spinal cord, and nerve appear to be less sensitive to hypoperfusion, explaining why the SSEP persists at blood pressures below which the EEG routinely disappears. Because of this differential sensitivity to cortical blood flow, the SSEP is used to monitor during surgical procedures such as carotid endarterectomy. Intraoperative SSEP changes are used as an indication for shunt placement and to predict postoperative morbidity. In some respects, use of the EEG and SSEP in CEA are complimentary because the SSEP is able to detect ischemia in deep cortical structures, and the EEG assesses a wider area of surface cortex.[14] The SSEP is employed during intracranial vascular procedures to determine the adequacy of collateral blood flow, tolerance to temporary vessel occlusion, or the adequacy of systolic blood pressure in the sensory cortex producing the response. The most specific use for ischemia monitoring is during intracranial vascular surgery involving aneurysms. Because the SSEP from the upper extremity is generated in the cerebral cortex supplied by the middle cerebral artery, it can be utilized during surgery for aneurysms of the internal carotid and middle cerebral arteries. Similarly, the SSEP from the lower extremity can be used to evaluate ischemia during vascular procedures on the anterior cerebral artery. Monitoring of these arteries may require both upper and lower SSEPs, depending on the vascular perforators and their impact on the subcortical pathways (e.g., lenticulate striate perforators).

Monitoring during temporary clipping in aneurysm surgery has shown that a very prompt loss of cortical SSEP response (less than 1 minute after clipping) is associated with development of permanent neurologic deficit. However, a delayed loss with prompt recovery after release of the clip is associated with the presence of collateral circulation, with a markedly reduced incidence of neural morbidity. Symon and colleagues[15] have suggested that when the N_{20} of the median nerve SSEP disappears slowly (over 4 minutes), 10 additional minutes of occlusion can be tolerated safely. A correlation between outcome and monitoring during anterior circulation aneurysms has been observed.[16] Studies suggest that a change in SSEP cortical amplitude is the most sensitive indication of ischemia.

In addition to its obvious intraoperative use to determine tolerance of cortical tissue to temporary aneurysm clipping or identification of inadvertent occlusion of a collateral vessel by a clip, monitoring can be used to identify ischemia from vasospasm or when a combination of factors produces unexpected ischemia (e.g., retractor pressure, hypotension, temporary clipping, and hyperventilation). Other applications are ischemia monitoring during neuroradiologic procedures, such as occlusion of vessels, and during streptokinase dissolution of blood clots.

Monitoring for Identification of Sensory Cortex

Evoked potentials have been termed "indispensable" for localization of the sensory-motor cortex in the anesthetized patient.[17] Localization is accomplished by recording of the cortical component (N_{20}) of the median nerve SSEP with use of bipolar recording strips placed on the cortex. The central gyrus separating the motor and sensory strips is identified from a phase reversal (initial wave changes from positive to negative) of the response, which is probably due to the horizontal nature of the dipole generator located in the gyrus.[18]

Somatosensory Evoked Potential Monitoring in Spinal Surgery

When the SSEP is used during spinal cord or axial surgery, it can identify mechanical or ischemic insults when they result in alteration or loss of transmission through the surgical field (Fig. 7-3). Current risks of neurologic morbidity in spinal surgery without monitoring are not minimal; the risk for anterior cervical diskectomy is 0.46%, that for scoliosis correction 0.25% to 3.2%, and that for intramedullary spinal cord tumor surgery 23.8% to 65.4%; monitoring is estimated to reduce the morbidity in spinal surgery by 50% to 80%.[19]

The basis of monitoring in humans is founded in studies in animals, in which generalized insults to the spinal cord (e.g., distraction, graded weights applied directly on the spinal cord,[20] or narrowing of the spinal canal anteriorly at C5 using an epidural screw[21]) are associated with SSEP latency and amplitude changes simultaneous to loss of clinical motor function. Because current spinal instrumentation techniques present multiple potential insults throughout the course of the operation, a nearly continuous monitoring technique (e.g., SSEP) is advantageous for ascertaining which insult contributed to neurologic dysfunction. In addition, the SSEP may be used to identify physiologic insults (e.g., hypotension) or positioning problems, especially those related to the brachial plexus. The once frequently used wake-up test is now often reserved for assessment of motor function when motor evoked potentials (MEPs) are not recordable or to confirm motor function when evoked responses deteriorate.[22-25]

Studies in humans undergoing spinal surgery indicate that the SSEP is predictive of neural outcome.[26-28] However, as with the wake-up test, the correlation of SSEP and neural injury is not exact; cases of motor injury without intraoperative SSEP warning have occurred. A major reason for dissociation of the SSEP from motor injury is the fact that the SSEP is transmitted predominantly via the posterior columns, where the blood supply is from the posterior spinal artery. The motor tracts are more anteriorly located, and their blood supply is via the anterior spinal arteries. Therefore the ability of the SSEP to predict most motor deficits probably results from insults that affect the entire spinal cord.

The utility of the SSEP in spinal surgery was shown in an analysis conducted by the Scoliosis Research Society and European Spinal Deformities Society in 1995. They evaluated the results of monitoring during correction of spinal deformity in 51,263 operations (scoliosis, kyphosis, fractures, and spondylolisthesis) performed by 173 surgeons.[29] In these cases, the overall injury incidence was 0.55% (1 in 182 cases), well below the 0.7% to 4% historical average expected for instrumentation without monitoring. The incidence of definite false-negative response (i.e., in which the patient sustained a major motor neurologic injury without SSEP warning)

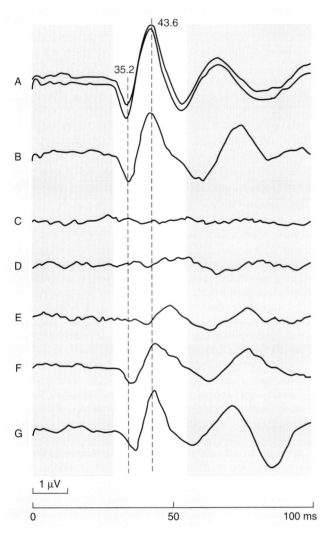

Figure 7–3 Example of somatosensory evoked potential monitoring for a patient undergoing surgery. Baseline recordings the afternoon prior to operation were normal (A). B shows recordings after the induction of anesthesia. Responses were abolished after passing through the wires around the laminae (C). The wake-up test result was positive (D). After 15 minutes, the poorly defined potentials reappeared (E). After closure of the wound, evoked potentials showed a little increased latency, P_{40} and N_{50} measuring 4.1 and 2.0 msec, respectively (F), with normal overall waveform (G). *(From Mostegl A, Bauer R, Eichenauer M: Intraoperative somatosensory potential monitoring: A clinical analysis of 127 surgical procedures. Spine 1988;13:396.)*

was very low (0.063%, or about 1 case in 1500 procedures). The economic impact of monitoring was assessed by Nuwer and colleagues,[12,29] who estimated that the cost of monitoring enough cases (200 cases) to prevent one major, persistent neurologic deficit is $120,000 (1995 dollars), which is small compared with the cost of lifelong medical care. Other writers have conducted similar cost analyses and concluded that properly applied monitoring can be cost effective.[30]

Numerous other studies demonstrate an improvement in outcome after spinal surgery with monitoring; the Scoliosis Research Society has developed a position statement that makes monitoring a virtual standard of care during axial skeletal and spinal cord procedures. The statement concludes that "neurophysiological monitoring can assist in the early detection of complications and possibly prevent post-operative morbidity in patients undergoing operations on the spine."[31] This principle has been echoed in the British literature by

Loughman and colleagues, who wrote, "Today, it is standard practice to conduct some form of monitoring when performing any spinal operation that is associated with a high risk of neurological injury. Generally operations are considered to carry such a risk when corrective forces are applied to the spine, the patient has pre-existing neurological damage, the cord is being invaded, or an osteotomy or other procedure is being carried out in immediate juxtaposition to the cord."[32] Hence SSEP monitoring has become commonplace and almost a de facto standard of care during a wide variety of procedures involving the spinal column.

Recording Somatosensory Evoked Potentials from the Spinal Column

As discussed later, anesthetic agents can decrease the SSEP cortical amplitude with minimal effect on responses recorded from the spinal cord; consequently, there has been substantial interest in monitoring from recording electrodes placed in the spinal bony elements or in the subdural or epidural space. Recording from epidural electrodes is commonplace in Japan and Europe, and despite its invasive nature, the technique appears remarkably safe.[26,32,33] One monitoring technique utilizes epidural recordings to monitor both descending motor evoked responses from cortical stimulation (see later) and ascending responses from the SSEP.[34] Although the actual neural tracts monitored with these techniques is not known, they have been used in an attempt to record responses that travel through the motor pathways. One technique, initially termed "neurogenic MEPs (NMEPs),"[35] is now thought to involve monitoring of both sensory and motor tracts, with the relative contributions to the response depending on the type of anesthesia and the specific type of stimulation employed.[4,25,36] Unfortunately recording a muscle response does not guarantee pure muscle tract stimulation, because antidromic, descending sensory tract stimulation can activate the motor pathway at the anterior horn cell by sensory to motor reflex pathways. Despite the uncertainty of the exact tract monitored, NMEP responses appear useful for monitoring, and the method has been advocated as a safe and effective way to perform monitoring in children and young adults with idiopathic or neuromuscular scoliosis.[25,36,37]

AUDITORY BRAINSTEM RESPONSES

Another commonly used sensory evoked potential is the auditory brainstem response (ABR), which is produced when sound activates the auditory pathway after being transmitted through the external and middle ear. Stimulation is usually performed with "clicks," but tone "pips" can be used when stimulation with specific frequencies is required. The clicks have a broad spectrum of frequency content, with significant stimulation in the 1000 to 4000 Hertz (Hz) range. In order to reduce responses from the nonstimulated ear by sound conducted through bone, "white" noise is delivered to the other ear.

The term *auditory brainstem response* refers to the responses recorded from the brainstem, usually in the first 10 msec after stimulation (Fig. 7-4). This early evoked potential has also been referred to as the "brainstem auditory evoked response (BAER)" and "brainstem auditory evoked potential (BAEP)." Sound stimulation activates the middle ear, producing vibrations that activate the hair cells in the cochlea; the resulting

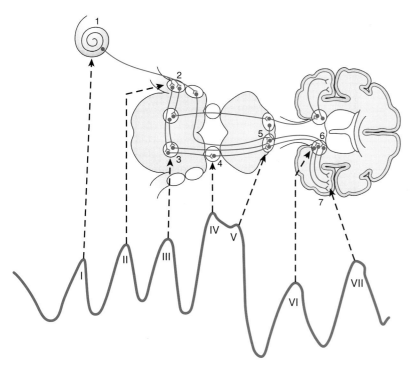

Figure 7–4 Normal auditory brainstem response tracing and corresponding region of brainstem generating the response peaks (labeled by Roman numerals by convention). 1. organ of Corti and extracranial cranial nerve VII; II. cochlear nucleus; III. superior olivary complex; IV. lateral lemniscus; V. inferior colliculus; VI. medial geniculate body; VII. auditory radiation. *(From Aravabhumi S, Izzo KL, Bakst BL, et al: Brainstem auditory evoked potentials: Intraoperative monitoring technique in surgery of posterior fossa tumors. Arch Phys Med Rehabil 1987;68:142.)*

nerve impulses travel to the brainstem via the eighth cranial nerve. The nerve impulse travels via the brainstem acoustic relay nuclei and lemniscal pathways to activate neurons in the auditory cortex. The responses are thought to be produced by neurologic structures in the auditory pathway. Three major peaks are usually seen in the ABR: waves I, III, and V.[8,38] Wave I is produced by the extracranial portion of cranial nerve (CN) VIII, wave III by acoustic relay nuclei and tracts deep in the midline of the lower pons, and wave V by the lateral lemniscus and inferior colliculus in the contralateral pons. Occasionally waves II and IV are seen.

Response to auditory stimulation can also be recorded over the sensory cortex; it is termed the midlatency auditory evoked response. This modality has been used infrequently to monitor cerebral viability, but it has been utilized as an index of anesthetic effect.[39] Later responses of the cortex, notably the positive peak at 300 msec (P_{300}), which appears to correlate with cognitive function, is not usually recordable with general anesthesia.

ABR is used extensively for monitoring during surgery involving the posterior fossa, perhaps because of its importance for hearing and the frequent involvement of the cochlear nerve by tumors in this region.[8,38,40-44] A variety of factors can cause alteration in the amplitude or latency of the ABR waves. They include sound conduction problems in the external or middle ear, ischemia of the cochlea, traction on cranial nerve VIII, and ischemia or neural damage to the auditory pathways in the brainstem.

Perhaps the most common changes seen intraoperatively with ABR recordings are increases in the latency of wave V and increases in the interpeak latency of I through V with retractor placement in the posterior fossa. Many of these changes, if mild, are reversible and are considered part of a routine procedure. Complete loss of wave I can be due to loss of cochlear blood supply by vascular obstruction or vasospasm[44] or transection of the nerve by the surgeon with subsequent loss of useful hearing. Changes in wave V are less clearly correlated with outcome; wave V can be lost because of desynchronization in

the pathways, and hearing may be retained even with its loss.[44] In general, if waves I and V are preserved, hearing is usually preserved, but if they are both lost, there is little chance of preservation of hearing postoperatively.

Responses to auditory stimuli can also be monitored by direct recordings from the neural pathway in the brainstem. Cochlear microphonics are recordings directly from the capsule (promontorium). Recordings from the exposed intracranial portion of CN VIII (cochlear nerve action potentials) have also been used. Studies suggest that these direct recording sites may be superior to ABR for monitoring and for predicting useful postoperative hearing in surgery peripheral to the recording location.[44-48]

ABR monitoring has also been used to evaluate brainstem viability during procedures in which the brainstem may be injured by direct manipulation, by positioning, or by changes in vascular supply. Examples are decompression of space-occupying defects in the cerebellum, removal of cerebellar vascular malformations, and monitoring (along with facial nerve monitoring) during microvascular decompression for relief of hemifacial spasm or trigeminal neuralgia.

VISUAL EVOKED POTENTIALS

Visual evoked potentials (VEPs) are produced in response to light stimulation of the eyes (see Fig. 7-1). The most commonly recorded responses appear to be generated bilaterally in the visual (occipital) cortex, which is supplied by the posterior cerebral artery. Diagnostic stimulation in awake subjects is usually performed with an alternating high-contrast checkerboard pattern, but with patients under anesthesia, flash stimulation is utilized through closed eyelids or via stimulators mounted on scleral caps. The response of the retina (electroretinogram [ERG]) can also be measured by means of electrodes placed near the eye. VEPs can be used to monitor the anterior visual pathways during craniofacial procedures, pituitary surgery, and surgery in the retrochiasmatic visual tracts and occipital cortex. VEPs are considered less useful in surgical monitoring for several reasons; flash stimulation may not measure the pathways of useful clinical vision, the large, bulky "goggles" usually used for stimulation pose technical problems, the bilateral nature of the response may obscure some focal changes, and anesthetic sensitivity makes recording difficult.[49]

BASIC ELECTROMYOGRAPHIC MONITORING

Using muscle responses to monitor neural tracts is called electromyography (EMG). Two types of EMG monitoring are common, recording spontaneous activity and recording responses subsequent to stimulation of the motor nerves or motor pathways. The motor unit potentials which constitute the EMG response are of sufficiently greater amplitude relative to background electrical activity and interference that averaging (such as employed with SSEPs) is not necessary thereby allowing immediate feedback. Recording for observing spontaneous activity can be done continuously, but some techniques using intentional stimulation may produce patient motion that may have to be integrated into the surgical procedure and are therefore not continuous. To record the muscle activity, needle pairs are placed near the muscles of interest, and the electrical activity is recorded. Direct feedback to the surgeon can be achieved by the playing of these responses through a loudspeaker.

The EMG response that results from irritation of a nerve is a recording of the generated motor unit potentials of individual axon-muscle fiber groups of that nerve. Neurotonic discharges, caused by mechanical or metabolic stimuli, are high-frequency intermittent or continuous bursts of motor unit potentials (Fig. 7-5) and are a sensitive indicator of nerve irritation. Activity can be bursts lasting less than 200 msec with single or multiple motor unit potentials firing at 30 to 100 Hz, or they can be long trains of activity lasting

1 to 30 seconds or more.[50] Short bursts (heard as brief "blurps" on the loudspeaker) represent relatively synchronous motor unit discharges that result from a single discharge of multiple axons from nerve irritation. When these are of sufficient amplitude they raise concern. Causes of irritation include mechanical stimulation (e.g., nearby dissection, ultrasonic aspiration or drilling), nerve retraction, thermal irritation (e.g., heating from irrigation, lasers, drilling, or electrocautery), and chemical or metabolic insults. Unfortunately, sharp transection of nerves may fail to provoke a discharge.[51] Long trains of continuous, synchronous motor unit discharges are associated with impending nerve injury (nerve compression, traction, or ischemia of the nerve). Their audible sounds have a more musical quality and have been likened to the sound of an outboard motor boat engine, swarming bees, popping corn ("popcorn"), or an aircraft engine ("bomber").

Direct stimulation can also be used to locate the nerve of interest or to assess its function. EMG responses recorded from intentional nerve stimulation (to determine whether the neural tract is intact) or MEPs (see later) are referred to as *compound muscle action potentials* (CMAPs). Stimulation is given by bipolar or monopolar electrodes with fine tips applied to the nerve. The EMG response that results from single or multiple stimuli of low-intensity current (0.5-5 milliamperes [mA]) and short duration (0.5-1 msec) are used for identifying cranial nerves or to identify damaged peripheral nerves. A response may be possible when as few as 1% to 2% of the nerve fibers remain intact.[51]

EMG responses are resistant to the effects of anesthetics and other physiologic variables (temperature, blood pressure) manipulated during surgery except for neuromuscular blockade (NMB), although appropriate response can still be monitored with 75% suppression of baseline CMAPs.[48] However, some writers have indicated that the small-amplitude responses from irritation, especially in damaged or poorly functioning nerves, are difficult to detect during controlled relaxation, making use of NMB controversial.

Cranial Nerve Monitoring

Cranial nerve monitoring is of particular interest because these nerves are susceptible to intraoperative damage owing to their small size, limited epineurium, and complicated course. As with all nerve injury, the damage occurs from either trauma (surgical disruption, manipulation) or ischemia and leads to paresis or paralysis (with subsequent disability or deformity) and, possibly, chronic pain. All cranial nerves with a motor component are monitored from their EMG activity in their respectively innervated muscles (Table 7-1).

Facial Nerve

The most common cranial nerve monitored during surgery is the facial nerve (CN VII). Because this nerve may be intertwined within brainstem tumors (e.g., acoustic neuroma), monitoring of the facial nerve allows identification of the nerve in the operative site and warning of the unrecognized proximity of the nerve to surgical activity. This identification is particularly helpful during surgery for vestibular schwannoma (acoustic neuroma), in which monitoring increases the likelihood that the anatomic integrity of the nerve will be maintained during surgery. In such cases, more than 60% of patients who have intact facial nerves at the conclusion of surgery will regain at least partial function several months postoperatively.[44] Reduction in the size of stimulated CMAPs of the facial nerve

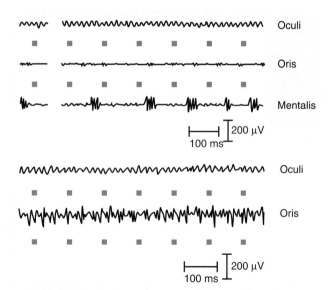

Oculi

Oris

Mentalis

200 µV
100 ms

Oculi

Oris

200 µV
100 ms

Figure 7–5 Examples of continuously recorded muscle potentials during posterior fossa surgery. Responses are recorded from the orbicularis oculi, orbicularis oris, and mentalis muscles. *Top,* Multiple short responses (neurotonic bursts) in the mentalis muscle from dissection near the fifth cranial nerve. *Bottom,* Prolonged neurotonic discharges in the other muscles after irrigation with cool fluids. *(From Cheek JC: Posterior fossa intraoperative monitoring. J Clin Neurophysiol 1993;10:412.)*

Table 7-1 Monitoring of Cranial Nerves

Cranial Nerve		Monitoring Site or Method*
I	Olfactory	No monitoring technique
II	Optic	Visual evoked potentials
III	Oculomotor	Inferior rectus muscle
IV	Trochlear	Superior oblique muscle
V	Trigeminal	Masseter muscle and/or temporalis muscle [sensory responses can also be monitored]
VI	Abducens	Lateral rectus muscle
VII	Facial	Orbicularis oculi and/or orbicularis oris muscles
VIII	Auditory	Auditory brainstem responses
IX	Glossopharyngeal	Stylopharyngeus muscle (posterior soft palate)
X	Vagus	Vocal folds, cricothyroid muscle
XI	Spinal accessory	Sternocleidomastoid and/or trapezius muscles
XII	Hypoglossal	Genioglossus muscle (tongue)

*Unless otherwise specified, monitoring is performed via electromyographic activity of the muscle(s) listed.

(CN VII) during posterior fossa surgery correlates with immediate and long-term outcomes of neurologic function.[53]

Because of the improvement in outcome in posterior fossa surgery seen with facial nerve monitoring,[54,55] a National Institutes of Health (NIH) consensus panel concluded, "The benefits of routine intraoperative monitoring of the facial nerve have been clearly established [in vestibular schwannoma]. This technique should be included in surgical therapy."[56] Therefore, facial nerve monitoring has become a standard of care in surgery for vestibular schwannoma (also known as acoustic neuroma), and this nerve is commonly monitored in other operations in the cerebellopontine angle.

The muscles used for monitoring are the orbicularis oculi and orbicularis oris muscles ipsilateral to the surgical site. To differentiate the response of the facial nerve from that of other motor cranial nerves, the adjacent muscles should also be monitored. Mechanical stimulation of other cranial nerves may activate nearby facial muscles, producing an artifact that may be misinterpreted as facial nerve activation. For example, contraction of the masseter or temporalis muscle (trigeminal nerve) can be seen as artifact in the orbicularis oris or orbicularis oculi muscle, respectively. These other cranial nerves can be differentiated by means of the distribution of the response in several recording locations and from the time interval between stimulation and response. The latency for true facial nerve response is 6 to 8 msec, whereas the latency for a trigeminal nerve response is 3 to 4 msec. Because of its course and location, facial nerve EMG monitoring is also utilized in surgery of the head and neck, particularly with parotid tumors, which may encase branches of the nerve.

Other Cranial Nerves

Monitoring of other cranial nerves may also involve EMG activity and can be performed, depending on the specific surgical risks. Such monitoring has been used extensively in surgery on the base of the skull, cavernous sinus, and posterior fossa[8,10,42,44,51,57] Stimulation of cranial nerves IX and X to determine whether they are intact produces cardiovascular changes, and trapezius and sternocleidomastoid activation with CN XI stimulation can cause potentially harmful head movement.

Vagus nerve (CN X) monitoring by vocal cord EMG is becoming common in skull base (large brainstem tumors) and anterior neck procedures. Monitoring of the recurrent laryngeal and superior laryngeal branches uses electrodes in the cricothyroid or vocalis muscles or contact electrodes mounted on an endotracheal tube. This technique is used in procedures such as neck dissections, thyroid and parathyroid removal, and anterior cervical spine fusions.[8,42,57] The risk of injury with thyroid surgery (2.3%-5.2%[58]) is higher in malignancy; such monitoring is common with reexploration for hemorrhage, during a second operation, and when anatomic distortion is present.

In surgery on tumors of the posterior fossa, monitoring of EMG events has been shown to correlate with postoperative neurologic status. In a study of pediatric patients undergoing removal of tumors in the brainstem in which the lower cranial nerves (IX, X, XII) were monitored, a positive EMG event in one nerve resulted in a postoperative deficit in 73% of patients, and neuropraxic EMG activity from all three nerves was always associated with a deficit. Postoperative aspiration pneumonia or a need for tracheotomy was always associated with abnormal intraoperative EMG activity in at least one of these nerves.[59]

Monitoring of the Peripheral Nervous System

EMG techniques can be used to assess the peripheral nervous system. It can be used for identifying peripheral nerves, localizing preexisting disease along the course of a nerve, determining the functional continuity across lesions, determining the likelihood of nerve root avulsion, identifying targets for nerve biopsy, and monitoring intact nerves to prevent inadvertent surgical injury.[60] This is typically performed to prevent surgical injury or guide surgical repair in these structures. In operations for repair of nerves damaged by trauma, EMG monitoring is considered indispensible because it guides the surgeon's decision about whether to perform graft repair.[61] Blunt trauma typically leaves nerves in continuity with varying degrees of internal disruption. If the damage is neuropraxic or axonotmetic, continuity will be detected, and the nerve can be expected to recover over time through remyelination or axon growth. Absence of continuity, signified by loss of action potentials, indicates complete disruption of the axon, sheath, and connective tissue (neurotmesis) and requires grafting for satisfactory outcome. In the case of a nerve root avulsion, action potentials can still be recorded because the injury is proximal to the dorsal root ganglion. In some cases the EMG response can be combined with sensory response to define an area of lesion. For example, recording of cortical sensory responses after stimulation of the proximal segment of a mixed motor and sensory nerve will indicate that the injury is distal to the ganglion.[62]

Monitoring of nerve roots with EMG is used when injury to the nerve root may occur during procedures on the spinal column with or without in situ instrumentation and for removal of tumors from or untethering of the cauda equina. As with cranial nerve monitoring, neurotonic EMG discharges alert the neurophysiologist and hence the surgeon to irritation of neural tissue. In addition, CMAPs from intentional

Table 7–2 Nerve Roots and Muscles Most Commonly Monitored

	Spinal Cord Nerve(s)	Muscle(s)
Cervical	C2-C4	Trapezoids, sternocleidomastoid
	C5, C6	Biceps, deltoid
	C6, C7	Flexor carpi radialis
Thoracic	C8-T1	Adductor pollicis brevis, abductor digiti minimi
	T5-T6	Upper rectus abdominis
	T7-T8	Middle rectus abdominis
	T9-T11	Lower rectus abdominis
	T12	Inferior rectus abdominis
Lumbar	L2	Adductor longus
	L2-L4	Vastus medialis
Lumbosacral	L4-S1	Tibialis anterior
	L5-S1	Peroneus longus
Sacral	S1-S2	Gastrocnemius
	S2-S4	Anal sphincter

stimulation allow identification of individual nerve roots and bony pedicles. For monitoring the EMG of the spinal nerve roots, it is important to select muscles that allow identification of discrete myotomes covering the area of nerve roots at risk (Table 7-2).[43,63,65,66]

Electromyography during spinal column surgery is more sensitive than SSEP for detecting nerve root injury, because multiple nerve roots contribute to the SSEP cortical response; monitoring of individual roots of the SSEP is not possible, and injuries have been reported with no change in cortical SSEP tracings. Dermatomal sensory responses have been used with cortical recording after cutaneous stimulation of the appropriate dermatome (dermatomal evoked potentials [DEPs]); however, these have not been used as commonly as EMG recording.

EMG recording in spinal column surgery is commonly used when spinal nerve roots are at risk owing to placement of instrumentation such as pedicle screws that may violate the bony pedicle wall and exert pressure on adjacent nerve roots Such violation has been reported to occur often as 15%-25% of cases.[64,67-69] EMG monitoring can be used to test screw placement through stimulation of the screw or screw-hole with a monopolar probe. Because the bone cortex has a higher resistance to current flow than soft tissue, a low threshold of stimulus to evoke a muscle response indicates a breach in the wall and prompts either exploration of the screw placement or removal and repositioning of the screw.[70] Stimulus thresholds vary according to the circumstance,[62] but in a normal nerve root, the threshold when a screw touches the nerve is less than 6 mA; when a screw has only broken through the medial pedicle wall, the threshold is 6 to 10 mA; and when the screw is entirely within the pedicle, the threshold exceeds 10 mA. Hence, stimulus thresholds less than 6 to 10 mA usually raise concern that the screw should be redirected.[71] It is important to note that abnormal nerves (e.g., diabetes, chronically compressed), through mechanisms of axonotmesis, have a much higher threshold at which they respond to stimulation than normal nerves, such that direct nerve root stimulation distal to the pedicle should be employed to establish a control threshold.[72]

Electromyography has also proven useful in monitoring the nerve roots that collectively form the cauda equina. Procedures such as release of tethered cord and tumor excision carry the risk of damage to nerve roots innervating the muscles of the leg as well as anal and urethral sphincters. Damage to these roots is extremely debilitating, and every effort is made to avoid this complication. It may be difficult, even with microscope assistance, to separate nervous from nonfunctional tissue. Spontaneous and evoked EMG recordings of the cord and tumor aid in differentiating nerves from non-neural tissue. For example, the stimulation threshold for filum terminale fibers may be 100 times that for motor nerve fibers.[73]

As with other spinal surgery, a multimodality approach is used. Suggested techniques to employ include spontaneous and evoked EMG (including anal and urethral sphincters), bladder pressure, tibial nerve SSEP, and motor pathway monitoring (see later). Urethral sphincter EMG may be recorded using a bladder catheter with electrodes attached 2 cm from the inflating balloon.[74] Although simple to perform, bladder pressure measurement primarily assesses stimulated responses and therefore does not provide the immediate and continuous feedback desired. It can be argued that anal sphincter EMG provides the needed information about the bladder because the innervation of both sphincters arises from the second through fourth sacral segments.[75] The cauda equina can be mapped during surgery with use of stimulated EMG, peripheral sensory stimulation with surgical field recording, MEPs, cortical sensory evoked potentials, and the bulbocavernosus reflex.[76] Data derived from multiple prospective studies and case series obtained during cervical, thoracic, and lumbosacral procedures of the spinal column support the sensitivity of EMG monitoring in preventing nerve root injury.[77-83]

Monitoring of Reflex Responses

Another method of monitoring the cauda equina, nerve roots, and spinal cord is to monitor the reflex responses that can be recorded in the peripheral nerve and muscle after stimulation of the peripheral nerve. When a motor nerve is activated, an initial CMAP, termed the M response, can be recorded. At low stimulation intensities a response termed the H response occurs after the M response. The H response results from a sensory to motor reflex (Fig. 7-6). This is the electrical equivalent of reflex activity from tapping of the knee with a reflex hammer. A second type of later wave is produced because nerve stimulation also causes a wave of depolarization in the motor nerve that travels centrally toward the spinal cord in the motor components of the nerve and is reflected, resulting in an outgoing response that produces a muscle contraction termed the F wave. The more commonly monitored H reflex therefore monitors the sensory *and* motor efferents in the nerve as well as the spinal gray matter and components of the reflex arc.

In addition to monitoring the sensory and motor nerves, these reflexes also monitor the spinal cord at the level of the reflex and more cephalad. The reason is that several descending pathways contribute to the excitability of the anterior horn cell and the reflex (descending suprasegmental systems [corticospinal, rubrospinal, vestibulospinal and reticulospinal systems] and propriospinal systems). Changes in these pathways can alter the reflex response. Because H reflexes are lost within minutes with more cephalad spinal injury owing to the phenomenon of spinal shock, they have been shown to be more sensitive than SSEPs to spinal cord injury, changing before or in the absence of SSEP changes. Although recordable from many nerve-muscle combinations, the H reflex in the lower extremity is frequently recorded from the gastrocnemius after stimulation of the posterior tibial nerve (S1 spinal segmental function). The extent of H reflex suppression correlates with the degree of spinal injury, a 90% depression correlating with a postoperative neurologic deficit.[84,85] As such, the H reflex is becoming more commonly used with SSEP and MEP monitoring in spinal surgery.

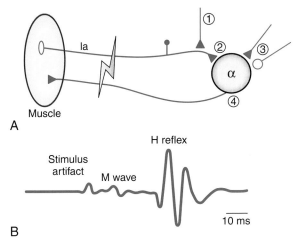

Figure 7–6 H reflex pathway and typical muscle response. The reflex arc is initiated by stimulation of the peripheral nerve (which produces the M wave) and activates the alpha motor neuron (α) in the spinal gray matter, producing the second muscle activity (the H reflex). Modulation of the response involves presynaptic inhibition (1), homosynaptic depression (2), descending spinal tract influences (3), and intrinsic alpha motor neuron membrane excitability (4). *(From Misiaszek JE, Misiaszek JE: The H-reflex as a tool in neurophysiology: Its limitations and uses in understanding nervous system function. Muscle Nerve 2003;28:144.)*

MOTOR EVOKED POTENTIALS

Motor pathway monitoring using MEPs is becoming commonplace, particularly in spinal surgery, because MEP has a better correlation with postoperative motor outcome. This is due in part to the fact that the MEP is inherently more sensitive to ischemic vascular insults. Pure motor monitoring was developed when it was demonstrated that transcranial stimulation of the motor cortex by electrical or magnetic means produces a descending response that traverses the corticospinal tract and produces a muscle response in the form of a CMAP.[86] As such, an MEP allows differentiation of the motor pathways from the monitoring of other pathways, particularly the SSEP. MEPs and SSEPs are located in a different topographic and vascular region of the cerebral cortex, brainstem, and spinal cord. MEP monitoring has become important during surgery for correction of axial skeletal deformity,[87-89] intramedullary spinal cord tumors,[90-92] intracranial tumors,[93-95] and vascular lesions.[96,97] It has also been used for preemptive assessment of outcome in stroke[98,99] and spinal cord function during thoracoabdominal aneurysm repair.[100]

Not surprisingly, the MEP has been particularly important in cases in which surgery can selectively injure the motor pathways of the anterior spinal artery blood supply. Although several stimulation techniques have been tried, reliable monitoring of the motor pathways has been accomplished only by electrical stimulation of the motor cortex via electrodes placed either on the scalp over the motor cortex (transcranial) or directly on the motor cortex.[4,101] The most common technique used is transcranial electrical stimulation, in which current directly stimulates pyramidal cells of the motor cortex, resulting in a wave of depolarization that often only involves 4% to 5% of the corticospinal tract. When this wave of depolarization is measured by electrodes in the epidural space it is termed the *D (direct) wave* (Fig. 7-7). Additional transsynaptic

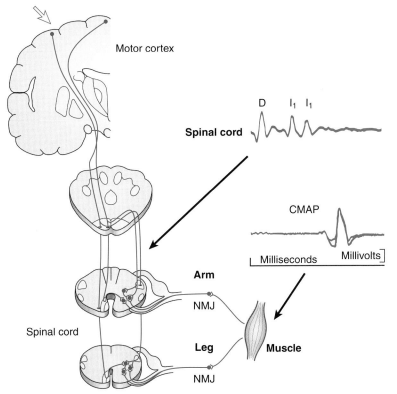

Figure 7–7 Motor evoked potentials are produced by stimulation of the motor cortex (hollow arrow). The response can be recorded epidurally over the spinal column as a D wave followed by a series of I waves. The pathway synapses in the anterior horn of the spinal cord and the response travels to the muscle via the neuromuscular junction (NMJ). The response is typically recorded near the muscle as a compound muscle action potential (CMAP). *(From Jameson LC, Sloan TB, Jameson LC, et al: Monitoring of the brain and spinal cord. Anesthesiol Clin 2006; 24:777.)*

activation of internuncial pathways in the cortex results in a series of smaller waves, called *I (indirect) waves,* which follow the D wave. The motor pathway descends from the motor cortex, crossing the midline in the lower lateral brainstem and descending in the ipsilateral and anterior funiculi of the spinal cord. The electrical activity of the D and I waves summate in the anterior horn cell, resulting in activation of the peripheral nerve, which produces a CMAP.

Hence, monitoring can be performed in the epidural space using the D wave and in a muscle with the CMAP response. The disadvantage of epidural recordings is that they do not differentiate laterality of injury; however, the amplitude of the D wave is usually stable and correlates inversely with the functioning fibers of the corticospinal tract. Muscle recordings, in contrast, can differentiate unilateral changes and can assesses specific nerves.[4] For spinal surgery, MEP responses are usually recorded in the lower extremity (tibialis anterior, lateral or medial gastrocnemius, and anterior hallicis muscles) and upper extremity (adductor pollicis brevis muscle).

MEP monitoring is commonly used during corrective axial skeletal procedures and neural parenchymal disease (spinal cord tumor, brain tumor, neurovascular lesions), and when cerebral or spinal cord perfusion is at risk (middle cerebral artery aneurysm, thoracoabdominal aneurysm). The most common use of MEP monitoring is in corrective axial skeletal surgery as part of a multimodality protocol that also includes SSEP and EMG monitoring. Several studies have examined the effect of MEP monitoring in spinal corrective surgery on outcome, and all reported that a transient or permanent loss of MEPs had a high correlation with long-term motor dysfunction. [87,102-104]

Consensus opinion and new studies strongly suggest that use of intraoperative spinal cord motor mapping improves long-term motor function after intramedullary spinal cord tumor resection.[90-92,105,106] The MEP is the only reliable monitor of motor pathways and is an earlier predictor of impending damage to the cord than the SSEP owing to the more precarious nature of the blood supply to the spinal gray matter. As such, in an anterior approach to an intramedullary spinal cord tumor resection, focal injury to the anterior spinal vasculature or motor tracts is often not detected (or is detected many minutes after injury) with SSEP monitoring alone.[86,89,96,107] MEP monitoring and spinal cord stimulation have been used successfully to define the "edge" of the intramedullary spinal tumor, thus maximizing the resection and minimizing motor impairment. During intramedullary spinal tumor mapping, use of the D wave as well as the CMAP may allow better correlation with motor outcome.[108]

MEP monitoring has also been useful during surgery in which the vasculature of the spinal cord is at risk. This includes surgical or interventional radiologic treatment for thoracoabdominal aneurysm[109] and corrective anterior thoracic spine surgery.[110] In these cases interruption of the radicular perforators from the aorta (especially the artery of Adamkiewicz) and inadequate perfusion via the pelvic supply to the caudal spinal cord may place the spinal cord at risk for ischemia. The anterior and posterior spinal arteries may not be continuous, especially in the mid-cervical spine, upper thoracic spine, and a narrowed region just cephalad to the lumbar enlargement, thus placing the blood flow distribution from the anterior spinal arteries to the motor tracts at risk for ischemic injury. The MEP allows rapid detection of ischemia because the gray matter, with its higher metabolic rate, is more sensitive to hypoperfusion (Fig. 7-8).[109,111]

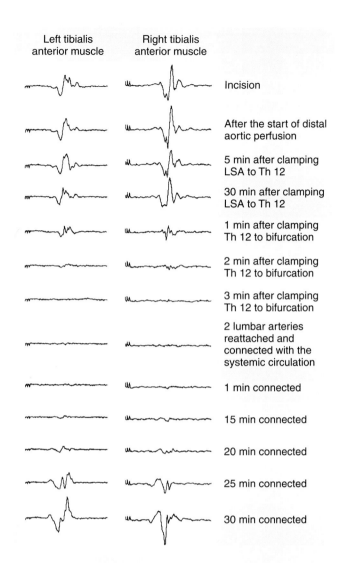

Left tibialis anterior muscle	Right tibialis anterior muscle	
		Incision
		After the start of distal aortic perfusion
		5 min after clamping LSA to Th 12
		30 min after clamping LSA to Th 12
		1 min after clamping Th 12 to bifurcation
		2 min after clamping Th 12 to bifurcation
		3 min after clamping Th 12 to bifurcation
		2 lumbar arteries reattached and connected with the systemic circulation
		1 min connected
		15 min connected
		20 min connected
		25 min connected
		30 min connected

Figure 7–8 Effect of ischemia on muscle evoked potential (MEP) response and recovery after reperfusion during a type II thoracoabdominal aneurysm. During the thoracic part of the operation, no MEP changes were observed, and eight intercostal arteries were ligated. During the abdominal part of the operation, MEP changes were observed within 2 minutes after placement of the clamps between T12 and the bifurcation. Two large lumbar spinal arteries (LSA) were identified and reattached to the graft. MEPs returned 15 minutes after the blood flow in the reattached lumbar spinal arteries was restored. *(From de Haan P, Kalkman CJ: Spinal cord monitoring: Somatosensory- and motor-evoked potentials. Anesthesiol Clin N Am 2001;19:923.)*

Like SSEP monitoring, MEP monitoring has also been found useful in cortical surgery. During middle and anterior cerebral aneurysm clipping several neural structures in the motor pathway are at risk for hypoperfusion (including the motor cortex, the pyramidal cells, corticospinal tracts, and internal capsule). MEPs have been reported to identify vasospasm, incorrect placement of the aneurysm clip, and inadequate clip placement.[96,97] A similar correlation of MEPs with outcome has been seen with aneurysm clipping in the basilar, carotid, and middle cerebral circulations. With tumor surgery near the motor cortex, direct motor cortex stimulation[112] has been successfully used to define the "edge" of motor cortex to limit undue motor injury. In brain tumor resection, reversible MEP change was usually associated with transient postoperative motor weakness. Irreversible MEP change was associated with permanent disabling paresis. The extent of MEP change correlates with the severity of postoperative paresis.[94,113]

MEP monitoring is not without risk; the U.S. Food and Drug Administration (FDA) approved MEP technology, noting relative contraindications to the method. The most common concern was direct cortical thermal injury (known as "kindling"), but over the last 15 years, even though hundreds of thousand of patients have undergone MEP monitoring, only two cases of kindling have been reported.[86] In a 2002 survey of the literature, published complications included were as follows: tongue laceration (n = 29), cardiac arrhythmia (n = 5), scalp burn at the site of stimulating electrodes (n = 2), jaw fracture (n = 1), and awareness (n = 1).[114] Notably, no new-onset seizures, epidural hematomas, or infections from epidural electrodes or movement injuries (e.g., surgical, joint dislocation), neuropsychiatric disease, headaches, or endocrine abnormalities have been reported. Common relative contraindications to MEP monitoring include epilepsy, cortex lesion, skull defects, high intracranial pressure, intracranial apparatus (electrodes, vascular clips, shunts), cardiac pacemakers, and other implanted pumps. Well-recognized and relatively more common complications are limited to sore muscles and tongue lacerations.[86] The absolute number and, certainly, the incidence of even minor complications are astonishingly low.[115] The movement associated with the MEP requires close coordination with the surgeon prior to performance of an MEP, so MEP monitoring is not nearly as continuous as SSEP or EMG monitoring.

ANESTHETIC CONSIDERATIONS DURING MONITORING

Each monitoring technique adds intraoperative vigilance to a different portion of the nervous system; consequently, it is common for several intraoperative neuromonitoring techniques to be employed during a surgical procedure. In order to facilitate the monitoring, the anesthesia provider must take into consideration the various effects of anesthesia management on the different modalities used. During monitoring, several factors can alter the responses in addition to the surgical procedure. Both physiologic management and anesthetic choices affect neural functioning and monitoring responses.

A variety of physiological alterations can alter neuronal functioning and after the monitoring so as to simulate surgically induced neuronal dysfunction.[116] These include conditions leading to inadequate oxygen delivery (e.g., relative hypotension, raised infracranial pressure, regional ischemia, anemia, tissue or systemic hypoxia), hypothermia, electrolyte abnormalities, and hypoglycemia. Although hypothermia may not be deleterious to the neural system, it can mimic surgical change, increased latency, and decreased amplitude. Hypotension is of particular interest, because some anesthetic plans include deliberate induction of hypotension to reduce blood loss. There is a growing appreciation that the presumed lower limit of autoregulation is not always adequate in tissues undergoing surgical stress.[117] Hence monitoring may allow a more optimal assessment of adequate blood pressure and tissue perfusion. Other factors, such as pathology, hyperventilation, and direct surgical manipulation, may alter the acceptable lower limit of blood pressure. Raising the blood pressure is one of the most common physiologic changes made when neurologic monitoring signals deteriorate.[118]

Anesthesia management involves choice of a favorable drug combination and maintenance of a steady state (e.g., avoiding changes in concentration or bolus drug delivery during critical monitoring periods). In general, the impact of anesthesia can be understood if one examines the mechanisms of action of anesthetic agents on the central nervous system.

For the SSEP, anesthetic agents appear to have two major mechanisms of action. First, anesthetic agents act to reduce synaptic transmission. Because the first synapse in the neural pathway is at the nucleus cuneatus in the brainstem, anesthetic agents have little effect on responses recorded at the cervical spine and more peripherally (i.e., peripheral nerve and epidural space). However, cortical responses are markedly affected. Second, anesthetic agents appear to produce gating of sensory information at the level of the thalamus through mechanisms activated in the brainstem.[119] This may explain why inhalational agents produce a dramatic nonlinear, dose-dependent reduction in cortical responses as their concentrations rise. Similar mechanisms appear to apply to ABR monitoring, in which small, progressively increasing effects are seen in the brainstem responses. As in SSEP, the dramatic decrease in response to increasing an inhalational agent occurs primarily in the cortical midlatency auditory evoked response.[116] Volatile anesthetics produce an increase in latency and a decrease in amplitude of cortical sensory responses until they cannot reliably be detected (at about 1-1.5 minimal alveolar concentration).

The effects on MEP can similarly be explained by anesthetic action. Because no synapses are involved in the production of the D wave, recordings of the D wave in the epidural space are altered little by anesthetics. However, the I waves are generated by synaptic mechanisms, so they are progressively reduced by increasing doses of anesthetic agents.[120] With the loss of I waves, the activation of the anterior horn cell and the production of a CMAP is blocked.[121] One method to overcome this effect is the use of multiple, usually four to six, electrical pulses spaced 2 to 3 msec apart. The temporal summation that occurs at the anterior horn cell overcomes some of the anesthetic effect.[121,122] This is currently the basis of the commonly used, FDA-approved technique of transcranial electrical stimulation. Further, anesthetic effects on the anterior horn cell synapse reduce the ability to produce a motor nerve response.[123] This effect may be more than a simple synaptic effect, because several other descending pathways are known to influence the excitability of the anterior horn cell and may explain why small concentrations of inhalational agents (0.5 MAC) can prevent production of a reproducible CMAP, especially in patients with abnormal neurologic function.[124]

The impact of these mechanisms varies according to the specific anesthetic agent, the agent's mechanism of action, and the synaptic receptors involved. In general, the inhalational anesthetic agents which have drug effects at multiple synaptic receptor types appear to have the most profound effect on monitoring. Not surprisingly, because of the effect on synapses, the effects and potency of specific agents parallel their effects on the EEG, which is also produced by synaptic activity.[116] Among the inhalational agents, isoflurane is the most potent and halothane the least potent (with enflurane being intermediate). Sevoflurane and desflurane appear similar to isoflurane at steady state, but owing to their relative insolubility, they may appear to be more potent during periods when concentrations are increasing.[125]

In the sensory responses, anesthetic effects of the inhalational anesthetics are prominent on the cortical responses, with increased latency, decreased amplitude, and marked depression of amplitude with concentrations above 0.5 to 1 MAC.[116,125] Smaller effects are seen on the ABR and SSEP responses recorded over the cervical spine, in the epidural space, or near peripheral nerves. The inhalational agents produce minimal changes in the epidurally recorded D wave of the MEP with dramatic depression of the muscle response (CMAP). Nitrous oxide (N_2O) also produces amplitude reduction and latency increases in cortical sensory responses or MEP CMAP responses when used alone or when combined with halogenated inhalational agents or opioid agents. As with halogenated agents, effects on subcortical, epidural, and peripheral nerve responses are minimal. Studies suggest that the effect of nitrous oxide may be "context sensitive," similar to its effects on the EEG (i.e., the actual effect may vary depending on the other anesthetics already present). Both nitrous oxide and desflurane have the advantage of insolubility, which facilitates their elimination when a low concentration is used and must be eliminated because of excessive anesthetic depression of monitoring.

The CMAP response of the MEP appears most easily abolished by low concentrations of halogenated inhalational agents (e.g., < 0.2%-0.5% isoflurane). Even in multiple stimuli protocols, 0.5 MAC isoflurane and sevoflurane may prevent detection of the CMAP response, especially in the presence of neurologic disease. Multiple studies have reported that with 0.5 MAC isoflurane, only about 60% of patients have MEPs, and at 0.8% isoflurane only 20% of patients have detectable MEPs.[86,89,126] Desflurane appears to have advantages over other volatile anesthetics.[127] Comparisons between 0.5 MAC desflurane-N_2O and propofol-N_2O show that these concentrations produce comparable MEP responses in scoliosis surgery.[127] N_2O has a similar but less profound depressant effect on MEP responses.[128] However, MEP monitoring of neurologically normal individuals undergoing spine surgery can frequently be accomplished with the use of 0.5 MAC of desflurane or sevoflurane.

Opioids cause only mild depression of all responses, with loss of late sensory evoked response peaks (> 100 msec) at doses producing sedation. Its effects on sensory and motor responses are otherwise minimal. As such, opioid analgesia is commonly used during recording of cortical sensory responses and MEPs, and opioid-based anesthesia with fentanyl, remifentanil, or sufentanil is often used to supplement low-dose inhalational agents or in total intravenous anesthesia.[129-132] The effects of ketamine on subcortical and peripheral responses are also minimal; this agent enhances the effect of the cortical SSEP amplitude[133] and CMAP response of the MEP.[134] This feature has made ketamine a desirable agent for monitoring responses that are usually difficult to record during anesthesia and in children. Use of ketamine with propofol reduces the depressant effect of propofol while providing an enhancement effect on responses.

Thiopental and midazolam produce mild depression of cortical sensory responses but long-lasting depression of MEPs.[135] Hence these agents are not commonly used with MEP monitoring. The ABR is virtually unaffected by doses of phenobarbital that produce coma, and the SSEP is unaffected at doses that produce a silent EEG; changes are not seen until doses high enough to produce cardiovascular collapse are used.[136] For this reason, SSEPs have been used successfully to monitor neurologic function during barbiturate-induced coma. Etomidate also produces an amplitude increase of cortical sensory components following injection,[137] with no changes in subcortical and peripheral sensory responses. This amplitude increase appears coincident with the myoclonus seen with the drug, suggesting a heightened cortical excitability. Etomidate has been used with SSEP recording but not commonly with MEP monitoring.

Droperidol and dexmedetomidine appear to have minimal effects on responses when combined with opioids. Dexmedetomidine has been successfully used with MEP, but occasional case reports have appeared suggesting that it may prevent MEP monitoring in some cases.[138] Further experience is currently evolving to clarify its role with monitoring.

Propofol is currently the most commonly used sedative component of total intravenous anesthesia when SSEPs and MEPs are monitored. Induction produces amplitude depression in cortical SSEPs, with rapid recovery after termination of infusion.[116] Recordings in the epidural space are unaffected, consistent with the site of anesthetic action of propofol in the cerebral cortex. The rapid metabolism of propofol makes it an excellent drug for infusion, because its sedative effect and its related effects on evoked responses can be adjusted quickly. An infusion of propofol can often be chosen that allows cortical SSEP and CMAP MEP monitoring, although depression of MEP can occur at higher doses.

In general, intravenous anesthetics suppress MEP responses much less than inhalational agents, so total intravenous anesthesia is preferred when MEPs are to be monitored in patients with neurologic disease.[139-141] Hence propofol[89] with or without ketamine is frequently combined with opioids.[140,125,142] With use of total intravenous anesthesia, MEPs are successfully obtained in more than 90% of patients, failures being associated with preexisting neurologic disorders or equipment failure.[114]

Depression of the neuromuscular junction by neuromuscular blocking agents impairs or prevents MEP and EMG monitoring. Muscle relaxants are generally thought to have no effect on the SSEPs; they may actually improve the cervically recorded sensory responses or epidural recordings of SSEPs and MEPs because EMG interference is reduced in nearby muscle groups. Stimulated EMG responses have been monitored successfully during NMB with 75% suppression of baseline CMAPs (one of four twitches in train-of-four twitch monitors).[50] Fluctuations in partial NMB could result in changes similar to those caused by adverse surgical manipulation or physiologic change. Further, because muscles vary in sensitivity to NMB, the extent of blockade must be assessed in the muscles monitored to clarify which changes are due to the NMB. Finally, partial NMB reduces the amplitude of motor unit potentials and might therefore change the ability to detect impending axonal injury from nerve irritation. For this reason, many anesthetists prefer to avoid NMB after anesthesia induction and during EMG and MEP monitoring. A new technique called post-tetanic MEPs enhances conventional MEPs by delivering a tetanic stimulus to a peripheral nerve before the MEP (e.g., 5-second 50-Hz tetanic stimulus to the posterior tibial nerve 6 seconds prior to transcranial MEP recorded in the abductor hallucis muscle).[143] This technique may facilitate MEP recording in patients in whom partial paralysis is desired (e.g., to reduce patient movement).

CONCLUSION

Neurophysiologic monitoring with EMG and evoked sensory and motor responses has become an important tool in the surgical management of some central and peripheral nervous system disorders. In general, multiple monitoring modalities

Table 7–3   Recommended Monitoring Modalities and Anesthetic Regimens for Surgical Procedures

Type of Procedure	Monitoring Modalities					Anesthetic Recommendation	
	Somatosensory Evoked Potentials	Transcranial Motor Evoked Potentials	Electromyography		Auditory Brainstem Responses	Volatile (Inhalational Anesthetics)	Total Intravenous Anesthesia
			Free Run	Stimulated			
Spine Skeletal							
Cervical	•	•	•				•
Thoracic	•	•	•	•			•
Lumbar instrumentation	•		•	•		•	
Lumbar disc			•	•		•	
Head and Neck							
Parotid			•			•	
Radical neck			•	•		•	
Thyroid			•	•		•	
Cochlear implant			•	•		•	
Mastoid			•	•		•	
Neurosurgery							
SPINE							
Vascular	•	•					•
Tumor	•	•					•
POSTERIOR FOSSA							
Acoustic neuroma			•	•	•	•	
Cerebellopontine	•	±	•	•	±		•
Vascular	•	•	•		±		•
SUPRATENTORIAL							
Middle cerebral artery aneurysm		•					•
Tumor in motor cortex	•	•					•

• Recommended for most surgeries, ± recommended for some procedures (depending on specific location of pathology)
Adapted from Jameson LC, Sloan TB, Jameson LC, et al: Monitoring of the brain and spinal cord. Anesthesiol Clin 2006; 24:777.

are used with each operation to provide the greatest assistance to the surgeon (Table 7-3). In some procedures, these methods have been demonstrated to reduce morbidity and have become a standard of care. They have been shown to be cost effective and have become part of routine management. For many surgeons and anesthesiologists, these methods have become an indispensable intraoperative diagnostic tool. The anesthesiologist, as a member of the surgical team, can make an important contribution to the success of the monitoring and can use the responses to guide physiologic management.

REFERENCES

1. Owen JH: Applications of neurophysiological measures during surgery of the spine. In Frymoyer JW, editor: *The Adult Spine: Principles and Practice*, ed 2, Philadelphia, 1997, Lippincott-Raven Publishers, p 673.
2. Sloan TB, Jameson LC, Sloan TB, et al: Electrophysiologic monitoring during surgery to repair the thoraco-abdominal aorta, *J Clin Neurophysiol* 24:316, 2007.
3. Aminoff MJ, Eisen AA, Aminoff MJ, et al: AAEM minimonograph 19: Somatosensory evoked potentials, *Muscle Nerve* 21:277, 1998.
4. Deletis V: Intraoperative monitoring of the functional integrity of the motor pathways, *Adv Neurol* 63:201, 1993.
5. Erwin CW, Linnoila M, Hartwell J: Effect of buspirone and diazepam, alone and in combination with alcohol, on skilled performance and evoked potentials, *J Clin Psychopharmacol* 55:199, 1986.
6. Grundy BL: Intraoperative monitoring of sensory-evoked potentials, *Anesthesiology* 58:72, 1983.
7. Jacobson GP, Tew JM Jr: Intraoperative evoked potential monitoring, *Intraoperative evoked potential monitoring* 4:145, 1987:[erratum appears in *J Clin Neurophysiol* 1987;4:420].
8. Moller AR: *Intraoperative neurophysiologic monitoring*, ed 2, Totowa, NJ, 2006, Humana Press.
9. Moller AR: Neurophysiological monitoring in cranial nerve surgery, *Neurosurg Q* 55:55, 1995.
10. Nuwer MR: *Evoked potential monitoring in the operating room*, New York, 1986, Raven Press.
11. Nuwer MR: Spinal cord monitoring, *Muscle Nerve* 22:1620, 1999.
12. Nuwer MR: Spinal cord monitoring with somatosensory techniques, *J Clin Neurophysiol* 15:183, 1998.
13. Branston NM, Symon L, Crockard HA: Recovery of the cortical evoked response following temporary middle cerebral artery occlusion in baboons: Relation to local blood flow and PO$_2$, *Stroke* 7:151, 1976.

14. Lam AM, Manninen PH, Ferguson GG, et al: Monitoring electrophysiologic function during carotid endarterectomy: A comparison of somatosensory evoked potentials and conventional electroencephalogram, *Anesthesiology* 75:15, 1991.

15. Symon L, Momma F, Murota T: Assessment of reversible cerebral ischaemia in man: Intraoperative monitoring of the somatosensory evoked response, *Acta Neurochir Suppl* 42:3, 1988.

16. Schramm J, Zentner J, Pechstein U, et al: Intraoperative SEP monitoring in aneurysm surgery, *Neurol Res* 16:20, 1994.

17. Firsching R, Klug N, Borner U, et al: Lesions of the sensorimotor region: Somatosensory evoked potentials and ultrasound guided surgery, *Acta Neurochir* 118:87, 1992.

18. Emerson RG, Turner CA: Monitoring during supratentorial surgery, *J Clin Neurophysiol* 10:404, 1993.

19. Costa P, Bruno A, Bonzanino M, et al: Somatosensory- and motor-evoked potential monitoring during spine and spinal cord surgery, *Spinal Cord* 45:86, 2007.

20. Croft TJ, Brodkey JS, Nulsen FE, et al: Reversible spinal cord trauma: A model for electrical monitoring of spinal cord function, *J Neurosurg* 36:402, 1972.

21. Kojima Y, Yamamoto T, Ogino H, et al: Evoked spinal potentials as a monitor of spinal cord viability, *Spine* 4:471, 1979.

22. Burke D, Hicks RG: Surgical monitoring of motor pathways, *J Clin Neurophysiol* 15:194, 1998.

23. Eggspuehler A, Sutter MA, Grob D, et al: Multimodal intraoperative monitoring during surgery of spinal deformities in 217 patients, *European Spine Journal* 16(Suppl 2)2007:S188.

24. Lenke LG: The clinical utility of intraoperative evoked-potential monitoring from a spinal surgeon's perspective, *Semin Spine Surg* 9:288, 1997.

25. Schwartz DM, Sestokis AK, Wierzbowski LR: Intraoperative neurophysiological monitoring during surgery for spinal instability, *Semin Spine Surg* 8:318, 1996.

26. Ben-David B: Spinal cord monitoring, *Orthop Clin N Am* 19:427, 1988.

27. Meyer PR Jr, Cotler HB, Gireesan GT: Operative neurological complications resulting from thoracic and lumbar spine internal fixation, *Clin Orthop Relat Res* 237:125, 1988.

28. Wilber RG, Thompson GH, Shaffer JW, et al: Postoperative neurological deficits in segmental spinal instrumentation: A study using spinal cord monitoring, *J Bone Joint Surg Am* 66:1178, 1984.

29. Nuwer MR, Dawson EG, Carlson LG, et al: Somatosensory evoked potential spinal cord monitoring reduces neurologic deficits after scoliosis surgery: Results of a large multicenter survey, *Electroencephalogr Clin Neurophysiol* 96:6, 1995.

30. Owen J: Cost efficacy of intraoperative monitoring, *Semin Spine Surg* 9:348, 1997.

31. Scoliosis Research Society: Somatosensory Evoked Potential Monitoring of Neurological Spinal Cord Function during Spinal Surgery, *SRS Position Statement on Somatosensory Evoked Potential Monitoring of Neurological Spinal Cord Function*, Park Ridge, IL, 1992, Scoliosis Research Society.

32. Loughman BA, Fennelly ME, Henley M, et al: The effects of differing concentrations of bupivacaine on the epidural somatosensory evoked potential after posterior tibial nerve stimulation, *Anesth Analg* 81:147, 1995.

33. Jones SJ, Edgar MA, Ransford AO, et al: A system for the electrophysiological monitoring of the spinal cord during operations for scoliosis, *J Bone Joint Surg Br* 65:134, 1983.

34. Stephen JP, Sullivan MR, Hicks RG, et al: Cotrel-Dubousset instrumentation in children using simultaneous motor and somatosensory evoked potential monitoring, *Spine* 21:2450, 1996.

35. Owen JH, Bridwell KH, Grubb R, et al: The clinical application of neurogenic motor evoked potentials to monitor spinal cord function during surgery, *Spine* 16(Suppl):S385, 1991.

36. Pereon Y, Bernard JM, Fayet G, et al: Usefulness of neurogenic motor evoked potentials for spinal cord monitoring: Findings in 112 consecutive patients undergoing surgery for spinal deformity, *Electroencephalogr Clin Neurophysiol* 108:17, 1998.

37. Accadbled F, Henry P, de Gauzy JS, et al: Spinal cord monitoring in scoliosis surgery using an epidural electrode. Results of a prospective, consecutive series of 191 cases [see comment], *Spine* 31:2614, 2006.

38. Aravabhumi S, Izzo KL, Bakst BL, et al: Brainstem auditory evoked potentials: Intraoperative monitoring technique in surgery of posterior fossa tumors, *Arch Phys Med Rehabil* 68:142, 1987.

39. Bruhn J, Myles PS, Sneyd R, et al: Depth of anaesthesia monitoring: What's available, what's validated and what's next?, *Br J Anaesth* 97:85, 2006.

40. Fischer G, Fischer C, Remond J: Hearing preservation in acoustic neuroma surgery [see comment], *J Neurosurg* 76:910, 1992.

41. Harper CM, Harner SG, Slavit DH, et al: Effect of BAEP monitoring on hearing preservation during acoustic neuroma resection, *Neurology* 42:1551, 1992.

42. Moller AR: *Intraoperative Neurophysiologic Monitoring*, Luxembourg, 1995, Harwood.

43. Nadol JB Jr, Chiong CM, Ojemann RG, et al: Preservation of hearing and facial nerve function in resection of acoustic neuroma, *Laryngoscope* 102:1153, 1992.

44. Yingling CD: Intraoperative monitoring of cranial nerves in skull base surgery. In Jackler RK, Brackman DE, editors: *Neurotology*, St. Louis, 1994, Mosby, p 967.

45. Lenarz T, Ernst A: Intraoperative monitoring by transtympanic electrocochleography and brainstem electrical response audiometry in acoustic neuroma surgery, *Eur Arch Otorhinolaryngol* 249:257, 1992.

46. Rowed DW, Nedzelski JM, Cashman MZ: Intraoperative monitoring of cochlear and auditory nerve potentials in operations in the cerebellopontine angle: an aid to hearing preservation. In Schramm J, Moller AR, editors: *Intraoperative neurophysiological monitoring*, Berlin, 1991, Springer-Verlag, p 214.

47. Silverstein H, McDaniel A, Norrell H, et al: Hearing preservation after acoustic neuroma surgery with intraoperative direct eighth cranial nerve monitoring. Part II: A classification of results, *Otolaryngol Head Neck Surg* 95:285, 1986.

48. Symon L, Jellinek D: Monitoring of auditory function in acoustic neuroma surgery. In Schramm J, Moller AP, editors: *Intraoperative neurophysiological monitoring*, Berlin, 1991, Springer-Verlag, p 173.

49. Cedzich C, Schramm J: Monitoring of flash visual evoked potentials during neurosurgical operations, *Int Anesthesiol Clin* 28:165, 1990.

50. Harper CM: Intraoperative cranial nerve monitoring, *Muscle Nerve* 29:339, 2004.

51. Harper CM, Daube JR: Facial nerve electromyography and other cranial nerve monitoring [see comment], *J Clin Neurophysiol* 15:206, 1998.

52. Gantz BJ: Intraoperative facial nerve monitoring, *Am J Otol* (Suppl 58)1985.

53. Harner SG, Daube JR, Ebersold MJ, et al: Improved preservation of facial nerve function with use of electrical monitoring during removal of acoustic neuromas, *Mayo Clinic Proc* 62:92, 1987.

54. Jackler RK, Selesnick SH: Indications for cranial nerve monitoring during otologic and neurotologic surgery, *Am J Otol* 55:611, 1994.

55. Cheek JC: Posterior fossa intraoperative monitoring, *J Clin Neurophysiol* 10:412, 1993.

56. Acoustic neuroma: *NIH Consens Statement* 9:1, 1991.

57. Kawaguchi M, Ohnishi H, Sakamoto T, et al: Intraoperative electrophysiologic monitoring of cranial motor nerves in skull base surgery, *Surg Neurol* 43:177, 1995.

58. Petro ML, Schweinfurth JM, Petro AB, et al: Transcricothyroid, intraoperative monitoring of the vagus nerve, *Arch Otolaryngol Head Neck Surg* 132:624, 2006.

59. Glasker S, Pechstein U, Vougioukas VI, et al: Monitoring motor function during resection of tumours in the lower brain stem and fourth ventricle, *Childs Nerv Syst* 22:1288, 2006.

60. Crum BA, Strommen JA: Peripheral nerve stimulation and monitoring during operative procedures, *Muscle Nerve* 35:159, 2007.

61. Turkof E, Millesi H, Turkof R: Intraoperative electroneurodiagnostics (transcranial electrical motor evoked potentials) to evaluate the functional status of anterior spinal roots and spinal nerves during brachial plexus surgery, *Plast Reconstr Surg* 99:1632, 1997.

62. Holland NR: Intraoperative electromyography, *J Clin Neurophysiol* 19:444, 2002.

63. Hormes JT, Chappuis JL: Monitoring of lumbosacral nerve roots during spinal instrumentation, *Spine* 18:2059, 1993.

64. Leppanen RE: Intraoperative monitoring of segmental spinal nerve root function with free-run and electrically-triggered electromyography and spinal cord function with reflexes and F-responses: A position statement by the American Society of Neurophysiological Monitoring, *J Clin Monit Comput* 19:437, 2005.

65. Owen JH, Kostuik JP, Gornet M, et al: The use of mechanically elicited electromyograms to protect nerve roots during surgery for spinal degeneration, *Spine* 19:1704, 1994.

66. Welch WC, Rose RD, Balzer JR, et al: Evaluation with evoked and spontaneous electromyography during lumbar instrumentation: A prospective study, *J Neurosurgery* 87:397, 1997.

67. Calancie B, Madsen P, Lebwohl N, et al: Stimulus-evoked EMG monitoring during transpedicular lumbosacral spine instrumentation: Initial clinical results, *Spine* 19:2780, 1994.

68. Liljenqvist UR, Halm HF, Link TM, et al: Pedicle screw instrumentation of the thoracic spine in idiopathic scoliosis, *Spine* 22:2239, 1997.

69. Rose RD, Welch WC, Donaldson WF 3rd, et al: Correlation of late intraforaminal screw removal with somatosensory evoked potentials and neurologic improvement, *Arch Physical Med Rehabil* 79:226, 1998.

70. Pajewski TN, Arlet V, Phillips LH, et al: Current approach on spinal cord monitoring: The point of view of the neurologist, the anesthesiologist and the spine surgeon, *Eur Spine J* 16(Suppl 2):S115, 2007.

71. Toleikis JR: Neurophysiological monitoring during pedicle screw placement. In Deletis V, Shils JL, editors: *Neurophysiology in Neurosurgery,* New York, 2002, Academic Press, p 231.

72. Holland NR: Intraoperative electromyography during thoracolumbar spinal surgery, *Spine* 23:1915, 1998.

73. Quinones-Hinojosa A, Gadkary CA, Gulati M, et al: Neurophysiological monitoring for safe surgical tethered cord syndrome release in adults, *Surg Neurol* 62:127, 2004.

74. Paradiso G, Lee GY, Sarjeant R, et al: Multi-modality neurophysiological monitoring during surgery for adult tethered cord syndrome, *J Clin Neuroscience* 12:934, 2005.

75. Kothbauer K, Schmid UD, Seiler RW, et al: Intraoperative motor and sensory monitoring of the cauda equina, *Neurosurgery* 34:702, 1994.

76. Kothbauer KF, Novak K: Intraoperative monitoring for tethered cord surgery: An update, *Neurosurg Focus* 16:E8, 2004.

77. Balzer JR, Rose RD, Welch WC, et al: Simultaneous somatosensory evoked potential and electromyographic recordings during lumbosacral decompression and instrumentation, *Neurosurgery* 42:1318, 1998.

78. Bose B, Wierzbowski LR, Sestokas AK, et al: Neurophysiologic monitoring of spinal nerve root function during instrumented posterior lumbar spine surgery, *Spine* 27:1444, 2002.

79. Djurasovic M, Dimar JR 2nd, Glassman SD, et al: A prospective analysis of intraoperative electromyographic monitoring of posterior cervical screw fixation [see comment], *J Spinal Disord Tech* 18:515, 2005.

80. Gunnarsson T, Krassioukov AV, Sarjeant R, et al: Real-time continuous intraoperative electromyographic and somatosensory evoked potential recordings in spinal surgery: Correlation of clinical and electrophysiologic findings in a prospective, consecutive series of 213 cases, *Spine* 29:677, 2004.

81. Krassioukov AV, Sarjeant R, Arkia H, et al: Multimodality intraoperative monitoring during complex lumbosacral procedures: Indications, techniques, and long-term follow-up review of 61 consecutive cases [see comment], *J Neurosurg Spine* 1:243, 2004.

82. Reidy DP, Houlden D, Nolan PC, et al: Evaluation of electromyographic monitoring during insertion of thoracic pedicle screws, *J Bone Joint Surg Br* 83:1009, 2001.

83. Shi YB, Binette M, Martin WH, et al: Electrical stimulation for intraoperative evaluation of thoracic pedicle screw placement, *Spine* 28:595, 2003.

84. Leis AA, Zhou HH, Mehta M, et al: Behavior of the H-reflex in humans following mechanical perturbation or injury to rostral spinal cord, *Muscle Nerve* 19:1373, 1996.

85. Leppanen RE: Intraoperative applications of the H-reflex and F-response: A tutorial, *J Clin Monit Comput* 20:267, 2006.

86. MacDonald DB: Intraoperative motor evoked potential monitoring: Overview and update, *J Clin Monit Comput* 20:347, 2006.

87. MacDonald DB, Al Zayed Z, Khoudeir I, et al: Monitoring scoliosis surgery with combined multiple pulse transcranial electric motor and cortical somatosensory-evoked potentials from the lower and upper extremities, *Spine* 28:194, 2003.

88. Minahan RE, Sepkuty JP, Lesser RP, et al: Anterior spinal cord injury with preserved neurogenic 'motor' evoked potentials [see comment], *Clin Neurophysiol* 112:1442, 2001.

89. Pelosi L, Lamb J, Grevitt M, et al: Combined monitoring of motor and somatosensory evoked potentials in orthopaedic spinal surgery, *Clin Neurophysiol* 113:1082, 2002.

90. Lang EW, Chesnut RM, Beutler AS, et al: The utility of motor-evoked potential monitoring during intramedullary surgery, *Anesth Analg* 83:1337, 1996.

91. Morota N, Deletis V, Constantini S, et al: The role of motor evoked potentials during surgery for intramedullary spinal cord tumors, *Neurosurgery* 41:1327, 1997.

92. Sala F, Palandri G, Basso E, et al: Motor evoked potential monitoring improves outcome after surgery for intramedullary spinal cord tumors: A historical control study, *Neurosurgery* 58:1129, 2006.

93. Mikuni N, Okada T, Enatsu R, et al: Clinical impact of integrated functional neuronavigation and subcortical electrical stimulation to preserve motor function during resection of brain tumors, *J Neurosurg* 106:593, 2007.

94. Mikuni N, Okada T, Nishida N, et al: Comparison between motor evoked potential recording and fiber tracking for estimating pyramidal tracts near brain tumors, *J Neurosurg* 106:128, 2007.

95. Neuloh G, Pechstein U, Cedzich C, et al: Motor evoked potential monitoring with supratentorial surgery, *Neurosurgery* 54:1061, 2004.

96. Neuloh G, Schramm J, Neuloh G, et al: Monitoring of motor evoked potentials compared with somatosensory evoked potentials and microvascular Doppler ultrasonography in cerebral aneurysm surgery, *J Neurosurg* 100:389, 2004.

97. Szelenyi A, Langer D, Kothbauer K, et al: Monitoring of muscle motor evoked potentials during cerebral aneurysm surgery: Intraoperative changes and postoperative outcome, *J Neurosurg* 105:675, 2006.

98. Nascimbeni A, Gaffuri A, Imazio P, et al: Motor evoked potentials: Prognostic value in motor recovery after stroke, *Funct Neurol* 21:199, 2006.

99. Woldag H, Gerhold LL, de Groot M, et al: Early prediction of functional outcome after stroke, *Brain Injury* 20:1047, 2006.

100. Hendricks HT, Zwarts MJ, Plat EF, et al: Systematic review for the early prediction of motor and functional outcome after stroke by using motor-evoked potentials, *Arch Phys Med Rehabil* 83:1303, 2002.

101. Amassian VE, Stewart M, Quirk GJ, et al: Physiological basis of motor effects on a transient stimulation to cerebral cortex, *Neurosurgery* 20:74, 1987.

102. Devlin VJ, Schwartz DM: Intraoperative neurophysiologic monitoring during spinal surgery, *J Am Acad Orthop Surg* 15:549, 2007.

103. Langeloo DD, Lelivelt A, Louis Journée H, et al: Transcranial electrical motor-evoked potential monitoring during surgery for spinal deformity: A study of 145 patients, *Spine* 28:1043, 2003.

104. Weinzierl MR, Reinacher P, Gilsbach JM, et al: Combined motor and somatosensory evoked potentials for intraoperative monitoring: intra- and postoperative data in a series of 69 operations, *Neurosurg Rev* 30:109, 2007.

105. Quinones-Hinojosa A, Gulati M, Lyon R, et al: Spinal cord mapping as an adjunct for resection of intramedullary tumors: surgical technique with case illustrations, *Neurosurgery* 51:1199, 2002.

106. Sala F, Lanteri P, Bricolo A, et al: Motor evoked potential monitoring for spinal cord and brain stem surgery, *Adv Tech Stand Neurosurg* 29:133, 2004.

107. de Haan P, Kalkman CJ, Ubags LH, et al: A comparison of the sensitivity of epidural and myogenic transcranial motor-evoked responses in the detection of acute spinal cord ischemia in the rabbit, *Anesth Analg* 83:1022, 1996.

108. Deletis V: Intraoperative neurophysiology and methodologies used to monitor the functional integrity of the motor system. In Deletis V, Shils JL, editors: *Neurophysiology in neurosurgery,* New York, 2002, Academic Press, p 25.

109. Sloan TB, Jameson LC: Electrophysiologic monitoring during surgery to repair the thoraco-abdominal aorta, *J Clin Neurophysiol* 24:316, 2007.

110. Leung YL, Grevitt M, Henderson L, et al: Cord monitoring changes and segmental vessel ligation in the "at risk" cord during anterior spinal deformity surgery, *Spine* 30:1870, 2005.

111. Jacobs MJ, Mess W, Mochtar B, et al: The value of motor evoked potentials in reducing paraplegia during thoracoabdominal aneurysm repair, *J Vasc Surg* 43:239, 2006.

112. Neuloh G, Schramm J: Motor evoked potential monitoring for the surgery of brain tumours and vascular malformations, *Adv Tech Stand Neurosurg* 29:171, 2004.

113. Zhou H, Kelly P: Transcranial electrical motor evoked potential monitoring for brain tumor resection, *Neurosurgery* 48:1075, 2001.

114. Legatt A: Current practice of motor evoked potential monitoring: Results of a survey, *J Clin Neurophysiol* 19:454, 2002.

115. MacDonald D: Safety of intraoperative transcranial electrical stimulation motor evoked potential monitoring, *J Clin Neurophysiol* 19:416, 2002.

116. Sloan TB: Evoked Potentials. In Albin MA, editor: *Textbook of neuroanesthesia with neurosurgical and neuroscience perspectives,* New York, 1997, McGraw-Hill, p 221.

117. Edmonds HL: Multi-modality neurophysiologic monitoring for cardiac surgery, *Heart Surg Forum* 5:225, 2002.

118. Edmonds HL, Rodriguez RA, Audenaert SM, et al: The role of neuromonitoring in cardiovascular surgery, *J Cardiothorac Vasc Anesth* 10:15, 1996.

119. John ER: The anesthetic cascade: a theory of how anesthesia suppresses consciousness [see comment], *Anesthesiology* 102:447, 2005.

120. Hicks RG, Woodforth IJ, Crawford MR, et al: Some effects of isoflurane on I waves of the motor evoked potential, *Br J Anaesth* 69:130, 1992.

121. Ubags LH, Kalkman CJ, Been HD: Influence of isoflurane on myogenic motor evoked potentials to single and multiple transcranial stimuli during nitrous oxide/opioid anesthesia, *Neurosurgery* 43:90, 1998.

122. Taniguchi M, Cedzich C, Schramm J: Modification of cortical stimulation for motor evoked potentials under general anesthesia: Technical description, *Neurosurgery* 32:219, 1993.

123. Zentner J, Albrecht T, Heuser D: Influence of halothane, enflurane, and isoflurane on motor evoked potentials [see comment], *Neurosurgery* 31:298, 1992.

124. Zhou HH, Zhu C: Comparison of isoflurane effects on motor evoked potential and F wave, *Anesthesiology* 93:32, 2000.

125. Sloan TB: Anesthetic effects on electrophysiologic recordings, *J Clin Neurophysiol* 15:217, 1998.

126. Chen Z: The effects of isoflurane and propofol on intraoperative neurophysiological monitoring during spinal surgery, *J Clin Monit Comput* 18:303, 2004.

127. Lo YL, Dan YF, Tan YE, et al: Intraoperative motor-evoked potential monitoring in scoliosis surgery: Comparison of desflurane/nitrous oxide with propofol total intravenous anesthetic regimens, *J Neurosurgical Anesthesiology* 18:211, 2006.

128. van Dongen EP, ter Beek HT, Schepens MA, et al: The influence of nitrous oxide to supplement fentanyl/low-dose propofol anesthesia on transcranial myogenic motor-evoked potentials during thoracic aortic surgery, *J Cardiothorac Vasc Anesth* 13:30, 1999.

129. Hargreaves SJ, Watt JW: Intravenous anaesthesia and repetitive transcranial magnetic stimulation monitoring in spinal column surgery, *Br J Anaesth* 94:70, 2005.

130. Langeron O, Vivien B, Paqueron X, et al: Effects of propofol, propofol-nitrous oxide and midazolam on cortical somatosensory evoked potentials during sufentanil anaesthesia for major spinal surgery, *Br J Anaesth* 82:340, 1999.

131. Scheufler KM, Zentner J: Total intravenous anesthesia for intraoperative monitoring of the motor pathways: An integral view combining clinical and experimental data, *J Neurosurg* 96:571, 2002.

132. Thees C, Scheufler KM, Nadstawek J, et al: Influence of fentanyl, alfentanil, and sufentanil on motor evoked potentials, *J Neurosurg Anesthesiol* 11:112, 1999.

133. Schubert A, Licina MG, Lineberry PJ: The effect of ketamine on human somatosensory evoked potentials and its modification by nitrous oxide, *Anesthesiology* 72:33, 1990:[erratum appears in Anesthesiology 1990;721104].

134. Kano T, Shimoji K: The effects of ketamine and neuroleptanalgesia on the evoked electrospinogram and electromyogram in man, *Anesthesiology* 40:241, 1974.

135. Glassman SD, Shields CB, Linden RD, et al: Anesthetic effects on motor evoked potentials in dogs, *Spine* 18:1083, 1993.

136. Marsh RR, Frewen TC, Sutton LN, et al: Resistance of the auditory brain stem response to high barbiturate levels, *Otolaryngol Head Neck Surg* 92:685, 1984.

137. Kochs E, Treede RD: Schulte am Esch J: Increase in somatosensory evoked potentials during anesthesia induction with etomidate [German], *Anaesthesist* 35:359, 1986.

138. Mahmoud M, Sadhasivam S, Sestokas AK, et al: Loss of transcranial electric motor evoked potentials during pediatric spine surgery with dexmedetomidine, *Anesthesiology* 106:393, 2007.

139. Kalkman CJ, Drummond JC, Ribberink AA, et al: Effects of propofol, etomidate, midazolam, and fentanyl on motor evoked responses to transcranial electrical or magnetic stimulation in humans, *Anesthesiology* 76:502, 1992.

140. Kawaguchi M, Sakamoto T, Inoue S, et al: Low dose propofol as a supplement to ketamine-based anesthesia during intraoperative monitoring of motor-evoked potentials, *Spine* 25:974, 2000.

141. Taniguchi M, Nadstawek J, Langenbach U, et al: Effects of four intravenous anesthetic agents on motor evoked potentials elicited by magnetic transcranial stimulation, *Neurosurgery* 33:407, 1993.

142. Ubags LH, Kalkman CJ, Been HD, et al: The use of ketamine or etomidate to supplement sufentanil/N2O anesthesia does not disrupt monitoring of myogenic transcranial motor evoked responses, *J Neurosurg Anesthesiol* 9:228, 1997.

143. Yamamoto Y, Kawaguchi M, Hayashi H, et al: The effects of the neuromuscular blockade levels on amplitudes of posttetanic motor-evoked potentials and movement in response to transcranial stimulation in patients receiving propofol and fentanyl anesthesia, *Anesth Analg* 106:930, 2008.

Chapter 8

TRANSCRANIAL DOPPLER ULTRASONOGRAPHY IN ANESTHESIA AND NEUROSURGERY

Basil Matta • Marek Czosnyka

Introduced in 1982 by Aaslid and colleagues,[1] transcranial Doppler (TCD) ultrasonography has become one of the most useful methods of noninvasively examining the cerebral circulation. Provided that the limitations of this technology are recognized, information about cerebral hemodynamics can be obtained that can be used in the perioperative and intensive care of neurologically injured patients (those with head injury) and in the prevention of neurologic insult in patients at risk for cerebral ischemia (those undergoing carotid endarterectomy). This chapter discusses the principles and limitations that govern the use of TCD and describes current and potential future applications of this reliable, indirect, noninvasive continuous measure of cerebral blood flow (CBF) and its regulation.

PRINCIPLES OF TCD ULTRASONOGRAPHY

Transcranial Doppler ultrasonography calculates the velocity of red blood cells (FV) flowing through the large vessels at the base of the brain by means of the Doppler principle. This principle, first described by Christian Doppler in 1843, relates the shift in the frequency of a sound wave when either the transmitter or the receiver is moving with respect to the wave-propagating medium. The change in the frequency of emitted pulse of ultrasound reflected by red blood cells is proportional to blood flow velocity. By convention, the shift in Doppler frequency is expressed in centimeters per second to allow comparison of readings from instruments that operate at different emission frequencies. The frequency best suited for TCD applications is on the order of 2 MHz.[2]

A constant vessel diameter and an unchanged angle of insonation are the two main assumptions that govern the use of TCD as an indirect measure of CBF. The velocity detected by the probe as a fraction of the real velocity depends on the cosine of the angle of red cell insonation (measured velocity = real velocity × cosine of angle of incidence). Therefore at 0 angle, the detected and true red cell velocities are equal (cosine of 0 = 1), whereas at 90 degrees, no detection of velocity is possible. Fortunately, the anatomic limitations of transtemporal insonation of the middle cerebral artery (MCA) are such that signal capture is possible only at narrow angles (<30 degrees). Thus the detected velocity is a very close approximation of the true velocity (87% to 100%). Furthermore, as long as the angle of insonation is kept constant by fixing the probe in position (and vessel diameter remains constant during examination—see later comments), changes in the detected velocity closely reflect changes in the true velocity.

The other main factor that affects the interpretation of TCD measurements is the diameter of the insonated vessel. The volume passing through a particular segment of a vessel depends on the velocity of red cells and the diameter of the vessel. Therefore for velocity to be a true reflection of flow, the diameter of the vessel must not change significantly during the measurement period. Factors that may affect the diameter of vessels are arterial carbon dioxide tension (Pa_{CO_2}), blood pressure, anesthetic agents, and vasoactive drugs. The basal cerebral arteries, being conductance vessels, do not dilate or constrict as the vascular resistance changes. It has been shown angiographically and through direct observation during brain surgery that change in Pa_{CO_2}, one of the most important determinants of cerebrovascular resistance (CVR), has no effect on the diameter of the basal arteries.[3] Moreover, CO_2 reactivity studies using TCD have demonstrated values similar to those obtained with conventional CBF measurements.[4-6] Similarly, changes in blood pressure have negligible influence on the diameter of the proximal segments of the basal arteries.[6,7] The effect of vasoactive drugs on cerebral conductance vessels is variable. Although sodium nitroprusside and phenylephrine do not significantly affect the proximal segments of the MCA,[8,9] significant vasodilation occurs when nitroglycerine is administered to healthy volunteers.[10]

The effect of anesthetic agents on the diameter of the basal vessels remains controversial. The intravenous agents are devoid of direct cerebrovascular effects, and it is accepted that these agents do not affect the diameter of the conductance vessels.[11] The situation is less clear-cut with the inhalational agents, with most but not all the evidence suggesting that they have negligible effects on the diameter of the conductance vessels.[12-15] It is generally accepted that during steady-state anesthetic conditions, changes in FV can be interpreted to mean corresponding changes in cortical CBF.[16-20]

A factor that may affect the reliability of TCD measurements as true representations of CBF variation is the presence of intracranial pathology. Intracranial lesions, increases in intracranial pressure (ICP), and cerebral vasospasm have all been identified as factors that affect the accuracy of FV measurements.[20,21]

MEASUREMENTS USING TRANSCRANIAL DOPPLER ULTRASONOGRAPHY

The Examination

Three main pathways for accessing the intracranial arteries are (1) the transtemporal route through the thin bone above the zygomatic arch to the anterior, middle, and posterior cerebral arteries, (2) the transorbital approach to the carotid siphon, and (3) the suboccipital route to the basilar and vertebral arteries. Although a complete diagnostic examination usually incorporates all three approaches, because the probe can be easily secured in position once a signal is obtained, intraoperative monitoring usually utilizes the transtemporal route. In expert hands, it is possible to transtemporally insonate the proximal segment (M1) of the MCA in more than 90% of people.[2,22-24] The MCA carries about 60% to 70% of the ipsilateral carotid artery blood flow and can be regarded as representative of hemispheric CBF. However, because the successful transmission of ultrasound through the skull depends on the thickness of the skull, which varies with gender, race, and age, the failure rate can be as high as 10% to 30%.[25-27] The incidence of failure can be decreased by increasing the power and, in some instances, with the use of 1-MHz probes.[28] The theoretical risk of eye damage limits the use of the transorbital route, and the lack of suitable means to secure the probe in position makes the suboccipital route impractical.

Through the temporal window, the MCA, anterior cerebral artery (ACA), and posterior cerebral artery (PCA) can be readily examined. In each patient, the same insonation window should be used throughout the entire study period. This can be accomplished by putting a small marker at the patient's temporal region. The TCD examination begins with the identification of the bifurcation of the intracranial portion of the internal carotid artery (ICA) into the MCA and ACA according to the method described by Aaslid.[2] This bifurcation can usually be identified at a depth of 60 to 65 mm. The typical Doppler signal from the carotid bifurcation, which consists of images above and below the zero line of reference, represents the flow directions toward and away from the ultrasound probe of the MCA and ACA, respectively. The depth of insonation is then reduced to follow the upward deflection image of the MCA flow velocity as the vessel runs toward the skull. The MCA can usually be traced up to a depth of 30 mm, which is beyond the bifurcation of the MCA into the peripheral branches. The proximal portion of the main trunk of the MCA (the M1 segment) can be located at a depth of around 45 to 55 mm. The depth that gives the highest velocity is usually chosen for measurement. In children, this depth is usually 10 mm less than that in adults, but the same principles apply. This method of obtaining the MCA signal eliminates the possibility of mistaking the PCA for the MCA, because for anatomic reasons, the PCA signal cannot be obtained at a depth less than 55 mm.

After the MCA signal is obtained, the depth of insonation is increased so that the image of the carotid bifurcation can be seen again. The depth is increased further with the probe directed slightly anteriorly so that the ACA image can be found. The first part of the ACA (the A1 segment) is recognized from a direction of flow away from the probe. With the identification of the ACA, the depth of insonation is decreased until the carotid bifurcation signal is obtained. The probe is then angled slightly posteriorly until the signal of the PCA is seen. The PCA can be distinguished from the MCA signal because it has a lower flow velocity and because the PCA signal cannot be obtained when the depth of insonation is decreased to less than 55 mm. A more detailed description of the TCD examination can be found in a standard textbook.[24] Figure 8-1 illustrates various signals obtained from the most commonly insonated vessels.

Velocity Measurements

Although the most physiologic correlate with actual CBF is the weighted mean velocity (FV_{mean}), which takes into consideration the different velocities of the formed elements in the blood vessel insonated, the maximal flow velocity (FV_{max} as depicted by the spectral outline) is generally used because of the higher signal-to-noise ratio. A good correlation also exists between the FV_{max} and FV_{mean}, as in the basal cerebral arteries, where the flow is usually laminar. The mean flow velocity with time-averaged FV usually refers to the mean velocity of FV_{max}. The time-averaged FV_{max} is determined from area under the spectral curve.

Volume of blood flowing through a vessel depends on the velocity of the moving cells and the diameter of vessel concerned. For a given blood flow, the narrower the vessel, the higher the velocity. Although CBF in millimeters per minute per 100 g of brain tissue is relatively constant under conditions of constant brain metabolism and arterial content of carbon dioxide and oxygen, FV in the MCA ranges from 35 to 90 cm/sec in the awake resting state.[2] This range is due to inter-individual variations in vessel diameter and angles of insonation and probably accounts for the poor correlation between absolute FV and CBF in any given population. However, relative changes in FV accurately reflect variations in CBF.[5-19]

Mean FV varies with age. MCA red cell velocity (FV_{MCA}) rises from 24 cm/sec at birth to a peak of 100 cm/sec at age 4 to 6 years.[25,26] Thereafter the FV_{MCA} decreases steadily to about 40 cm/sec during the seventh decade of life.[1,22,29] This reduction can be explained partly by the increase in the diameter of basal arteries that occurs with age.[30] However, some of the reduction is the result of the genuine decrease in hemispheric CBF, which has been reported by several investigators.[31,32] Overall, the velocity trend seen in the MCA with age is similar to that in hemispheric CBF.

Mean FV is higher in females and during hemodilution. A reduction in hematocrit has been shown to increase CBF in a linear fashion and probably accounts for the greater velocities reported in low hematocrit states.[33-35] However, low hematocrit may present diagnostic difficulties in patients with potential arterial stenotic lesions because the increase in velocity observed may be incorrectly interpreted as vessel stenosis. An example is subarachnoid-related vasospasm. Women have higher hemispheric CBF than men, which is reflected in 3% to 5% higher mean FV_{MCA} values.[35,36] Although a convincing explanation for this difference in velocity has not yet been found, a lower hematocrit and slightly higher arterial CO_2 tension found in premenopausal women may partly explain this increase in velocity.[29,37]

Waveform Pulsatility

Pulsatility describes the shape of the maximal shift (the envelope) of the Doppler spectrum from peak systolic pressure to end-diastolic pressure with each cardiac cycle.[38] The FV waveform depends on the arterial blood pressure (ABP) waveform and the viscoelastic properties of the cerebrovascular bed, provided that blood rheology remains constant. Thus in the absence of vessel stenosis or vasospasm, with constant pulsatility of ABP and during constant cerebral perfusion pressure (CPP), changes in pulsatility reflect the changes in distal CVR.[38,39] Two derived indices have been used to quantify

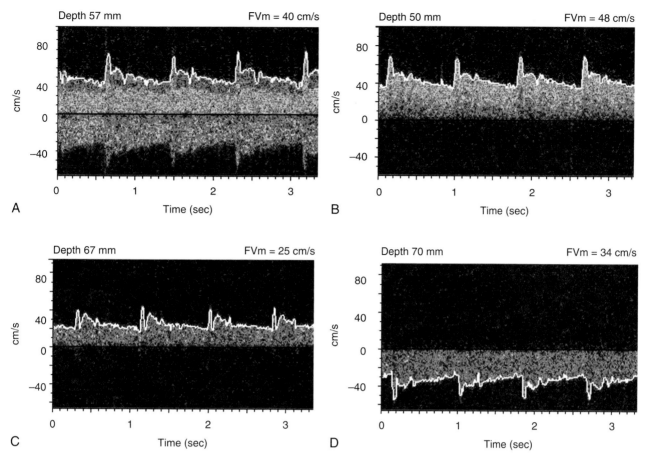

Figure 8–1 Schematic representations of blood flow velocity (FV) traces obtained from the internal carotid artery bifurcation at 5.5 to 6.5 cm **(A)**, the M1 segment of the middle cerebral artery (MCA) at 3 to 6 cm **(B)**, the posterior cerebral artery (P1) at 6 to 8 cm **(C)**, and the anterior cerebral artery (A1) at 6 to 8 cm **(D)**. Flow above the horizontal is toward the probe, and flow below the horizontal is away from the probe.

pulsatility. The pulsatility index (PI), or Gosling index, is calculated as follows[39]:

$$PI = \frac{(FV_{sys} - FV_{dias})}{FV_{mean}}$$

where FV_{dias} is diastolic blood flow velocity and FV_{sys} is systemic blood flow velocity. The resistance index (RI), or Pourcelot index, is calculated with the following equation[40]:

$$RI = \frac{(FV_{sys} - FV_{dias})}{FV_{sys}}$$

In a highly pulsatile spectrum, FV_{sys} is peaked and much greater than end-FV_{dias}, whereas FV_{dias} greater than 50% of FV_{sys} gives a "damped" waveform. Normal PI ranges from 0.5 to 1 with no significant side-to-side or cerebral interarterial differences.[41]

In general, PI and RI correspond to each other, reflecting changes in central or cerebral hemodynamics. However, neither index provides meaningful information about the cause of the change; for example, an increase in PI can be caused by cerebral vasoconstriction (intrinsic, as in hyperventilation) or vasodilatation happening at low CPP, when vessels dilate because of the autoregulatory response.[38] Furthermore, PI is very sensitive to changes in heart rate and its values are best compared when measured during periods of similar heart rates. The advantage of PI is that it is dimensionless and therefore is not affected by the angle of insonation because the

equation used to calculate PI has the cosine of the angle of incidence in both the numerator and the denominator. A PI value above 1.5 with normal or increased mean arterial pressure (MAP) in a normocapnic patient may indicate elevated ICP. Also, asymmetry in PI values greater than 0.5 between the left and right hemispheres may give rise to concern about clinically relevant asymmetry of cerebral hemodynamics (unilateral carotid artery stenosis, acute subdural hematoma, etc.). PI is only superficially simple. It depends on numerous interrelated factors: ABP pulsatility, heart rate, Pa_{CO_2}, CPP, hematocrit, body temperature, CVR, compliance of the proximal cerebral vessels, ICP, and compliance of the cerebrospinal space.

REGULATION OF CEREBRAL BLOOD FLOW: TESTING AND MONITORING

Cerebrovascular Reactivity to CO_2

Cerebrovascular reactivity to CO_2 describes the relationship between arterial CO_2 tension and CBF. Within limits from mild hypocapnia to mild hypercapnia, change in Pa_{CO_2} produces almost proportional change in CBF and FV. In deep hypocapnia and hypercapnia, this linear relationship saturates. This relationship can be tested by observation of the change in CBF in response to a change in Pa_{CO_2}. If we accept that the diameter of the basal arteries is unaffected or is affected to a negligible degree by changes in arterial CO_2 tension, then TCD is particularly suitable for such investigations because multiple paired measurements are taken and regression lines can be constructed more accurately than with a limited number of conventional blood flow measurements.[4,42,43] Moreover, both the absolute and the relative FV-Pa_{CO_2} (percentage change in FV from baseline) relationships can be examined. The absolute CO_2 reactivity will depend on the baseline FV. Therefore when the baseline FV is low, such as during intravenous anesthesia, the change per mm Hg change in Pa_{CO_2} is similarly reduced. However, when the values are normalized to an FV at Pa_{CO_2} of 40 mm Hg, the relative slope expressed in percentage approximates the awake value.[44] Compared with the absolute change, the percentage change in FV with change in Pa_{CO_2} shows less dependence on baseline value and is therefore a more valid indicator of CO_2 reactivity and a more appropriate variable for use in comparing clinical conditions.[42-46]

In normal individuals CBF (or FV) changes by approximately 2.5% to 3% for every mm Hg change in Pa_{CO_2}. TCD can therefore be used in many clinical situations to assess cerebrovascular reserve, such as in patients with carotid artery stenosis and after head injury. The effect of anesthetics and vasoactive drugs on cerebral vasoreactivity to CO_2 can also be easily examined with use of TCD.[5,9,42,43,47] Induced change in Pa_{CO_2} usually provokes changes in ABP. In such cases CO_2 reactivity values should be adjusted accordingly (Fig. 8-2).[48]

Another method of examining the cerebral vasoreactivity to CO_2 involves the use of carbonic anhydrase inhibitors. Intravenous administration of 1 g of acetazolamide produces vasodilatation with a concomitant rise in FV. Although this method has its advantages in patients with cardiac and respiratory disease, in that it obviates the need for hyperventilation,

it provides only a unidirectional, crude estimate of cerebral vasomotor reactivity. Increasing and decreasing CO_2 tension test both the vasodilatory and vasoconstrictive capabilities of the cerebral circulation.

Cerebral Pressure Autoregulation

Cerebral autoregulation, a sensitive mechanism that can be impaired by pathologic processes and inhalational anesthesia, minimizes deviations in CBF when CPP changes between 50 and 170 mm Hg.[49-55] Cerebral autoregulation has been traditionally assessed by repeated static measurements of CBF during a period of hypotension or hypertension. In addition to the bulky equipment or radioactive material necessary for these measurements, the process is labor intensive and assumes that cerebral autoregulation is a uniform and slow-acting process. Furthermore, drugs used to induce hypertension or hypotension may influence cerebrovascular tone.[50]

Cerebral autoregulation is a complex process composed of several physiologic mechanisms operating possibly at different rates. Observations of the reaction of the CBF to different levels of perfusion pressure suggest that pressure-induced changes in CVR consist of two components: a rapid response sensitive to pressure oscillations (20 sec to 3 min) followed by a slow response to changes in mean pressure.[56] TCD studies have estimated time constant of fast autoregulatory responses; FV_{MCA} as an index of CBF was fully restored to the baseline value as early as 5 to 16 seconds after a step decrease in blood pressure.[57] Conventional CBF measurement techniques, with the inability to record instantaneous changes, probably would

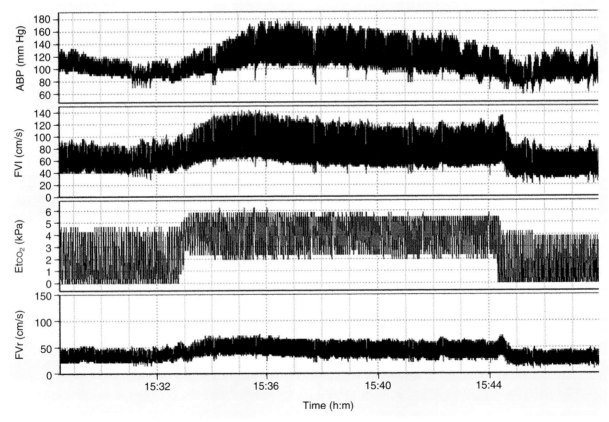

Figure 8–2 CO_2 reactivity test performed in patient with right side common carotid artery stenosis (90%). Right side reactivity was 27%/kPa, and left side reactivity 14%/kPa. After corrections for change in arterial pressure, reactivity at left was 19%/kPa and right 9%/kPa, indicating that right side reactivity was severely depleted. ABP, arterial blood pressure; FVl, blood flow velocity in left middle cerebral artery (MCA); FVr, blood flow velocity in right MCA; Et_{CO_2}, end-tidal CO_2 pressure.

miss these initial fast components and therefore at best can be characterized as an incomplete assessment of the cerebral autoregulatory response. Hence, TCD allows noninvasive measurement of the autoregulatory response and can provide insight into both rapid and delayed components of cerebral autoregulatory mechanisms. Other continuous techniques, such as laser Doppler flowmetry and thermal methods, are invasive.[58,59] Near infrared spectroscopy seems to be the only competitor of TCD in this implementation,[60,61] but its clinical use needs more validation.

Although many methods for the assessment of cerebral autoregulation have been described, only the methods most commonly employed are described here. Examples of testing dynamic and static autoregulation are shown in Figure 8-3.

Leg-Cuff Test

Dynamic autoregulation is tested by measurement of the recovery in FV after a rapid transient decrease in mean blood pressure (MBP) induced by deflation of large thigh cuffs. These large blood pressure cuffs modified with larger tubes are placed around one or both thighs, inflated to 50 mm Hg above

systolic pressure for 3 minutes, and then deflated to produce an approximately 20–mm Hg drop in MBP. Through the use of an algorithm previously validated,[57-62] the FV response to the drop in blood pressure is fitted to a series of curves to determine the rate of dynamic cerebral autoregulation (dRoR) or autoregulation index (ARI). These curves are generated by a computer model of cerebral autoregulation that predicts the autoregulatory response on the basis of the continuous blood pressure record and compares its predictions with the measured response.[56] The dRoR describes the rate of restoration of FV (percentage per second) with respect to the drop in MBP. The normal dRoR is 20%/sec (i.e., the process is complete within approximately 5 seconds).[57]

The time for autoregulation to normalize FV during normocapnia occurs well within the period of hypotension achieved with cuff deflation before the MAP returns to baseline (10 to 20 sec).[57,62] Collection of autoregulation data in the first 10 seconds avoids the influence of CO_2-rich blood from the legs after thigh cuff deflation. Hypercapnia increases CBF through vasodilation of cerebral blood vessels and reduces autoregulatory capacity, therefore "normal" dRoR strongly depends on Pa_{CO_2}.[23]

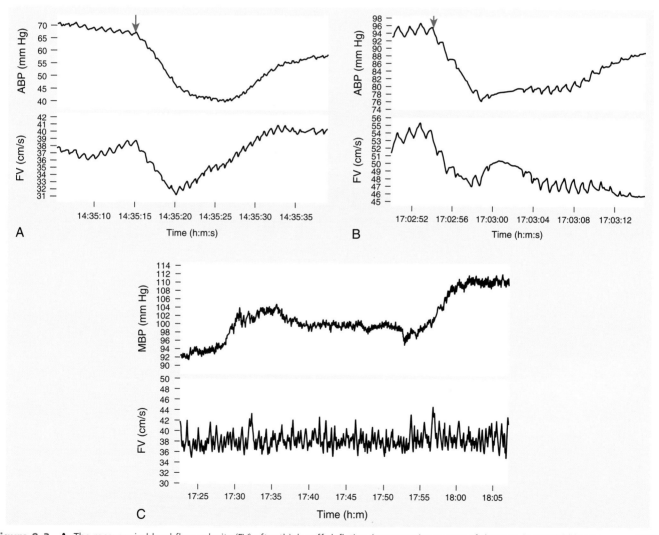

Figure 8–3 **A,** The recovery in blood flow velocity (FV) after thigh cuff deflation (*arrows* point to start of decrease in arterial blood pressure [ABP] after deflation) is "steeper" in patients with intact dynamic autoregulation than the increase in ABP. **B,** In contrast, FV remains depressed after cuff deflation in patients with impaired autoregulation. **C,** Testing of static autoregulation during propofol anesthesia. *Top trace* represents mean blood pressure (MBP) in mm Hg; *bottom trace* represents middle cerebral artery. There is virtually no change in FV despite the increase in MBP as a result of dopamine infusion.

Static Autoregulation

Static autoregulation can be tested by induction of an approximately 20–mm Hg increase in MBP through the use of a 0.01% phenylephrine infusion with simultaneous recording of the FV. The FV and MBP recorded are then used for subsequent calculation of the estimated CVR (CVRe; CVRe = MBP/FV). The static rate of autoregulation (SRoR) is the ratio of percentage change in estimated CVRe to percentage change in MBP.[42] Theoretically, no change in the FV would occur if the percentage change in CVRe was equal to the percentage change in MBP. Thus an SRoR of 1 implies perfect autoregulation, and an SRoR of 0 implies a complete disruption of autoregulation. When ICP is elevated and measured, CPP should be substituted for MBP. Measurement of SRoR with MBP instead of CPP may cause an error called "false autoregulation." It happens when a non-autoregulating brain change in MBP produces a 1:1 increase in ICP, leaving CPP constant. This obviously does not produce any change in CBF, giving a false SRoR value equal to 1.

Transient Hyperemic Response Test

The transient hyperemic response test is performed by compression of the common carotid artery for 5 to 8 seconds and observation of the change in FV after compression is released. When the carotid artery is compressed, the distal cerebrovascular bed dilates in response to the drop in perfusion pressure. When the compression is released, an increase in FV_{MCA} is observed as a result of this dilation that persists until the distal cerebrovascular bed constricts to its former diameter. The compression results in this "transient hyperemia" only when autoregulation is intact. When autoregulation is impaired, no dilation of the distal cerebrovascular beds occurs in response to the compression, and hence no transient hyperemia is detected (Fig. 8-4).

Although the transient hyperemic response test is reproducible, is easy-to-perform, and can be used to assess cerebral autoregulation in the neurologically injured patient, the results depend heavily on the compression technique.[63-65] Furthermore, it is contradicted in patients with carotid disease, in whom there are theoretical risks associated with the maneuver, including the possibility of dislodging atheroma. Nevertheless results indicate that the test may be useful in the assessment of outcome after head injury[65] or in management after subarachnoid hemorrhage.[66]

Continuous Monitoring of Cerebral Autoregulation

PHASE SHIFT BETWEEN THE SUPERIMPOSED RESPIRATORY AND ARTERIAL BLOOD PRESSURE WAVES

An interesting noninvasive method of deriving autoregulatory status from natural fluctuations in MCA flow velocity involves the assessment of the angle of the phase shift

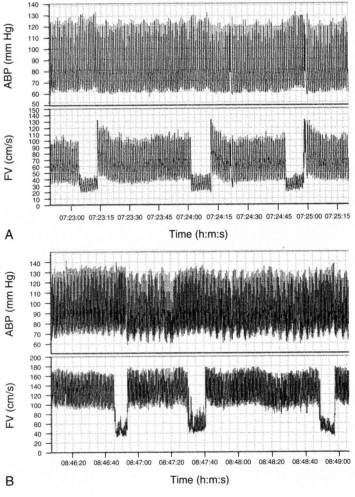

Figure 8–4 Autoregulation testing using the transient hyperemic response test in two patients receiving intensive care. **A,** Transient hyperemia of blood flow velocity (FV) in the middle cerebral artery FV following short-term compression of the common carotid artery indicates intact autoregulation. **B,** The lack of response suggests impaired autoregulation. In clinical practice the test is repeated to improved accuracy, after scanning of the carotid artery to confirm that it is free of atherosclerotic plaque. ABP, arterial blood pressure.

between the superimposed respiratory and ABP waves during slow and deep breathing. A 0-degree phase shift angle indicates absence of autoregulation, whereas a positive phase shift angle (>30 degrees) indicates intact autoregulation.[67]

CALCULATION OF THE AUTOREGULATION INDEX

For assessment of dynamic cerebral autoregulation based on spontaneous fluctuations of ABP, more reliable values of the ARI are obtained by fitting the models proposed by Tiecks and colleagues[68] to the CBFV step response to a change in ABP.[57] These researchers used transfer function analysis to quantify the dynamic relationship between mean ABP (input) and mean CBFV (output). A fast Fourier transform (FFT) algorithm was applied to the time-series of beat-to-beat changes in mean ABP and mean CBFV, and the auto- and cross-spectra were calculated. The inverse Fourier transform was used to obtain the CBFV impulse response in the time domain, which was integrated to yield an estimate of the CBFV response to a hypothetical step change in ABP. Each of the 10 models proposed by Tiecks and colleagues,[68] corresponding to ARI values from 0 (absence of autoregulation) to 9 (best autoregulation), was fitted to the first 10 seconds of the CBFV step response, and the best fit, as selected by the minimum squared error, was selected as the representative value of ARI for that segment of data. Values of ARI are averaged for patients with more than one segment of data.

TIME CORRELATION METHOD

Continuous monitoring over consecutive time-averaged samples of flow velocity and CPP (thirty to sixty 5- to 10-second averages are usually taken) enables a correlation coefficient between mean CPP and mean FV to be calculated. This coefficient has been termed the mean index (Mx index).[69] A positive coefficient signifies a positive association between BFV and CPP, that is, disturbed autoregulation. A zero or negative correlation coefficient signifies absence of or a negative association, implying intact autoregulation. The calculation may be repeated with a moving time window, so the Mx index may form new variables, indicating changes of cerebral autoregulation with time.

This index seems to be ideal to monitor transient changes in autoregulation that occur in response to a cerebral intrinsic phenomenon. Group analysis has demonstrated that the autoregulation index averaged daily was related to clinical outcome after head injury; a positive Mx value (disturbed autoregulation) was associated with worse outcome.[70] The method has been positively cross-validated with the "gold standard," static rate of autoregulation, as well as with the leg-cuff test, ARI, phase shift analysis, and the transient hyperemic response test. Continuous monitoring of autoregulation is possible (however, probe positioning over a longer period is still a technical challenge). Following head injury, autoregulation fluctuates in time in response to changing clinical conditions. "Optimization" of CPP—that is, choosing a CPP value at which conditions for regulation of CBF are the best—is possible (Fig. 8-5).

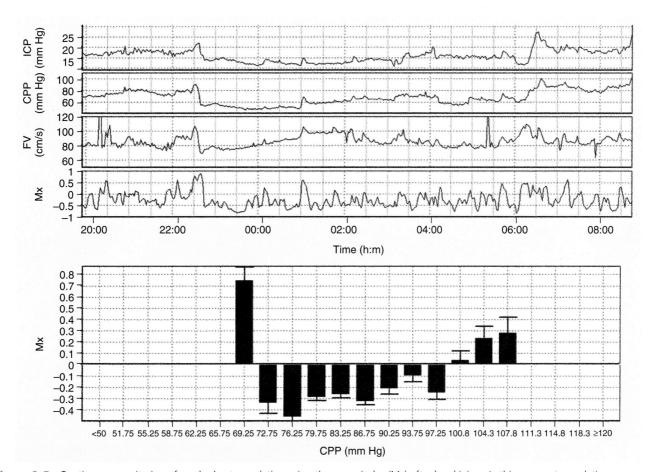

Figure 8–5 Continuous monitoring of cerebral autoregulation using the mean index (Mx) after head injury. In this case, autoregulation was generally preserved (Mx value was negative) with the exception of short episodes around 22:30 and 1:00. Plotting of averaged Mx values against cerebral perfusion pressure (CPP) shows that the "optimal" CPP for this period (value of CPP for minimal Mx) was around 75 mm Hg. FV, blood flow velocity; ICP, intracranial pressure.

Similar techniques based on optimization of pressure reactivity (index based on changes in ICP and ABP) are already used in clinical practice.

NONINVASIVE ASSSESSMENT OF BRAIN PRESSURES AND MULTIMODAL MONITORING

Noninvasive Assessment of Cerebral Perfusion Pressure and Intracranial Pressure

As ICP increases and CPP correspondingly decreases, a highly pulsatile flow velocity pattern is seen. In deep intracranial hypertension, a progressive loss of diastolic flow to systolic spike and eventually to an oscillating flow pattern is observed. This oscillating flow pattern signifies the onset of intracranial circulatory arrest and, if not reversed, is terminal.[71-74]

The PI, defined either as Gosling PI (GPI)—that is, the peak-to-peak amplitude of FV pulsations divided by time-averaged FV—or as "spectral" PI (SPI)—that is, the first harmonic component of FV pulsations divided by mean FV—is inversely proportional to reductions in CPP.[75,76] This inverse relationship between CPP and PI has been proposed as a method of estimating CPP noninvasively.[77] By relating the first harmonic component of the ABP pulse waveform to SPI, Aaslid and coworkers[77] demonstrated the ability to estimate CPP with a 95% confidence limit for prediction of around ± 25 mm Hg. An improved method of estimating CPP using mean arterial pressure and diastolic and mean blood velocities has also been reported. Czosnyka and associates[78] were able

to estimate CPP noninvasively with errors of estimation less than 10 mm Hg in more than 85 % of the measurements. Furthermore, when this method was used as a continuous monitor, the author's group was able to detect real-time changes in "true" CPP. Bilateral monitoring may also provide useful information about side-to-side variations in perfusion that, in turn, may allow clinical decisions to be made earlier. An example of noninvasive estimation of CPP is illustrated in Figure 8-6.

The ability to estimate CPP noninvasively has obvious advantages. This form of monitoring is particularly useful in centers where ICP monitoring is not routinely used or in the patient for whom ICP monitoring is not indicated but who may have decreased intracranial compliance (e.g., after a concussion or mild closed-head injury). The role of TCD in noninvasive estimation of cerebral perfusion is promising.[79]

A more complex method aimed at the noninvasive assessment of ICP has been introduced and tested by Schmidt and associates.[80,81] The method is based on the presumed transformation between arterial pressure and ICP waveforms. Coefficients of these transformations are derived from the database of real ABP and ICP recordings. Similar linear transformation is built, using the same database between flow velocity and arterial pressure. Then, the model assumes a linear relationship between arterial pressure and flow velocity and arterial pressure to ICP transformations. Multiple regression coefficients are calculated. Finally, for each prospective study, ICP is calculated using ABP to ICP transformation, formed from ABP to flow velocity transformation transposed using precalculated regression coefficients (see Fig. 8-6).

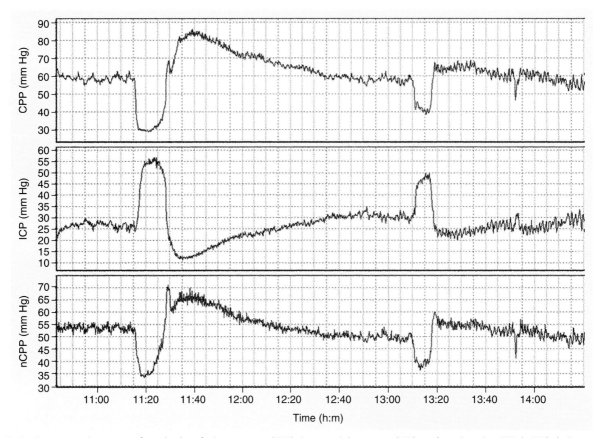

Figure 8–6 Representative traces of cerebral perfusion pressure (CPP), intracranial pressure (ICP), and noninvasive CPP (nCPP) during an episode of intracranial hypertension (plateau waves) in a head-injured patient.

Critical Closing Pressure

Critical closing pressure (CCP) was first described by means of a mathematical model showing that small vessels can collapse when the ABP approaches a critical value, defined as the *critical closing pressure*.[82] In cerebrovascular circulation this value was postulated to be equal to the sum of intracranial pressure (ICP) and a component proportional to the active tension of vascular smooth muscle, as follows:

$$CCP = ICP + \text{tension of arterial walls}$$

For prediction of CCP, arterial pressure should be first decreased below the lower limit of autoregulation with parallel measurements of CBF. A linear relationship between CBF and arterial pressure can be then extrapolated to the value of pressure at which flow reaches zero. Aaslid and colleagues[83] and Panerai and associates[84] proposed a method for the calculation of CCP using TCD. In this method the intercept point of a regression line between single pulse pressure plotted along the x-axis and the of blood flow velocity in the middle cerebral artery plotted along the y-axis can be used for the estimation of CCP. Alternative methods have been suggested that use ratios of first harmonics of flow velocity pulse and arterial pressure pulse.[85] These methods are attractive from a clinical standpoint because they make a continuous, noninvasive prediction of CCP possible without the need to decrease arterial pressure. CCP is useful for detection of changes in ICP (however, accuracy is worse than for noninvasive ICP; see the previous section) and cerebrovascular resistance.

Transcranial Doppler Ultrasonography in Multimodality Monitoring

TCD is an integral component of multimodality monitoring. Together with ICP measurement, jugular venous bulb oximetry (Sjo_2), near-infrared spectroscopy, laser Doppler flowmetry (LDF), and brain microelectrodes, TCD enables important minute-by-minute information to be obtained in the neurologically injured patient. Multimodal data are captured and examined at the bedside or subsequently in the light of available clinical information. The effect of interventions or pathologic processes on cerebral hemodynamics can be viewed from several angles. The main factor controlling the ability to process such information is data acquisition. Up to 50% of data collected are often discarded because of poor quality (B. Matta, unpublished data). Nevertheless, being able to see time trends for multiple parameters brings us one step closer to observing the "whole picture" of secondary ischemic brain insults.[85]

TRANSCRANIAL DOPPLER ULTRASONOGRAPHY IN CLINICAL PRACTICE

Carotid Artery Disease

Stroke is both the principal indication for and the major complication of carotid endarterectomy. The majority of perioperative strokes are embolic, but hypoperfusion, hyperperfusion, or both may be responsible for more than 40% of perioperative strokes.[86,87] Therefore the maximum benefit of this procedure can be realized only if perioperative cerebral perfusion is optimized and embolic phenomena are minimized. TCD is

an attractive technique for the detection of cerebral ischemia during cross-clamping of the carotid artery because it is continuous and noninvasive and the transducer probes can be used successfully without impinging on the surgical field. It is also an important tool in the preoperative assessment and postoperative care of patients with carotid disease.[85-105] In addition to providing the means for the preoperative assessment of cerebrovascular reserve and, possibly, for determining the need for shunting by examination of CO_2 reactivity, TCD is being increasingly used for detection of preoperative and postoperative embolic phenomena and for testing the integrity of cerebral autoregulation.[97,100,101,103-105] Also, pressure autoregulation can be tested; it is commonly impaired in any state in which collateral blood supply is poor[106] and improves gradually after surgery or stenting.[107]

Cerebral ischemia following clamping of the ICA is considered severe if FV_{MCA} is 15% or less of preclamping value, mild if FV_{MCA} is 16% to 40% of preclamping value, and absent if FV_{MCA} is greater than 40% of preclamping value.[94] This criterion correlates well with subsequent ischemic electroencephalographic changes and hence can be used as an indication for shunt placement.[89-94] An intravascular shunt used to bypass the clamped ICA is effective in restoring blood flow but has its own inherent problems, namely, potential dislodgment of embolus from the distal ICA, traumatic dissection of the vessel wall resulting in an occluding intimal flap, and a technically more difficult endarterectomy. Furthermore, in a nonrandomized multicenter study involving more 1400 patients, Halsey[94] showed that the placement of shunts in patients with post–ICA clamping velocities greater than 40% of preclamping value is associated with a higher risk of stroke (presumably embolic). Although there is no universal consensus on the magnitude of FV_{MCA} change that necessitates shunt placement, a reduction in FV_{MCA} to less than 40% of baseline before clamping is the most commonly accepted indication. Unnecessary shunting is best avoided. TCD can also instantly detect shunt malfunction caused by kinking or thrombosis.[96]

Emboli are detected on TCD as short-duration, high-intensity "chirps," and waveform analysis can help differentiate air from particulate emboli.[108] Nevertheless, there are currently no automatic detection systems that have the required sensitivity and specificity for clinical use.[109] Emboli can occur throughout the procedure but are more common during dissection of the carotid arteries, on release of ICA cross-clamping, and during wound closure.[97,98,110] Although the clinical significance of TCD-detected emboli is not yet fully understood, they probably represent adverse embolic events during surgery.[97,102,109,111] The rate of microembolus generation can indicate incipient carotid artery thrombosis, has been related to intraoperative infarcts, and has been correlated to postoperative neuropsychological morbidity.[98,102,111]

At operation, emboli are clearly audible, and interestingly, surgeons tend to adapt their operative technique to minimize embolus generation. After the introduction of intraoperative TCD monitoring, some centers have reported a reduction in operative stroke rates.[87,93] Although it is tempting to attribute this reduction to the introduction of TCD monitoring, many other factors also have changed during the same period.

After closure of the arteriotomy and release of carotid clamps, FV typically rises immediately to levels above baseline (preclamping) value and gradually corrects back to the preclamping value over a few minutes.[102] This hyperemic response is to be expected as the dilated vascular bed vasoconstricts in autoregulatory response to an increased perfusion pressure.

However, approximately 10% of patients are at greater risk of cerebral edema or hemorrhage because of gross hyperemia, with FV at values 230% of baseline value lasting from several hours to days.[99-101,104,112] This persistent postoperative hyperemia, which is likely to occur in patients with high-grade stenosis, probably results from defective autoregulation in the ipsilateral hemisphere, because a reduction in blood pressure is effective in both normalizing FV and alleviating the symptoms.[103] TCD provides the means of early detection and effective treatment of this potentially fatal complication.

Finally, a progressive postoperative drop in FV to below the preclamping baseline value can indicate postoperative occlusion of the ipsilateral carotid artery and has been used as an indication for reexploration of the endarterectomy.[104] Clinically, postoperative development of sudden symptoms should prompt an immediate TCD examination. This step avoids invasive angiographic procedures and allows early reexploration. Figure 8-7 shows monitoring of FV during carotid endarterectomy.

Intracranial Vascular Disease

Subarachnoid Hemorrhage

Cerebral vasospasm is the leading cause of morbidity and mortality in patients who survive a subarachnoid hemorrhage (SAH). Although radiologic evidence of vasospasm has been reported in up to 70% of angiograms performed within the first week of aneurysmal rupture, the incidence of clinically significant vasospasm approximates 20%.[113,114] The cause remains uncertain but appears to be related to the amount and distribution of blood in the subarachnoid space. Results of one study suggest that nitric oxide levels are reduced by extravascular oxyhemoglobin or the presence of the potent vasoconstrictor endothelin.[115] In the patient with SAH, the appearance of new focal neurologic signs or a decrease in level of consciousness may be an early sign of vasospasm. This finding is normally confirmed by computed tomography and angiography.

A constant vessel diameter is one of the main assumptions that govern the use of TCD as an indirect measure of CBF. Therefore, although TCD is unreliable as a measure of CBF in patients with SAH because of changes in vessel diameter, it has become valuable for diagnosing vasospasm noninvasively before the onset of clinical symptoms. As the vessel diameter is reduced for the same blood flow, the FV increases. Hence cerebral vasospasm is generally considered present if the FV_{MCA} is greater than 120 cm/sec or the ratio between FV_{MCA} and FV in the ICA (FV_{ICA}) exceeds 3.[98,99] In the sedated patient, the diagnosis of cerebral vasospasm relies on gross neurologic signs as well as findings on computed tomography, cerebral angiography, and TCD. Cerebral angiography and computed tomography can be performed only intermittently, leaving TCD as the only way of diagnosing and judging the severity and efficacy of treatment of cerebral vasospasm.[116,117] The ratio of FV_{MCA} to FV_{ICA} should decrease with effective treatment. Needless to say, to rule out cerebral vasospasm with TCD, one must perform a thorough examination of the basal arteries. Unfortunately, detection of small vessel spasm is not possible. Our policy is to perform daily TCD examinations in all patients with SAH. Initial impressions suggest that the incidence of TCD-diagnosed vasospasm is much higher

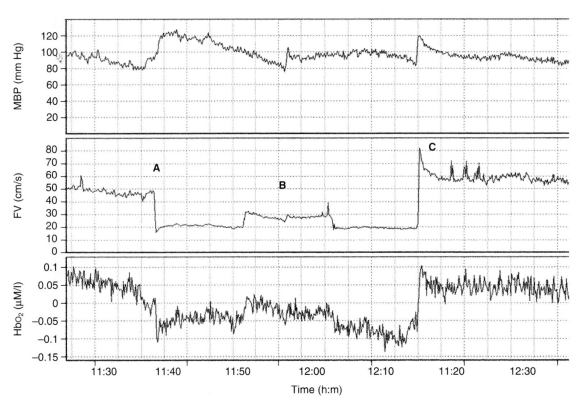

Figure 8–7 Monitoring during carotid endarterectomy. At time of carotid cross-clamping (A), there was a rapid fall in blood velocity (FV), which was accompanied by a sustained fall in the cerebral oxygenation (Hbo_2 monitoring using near infrared spectroscopy). These changes were independent of any change in mean blood pressure (MBP). Signals recovered with the insertion of an intravascular shunt, with a second fall seen during shunt removal (B). Hyperemia occurred at the end of the procedure (C).

than that of clinically significant vasospasm, and therefore therapy is not usually escalated on the basis of TCD findings alone. Cerebral autoregulation dysfunction that is overlapped by or precedes cerebral vasospasm correlates with neurologic deterioration.[118,119] Administration of statins in the acute phase after SAH improves autoregulation and decreases the incidence of vasospasm.[76] The transient hyperemic response test is particularly useful for testing cerebral autoregulation in patients with SAH.

In addition to the detection and treatment of vasospasm, TCD has been successfully used in the perioperative management of patients with cerebral aneurysms in a variety of other situations. Eng and coworkers[120] reported the advantages of TCD monitoring for the perioperative management of a patient in whom the aneurysm ruptured before dural incision. Giller and associates[121] highlighted the relatively rare but important incidence of embolic cerebral ischemia after aneurysm surgery. Over a 2-year period, 9 of their 11 patients in whom TCD demonstrated emboli after aneurysm surgery also had low-density areas on computed tomography, and credible sources for emboli were identified in all the patients studied.[121] The advantage of detecting embolic sources is self-evident.

The treatment of giant aneurysms and certain vascular masses often necessitates ligation of the carotid artery. The ability to predict tolerance to carotid artery occlusion is therefore beneficial to the planning of such procedures. Although a trial angiographic balloon occlusion of the carotid artery while the patient is awake, with concurrent blood flow studies, is an accepted method for testing tolerance, it is invasive and cannot be performed at the bedside. TCD has been used to observe change in FV_{MCA} during manual compression of the ICA at the bedside. When the drop in FV_{MCA} does not exceed 65% of baseline value, ICA occlusion is generally well tolerated. However, when the FV_{MCA} falls below 65% of baseline, focal neurologic deficit with ICA occlusion can be expected in more than 85% of patients tested.[122]

Arteriovenous Malformations

Arteries leading to an arteriovenous malformation (AVM), a developmental anomaly with abnormal embryonic vascular network, shunt blood to the venous side with flow rates out of proportion to the low metabolism within the AVM. These "feeder" vessels are characterized by high blood velocity, low pulsatility, low perfusion pressure, and decreased CO_2 reactivity.[123-128] Lindegaard and associates[125] were able to diagnose AVMs in 26 of 28 patients from the characteristic findings of blood velocity, waveform pulsatility, and CO_2 reactivity outside the ranges for expected normal variation. Embolization or resection of AVMs results in normalization of FV, pulsatility, and CO_2 reactivity.[129-132] The potential use of intraoperative TCD with AVM resection lies with estimating the completeness of resection and the diagnosis and treatment of the hyperperfusion syndrome,[133,134] provided that the feeding vessel can be monitored. With simultaneous monitoring of both the feeding vessel and the contralateral nonfeeding vessel, theoretically, the preoperative difference in velocity and in pulsatility between the two sides should progressively disappear.

Closed-Head Injury

Although many factors affect outcome after head injury, episodes of hypoxemia, hypotension, and reduced cerebral perfusion caused by high ICP are predictive of poor outcome.[135,136] Because these episodes may only last a few minutes, their reliable detection and quantification requires real-time measurement. The greater availability of multimodal monitoring—simultaneous monitoring of ICP, CPP, jugular bulb oxygen saturation (Sjo_2), and TCD—has made the detection of such pathophysiologic episodes possible. Furthermore, as more of the "picture" is seen with several monitors reflecting the changes at the same time, appropriate therapeutic interventions are made early. For example, Kirkpatrick and colleagues[137] demonstrated that it is possible to distinguish between rises in ICP due to low CPP and those due to hyperemia through the use of TCD as part of a multimodality setup. An example of multimodal monitoring in head injury is shown in Figure 8-8.

TCD monitoring can be used to observe changes in FV and waveform pulsatility as well as for testing cerebrovascular reserve. Cerebral autoregulation is often impaired after head injury with an increased susceptibility to secondary ischemic insults and possible correlation with poor outcome.[69,135,138-140] The transient hyperemic response test,[66] cuff deflation–induced drops in MBP (both dynamic tests), and vasopressor-induced increases in MBP (static test) have all been used to test autoregulation after head injury.[139-142] However, the most noninvasive and most continuous assessment of autoregulation relies on correlation of the spontaneous fluctuations in FV_{MCA} waveform and CPP (Mx index). When autoregulation is present, little change is observed in FV_{MCA} during changes in CPP. Conversely, in the patient with impaired autoregulation, a positive linear correlation between FV_{MCA} and CPP is observed.[121] In addition, continuous recording of the FV_{MCA} enables easy detection of the autoregulatory "threshold" or "breakpoint," the CPP at which autoregulation fails, thus providing a target CPP value for treatment.

Cerebral vasospasm causing ischemia or non–contusion-related infarction remains an important cause of morbidity and mortality after head injury.[143-145] The appearance of new focal neurologic signs or a decrease in the level of consciousness after head injury may be an early sign of vasospasm. TCD can be used to diagnose and treat cerebral vasospasm with use of the same criteria as for patients with SAH. Increased FV in combination with high Sjo_2 and a ratio of FV_{MCA} to FV_{ICA} less than 2 indicates hyperemia, whereas high FV in the presence of low or normal Sjo_2 values and a ratio of FV_{MCA} to FV_{ICA} greater than 3 suggests cerebral vasospasm.[143-146]

Although clinical decisions on outcome after head injury cannot be based solely on TCD findings, the information obtained may provide guidance for further therapy and likely outcome. Cerebral autoregulation and CO_2 vasoreactivity can be repeatedly tested in the intensive care unit. The loss of these hallmarks of a normal cerebral vasculature suggests poor prognosis.[141,147] Similarly, the oscillating FV pattern typically seen before complete circulatory arrest can be used to confirm the diagnosis of brain death.[148,149] The use of TCD for noninvasive estimation of CPP has already been addressed.

Stroke

The development of fibrinolytic agents such as streptokinase and recombinant tissue-type plasminogen activator (rTPA) has raised the need for more precise knowledge of the pathophysiology of acute ischemic stroke. TCD can be used to identify cerebral arterial occlusion[149,150] and recanalization,[151-153] as well as to help determine the risk of hemorrhagic transformations of large-volume ischemic lesions.[154] Repeated TCD examinations within 6, 24, and 48 hours after admission with

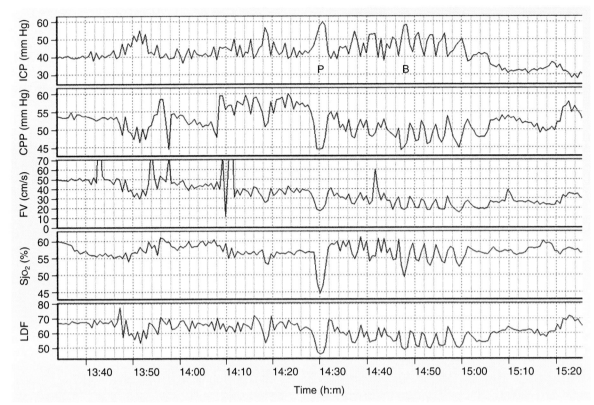

Figure 8–8 Recording of events characterized by intracranial hypertension in a head-injured patient receiving intensive care. Using multimodality monitoring makes it possible to identify the cause of this increase. Increase in intracranial pressure (ICP) (plateau wave [P]) is secondary to a fall in cerebral perfusion pressure (CPP), as the blood velocity (FV), the jugular bulb oxygen saturation values (SjO$_2$) and cortical blood flow (LDF, in arbitrary units) also fall, indicating hypoperfusion. Repetitive vasogenic waves of ICP (B waves [B]) are secondary to fluctuations of cerebral blood flow as SjO$_2$, and FV, and LDF increase and decrease in phase with ICP.

acute stroke can help identify both those patients at risk for further ischemic episodes and the sources of emboli.[155] Unilateral emboli most commonly originate from the carotid arteries, whereas bilateral emboli most commonly arise from cardiac sites. The effect of anticoagulation on reperfusion, recanalization, and outcome after acute stroke can also be evaluated with TCD.[156] In patients with stroke and poor status, in whom the possibility of brain edema and rise in ICP increases, noninvasive assessment of CPP and ICP using TCD seemed to be useful. Also, assessment of cerebral autoregulation with TCD is promising, although this area requires intensive clinical trials.

Miscellaneous Nonneurosurgical Applications

Because of its noninvasive nature, TCD has found many applications in fields other than neurosurgery and neurointensive care, mainly in patients at risk for neurologic injury secondary to primary pathologic conditions outside the central nervous system.

Cardiac Surgery

Detection of microemboli and the estimation of cerebral perfusion during cardiac surgery are probably the most important applications of TCD outside neurosurgery and neurointensive care. Although the incidence of stroke after cardiac surgery is estimated at 5%, subtler cognitive dysfunction has been reported in more than 60% of patients.[157]

Although changes in FV do not always accurately reflect changes in CBF during cardiopulmonary bypass,[158,159] there

is little doubt about the benefits that TCD offers in detecting emboli both during and after cardiopulmonary bypass,[160-162] in testing cerebral autoregulation and CO$_2$ reactivity,[163] in comparing the effects of different techniques of blood gas management during cardiopulmonary bypass,[164] and in detecting hyperperfusion during cardiac surgery.[165] Furthermore, with the increase in minimally invasive cardiac surgery, TCD has been used to ensure correct positioning of endovascular aortic balloon clamps.[166]

Orthoptic Liver Transplantation

Portal-systemic encephalopathy, a major complication of acute and chronic liver disease, has clinical and subclinical manifestations.[167] Alterations in CBF are implicated in the etiology of portosystemic encephalopathy, with possible cerebral vasodilation resulting in cerebral edema and reduced CPP.

TCD has been used successfully in patients with hepatic failure to assess CO$_2$ reactivity and cerebral autoregulation. Although cerebral autoregulation is often impaired in acute liver failure and may be restored by mechanical hyperventilation, CO$_2$ reactivity seems to be less affected.[168,169] TCD may also provide the means to noninvasively estimate CPP in patients with liver failure with the use of methods similar to those described for head-injured patients. The advantages of not inserting ICP measuring devices in patients with liver failure, who are often coagulopathic, are self-evident. An example of TCD monitoring during liver transplantation with continuous assessment CPP by means of noninvasive CPP monitoring and of autoregulation using the Mx index is presented in Figure 8-9.

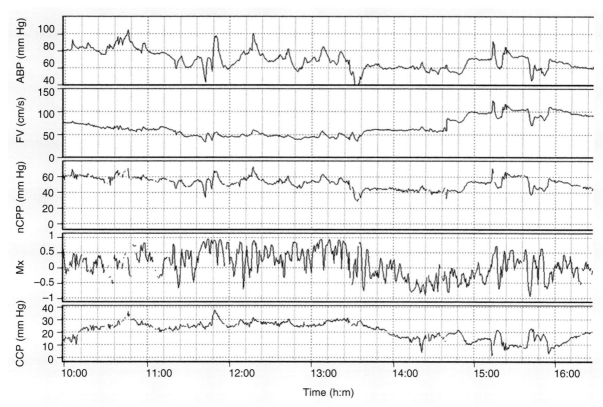

Figure 8–9 Example of arterial blood pressure (ABP) and transcranial Doppler ultrasonography (TCD) monitoring during liver transplantation. Note worsening of autoregulation (positive mean index [Mx] value) during anhepatic phase, which improves during reperfusion (after 14:30). During reperfusion, noninvasive cerebral perfusion pressure (nCPP) and blood flow velocity (FV) values gradually improve, and critical closing pressure (CCP) decreases (which may indicate either a decrease in intracranial pressure or gradual vasodilation).

Pregnancy and Eclampsia

Abnormal pregnancies are usually associated with impairment of the maternal cerebral circulation. TCD has been used in two studies to measure FV in normal pregnancies and in mothers with preeclampsia.[170,171] Up to 70% of abnormal pregnancies were found to be associated with higher FV than those in normal pregnancies.[170] Furthermore, the extent of toxemia was significantly correlated to the increase in FV, with progressive increases in FV often preceding neurologic symptoms.[170,171] Although the significance of cerebral vasospasm in preeclampsia remains controversial, the cause of this increase in FV requires further investigation. Noninvasive assessments of ICP, CPP, and autoregulatory reserve remain to be rediscovered in this pathology.

SUMMARY

TCD is a useful noninvasive means of monitoring cerebral hemodynamics, for which benefits have been demonstrated in many specific instances. This "window" on the brain has been severely disadvantaged by the lack of means for fixing the probe in position. Most fixation devices require constant adjustment and often interfere with the surgical field or the intensive care of the patient. Although the "Lam Frames," holders that attach to the ear canals and the bridge of the nose, seem to provide the most reliable intraoperative recordings (DWL Elektronische Systeme GmbH, Sipplingen, Germany), earplugs do not allow proper patient care and therefore make the frames unsuitable for long-term monitoring in intensive care. As manufacturers and clinicians continue to address the problem, more successful solutions will increase the use of this exciting technology, thereby improving our understanding of cerebral pathophysiology, and one hopes, patient care.

Indirect measurement of CBF using TCD is extremely useful. Not absolute values but the dynamical changes in CBF values contain enormous amounts of information about cerebrovascular reactivity, autoregulation, abnormalities within the circle of Willis and also small vessel behavior, transmural pressures (often compared with CPP), and ICP.

REFERENCES

1. Aaslid R, Markwalder TM, Nornes H: Non-invasive transcranial Doppler ultrasound recording of flow velocity in basal cerebral arteries, *J Neurosurg* 57:769, 1982.
2. Aaslid R: Transcranial Doppler examination techniques. In Aaslid R, editor: *Transcranial Doppler Sonography*, New York, 1986, Springer-Verlag, p 39.
3. Huber P, Handa J: Effect of contrast material, hypercapnia, hyperventilation, hypertonic glucose and papaverine on the diameter of the cerebral arteries: Angiographic determination in man, *Invest Radiol* 2:17, 1967.
4. Markwalder TM, Grolimund P, Seiler RW, et al: Dependency of blood flow velocity in the middle cerebral artery on end-tidal carbon dioxide partial pressure: A transcranial ultrasound Doppler study, *J Cereb Blood Flow Metab* 4:368, 1984.
5. Eng CC, Lam AM, Mayberg TS, et al: Influence of propofol and propofol-nitrous oxide anesthesia on cerebral blood flow velocity and carbon dioxide reactivity in humans, *Anesthesiology* 77:872, 1992.
6. Newell WD, Aaslid R, Lam AM, et al: Comparison of flow and velocity during dynamic autoregulation testing in humans, *Stroke* 25:793, 1994.

7. Giller CA, Bowman G, Dyer H, et al: Cerebral arterial diameters during changes in blood pressure and carbon dioxide during craniotomy, *Neurosurgery* 32:737, 1993.

8. Strebel SP, Kindler C, Bissonnette B, et al: The impact of systemic vasoconstrictors on the cerebral circulation of anesthetized patients, *Anesthesiology* 89:67, 1998.

9. Matta BF, Lam AM, Mayberg TS, et al: The cerebrovascular response to carbon dioxide during sodium nitroprusside- and isoflurane-induced hypotension, *Br J Anaesth* 74:296, 1995.

10. Dahl A, Russell D, Nyberg-Hansen R, et al: Effect of nitroglycerin on cerebral circulation measured by transcranial Doppler and SPECT, *Stroke* 20:1733, 1989.

11. Schregel W, Schafermeyer H, Muller C, et al: The effect of halothane, alfentanil and propofol on blood flow velocity, blood vessel cross section and blood volume flow in the middle cerebral artery, *Anaesthesist* 41:21, 1992.

12. Kochs E, Hoffman WE, Werner C, et al: Cerebral blood flow velocity in relation to cerebral blood flow, cerebral metabolic rate for oxygen, and electroencephalogram analysis during isoflurane anesthesia in dogs, *Anesth Analg* 76:1222, 1993.

13. Matta BF, Lam AM: Isoflurane and desflurane do not dilate the middle cerebral artery appreciably, *Br J Anaesth* 74:486P, 1995.

14. Schregel W, Schafermeyer H, Muller C, et al: The effect of halothane, alfentanil and propofol on blood flow velocity, blood vessel cross section and blood volume flow in the middle cerebral artery, *Anaesthesist* 41:21, 1992.

15. Matta BF, Mayberg TS, Lam AM: Direct cerebrovasodilatory effects of halothane, isoflurane and desflurane during propofol-induced isoelectric encephalogram in humans, *Anesthesiology* 83:980, 1995.

16. Schregel W, Schaefermeyer H, Sihle-Wissel M, et al: Transcranial Doppler sonography during isoflurane/N2O anesthesia and surgery: Flow velocity, "vessel area" and "volume flow.", *Can J Anaesth* 41:607, 1994.

17. Werner C, Kochs E, Reimer R, et al: The effect of postural changes on cerebral hemodynamics during general anesthesia, *Anaesthesist* 39:429, 1990.

18. Bissonette B, Leon JE: Cerebrovascular stability during isoflurane anaesthesia in children, *Can J Anaesth* 39:128, 1992.

19. Lam AM, Mayberg TS, Cooper JO, et al: Nitrous oxide is a more potent cerebrovasodilator than isoflurane in humans, *Anesth Analg* 78:462, 1994.

20. Kontos HA: Validity of cerebral arterial blood calculations from velocity measurements, *Stroke* 20:1, 1989.

21. Brauer P, Kochs E, Werner C, et al: Correlation of transcranial Doppler sonography mean flow velocity with cerebral blood flow in patients with intracranial pathology, *J Neurosurg Anesthesiol* 10:80, 1998.

22. Harders A: *Neurosurgical Applications of Transcranial Doppler Sonography*, Vienna, 1986, Springer-Verlag.

23. Harders A, Gilsbach J: Transcranial Doppler sonography and its application in extracranial-intracranial bypass surgery, *Neurol Res* 7:129, 1985.

24. Newell DW, Aaslid R: *Transcranial Doppler*, New York, 1992, Raven Press.

25. Bode H, Wais U: Age dependence of flow velocity in basal cerebral arteries, *Arch Dis Child* 63:606, 1988.

26. Adams RJ, Nichols FT, Stephens S: Transcranial Doppler: The influence of age and hematocrit in normal children, *J Cardiovasc Ultrasound* 7:201, 1988.

27. Arnolds BJ, von Reuten GM: Transcranial Doppler sonography: Examination technique and normal reference values, *Ultrasound Med Biol* 12:115, 1986.

28. Klotzsch C, Popescu O, Berlit P: A new 1 NHz probe for transcranial Doppler sonography in patients with inadequate temporal bone windows, *Ultrasound Med Biol* 24:101, 1998.

29. Grolimund P, Seiler RW: Age dependence of the flow velocity in the basal cerebral arteries: A transcranial Doppler ultrasound study, *Ultrasound Med Biol* 14:191, 1988.

30. Gabrielsen TO, Greitz T: Normal size of the internal carotid, middle cerebral and anterior cerebral arteries, *Acta Radiol* 10:1, 1970.

31. Kennedy C, Sokoloff L: An adaptation of nitrous oxide method to the study of the cerebral circulation in children: Normal values for cerebral blood flow and metabolic rate in childhood, *J Clin Invest* 36:1130, 1957.

32. Leenders KL, Perani D, Lammertsma AA, et al: Cerebral blood flow, blood volume and oxygen utilisation: Normal values and effect of age, *Brain* 113:27, 1990.

33. Heyman A, Patterson JL, Duke TW: Cerebral circulation and metabolism in sickle cell and other chronic anemias, with observations on the effects of oxygen inhalation, *J Clin Invest* 31:824, 1952.

34. Brass L, Pavlakis S, DeVivo D, et al: Transcranial Doppler measurements of the middle cerebral artery: Effect of hematocrit, *Stroke* 19:1466, 1988.

35. Thomas DJ, Marshall J, Ross Russell RW, et al: Effects of hematocrit on cerebral blood flow in man, *Lancet* 2(8564):941, 1987.

36. Vriens EM, Kraier V, Musbach M, et al: Transcranial pulsed Doppler measurements of blood velocity in the middle cerebral artery: Reference values at rest and during hyperventilation in healthy volunteers in relation to age and sex, *Ultrasound Med Biol* 15:1, 1989.

37. Brouwers P, Vriens EM, Musbach M, et al: Transcranial pulsed Doppler measurements of blood velocity in the middle cerebral artery: Reference values at rest and during hyperventilation in healthy children and adolescents in relation to age and sex, *Ultrasound Med Biol* 16:1, 1990.

38. Czosnyka M, Richards HK, Whitehouse HE, Pickard JD: Relationship between transcranial Doppler-determined pulsatility index and cerebrovascular resistance: An experimental study, *J Neurosurg* 84:79, 1996.

39. Gosling RG, King DH: Arterial assessment by Doppler shift ultrasound, *Proc R Soc Med* 67:447, 1974.

40. Planiol T, Purcelot L, Itti R: The carotid and cerebral circulations: Advances in its study by external physical methods. Principles, normal recordings, adopted parameters [French], *Nouv Presse Med* 37:2451, 1973.

41. Sorteberg W, Langmoen IA, Lindergaard KF, et al: Side to side differences and day to day variations of transcranial Doppler parameters in normal subjects, *J Ultrasound Med* 1009;9:403

42. Matta BF, Lam AM, Strebel S, et al: Cerebral pressure autoregulation and CO2-reactivity during propofol-induced EEG suppression, *Br J Anaesth* 74:159, 1995.

43. Strebel S, Kaufmann M, Guardiola P-M, et al: Cerebral vasomotor responsiveness to carbon dioxide is preserved during propofol and midazolam anesthesia in humans, *Anesth Analg* 78:884, 1994.

44. Hirst RP, Slee TA, Lam AM: Changes in cerebral blood flow velocity after release of intraoperative tourniquets in humans: A transcranial Doppler study, *Anesth Analg* 71:503, 1990.

45. Kirkham FJ, Padayachee TS, Parsons S, et al: Transcranial measurements of blood flow velocities in the basal arteries using pulsed Doppler ultrasound: Velocity as an index of flow, *Ultrasound Med Biol* 12:15, 1986.

46. Kaiser L: Adjusting for baseline: Change or % change? *Stat Med* 8:1183, 1989.

47. Dumville J, Panerai RB, Lennard NS, et al: Can cerebrovascular reactivity be assessed without measuring blood pressure in patients with carotid artery disease? *Stroke* 30:1293, 1999.

48. Cho S, Fujigaki T, Uchiyama Y, et al: Effects of sevoflurane with and without nitrous oxide on human cerebral circulation, *Anesthesiology* 85:755, 1996.

49. Paulson OB, Strandgaard S, Edvinsson L: Cerebral autoregulation, *Cerebrovasc Brain Metab Rev* 2:161, 1990.

50. Strandgaard S, Paulson OB: Cerebral autoregulation, *Stroke* 15:413, 1984.

51. Lassen NA: Cerebral blood flow and oxygen consumption in man, *Physiol Rev* 39:183, 1959.

52. Harper AM: Autoregulation of cerebral blood flow: influence of arterial blood pressure on the blood flow through the cerebral cortex, *J Neurol Neurosurg Psychiatry* 29:398, 1966.

53. Agnoli A, Fieschi C, Bozzao L, et al: Autoregulation of cerebral blood flow: Studies during drug-induced hypertension in normal subjects and in patients with cerebral vascular diseases, *Circulation* 38:800, 1968.

54. Smith AL, Neigh JL, Hoffman JC, et al: Effects of general anesthesia on autoregulation of cerebral blood flow in man., *J Appl Physiol* 29:665, 1970.

55. Miletich DJ, Ivankovich AD, Albrecht RF, et al: Absence of autoregulation of cerebral blood flow during halothane and enflurane anesthesia, *Anesth Analg* 55:100, 1976.

56. Held K, Niedermayer W, Gottstein U: Reactivity of cerebral blood flow to variations of transmural pressure, *Circulation* 43/44:11, 1971.

57. Aaslid R, Lindegaard KF, Sorteberg W, et al: Cerebral autoregulation in humans, *Stroke* 20:45, 1989.

58. Lam JM, Hsiang JN, Poon WS: Monitoring of autoregulation using laser Doppler flowmetry in patients with head injury, *J Neurosurg* 86:438, 1997.

59. Keller E, Wietasch G, Ringleb P, et al: Bedside monitoring of cerebral blood flow in patients with acute hemispheric stroke, *Crit Care Med* 28:511, 2000.

60. Reinhard M, Wehrle-Wieland E, Grabiak D, et al: Oscillatory cerebral hemodynamics—the macro- vs. microvascular level, *J Neurol Sci* 250:103, 2006.

61. Brady KM, Lee JK, Kibler KK, et al: Continuous time-domain analysis of cerebrovascular autoregulation using near-infrared spectroscopy, *Stroke* 38:2818, 2007.

62. Aaslid R, Newell DW, Stooss R, et al: Assessment of cerebral autoregulation dynamics from simultaneous arterial and venous transcranial Doppler recordings in humans, *Stroke* 22:1148, 1991.

63. Giller CA: A bedside test for cerebral autoregulation using transcranial Doppler ultrasound, *Acta Neurochir* 108:7, 1991.

64. Smielewski P, Czosnyka M, Kirkpatrick P, et al: Assessment of cerebral autoregulation using carotid artery compression, *Stroke* 27:2197, 1996.

65. Smielewski P, Czosnycka M, Kirkpatrick PJ, et al: Validation of the computerised transient hyperemic response test as a method of testing autoregulation in severely head injured patients, *J Neurotrauma* 12:420, 1995.

66. Tseng MY, Czosnyka M, Richards H, et al: Effects of acute treatment with pravastatin on cerebral vasospasm, autoregulation, and delayed ischemic deficits after aneurysmal subarachnoid hemorrhage: A phase II randomized placebo-controlled trial, *Stroke* 36:1627, 2005.

67. Diehl RR, Linden D, Lucke D, Berlit P: Phase relationship between cerebral blood flow velocity and blood pressure: A clinical test of autoregulation, *Stroke* 26:1801, 1995.

68. Tiecks FP, Lam AM, Aaslid R, Newell DW: Comparison of static and dynamic cerebral autoregulation measurements, *Stroke* 26:1014, 1995.

69. Czosnyka M, Smielewski P, Kirkpatrick P, et al: Monitoring of cerebral autoregulation in head-injured patients, *Stroke* 27:1829, 1996.

70. Czosnyka M, Smielewski P, Piechnik S, et al: Cerebral autoregulation following head injury, *J Neurosurg* 95:756, 2001.

71. Hassler W, Steinmetz H, Gawlowske J: Transcranial Doppler ultrasonography in raised intracranial pressure and in intracranial circulatory arrest, *J Neurosurg* 68:745, 1988.

72. Hassler W, Steinmetz H, Pirschel J: Transcranial Doppler study of intracranial circulatory arrest, *J Neurosurg* 71:195, 1989.

73. Am Homburg, Jakobsen M, Enevoldsen E: Transcranial Doppler recordings in raised intracranial pressure, *Acta Neurol Scand* 87:488, 1993.

74. Sanker P, Richard KE, Weigl HC, et al: Transcranial Doppler sonography and intracranial pressure monitoring in children and juveniles with acute brain pressure monitoring in children and juveniles with acute brain injuries or hydrocephalus, *Childs Nerv Syst* 7:391, 1991.

75. Chan KH, Miller DJ, Dearden M, et al: The effect of changes in cerebral perfusion pressure upon middle cerebral artery blood flow velocity and jugular bulb venous oxygen saturation after severe brain trauma, *J Neurosurg* 77:55, 1992.

76. Czosnyka M, Richards HK, White-house H, et al: Relationship between transcranial Doppler-determined pulsatility index and cerebrovascular resistance: An experimental study, *J Neurosurg* 84:79, 1996.

77. Aaslid R, Lundar T, Lindergaard KF, et al: Estimation of cerebral perfusion pressure from arterial blood pressure and transcranial Doppler recordings. In Miller JD, Teasdale GM, Rowan JO, et al, editors: *Intracranial Pressure* vol VI, Berlin, 1986, Springer-Verlag, p 226.

78. Czosnyka M, Matta BF, Smielewski P, et al: Cerebral perfusion pressure in head injured patients: A noninvasive assessment using transcranial Doppler ultrasonography, *J Neurosurg* 88:802, 1998.

80. Schmidt EA, Czosnyka M, Gooskens I, Piechnik, et al: Preliminary experience of the estimation of cerebral perfusion pressure using transcranial Doppler ultrasonography, *J Neurol Neurosurg Psychiatry* 70:198, 2001.

81. Schmidt B, Czosnyka M, Raabe A, et al: Adaptive noninvasive assessment of intracranial pressure and cerebral autoregulation, *Stroke* 34:84, 2003.

82. Dewey RC, Pieper HP, Hunt WE: Experimental cerebral hemodynamics: Vasomotor tone, critical closing pressure, and vascular bed resistance, *Neurosurgery* 41:597, 1974.

83. Aaslid R, Lash SR, Bardy GH, et al: Dynamic pressure—flow velocity relationships in the human cerebral circulation, *Stroke* 34:1645, 2003.

84. Panerai RB, Sammons EL, Smith SM, et al: Cerebral critical closing pressure estimation from Finapres and arterial blood pressure measurements in the aorta, *Physiol Meas* 27:1387, 2006.

85. Czosnyka M, Kirkpatrick E, Guazzo H, et al: Assessment of the autoregulatory reserve using continuous CPP and TCD blood flow velocity measurement in head injury. In Nagai H, Kamiya K, Ishii S, editors: *Intracranial Pressure IX (International Symposium on Intracranial Pressure)*, Berlin, 1994, Springer-Verlag, p 593.

86. Krul JMJ, van Gijn J, Ackerstaff RGA, et al: Site and pathogenesis of infarcts associated with carotid endarterectomy, *Stroke* 20:324, 1989.

87. Spencer MP: Transcranial Doppler monitoring and causes of stroke from carotid endarterectomy, *Stroke* 28:685, 1997.

88. Halsey JH, McDowell HA, Gelman S, et al: Blood velocity in the middle cerebral artery and regional cerebral blood flow during carotid endarterectomy, *Stroke* 20:53, 1989.

89. Jorgensen LG, Schroeder TV: Transcranial Doppler for detection of cerebral ischemia during carotid endarterectomy, *Eur J Vasc Surg* 6:142, 1992.

90. Powers AD, Smith RR, Graeber MC: Transcranial Doppler monitoring of cerebral flow velocities during surgical occlusion of the carotid artery, *Neurosurgery* 25:383, 1989.

91. Spencer MP, Thomas GI, Moehring MA: Relationship between middle cerebral artery blood flow velocity and stump pressure during carotid endarterectomy, *Stroke* 23:1439, 1992.

92. Steiger HJ, Schaffler L, Boll J, et al: Results of microsurgical carotid endarterectomy: A prospective study with transcranial Doppler sonography and EEG monitoring and elective shunting, *Acta Neurochir* 100:31, 1989.

93. Jansen C, Vriens EM, Eikelboom BC, et al: Carotid endarterectomy with transcranial Doppler and electroencephalographic monitoring: A prospective study in 130 operations, *Stroke* 24:665, 1993.

94. Halsey JH: Jr: Risks and benefits of shunting in carotid endarterectomy: The International Transcranial Doppler Collaborators, *Stroke* 23:1583, 1992.

95. Kalra M, al-Khaffaf H, Farrell A, et al: Comparison of measurement of stump pressure and transcranial measurement of flow velocity in the middle cerebral artery in carotid surgery, *Ann Vasc Surg* 8:225, 1994.

96. Naylor AR, Wildsmith JA, McClure J, et al: Transcranial Doppler monitoring during carotid endarterectomy, *Br J Surg* 78:1264, 1991.

97. Spencer MP, Gl Thomas, Nicholls SC, et al: Detection of middle cerebral artery emboli during carotid endarterectomy using transcranial Doppler ultrasonography, *Stroke* 21:415, 1990.

98. Jansen C, Ramos LM, van-Heesewijk JP, et al: Impact of microembolism and hemodynamic changes in the brain during carotid endarterectomy, *Stroke* 25:992, 1994.

99. Piepgras DG, Morgan MK, Sundt TM, et al: Intracerebral hemorrhage after carotid endarterectomy, *J Neurosurg* 68:532, 1988.

100. Sbarigia E, Speziale F, Giannoni MF, et al: Post-carotid endarterectomy hyperperfusion syndrome: Preliminary observations for identifying at risk patients by transcranial Doppler sonography and the acetazolamide test, *Eur J Vasc Surg* 7:252, 1993.

101. Powers AD, Smith RR: Hyperperfusion syndrome after carotid endarterectomy: A transcranial Doppler evaluation, *Neurosurgery* 26:56, 1990.

102. Naylor AR, Whyman M, Wildsmith JAW, et al: Immediate effects of carotid clamp release on middle cerebral artery blood flow velocity during carotid endarterectomy, *Eur J Vasc Surg* 7:308, 1993.

103. Jorgensen LG, Schroeder TV: Defective cerebrovascular autoregulation after carotid endarterectomy, *Eur J Vasc Surg* 7:370, 1993.

104. Jansen C, Sprengers AM, Moll FL, et al: Prediction of intracerebral haemorrhage after carotid endarterectomy by clinical criteria and intraoperative transcranial Doppler monitoring, *Eur J Vasc Surg* 8:303, 1994.

105. Gaunt ME, Ratliff DA, Martin PJ, et al: On-table diagnosis of incipient carotid artery thrombosis during carotid endarterectomy by transcranial Doppler scanning, *J Vasc Surg* 20:104, 1994.

106. Gooskens I, Schmidt EA, Czosnyka M, et al: Pressure-autoregulation, CO2 reactivity and asymmetry of haemodynamic parameters in patients with carotid artery stenotic disease: A clinical appraisal, *Acta Neurochir (Wien)* 145:527, 2003.

107. Reinhard M, Roth M, Müller T, et al: Effect of carotid endarterectomy or stenting on impairment of dynamic cerebral autoregulation, *Stroke* 35:1381, 2004.

108. Marcus HS, Tegeler CH: Experimental aspects of high intensity transient signals in the detection of emboli, *J Clin Ultrasound* 23:81, 1995.

109. Ringelstein EB, Droste DW, Babikian VL, et al: Consensus on microembolus detection by TCD: International consensus group on microemboli detection, *Stroke* 29:725, 1998.

110. Gravilescu T, Babikian VL, Cantelmo NL, et al: Cerebral microembolism during carotid endarterectomy, *Am J Surg* 170:159, 1995.

111. Gaunt ME, Martin PJ, Smith JJ, et al: Clinical relevance of intraoperative embolization detected by transcranial Doppler ultrasonography during carotid endarterectomy: A prospective study of 100 patients, *Br J Surg* 81:1435, 1994.

112. Schroeder T, Sillesen H, Sorensen O, et al: Cerebral hyperperfusion syndrome following carotid endarterectomy, *J Neurosurg* 28:824, 1987.

113. Weir B, Grace M, Hansen J, et al: Time course of vasospasm in man, *J Neurosurg* 48:173, 1978.

114. Kassell NF, Torner JC, Jane JA, et al: The international co-operative study on the timing of aneurysm surgery. Part 1: Overall management results, *J Neurosurg* 73:18, 1990.

115. Macdonald RL, Weir BKA: A review of hemoglobin and the pathogenesis of cerebral vasospasm, *Stroke* 22:971, 1991.

116. Aaslid R, Huber P, Nornes H: Evaluation of cerebrovascular spasm with transcranial Doppler ultrasound, *J Neurosurg* 60:37, 1984.

117. Lindegaard KF, Nornes H, Bakke SJ, et al: Cerebral vasospasm after subarachnoid hemorrhage investigated by means of transcranial Doppler ultrasound, *Acta Neurochirurg* 24:81, 1988.

118. Lam JM, Smielewski P, Czosnyka M, et al: Predicting delayed ischemic deficits after aneurysmal subarachnoid hemorrhage using a transient hyperemic response test of cerebral autoregulation, *Neurosurgery* 47:819, 2000.

119. Soehle M, Czosnyka M, Pickard JD, Kirkpatrick PJ: Continuous assessment of cerebral autoregulation in subarachnoid hemorrhage, *Anesth Analg* 98:1133, 2004.

120. Eng CC, Lam AM, Byrd S, et al: The diagnosis and management of a perianesthetic cerebral aneurysmal rupture aided with transcranial Doppler ultrasonography, *Anesthesiology* 78:191, 1993.

121. Giller CA, Giller AM, Landreneau F: Detection of emboli after surgery for intracerebral aneurysms, *Neurosurgery* 42:490, 1998.

122. Giller CA, Mathews D, Walker B, et al: Prediction of tolerance to carotid artery occlusion using transcranial Doppler ultrasound, *J Neurosurg* 81:15, 1994.

123. Hassler W, Steinmetz H: Cerebral hemodynamics in angioma patients: An intraoperative study, *J Neurosurg* 67:822, 1987.

124. Fleischer LH, Young WL, Pile-Spellman J, et al: Relationship of transcranial Doppler flow velocities and arteriovenous malformation feeding artery pressures, *Stroke* 24:1897, 1993.

125. Lindegaard KF, Grolimund P, Aaslid R, et al: Evaluation of cerebral arteriovenous malformations using transcranial Doppler ultrasound, *J Neurosurg* 65:335, 1986.

126. Massaro AR, Young WL, Kader A, et al: Characterisation of arteriovenous malformation feeding vessels by carbon dioxide reactivity, *Am J Neuroradiol* 15:55, 1994.

127. Diehl RR, Henkes H, Nahser HC, et al: Blood flow velocity and vasomotor reactivity in patients with arteriovenous malformations: A transcranial Doppler study, *Stroke* 25:1574, 1994.

128. De Salles AA, Manchola I: CO2 reactivity in arteriovenous malformations of the brain: A transcranial Doppler ultrasound study, *J Neurosurg* 80:624, 1994.

129. Chioffi F, Pasqualin A, Beltramello A, et al: Hemodynamic effects of preoperative embolization in cerebral arteriovenous malformations: Evaluation with transcranial Doppler sonography, *Neurosurgery* 31:877, 1992.

130. Petty GW, Massaro AR, Tatemichi TK, et al: Transcranial Doppler ultrasonographic changes after treatment for arteriovenous malformations, *Stroke* 21:260, 1990.

131. Kader A, Young WL, Massaro AR, et al: Transcranial Doppler changes during staged surgical resection of cerebral arteriovenous malformations: A report of three cases, *Surg Neurol* 39:392, 1993.

132. Pasqualin A, Barone G, Cioffi F, et al: The relevance of anatomic and hemodynamic factors to a classification of cerebral arteriovenous malformations, *Neurosurgery* 28:370, 1991.

133. Spetzler RF, Wilson CB, Weinstein P: Normal perfusion pressure breakthrough theory, *Clin Neurosurg* 25:651, 1978.

134. Matta BF, Lam AM, Winn HR: The intraoperative use of transcranial Doppler ultrasonography during resection of arteriovenous malformations, *Br J Anaesth* 75:242P, 1995.

135. Marmarou A, Anderson RL, Ward JD, et al: Impact of ICP instability and hypotension on outcome in patients with severe head trauma, *J Neurosurg* 75:S59, 1991.

136. Andrews PJD: What is the optimal cerebral perfusion pressure after brain injury: A review of the evidence with an emphasis on arterial pressure, *Acta Anaesthesiol Scand* 39:112, 1995.

137. Kirkpatrick PJ, Czosnyka M, Pickard JD: Multimodality monitoring in intensive care, *J Neurol Neurosurg Psychiatry* 60:131, 1996.

138. Miller JD: Head injury and rain ischemia: Implications for therapy, *Br J Anaesth* 57:120, 1985.

139. Junger EC, Newell DW, Grant GA, et al: Cerebral autoregulation after minor head injury, *J Neurosurg* 86:425, 1997.

140. Strebel S, Lam AM, Matta BF, et al: Impaired cerebral autoregulation after mild brain injury, *Surg Neurol* 47:128, 1997.

141. Czosnycka M, Smielewski P, Kirkpatrick P, et al: Monitoring of cerebral autoregulation in head injured patients, *Stroke* 27:1829, 1996.

142. Matta BF, Risdall J, Menon DK, et al: The effect of propofol on cerebral autoregulation after head injury: A preliminary report, *Br J Anaesth* 78:A237, 1997.

143. Chan KH, Dearden NM, Miller JD: The significance of posttraumatic increase in cerebral blood flow velocity: A transcranial Doppler ultrasound study, *Neurosurgery* 30:697, 1992.

144. Martin NA, Patwardhan RV, Alexander MJ, et al: Characterisation of cerebral hemodynamic phases following severe head trauma: Hypoperfusion, hyperemia, and vasospasm, *J Neurosurg* 87:9, 1997.

145. Lee JH, Martin NA, Alsinda G, et al: Hemodynamically significant cerebral vasospasm and outcome after head injury, *J Neurosurg* 87:221, 1997.

146. Rommer B, Bellner J, Kongstad P, et al: Elevated transcranial Doppler flow velocities after severe head injury: Cerebral vasospasm or hyperemia? *J Neurosurg* 85:90, 1996.

147. Schalöen W, Messeter K, Nordstrom CH: Cerebral vasoreactivity and the prediction of outcome in severe traumatic brain lesions, *Acta Anaesthesiol Scand* 35:113, 1991.

148. Werner C, Kochs E, Rau M, et al: Transcranial Doppler sonography as a supplement in the detection of cerebral circulatory arrest, *J Neurosurg Anesthesiol* 2:159, 1990.

149. Feri M, Ralli L, Felici M, et al: Transcranial Doppler and brain death diagnosis, *Crit Care Med* 22:1120, 1994.

150. Zanette EM, Fieschi C, Bozzao L, et al: Comparison of cerebral angiography and transcranial Doppler sonography in acute stroke, *Stroke* 20:899, 1989.

151. Toni D, Fiorelli M, Zanette EM, et al: Early spontaneous improvement and deterioration of ischemic stroke patients: A serial study with transcranial Doppler ultrasonography, *Stroke* 29:1144, 1998.

152. Fieschi C, Argentino C, Lenzi GL, et al: Clinical and instrumental evaluation of patients with ischemic stroke within 6 hours, *J Neurol Sci* 91:311, 1989.

153. Zanette EM, Roberti C, Mancini G, et al: Spontaneous middle cerebral artery reperfusion in ischemic stroke: A follow up study with transcranial Doppler, *Stroke* 26:430, 1995.

154. Alexandrov AV, Black SE, Ehrlich LE, et al: Prediction of hemorrhagic transformation occurring spontaneously and on anticoagulants in patients with acute ischemic stroke, *Stroke* 28:1198, 1997.

155. Sliwa U, Lingnau A, Stohlman WD, et al: Prevalence and time course of microembolic signals in patients with acute stroke: A prospective study, *Stroke* 28:358, 1997.

156. Yasaka M, O'Keefe GJ, Chambers BR, et al: Streptokinase in acute stroke: Effect on reperfusion and recanalization. Australian Streptokinase Trial Study Group, *Neurology* 50:626, 1998.

157. Murkin JM: Anesthesia, the brain, and cardiopulmonary bypass, *Ann Thorac Surg* 56:1461, 1993.

158. Vander Linden J, Wesslen O, Ekroth R, et al: Transcranial Doppler estimated versus thermodilution-estimated cerebral blood flow during cardiac operations, *J Thorac Cardiovasc Surg* 102:95, 1991.

159. Grocott HP, Amory DW, Lowry E, et al: Transcranial Doppler blood flow velocity versus 133Xe clearance cerebral blood flow during mild hypothermic cardiopulmonary bypass, *J Clin Monit Comput* 14:35, 1998.

160. Van der Linden J, Casmir-Ahn H: When do cerebral emboli appear during open heart operations? A transcranial Doppler study, *Ann Thorac Surg* 51:237, 1991.

161. Clarke RE, Brillman J, Davis DA, et al: Microemboli during coronary artery bypass grafting: Genesis and effect on outcome, *J Thorac Cardiovasc Surg* 109:249, 1995.

162. Grocott HP, Croughwell ND, Amory DW, et al: Cerebral emboli and serum S100beta during cardiac operations, *Ann Thorac Surg* 65:1645, 1998.

163. Lundar T, Lindegaard KF, Froysaker T, et al: Dissociation between cerebral autoregulation and carbon dioxide reactivity during non pulsatile cardiopulmonary bypass, *Ann Thorac Surg* 40:582, 1985.

164. Venn GE, Patel RL, Chambers DJ: Cardiopulmonary bypass: Perioperative cerebral blood flow and postoperative cognitive deficit, *Ann Thorac Surg* 59:1331, 1995.

165. Briliman J, Davis D, Clark RE, et al: Increased middle cerebral artery flow velocity during the initial phase of cardiopulmonary bypass may cause neurological dysfunction, *J Neuroimaging* 5:135, 1995.

166. Grocott HP, Smith MS, Glower DD, et al: Endovascular aortic balloon clamp malposition during minimally invasive cardiac surgery: Detection by transcranial Doppler monitoring, *Anesthesiology* 88:1396, 1998.

167. Gitlin N, Lewis DC, Hinckley L: The diagnosis and prevalence of subclinical hepatic encephalopathy in apparently healthy, ambulant, nonshunted patients with cirrhosis, *J Hepatol* 3:75, 1986.

168. Katz JJ, Mandell MS, House RM, et al: Cerebral blood flow velocity in patients with subclinical portal-systemic encephalopathy, *Anesth Analg* 86:1005, 1998.

169. Strauss G, Hansen BA, Knudsen GM, et al: Hyperventilation restores cerebral blood flow autoregulation in patients with acute liver failure, *J Hepatol* 28:199, 1998.

170. Demarin V, Rundek T, Hodek B: Maternal cerebral circulation in normal and abnormal pregnancies, *Acta Obstet Gynecol Scand* 76:619, 1997.

171. Hansen WF, Burnham SJ, Svendsen TO, et al: Transcranial Doppler findings of cerebral vasospasm in preeclampsia, *J Matern Fetal Med* 5:194, 1996.

Chapter 9

FLUID MANAGEMENT DURING CRANIOTOMY

Renata Rusa • Mark H. Zornow

The intraoperative fluid management of neurosurgical patients presents special challenges for the anesthesiologist. Neurosurgical patients often experience rapid changes in intravascular volume caused by hemorrhage, the administration of potent diuretics, or the onset of diabetes insipidus. The administration of volatile anesthetics and potent vasodilators during surgery may contribute to decreased cardiac filling pressures without causing actual changes in intravascular volume. In the midst of this dynamic situation, the anesthesiologist often faces the additional concern of minimizing increases in cerebral water content and, thus, intracranial pressure. Intracranial hypertension secondary to cerebral edema is now known to be one of the most common causes of morbidity and mortality in the intraoperative and postoperative periods.

In this chapter, we examine some of the physical determinants of water movement between the intravascular space and the central nervous system. Then we address specific clinical situations and make suggestions for the types and volumes of fluids to be administered.

OSMOLALITY, ONCOTIC PRESSURE, AND INTRAVASCULAR VOLUME

Osmolality

Osmolality is one of the four colligative properties of a solution. (The other three are vapor pressure, freezing point depression, and boiling point elevation.) The addition of 1 osmole of any solute to 1 kg of water causes the vapor pressure to fall by 0.3 mm Hg, the freezing point to drop by 1.85° C, and the boiling point to rise by 0.52° C.[1] The colligative properties are determined solely by the *number* of particles in solution and are independent of the chemical structure of the solute. The solute may exist in either an ionized or a nonionized state, and the size (molecular weight) of the solute is of no importance. Although it may seem counterintuitive, equimolar concentrations of glucose, urea, and mannitol have the same effect on the colligative properties of a solution. Osmolality is strictly a function of the number of particles in solution.

For physiologic solutions, *osmolality* is commonly expressed as milliosmoles (mOsm) *per kilogram of solvent*, whereas the units of measure for *osmolarity* are milliosmoles *per liter of solution*. For dilute solutions (including most of those of physiologic importance), the two terms may be used interchangeably. Osmolarity can be calculated if the molecular weight of the solute and its tendency to disassociate in solution are known (Boxes 9-1 and 9-2). The osmolarities of some commonly used intravenous fluids are listed in Table 9-1.

Osmolarity is important in determining fluid movement between various physiologic compartments because of the osmotic pressure that is generated when solutions of unequal osmolarity are separated by a membrane permeable to water but not to solutes. According to the second law of thermodynamics, which states that all systems spontaneously change to maximize entropy, water has a tendency to move from the solution of lower osmolarity, across the membrane, and into the solution of higher osmolarity (Fig. 9-1).

This process continues until the solutions are of equal osmolarity or the hydrostatic pressure is sufficient to preclude any further net flow of water across the membrane. The hydrostatic pressure that can be generated by osmolar differences is formidable and may be calculated by the following equation:

$$\pi = CRT$$

where π is osmotic pressure in atmospheres, C is concentration of all osmotically active solutes in the solution (in moles per liter), R is gas constant (0.08206 liter-atm/mole-degree), and T is temperature in degrees Kelvin (° K).

BOX 9–1 *Calculate the Osmolarity of a 0.9% Solution of Saline*

Fact: The molecular weight of NaCl is 58.43 g/mol.

Fact: A 0.9% solution of NaCl contains 9 g of NaCl per 1000 mL of solution.

The first step is to calculate the molarity of the 0.9% solution. To do this, we divide 9 g/L by 58.43 g/mol, which equals 0.154 mol/L or a 154 mmol/L solution of NaCl. Because each molecule of NaCl disassociates in water into a Na^+ and a Cl^- ion, we multiply the molar value by 2 to get an osmolarity of 308 mOsm/L. This value corresponds to the osmolarity listed on any container of 0.9% saline.

BOX 9–2 *Calculation of Osmotic Pressure*

Calculate the osmotic pressure generated by a 1 mOsm difference in osmolarity at body temperature and express the results in millimeters of mercury.

Formula for calculation of osmotic pressure is as follows:

$$\pi = CRT$$

where:

$C = 0.001$ mol/L (i.e., 1 mOsm/L)
$R = 0.08206$
$T = 273°$ K $+ 36°$ K $= 309°$ K (body temperature)

Therefore:

$$\pi = 0.001 \times 0.08206 \times 309° = 0.02535 \text{ atm}$$
$$\text{or } 19.27 \text{ mm Hg}$$

Table 9–1 Osmolarity of Commonly Used Intravenous Fluids

Fluid	Osmolarity (mOsm/L)	Oncotic Pressure (mm Hg)
Lactated Ringer's solution	273	0
D$_5$ lactated Ringer's solution	525	0
0.9% saline	308	0
D$_5$ 0.45% saline	406	0
0.45% saline	154	0
20% mannitol	1098	0
Hetastarch (6%)	310	31[2]
Dextran 40 (10%)	≈300	169[3]
Dextran 70 (6%)	≈300	69[3]
Albumin (5%)	290	19
Plasma	295	26

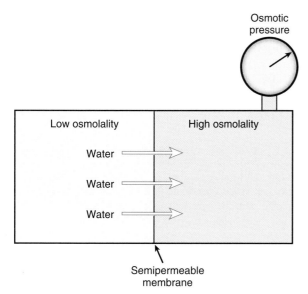

Figure 9–1 When solutions of unequal osmolality are separated by a semipermeable membrane, water moves from the solution of lower osmolality through the membrane and into the more concentrated solution. This process continues until the solutions are of equal osmolality or the osmotic pressure reaches the point that no further net flux of water across the membrane is possible.

On the basis of this formula, a pressure of more than 19 mm Hg is generated for each milliosmole difference across a semipermeable membrane (see Box 9-2). Thus, osmolar differences can provide a potent driving force for the movement of water between the intracellular and extracellular spaces and, as seen later, across the blood-brain barrier. Although osmolar gradients can be produced by administering hypo-osmolar or hyperosmolar fluids, these gradients are fleeting; and water moves from one compartment to another so that all body fluids are again of equal osmolarity.

Oncotic Pressure

Oncotic pressure is the osmotic pressure generated by solutes larger than an arbitrary limit (usually 30,000 molecular weight [MW]). Albumin (69,000 approximate MW), heta-starch (480,000 mean MW), dextran 40 (40,000 mean MW),

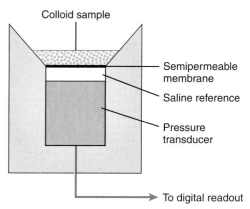

Figure 9–2 Oncotic pressure of various fluids can be measured with the use of a simple device constructed from a pressure transducer and semipermeable membrane. The chamber containing a saline reference is positioned above the pressure transducer and is separated from the sample well by a semipermeable membrane. The colloidal fluid being tested is placed in the sample well. Oncotic pressure of the colloidal fluid draws a small volume of saline across the semipermeable membrane, thereby creating a negative pressure above the pressure transducer. This pressure, which is digitally displayed, represents the oncotic pressure of the colloidal sample.

and dextran 70 (70,000 mean MW) are compounds of clinical interest that are capable of exerting oncotic pressure. Reported values for the oncotic pressures of plasma, mannitol, albumin, and hetastarch are listed in Table 9-1.[2,3] The oncotic pressure produced by all plasma proteins (e.g., albumin, globulins, fibrinogen) accounts for less than 0.5% of total plasma osmotic pressure. The oncotic pressure of various solutions can be easily measured with an electronic pressure transducer and a membrane that is freely permeable to low-molecular-weight (LMW) solutes but that prevents the passage of particles greater than 30,000 MW (Fig. 9-2).

Determinants of Fluid Movement between Vasculature and Tissues

Nearly 100 years ago, Ernest Starling described the forces that determine the movement of water between tissues and the intravascular space.[4] This description was subsequently formalized in what is now known as the Starling equation, as follows[5]:

$$Q_f = K_f S [(P_c - P_t) - \sigma(\pi_c - \pi_t)]$$

where Q_f is net amount of fluid that moves between the capillary lumen and the surrounding extracellular space (interstitium)

K_f is filtration coefficient for the membrane, S is surface area of the capillary membrane

P_c is hydrostatic pressure in the capillary lumen

P_t is hydrostatic pressure (usually negative) in the extracellular space of the surrounding tissue, σ is the coefficient of reflection—this number, which can range from 1 (no movement of the solute across the membrane) to 0 (free diffusion of the solute across the membrane), quantitates the "leakiness" of the capillary and is different for vessels in the brain and those in peripheral tissues—π_c is oncotic pressure of the plasma

π_t is oncotic pressure of the fluid in the extracellular space.[5]

Capillary pressure, tissue pressure (negative in nonedematous tissues), and tissue oncotic pressure all act to draw fluid from the capillaries and into the extracellular space of the tissue (Fig. 9-3). In peripheral tissues, the only factor that serves to maintain intravascular volume is the plasma oncotic

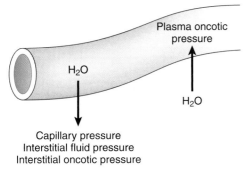

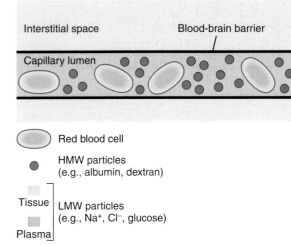

Red blood cell

HMW particles
(e.g., albumin, dextran)

Tissue

LMW particles
(e.g., Na⁺, Cl⁻, glucose)

Plasma

Figure 9–3 In peripheral tissues, four forces act on intravascular water: Capillary hydrostatic pressure, interstitial fluid pressure (negative in most tissues), and interstitial oncotic pressure (exerted by proteins in the interstitial space) act to draw water from the intravascular space into the interstitium. The only force that acts to maintain intravascular volume is plasma oncotic pressure. This last force is produced by the presence in plasma of high-molecular-weight proteins that cannot cross the capillary wall.

Figure 9–5 In cerebral capillaries, the blood-brain barrier (estimated pore size of 7-9 Å) prevents movement of even very small particles between the capillary lumen and the brain's interstitial space. Increasing plasma osmolality by intravenous infusion of mannitol or hypertonic saline can therefore establish an osmotic gradient between the brain and intravascular space that acts to move water from the brain into capillaries. HMW, high-molecular-weight; LMW, low-molecular-weight.

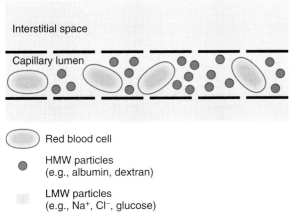

Red blood cell

HMW particles
(e.g., albumin, dextran)

LMW particles
(e.g., Na⁺, Cl⁻, glucose)

Figure 9–4 In peripheral capillaries, free movement of most low-molecular-weight (LMW) particles (including sodium and chloride ions, glucose, and mannitol) occurs between the capillary lumen and the interstitial space. Intravenous administration of low-molecular-weight solutes cannot affect the movement of water between the interstitium and vasculature because no osmotic gradient can be established. In contrast, a rise in plasma oncotic pressure from the administration of concentrated albumin, hetastarch, or dextran may draw water from the interstitium into the vessels because these high-molecular-weight (HMW) particles are precluded from passing through the capillary wall. Hypertonic saline solutions create an osmotic gradient across cell membranes and thus transfer fluid from the intracellular to the extracellular compartment, including the intravascular space.

flux exceeds the drainage capacity of the lymphatics, clinically apparent edema results.

Another example of the Starling equation in action is the facial edema that is often seen in patients who have been placed in the Trendelenburg position for prolonged periods. In this case, the edema is due not to a decrease in plasma oncotic pressure but rather to an increase in the capillary hydrostatic pressure (P_c), favoring an increased transudation of fluid into the tissue.

Fluid Movement between Capillaries and the Brain

The Starling equation describes the factors that govern fluid movement between the intravascular and peripheral extracellular spaces (e.g., the interstitium of lung, bowel, and muscle). However, the brain and spinal cord are unlike most other tissues in the body in that they are isolated from the intravascular compartment by the blood-brain barrier. Morphologically, this barrier is now thought to be composed of endothelial cells that form tight junctions in the capillaries supplying the brain and spinal cord. In normal brain, these tight junctions severely limit the diffusion of molecules between the intravascular space and the brain. By measuring the movement of water out of the central nervous system after abrupt changes in plasma osmolality, Fenstermacher and Johnson[6] calculated the effective pore radius for the blood-brain barrier to be only 7 to 9 Å. This small pore size of the blood-brain barrier prevents movement not only of plasma proteins but also of sodium, chloride, and potassium ions between the intravascular compartment and the brain's extracellular space (Fig. 9-5). In effect, the blood-brain barrier acts like the semipermeable membrane of an osmometer, and movement of water across this membrane is determined by the relative concentrations of impermeable solutes.

This situation is markedly different in peripheral tissues, where endothelial cells do not form tight junctions and pore sizes in the capillaries may be as much as several orders of magnitude greater. Although these pores are small enough

pressure, which is produced predominantly by albumin and to a lesser extent by immunoglobulins, fibrinogen, and other high-molecular-weight (HMW) plasma proteins (Fig. 9-3).

Under most circumstances, the sum of the forces results in a Q_f value that is slightly greater than zero, indicating a net outward flux of fluid from the vessels into the tissue extracellular space. This fluid is cleared from the tissue by the lymphatic system, thereby preventing the development of edema (Fig. 9-4).

The clinical effects of altering one or more of the variables in the Starling equation may frequently be observed in the operating room. Many patients who have been resuscitated from hemorrhagic hypovolemia with large volumes of crystalloid solutions demonstrate pitting edema, caused by a dilution of plasma proteins. This results in a decrease in intravascular oncotic pressure (π_c). In the presence of relatively unchanged capillary hydrostatic pressure, an increased movement of fluid from the vasculature into the tissues occurs. When this fluid to preclude the movement of most protein components of plasma, electrolytes pass freely from the capillary lumen into the extracellular space. Thus, in peripheral tissues, movement of water between the intravascular space and the extravascular space is governed by the plasma concentration of large macromolecules (oncotic gradient) as defined by the Starling equation. In contrast, fluid moves in and out of the central nervous system according to the *osmolar* gradient (determined by relative concentrations of all osmotically active particles, including most electrolytes) between the plasma and the extracellular fluid. This difference in the determinants of fluid flux explains why the administration of large volumes of iso-osmolar crystalloid results in peripheral edema caused by dilutional reduction of plasma protein content but does not increase brain water content or intracranial pressure (ICP).

There can be little doubt that osmolarity is the primary determinant of water movement across the intact blood-brain barrier.[7] The administration of excess free water (either iatrogenically or as a result of psychogenic polydipsia) can result in an increased ICP and an edematous brain.[8] Conversely, the intravenous administration of markedly hyperosmolar crystalloids (e.g., mannitol) to increase plasma osmolarity results in a decrease in brain water content and ICP. Hyperosmolar solutions are used daily in operating rooms throughout the world as standard therapeutic agents to treat intracranial hypertension.

In the presence of an intact blood-brain barrier, plasma osmolarity is the key determinant of water movement between the central nervous system and the intravascular space. However, what occurs when the brain is injured with disruption of the barrier? If the blood-brain barrier is partially disrupted, will blood vessels in the brain start to act more like peripheral capillaries? Experimental evidence is not conclusive, but if the injury is of sufficient severity to allow extravasation of plasma proteins into the interstitial space (i.e., capillaries have become "leaky"), plasma oncotic pressure does not affect water movement, because no oncotic gradient between the plasma and the brain interstitial space can be produced (i.e., the proteins leak out of the capillaries and into the brain tissue) (Fig. 9-6). In an animal study using a cryogenic lesion as a model of acute brain injury, a 50% decrease in plasma oncotic pressure had no effect on regional water content or ICP.[9] These results were confirmed in a subsequent study that demonstrated that reducing the plasma oncotic pressure from approximately 21 mm Hg to 10 mm Hg for 8 hours had no effect on ICP or brain water content in animals with a cryogenic brain injury despite the fact that the anticipated increase in water content was documented in peripheral tissues (muscle and jejunum).[10]

Despite a lack of convincing experimental evidence that iso-osmolar crystalloids are detrimental, the neurosurgical literature is filled with admonitions to restrict the use of crystalloids in patients at risk for intracranial hypertension.[11] The infusion of colloids is often recommended to maintain intravascular volume in such patients, implying that maintaining or increasing plasma oncotic pressure reduces cerebral edema. In the case of the intact blood-brain barrier, neither theoretical nor experimental evidence suggests that colloids are more beneficial than crystalloids for either brain water content or ICP. The crystalloid-colloid question has been addressed in animal models of cerebral injury, with varying and sometimes conflicting results. Warner and Boehland[12] studied the effects of hemodilution with either saline or 6% hetastarch in rats subjected to 10 minutes of severe forebrain ischemia. Despite an approximately 50% reduction in plasma oncotic pressure

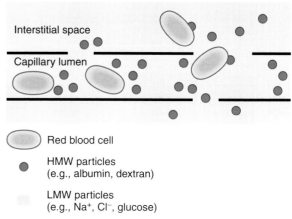

Figure 9–6 After a variety of brain injuries (e.g., ischemia, contusion), breakdown of the blood-brain barrier may occur, allowing both low-molecular-weight (LMW) and high-molecular-weight (HMW) particles to escape from the capillary lumen (i.e., the capillaries become "leaky"). In severe cases, extravasation of red blood cells into the interstitium may even occur. In this situation, neither hyperosmolar nor hyperoncotic solutions will help reduce edema formation in the area of the injury. Hyperosmolar solutions may still be beneficial in areas remote from the injury, where the blood-brain barrier remains intact.

in the saline group (from 17.2 ± 0.8 to 9 ± 0.6 mm Hg), no beneficial effect in terms of decreased edema formation was demonstrated in the hetastarch group. Similarly, in a study that used a cryogenic lesion as a model of cerebral injury, Zornow and colleagues[9] found no differences in regional water content or ICP between animals that received saline, those that received 6% hetastarch, and those that received albumin.

In contrast, Korosue and associates[13] found a smaller infarct volume and better neurologic status in dogs undergoing hemodilution with a colloid (LMW dextran) than in animals undergoing hemodilution with lactated Ringer's solution after ligation of the middle cerebral artery. The researchers speculated (but did not provide evidence) that this beneficial effect was due to decreased edema formation in the ischemic zone. They further speculated that, in this model of moderate ischemic injury, the blood-brain barrier may become selectively permeable to ions with preservation of its impermeability to high-molecular-weight compounds (e.g., dextran and proteins). If this is the case, then the brain tissue in the ischemic region may act very much like tissues in the periphery (i.e., decreases in plasma oncotic pressure result in increased water movement into the tissue). A study by Drummond and coworkers[14] suggests that a similar situation may occur after traumatic brain injury. They subjected anesthetized rats to a 2.7 atm fluid percussion injury and then hemodilution with normal saline or a colloid. Brain water content was increased in the animals that received the normal saline. Thus, although the osmolality of the infused solution is the primary determinant of water movement between the vasculature and brain tissue in the noninjured state, apparently in cases of ischemic or traumatic injury, colloids may or may not be beneficial, depending on the severity and extent of the injury as well as the time at which brain water content is measured.

Beneficial effects of hypertonic solutions in cases of localized brain injury with disruption of the blood-brain barrier appear to be derived primarily from the ability of hypertonic solutions to cause a fluid flux out of brain tissue where the blood-brain barrier remains intact. In effect, normal brain is dehydrated to compensate for the edema that forms in the vicinity of the lesion. Using a cryogenic lesion to model brain injury in the laboratory, Zornow and associates[15] found that the infusion of a hypertonic solution attenuated the increase in ICP associated with this lesion but did not have a significant effect on the water content of brain tissue at the lesion site or in its immediate vicinity. The most likely mechanism for this beneficial effect is a decrease in brain water content in regions remote from the lesion.

SOLUTIONS FOR INTRAVENOUS USE

The anesthesiologist may choose from among a variety of fluids suitable for intravenous administration. These fluids may be categorized conveniently on the basis of osmolality, oncotic pressure, and dextrose content. The term *crystalloid* is commonly applied to solutions that do not contain high-molecular-weight compounds and thus have an oncotic pressure of zero. Crystalloids may be hyperosmolar, hypo-osmolar, or iso-osmolar and may or may not contain dextrose. Some commonly used crystalloid solutions are listed in Table 9-1. Crystalloids may be made hyperosmolar by the inclusion of electrolytes (e.g., Na^+ and Cl^-, as in hypertonic saline) or LMW solutes, such as mannitol (182 MW), glycerol (92 MW), glucose (180 MW), or urea (60 MW). Urea and glycerol are now rarely used because over time they penetrate the blood-brain barrier and may cause worsening of intracranial hypertension hours after their initial beneficial effect.[16]

The term *colloid* denotes solutions that have an oncotic pressure similar to that of plasma. Some commonly administered colloids are 6% hetastarch (Hespan), 5% and 25% albumin, the dextrans (40 and 70), and plasma. Dextran and hetastarch are dissolved in normal saline, so the osmolarity of the solution is approximately 290 to 310 mOsm/L with a sodium and chloride ion content of about 145 mEq/L.

Hyperosmolar Solutions

There is renewed interest in using hyperosmotic fluids to resuscitate patients with hemorrhagic hypovolemia. The reputed advantages of such solutions include a more rapid resuscitation with smaller infused volumes, improved cardiac output, decreased peripheral resistance, and lower ICP.[17] Benefits of a variety of hypertonic solutions in terms of ICP and cerebral blood flow have been demonstrated in a number of animal models.[15,18-21] Clearly, these solutions exert at least part of their beneficial effects by osmotically shifting water from the interstitial and intracellular spaces of the central nervous system to the intravascular space. Additional benefit may be derived from a reported reduction in cerebrospinal fluid production.[22]

Although an acute beneficial effect has been demonstrated, the longer-term (24-48 hours) effect of such hyperosmotic fluid therapy remains unknown. One primary area of concern is the hypernatremia that results from many of these solutions. Although survival has been reported with serum sodium levels as high as 202 mEq/L, acute increases to values that exceed 170 mEq/L are likely to result in a depressed level of consciousness or seizures.[23] Even with the administration of relatively small volumes (4.5 L) of moderately hypertonic saline (Na, 250 mEq/L; osmolarity, 514 mOsm/L), Shackford and coworkers[24,25] reported that serum sodium levels peaked at over 155 mEq/L in the postoperative period.

Several studies have reported a beneficial effect of hypertonic saline solutions in patients with intracranial hypertension. In one report, the administration of small volumes of markedly hypertonic saline in two patients resulted in a striking and sustained diminution in ICP. Both patients had suffered closed-head injuries with ICPs in the range of 30 to 50 mm Hg. After conventional therapy with repeated doses of mannitol and hyperventilation had failed, 100 to 250 mmol of hypertonic saline was administered, resulting in prompt control of the intracranial hypertension.[26] In a second study involving eight patients with a total of 20 episodes of intracranial hypertension that was resistant to standard forms of management (including hyperventilation and mannitol), 30 mL of 23.4% saline brought prompt and sustained decreases in ICP.[27] In 80% of the cases, ICP dropped by more than 50% of the pretreatment value within 21 ± 10 minutes. Associated with this decrease in ICP, a significant rise in cerebral perfusion pressure from 64 ± 19 to 85 ± 18 mm Hg occurred 1 hour after hypertonic saline administration. Despite these impressive results, it is unclear why hypertonic saline should be more effective than mannitol. In a controlled animal study designed to directly compare the cerebral effects of mannitol (20%) and hypertonic saline (3.2%), rabbits were randomly allocated to receive an equiosmolar load of one of these two solutions (10 mL/kg). Plasma osmolality increased to a similar extent in both groups, and no differences in ICP reduction or regional water content were identified (Fig. 9-7).[28]

The possible benefit of adding furosemide to treatment with hypertonic solutions is controversial. In rats subjected to a closed-head injury, Mayzler and colleagues[29] demonstrated an additional decrease in brain water content when furosemide was added to treatment with 3% hypertonic saline. However, this additional benefit was not seen when furosemide was added to treatment with mannitol.[30] Although the protocols for these two studies differed in both the timing and the type of osmotic solutions administered, the findings suggest that the benefit of furosemide for a given patient is likely to be small, if it exists at all.

In a prospective controlled trial in children with head trauma, patients received a bolus (approximately 10 mL/kg) of either 0.9% or 3% saline. Baseline ICP values were similar in both groups (20 mm Hg). No significant change in ICP was demonstrated in patients who received 0.9% saline. However, after a bolus of 3% saline, ICP decreased significantly and averaged 15.8 mm Hg for the next 2 hours. In patients who received 3% saline, serum sodium concentrations increased from a mean of 147 mEq/L to 151 mEq/L.[31]

In a later study, Rozet and associates[32] compared the effect of 5 mL/kg of 20% mannitol (1 g/kg) with that of an equiosmolar volume of 5 mL/kg of 3% hypertonic saline on brain relaxation in patients undergoing craniotomy. Both mannitol and hypertonic saline resulted in a similar increase in serum and CSF osmolalities and achieved a comparable degree of brain relaxation as assessed by the surgeon. Compared with 3% hypertonic saline, mannitol caused more diuresis ($P < .03$) with less pronounced positive fluid balance at 3 hours (hypertonic saline group, 3230 ± 1543 mL; mannitol group, 1638 ± 1620 mL; $P < .004$); however, fluid balance values were not statistically different at 6 hours. The investigators suggested that hypertonic saline may be recommended as a safe alternative to mannitol for brain relaxation in patients undergoing craniotomy, especially those who are hemodynamically unstable.[32] It must be noted that the study involved only 20 patients randomly assigned to receive 3% hypertonic saline and may have been insufficiently powered to allow direct comparison of adverse events, which are infrequent.[33]

In summary, hypertonic saline solutions can exert a beneficial effect on intracranial hypertension while providing rapid volume resuscitation. The sodium load and consequent hypernatremia may be a concern in patients with neurologic injury who are at risk for seizures and who may have altered mental status due to an underlying injury. Whether hyperosmolar saline solutions provide significant advantages over the more conventional mannitol awaits further investigation.

Dextrose Solutions and Hyperglycemia

The belief that hyperglycemia before or during an episode of ischemia worsens neurologic outcome is now fairly well established. Several independent investigators using

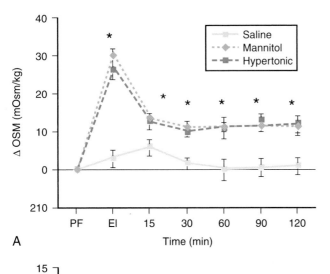

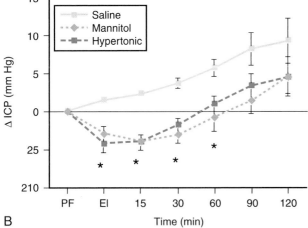

Figure 9–7 **A,** Changes in plasma osmolality after intravenous administration of 0.9% saline or 11 mOsm/kg of either 20% mannitol or 3.2% (hypertonic) saline (Hypertonic). Note the prompt and equal increase (approximately 29 mOsm/kg) in plasma osmolality after administration of either of these two osmotic agents. No differences in plasma osmolality were noted between the hypertonic saline and mannitol groups at any time during the study. **B,** Effect of hypertonic saline and mannitol on intracranial pressure. Both of these osmotic agents produced transient decreases in intracranial pressure when compared with an equal volume of 0.9% saline. Δ ICP, Change in ICP from PF value; Δ OSM, Change in OSM from PF value; EI, end of infusion of 0.9% saline, mannitol, or hypertonic saline; PF, 45 minutes after induction of a cryogenic brain lesion; *, p < 0.05 mannitol and hypertonic saline groups vs. 0.9% saline group.) *(From Scheller MS, Zornow MH, Oh YS: A comparison of the cerebral and hemodynamic effects of mannitol and hypertonic saline in a rabbit model of acute cryogenic brain injury. J Neurosurg Anesth 1991;3:291-296.)*

a variety of animal models have reached this conclusion. Worsened neurologic outcome has been repeatedly demonstrated after global ischemia of either the brain or the spinal cord. Elevations in plasma glucose do not have to be marked to produce a significant worsening of neurologic outcome. In an early study using a primate model, Lanier and associates[34] showed that dextrose infusions (50 mL of 5% dextrose in 0.45% saline) markedly worsened the neurologic score after 17 minutes of global cerebral ischemia. Although plasma glucose levels were slightly higher in animals that received the dextrose infusion (181 ± 19 vs. 140 ± 6 mg/dL), this elevation did not even reach statistical significance. Drummond and Moore[35] demonstrated a similar detrimental effect of hyperglycemia on spinal cord function after transient ischemia. Elevation of plasma glucose by either the infusion of 5% dextrose in water or the bolus administration of 50% dextrose resulted in substantially worsened outcome. In animals that received dextrose by infusion before the ischemic event, plasma glucose was only mildly elevated (177 vs. 137 mg/dL). Nonetheless, 9 of these 10 animals were rendered paraplegic compared with 3 of the 10 in the control group.[35]

Although the apparent consensus is that hyperglycemia during transient global ischemia is detrimental, both beneficial and adverse effects of glucose have been shown in models of focal ischemia. Ginsberg and colleagues[36] have demonstrated a decrease in infarct volume from 12.5 ± 4 mm³ (normoglycemic controls) to 9.3 ± 3.3 mm³ in rats made hyperglycemic before the ischemic event. Even greater beneficial effects (approximately 50% reduction in ischemic area) have been reported in a short-term study of hyperglycemia in cats after ligation of the middle cerebral artery.[37] The significance of these findings is uncertain because in a long-term cat study (survival time of 14 days), the hyperglycemic animals sustained infarcts twice the size of normoglycemic controls.[38]

The mechanism by which hyperglycemia worsens neurologic outcome is not clear. One hypothesis is that the glucose loading that occurs in central nervous system tissue during periods of hyperglycemia provides additional substrate for the production of lactic acid during the ischemic period. This increase in intracellular lactate is postulated to have a neurotoxic effect resulting in neuronal death. Although there is little doubt that lactate production increases in brains of hyperglycemic animals, the neurotoxic effect is less firmly established. Indeed, in neuronal cell cultures, lactic acidosis has been shown to be neuroprotective.[39,40] Another mechanism by which hyperglycemia may exacerbate neuronal injury is by enhancing glutamate release in the neocortex, but probably not in the hippocampus.[41,42]

In clinical studies, hyperglycemia has been associated with worsened neurologic outcome after traumatic brain injury (glucose > 200 mg/dL),[43] acute ischemic stroke,[44-46] and subarachnoid hemorrhage.[47] Hyperglycemia and worse neurologic outcome, however, may be parallel reflections of a stress response to tissue injury and its severity rather than the direct effects of excess glucose on ischemic neuronal tissue.[48,49] Furthermore, the effects of hyperglycemia may differ in diabetic and nondiabetic patients.[50]

So, does treating hyperglycemia indeed make a difference in morbidity and mortality? A frequently cited study by Van den Berghe,[51] demonstrating reduced morbidity and mortality in postoperative patients managed with "tight" (80-110 mg/dL) versus conventional (180-200 mg/dL) glucose control, stimulated interest in a more aggressive approach to treating hyperglycemia in the perioperative period. However, concerns about the efficacy and safety of such tight glucose control have been raised. In a randomized controlled trial of patients undergoing cardiac surgery,[52] intensive intraoperative insulin therapy (glucose, 80-100 mg/dL) did not result in significantly lower morbidity or mortality than a conventional approach of treating glucose levels above 200 mg/dL. Furthermore, two large prospective multicenter trials in Europe comparing patients managed with tight glucose control and patients treated with conventional glycemic control were halted owing to a threefold to fourfold increase in incidence of severe hypoglycemia (glucose < 40 mg/dL) in patients being treated in intensive care units (ICUs)[53,54] and a fourfold to fivefold increase in patients with sepsis[55] (17% vs. 4.1%, $P < .001$) without demonstrating any reduction in death rate or organ failure.[55] Recently published results of a large, multicenter, prospective trial (NICE-SUGAR)[56] suggest that tight glycemic control may increase mortality in the critically ill patient population. In this study, 6104 ICU patients were randomized to undergo either intensive glucose control (target blood glucose levels 81-108 mg/dl) or conventional glucose control (target blood glucose levels ≤180 mg/dl). Mortality at 90 days was higher in the intensive-control group (27.5%) compared to the conventional-control group (24.9%; OR for intensive control 1.14; 95% CI, 1.02-1.28; p=0.02), and the treatment effect did not differ between medical and surgical patients. The incidence of severe hypoglycemia (glucose ≤40 mg/dL) was also higher in patients assigned to intensive glucose control (6.8%) vs. conventional control (0.5%). New single or multiple organ failure and hospital or ICU lengths of stay were no different between the groups.

Therefore, it appears that tight glucose control may carry a significant risk of hypoglycemic events and reduced survival, at least in the critically ill; and the question becomes how to minimize the very real risks associated with the treatment of hyperglycemia while maximizing the potential benefits. In many cases, the answer to this question is institution-specific and depends on the staffing and resources available to provide safe and effective care. Krinsley[55] compared outcomes in 800 patients with intensive glucose management (target plasma glucose <140 mg/dL) who were consecutively admitted to a medical-surgical ICU to outcomes in a historical control group of 800 ICU patients without standardized glycemic control. The incidence of hypoglycemia (glucose < 40 mg/dL) was similar (0.34% vs. 0.35%, respectively) in the two groups of patients. However, hospital mortality decreased 29.3% ($P = .002$) in the protocol group. Although the study was not adequately powered to allow a robust subgroup analysis, the decrease in mortality was especially marked in the neurologic patients (mortality 8.5% in the protocol group vs. 21% in the historical control group, $P = .007$).[56] The weaknesses of this study are all those associated with nonrandomized clinical trials using historical controls. A randomized prospective pilot trial on the effect of intensive insulin therapy in patients after intracranial aneurysm clipping with acute subarachnoid hemorrhage showed reduced infection rates (27% vs. 42%, respectively; $P < .001$) when glucose was maintained in a range of 80 to 120 mg/dL than a range of 80-220 mg/dL.[57] However, the study was not intended to be sufficiently powered to address questions about the incidence of vasospasm, overall mortality, and neurologic outcome.

In summary, hyperglycemia should be avoided in patients who are at risk for an ischemic event. Dextrose solutions should not be infused in the patient undergoing a neurosurgical procedure unless they are needed for the treatment or prevention of hypoglycemia. A more complex question is how to proceed when a patient enters the operating room with hyperglycemia. Although normalizing this patient's plasma glucose level with insulin infusion is tempting, the effect of this intervention in reducing the risk of adverse outcome in a patient with neurologic injury is not clear. The preceding evidence suggests that tight glucose control carries a definite risk for hypoglycemia and may be harmful in the critically ill patient. The results of the NICE-SUGAR trial suggest that a target blood glucose level of < 180 mg/dL is a reasonable approach to glucose management until further evidence specifically related to patients with neurologic injury becomes available.[58]

FLUID ADMINISTRATION DURING CRANIOTOMY

Preoperative Deficits

The preoperative intravascular volume deficit of neurosurgical patients may be estimated in a manner similar to that used for patients undergoing other types of surgical procedures. For the nonfebrile adult patient, daily water loss averages approximately 100 mL/hr (Table 9-2) and occurs by evaporation from the skin and airways (insensible losses) and in urine, sweat, and feces.[59]

In addition to these obligatory losses, fluid loss caused by nasogastric suction, diarrhea, emesis, and phlebotomy must be considered. Patients who have undergone angiographic studies with intravenous contrast agents have excessive urinary losses from the diuresis produced by these hyperosmotic agents. Respiratory and insensible losses are higher in patients who are febrile from any cause in the preoperative period. To determine the net deficit, one must add whatever fluids have been administered to the patient. These usually consist of intravenous intake or intake by mouth. Consideration of these values, in combination with physical examination, gives an estimate of the net volume deficit for a given patient.

Intraoperative Fluids

Crystalloids

Intraoperative maintenance fluid administration usually consists of lactated Ringer's or normal saline solution. As stated previously, these fluids are crystalloids and are approximately equiosmolar to normal plasma. As a general rule,

Table 9–2	**Daily Water Loss for an Adult**
Type/Location	Amount (mL/day)
Insensible losses:	
Skin	350
Lungs	350
Urine	1400
Sweat	100
Feces	200
TOTAL	2400

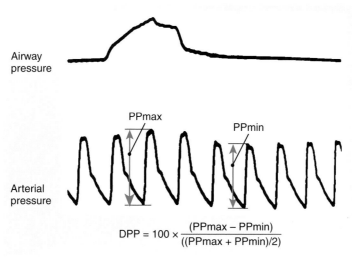

$$DPP = 100 \times \frac{(PPmax - PPmin)}{((PPmax + PPmin)/2)}$$

Figure 9–8 Illustration of delta pulse pressure measurement from arterial blood pressure tracing during positive-pressure ventilation. *Delta pulse pressure* (DPP) is the difference between the maximal (PPmax) and minimal (PPmin) pulse pressures during one breath cycle, divided by the mean. *(From Deflandre E, Bonhomme V, Hans P: Delta down compared with delta pulse pressure as an indicator of volaemia during intracranial surgery. Br J Anaesth 2008;100:245-250. By permission of Oxford University Press/British Journal of Anaesthesia.)*

hypo-osmolar solutions and dextrose-containing solutions should be avoided. Iso-osmolar crystalloids are given at a rate sufficient to replace the patient's urine output and insensible losses milliliter for milliliter. Blood loss is replaced at about a 3:1 ratio (crystalloid/blood) down to a hematocrit value of approximately 25% to 30%, depending on the rate of hemorrhage and the patient's physical status. During procedures in which marked brain swelling is present, requests are often made to keep the patient "dry" in the unsubstantiated belief that fluid restriction lessens brain edema formation. Complete water restriction in dogs for 72 hours, however, results in an 8% loss of body weight but only a 1% decrease in brain water content.[60] Such severe water restriction imposes severe physiologic stress, and the benefit of the minimal decrease in brain water content is unwarranted. Under no circumstances should iso-osmolar fluids be withheld to the point that the patient manifests hemodynamic instability caused by hypovolemia.

Ideally, sufficient intravenous fluids should be administered to maintain an adequate cardiac output but should avoid excessive fluid resuscitation. A great deal of evidence has accumulated in the critical care literature showing that the "dynamic" hemodynamic parameters (e.g., changes in stroke volume, arterial pulse pressure [Fig. 9-8], and delta down [Fig. 9-9; see later] during positive-pressure ventilation) provide a more accurate picture of volume status and responsiveness to fluid expansion than static hemodynamic parameters (e.g., right atrial pressure or pulmonary artery occlusion pressure, right-ventricular end-diastolic volume, and left ventricular end-diastolic area).[61-63]

In a study of 40 septic patients, Michard and associates[64] found that a delta pulse pressure (calculated as the difference between the maximal and minimal pulse pressure during one mechanical breath cycle, divided by their mean) greater than or equal to 13% during one respiratory cycle predicted a positive response (15% improvement in cardiac index) to a 500-mL colloid bolus with 94% sensitivity and 96% specificity. There was no difference in right atrial pressure and pulmonary artery occlusion pressure between responders and nonresponders to fluid challenge and the pressure values did not correlate with changes in cardiac index. Tavernier and coworkers[63] showed

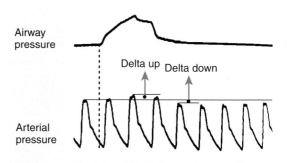

Figure 9–9 Illustration of delta down measurement from arterial blood pressure tracing during positive-pressure ventilation. *Delta down* is the difference between baseline apneic systolic blood pressure and minimum systolic blood pressure. Delta up, the difference between baseline apneic systolic blood pressure and maximal systolic blood pressure during one mechanical respiratory cycle. *(Illustration from Deflandre E, Bonhomme V, Hans P: Delta down compared with delta pulse pressure as an indicator of volaemia during intracranial surgery. Br J Anaesth 2008;100:245-250. By permission of Oxford University Press/British Journal of Anaesthesia.)*

that a delta down value (the difference between the systolic arterial pressure at end-expiration and its minimal value during the course of one mechanical breath) greater than 5 mm was a better predictor of positive response to volume expansion than pulmonary artery occlusion pressure or an end-diastolic area index assessed by transesophageal echocardiography. This study involved septic patients requiring catecholamine therapy. It is important to note that the patients in these studies were mechanically ventilated with relatively constant tidal volumes (8-12 mL/kg) and positive end-expiratory pressure levels up to 10 to 11 cm H_2O, and that patients with history of congestive heart failure or presence of dysrhythmia were excluded. Similarly, the delta down value was superior to pulmonary artery occlusion pressure in predicting fluid responsiveness in patients after aortic surgery.[65] Further clinical studies of dynamic hemodynamic parameters suggest that pulse pressure variation and delta down indices obtained from arterial blood pressure measurements correlate well with analogous indices obtained from plethysmography measured by the pulse oximeter in hypotensive patients[66] and in patients undergoing surgery.[67,68]

In terms of the neurosurgical patient population, Deflandre and associates[69] examined 26 patients undergoing scheduled intracranial surgery and concluded that a delta down value greater than 5 mm Hg highly predicted a pulse pressure variation below or above a threshold of 13%, which served as a surrogate for fluid responsiveness. Berkenstadt and colleagues[61] reported that a stroke variation of 9.5% or more was highly predictive of an increase in stroke volume in response to a volume load as low as 100 mL of 6% hydroxyethyl starch in patients undergoing brain surgery.

To summarize, the studies previously described suggest that dynamic hemodynamic parameters are more accurate in predicting hypovolemia and positive response to fluid challenge than static parameters; and evidence in the literature also suggests using thresholds of 13% for arterial pulse pressure variation (or delta pulse pressure) and 5 mm Hg for delta down during positive-pressure ventilation for the administration of additional volume. Further studies are needed to validate these results in larger numbers of patients undergoing general as well as neurosurgical procedures and to examine the accuracy of indices obtained from plethysmography.

MANNITOL

Mannitol, a six-carbon sugar with an MW of 182, is the most commonly administered hyperosmolar solution. It is available in 20% and 25% solutions with osmolalities of 1098 and 1372, respectively. Mannitol is often administered when significant brain swelling occurs or when it becomes necessary to decrease brain volume to facilitate exposure and thereby reduce brain retractor ischemia. It should be given only after other potential causes of increased brain volume have been considered (e.g., hypercapnia, vasodilators, obstruction to venous outflow). Mannitol is commonly administered as a rapid intravenous infusion in doses of 0.25 to 1 g/kg. Manninen and coworkers[70] examined the effects of 1- and 2-g/kg doses on serum electrolytes and plasma osmolality in neurosurgical patients. In addition to the anticipated transient increase in plasma osmolality, these researchers observed an associated decrease in serum sodium and bicarbonate concentrations, probably due to osmotically induced expansion of the extracellular volume. Patients who received the high dose of mannitol (i.e., 2 g/kg) also manifested a marked increase in serum potassium concentration (maximum mean increase of 1.5 mmol/L). Possible explanations include solvent drag (i.e., as water leaves the intracellular compartment, potassium is carried with it) and hemolysis of red cells near the tip of the infusion catheter caused by the locally high concentration of mannitol. Although transient, the hyperkalemia is reportedly associated with characteristic electrocardiographic changes.[71]

Mannitol may have a biphasic effect on ICP. Concomitant with the infusion, ICP may transiently increase, presumably because of vasodilation of cerebral vessels in response to the sudden increase in plasma osmolality.[16] Subsequent reduction in ICP is achieved by the movement of water from the brain's interstitial and intracellular spaces into the vasculature.

Colloids

HETASTARCH

The commonly used non–blood-derived colloids available for infusion are hetastarch, dextran 40, and dextran 70. Hetastarch (Hespan) is a 6% solution of hydroxyethyl starch (HES) in normal (0.9%) saline. HES is an enzymatically hydrolyzed amylopectin, which is chemically modified by hydroxyethylation of glucose subunits at carbon positions C2, C3 or C6. The metabolism and plasma clearance of HES is determined by the molecular weight (MW), degree of molar hydroxyethyl substitution (number of moles of hydroxyethyl groups present per mole of glucose subunits) and the pattern of this substitution (C2/C6 ratio). HES with lower MW, molar substitution, and C2/C6 ratio are degraded faster, resulting in faster renal elimination, shorter volume effect, and fewer adverse effects on coagulation.[72]

The mean MW for hetastarch is approximately 450,000 with a molar substitution of 0.7 (HES 450/0.7). The polymerized glucose molecules are nonuniform in size, and 80% fall within MW range of 30,000 to 2,400,000. The smaller molecules (less than 50,000 MW) are rapidly filtered by the kidneys, so that approximately 30% of the administered dose is excreted into the urine within the first 24 hours. Hetastarch, unlike dextran, is associated with an extremely low reported incidence of anaphylactic reactions and is useful when rapid intravascular volume expansion is required. The volume expansion produced by hetastarch is approximately equal to that produced by an equal volume of 5% albumin. Hetastarch may be contraindicated in patients with coagulopathies because administration of large volumes of this colloid may result in prolongation of prothrombin and partial thromboplastin times. These adverse effects on the ability of the blood to clot have limited the use of hetastarch in neurosurgery. Sporadic case reports of cerebral hemorrhage after hetastarch infusion have made some anesthesiologists and neurosurgeons reluctant to use it.

MEDIUM MW HYDROXYETHYL STARCH PRODUCTS

A wide variety of medium MW hydroxyethyl starch products (mean MW 200,000) have been available as volume expanders in Europe and for research purposes in the United States. These colloidal solutions differ from hetastarch primarily in their lower MW (130,000 – 264,000 vs. 450,000 for hetastarch) and molar substitution (0.4-0.62 vs. 0.7 for hetastarch). Results of clinical studies suggest that HES solutions of lower MW and molar substitution have fewer adverse effects on coagulation and hemostasis than solutions with higher MW and molar substitution. In a study of 24 healthy adults, infusion of clinically relevant doses of pentastarch (90 g of HES 264/0.45) led to a smaller reduction in Factor VIII activity and von Willebrand antigen and lesser effect on bleeding time than intravenous hetastarch.[73] In a prospective, randomized trial of patients undergoing major orthopedic surgery, the nadir Factor FVIII activity within two hours of the end of surgery was lower in subjects who received hetastarch (HES 670/0.75) compared to Voluven (HES 130/0.4), with similar volumes of respective colloids and crystalloids infused intraoperatively according to the study protocol. The estimated blood loss did not differ between the groups.[74] Langeron and his associates studied the effectiveness of Voluven vs. HAES-steril (HES 200/0.5) in treating severe hypovolemia in another study of patients undergoing major orthopedic surgery with expected blood loss of more than 2 liters. On average, the two groups of patients received similar volumes of colloid and crystalloid solutions to achieve pre-defined hemodynamic targets. The total blood loss and the total amount of autologous and homologous red blood cells transfused were not significantly different between groups. However, patients who received Voluven required fewer homologous blood transfusions. Factor VIII concentration and partial thromboplastin time were less compromised in the Voluven patients than in the HAES-steril patients at five hours after surgery.[75] In summary, these studies suggest that Voluven is an equally effective volume expander compared to hetastarch or HES 200/0.5 in the patient populations described. Whether hydroxyethyl starches of lower MW and molar substitution will prove to be useful for volume replacement in neurosurgical patients depends on results of ongoing investigations into their effects on hemostasis and brain water content in patients with neurologic injury.

DEXTRANS

Dextran solutions are colloids composed of glucose polymers with predominantly 1-6 glycosidic linkages. Although dextran 70 has an oncotic pressure about twice that of plasma, the oncotic pressure of dextran 40 is significantly greater; thus, infusion of dextran 40 can actually draw water from the interstitial space into the intravascular compartment. Effective volume expansion may therefore be greater than the volume of dextran infused. This volume expansion lasts approximately 3 to 4 hours for LMW preparations (dextran 40, 10% solution; mean MW 40,000) and approximately 6 to 8 hours for the high-molecular-weight form (dextran 70, 6% solution; mean MW 70,000). Within 24 hours of intravenous injection, 60% of dextran 40 and 35% of dextran 70 are cleared from the intravascular space, predominantly by renal excretion of the lower-molecular-weight fractions of these compounds.[76]

Dextrans are associated with a variety of adverse effects that have limited their clinical use. In a manner analogous to the effect of hetastarch, dextrans interfere with normal blood coagulation. It is recommended that infusions not exceed 20 ml/kg of dextran per kg body weight in the first 24 hours.[77] Dextrans are also associated with pseudoallergic reactions in approximately 0.032% of patients. In severe cases, patients may experience bronchospasm and circulatory collapse. To reduce the likelihood of such occurrences, the recommendation was made to administer 20 mL of very LMW dextran (dextran 1, 15% solution) intravenously immediately before the infusion of dextran 40 or 70. However, Dextran 1 is no longer available in the United States.

Dextran may also interfere with blood typing and crossmatching. When more than 20% of the blood volume has been replaced by dextran, determining the ABO type may be difficult. With smaller blood volumes, Rh and various minor antigenic markers may also be difficult to identify.[78] In addition, circulating dextrans can interfere with a number of clinical laboratory tests, including blood glucose, bilirubin, and protein measurements. Finally, acute renal failure was reported following the overzealous administration of dextran 40 that resulted in a hyperoncotic state (plasma oncotic pressure 33.1 mm Hg).[79]

ALBUMIN

Human albumin is available for infusion in 5% and 25% solutions. These solutions do not contain any of the clotting factors found in fresh whole blood or fresh plasma. Because all of the isoagglutinins are also removed in the processing, albumin may be given without regard to the patient's blood type. The albumin is derived from the plasma of volunteer donors, pooled, heat-treated at 60° C for 10 hours to inactivate possible viral contamination, and finally sterilized by ultrafiltration. Albumin has an MW of approximately 69,000 and constitutes 50% of the total plasma proteins by weight. Intravenously infused albumin has a plasma half-life of 16 hours in nonedematous patients. Although albumin is useful as a volume expander, it is expensive. At our institution, the current cost to the patient for 500 mL of 5% albumin is $434, whereas an equal volume of hetastarch is only $68.

Plasma and Red Blood Cells

Greater professional and public awareness of the hazards associated with infusing blood products has markedly curtailed their use. Currently, red blood cells should be given only to keep hematocrit at a "safe" level. This level varies from patient to patient; and even in a specific circumstance, it may be difficult to objectively define what constitutes "safe." Thus, no specific recommendation can be made regarding how far the hematocrit may fall before initiation of transfusion. However, in general, healthy individuals easily tolerate hematocrits in the 20% to 25% range. In vitro studies have shown that oxygen delivery to the tissues is maximal at a hematocrit of approximately 30%. At higher hematocrits, oxygen delivery is compromised by increased viscosity of the blood, whereas at hematocrits much below 25%, delivery falls off because of decreased carrying capacity of the blood.

Plasma should be administered only in an attempt to correct a coagulation defect caused by a deficiency of one or more of the coagulation factors. Volume expansion is no longer considered an appropriate use of this blood product. Coagulation defects may arise in neurosurgical patients for a variety of reasons. In one study, an abnormality in the prothrombin time, partial thromboplastin time, or platelet count at admission was present in 55% of patients with head injuries and computed tomography evidence of new or progressive lesions.[80] Victims of traumatic injury may require massive fluid resuscitation because of hemorrhagic hypovolemia. If this initial fluid resuscitation is achieved with asanguinous fluids, a dilutional coagulopathy may aggravate a preexisting clotting disorder.

SPECIFIC NEUROSURGICAL CHALLENGES

Fluid Management in Patients with Cerebral Aneurysms

Patients who require surgery after rupture of a cerebral aneurysm pose additional problems in fluid management. Cerebral vasospasm is a leading cause of morbidity in these patients and produces death or severe disability in approximately 14% of patients who survive rupture of the aneurysm. Angiographic evidence of vasospasm occurs in as many as 60% to 80% of patients after subarachnoid hemorrhage, and the incidence of symptomatic vasospasm reaches a peak at 4 to 10 days after the rupture of the aneurysm. The mechanism by which blood in the subarachnoid space provokes this arterial luminal narrowing is the subject of intense investigation and debate. We know that vasospasm after aneurysm rupture can be so severe that it causes cerebral ischemia and infarction.

Currently, two accepted therapeutic interventions may reduce the incidence or severity of vasospasm. The first is hypervolemic/hyperdynamic therapy. Observational studies have shown that volume loading of patients suffering from neurologic impairment secondary to vasospasm in conjunction with inotropic support can reverse or reduce neurologic morbidity. This approach can be used only when the aneurysm has been secured and the patient is no longer at risk for its rerupture. Institution of hypervolemic/hyperdynamic therapy should be guided by hemodynamic data provided by an index of central volume, such as a central venous pressure line, a pulmonary artery catheter, or echocardiography. In previously healthy individuals, maximum cardiac performance occurs at a pulmonary capillary wedge pressure of 14 mm Hg. Volume expansion beyond this point results in higher wedge pressures but no further rise in cardiac index.[81] Volume loading may be accomplished by infusing iso-osmolar crystalloids, colloids, or red blood cells in order to achieve hemodilution to a hematocrit of approximately 30%. Frequent assessment of pulmonary function with arterial blood gas measurements, chest radiographs, and physical examination is essential, because onset of pulmonary edema with hypoxia will negate any possible beneficial effects of greater flow to ischemic brain tissue.

The efficacy of the prophylactic use of hypervolemic/hyperdynamic therapy to prevent cerebral vasospasm has been questioned by several studies.[82,83] In a prospective trial, Lennihan and associates[84] randomly allocated 82 patients who had undergone subarachnoid hemorrhage and aneurysm repair to a hypervolemic (pulmonary artery diastolic pressure, 14 mm Hg; central venous pressure, 8 mm Hg) or normovolemic (pulmonary artery diastolic pressure, 7 mm Hg; central venous pressure, 5 mm Hg) protocol. Fluid management consisted of infusing crystalloid (5% dextrose and 0.9% saline) and 5% albumin to maintain either normal (normovolemic group) or elevated (hypervolemic group) cardiac filling pressures. There was no difference between the treatment groups in mean global CBF, as assessed by xenon ^{133}Xe clearance, or rate of vasospasm (20% in both groups) during the treatment period.

The second therapy for vasospasm is calcium channel blockers. For example, nimodipine (Nimotop) has been in use for the longest and has been shown to decrease the incidence of severe neurologic impairment caused by vasospasm. Nimodipine has an advantage over hypervolemic/hyperdynamic therapy, in that it can be administered before aneurysm clipping because it has no adverse hemodynamic effects that may provoke rerupture.[85-87]

Fluid Management of Diabetes Insipidus

Neurogenic diabetes insipidus may occur in patients with lesions in the vicinity of the hypothalamus after pituitary surgery or traumatic head injury. This syndrome results when the neurons located in the supraoptic nuclei of the hypothalamus fail to release sufficient quantities of vasopressin into the systemic circulation. Diabetes insipidus is characterized by the production of large volumes of dilute urine and normal or elevated plasma osmolality. In severe cases, urinary output can be as great as a liter per hour. Left untreated or unrecognized, diabetes insipidus can quickly result in severe dehydration, hypovolemia, and hypotension.[88] To promptly diagnose diabetes insipidus, one must have a high index of suspicion when dealing with patients who are at risk. Confirmation may be obtained by documenting elevated serum osmolality and sodium concentration in conjunction with a low urine specific gravity or osmolality. The patient should be vigorously rehydrated with 0.45% saline until euvolemia is established. Because of the preexisting hyperosmolar/hypernatremic state, normal saline should *not* routinely be used for the initial rehydration of these patients. Concomitantly, replacement therapy should be initiated with either aqueous vasopressin (5-10 units by intramuscular or subcutaneous injection) or desmopressin (1-2 μg intravenously or subcutaneously).

Fluid Management of the Trauma Patient with Head Injuries

Victims of traumatic injury often have associated closed-head injuries. Some of these patients are in hemorrhagic shock and require immediate volume resuscitation. The anesthesiologist is confronted by a variety of concerns about such a patient, including how to rapidly restore intravascular volume and organ perfusion while minimizing cerebral edema formation. Although a variety of hypertonic, hyperoncotic solutions appear ideally suited for this purpose on the basis of animal studies, none is commercially available in the United States, and their use in humans is not currently considered the standard of care. In a meta-analysis of hypertonic versus near-isotonic crystalloids for fluid resuscitation in critically ill patients, reviewers for the Cochrane Database analyzed 14 trials and concluded that data was insufficient to determine whether hypertonic fluid is better than isotonic for resuscitating patients with trauma or burns or patients undergoing surgery.[89] Furthermore, an Australian randomized controlled trial attempted to determine whether early resuscitation with a bolus of hypertonic saline or standard crystalloid therapy better improves neurologic outcome in comatose, hypotensive patients with traumatic brain injury.[90] Patients received either a bolus of 250 mL of 7.5% hypertonic saline or 250 mL of Ringer's lactate in the prehospital setting. Subsequent fluid management was left to paramedic and hospital resuscitation protocols. Patients in both groups had favorable systolic blood pressure on arrival at the emergency department. Cerebral perfusion pressures and ICPs measured in the ICU were similar in the groups, as were rates of survivability to hospital discharge (55% vs. 50% controls, $P = .32$) and neurologic function at 6 months ($P = .45$). A potential flaw in this study is that a beneficial effect of hypertonic saline could have been obscured by subsequent resuscitation with isotonic crystalloid and/or colloid.[91]

Currently, the ideal resuscitation fluid for patients who are hypovolemic with ongoing blood loss is fresh whole blood. Because whole blood is a colloid rather than a crystalloid, smaller volumes of whole blood are required to restore intravascular volume, thus producing a more rapid resuscitation. Whole blood replaces clotting factors and platelets that have been lost and may therefore prevent the emergence of a dilutional coagulopathy. Unfortunately, because blood banks now fractionate all donor units and because donor units must be tested for infectious agents, few, if any, institutions in the United States have fresh whole blood available. Hetastarch is not widely used because of its potential to induce a coagulopathy when given in large volumes. Dextrans have also been implicated as causing increased bleeding and carry the risk (although slight) of an anaphylactoid reaction.

Albumin is expensive and results in no better reduction in cerebral edema or ICP when compared with isotonic crystalloids during the initial resuscitative efforts.[92] Safety concerns about the use of albumin in critically ill patients were partly alleviated by the results of a large, prospective, multi-center trial: the Saline versus Albumin Fluid Evaluation (SAFE) Study.[93] In this study, a total of 6997 critically ill patients admitted to multidisciplinary ICUs in Australia and New Zealand were randomly assigned to receive either 0.9% saline or 4% albumin for volume resuscitation. Patients who had undergone cardiac surgery or liver transplantation or who had burns were excluded. The primary outcomes of all-cause mortality during a 28-day period were similar in the groups ($P = .87$). Furthermore, there was no significant difference in the number of new organ failures ($I = 0.85$), duration of mechanical ventilation ($p = 0.74$), days of renal replacement therapy ($P = .41$), duration in ICU ($P = .44$), or days spent in the hospital ($P = .30$). There was a trend toward higher mortality in trauma patients assigned to the albumin group (relative risk [RR] of death, 1.36; 95% confidence interval [CI], 0.99-1.86; $P = .06$), primarily owing to patients with traumatic brain injury (RR of death, 1.62 in albumin group; 95% CI, 1.12-2.34; $P = .009$). Mortality rates in trauma patients without brain injury were no different whether they were given albumin or saline (RR of death, 1.00; 95% CI, 0.56-1.79; $P = 1.00$). The study was insufficiently powered to detect differences in mortality in various predefined subgroups of patients, such as those with traumatic brain injury. Nevertheless, the use of albumin in patients with traumatic brain injury cannot be recommended until a properly powered trial determines its safety and benefit, if any, in this patient population.

In pragmatic terms, this discussion leaves isotonic crystalloid solutions as the first choice for volume resuscitation of trauma patients with head injuries. Normal saline is a good choice because it is inexpensive, can be given with packed red blood cells when they become available, has a long shelf-life, and is mildly hyperosmolar in comparison with normal plasma. A disadvantage is the development of hyperchloremic acidosis in large-volume resuscitation settings; many trauma centers use other balanced salt solutions. Fluids to be avoided include hypotonic solutions (i.e., 0.45% saline) and any solution containing dextrose.

SUMMARY

The movement of water between the vasculature and the brain's extracellular space is driven primarily by the presence of osmotic gradients. Clinically, these gradients can be established by administration of either hyperosmolar (e.g., mannitol) or hypo-osmolar (e.g., 5% dextrose in water) solutions. In the brain (unlike peripheral tissues), plasma oncotic pressure has little impact on cerebral edema formation. Attempts to minimize cerebral edema formation by fluid restriction are unlikely to be successful and, if overzealously pursued, may lead to hemodynamic instability. Although no single intravenous solution is best suited for the neurosurgical patient who is at risk for intracranial hypertension, the use of iso-osmolar crystalloids is widely accepted and can be justified on a scientific basis.

Acknowledgment

The authors wish to thank Dr. Michael M. Todd for the inspiration for Figures 9-4, 9-5, and 9-6 and Kathy Gage, Grant and Publications Writer in the Department of Anesthesiology and Peri-Operative Medicine at Oregon Health & Science University, for providing editorial assistance for the final version of this chapter.

REFERENCES

1. Bevan DR: Osmometry I: Terminology and principles of measurement, *Anaesthesia* 33:794–800, 1978.
2. Haupt MT, Rackow EC: Colloid osmotic pressure and fluid resuscitation with hetastarch, albumin, and saline solutions, *Crit Care Med* 10:159–162, 1982.
3. Marty AT, Zweifach BW: The high oncotic pressure effects of dextrans, *Arch Surg* 101:421–424, 1970.
4. Starling EH: On the absorption of fluids from the connective tissue spaces, *J Physiol* 19:312–326, 1896.
5. Peters RM, Hargens AR: Protein vs. electrolytes and all of the Starling forces, *Arch Surg* 116:1293–1298, 1981.
6. Fenstermacher JD, Johnson JA: Filtration and reflection coefficients of the rabbit blood-brain barrier, *Am J Physiol* 211:341–346, 1966.
7. Zornow MH, Todd MM, Moore SS: The acute cerebral effects of changes in plasma osmolality and oncotic pressure, *Anesthesiology* 67:936–941, 1987.
8. Dodge PR, Crawford JD, Probst JH: Studies in experimental water intoxication, *Arch Neurol* 5:513–529, 1960.
9. Zornow MH, Scheller MS, Todd MM, et al: Acute cerebral effects of isotonic crystalloid and colloid solutions following cryogenic brain injury in the rabbit, *Anesthesiology* 69:180–184, 1988.
10. Kaieda R, Todd MM, Warner DS: Prolonged reduction in colloid oncotic pressure does not increase brain edema following cryogenic injury in rabbits, *Anesthesiology* 71:554–560, 1989.
11. Shenkin HA, Bezier HS, Bouzarth W: Restricted fluid intake: Rational management of the neurosurgical patient, *J Neurosurg* 45:432–436, 1976.
12. Warner DS, Boehland LA: Effects of iso-osmolal intravenous fluid therapy on post-ischemic brain water content in the rat, *Anesthesiology* 68:86–91, 1988.
13. Korosue K, Heros RC, Ogilvy CS, et al: Comparison of crystalloids and colloids for hemodilution in a model of focal cerebral ischemia, *J Neurosurg* 73:576–584, 1990.
14. Drummond JC, Patel PM, Cole DJ, et al: The effect of the reduction of colloid oncotic pressure, with and without reduction of osmolality, on posttraumatic cerebral edema, *Anesthesiology* 88:993–1002, 1998.
15. Zornow MH, Scheller MS, Shackford SR: Effect of a hypertonic lactated Ringer's solution on intracranial pressure and cerebral water content in a model of traumatic brain injury, *J Trauma* 29:484–488, 1989.
16. Shenkin HA, Goluboff B, Haft H: Further observations on the effects of abruptly increased osmotic pressure of plasma on cerebrospinal-fluid pressure in man, *J Neurosurg* 22:563–568, 1964.
17. Kien ND, Kramer GC, White DA: Acute hypotension caused by rapid hypertonic saline infusion in anesthetized dogs, *Anesth Analg* 73:597–602, 1991.
18. Gunnar W, Jonasson O, Merlotti G, et al: Head injury and hemorrhagic shock: Studies of the blood brain barrier and intracranial pressure after resuscitation with normal saline solution, 3% saline solution, and dextran-40, *Surgery* 103:398–407, 1988.
19. Gunnar WP, Merlotti GJ, Jonasson O, et al: Resuscitation from hemorrhagic shock: Alterations of the intracranial pressure after normal saline, 3% saline and Dextran-40, *Ann Surg* 204:686–692, 1986.
20. Shackford SR, Zhuang J, Schmoker J: Intravenous fluid tonicity: Effect on intracranial pressure, cerebral blood flow, and cerebral oxygen delivery in focal brain injury, *J Neurosurg* 76:91–98, 1992.
21. Todd MM, Tommasino C, Moore S: Cerebral effects of isovolemic hemodilution with a hypertonic saline solution, *J Neurosurg* 63:944–948, 1985.
22. Sahar A, Tsiptstein E: Effects of mannitol and furosemide on the rate of formation of cerebrospinal fluid, *Exp Neurol* 60:584–591, 1978.
23. Sotos JF, Dodge PR, Meara P, et al: Studies in experimental hypertonicity I: Pathogenesis of the clinical syndrome, biochemical abnormalities and cause of death, *Pediatrics* 26:925–938, 1960.
24. Shackford SR, Fortlage DA, Peters RM, et al: Serum osmolar and electrolyte changes associated with large infusions of hypertonic sodium lactate for intravascular volume expansion of patients undergoing aortic reconstruction, *Surg Gynecol Obstet* 164:127–136, 1987.
25. Shackford SR, Sise MJ, Fridlund PH, et al: Hypertonic sodium lactate versus lactated Ringer's solution for intravenous fluid therapy in operations on the abdominal aorta, *Surgery* 94:41–51, 1983.
26. Worthley LIG, Cooper DJ, Jones N: Treatment of resistant intracranial hypertension with hypertonic saline, *J Neurosurg* 68:478–481, 1988.
27. Suarez JI, Qureshi AI, Bhardwaj A, et al: Treatment of refractory intracranial hypertension with 23.4% saline, *Crit Care Med* 26:1118–1122, 1998.
28. Scheller MS, Zornow MH, Oh YS: A comparison of the cerebral and hemodynamic effects of mannitol and hypertonic saline in a rabbit model of acute cryogenic brain injury, *J Neurosurg Anesth* 3:291–296, 1991.
29. Mayzler O, Leon A, Eilig I, et al: The effect of hypertonic (3%) saline with and without furosemide on plasma osmolality, sodium concentration, and brain water content after closed head trauma in rats, *J Neurosurg Anesth* 18:24–31, 2006.
30. Todd MM, Cutkomp J, Brian JE: Influence of mannitol and furosemide, alone and in combination, on brain water content after fluid percussion injury, *Anesthesiology* 105:1176–1181, 2006.
31. Fisher B, Thomas D, Peterson B: Hypertonic saline lowers raised intracranial pressure in children after head trauma, *J Neurosurg Anesth* 4:4–10, 1992.

32. Rozet I, Tontisirin N, Muangman S, et al: Effect of equiosmolar solutions of mannitol versus hypertonic saline on intraoperative brain relaxation and electrolyte balance, *Anesthesiology* 107:697–704, 2007.

33. McDonagh DL, Warner DS: Hypertonic saline for craniotomy [editorial]? *Anesthesiology* 107:91–89, 2007.

34. Lanier WL, Stangland KJ, Scheithauer BW, et al: The effects of dextrose infusion and head position on neurologic outcome after complete cerebral ischemia in primates: Examination of a model, *Anesthesiology* 66:39–48, 1987.

35. Drummond J, Moore S: The influence of dextrose administration on neurologic outcome after temporary spinal cord ischemia in the rabbit, *Anesthesiology* 70:64–70, 1989.

36. Ginsberg MD, Prado R, Dietrich WD, et al: Hyperglycemia reduces the extent of cerebral infarction in rats, *Stroke* 18:570–574, 1987.

37. Zasslow MA, Pearl RG, Shuer LM, et al: Hyperglycemia decreases acute neuronal ischemic changes after middle cerebral artery occlusion in cats, *Stroke* 20:519–523, 1989.

38. De Courten-Meyers G, Myers RE, Schoolfield L: Hyperglycemia enlarges infarct size in cerebrovascular occlusion in cats, *Stroke* 19:623–630, 1988.

39. Choi DW, Monyer H, Giffard RG, et al: Acute brain injury, NMDA receptors, and hydrogen ions: Observations in cortical cell cultures, *Adv Exp Med Biol* 268:501–504, 1990.

40. Giffard RG, Monyer H, Christine CW, et al: Acidosis reduces NMDA receptor activation, glutamate neurotoxicity, and oxygen-glucose deprivation neuronal injury in cortical cultures, *Brain Res* 506:339–342, 1990.

41. Ping-An L, Shuaib A, Miyashita H, et al: Hyperglycemia enhances extracellular glutamate accumulation in rats subjected to forebrain ischemia, *Stroke* 31:183–192, 2000.

42. Choi KT, Illievich UM, Zornow MH, et al: Effect of hyperglycemia on peri-ischemic neurotransmitter levels in the rabbit hippocampus, *Brain Res* 642:104–110, 1994.

43. Lam AM, Winn RH, Cullen BF, et al: Hyperglycemia and neurological outcome in patients with head injury, *J Neurosurg* 75:545–551, 1991.

44. Bruno A, Biller J, Adams HP, et al: Acute blood glucose level and outcome from ischemic stroke, *Neurology* 52:280–284, 1999.

45. Weir CJ, Murray GD, Dyker AG, et al: Is hyperglycaemia an independent predictor of poor outcome after acute stroke? Results of a long term follow up study, *BMJ* 314:1303–1306, 1997.

46. Capes SE, Hunt D, Malmberg K, et al: Stress hyperglycemia and prognosis of stroke in nondiabetic and diabetic patients, *Stroke* 32:2426–2432, 2001.

47. Frontera JA, Fernandez A, Claassen J, et al: Hyperglycemia after SAH, predictors, associated complications, and impact on outcome, *Stroke* 37:199–203, 2006.

48. Murros K, Fogelholm R, Kettunen S, et al: Blood glucose, glycosylated haemoglobin, and outcome of ischemic brain infarction, *J Neurol Sci* 111:59–64, 1992.

49. Tracey F, Crawford VLS, Lawson JT, et al: Hyperglycaemia and mortality from acute stroke, *Q J Med* 86:439–446, 1993.

50. Puskas F, Grocott HP, White WD, et al: Intraoperative hyperglycemia and cognitive decline after CABG, *Ann Thorac Surg* 84:1467–1473, 2007.

51. Van den Berghe G, Wouters P, Weekers F, et al: Intensive insulin therapy in critically ill patients, *N Engl J Med* 345:1359–1367, 2001.

52. Gandhi GY, Nuttall GA, Abel MD, et al: Intensive intraoperative insulin therapy versus conventional glucose management during cardiac surgery, *Ann Intern Med* 146:233–243, 2007.

53. National Institutes of Health: Glucontrol Study: A Multi-Center Study Comparing the Effects of Two Glucose Control Regimens by Insulin in Intensive Care Unit Patients Available at http://www.clinicaltrials.gov/ct/gui/show/NCT00107601.

54. Devos P, Preiser J-C: Current controversies around tight glucose control in critically ill patients, *Curr Opin Clin Nutr Metab Care* 10:206–209, 2007.

55. Brunkhorst FM, Engel C, Bloos F, et al: German Competence Network Sepsis (SepNet). Intensive insulin therapy and pentastarch resuscitation in severe sepsis, *N Engl J Med* 358:125–139, 2008.

56. Finfer S, Chittock DR, Su SY, et al: The NICE-SUGAR Study Investigators: Intensive verus Conventional Glucose Control in Critically Ill Patients. *N Engl J Med* 360:1283–1297, 2009.

57. Krinsley JS: Effect of an intensive glucose management protocol on the mortality of critically ill adult patients, *Mayo Clin Proc* 79:992–1000, 2004.

58. Bilotta F, Spinelli A, Giovannini F, et al: The effect of intensive insulin therapy on infection rate, vasospasm, neurologic outcome, and mortality in neurointensive care unit after intracranial aneurysm clipping in patients with acute subarachnoid hemorrhage: A randomized prospective pilot trial, *J Neurosurg Anesth* 19:156–160, 2007.

59. Guyton AC: *Textbook of Medical Physiology*, ed 5, Philadelphia, 1976, WB Saunders.

60. Jelsma LF, McQueen JD: Effect of experimental water restriction on brain water, *J Neurosurg* 26:35–40, 1967.

61. Berkenstadt H, Margalit N, Hadani M, et al: Stroke volume variation as a predictor of fluid responsiveness in patients undergoing brain surgery, *Anesth Analg* 92:984–989, 2001.

62. Michard F, Teboul J-L: Predicting fluid responsiveness in ICU patients: A critical analysis of the evidence, *Chest* 121:2000–2008, 2002.

63. Tavernier B, Makhotine O, Lebuffe G, et al: Systolic pressure variation as a guide to fluid therapy in patients with sepsis-induced hypotension, *Anesthesiology* 89:1313–1321, 1998.

64. Michard F, Boussat S, Chemla D, et al: Relation between respiratory changes in arterial pulse pressure and fluid responsiveness in septic patients with acute circulatory failure, *Am J Respir Crit Care Med* 162:134–138, 2000.

65. Coriat P, Vrillon M, Perel A, et al: A comparison of systolic blood pressure variations and echocardiographic estimates of end-diastolic left ventricular size in patients after aortic surgery, *Anesth Analg* 78:46–53, 1994.

66. Natalini G, Rosano A, Taranto M, et al: Arterial versus plethysmographic dynamic indices to test responsiveness for testing fluid administration in hypotensive patients: A clinical trial, *Anesth Analg* 103:1478–1484, 2006.

67. Natalini G, Rosano A, Franceschetti ME, et al: Variations in arterial blood pressure and photoplethysmography during mechanical ventilation, *Anesth Analg* 103:1182–1188, 2006.

68. Cannesson M, Attof Y, Rosamel P, et al: Respiratory variations in pulse oximetry plethysmographic waveform amplitude to predict fluid responsiveness in the operating room, *Anesthesiology* 106:1105–1111, 2007.

69. Deflandre E, Bonhomme V, Hans P: Delta down compared with delta pulse pressure as an indicator of volaemia during intracranial surgery, *Br J Anaesth* 100:245–250, 2008.

70. Manninen PH, Lam AM, Gelb AW, et al: The effect of high-dose mannitol on serum and urine electrolytes and osmolality in neurosurgical patients, *Can J Anaesth* 34:442–446, 1987.

71. Moreno M, Murphy C, Goldsmith C: Increase in serum potassium resulting from the administration of hypertonic mannitol and other solutions, *J Lab Clin Med* 73:291–298, 1969.

72. Treib J, Baron J-F, Grauer MT, et al: An international view of hydroxyethyl starches, *Intensive Care Med* 25: 258–268, 1999.

73. Strauss RG, Pennell BJ, Stump DC: A randomized, blinded trial comparing the hemostatic effects of pentastarch versus hetastarch, *Transfusion* 42: 27–36, 2002.

74. Gandhi SD, Weiskopf RB, Jungheinrich C, et al: Volume replacement therapy during major orthopedic surgery using Voluven (Hydroxyethyl Starch 130/0.4) or Hetastarch, *Anesthesiology* 106: 1120–1127, 2007.

75. Langeron O, Doelberg M, Ang E-T, et al: Voluven, a lower substituted novel hydroxyethyl starch (HES 130/0.4), causes fewer effects on coagulation in major orthopedic surgery than HES 200/0.5, *Anesth Analg* 92: 855–862, 2001.

76. Nearman HS, Herman ML: Toxic effects of colloids in the intensive care unit, *Crit Care Clin* 7:713–723, 1991.

77. Lacy Ch, Armstrong L, Goldman M, Lance L (eds): Dextran. In Drug Information Handbook, 17th Edition. Hudson, Lexi-comp, 2008, p 445.

78. Lutz H, Georgieff M: Effects and side effects of colloid plasma substitutes as compared to albumin, *Curr Stud Hematol Blood Transfus* 53:145–154, 1986.

79. Moran M, Kapsner C: Acute renal failure associated with elevated plasma oncotic pressure, *N Engl J Med* 317:150–153, 1987.

80. Stein SC, Young GS, Talucci RC, et al: Delayed brain injury after head trauma: Significance of coagulopathy, *Neurosurgery* 30:160–165, 1992.

81. Levy ML, Giannotta SL: Cardiac performance indices during hypervolemic therapy for cerebral vasospasm, *J Neurosurg* 75:27–31, 1991.

82. Treggiari MM, Walder B, Suter PM, et al: Systematic review of the prevention of delayed ischemic neurological deficits with hypertension, hypervolemia, and hemodilution therapy following subarachnoid hemorrhage, *J Neurosurg* 98:978–984, 2003.

83. Rinkel GJ, Feigin VL, Algra A, et al: Circulatory volume expansion therapy for aneurysmal subarachnoid haemorrhage, *Cochrane Database Syst Rev* (4):CD000483, 2004.

84. Lennihan L, Mayer SA, Fink ME, et al: Effect of hypervolemic therapy on cerebral blood flow after subarachnoid hemorrhage: A randomized controlled trial, *Stroke* 31:383–391, 2000.

85. Allen GS, Ahn HS, Preziosi TJ, et al: Cerebral arterial spasm: A controlled trial of nimodipine in patients with subarachnoid hemorrhage, *N Engl J Med* 308:619–624, 1983.

159

86. Ohman J, Heiskanen O: Effect of nimodipine on the outcome of patients after aneurysmal subarachnoid hemorrhage and surgery, *J Neurosurg* 69:683–686, 1988.

87. Petruk KC, West M, Mohr G, et al: Nimodipine treatment in poor-grade aneurysm patients, *J Neurosurg* 68:505–517, 1988.

88. Wilson JD, Braunwald E, Isselbacher KJ, et al: *Harrison's Principles of Internal Medicine*, ed 12, New York, 1991, McGraw-Hill, pp 1684–1689.

89. Bunn F, Roberts I, Tasker R: Hypertonic versus near isotonic crystalloid for fluid resuscitation in critically ill patients, *Cochrane Database Syst Rev* (4):CD002045, 2000.

90. Cooper DJ, Myles PS, McDermott FT, et al: Prehospital hypertonic saline resuscitation of patients with hypotension and severe traumatic brain injury, *JAMA* 291:1350–1357, 2004.

91. Lewis RJ: Prehospital care of the multiply injured patient: The challenge of figuring out what works [editorial], *JAMA* 17:1382–1384, 2004.

92. Wisner D, Busche F, Sturn J, et al: Traumatic shock and head injury: Effects of fluid resuscitation on the brain, *J Surg Res* 46:49–59, 1989.

93. Finfer S, Bellomo R, Boyce N, et al: SAFE Study Investigators: A comparison of albumin and saline for fluid resuscitation in the intensive care unit, *N Engl J Med* 350:2247–2256, 2004.

Chapter 10

CARE OF THE ACUTELY UNSTABLE PATIENT

Irene Rozet • Karen B. Domino

Most neurologic emergencies that require the acute care of an anesthesiologist are caused by head and spinal cord trauma. On occasion, patients with ruptured cerebral aneurysms or arteriovenous malformations, acute hydrocephalus, intracerebral hematomas, and intracranial tumors arrive for treatment with impending brain herniation. Likewise, tumors or hematomas compressing the spinal cord may cause acute spinal cord injury (SCI).

The aim of the acute care of patients with either brain injury or SCI is prevention of secondary neurologic injury. Secondary insults to other organs and systems as a result of the primary neurologic injury and coexisting injuries also contribute to development of the secondary injury of the neurologic system, adversely affecting outcome.

This chapter focuses on the acute care of the neurologically unstable patient with brain and spinal cord injuries, regardless of the cause. We discuss the initial neurologic evaluation, the evaluation of other organ systems, and the aims in the acute care of the unstable patient.

BRAIN INJURY

Neurologic Evaluation

The Glasgow Coma Scale (GCS)[1] is used to quickly evaluate the neurologic status of the patient with a brain injury (Box 10-1). It evaluates the best verbal response, best motor response, and presence of eye opening with a scale from 3 to 15. The scaling system is effective because it is easy to use, has good interobserver reliability, helps guide diagnosis and therapy, and has prognostic significance. Morbidity and mortality are closely related to the initial GCS score irrespective of the cause of the head injury.[2] Another factor that predicts the severity of the head injury is age, with a better prognosis noted among pediatric patients.[2]

Respiratory pattern, pulse, blood pressure, pupillary responses, and gag reflexes are also evaluated in the initial neurologic examination. If the patient is comatose (e.g., no eye opening, verbal response, or ability to follow commands), evaluation of midbrain and brainstem reflexes (e.g., pupillary response, corneal reflexes, oculomotor movements, and gag reflex) may aid in localization of the lesion. In the acute setting, examination of the size and reactivity of the pupils is particularly important (Box 10-2). A dilated, unresponsive ("blown") pupil may be a sign of ipsilateral uncal herniation, in which the medial aspect of the temporal lobe (uncus) herniates through the tentorium, thereby compressing the midbrain and nucleus of the third cranial nerve.[3] Anisocoria is also associated with mechanical brain compensation.[4] Bilateral pupillary dilation may be due to bilateral uncal herniation or injury (e.g., ischemic or metabolic) to the midbrain. Local eye trauma

---

BOX 10–1 *Neurologic Evaluation of the Brain-Injured Patient*

Glasgow Coma Scale Score (points):
  Eye opening:
    Spontaneous (4)
    To speech (3)
    To pain (2)
    None (1)
  Best verbal response:
    Oriented (5)
    Confused (4)
    Inappropriate (3)
    Incomprehensible (2)
    None (1)
  Best motor response:
    Obeys commands (6)
    Localizes pain (5)
    Withdraws (4)
    Flexion to pain (3)
    Extension to pain (2)
    None (1)
Pupillary size and reactivity
CT scan:
  Mass lesion
  Cerebral edema
  Midline shift/absent basal cisterns

BOX 10–2 *Pupillary Assessment in the Patient with Brain Injury*

1. The pupil is considered "dilated" if pupillary diameter is > 4 mm.
2. The pupil is considered "fixed" in the absence of constrictor response to bright light.
3. Bilateral pupillary light reflex should be assessed and used as a prognostic factor.
4. The duration of pupillary dilation and fixation should be documented.
5. Any asymmetry of pupils should be documented.
6. Hypotension and hypoxia should be corrected before pupillary assessment.
7. Orbital trauma should be excluded.
8. Pupils should be reassessed after surgical intervention (e.g., evacuation of hematoma).

Modified from The Brain Trauma Foundation, The American Association of Neurological Surgeons, The Joint Section on Neurotrauma and Critical Care: Pupillary diameter and light reflex. J Neurotrauma 2000;17:583-590.

---

or third nerve compression may cause a dilated, nonreactive pupil in the absence of a brain injury. In head-injured patients with systolic blood pressures greater than 60 mm Hg, clinical signs of tentorial herniation or upper brainstem dysfunction are valid indicators of possible mechanical compression.[5]

Figure 10–1 Computed tomography (CT) of epidural hematoma. **A,** Plain CT scan shows parietal epidural hematoma. **B,** Contrast-enhanced CT scan shows enhancing dural rim (*arrow*). (*From Haaga JR, Alfidi RJ [eds]: Computed Tomography of the Whole Body, Vol 1. St. Louis, Mosby, 1983, p 185.*)

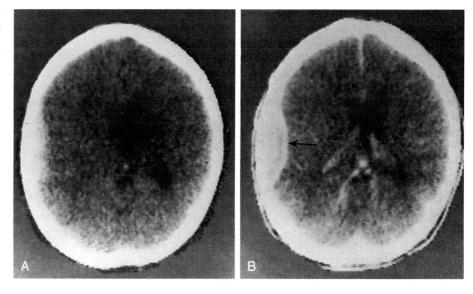

Figure 10–2 Computed tomography (CT) of subdural hematoma. **A,** Acute subdural hematoma can be seen (*arrow*). **B,** Note the marked midline shift, with displacement of lateral ventricles toward the left. (*From Haaga JR, Alfidi RJ [eds]: Computed Tomography of the Whole Body, Vol 1. St. Louis, Mosby, 1983, p 187.*)

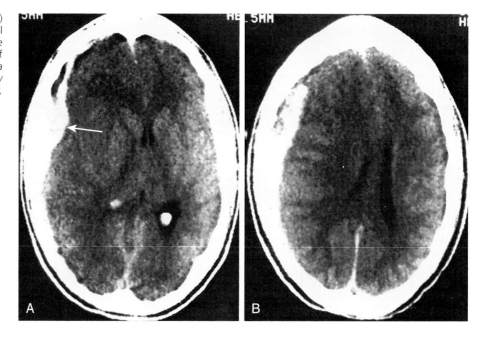

However, in patients with systolic blood pressure less than 60 mm Hg or with cardiac arrest, pupillary signs are unreliable indicators of mechanical compression.[5]

Radiologic Evaluation

After neurologic evaluation and initial stabilization, radiologic evaluation with computed tomography (CT) is performed to diagnose the underlying disease process. If the patient is hemodynamically unstable with intra-abdominal or intrathoracic bleeding, the head CT scan is delayed until the life-threatening surgical bleeding is stopped. If the physical examination indicates high likelihood of a brain injury, an intracranial pressure (ICP) monitor may be placed concurrently with the laparotomy or thoracotomy. Intracranial mass lesions that require rapid surgical treatment, such as epidural, subdural, or large intracerebral hemorrhages, are readily identified on CT scan (Figs. 10-1 and 10-2).

Nonsurgical lesions, such as cerebral edema and hemorrhagic contusion, are also identified (Fig. 10-3). Diffuse cerebral swelling may develop after head trauma, especially in children.[6] The severity of the brain injury can be correlated with the magnitude of the midline shift (see Fig. 10-2) and compression of the basal cisterns (see Fig. 10-3).[7] In one study, patients with GCS scores of 6 to 8 in whom initial CT scan showed absence of or compression of the basal cisterns had a fourfold higher risk of poor outcome than those with normal cisterns.[7] Because patients may often have delayed neurologic deterioration, a repeat CT scan is indicated after any deterioration in neurologic status. Of patients whose conditions deteriorated after a mild head injury, 80% had a mass lesion that potentially required surgery.[7] In contrast, cerebral swelling is more likely to be the cause of deterioration in patients with severe head injury. Occasionally, manifestation of an intracerebral hematoma after head trauma is delayed.

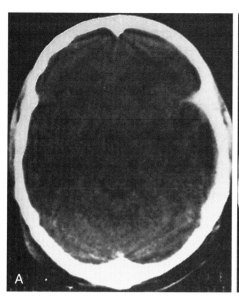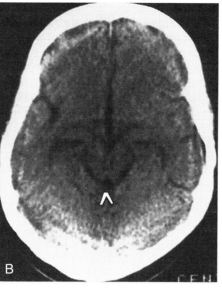

Figure 10–3 Computed tomography scans showing compressed basal cisterns (**A**) and normal basal cisterns (**B**, *arrow*). The presence of compressed basal cisterns after head trauma increases the risk of poor outcome. *(From Toutant SM, Klauber MR, Marshall LF, et al: Absent or compressed basal cisterns on first CT scan: Ominous predictors of outcome in sever head injury. J Neurosurg 1984;61:691-694.)*

Evaluation of Other Organ Systems

In addition to the neurologic evaluation, an evaluation of other organ systems should be performed (Box 10-3).

Respiratory System

Chest radiography should be performed soon after the patient arrives in the emergency department. Many patients are hypoxemic after head trauma, and an increased degree of pulmonary shunting is associated with a worsened neurologic outcome.[8,9] Hypoxemia may be due to airway obstruction, hypoventilation from the brain injury, atelectasis, aspiration, pneumothorax, or pulmonary contusion. On rare occasions, neurogenic pulmonary edema may occur, often in the more devastating injuries. Neurogenic pulmonary edema has been reported after a variety of central nervous system insults, including subarachnoid hemorrhage (SAH), intracranial hemorrhage, head trauma, spinal cord trauma, acute hydrocephalus, colloid cyst of the third ventricle, seizures, and hypothalamic lesions. An acute rise in ICP often, but not always, accompanies the development of pulmonary edema. Increases in ICP may elicit only the sympathetic activation and cardiopulmonary responses that are essential for the development of edema. The mechanism of neurogenic pulmonary edema is not completely understood.[10] Marked sympathetic activation at the time of the injury may damage the pulmonary capillary endothelium by both hydrostatic and increased permeability mechanisms.[10,11] Increased pulmonary shunting may also be observed in patients with head trauma in the absence of distinct pulmonary edema or pathologic condition.[12,13] The increased alveolar-arterial oxygen tension gradient in these patients may be related to airway closure caused by a decreased functional residual capacity in a comatose patient or by neurogenic alterations in ventilation-perfusion matching.[14]

Cardiovascular System

Severe brain injury activates the autonomic nervous system and causes a hyperdynamic cardiovascular response consisting of hypertension, tachycardia, increased cardiac output, and electrocardiogram changes that may mimic myocardial ischemia.[15-17] A Cushing response, in which bradycardia accompanies the hypertension, may occur.[18] This response is thought to occur because marked intracranial hypertension

---

BOX 10–3 *Brain Injury: Effects on Other Organ Systems*

1. Respiratory system:
   a. Upper airway obstruction, inability to protect airway.
   b. Increased pulmonary shunting.
   b. Neurogenic pulmonary edema.
   c. Associated pulmonary injuries: atelectasis, aspiration, pneumothorax, hemothorax, flail chest, pulmonary contusion.
2. Cardiovascular system:
   a. Sympathetic nervous system overactivity.
   b. Hemorrhagic shock.
   c. Cushing response (hypertension, bradycardia).
   d. Hypotension (another cause should be sought).
3. Musculoskeletal system:
   a. Cervical spine injury in 10% of cases.
   b. Long bone or pelvic fractures.
4. Gastrointestinal system:
   a. "Full stomach."
   b. Blood alcohol levels.
   c. Possible intra-abdominal injury.
5. Other systems:
   a. Disseminated intravascular coagulation.
   b. Hypokalemia.
   c. Hyperglycemia.
   d. Diabetes insipidus.
   e. Hyponatremia.

---

causes medullary ischemia as a result of decreased cerebral perfusion pressure (CPP) and brainstem distortion, resulting in activation of medullary sympathetic and vagal centers.[18] Although bradycardia accompanies the hypertension in a classic Cushing response, the presence of a relative tachycardia in a patient with a "blown" pupil may indicate that the patient is hypovolemic. If the patient has outright hypotension, other sources of blood loss (e.g., pelvic, thoracic, abdominal) should be sought. An isolated head injury is not generally associated with hypotension because the blood loss from the head wound is usually insufficient to cause hypotension in adults.

Musculoskeletal System

A lateral cervical spine (C-spine) radiography study should be performed immediately because approximately 10% of patients with head injuries have associated cervical spine injuries. The lateral cervical spine film picks up approximately 80% of cervical spine fractures[19] and can display lethal injuries such as atlanto-occipital separation. The remainder of the spine series that is required to "clear the neck" (confirm absence of vertebral injuries) should be performed later, after complete evaluation of the head injury. Many patients with head trauma also have long-bone or pelvic fractures that may cause significant blood loss or fat emboli.

Gastrointestinal System

Every patient with a neurosurgical emergency should be assumed to have a full stomach and to be at risk for aspiration. Patients with acute head trauma may also have intra-abdominal injuries. Delayed gastric emptying may persist for several weeks after severe head injury.[20] Significant blood alcohol levels have been found in more than 50% of head-injured patients.[21]

Other Systems

Patients with head trauma may also have disseminated intravascular coagulation, possibly caused by release of brain thromboplastin into the systemic circulation.[22,23] Outcome is poorer in patients in whom the condition develops.[22] An increase in fibrin split products may identify patients with head injury who are at high risk for adult respiratory distress syndrome.[24] Coagulation factor levels should be checked in the emergency department, and aggressive replacement of platelets and clotting factors may be required. Use of recombinant factor VII has been advocated in patients with polytrauma that includes traumatic brain injury (TBI)[25-27] and with spontaneous intracranial hemorrhages.[28] However, this agent cannot be recommended as prophylactic therapy in patients without acute bleeding because of the serious risk of thromboembolic events.[29]

The patient may demonstrate hypokalemia and hyperglycemia in response to stress and trauma.[30] β-adrenergic receptor stimulation from epinephrine causes a decrease in serum potassium by driving potassium into the cells. Similarly, when pH is elevated, as is common in the brain-injured patient in whom hyperventilation is used to reduce ICP, potassium is driven into cells as hydrogen ions are released. Decreases in serum potassium values associated with acute hyperventilation and stress do not need to be treated, because total body potassium is unchanged. However, diuretic-induced renal losses of potassium do require replacement to avoid complications of acute intracellular potassium depletion, including potentiation of neuromuscular blockade and cardiac dysrhythmias. Often, in the acutely brain-injured patient, the cause of hypokalemia is multifactorial. Initiation of treatment depends on the predominant clinical circumstances.

Diabetes insipidus may occur in the patient with basilar skull fracture or severe head injury involving the hypothalamus or posterior pituitary. Antidiuretic hormone (ADH) is synthesized in the hypothalamus and secreted by the posterior pituitary. ADH enhances the permeability of free H_2O in the distal convoluted tubule and collecting duct of the kidney. Patients with diabetes insipidus can lose large volumes (25 L/day) of dilute urine, resulting in marked increases in serum sodium and osmolality values.

Diabetes insipidus should be considered in the differential diagnosis of polyuria in any patient with head trauma or pituitary and hypothalamic lesions. The differential diagnosis of intraoperative polyuria includes excessive fluid administration, osmotic agents (e.g., hyperglycemia with serum glucose level greater than 180 mg/dL, mannitol), diuretics, paradoxic diuresis in patients with brain tumor,[31] and nephrogenic and central diabetes insipidus. Diabetes insipidus is diagnosed intraoperatively by the ruling out of iatrogenic causes and hyperglycemia and through demonstration of marked increases in serum sodium and osmolality with low urine osmolality.

Treatment of diabetes insipidus involves adequate fluid replacement with half-normal (0.45%) saline and administration of ADH. Five percent dextrose in water may alternatively be used; however, caution should be applied to avoid hyperglycemia. Aqueous vasopressin may be given subcutaneously or intramuscularly (5 to 10 U) every 6 hours or as a slow intravenous infusion (up to 0.01 U/kg/hr) for rapid control of intraoperative or postoperative diabetes insipidus.[32] Larger doses may cause hypertension. For less frequent dosage, desmopressin (DDAVP) 1 to 4 mcg intravenously or subcutaneously every 12 hours may be administered. Desmopressin may be given more frequently if the diabetes insipidus is not controlled. This agent has less vasopressor activity than aqueous vasopressin and is preferable to vasopressin in patients with coronary artery disease and hypertension.

Hyponatremia may also occur in the acutely brain-injured patient. Hyponatremia may be associated with diminished (e.g., diuretic usage, adrenal insufficiency, salt-losing nephritis), expanded (e.g., congestive heart failure, renal failure), or normal (e.g., hypothyroidism, syndrome of inappropriate ADH secretion) extracellular fluid volumes. Rapid reduction of the serum sodium value to less than 125 to 130 mEq/L may cause changes in mental status and seizures. The first step in diagnosis is to establish the category to which the patient belongs. Although many clinicians are quick to suggest syndrome of inappropriate ADH secretion in patients with brain injury, this diagnosis should be made only after exclusion of other possible causes. In neurosurgical patients, hyponatremia is most commonly associated with intravascular volume depletion caused by diuretic administration or a loss of sodium via the kidney. After subarachnoid hemorrhage, patients may have a primary natriuresis ("cerebral salt wasting"), which, unlike syndrome of inappropriate ADH secretion, is associated with a decreased intravascular volume.[33] Aggressive fluid therapy is required in patients with SAH to maintain a normal intravascular volume.

Airway Management of the Brain-Injured Patient

Patients with a GCS score of 8 or less or with impending herniation require endotracheal intubation in the emergency department. Uncooperative patients who require sedation for CT and other radiologic studies also require intubation, because patients with suspected head injury should not be sedated without an endotracheal tube in place and control of ventilation ensured. Trauma patients should be assumed to have a cervical spine injury until proven otherwise. Nasal intubation should be avoided in patients with suspected basilar skull fractures and sinus injuries.

The patient's airway and hemodynamic status should be quickly assessed before a plan for endotracheal intubation is chosen (Fig. 10-4). If the airway is difficult, hypnotic drugs and muscle relaxants are contraindicated unless the ability to ventilate has been established. Direct laryngoscopy is usually performed with minimal sedation. Newer airway equipment,

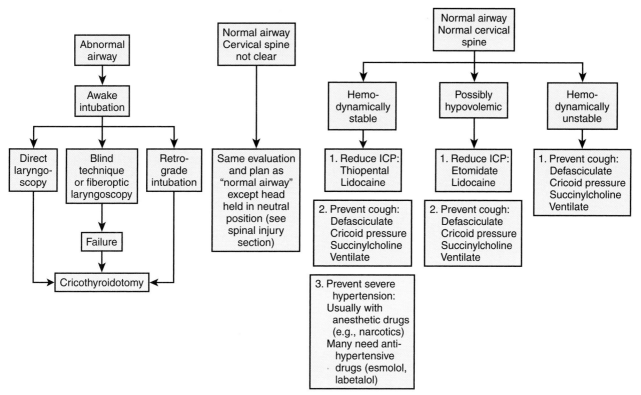

Figure 10–4 Airway management of the brain-injured patient. ICP, intracranial pressure.

such as optical and video laryngoscopes (AirTraq, GlideScope, McGrath) and stylets (Shikani Seeing Stylet), may be utilized to improve visualization of the glottic opening. However, fiberoptic laryngoscopy is still considered the "gold standard" for management of the difficult airway, especially if concomitant cervical spine injury is suspected. In some cases, a cricothyroidotomy may be required.

If the airway appears normal, a muscle relaxant should be given to facilitate glottic exposure and reduce coughing.[34] The prevention of the cough by the prior administration of a muscle relaxant appears to be most important in preventing significant increases in ICP with endotracheal intubation. White and colleagues[35] found that succinylcholine, but not thiopental, fentanyl, or lidocaine, prevented marked rises in ICP with endotracheal suctioning in comatose head-injured patients, because of the greater reduction in coughing after administration of succinylcholine. However, barbiturates and lidocaine were effective in attenuating the increase in ICP due to tracheal stimulation in patients who also received a muscle relaxant.[5,36-39] These drugs and narcotics may also be necessary to prevent increases in mean arterial pressure and ICP with endotracheal intubation.

One should assess the patient's hemodynamic status to choose an anesthesia induction agent that reduces the increase in ICP that accompanies endotracheal intubation. The primary goal is to maintain adequate CPP by ensuring hemodynamic stability while reducing ICP. Severe hypotension from the inappropriate administration of a large dose of thiopental in a hypovolemic patient may be worse for the patient than the transient rise in ICP that accompanies endotracheal intubation. If the patient is hypertensive or hemodynamically stable, a rapid-sequence induction with head and neck stabilization, defasciculation, cricoid pressure, and administration of thiopental, lidocaine, and suc-

cinylcholine can be used. To avoid hypoxemia and excessive increases in $Paco_2$, the patient is manually hyperventilated while cricoid pressure is maintained before intubation. If the patient is hypertensive, administration of narcotics (such as fentanyl), antihypertensive agents, or both may be necessary to prevent severe hypertension and increases in ICP with endotracheal intubation, but extreme caution is required to prevent untoward reductions in CPP in this setting. Esmolol and labetalol have less potential to raise ICP than sodium nitroprusside, which is a marked cerebrovasodilator.[40-42] If the patient is somewhat hypovolemic (as is common in the patient with multiple injuries), etomidate (0.2-0.4 mg/kg) should be used as an alternative to thiopental because it is effective in reducing cerebral blood flow (CBF) and ICP.[43] If the patient is severely hypovolemic, a hypnotic agent is contraindicated, and defasciculation followed by succinylcholine should be used. Ketamine should be avoided because it raises ICP.[44]

The use of succinylcholine as the muscle relaxant of choice in endotracheal intubation of the acutely brain-injured patient is somewhat controversial. Succinylcholine may transiently increase ICP because of greater CO_2 production or cerebral stimulation from the fasciculations.[45] Defasciculation with metocurine appears to prevent succinylcholine-induced rises in ICP.[46] In addition, thiopental, etomidate, and lidocaine reduce ICP and minimize the succinylcholine effect. Therefore the benefits of rapid intubation and hyperventilation outweigh the disadvantages in the acutely injured patient. However, in the patient recovering from a closed-head injury even without residual neurologic deficit, use of succinylcholine can potentially cause hyperkalemia and subsequent cardiac arrest, and so should be avoided. The exact mechanism of this phenomenon is not clear. Rocuronium (0.6-1.2 mg/kg) should be chosen in this circumstance,

> **BOX 10–4** *Major Goals in the Acute Care of the Brain-Injured Patient*
>
> A. Prevention of hypoxemia—maintain PaO_2 > 60 mm Hg or SaO_2 > 90%:
>   1. Increase inspired oxygen tension.
>   2. Treat pulmonary pathologic condition.
>   3. Consider positive end-expiratory pressure (10 cm H_2O or less).
> B. Maintenance of blood pressure:
>   1. Prevent hypotension—maintain systolic blood pressure (SBP) > 90 mm Hg:
>   a. Avoid glucose-containing solutions.
>   b. Maintain intravascular volume status—aim for euvolemia.
>   2. Treat hypertension:
>   a. Sympathetic nervous system overactivity.
>   b. Increased intracranial pressure.
>   c. Light anesthesia.
> C. Reduction in intracranial pressure:
>   1. Head position.
>   2. Brief periods of hyperventilation.
>   3. Hyperosmolar therapy.
>   4. Sedation.
>   5. Hypothermia.
>   6. Surgical procedures: drainage of cerebrospinal fluid and evacuation of hematoma.

assuming that the airway is not difficult and the patient can receive ventilation.

Aims in the Acute Care of the Brain-Injured Patient

The principal aim in the acute medical management of the brain-injured patient is to prevent secondary neurologic injury. Over the last 30 years, an understanding of the pathophysiology and goals of an early treatment of the potential causes of secondary neurologic injury led to a significant decrease in mortality of patients with severe traumatic brain injury, from 50% to 25% to 30%.[47]

Secondary brain injury is an important determinant of outcome from severe head injury. Factors contributing to the development of secondary neurologic injury include hypoxia, hypercapnia, hypotension, intracranial hypertension, and transtentorial or cerebellar herniation. Durations of systemic hypotension with systolic blood pressure (SBP) 90 mm Hg or higher, hypoxia with arterial O_2 saturation (SaO_2) 90% or higher, and pyrexia with core temperature 38° C or higher have been found to be strongly associated with mortality after head injury.[48] Many of these factors are potentially treatable. Rose and associates[49] found that an avoidable factor (such as hypoxia, hypotension, and delay in the treatment of an intracranial hematoma) was identified in 54% of 116 patients who had been known to have talked before dying. Both CPP greater than 90 mm Hg and higher GCS scores correlated with better neurologic outcome,[50] whereas CPP lower than 50 mm Hg is independently associated with poor outcome after head trauma.[48] Box 10-4 summarizes the aims in the acute care of patients with head injuries.

High-dose steroids do not reduce ICP in head trauma[51] and do not affect outcome from severe head injury.[52] They are therefore not recommended for the treatment of acute TBI. Steroids may be useful in reducing edema in the rare patient who presents with impending brain herniation from a brain tumor.[53] In such a patient, clinical improvement occurs within hours of the initiation of steroid therapy.

Prevention of Hypoxemia

Prompt and aggressive treatment of hypoxemia in head-injured patients is imperative because hypoxemia is associated with development of secondary brain injury, worsening neurologic outcome,[8] and increasing mortality, especially when associated with systemic hypotension.[48,54] Stocchetti and colleagues[55] reported that hypoxemia was present at the accident in 55% of patients with TBI and was strongly associated with the poor outcome.[55] According to a study of 717 cases in the Traumatic Coma Data Bank, hypoxemia was identified in 22.4% patients with severe TBI and was associated with increases in morbidity and mortality.[54]

Every patient with brain injury should be assessed according to general "ABC" principles of trauma management (airway, breathing, circulation), which is initiated with providing an adequate airway and breathing/ventilation. Every brain-injured patient should receive supplemental oxygen regardless of initial GCS score. Oxygenation should be monitored whenever possible with pulse oximeter or by measurement of arterial blood gas levels. The minimum goal of oxygenation in patients with brain injury should be to maintain SaO_2 at 90% or higher or PaO_2 at 60 mm Hg or higher.[56] Patients with severe brain injury should be intubated and ventilated with 100% oxygen until adequate oxygenation is verified.

The possibility has been raised that positive end-expiratory pressure (PEEP) may increase ICP in the brain-injured patient because it may increase cerebral venous volume by reducing cerebral venous outflow.[57] However, most later studies suggest that 10 cm H_2O PEEP improves oxygenation and usually causes clinically inconsequential increases in ICP in patients with severe head trauma.[58-60] PEEP may affect ICP less in patients with the stiffest lungs, who are presumably the ones who need PEEP the most.[58,59]

Maintenance of Blood Pressure

HYPOTENSION

When systemic hypotension is defined as SBP less than 90 mm Hg, even a single recorded prehospital episode has been shown to correlate with higher morbidity and mortality in patients with TBI.[54] While patients are in the intensive care unit, the duration of hypotension (SBP < 90 mm Hg) strongly correlates with worsening of neurologic outcome as assessed by the GCS and with an increase in mortality.[48] Blood pressure should be monitored and SBP should be kept higher than 90 mm Hg.[56]

The most common hemodynamic problem in the patient with head trauma and multiple injuries is hypovolemia caused by blood loss, profound diuresis from mannitol, and inappropriate attempts to restrict fluid intake. Because the damaged brain tolerates hypotension poorly, intravenous fluids should be administered in sufficient quantities to rapidly restore intravascular volume and CBF. Intraoperative blood loss may be severe in vascular injuries and skull fractures. Massive volume replacement may be required intraoperatively if a dural sinus is injured. In addition, blood loss may be difficult to quantify because it spills on the drapes and on the floor. Patients with large intracranial hemorrhages, with normal blood pressures in the lower range (SBP 100-120 mm Hg), or with relative tachycardia (heartbeat > 100 beats/min), should be considered to be hypovolemic unless proven otherwise. The hypovolemia may manifest as severe hypotension when the brain is decompressed. With the acute reduction of ICP,

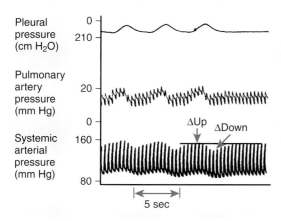

Pleural pressure (cm H₂O)

Pulmonary artery pressure (mm Hg)

ΔUp   ΔDown

Systemic arterial pressure (mm Hg)

5 sec

Figure 10–5 Continuous record from mechanically ventilated dog after hemorrhage of 10% of blood volume. Pleural, pulmonary arterial, and systemic pressures are shown. Note the fluctuation in systolic blood pressure with positive-pressure ventilation. The difference between maximum and minimum systolic blood pressure is divided into delta up (ΔUp) and delta down (ΔDown) components. The delta up component is the difference between maximum systolic and end-expiratory systolic blood pressure during a 5-second period of apnea; the delta down component is the difference between end-expiratory and minimum systolic blood pressures. The systolic blood pressure variation and delta up and delta down components correlate with the severity of hypovolemia better than central venous pressure. *(From Perel A, Pizov R, Cotev S: Systolic blood pressure variation is a sensitive indicator of hypovolemia in ventilated dogs subjected to graded hemorrhage. Anesthesiology 1987;67:498-502.)*

sympathetic tone and systemic vascular resistance are diminished, revealing profound intravascular volume depletion. Vasopressors may be helpful in restoring blood pressure while fluid is being given to restore intravascular volume to normal. However, overzealous fluid administration that elevates cerebral venous pressure may exacerbate brain edema.

The presence of hypovolemia is best assessed from clinical signs such as hypotension, tachycardia, inability to tolerate anesthetic agents, and SBP variations with positive-pressure ventilation. A drop in SBP greater than 10 mm Hg with positive-pressure ventilation is a sensitive indicator of a 10% reduction in blood volume (Fig. 10-5).[61] This decrease in SBP is a significantly better indicator than the central venous pressure.[62,63]

The variation in SBP correlates well with the degree of hemorrhage in dogs and humans. However, placement of a central venous line may be helpful in the acute setting, especially to prevent overhydration, and should ultimately be performed to help guide fluid replacement. Timely evacuation of the brain mass must be accomplished first, with placement of central line performed later, after surgery has begun and the patient has been stabilized.

HYPERTENSION

Patients are often hypertensive after an isolated brain injury, because of an increase in catecholamines from stress-induced activation of the sympathetic nervous system.[15,16] Because autoregulation may be impaired after head trauma,[64] hypertension may cause brain hyperemia, promote the development of vasogenic edema, and further increase ICP. However, before immediate treatment of the blood pressure elevation with an antihypertensive agent, other causes of hypertension (such as increased ICP and inadequate anesthesia) should be first eliminated. Ensuring adequate oxygenation and ventilation, placing the head up slightly in neutral position,

preventing coughing, or administering barbiturates alone or together with narcotics may help reduce ICP and provide greater anesthesia. Usually these measures are effective to control blood pressure in the acute management of the brain-injured patient. However, in the patient with preexisting hypertension or the severely hyperdynamic patient, control of hypertension with β-adrenergic antagonists (e.g., metoprolol, labetalol, esmolol) may also be indicated.[42] These drugs specifically treat the cause of hypertension (e.g., sympathetic overactivity), and they are not cerebral vasodilators. Prophylactic β-adrenergic receptor blockade may also be useful in reducing supraventricular tachycardia, ST-segment and T-wave changes, and myocardial necrosis associated with severe head injury. Systemic vasodilators, such as sodium nitroprusside, nitroglycerin, and hydralazine, may increase ICP and should be avoided.[40,41,65-67]

FLUID MANAGEMENT

Iso-osmolar crystalloid solutions should be used to replace intravascular volume. These include Plasma-Lyte, Normosol-R, and 0.9% normal saline. Although use of any of these solutions may considerably raise ICP after resuscitation from shock,[68] ICP would be higher after inadequate resuscitation because of the development of cytotoxic edema from cerebral ischemia. The blood-brain barrier may be damaged by head trauma, allowing all fluids to cross the blood-brain barrier. Overhydration, causing increases in central venous pressure, should be avoided. Therefore the aim of fluid management is to maintain a euvolemic patient. Bloody, less urgent procedures (e.g., many orthopedic procedures) should be delayed several days, until the brain injury has stabilized, because of the potential for exacerbation of cerebral edema. Lactated Ringer's solution should be avoided because of its hypo-osmolarity.[69]

The choice between *colloid* and *crystalloid* solutions for fluid replacement remains controversial. Water movement across the blood-brain barrier depends primarily on the difference in osmolality between plasma and brain. Decreases in oncotic pressure may not affect brain water content much because oncotic pressure makes only a small contribution to total plasma osmolality. Most experimental studies suggest that brain water content and ICP are no different whether isotonic colloid or crystalloid solutions are administered.[70] Although there is experimental evidence that colloids may result in less brain edema in a model of head trauma,[71] this finding has not been supported by human studies. Investigators of the SAFE (Saline versus Albumin Fluid Evaluation) trial[72] analyzed results from a subgroup of 460 patients with TBI who were randomized to receive albumin or 0.9% saline for the initial fluid resuscitation.[73] The authors demonstrated a strong association of albumin administration with the poor neurologic outcome (52.7% in albumin versus 39.4% in saline group) and death (33.2% in albumin versus 20.4% in saline group) at 24 months after TBI.[73] Significantly higher morbidity and mortality with albumin than with saline was found for patients with severe TBI, with GCS score 3 to 8 at admission, but not with moderate TBI. The mechanism of such a dramatic influence of albumin on the outcome after TBI is not clear; however, aggravation of brain edema following movement of albumin across the disrupted blood-brain barrier has been hypothesized.[73] This theory is also supported by another randomized clinical trial,[74] in which 90 patients with TBI were randomly assigned to receive initial fluid resuscitation with either fresh frozen plasma or 0.9% saline, which demonstrated a higher incidence of intracerebral hematoma formation and an increased 1-month mortality after the use of fresh frozen plasma.[74]

Large volumes (>500 mL) of 6% hetastarch also should not be administered because they may cause a coagulopathy that may manifest as an intracranial hematoma.[75] Hetastarch prolongs the partial thromboplastin time (PTT) through a decrease in factor VIII coagulant activity and von Willebrand factor level.

Hypertonic saline (HS) solutions have potential advantage over other solutions in the resuscitation of hypotensive brain-injured patients because of their ability to reduce brain water content and ICP[68,76,77] and to stabilize blood pressure. Small-volume (bolus of 250 mL) resuscitation with 7.5% HS in hypotensive patients with multiple trauma and TBI has been shown to be safe[78] and tends to better stabilize blood pressure and to improve in-hospital survival in patients with severe TBI (GCS score < 8) than lactated Ringer's solution.[79,80] However, when the same regimens of fluid resuscitation were compared in patients with GCS scores less than 9 and SBP lower than 100 mm Hg, the neurologic outcome at 6 months after injury in patients who received HS did not differ from that in the patients who received lactated Ringer's solution.[81] There are no current data about an optimal concentration and volume of HS that can be recommended for fluid resuscitation. However, with safety and potential benefits taken into account, use of HS for fluid resuscitation in a hemodynamically unstable patient with brain injury represents one of the reasonable options. Other concentrations of HS—1.6%[82] or 3%[83]—may be used as well. Because the osmolality values of 3% HS and 20% mannitol are close, 5 mL/kg of 3% HS will provide the same osmolar load as 1 g/kg of 20% mannitol. To date, there are very few clinical situations in which use of HS is of major concern. Although rapid correction of sodium in a patient with chronic hyponatremia may potentially predispose to development of central pontine myelinolysis,[84] the later literature does not reveal any cases of central pontine myelinolysis after resuscitation with HS, even after repeated boluses. On the other hand, continuous administration of HS in patients with syndrome of inappropriate ADH secretion may potentially aggravate hyponatremia owing to accumulation of fluid, so HS should not be used as a first-line drug; it should be given only after water restriction and a diuretic regimen have been initiated.

In summary, 0.9% saline remains the "gold standard" for fluid resuscitation after brain injury. Other iso-osmotic solutions (e.g., Plasma-Lyte) are appropriate choices, but levels of blood electrolytes should be monitored with their use. Albumin is not recommended and, most probably, can be considered contraindicated in patients with severe TBI. Prophylactic administration of fresh frozen plasma is not recommended and should be used judiciously in patients with signs of coagulopathy.

Blood Glucose Control

In critically ill neurologic patients stress-induced hyperglycemia is common, and has been strongly associated with increased morbidity and mortality after stroke,[85-87] subarachnoid hemorrhage[88] head trauma,[89,90] and cardiac arrest.[89,91] In these human studies, whether the hyperglycemia was the cause or the result of the increased severity of the neurologic damage is unclear.

Although cellular mechanisms of hyperglycemia, such as an impaired immunity and an increased risk of infection, mitochondrial damage, intracellular acidosis, endothelial injury and inflammation, have been described, the exact mechanisms for the enhanced neurologic damage are unclear. How glucose administration affects outcome after brain injury also is not known. In a rat model of head trauma, glucose administration did not alter neurologic outcome or the formation of brain edema.[92]

The exact threshold level of blood glucose value above which ischemic neurologic damage is increased is also not known; however, it appears to be less than 200 mg/dL. On the other hand, tight glycemic control (maintaining of blood glucose level at 80-100 mg/dL) using intensive insulin therapy, which has been broadly advocated in the surgical critically ill population,[93] has been recently shown to be detrimental.[94] Tight glycemic control may be particularly dangerous in patients who had experienced some degree of brain injury, such as cardiac arrest,[95] and subarachnoid hemorrhage[96] because of high incidence of hypoglycemia, lack of benefit, or worsening of outcome.

Glucose-containing solutions should not be administered acutely to the brain-injured patient because they may exacerbate neurologic damage. Numerous animal studies provide convincing evidence that glucose administration, with or without marked hyperglycemia, enlarges infarct size and augments neurologic damage from global and regional cerebral ischemia.[97]

Part of the difficulty in determining a "safe" level of blood glucose in patients is that blood glucose levels may not accurately reflect brain glucose levels during periods of transient hyperglycemia. Brain glucose values remain elevated after glucose infusion, whereas blood glucose values decrease in response to insulin. Experimental evidence has suggested that postischemic treatment of acute hyperglycemia with insulin reduces neurologic damage.[98] Rats that received low doses of insulin to lower blood glucose to 67 mg/dL after an ischemic brain insult had lower seizure incidence, cortical infarction size, and mortality than control animals that remained hyperglycemic (212 mg/dL). These data suggest that at least acute elevations (as associated with stress caused by the neurologic injury) in blood glucose should be treated. Chronic elevations in blood glucose should also presumably be treated. However, the actual benefits and risks of acute reductions of blood glucose in patients with chronic hyperglycemia are unclear from current experimental and clinical evidence.

Temperature Control

Hyperthermia (temperature > 38° C) is known to be detrimental for patients with brain injury and is strongly associated with worsening neurologic outcome and increasing mortality in patients with TBI,[48] SAH,[99] and stroke.[100] Undoubtedly, hyperpyrexia in patients with brain injury should be avoided and treated. Aggressive warming up of patients with traumatic brain injury who were hypothermic at arrival has been shown to be detrimental[101]; therefore fast infusion of warmed fluids should be performed cautiously, especially in the operating room setting in cases of hypovolemia and hemorrhage, with the danger of hyperpyrexia in mind.

Treatment options to reduce temperature in patients with acute brain injury include (1) antipyretic medications (aspirin, acetaminophen, ibuprofen, diclofenac), which can be used in patients with stroke but not in those with TBI because of potential worsening of coagulation, (2) external devices such as cooling blankets, which are the most safe and useful tools, and (3) internal cooling such as an intravenous infusion of cold saline and, in resistant hyperpyrexia, endovascular cooling. Currently, there are no data available demonstrating the optimal treatment of the febrile patient with acute neurologic injury, so the treatment approach should be specifically chosen for each patient.

From the physiologic point of view, induction of hypothermia in the patient with brain injury offers the potential benefit of reducing the cerebral metabolic rate of oxygen. Currently there are no sufficient data for a strong recommendation of inducing mild hypothermia in brain-injured patients. Based on the analysis of six randomized control trials[101-106] performed during the last 15 years (target cooling temperature between 32° and 35° C), Brain Trauma Foundation 2007 Guidelines suggested recently that moderate hypothermia may potentially improve outcome after traumatic brain injury, suggesting that initiation of hypothermia targeted to 32° to 33° C should be induced and maintained for at least 48 hours after injury to decrease the mortality rate.[107] However, concomitant use of barbiturates and hypothermia can significantly raise the incidence of pneumonia, and therefore, in patients with increased ICP, the conventional treatment including barbiturates should be applied first, before hypothermia is considered.

Monitoring and Treatment of Intracranial Hypertension

A major goal in the acute treatment of the brain-injured patient is to reduce ICP, which may be accomplished through head position, hyperventilation, hyperosmotic solutions and diuretics, barbiturates, and surgical treatment. Monitoring of ICP, CPP, oxygen saturation in the jugular bulb (Sjo_2), and brain tissue oxygen (Pbo_2) are useful tools for the bedside assessment of the patients with brain injury.

HEAD POSITION

A slightly head-up position (up to 30-degree head-up tilt) with the neck in neutral position promotes cerebral venous drainage and reduces ICP if the cerebrospinal fluid pathways are still patent.[108] Lateral turning of the head, tight endotracheal or tracheostomy tube ties around the neck, and the Trendelenburg position may dramatically raise ICP because they restrict venous return from the brain. The patient's respiratory muscles should be paralyzed to prevent coughing and bucking on the endotracheal tube, which also increases ICP. On the other hand, marked elevation of the head in a hypovolemic patient, if it diminishes mean arterial pressure, may cause decreased brain perfusion and cerebral ischemia.

HYPERVENTILATION

Hyperventilation-induced hypocapnia is a powerful therapeutic tool in treatment of intracranial hypertension. Although hypocapnia may acutely lower ICP by causing an extracellular alkalosis and cerebral vasoconstriction, it may increase cerebral ischemia.[109,110] Excessive hyperventilation causes profound cerebral vasoconstriction and a decrease in CBF, which may be detrimental if CBF was already impaired as a result of brain injury. Taking into account that a majority of brain-injured patients suffer a dramatic decrease in CBF to less than 50% of normal in the first 24 to 48 hours after injury,[111,112] the Brain Trauma Foundation's 2007 guidelines recommend avoiding hyperventilation in the first 24 hours after brain injury and avoiding prophylactic hyperventilation.[113]

A randomized, controlled trial of prophylactic hyperventilation therapy for 5 days after severe head trauma also found that outcome was worse in the hyperventilated group, but only in patients with relatively intact motor function.[114] This result may reflect the ability of hypocapnic vasoconstriction to exacerbate cerebral ischemia in the injured brain. Global CBF and regional CBF are severely reduced and metabolism is increased during the first few hours and days after brain injury. Focal cerebral ischemia is common after head trauma.[115,116] Hyperventilation causes a further drop in CBF, often without a decrease in ICP, which may further exacerbate cerebral ischemia.

Mechanical hyperventilation may also have significant adverse cardiopulmonary effects. It may lower systemic blood pressure by reducing venous return, sympathetic stimulation, and cardiac output. It results in a leftward shift of the oxyhemoglobin dissociation curve, causing lower mixed venous and arterial oxygen tension values for any given oxygen saturation. Hypocapnia inhibits hypoxic pulmonary vasoconstriction and causes bronchoconstriction. Increases in pulmonary shunt may occur in hyperventilated patients.[117]

Because of these concerns, $Paco_2$ generally should be kept at normocapnic levels in the patient with head trauma. Brief periods of hypocapnia may be useful and have not been shown to be harmful in the acutely decompensating patient until definitive surgical treatment takes place. According to the Brain Injury Foundation's guidelines for the management of severe traumatic brain injury,[113] if hyperventilation is considered for treatment, a jugular venous bulb catheter should be inserted for monitoring of Sjo_2. Jugular desaturation is common after head injury and traumatic intracranial hematoma, and it may be exacerbated by hyperventilation.[115,116] High interpersonal variability in normal levels of Sjo_2 (55%-75%) may make interpretation of the parameter difficult in the brain-injured patient. However, the majority of experts believe that decrease in Sjo_2 to less than 50% reflects a profound decrease in CBF, which could potentially lead to brain ischemia and should be avoided.

HYPEROSMOLAR THERAPY

Mannitol decreases brain water content and ICP primarily by increasing plasma osmolality, thereby creating an osmotic gradient across the intact blood-brain barrier. The amount of water that can be withdrawn from the brain depends on the magnitude of the osmotic gradient, the total time the gradient exists, and the integrity of the blood-brain barrier. Mannitol is less effective with larger lesions because with damaged blood-brain barriers, mannitol moves down its concentration gradient into the brain. This movement may account for a rebound increase in ICP occasionally seen after mannitol infusion.

Administration of mannitol may cause a triphasic hemodynamic response. Transient (1 to 2 minutes) hypotension may occur after rapid administration of mannitol.[17] Mannitol then increases blood volume, cardiac index, and pulmonary capillary wedge pressure, with a maximum increase shortly after termination of the infusion.[118] ICP may rise transiently because of increases in cerebral blood volume and CBF.[119] ICP increases are attenuated by slow infusion of mannitol, which tends to occur naturally when a bag of 20% mannitol is administered by gravity, as opposed to administration of more concentrated solutions under pressure. Transient rises in ICP are uncommon in the patient with elevated ICP.[120] At 30 minutes after mannitol administration, blood volume returns to normal, and pulmonary capillary wedge pressure and cardiac index drop to below normal levels because of peripheral vascular pooling.[118]

Mannitol reduces blood viscosity and red blood cell rigidity, which may enhance perfusion of the brain microcirculation.

This agent transiently reduces hematocrit and increases serum osmolality. It also causes hyponatremia, hyperkalemia, and decreases in pH caused by HCO_3 dilution. Prolonged and marked hyperosmolality with hyponatremia can occur in patients with acute or chronic renal failure.[121]

Doses of mannitol from 0.25 to 2 g/kg are usually administered; a typical dose is 1 g/kg. Lower doses are effective in reducing ICP acutely and cause fewer electrolyte abnormalities; however, they must be given more frequently. Rapid administration of mannitol causes a more profound reduction in ICP but may transiently cause hypotension and more marked increases in intravascular and cerebral blood volumes. The benefits and disadvantages of a particular dose and speed of administration must be weighed carefully in any patient. Giving more mannitol when the patient's serum osmolality value is higher than 330 mOsm/L is seldom effective.

Mechanisms of action of *hypertonic saline* on the cerebral physiology resemble those of mannitol. Equiosmolar boluses of HS and mannitol have been shown to have similar effects on brain shrinkage in patients undergoing craniotomy with and without SAH[83] as well as on the decrease in ICP in patients with TBI.[122] However, HS does not cause as profound a diuresis or as negative a fluid balance as mannitol does. Therefore, administration of HS can be beneficial and should be considered in hemodynamically unstable or hypovolemic patients or patients with heart disease. Boluses of HS may be administered intravenously over 15 to 20 minutes. No exact bolus volume or concentration of HS solution can be strongly recommended. A wide range of HS solution concentrations, between 1.6% and 7.5%, have been successfully administered peripherally without significant complications. Administration of 5 mL/kg of 3% HS will provide the same osmolar load as 1g/kg of 20% mannitol.

DIURETICS

Furosemide has been reported to lower ICP and brain water content when used alone in large (1 mg/kg) doses[123] or in combination with mannitol in smaller doses.[124] In contrast to mannitol, in some studies, furosemide alone did not reduce ICP. Clinical impressions are that mannitol produces a better reduction of brain bulk than furosemide. However, furosemide may be advantageous to patients with heart and renal diseases because unlike mannitol, it does not increase blood volume or ICP or cause severe electrolyte abnormalities.

The mechanism of furosemide's action on reducing ICP is unknown. It is not related to the agent's diuretic effect. Furosemide may reduce cerebrospinal fluid formation and water and ion penetration across the blood-brain barrier. It also potentiates mannitol by sustaining the increase in serum osmolality induced by mannitol. Therefore reductions in ICP and brain shrinkage are consistently greater and longer in duration with mannitol plus furosemide than with either agent alone.[124] However, hyponatremia, hypokalemia, hypochloremia, hyperosmolality, and a significantly greater rate of water and electrolyte excretion occur with this combination of diuretics. Water excretions of up to 42 mL/min have been reported with the combination of drugs, compared with 17 mL/min with mannitol alone.

Low doses of furosemide (5 to 20 mg) added to mannitol (0.25 to 1 g/kg) are very effective in reducing brain bulk. Larger doses of furosemide may be required to produce the same effect in the patient who had been undergoing long-term diuretic therapy. Mannitol-induced increases in blood volume and ICP may also be attenuated when furosemide is administered before mannitol. However, with administration of combined diuretics, vigorous intravascular fluid and electrolyte replacement are required. A urine loss of 2 to 3 L over 2 hours is common with combined diuretic therapy.

BARBITURATES AND OTHER SEDATIVES AND ANALGETICS

Barbiturates reduce cerebral metabolism, CBF, cerebral blood volume, and ICP. In the acute management of the brain-injured patient, barbiturates are useful to reduce the intracranial response to noxious stimuli, such as endotracheal intubation, tracheal suctioning, and surgical stimulation.[38,39] They may also acutely reduce intraoperative brain swelling. High-dose barbiturates have been used successfully to reduce ICP in patients with head trauma refractory to other treatments[125] and are considered the gold standard for sedation in patients with refractory intracranial hypertension.[126] However, long-term barbiturate therapy probably does not affect long-term outcome after head trauma.[127]

Although barbiturates may aid in the acute control of ICP, their use is limited by the fact that they may cause cardiac depression as well as reduce arterial blood pressure and CPP. Because hypotension is a definite risk factor for worsened neurologic outcome in the brain-injured patient, maintaining a normal blood pressure is particularly important. Thus barbiturates should be carefully titrated (e.g., thiopental in 1- to 4-mg/kg doses), and blood pressure supported with vasopressors or inotropic agents as necessary. Barbiturates should not be administered to hypovolemic or hypotensive patients. Likewise, high doses of barbiturates (e.g., greater than 8 to 10 mg/kg of thiopental) are contraindicated before the surgical evacuation of an intracranial mass, because blood pressure may severely decrease with the reduction in sympathetic tone that accompanies brain decompression. Pentobarbital is the most useful barbiturate for the control of ICP. The classic regimen, which was recommended for inducing barbiturate coma, consisted of a loading dose of pentobarbital, 10 mg/kg over 30 minutes, followed by 5mg/kg/hour for 3 hours, followed by a maintenance infusion of 1 mg/kg/hour.[128] However, other regimens may be successfully used, especially if burst suppression is controlled by EEG. Given the instability of the acutely injured patient, high doses of barbiturates are best reserved for use in the intensive care unit.

Propofol can also be recommended for sedation and control of ICP.[126] Like barbiturates, propofol may cause a decrease in blood pressure; however, the major advantage of propofol is the fast recovery from its effect, which provides a favorable condition for neurologic examination. The dose of propofol required for the burst suppression is high (about 200 µg/kg/min) and therefore provides a high lipid load to the patient. Long-term high-dose (>5 mg/kg/hour) propofol sedation is dangerous because of the potential for development of the fatal propofol-infusion syndrome. This condition is characterized by lactic acidosis, rhabdomyolysis, renal failure, lipemia, fatty infiltration of liver, and fatal cardiac failure.[129-131] It has been shown to have a strong association with neurologic disease, particularly traumatic brain injury. The onset of propofol-infusion syndrome may be short—less than 24 hours—so when a patient is in the intensive care unit, the choice of sedative agent should be reconsidered daily.

Midazolam also reduces cerebral metabolism, blood flow, and blood volume but preserves cerebral autoregulation and can be successfully used for sedation. Usually, continuous infusion of midazolam (2-4 mg/hour) is combined with opioids (morphine sulfate 4 mg/hour, fentanyl 2-5 µg/kg/hour, or sufentanil 0.05-2 µg/kg/hour). Because opioids generally do not affect cerebral metabolism and blood flow and do provide hemodynamic stability, these regimens are well tolerated. However, slow recovery after cessation of infusion makes midazolam-opioid sedation less desirable for patients with brain injury. Reversal of benzodiazepine effects with flumazenil cannot be recommended and should be avoided because flumazenil raises ICP.[132]

SURGICAL TREATMENT

Surgical treatment may be required to lower ICP acutely. If hydrocephalus is present, as it commonly is after an SAH, a ventriculostomy with drainage of cerebrospinal fluid is indicated to reduce ICP. Ventriculostomies are seldom helpful in patients with head trauma because the extent of brain swelling may prevent localization of the ventricles.

Prompt removal of an acute subdural, epidural, or large solitary intracerebral hematoma is indicated. Mortality and morbidity are reduced by prompt diagnosis and surgical treatment of an epidural hematoma, especially if performed before signs of tentorial herniation occur. In addition, mortality from an acute subdural hematoma is reduced by rapid diagnosis and surgical treatment. Seelig and colleagues[133] reported that patients who underwent surgery within 4 hours of injury had a 30% mortality rate, compared with a 90% mortality for those who had surgery after 4 hours.[133]

SPINAL CORD INJURY

Spinal injuries occur in 5% to 10% of major trauma cases. The National Emergency X-Radiography Utilization Study (NEXUS) group, which prospectively enrolled 34,069 patients with blunt trauma who underwent cervical spine radiography at admission in 21 institutions, found an incidence of cervical spine injuries of 2.4%.[134] Risk factors for cervical spine injury included (1) male gender, (2) age older than 65 years, and (3) ethnicity (white, and "other" ethnicity, non-Hispanic, non-black).[135] Motor vehicle accidents are the most common cause of injury, followed by falls, sports injuries, and gunshot or stab wounds. People experiencing head-first falls and unrestrained (by seatbelts) drivers or passengers in high-speed, front-end motor vehicle accidents are at particularly high risk (6% to 10%) for cervical spine injury.[136] At moderate risk (1% to 3%) are drivers or passengers (unrestrained by seatbelts) in lower-speed motor vehicle accidents and people with blunt head trauma or with side-first or foot-first falls. Totally alert patients without any neck pain or tenderness are generally not at risk for spinal injury,[137] because a significant association is found between neck pain or tenderness and cervical injury. However, if a patient has even minimal spinal tenderness, has other painful injuries, or is intoxicated, the cervical spine should be considered unstable and should be fully evaluated.

Only about 5% of all spinal cord injuries are observed in children. In childhood, fractures are less common because spine mobility is greater than that in adulthood as a result of ligamentous laxity and incompletely ossified wedge-shaped vertebrae.[138] However, these anatomic features make children prone to extremely high cervical lesions and increase the incidence of SCI without radiographic abnormality.[139]

Neurologic Evaluation

Evaluation of the Extent of Spinal Cord Injury

A convenient way to visualize the structure of the vertebral column uses the three-column concept.[140] The anterior column contains the anterior longitudinal ligament and the anterior two thirds of the vertebral body and annulus fibrosus. The middle column contains the posterior one third of the vertebral body, annulus fibrosus, and posterior longitudinal ligament. The posterior column consists of the posterior neural arch, spinous processes, articular facet processes, and their corresponding posterior ligamentous column. The three-column concept is useful in localizing spinal injury, depending on the mechanism of injury.

Injuries to the spine may be classified as extension, flexion, compression, rotation, or some combination of these four basic mechanisms (Fig. 10-6). Extension injuries, such as those from blows under the chin or whiplash, mostly disrupt the posterior column. Flexion injuries, such as a diving injury, mostly disrupt the anterior column. The stability of the injured spine is variable and ranges from stable (e.g., burst fracture or wedge of a vertebral body) to very unstable (e.g., hangman's fracture). The primary factor that determines the stability of the injury is the integrity of the ligaments, intervertebral disks, and osseous articulators.[141] In addition, the spinal cord may or may not be injured. With a complete SCI, there is loss of all motor or sensory function below the level of the injury. With incomplete injuries, there is some preservation of

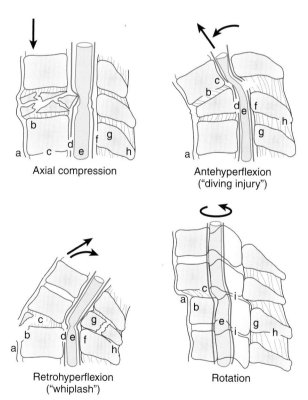

Axial compression

Antehyperflexion ("diving injury")

Retrohyperflexion ("whiplash")

Rotation

Figure 10–6 Mechanisms of spinal cord injury: axial compression, antehyperflexion (flexion injury), retrohyperflexion (extension injury), and rotation. The arrows show the direction of compression, flexion, or rotation injury to the spinal cord. a, Anterior spinal ligament; b, vertebral body; c, intervertebral disk; d, posterior spinal ligament; e, spinal cord; f, ligamentum flavum; g, spinal process; h, interspinous ligaments; i, intervertebral facet joint. Note compression of the anterior elements in flexion injury and compression of the posterior elements in extension injuries. *(From Fraser A, Edmonds-Seal J: Spinal cord injuries: A review of the problems facing the anaesthetist. Anesthesia 1982;37:1084-1098.)*

Table 10–1	**Spinal Cord Injury Syndromes**
Syndrome	Signs
Complete neurologic injury	Loss of all motor and sensory below the level of injury
Incomplete neurologic injury:	
Central cord	Motor loss (arms greater than legs) Bladder dysfunction Variable sensory loss
Brown-Séquard syndrome	Ipsilateral paralysis Ipsilateral loss of proprioception, touch, and vibration Contralateral loss of pain and temperature
Anterior cord syndrome	Bilateral motor loss Bilateral loss of pain and temperature Preservation of proprioception, touch, and vibration
Posterior cord syndrome	Loss of touch and temperature Motor function intact Proprioception and vibration intact

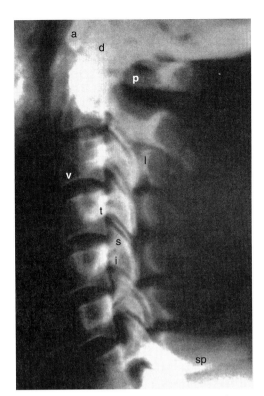

Figure 10–7 Cross-table radiograph of normal cervical spine. a, Anterior arch of C1; d, posterior arch of C1; i, inferior articulating facet of C5; l, lamina of C3; s, superior articulating facet of C5; sp, spinous process of C7; t, transverse process of C4; v, vertebral body of C3. *(From Ovassapian A: Fiberoptic Airway Endoscopy in Anesthesia and Critical Care. New York, Raven Press, 1990.)*

function. Incomplete lesions may result in one of several syndromes: central cord syndrome, Brown-Séquard syndrome, and anterior cord or posterior cord syndrome (Table 10-1). Of patients with significant spinal injury 30% to 70% have neurologic deficits.[142] About 70% of cervical spine injuries are considered potentially unstable or to be associated with clinically significant SCI.[134] Vertebrae C5 to C7 constitute the most vulnerable segment of cervical spine, and fractures, dislocations, or bony injuries in this segment are most likely to result in SCI. However, the degree of SCI cannot be correlated with the stability of the spine.

Extension injuries are twice as common as flexion injuries.[141] One third of extension injuries involve the atlantoaxial joint. Hyperextension with compression may cause fracture-dislocation disruption of both anterior and posterior columns and is highly unstable. A hangman's fracture, which occurs with violent hyperextension, fractures the pedicles of C2, causes anterior subluxation of C2 or C3, and is also highly unstable, with a variable severity of spinal cord damage. Flexion injuries may result in wedge fractures of the vertebral body without ligamentous injuries. These are often stable, except in severe injuries, in which greater disruption of the anterior and posterior columns may occur. The most severe flexion injury is a teardrop fracture, which is highly unstable. Compression injuries cause burst fractures, and posterior displacement of vertebral body fragments may cause SCI despite the relative stability of the fracture.

Spine Immobilization

Because patients with high-speed multiple trauma and head injury are at increased risk for SCI, their cervical spines should be immobilized, and they should be moved using the logroll technique until evaluation reveals no injury. The best way to immobilize the neck in the acute setting is with use of a rigid collar, sandbags on either side of the neck, and tape across the forehead.[143] Soft collars do not effectively limit neck motion; they actually permit 96% of normal flexion and 73% of normal extension, and they do not restrict motion in the lateral

or rotational directions.[143] Thus soft collars serve only as a reminder of the possibility of cervical spine injury. Rigid collars (e.g., Philadelphia collar, extrication collar) still allow about 30% of neck extension and flexion and about 45% of normal rotation or lateral movement. The Philadelphia collar is preferred because it is a two-piece collar that is easy to place without significantly moving the patient. In contrast, lateral sandbags and forehead tape effectively prevent flexion, reducing lateral and rotary motions to 5% of normal and extension to 35% of normal. After the initial diagnosis and work-up are completed, tong or halo fixation devices can be applied. These devices dramatically reduce neck motion, allowing only 4% of flexion or extension and 1% of normal rotation.[143]

Radiologic Evaluation

The standard radiologic evaluation of the cervical spine involves obtaining cross-table lateral, anteroposterior, and odontoid (open-mouth) radiographs of the cervical spine. Because 20% of all spinal fractures occur at C7,[134] all seven cervical vertebrae must be evident on the lateral spine film.[19,144] The cross-table lateral film (Fig. 10-7) allows evaluation of the alignment of the vertebrae, the bony structure of each vertebra, and the width of the prevertebral and intervertebral spaces.[144] A lordotic alignment should be present on each of the four anatomic lines on the cervical spine, (i.e., along the anterior and posterior margins of the vertebral border, the spinolaminar line, and the posterior margins of the spinous process; Fig. 10-8). The bony structure of each vertebra is examined for the structure of the vertebral body and spinous processes, the size of the intervertebral disk space, the relationship of the articular facet and joints, and the interspinous process distance.[144] Widening of the prevertebral space may indicate the presence of a severe and unstable spine injury, even on an otherwise normal C-spine radiograph, or it may be associated with airway obstruction (Fig. 10-9).[145,146] The cross-table lateral radiograph misses about 15% to 20% of cervical spine fractures.[144] Therefore, if a lateral film alone has been taken in a high-risk patient, the neck should continue to be treated as injured and potentially unstable. The sensitivity of the radiographs can be increased to 93% by adding an anteroposterior view and an odontoid view.[144] The anteroposterior view (Fig. 10-10) demonstrates the vertical alignment of the spinous and articular process and abnormalities in disk and joint spaces, such as disk space enlargement, which may indicate a severe ligamentous injury.[141] The open-mouth or odontoid view (Fig. 10-11) visualizes the atlanto-occipital and atlantoaxial joints and the odontoid process. Supplemental films, such as oblique and flexion-extension views, may be required for further detail.

CT may be used to rule out cervical spine injury when the plain radiograph findings are suspicious, equivocal, or negative in the patient with clinical signs of SCI. This modality is also used to evaluate the cervical spine in patients who cannot open their mouths (such as intubated patients). It is superior to the plain radiographs in diagnosing cervical spine trauma, especially at C1 or C2; however, ligamentous injuries may be missed on a CT scan.[142] In rare cases, magnetic resonance imaging or myelography may be required to determine the extent of spine injury.

It is important to identify and to differentiate cervical spine injuries that are not associated with clinical instability. Two large multicenter studies, performed by The National Emergency X-Radiography Utilization Study (NEXUS) group and the Canadian CT Head and Cervical Spine Study group, have identified the radiographic signs of clinically insignificant cervical spine injuries (Table 10-2).[134,147]

Evaluation of Other Organ Systems

Respiratory System

Respiratory complications represent the most common (80% in some studies) and serious complications in patients with SCI, significantly contributing to morbidity and mortality.

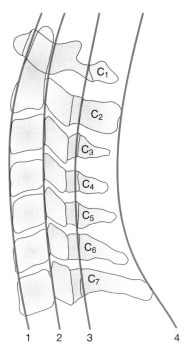

Figure 10–8 Diagram of the lateral view of the cervical spine demonstrating normal alignment. The "ABCs" of interpretation involve alignment, bones, cartilage, and soft tissue spaces. Four smooth, lordotic curves are drawn along the anterior margins of the vertebral border (1), the posterior margins (2), the junction between the lamina and the spinous processes (3), and the tips of the spinous process (4). Lines 2 and 3 are the approximate borders of the spinal canal. *(From Williams CF, Bernstein TW, Jalenko C: Essentiality of the lateral cervical spine radiograph. Ann Emerg Med 1981;10:198.)*

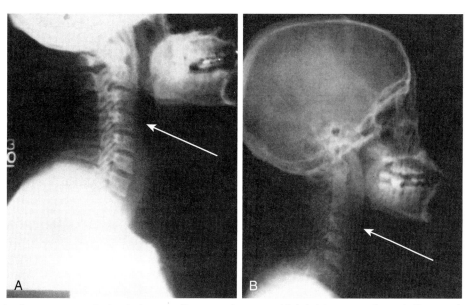

Figure 10–9 Example of severe prevertebral soft tissue swelling secondary to a whiplash injury. **A,** Radiograph illustrates lateral cervical spine in a normal patient. *Arrow* points to the prevertebral plane, which has a width of 3.2 mm at C2. **B,** Radiograph illustrates a patient with marked widening of the prevertebral plane (*arrow*), which measures 11 mm at C2. This patient presented with airway obstruction requiring endotracheal intubation with a fiberoptic technique. *(From Biby L., Santora AH: Prevertebral hematoma secondary to whiplash injury necessitating emergency intubation. Anesth Analg 1990;70:112.)*

10 • CARE OF THE ACUTELY UNSTABLE PATIENT

173

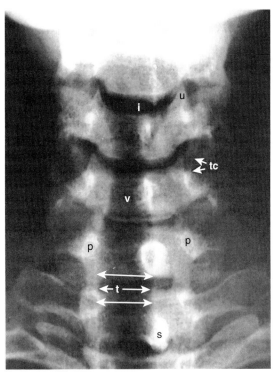

Figure 10–10 Anteroposterior radiograph of the normal cervical spine. i, Intervertebral foramen of C3-C4; p, pedicle of C6; s, spinous process of C7; t, trachea (arrows); tc, thyroid cartilage; u, uncinate process of C4; v, vertebral body of C5. (From Ovassapian A: Fiberoptic Airway Endoscopy in Anesthesia and Critical Care. New York, Raven Press, 1990, p 37.)

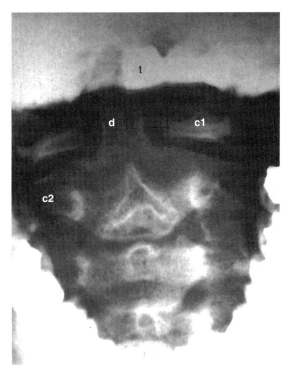

Figure 10–11 Open-mouth or odontoid radiograph of normal cervical spine. c1, Anterior arch of C1; c2, body of C2; D, Dens axis (C2); t, teeth. (From Ovassapian A: Fiberoptic Airway Endoscopy in Anesthesia and Critical Care. New York, Raven Press, 1990, p 37.)

174

The pathophysiologic changes of the breathing process and lung injury secondary to SCI occur early after SCI. Forced vital capacity and functional residual capacity are reduced in patients with SCIs, with the greatest respiratory impairment observed with cervical lesions (Box 10-5 and Table 10-3).[148] The diaphragm, which contributes 60% to normal vital capacity, is innervated by the phrenic nerve (C3 to C5). Lesions above this level cause total diaphragmatic paralysis and inability to ventilate (see Table 10-3). The patient with a lesion below C6 has an intact diaphragm but variable loss of intercostal and abdominal muscle function. Patients with C6 lesions have a significant decrease in vital capacity to 30% of predicted, associated with a reduction in functional residual capacity, caused primarily by loss of expiratory reserve volume. Paradoxical ventilation (chest retraction on inspiration and chest expansion during expiration), relaxation of the abdominal wall that interferes with the normal position and movement of the diaphragm, loss of cough, reduced ability to handle secretions, and associated chest injuries also contribute to respiratory compromise. Vital capacity is higher in the supine than in the head-up or prone position because of diaphragmatic mechanics. Postural hypoxemia may develop. In addition to impaired ventilation, other pulmonary injuries, such as atelectasis, aspiration, pulmonary contusion, hemothorax, pneumothorax, and neurogenic or nonneurogenic pulmonary edema, may contribute to respiratory failure in the acute setting. Like patients with head injury, patients with spinal cord trauma are at a particular risk for the development of neurogenic pulmonary edema.[9]

Although a patient's ventilation may be adequate on initial presentation in the emergency department, progressive atelectasis and pneumonia caused by inability to cough and clear secretions, sedative and narcotic administration, gastric atony and dilation, and spinal cord edema may contribute to the subsequent development of respiratory failure. Ledsome and Sharp[148] found that five patients with an injury at the C4 to C5 level had a vital capacity of 25% of predicted on admission, and all required ventilatory support 1 to 5 days after injury. Loss of sympathetic control may contribute to hypersecretion of bronchial mucus, which can occur just 1 hour after acute SCI with tetraplegia,[149] and also contributes to formation of plugs, atelectasis, and pneumonia. In the acute phase of SCI, neurogenic pulmonary edema can occur owing to systemic and pulmonary vasoconstriction with subsequent ventilation-perfusion mismatch and left heart failure.

Cardiovascular System

At the time of primary spinal cord injury, intense sympathetic nervous system activation causes a brief period of severe hypertension.[150] The excessive sympathetic discharge may raise ICP and cause ST-segment and T-wave changes that may mimic myocardial ischemia or dysrhythmias or may result in neurogenic pulmonary edema.

Currently a four-phase model of the spinal shock development has been proposed.[151] Phase 1, called "hyporeflexive," usually manifests during the first 24 hours after injury. It is characterized by areflexia or hyporeflexia due to loss of the descending pathways, causing flaccid paralysis, loss of deep tendon reflexes below the level of the lesion and autonomic dysfunction. This is followed by phase 2, which is characterized by some return of the initial reflexes and denervation supersensitivity. One week later, phase 2 transforms into phase 3, with the symptoms of the "initial" hyperreflexia, what is explained by the axon-related growth of synapses. Phase 3 usually takes a month, and is followed by phase 4,

Table 10–2 Radiologic Signs of Clinically Insignificant Cervical Spine Injuries

From the National Emergency X-Radiography Utilization Study (NEXUS) (21 hospitals; 34,069 patients)[134]	Spinous process fracture Wedge compression fractures with loss of ≤ 25% of vertebral body height Isolated osteophyte fractures Isolated transverse process fractures End-plate fractures Type 1 odontoid fracture Trabecular fractures Isolated avulsion fractures without ligament injury
From the Canadian CT Head and Cervical Spine Study (CCTHCSS) (10 hospitals; 8,924 patients)[147]	Spinous process fracture Compression fractures with loss of ≤ 25% of vertebral body height Simple osteophyte fractures Isolated transverse process fractures

---

BOX 10–5 *Spinal Cord Injury: Effects on Other Organ Systems*

1. Respiratory system:
   a. Decreased ability to ventilate, depending on level of injury.
   b. Associated pulmonary injuries: atelectasis, aspiration, pulmonary contusion, pneumothorax, neurogenic or nonneurogenic pulmonary edema.
2. Cardiovascular system:
   a. Initial sympathetic nervous system overactivity.
   b. Spinal shock: hypotension, bradycardia.
   c. Severe bradycardia (or asystole) with airway instrumentation.
3. Temperature control: poikilothermia.
4. Other systems: possible orthopedic, intrathoracic, intra-abdominal, or head injuries.

Table 10–3 Effects of Spinal Cord Injury on Respiratory Function

Damaged Cord Segment	Severity of Respiratory Compromise
C3-C5	Decrease in vital capacity to 20%-25% of normal or lower
	Paradoxical respiration
	Use of accessory muscles
	Variable loss of phrenic nerve function and paralysis of diaphragm
	Loss of intercostal and abdominal muscles
	Ventilatory support required
C5-C8	Decrease in vital capacity to 30% of normal
	Paradoxical respiration
	Use of accessory muscles
	No cough
	Ventilation improved in supine position
	Loss of intercostal and abdominal muscles
T1-T6	Variable intercostal muscle functions
	Partial loss of diaphragm effectiveness
	Weak cough
T6-T12	Weak cough
	Variable abdominal muscle strength

or "final hyperreflexia," with the underlying process of the soma-related growth of synapses.

If phase 1 of spinal shock is associated with profound peripheral vasodilatation and systemic hypotension, it is called *neurogenic shock*. The loss of sympathetic tone results in a decrease in systemic vascular resistance, an increase in venous capacitance with venous pooling, a reduced ability for vasoconstriction in response to changes in position and hypovolemia, and a poor hemodynamic response to surgical stimulation. Unopposed vagal tone with loss of cardioaccelerator fibers (T2 to T5) contributes to the bradycardia. Severe reflex bradycardia and asystole may occur in response to airway instrumentation and may be prevented by prophylactic administration of atropine. A relative tachycardia in a quadriplegic patient may indicate hypovolemia. Patients with high cervical injuries (C1-C5) or patients with complete motor deficit below the injury tend to have lower systolic blood pressure at admission than patients with C6-C7 injury or with mild or moderate motor deficit. When neurogenic shock is defined as systolic blood pressure lower than 90 mm Hg, there is an association between neurogenic shock and a delay in surgical intervention.[152]

Treatment of neurogenic shock involves the careful administration of isotonic fluids and possibly the administration of vasopressors to maintain spinal cord perfusion pressure. Some writers suggest using pulmonary artery catheters to gauge fluid requirements in all quadriplegic patients because even previously healthy patients may be susceptible to pulmonary edema and myocardial dysfunction.[153] In most patients, judicious fluid replacement alone is enough to raise blood pressure moderately in order to improve spinal cord perfusion. A pulmonary artery catheter should be placed in the patient who requires large volumes of fluid or vasopressors. Ephedrine, phenylephrine, and dopamine are commonly used as vasopressors, with the choice of drug depending on heart rate, cardiac output, and vascular resistance as measured by a pulmonary artery catheter.

Temperature Control

There is a loss of thermoregulatory ability below the level of the lesion. Patients with injury above T6 tend to become poikilothermic, assuming the temperature of their surroundings. Careful monitoring of temperature and warming efforts are required.

Associated Injuries

As with head trauma, multiple organ systems (e.g., orthopedic, intrathoracic, intra-abdominal, head) may be affected by the injury. Patients are assumed to have a full stomach (i.e., to be at risk for aspiration). Intravenous access should be established, and Foley catheters and a nasal gastric tube should be placed. Long-bone fractures should be immobilized.

Airway Management of the Patient with Suspected Cervical Spine Injury

In the airway management of a patient with a potentially unstable cervical spine, the goal of the anesthesiologist is to establish endotracheal intubation without causing further injury to the spinal cord. Unfortunately, there is little data on the safety of the various airway maneuvers and intubation techniques.[154] Unrestricted neck motion associated with excessive traction during spine fixation or the failure to detect a cervical spine fracture on initial work-up[155] has been associated with new neurologic deficits. Overall incidence of the development of secondary neurologic injury after cervical spine injury ranges between 2% and 10%.[154] In one study, secondary neurologic defect occurred in 10.5% of patients with a missed diagnosis of cervical spine fracture, compared with 1.4% of those correctly diagnosed.[155] Laryngoscopy, without neck stabilization, has also resulted in quadriplegia or death in several patients.[142,156] However, no studies have elucidated the actual risk of airway management techniques in patients with cervical spine injuries when standard cervical spine precautions, including in-line stabilization, are used.[148] Because of the lack of outcome data, no consensus has been reached regarding which technique for endotracheal intubation is safest in patients with suspected cervical spine injuries. Therefore the optimal technique must be chosen by the anesthesiologist, depending on the particular patient's medical condition, the urgency with which the airway must be secured, the patient's level of cooperation, and the anesthesiologist's skills.

Effects of Various Airway Maneuvers on Cervical Spine Mobility

BASIC AIRWAY MANEUVERS

Impressive radiographic evidence has shown that many airway maneuvers may increase distraction and subluxation at the site of a cervical spine injury.[154,157] However, no outcome studies are available to determine whether these maneuvers are, in fact, dangerous to living patients.[154] Aprahamian and colleagues[157] found that chin lift and jaw thrust in a cadaver model with an unstable C5 to C6 ligamentous injury caused a greater than 5-mm widening of the disk space. This widening was not prevented by a Philadelphia collar. Insertion of an esophageal obturator airway caused a 3- to 4-mm increase in disk space.[157] Anterior neck pressure used to stabilize the larynx for nasal tracheal intubation caused greater than 5-mm posterior subluxation. Single-handed cricoid pressure, with manual in-line stabilization of the neck but without posterior neck support, also caused a vertical displacement of the neck between 4.6 and 5 mm (range of 0 to 9 mm).[158] It is not known whether support to the posterior part of the neck with a hard collar or a second hand would also allow this posterior displacement. Head tilt, insertion of an oral airway, or insertion of a nasopharyngeal airway resulted in only a minimal change in the disk space.[157] Both the intubating laryngeal mask airway (LMA) and the regular LMA exert greater pressures against the cervical vertebrae than other intubation techniques and may produce posterior displacement of the cervical spine.[159] The rigid intubating LMA tube also compresses the posterior pharynx and has resulted in severe pharyngeal edema in patients undergoing anterior cervical spine fixation.[160] However, outcome data are not available.

There is also concern that the use of "manual in-line traction" to stabilize the neck, depending on the force of the traction and integrity of the surrounding tissues, may by itself cause significant subluxation and distraction of the disk space.[161] Cervical traction increases distraction of the vertebra, especially at the C5 to C6 level.[161] Whether traction may cause neurologic damage is not clear; however, deterioration of neurologic function has been reported in association with excessive traction during cervical spine stabilization procedures. Therefore, only "manual in-line stabilization" should be used, and traction should not be performed.

TECHNIQUES FOR URGENT AIRWAY CONTROL

The following sections discuss techniques for urgent airway control.

Direct Laryngoscopy. To secure the airway quickly, a rapid-sequence induction with direct laryngoscopy may be required. Unfortunately, direct laryngoscopy is associated with cervical spine movement in normal anesthetized volunteers[162-164] as well as in cadavers with unstable spines.[157,161] Horton and colleagues[163] found that direct laryngoscopy progressively increased extension from C4 to C1. Atlantoaxial (C1 to C2) extension was near the upper limit of normal, whereas the lower cervical spine was relatively straight. Laryngoscopy caused superior rotation of the occiput and C1 and extension at the occipitoatlantal and atlantoaxial joints. The subaxial cervical segments were displaced only minimally. Laryngoscopy with either a straight or curved blade caused a 3- to 4-mm widening of the C5 to C6 disk space in the cadaver model of an unstable C5 to C6 injury.[157] Extension of the cervical spine movement was not prevented by a Philadelphia collar; however, it was reduced 60% when in-line stabilization was provided by an assistant.[157,162]

Although direct laryngoscopy does result in motion of the cervical spine, especially at C1 to C2, the actual risk of exacerbating neurologic damage associated with laryngoscopy is not known. No large outcome studies have been performed on the safety of direct laryngoscopy in patients with unstable cervical spines. The available evidence suggests that neurologic deterioration after oral intubation with neck stabilization is very rare.[142,143,154,165-169] The widespread use of direct laryngoscopy with in-line stabilization in the trauma setting and the few cases of exacerbation of neurologic damage suggests that the 95% confidence interval for neurologic deterioration is smaller (2% or less). In case reports, neurologic deterioration with direct laryngoscopy has occurred in the absence of precautions taken for spine injury.[170,171]

In addition to the risks of causing secondary neurologic injury during endotracheal intubation, direct laryngoscopy may be difficult in the patient who is obese, has facial fractures, has blood in the pharynx, or has oral soft tissue injuries. Immobilization of the cervical spine also may make visualization of the larynx more difficult.[172,173] A poor view is obtained on laryngoscopy (grade 3 or 4) in 22% of patients with manual in-line stabilization.[173] However, visualization was even worse when the head was immobilized by a rigid collar with tape across the forehead and sandbags on either side of the neck, with a grade 3 to 4 laryngoscopy in 64% of the patients. Because the main limitation to laryngoscopy with a rigid collar is a reduction in mouth opening, the front portion of the cervical collar should be removed before laryngoscopy. The posterior portion should remain in place to provide neck support for cricoid pressure. The view at laryngoscopy can often be improved by application of *b*ackward pressure on the thyroid cartilage and by the addition of *u*pward and slightly *r*ightward *p*ressure on the thyroid cartilage (BURP maneuver).[174]

Other types of scopes and blades, including the Bullard laryngoscope, McCoy laryngoscope blade, and GlideScope, have been advocated by some for use in the cervical spine–injured patient. The McCoy laryngoscope blade consists of a Macintosh blade with hinged tip and standard laryngoscope handle. The blade tip lifts up the epiglottis, providing a better view of the vocal cords in patients with cervical spine immobilization. The Bullard laryngoscope causes less head extension and cervical spine extension than conventional laryngoscopes and also gives a better view. Cohn and Zornow[175] reported that with the Bullard laryngoscope, in trained hands, the glottis was visualized in an average of 10 seconds, compared with 30 seconds for the fiberoptic bronchoscope. Passage of the endotracheal tube required an average of 46 seconds with the Bullard laryngoscope, compared with 99 seconds with the fiberoptic bronchoscope.[175] In another report, movement at the C2 to C5 segment was 50% less with laryngoscopy using the GlideScope than with the Macintosh laryngoscope.[176] However, motion at the occiput to C2 was unchanged. In contrast, use of the light wand reduced movement at each level. The time to intubation was longest with the GlideScope (27 ± 12 sec) but times were similar with the light wand (14 ± 9 sec) and the Macintosh laryngoscope (16 ± 7 sec).[176] On occasion, the trachea may be difficult to intubate with the Bullard laryngoscope or GlideScope because the endotracheal tube is lateral to the blade. Prevertebral swelling may occur with cervical spine fractures, which may result in airway compromise and distortion of the larynx, causing difficult visualization.

Cricothyroidotomy. Cricothyroidotomy has been suggested as an alternative to direct laryngoscopy for rapid securing of the airway in the patient with suspected or actual cervical spine injury. In theory, cricothyroidotomy might allow intubation of the trachea without causing neck motion. In reality, lack of spinal motion has not been documented because radiographic studies on the risk of cervical spine motion during cricothyroidotomy and neurologic outcome studies have not been performed.[142] In addition, the complication rate for cricothyroidotomy is fairly high. When performed in the field or the emergency department, cricothyroidotomy has a very high immediate complication rate (32%),[177] including an execution time longer than 3 minutes (10%), incorrect (13%) or unsuccessful tracheostomy tube placement (8% to 25%), significant hemorrhage (5%), and subcutaneous emphysema. Long-term complications, such as infection and damage to the larynx, may also occur (2%). Cricothyroidotomy may also make definitive repair of the cervical spine by an anterior approach difficult or impossible because of the presence of the contaminated wound in the surgical field. Many of the complications can be attributed to the inexperience of the physician performing the procedure. However, the lack of documentation of any beneficial effect on neurologic outcome, the relative inexperience of most anesthesiologists, emergency department physicians, and surgeons in using the technique, and the usually high complication rate suggest that use of cricothyroidotomy should be reserved to secure the airway quickly in selected patients in whom direct laryngoscopy has failed or is anticipated to fail.

Transtracheal Jet Ventilation. Transtracheal jet ventilation may be used to temporarily oxygenate the patient during difficult direct laryngoscopy, cricothyroidotomy, or fiberoptic laryngoscopy. Use of a 14-gauge catheter placed through the cricothyroid membrane and connected to a high-pressure source of oxygen may provide adequate oxygenation and ventilation. However, it does not protect against aspiration, and it may be associated with barotrauma (10%) and catheter dislodgment. As such, it should only be used as a temporary measure to oxygenate a patient while definitive airway control is achieved.

TECHNIQUES FOR ELECTIVE AIRWAY CONTROL

The following sections discuss techniques for elective airway control.

Awake Intubation (Blind Nasal, Light Wand, or Fiberoptic Laryngoscopy). Awake nasotracheal or orotracheal intubation has been advocated as a safer technique for endotracheal intubation in the patient with an unstable cervical spine.[141,154] Meschino and coworkers[178] reported their institutional experience using awake tracheal intubation in patients with cervical spine injuries. These researchers found that neurologic outcomes with cervical spine injury were no different in the 136 patients who required endotracheal intubation from those in 233 patients who did not require intubation. Awake intubation was used; however, the report of this study did not supply details of how the intubations were performed, how the neurologic examination was assessed, and the location and degree of instability of the injury. The risk of secondary neurologic damage due to awake intubation is low.

Although awake intubation is often appropriate, especially for an elective intubation, it may not secure the airway quickly enough if rapid intubation is required, as in the hypoxemic, hemodynamically unstable, or head-injured patient. Nasal intubation should be avoided in the patient with a midface or basilar skull fracture, in whom it might allow entry of bacteria and foreign materials into the cranial cavity.[179] It also may induce a nosebleed, which is aggravated in the multiple-trauma victim by dilutional coagulopathy and which, with long-term intubation, may cause paranasal sinusitis and sepsis.[180] Uncooperative, inebriated, or head-injured patients may thrash about and cause even greater neck motion (and potential cervical spine damage) than if direct laryngoscopy were performed with the use of general anesthesia. Although blind nasotracheal intubation is often successful, it may be slower and may require multiple attempts. Ovassapian and colleagues[181] found that blind nasotracheal intubation required multiple attempts in 70% to 90% of patients.

Fiberoptic laryngoscopy has often been recommended for intubation in the patient with an unstable cervical spine because it allows intubation under direct vision without much neck motion. It has a high rate of success under elective conditions when performed by an anesthesiologist knowledgeable of the technique. However, in practice, fiberoptic laryngoscopy may be difficult to use in the acutely injured patient because of excessive salivation, airway bleeding, and edema in the pharyngeal space. It may be time consuming because it requires a cooperative patient and adequate topical anesthesia of the supraglottic and infraglottic regions to prevent gagging. Anesthetizing the area below the vocal cords is controversial. Although this step may prevent severe coughing and bucking (which potentially may exacerbate neurologic damage), it might increase the likelihood of aspiration. Ovassapian and colleagues,[181] however, found no evidence of aspiration 24 hours after fiberoptic intubation performed with laryngeal anesthesia in 105 patients at risk for aspiration. There is also no evidence that coughing raises the neurologic risk to the spinal cord.

Retrograde Tracheal Intubation. Another possible technique advocated to minimize neck motion in the patient with trauma is retrograde tracheal intubation over a wire passed through the cricothyroid membrane. Barriot and Riou[182] found that retrograde orotracheal intubation was easily and quickly (less than 5 minutes) performed in 19 trauma patients in whom conventional techniques failed or were expected to fail. However, large-scale assessment of the reliability and safety of this technique as the primary means to secure the airway has not been performed.

Management of Endotracheal Intubation

Because of the lack of outcome studies, no consensus has been reached regarding the relative safety of the various techniques to achieve endotracheal intubation.[154] Many techniques are feasible, and the specific choice often depends on the particular anesthesiologist's skills. However, the possible risk of secondary damage to the spinal cord with laryngoscopy (which varies with stability of the injuries) must be balanced by other considerations, such as the degree of urgency for achieving intubation, associated medical conditions (head trauma, airway trauma or pathologic condition, hypoxemia, and cardiovascular instability), and level of patient cooperation.

The first step of the airway management plan involves determination of the degree of urgency for securing the airway (Fig. 10-12). Immediate endotracheal intubation is required in patients with cardiovascular instability, hypoxemia, or elevated ICP. Oxygenation and ventilation are initially provided with bag and mask, with an airway or jaw thrust as required to open the airway. If the patient has an anatomically normal airway (i.e., one in which endotracheal intubation is expected to be easily achieved with the head and neck secured in neutral position), a modified rapid-sequence induction should be performed. The front half of the Philadelphia collar should be removed before laryngoscopy because it interferes with mouth opening. To prevent aspiration, cricoid pressure should be applied. Although this pressure may cause a posterior subluxation of the cervical cord,[158] adverse effects have not been documented (especially when the posterior portion of the neck is stabilized by the Philadelphia collar). Succinylcholine is the muscle relaxant of choice if the injury is less than 48 hours old, because hyperkalemia does not occur until later.[183] Ventilation should continue with cricoid pressure in place until the intubation is complete. During laryngoscopy, an assistant should stabilize the head in a neutral position without applying traction. Neck flexion should be avoided, and the minimum of neck extension necessary to visualize the glottis should be used. If conventional methods to place the endotracheal tube fail, an intubating LMA can be inserted and an endotracheal tube passed with or without fiberoptic guidance through the airway.[184]

If immediate control of the airway is required and the airway is anatomically abnormal, a cricothyroidotomy should be performed to secure the airway. Ventilation using an LMA or transtracheal jet ventilation may be required as a temporary measure if ventilation by bag and mask is difficult. Patients with severe facial fractures, soft tissue swelling or injuries, marked obesity, or airway obstruction due to massive prevertebral hematoma, in whom endotracheal intubation appears to be or is impossible, should be managed with cricothyroidotomy.

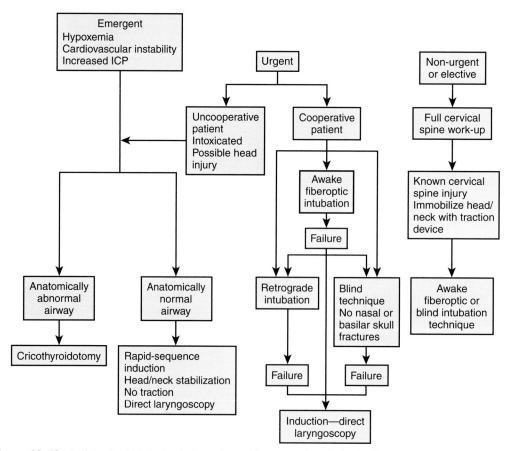

Figure 10–12 Endotracheal intubation in the patient with suspected cervical spine injury. ICP, intracranial pressure.

If the airway must be secured urgently, but not immediately, the other techniques for endotracheal intubation may be useful. Examples of such cases are the patient with a known or suspected cervical spine injury who is hemodynamically stable but has a ruptured spleen and the patient who is beginning to show signs of respiratory insufficiency but is not hypoxic. The key point in the decision for urgent endotracheal intubation is whether the patient is cooperative (see Fig. 10-12). If the patient is uncooperative or inebriated or has a possible significant head injury, the steps listed for emergent intubation—namely, a rapid-sequence induction—should be performed. In a cooperative patient, a retrograde intubation, awake fiberoptic intubation, or blind technique may be chosen. Fiberoptic intubations may seem desirable but may be difficult in patients with edema, blood, secretions, or emesis in the airway. Theoretically, these methods minimize cervical spine movement because they minimize atlanto-occipital extension. However, the safety of these techniques in comparison with direct laryngoscopy has not been unequivocally proven.[154]

In the non-urgent elective setting, such as requiring anesthesia for the repair of orthopedic or facial injuries, the patient should first undergo a full evaluation of the cervical spine. In the patient with a known cervical spine injury, the head and neck should be immobilized first with a traction device, such as tongs or halo traction, before endotracheal intubation. An awake fiberoptic or a blind intubation technique may then be used. Direct laryngoscopy is seldom useful because visualization of the glottis is difficult with the traction devices in place.

Aims in the Acute Care of the Spinal Cord–Injured Patient

As for patients with head trauma, the primary aim in the management of patients with SCI is to prevent secondary cord injury (Box 10-6). The principal way to prevent additional injury is immobilization of the spine. Treatment, therefore, has consisted of anatomic realignment and stabilization with or without surgery for decompression and stabilization.

Prevention of secondary neurologic damage by treating hypoxemia and maintaining spinal cord perfusion is also important in the acute management of these patients. Spinal cord blood flow is autoregulated in a fashion similar to blood flow in the brain,[185] and autoregulation may be impaired several hours after injury.[186] Maintenance of spinal cord perfusion pressure at greater than 60 mm Hg is advised to improve spinal cord blood flow after injury. In an experimental model of spinal injury, spinal cord blood flow was increased by infusion of phenylephrine but not of mannitol or hetastarch, although neurologic function was not improved.[187] However, the control blood pressure was 80 mm Hg, suggesting that elevation of blood pressure beyond a minimum of 60 mm Hg is not helpful. In addition, hypertension may cause hemorrhage and increase edema formation. No evidence has shown that hyperventilation to reduce Pa_{CO_2}

(and theoretically to decompress the spinal cord) improves outcome with experimentally induced SCI.[188]

Hyperglycemia should be avoided immediately after SCI. Drummond and Moore[189] found that minimally increased blood glucose levels (177 mg/dL), associated with intravenous infusions of glucose before experimentally induced spinal cord ischemia, worsened neurologic outcome.[190] Nine of ten animals in their study that received 5% glucose in water were paraplegic, compared with only three of ten control animals.[191] Reduction of blood glucose by insulin has also been found to improve recovery of electrophysiologic function after experimentally induced spinal cord ischemia.[192] These results suggest that infusion of glucose-containing solutions within the first 24 hours of injury should be avoided. In addition, hyperglycemia should be promptly treated.

Large doses of methylprednisolone (30 mg/kg followed by a continuous infusion of 5.4 mg/kg/hr for 23 hours) have been reported to improve neurologic outcome in patients with complete and incomplete lesions.[193] However, the effectiveness of this regimen has been recently questioned.[194] Currently, use of steroids in the acute SCI may be considered only as optional, but not standard care.

SUMMARY

The care of the acutely unstable patient involves neurologic and radiologic examination, evaluation of other organ systems, appropriate airway management, and treatment of associated problems. Brain and spinal cord injuries are both accompanied by physiologic derangements in other bodily functions, challenges in airway control, and the primary management goal of prevention of secondary injury and further neurologic damage. In head injury, management involves a reduction in ICP and treatment of hypoxemia. In SCI, immobilization of the spine, supportive care, and early administration of methylprednisolone are of paramount importance.

> **BOX 10–6** *Aims in Acute Care of Spinal Cord Injury*
>
> 1. Immobilize the spine.
> 2. Prevent subsequent damage associated with hypoxemia and decreased spinal cord perfusion pressure.
> 3. Treat hyperglycemia and avoid glucose-containing solutions in first 24 hours of the injury.

REFERENCES

1. Teasdale G, Jennett B: Assessment of coma and impaired consciousness: A practical scale, *Lancet* 2(7872):81–84, 1974.
2. Choi SC, Muizelaar JP, Barnes TY, et al: Prediction tree for severely head-injured patients, *J Neurosurg* 75:251–255, 1991.
3. Jennett WB, Stern WE: Tentorial herniation, the midbrain and the pupil: Experimental studies in brain compression, *J Neurosurg* 17:598–609, 1960.
4. Andrews BT, Levy ML, Pitts LH: Implications of systemic hypotension for the neurological examination in patients with severe head injury, *Surg Neurol* 28:419–422, 1987.
5. Bedford RF, Persing JA, Pobereskin L, et al: Lidocaine or thiopental for rapid control of intracranial hypertension? *Anesth Analg* 59:435–437, 1980.
6. Bruce DA, Alavi A, Bilaniuk L, et al: Diffuse cerebral swelling following head injuries in children: The syndrome of "malignant brain edema, *J Neurosurg* 54:170–178, 1981.
7. Toutant SM, Klauber MR, Marshall LF, et al: Absent or compressed basal cisterns on first CT scan: Ominous predictors of outcome in severe head injury, *J Neurosurg* 61:691–694, 1984.
8. Frost EAM, Arancibia CU, Shulman K: Pulmonary shunt as a prognostic indicator in head injury, *J Neurosurg* 50:768–772, 1979.
9. Poe RH, Reisman JL, Rodenhouse TG: Pulmonary edema in cervical spinal cord injury, *J Trauma* 18:71–73, 1978.
10. Malik AB: Mechanisms of neurogenic pulmonary edema, *Circ Res* 57:1–18, 1985.
11. McClellan MD, Dauber IM, Weil JV: Elevated intracranial pressure increases pulmonary vascular permeability to protein, *J Appl Physiol* 67:1185–1191, 1989.

12. Popp AJ, Shah DM, Berman RA, et al: Delayed pulmonary dysfunction in head-injured patients, *J Neurosurg* 57:784–790, 1982.

13. Schumacker PT, Rhodes GR, Newell JC, et al: Ventilation-perfusion imbalance after head trauma, *Am Rev Respir Dis* 119:33–43, 1979.

14. Cooper KR, Boswell PA: Reduced functional residual capacity and abnormal oxygenation in patients with severe head injury, *Chest* 84:29–35, 1983.

15. Clifton GL, Robertson CS, Kyper K, et al: Cardiovascular response to severe head injury, *J Neurosurg* 59:447–454, 1983.

16. Clifton GL, Ziegler MG, Grossman RG: Circulating catecholamines and sympathetic activity after head injury, *Neurosurgery* 8:10–14, 1981.

17. Cote CJ, Greenhow DE, Marshall BE: The hypotensive response to rapid intravenous administration of hypertonic solutions in man and in the rabbit, *Anesthesiology* 50:30–35, 1979.

18. Cushing H: Concerning a definite regulatory mechanism of the vasomotor center which controls blood pressure during cerebral compression, *Johns Hopkins Hosp Bull* 12:290, 1901.

19. Ross SE, Schwab CW, David ET, et al: Clearing the cervical spine: Initial radiologic evaluation, *J Trauma* 27:1055–1060, 1987.

20. Ott L, Young B, Phillips R, et al: Altered gastric emptying in the head-injured patient: Relationship to feeding intolerance, *J Neurosurg* 74:738–742, 1991.

21. Kraus JF, Morgenstern H, Fife D, et al: Blood alcohol tests, prevalence of involvement, and outcomes following brain injury, *Am J Public Health* 79:294–299, 1989.

22. Becker P, Zieger S, Rother U, et al: Complement activation following head and brain trauma, *Anaesthesist* 36:301–365, 1987.

23. Clark JA, Finelli RE, Netsky MG: Disseminated intravascular coagulation following cranial trauma: Case report, *J Neurosurg* 52:266–269, 1980.

24. Crone KR, Lee KS, Kelly DL Jr: Correlation of admission fibrin degradation products with outcome and respiratory failure in patients with severe head injury, *Neurosurgery* 21:532–536, 1987.

25. Boffard KD, Riou B, Warren B, et al: Recombinant factor VIIa as adjunctive therapy for bleeding control in severely injured trauma patients: Two parallel randomized, placebo-controlled, double-blind clinical trials, *J Trauma* 59:8–15, 2005.

26. Kluger Y, Riou B, Rossaint R, et al: Safety of rFVIIa in hemodynamically unstable polytrauma patients with traumatic brain injury: Post hoc analysis of 30 patients from a prospective, randomized, placebo-controlled, double-blind clinical trial, *Crit Care* 11:R85, 2007.

27. Dutton RP, McCunn M, Hyder M, et al: Factor VIIa for correction of traumatic coagulopathy, *J Trauma* 57:709–718, 2004.

28. Mayer SA, Brun NC, Begtrup K, et al: Recombinant activated factor VII for acute intracerebral hemorrhage, *N Engl J Med* 352:777–785, 2005.

29. Pickard JD, Kirkpatrick PJ, Melsen T, et al: Potential role of NovoSeven in the prevention of rebleeding following aneurysmal subarachnoid haemorrhage, *Blood Coagul Fibrinolysis* 11(Suppl 1):S117–S120, 2000.

30. Shin B, Mackenzie CF, Helrich M: Hypokalemia in trauma patients, *Anesthesiology* 65:90–92, 1986.

31. Mehta MP, Gergis SD, Sokoll M: Paradoxical diuresis in some neurosurgical patients under balanced anesthesia, *Anesthesiology* 59:585–587, 1983.

32. Harris AS: Clinical experience with desmopressin: Efficacy and safety in central diabetes insipidus and other conditions, *J Pediatr* 114:711–718, 1989.

33. Nelson PB, Seif S, Gutai J, et al: Hyponatremia and natriuresis following subarachnoid hemorrhage in a monkey model, *J Neurosurg* 60:233–237, 1984.

34. Burney RG, Winn R: Increased cerebrospinal fluid pressure during laryngoscopy and intubation for induction of anesthesia, *Anesth Analg* 54:687–690, 1975.

35. White PF, Schlobohm RM, Pitts LH, et al: A randomized study of drugs for preventing increases in intracranial pressure during endotracheal suctioning, *Anesthesiology* 57:242–244, 1982.

36. Donegan MF, Bedford RF: Intravenously administered lidocaine prevents intracranial hypertension during endotracheal suctioning, *Anesthesiology* 52:516–518, 1980.

37. Hamill JF, Bedford RF, Weaver DC, et al: Lidocaine before endotracheal intubation: Intravenous or laryngotracheal? *Anesthesiology* 55:578–581, 1981.

38. Shapiro HM, Galindo A, Wyte SR, et al: Rapid intraoperative reduction of intracranial pressure with thiopentone, *Br J Anaesth* 45:1057–1062, 1973.

39. Unni VKN, Johnston RA, Young HSA, et al: Prevention of intracranial hypertension during laryngoscopy and endotracheal intubation: use of a second dose of thiopentone, *Br J Anaesth* 56:1219–1223, 1984.

40. Cottrell JE, Patel K, Turndorf H, et al: Intracranial pressure changes induced by sodium nitroprusside in patients with intracranial mass lesions, *J Neurosurg* 48:329–331, 1978.

41. Marsh ML, Shapiro HM, Smith RW, et al: Changes in neurologic status and intracranial pressure associated with sodium nitroprusside administration, *Anesthesiology* 51:336–338, 1979.

42. Van Aken H, Puchstein C, Schweppe ML, et al: Effect of labetalol on intracranial pressure in dogs with and without intracranial hypertension, *Acta Anaesthesiol Scand* 26:615–619, 1982.

43. Moss E, Powell D, Gibson RM, et al: Effect of etomidate on intracranial pressure and cerebral perfusion pressure, *Br J Anaesth* 51:347–352, 1979.

44. Shapiro HM, Wyte SR, Harris AB: Ketamine anaesthesia in patients with intracranial pathology, *Br J Anaesth* 44:1200–1204, 1972.

45. Lanier WL, Milde JH, Michenfelder JD: Cerebral stimulation following succinylcholine in dogs, *Anesthesiology* 64:551–559, 1986.

46. Stirt JA, Grosslight KR, Bedford RF, et al: "Defasciculation" with metocurine prevents succinylcholine-induced increases in intracranial pressure, *Anesthesiology* 67:50–53, 1987.

47. Brain Trauma Foundation: American Association of Neurological Surgeons, Congress of Neurological Surgeons, Joint Section on Neurotrauma and Critical Care, AANS/CNS; Carney NA, Ghajar J: Guidelines for the management of severe traumatic brain injury, *Introduction. J Neurotrauma* 24(Suppl 1):S1–S2, 2007.

48. Jones PA, Andrews PJ, Midgley S, et al: Measuring the burden of secondary insults in head-injured patients during intensive care, *J Neurosurg Anesthesiol* 6:4–14, 1994.

49. Rose J, Valtonen S, Jennett B: Avoidable factors contributing to death after head injury, *BMJ* 2:615–618, 1977.

50. Changaris DG, McGraw CP, Richardson JD, et al: Correlation of cerebral perfusion pressure and Glasgow Coma Scale to outcome, *J Trauma* 27:1007–1013, 1987.

51. Gudeman SK, Miller JD, Becker DP: Failure of high-dose steroid therapy to influence intracranial pressure in patients with severe head injury, *J Neurosurg* 51:301–306, 1979.

52. Dearden NM, Gibson JS, McDowall DG, et al: Effect of high-dose dexamethasone on outcome from severe head injury, *J Neurosurg* 64:81–88, 1986.

53. Miller JD, Sakalas R, Ward JD, et al: Methylprednisolone treatment in patients with brain tumors, *Neurosurgery* 1:114–117, 1977.

54. Chesnut RM, Marshall LF, Klauber MR, et al: The role of secondary brain injury in determining outcome from severe head injury, *J Trauma* 34:216–222, 1993.

55. Stocchetti N, Furlan A, Volta F: Hypoxemia and arterial hypotension at the accident scene in head injury, *J Trauma* 40:764–767, 1996.

56. Bratton SL, Chestnut RM, Ghajar J, Brain Trauma Foundation, American Association of Neurological Surgeons, Congress of Neurological Surgeons, Joint Section on Neurotrauma and Critical Care, AANS/CNS, et al: Guidelines for the management of severe traumatic brain injury. I: Blood pressure and oxygenation, *J Neurotrauma* 24(Suppl 1):S7–S13, 2007.

57. Shapiro HM, Marshall LF: Intracranial pressure responses to PEEP in head-injured patients, *J Trauma* 18:254–256, 1978.

58. Burchiel KJ, Steege TD, Wyler AR: Intracranial pressure changes in brain-injured patients requiring positive end-expiratory pressure ventilation, *Neurosurgery* 8:443–449, 1981.

59. Cooper KR, Boswell PA, Choi SC: Safe use of PEEP in patients with severe head injury, *J Neurosurg* 63:525–552, 1985.

60. Frost EAM: Effects of positive end-expiratory pressure on intracranial pressure and compliance in brain-injured patients, *J Neurosurg* 47:195–200, 1977.

61. Perel A, Pizov R, Cotev S: Systolic blood pressure variation is a sensitive indicator of hypovolemia in ventilated dogs subjected to graded hemorrhage, *Anesthesiology* 67:498–502, 1987.

62. Godje O, Peyerl M, Seebauer T, et al: Central venous pressure, pulmonary capillary wedge pressure and intrathoracic blood volumes as preload indicators in cardiac surgery patients, *Eur J Cardiothorac Surg* 13:533–539, 1998.

63. Ornstein E, Eidelman LA, Drenger B, et al: Systolic pressure variation predicts the response to acute blood loss, *J Clin Anesth* 10:137–140, 1998.

64. Enevoldsen EM, Jensen FT: Autoregulation and CO2 responses of cerebral blood flow in patients with acute severe head injury, *J Neurosurg* 48:689–703, 1978.

65. Turner JM, Powell D, Gibson RM, et al: Intracranial pressure changes in neurosurgical patients during hypotension induced with sodium nitroprusside or trimethaphan, *Br J Anaesth* 49:419–425, 1977.

66. Cottrell JE, Gupta B, Rappaport H, et al: Intracranial pressure during nitroglycerin-induced hypotension, *J Neurosurg* 53:309–311, 1980.

67. James DJ, Bedford RF: Hydralazine for controlled hypotension during neurosurgical operations, *Anesth Analg* 61:1016–1019, 1982.

68. Gunnar W, Jonasson O, Merlotti G, et al: Head injury and hemorrhagic shock: Studies of the blood brain barrier and intracranial pressure after resuscitation with normal saline solution, 3% saline solution, and dextran-40, *Surgery* 103:398–407, 1988.

69. Poole GV Jr, Prough DS, Johnson JC, et al: Effects of resuscitation from hemorrhage shock on cerebral hemodynamics in the presence of an intracranial mass, *J Trauma* 27:18–23, 1987.

70. Zornow MH, Todd MM, Moore SS: The acute cerebral effects of changes in plasma osmolality and oncotic pressure, *Anesthesiology* 67:936–941, 1987.

71. Drummond JC, Patel PM, Cole DJ, et al: The effect of the reduction of colloid oncotic pressure, with and without reduction of osmolality, on post-traumatic cerebral edema, *Anesthesiology* 88:993–1002, 1998.

72. Finfer S, Bellomo R, Boyce N, et al: A comparison of albumin and saline for fluid resuscitation in the intensive care unit, *N Engl J Med* 350:2247–2256, 2004.

73. SAFE Study Investigators, Australian and New Zealand Intensive Care Society Clinical Trials Group, Australian Red Cross Blood Service, George Institute for International Health, Myburgh J, Cooper DJ, Finfer S, et al: Saline or albumin for fluid resuscitation in patients with traumatic brain injury, *N Engl J Med* 357:874–884, 2007.

74. Etemadrezaie H, Baharvahdat H, Shariati Z, et al: The effect of fresh frozen plasma in severe closed head injury, *Clin Neurol Neurosurg* 109:166–171, 2007.

75. Culley MD, Larson CP Jr, Silverberg GD: Hetastarch coagulopathy in a neurosurgical patient, *Anesthesiology* 66:706–707, 1987.

76. Prough DS, Johnson JC, Poole GV Jr, et al: Effects on intracranial pressure of resuscitation from hemorrhagic shock with hypertonic saline versus lactated Ringer's solution, *Crit Care Med* 13:407–411, 1985.

77. Todd MM, Tommasino C, Moore S: Cerebral effects of isovolemic hemodilution with a hypertonic saline solution, *J Neurosurg* 63:944–948, 1985.

78. Vassar MJ, Perry CA, Holcroft JW: Analysis of potential risks associated with 7.5% sodium chloride resuscitation of traumatic shock, *Arch Surg* 125:1309–1315, 1990.

79. Vassar MJ, Perry CA, Gannaway WL, Holcroft JW: 7.5% sodium chloride/dextran for resuscitation of trauma patients undergoing helicopter transport, *Arch Surg* 126:1065–1072, 1991.

80. Vassar MJ, Fischer RP, O'Brien PE, et al: A multicenter trial for resuscitation of injured patients with 7.5% sodium chloride: The effect of added dextran 70. The Multicenter Group for the Study of Hypertonic Saline in Trauma Patients, *Arch Surg* 128:1003–1011, 1993.

81. Cooper DJ, Myles PS, McDermott FT, et al: Prehospital hypertonic saline resuscitation of patients with hypotension and severe traumatic brain injury: A randomized controlled trial, *JAMA* 291:1350–1357, 2004.

82. Shackford SR, Bourguignon PR, Wald SL, et al: Hypertonic saline resuscitation of patients with head injury: A prospective, randomized clinical trial, *J Trauma* 44:50–58, 1998.

83. Rozet I, Tontisirin N, Muangman S, et al: Effect of equiosmolar solutions of mannitol versus hypertonic saline on intraoperative brain relaxation and electrolyte balance, *Anesthesiology* 107:697–704, 2007.

84. Kleinschmidt-DeMasters BK, Norenberg MD: Rapid correction of hyponatremia causes demyelination: Relation to central pontine myelinolysis, *Science* 211:1068–1070, 1981.

85. Pulsinelli WA, Levy DE, Sigsbee B, et al: Increased damage after ischemic stroke in patients with hyperglycemia with or without established diabetes mellitus, *Am J Med* 74:540–544, 1983.

86. Bruno A, Levine SR, Frankel MR, et al: Admission glucose level and clinical outcomes in the NINDS rt-PA Stroke Trial, *Neurology* 59:669–674, 2002.

87. Danaei G, Lawes CM, Vander Hoorn S, et al: Global and regional mortality from ischaemic heart disease and stroke attributable to higher-than-optimum blood glucose concentration: Comparative risk assessment, *Lancet* 368:1651–1659, 2006.

88. Badjatia N, Topcuoglu MA, Buonanno FS, et al: Relationship between hyperglycemia and symptomatic vasospasm after subarachnoid hemorrhage, *Crit Care Med* 33:1603–1609, 2005.

89. Lam AM, Winn HR, Cullen BF, et al: Hyperglycemia and neuro logical outcome in patients with head injury, *J Neurosurg* 75:545–551, 1991.

90. Rovlias A, Kotsou S: The influence of hyperglycemia on neurological outcome in patients with severe head injury, *Neurosurgery* 46:335–342, 2000.

91. Longstreth WT Jr, Inui TS: High blood glucose level on hospital admission and poor neurological recovery after cardiac arrest, *Ann Neurol* 15:59–63, 1984.

92. Shapira Y, Artru AA, Cotev S, et al: Brain edema and neurologic status following head trauma in the rat: No effect from large volumes of isotonic or hypertonic intravenous fluids, with or without glucose, *Anesthesiology* 77:79–85, 1992.

93. Van den Berghe G, Wouters P, Weekers F, et al: Intensive insulin therapy in the critically ill patients, *N Engl J Med* 345:1359–1367, 2001.

94. NICE-SUGAR Study Investigators, Finfer S, Chittock DR, Su SY, et al: Intensive versus conventional glucose control in critically ill patients, *N Engl J Med* 360:1283–1297, 2009.

95. Oksanen T, Skrifvars MB, Varpula T, et al: Strict versus moderate glucose control after resuscitation from ventricular fibrillation, *Intensive Care Med* 33:2093–2100, 2007.

96. Bilotta F, Spinelli A, Giovannini F, et al: The effect of intensive insulin therapy on infection rate, vasospasm, neurologic outcome, and mortality in neurointensive care unit after intracranial aneurysm clipping in patients with acute subarachnoid hemorrhage: A randomized prospective pilot trial, *J Neurosurg Anesthesiol* 19:156–160, 2007.

97. de Courten-Myers G, Myers RE, Schoolfield L: Hyperglycemia enlarges infarct size in cerebrovascular occlusion in cats, *Stroke* 19:623–630, 1988.

98. Voll CL, Auer RN: The effect of postischemic blood glucose levels on ischemic brain damage in the rat, *Ann Neurol* 24:638–646, 1988.

99. Oliveira-Filho J, Ezzeddine MA, Segal AZ, et al: Fever in subarachnoid hemorrhage: Relationship to vasospasm and outcome, *Neurology* 56:1299–1304, 2001.

100. Reith J, Jorgensen HS, Pedersen PM, et al: Body temperature in acute stroke: Relation to stroke severity, infarct size, mortality, and outcome, *Lancet* 347:422–425, 1996.

101. Clifton GL, Miller ER, Choi SC, et al: Lack of effect of induction of hypothermia after acute brain injury, *N Engl J Med* 344:556–563, 2001.

102. Marion DW, Penrod LE, Kelsey SF, et al: Treatment of traumatic brain injury with moderate hypothermia, *N Engl J Med* 336:540–546, 1997.

103. Clifton GL, Allen S, Barrodale P, et al: A phase II study of moderate hypothermia in severe brain injury, *J Neurotrauma* 10:263–271, 1993.

104. Aibiki M, Maekawa S, Yokono S: Moderate hypothermia improves imbalances of thromboxane A2 and prostaglandin I2 production after traumatic brain injury in humans, *Crit Care Med* 28:3902–3906, 2000.

105. Jiang J, Yu M, Zhu C: Effect of long-term mild hypothermia therapy in patients with severe traumatic brain injury: 1-year follow-up review of 87 cases, *J Neurosurg* 93:546–549, 2000.

106. Qiu WS, Liu WG, Shen H, et al: Therapeutic effect of mild hypothermia on severe traumatic head injury, *Chin J Traumatol* 8:27–32, 2005.

107. Bratton SL, Chestnut RM, Ghajar J, Brain Trauma Foundation, American Association of Neurological Surgeons, Congress of Neurological Surgeons, Joint Section on Neurotrauma and Critical Care, AANS/CNS, et al: Guidelines for the management of severe traumatic brain injury. III: Prophylactic hypothermia, *J Neurotrauma* 24(Suppl 1):S21–S25, 2007.

108. Kenning JA, Toutant SM, Saunders RL: Upright patient positioning in the management of intracranial hypertension, *Surg Neurol* 15:148–152, 1981.

109. Harp JR, Wollman H: Cerebral metabolic effects of hyperventilation and deliberate hypotension, *Br J Anaesth* 45:256–262, 1973.

110. Lassen NA: Brain extracellular pH: The main factor controlling cerebral blood flow, *Scand J Clin Lab Invest* 22:247–251, 1968.

111. Bouma GJ, Muizelaar JP, Stringer WA, et al: Ultra-early evaluation of regional cerebral blood flow in severely head-injured patients using xenon-enhanced computerized tomography, *J Neurosurg* 77:360–368, 1992.

112. Sioutos PJ, Orozco JA, Carter LP, et al: Continuous regional cerebral cortical blood flow monitoring in head-injured patients, *Neurosurgery* 36:943–949, 1995.

113. Brain Trauma Foundation, American Association of Neurological Surgeons, Congress of Neurological Surgeons, Joint Section on Neurotrauma and Critical Care, AANS/CNS, Bratton SL, Chestnut RM, Ghajar J, et al: Guidelines for the management of severe traumatic brain injury. XIV: Hyperventilation, *J Neurotrauma* 24(Suppl 1):S87–S90, 2007.

114. Muizelaar JP, Marmarou A, Ward JD, et al: Adverse effects of prolonged hyperventilation in patients with severe head injury: A randomized clinical trial, *J Neurosurg* 75:731–739, 1991.

115. Gopinath SP, Robertson CS, Contant CF, et al: Jugular venous desaturation and outcome after head injury, *J Neurol Neurosurg Psychiatry* 57:717–723, 1994.

116. Sheinberg M, Kanter MJ, Robertson CS, et al: Continuous monitoring of jugular venous oxygen saturation in head-injured patients, *J Neurosurg* 76:212–217, 1992.

117. Michenfelder JD, Fowler WS, Theye RA: CO2 levels and pulmonary shunting in anesthetized man, *J Appl Physiol* 21:1471–1476, 1966.

118. Rudehill A, Lagerkranser M, Lindquist C, et al: Effects of mannitol on blood volume and central hemodynamics in patients undergoing cerebral aneurysm surgery, *Anesth Analg* 62:875–880, 1983.

119. Ravussin P, Archer DP, Tyler JL, et al: Effects of rapid mannitol infusion on cerebral blood volume: A positron emission tomographic study in dogs and man, *J Neurosurg* 64:104–113, 1986.

120. Ravussin P, Abou-Madi M, Archer D, et al: Changes in CSF pressure after mannitol in patients with and without elevated CSF pressure, *J Neurosurg* 69:869–876, 1988.

121. Berry AJ, Peterson ML: Hyponatremia after mannitol administration in the presence of renal failure, *Anesth Analg* 60:165–167, 1981.

122. Francony G, Fauvage B, Falcon D, et al: Equimolar doses of mannitol and hypertonic saline in the treatment of increased intracranial pressure, *Crit Care Med* 36:795–800, 2008.

123. Cottrell JE, Robustelli A, Post K, et al: Furosemide- and mannitol-induced changes in intracranial pressure and serum osmolality and electrolytes, *Anesthesiology* 47:28–30, 1977.

124. Schettini A, Stahurski B, Young HF: Osmotic and osmotic-loop diuresis in brain surgery: Effects on plasma and CSF electrolytes and ion excretion, *J Neurosurg* 56:679–684, 1982.

125. Rea GL, Rockswold GL: Barbiturate therapy in uncontrolled intracranial hypertension, *Neurosurgery* 12:401–404, 1983.

126. Bratton SL, Chestnut RM, Ghajar J, Brain Trauma Foundation, American Association of Neurological Surgeons, Congress of Neurological Surgeons, Joint Section on Neurotrauma and Critical Care, AANS/CNS, et al: Guidelines for the management of severe traumatic brain injury. XI: Anesthetics, analgesics, and sedatives, *J Neurotrauma* 24(Suppl 1):S71–S76, 2007.

127. Ward JD, Becker DP, Miller JD, et al: Failure of prophylactic barbiturate coma in the treatment of severe head injury, *J Neurosurg* 62:383–388, 1985.

128. Eisenberg HM, Frankowsky RF, Contant CF, et al: High-dose barbiturate control of elevated intracranial pressure in patients with severe head injury, *J Neurosurg* 69:15–23, 1988.

129. Kang TM: Propofol infusion syndrome in critically ill patients, *Ann Pharmacother* 36:1453–1456, 2002.

130. Vasile B, Rasulo F, Candiani A, Latronico N: The pathophysiology of propofol infusion syndrome: A simple name for a complex syndrome, *Intensive Care Med* 29:1417–1425, 2003.

131. Wysowski DK, Pollock ML: Reports of death with use of propofol (Diprivan) for nonprocedural (long-term) sedation and literature review, *Anesthesiology* 105:1047–1051, 2006.

132. Chiolero RL, Ravussin P, Anderes JP, et al: The effects of midazolam reversal by RO 15-1788 on cerebral perfusion pressure in patients with severe head injury, *Intensive Care Med* 14:196–200, 1988.

133. Seelig JM, Becker DP, Miller JD, et al: Traumatic acute subdural hematoma: Major mortality reduction in comatose patients treated within four hours, *N Engl J Med* 304:1511–1518, 1981.

134. Goldberg W, Mueller C, Panacek E, et al: NEXUS Group: Distribution and patterns of blunt traumatic cervical spine injury, *Ann Emerg Med* 38:17–22, 2001.

135. Lowery DW, Wald MM, Browne BJ, et al: Epidemiology of cervical spine injury victims, *Ann Emerg Med* 38:12–16, 2001.

136. Kreipke DL, Gillespie KR, McCarthy MC, et al: Reliability of indications for cervical spine films in trauma patients, *J Trauma* 29:1438–1439, 1989.

137. Roberge RJ, Wears RC, Kelly M, et al: Selective application of cervical spine radiography in alert victims of blunt trauma: A prospective study, *J Trauma* 28:784–788, 1988.

138. Fesmire FM, Luten RC: The pediatric cervical spine: Developmental anatomy and clinical aspects, *J Emerg Med* 7:133–142, 1989.

139. Hadley MN, Zabramski JM, Browner CM, et al: Pediatric spinal trauma: Review of 122 cases of spinal cord and vertebral column injuries, *J Neurosurg* 68:18–24, 1988.

140. Denis F: The three column spine and its significance in the classification of acute thoracolumbar spinal injuries, *Spine* 8:817–831, 1983.

141. Crosby ET, Lui A: The adult cervical spine: Implications for airway management, *Can J Anaesth* 37:77–93, 1990.

142. Hastings RH, Marks JD: Airway management for trauma patients with potential cervical spine injuries, *Anesth Analg* 73:471–482, 1991.

143. Podolsky S, Baraff LJ, Simon RR, et al: Efficacy of cervical spine immobilization methods, *J Trauma* 23:461–465, 1983.

144. Williams CF, Bernstein TW, Jelenko C III: Essentiality of the lateral cervical spine radiograph, *Ann Emerg Med* 10:198–204, 1981.

145. Biby L, Santora AH: Prevertebral hematoma secondary to whiplash injury necessitating emergency intubation, *Anesth Analg* 70:112–114, 1990.

146. Meakem TD, Meakem TJ, Rappaport W: Airway compromise from prevertebral soft tissue swelling during placement of halo-traction for cervical spine injury, *Anesthesiology* 73:775–776, 1990.

147. Stiell IG, Wells GA, Vandemheen KL, et al: The Canadian C-spine rule for radiography in alert and stable trauma patients, *JAMA* 286:1841–1848, 2001.

148. Ledsome JR, Sharp JM: Pulmonary function in acute cervical cord injury, *Am Rev Respir Dis* 124:41–44, 1981.

149. Lanig IS, Peterson WP: The respiratory system in spinal cord injury, *Phys Med Rehabil Clin N Am* 11:29–43, 2000.

150. Piepmeier JM, Lehmann KB, Lane JG: Cardiovascular instability following acute cervical spinal cord trauma, *Cent Nerv Syst Trauma* 2:153–160, 1985.

151. Ditunno JF, Little JW, Tessler A, Burns AS: Spinal shock revisited: A four-phase model, *Spinal Cord* 42:383–395, 2004.

152. Tuli S, Tuli J, Coleman WP, et al: Hemodynamic parameters and timing of surgical decompression in acute cervical spinal cord injury, *J Spinal Cord Med* 30:482–490, 2007.

153. Mackenzie CF, Shin B, Krishnaprasad D, et al: Assessment of cardiac and respiratory function during surgery on patients with acute quadriplegia, *J Neurosurg* 62:843–849, 1985.

154. Crosby ET: Airway management in adults after cervical spine trauma, *Anesthesiology* 104:1293–1318, 2006.

155. Reid DC, Henderson R, Saboe L, et al: Etiology and clinical course of missed spine fractures, *J Trauma* 27:980–986, 1987.

156. Muckart DJJ, Bhagwanjee S, van der Merwe R: Spinal cord injury as a result of endotracheal intubation in patients with undiagnosed cervical spine fractures, *Anesthesiology* 87:418–420, 1997.

157. Aprahamian C, Thompson BM, Finger WA, et al: Experimental cervical spine injury model: Evaluation of airway management and splinting techniques, *Ann Emerg Med* 13:584–587, 1984.

158. Gabbott DA: The effect of single-handed cricoid pressure on neck movement after applying manual inline stabilization, *Anaesthesia* 52:586–588, 1997.

159. Keller C, Brimacombe J, Keller K: Pressures exerted against the cervical vertebrae by the standard and intubating laryngeal mask airways: A randomized, controlled, cross-over study in fresh cadavers, *Anesth Analg* 89:1296–1300, 1999.

160. Nakazawa K, Tanaka N, Ishikawa S, et al: Using the intubating laryngeal mask airway (LMA-Fastrach™) for blind endotracheal intubation in patients undergoing cervical spine operation, *Anesth Analg* 89:1319–1321, 1999.

161. Bivins HG, Ford S, Bezmalinovic Z, et al: The effect of axial traction during orotracheal intubation of the trauma victim with an unstable cervical spine, *Ann Emerg Med* 17:25–29, 1988.

162. Majernick TG, Bieniek R, Houston JB, et al: Cervical spine movement during orotracheal intubation, *Ann Emerg Med* 15:417–420, 1986.

163. Horton WA, Fahy L, Charters P: Disposition of cervical vertebrae, atlanto-axial joint, hyoid and mandible during x-ray laryngoscopy, *Br J Anaesth* 63:435–438, 1989.

164. Sawin PD, Todd MM, Traynelis VC, et al: Cervical spine motion with direct laryngoscopy and orotracheal intubation: An in vivo cinefluoroscopic study of subjects without cervical abnormality, *Anesthesiology* 85:26–36, 1996.

165. Doolan LA, O'Brien JF: Safe intubation in cervical spine injury, *Anaesth Intensive Care* 13:319–324, 1985.

166. Rhee KJ, Green W, Holcroft JW, et al: Oral intubation in the multiply injured patient: The risk of exacerbating spinal cord damage, *Ann Emerg Med* 19:511–514, 1990.

167. Shatney CH, Brunner RD, Nguyen TQ: The safety of orotracheal intubation in patients with unstable cervical spine fracture or high spinal cord injury, *Am J Surg* 170:676–679, 1995.

168. Talucci RC, Shaikh KA, Schwab CW: Rapid sequence induction with oral endotracheal intubation in the multiple injured patient, *Am Surg* 54:185–187, 1988.

169. Smith CE: Cervical spine injury and tracheal intubation: a never-ending conflict, *Trauma Care* 10:20–26, 2000.

170. Muckart DJ, Bhagwanjee S, van der Merwe R: Spinal cord injury as a result of endotracheal intubation in patients with undiagnosed cervical spine fractures, *Anesthesiology* 87:418–420, 1997.

171. Hastings RH, Kelley SD: Neurologic deterioration associated with airway management in a cervical spine-injured patient, *Anesthesiology* 78:580–583, 1993.

172. Hastings RH, Wood PR: Head extension and laryngeal view during laryngoscopy with cervical spine stabilization maneuvers, *Anesthesiology* 80:825–831, 1994.

173. Nolan JP, Wilson ME: Orotracheal intubation in patients with potential cervical spine injuries: An indication for the gum elastic bougie, *Anaesthesia* 48:630–633, 1993.

174. Knill RL: Difficult laryngoscopy made easy with a "burp, *Can J Anaesth* 40:279–282, 1993.

175. Cohn AI, Zornow MH: Awake endotracheal intubation in patients with cervical spine disease: A comparison of the Bullard laryngoscope and the fiberoptic bronchoscope, *Anesth Analg* 81:1283–1286, 1995.

176. Turkstra TP, Craen RA, Pelz DM, Gelb AW: Cervical spine motion: A fluoroscopic comparison during intubation with lighted stylet, Glidescope, and Macintosh laryngoscope, *Anesth Analg* 101:910–915, 2005.

177. McGill J, Clinton JE, Ruiz E: Cricothyrotomy in the emergency department, *Ann Emerg Med* 11:361–364, 1982.

178. Meschino A, Devitt JH, Koch JP, et al: The safety of awake tracheal intubation in cervical spine injury, *Can J Anaesth* 39:114–117, 1992.

179. Seebacher J, Nozik D, Mathieu A: Inadvertent intracranial introduction of a nasogastric tube, a complication of severe maxillofacial trauma, *Anesthesiology* 42:100–102, 1975.

180. Grindlinger GA, Niehoff J, Hughes SL, et al: Acute paranasal sinusitis related to nasotracheal intubation of head-injured patients, *Crit Care Med* 15:214–217, 1987.

181. Ovassapian A, Krejcie TC, Yelich SJ, et al: Awake fiberoptic intubation in the patient at high risk of aspiration, *Br J Anaesth* 62:13–16, 1989.

182. Barriot P, Riou B: Retrograde technique for tracheal intubation in trauma patients, *Crit Care Med* 16:712–713, 1988.

183. Gronert GA, Theye RA: Pathophysiology of hyperkalemia induced by succinylcholine, *Anesthesiology* 43:89–99, 1975.

184. Pennant JH, Pace NA, Gajraj NM: Role of the laryngeal mask airway in the immobile cervical spine, *J Clin Anesth* 1993;:226-230

185. Hickey R, Albin MS, Bunegin L, et al: Autoregulation of spinal cord blood flow: Is the cord a microcosm of the brain? *Stroke* 17:1183–1189, 1986.

186. Senter HJ, Venes JL: Loss of autoregulation and posttraumatic ischemia following experimental spinal cord trauma., *J Neurosurg* 50:198–206, 1979.

187. Dyste GN, Hitchon PW, Girton RA, et al: Effect of hetastarch, mannitol, and phenylephrine on spinal cord blood flow following experimental spinal injury, *Neurosurgery* 24:228–235, 1989.

188. Ford RWJ, Malm DN: Therapeutic trial of hypercarbia and hypocarbia in acute experimental spinal cord injury, *J Neurosurg* 61:925–930, 1984.

189. Drummond JC, Moore SS: The influence of dextrose administration on neurologic outcome after temporary spinal cord ischemia in the rabbit, *Anesthesiology* 70:64–70, 1989.

190. Robertson CS, Grossman RG: Protection against spinal cord ischemia with insulin-induced hypoglycemia, *J Neurosurg* 67:739–744, 1987.

191. Bracken MB, Shepard MJ, Collins WF, et al: A randomized, controlled trial of methylprednisolone or naloxone in the treatment of acute spinal cord injury: Results of the Second National Acute Spinal Cord Injury Study, *N Engl J Med* 322:1405–1411, 1990.

192. Rozet I: Methylprednisolone in acute spinal cord injury: Is there any other ethical choice? *J Neurosurg Anesthesiol* 20:137–139, 2008.

193. Miller SM: Methylprednisolone in acute spinal cord injury: A tarnished standard, *J Neurosurg Anesthesiol* 20:140–142, 2008.

194. Sayer FT, Kronvall E, Nilsson OG: Methylprednisolone treatment in acute spinal cord injury: the myth challenged through a structured analysis of published literature. *Spine J* 6:335–343, 2006.

Chapter 11

SUPRATENTORIAL MASSES: ANESTHETIC CONSIDERATIONS

Nicolas Bruder • Patrick A. Ravussin

ANESTHESIA FOR SUPRATENTORIAL TUMORS

According to the Central Brain Tumor Registry of the United States (CBTRUS), 51,410 new cases of primary nonmalignant and malignant brain and central nervous system tumors were diagnosed in the United States in 2007. It is estimated that these tumors are responsible for 12,740 deaths every year. The most common in adults are gliomas (36%), meningiomas (32.1%), and pituitary adenomas (8.4%).[1] Approximately half of the tumors are malignant. The majority of tumors (>80%) are supratentorial. For all primary brain tumors, the median age of diagnosis is 57 years. From 1985 to 1999, the incidence of primary brain tumors rose modestly (1.1% per year).[2] The exact incidence of brain metastases is unknown but certainly underestimated. In about 25% of patients who die from cancer, central nervous system metastases are detected at autopsy. For the five most common sources of brain metastases (breast, colorectal, kidney, lung, and melanoma), 6% of the patients suffer this complication within 1 year of diagnosis of the primary cancer.[3] Thus, these five cancers would cause approximately 37,000 cases of brain metastases per year in the United States. Conversely, about 10% of patients with lung cancer present to the physician with symptoms from a brain metastasis.

General Considerations

For patients the problems associated with supratentorial tumors result from local and generalized pressure, whereas for surgeons the difficulties arise during surgical exposure because the brain is particularly susceptible to damage from retraction and mobilization. Anesthesia for supratentorial tumors thus requires an understanding of the pathophysiology of localized or generalized rising intracranial pressure (ICP); the regulation and maintenance of intracerebral perfusion; how to avoid secondary systemic insults to the brain[4,5] (Box 11-1); the effects of anesthesia on ICP, perfusion, and metabolism; and the therapeutic options available for decreasing ICP, brain bulk, and tension perioperatively. Specific problems include massive intraoperative hemorrhage, seizures, and air embolism in the head-elevated or sitting position or if venous sinuses are traversed. Further questions are how to monitor the brain's function and environment and whether to aim for rapid anesthesia emergence or for prolonged postoperative sedation and ventilation. Finally, the concurrence of various intracranial and extracranial pathologic conditions should not be forgotten, such as the presence of cardiovascular or pulmonary disease or—in the case of metastases—the existence of

paraneoplastic phenomena and the effects of chemotherapy or radiotherapy. This concept can be summarized as follows:

The anesthetic goal:	To preserve brain from secondary insult
The anesthetic risk factors:	Hypoxemia, hypercapnia, anemia, hypotension
The anesthetic actions:	Conserve cerebral autoregulation and CO2 responsiveness
	Maximize brain elastance to decrease retractor pressure

Pathophysiology of Rising Intracranial Pressure

The main normal intracranial components of the brain (tissue, intravascular blood, cerebrospinal fluid [CSF]) are contained in an unyielding skull. Hence any increase in their volume—or the addition of an abnormal mass—must be compensated by a concurrent reduction in volume of one or more of these components, mainly CSF or blood (the brain is largely incompressible) (Fig. 11-1). The ability of these homeostatic mechanisms to compensate depends not only on the volume of the mass but also on the speed at which it arises: For rapidly expanding masses, the ICP volume curve shifts markedly to the left. Early but limited homeostasis is provided by extracranial shifts of intracranial blood, followed by larger-capacity displacement of CSF—which is ineffective if CSF flow is obstructed. Once these compensatory mechanisms are exhausted, ICP rises rapidly, followed by impairment of cerebral circulation[6] and,

---

BOX 11–1 *Secondary Insults to the Already Injured Brain*

Intracranial

Increased intracranial pressure
Midline shift: tearing of the cerebral vessels
Herniation: falx, transtentorial, trans–foramen magnum, transcraniotomy
Epilepsy
Vasospasm

Systemic

Hypercapnia
Hypoxemia
Hypotension or hypertension
Hypo-osmolality or hyperosmolality
Hypoglycemia
Hyperglycemia
Low cardiac output
Hyperthermia

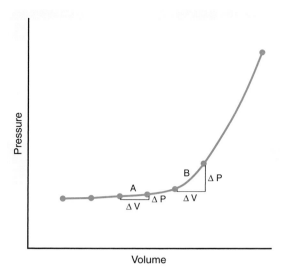

Figure 11–1 Idealized hyperbolic intracranial pressure-volume curve. **A,** high intracranial compliance: a change in volume produces minimal change in pressure; **B,** low intracranial compliance: a same change in volume as that in A produces a large change in intracranial pressure; ΔP, change in pressure; ΔV, change in volume.

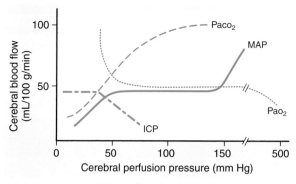

Figure 11–2 Cerebral blood flow (CBF) autoregulation: For a cerebral perfusion pressure (CPP) value between 50 and 150 mm Hg, CBF is maintained at 50 mL/100g/min (__ MAP). There is a linear relationship between PaCO₂ (20-80 mm Hg) and CBF (--- PaCO₂). Hypoxemia increases CBF and hyperoxia decreases CBF (.... PaO₂). If arterial pressure remains constant, CBF decreases when ICP increases (_ - _ - ICP). MAP mean arterial (blood) pressure.

ultimately, by brain herniation, generally subfalcine ("midline shift") or transtentorial, the end stage of compensation. This concept can be summarized as follows:

The cornerstone of neuroanesthesia:	Intracranial pressure-volume relationship
The main goal of neuroanesthesia:	Avoiding intracranial compartment volume increase, especially for cerebral blood volume (anesthetics, mean arterial pressure autoregulation, CO₂)

Volume Effects of Intracranial Tumors

The intracranial volume effects of tumors are due not only to the mass of the tumor itself but also to the surrounding vasogenic brain edema.[7,8] Such edema, commonly seen on preoperative computed tomography (CT) or magnetic resonance imaging, apparently results from secretory factors that increase vascular permeability in the nearby brain.[8] Peritumoral edema is particularly marked around fast-growing tumors, generally responds well to corticosteroid therapy, and can persist or even rebound after surgery for excision of the tumor.[8] Thus the areas surrounding large tumors suffer from ischemia resulting from compression (cerebral blood flow [CBF] in peritumoral tissue may be decreased by up to one third compared with normal tissue).[9] Treatment with steroids such as dexamethasone usually results in dramatic decreases in surrounding brain edema. The emergency and preoperative treatment of peritumoral vasogenic edema is the only good indication for steroid therapy in this context.

The Blood-Brain Barrier and Edema

The blood-brain barrier is also affected by intracranial pathologic conditions. Normally the blood-brain barrier is impermeable to large or polar molecules and variably permeable to ions and small hydrophilic nonelectrolytes. Thus any disruption of the blood-brain barrier permits water, electrolytes, and large hydrophilic molecules to enter perivascular brain tissues, leading to vasogenic brain edema. In this case, leakage—and the resulting brain edema—is directly proportional to the cerebral perfusion pressure (CPP). Vasogenic edema should be differentiated from osmotic edema (caused by a drop in serum osmolality) and cytotoxic edema (secondary to ischemia). Blood osmolality is a critical determinant of cerebral edema because a 19–mm Hg pressure gradient across the blood-brain barrier is generated for every milliosmole. In contrast, oncotic pressure plays a minor role. Neuroimaging shows disruption of the blood-brain barrier in many tumors. New strategies are being investigated to improve drug delivery to brain tumors. In the future, it is possible that new treatments to augment blood-brain barrier permeability (osmotic blood-brain barrier disruption, intra-arterial chemotherapy) will interfere with perioperative management.[10]

Intracerebral Perfusion and Cerebral Blood Flow

CBF is regulated at the level of the cerebral arteriole. It depends on the pressure gradient across the vessel wall (which in turn is the result of CPP) and PaCO₂ value (which depends on ventilation) (Fig. 11-2). CBF autoregulation, dominant to ICP homeostasis, keeps CBF constant in the face of changes in CPP or mean arterial pressure (MAP). It does this through alterations in cerebral vasomotor tone (i.e., cerebrovascular resistance [CVR]). Autoregulation is normally functional for CPP values of 50 to 150 mm Hg and is impaired by many intracranial (e.g., blood in CSF, trauma, tumors) and extracranial (e.g., chronic systemic hypertension) pathologic conditions. It is also affected by drugs used in anesthesia.

If CPP is inadequate, tissue perfusion will decrease when the lower limit of autoregulation is less than 50 mm Hg (if autoregulation is intact)). Ischemia results at levels of CBF below 20 mL/100 g/min unless CPP is restored (by increasing MAP or decreasing ICP) or cerebral metabolic demand is reduced (through deepened anesthesia or hypothermia). Increased ICP resulting in reduced CPP is met by cerebral arteriolar relaxation; in parallel, MAP is increased via the systemic autonomic response. As a result, a vicious cycle can be established, particularly in the presence of impaired intracranial homeostasis, as cerebral vessel relaxation increases cerebral blood volume (CBV), thus further raising ICP. In addition, an acute reduction in CPP or MAP tends to acutely increase ICP (the so-called vasodilatory cascade[11]). Reductions in PaCO₂ induce vasoconstriction,[12] reducing CBF, CBV, and thus ICP Conversely, hypercapnia increases ICP and should be prevented in the perioperative period. This makes hyperventilation a useful

185

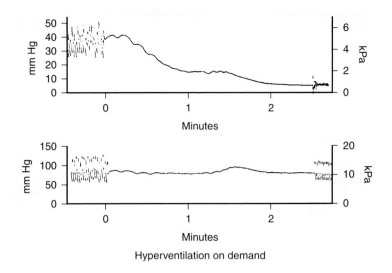

Figure 11-3 Beneficial effect of voluntary hyperventilation on intracranial pressure before anesthesia induction. The upper trace is the ICP trend. The bottom trace shows the stability of the mean arterial pressure *(Courtesy R Chiolero, MD)*

tool for the acute control of intracerebral hyperemia and elevated ICP (Fig. 11-3), as summarized here:

The anesthetic goal:	Hemodynamic stability
The reason:	Autoregulation takes 30 to 120 seconds to be established; thus sharp MAP fluctuations entrain undesirable CBF, CBV, and ICP changes
The formulas:	CBF= CPP/CVR
	CPP= MAP − ICP
	Normally, ICP < CVP

Anesthesia and Intracerebral Pressure, Perfusion, and Metabolism

Anesthesia exerts major effects on the intracranial environment through a variety of drug and nondrug effects. These effects are sensitive to the state of the intracranial and extracranial environment (e.g., cerebral compliance, presence or absence of intracranial pathologic condition, general volemic state).

INTRAVENOUS ANESTHETICS

Intravenous anesthetics include barbiturates, propofol, etomidate and ketamine. Apart from anesthesia induction, propofol is being increasingly used for maintenance as a continuous intravenous infusion (often computer controlled).[13] All the intravenous drugs mentioned are cerebral vasoconstrictors that act by depression of cerebral metabolic rate (CMR), except ketamine.[14-19] Ketamine increases whole brain CBF without changing CMR in healthy volunteers.[20] At subanesthetic doses, ketamine increases regional glucose metabolic rate and CBF.[21] The other agents decrease CBF, CBV, and ICP while leaving autoregulation and vessel reactivity to $Paco_2$ intact (see Fig. 11-3).[17,22-25] CMR reduction reflects brain activity[26] and is mediated through the electrical but not the basal metabolic activity of the neurons. Hence there is a ceiling effect for CMR reduction at electroencephalogram (EEG) burst suppression (Fig. 11-4). In contrast to volatile anesthetics, propofol has been shown capable of suppressing the cerebrostimulatory effects of nitrous oxide.[22] Etomidate directly inhibits adrenal cortisol secretion for 24 to 48 hours even after a single injection,[27] and its use is often associated with myoclonic (not epileptic) movements.

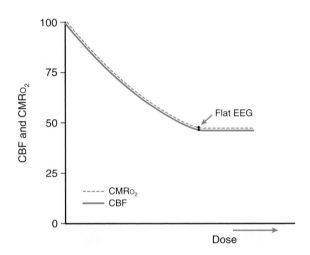

Figure 11-4 Parallel decrease in cerebral blood flow (CBF) and cerebral metabolic rate of O_2 (CMRo$_2$) produced by an intravenous agent. Change is dose dependent until the electroencephalogram (EEG) becomes isoelectric (flat).

VOLATILE ANESTHETICS

All volatile anesthetics are cerebral vasodilators,[28,29] but isoflurane, sevoflurane, and desflurane also reduce CMR. A flat EEG is obtained with these three agents at around 2 minimum alveolar concentrations (2 MAC), a concentration at which maximum metabolic depression is achieved. The response of cerebral metabolism to rising concentrations of volatile anesthetics is not linear. The decrease in CMR is steep from 0 to 0.5 MAC and then more gradual up to 2 MAC.[30] The effect of volatile anesthetics on CBF is the result of their vasodilatory properties and flow-metabolism coupling. At low concentrations (<1 MAC), CBF is lower than in the awake person.[31] But CBV is unchanged with isoflurane and decreased with propofol at comparable concentrations.[16] Among the newer volatile anesthetics, sevoflurane is the least vasodilating and desflurane the most.[32,33] The effects of xenon are more complex. This agent decreases CBF in gray matter, particularly in specific brain areas like the thalamus, the cerebellum, the cingulated gyrus, and the hippocampus, and increases CBF in white matter.[34] It does not impair flow-metabolism coupling.

For the normal brain and volatile concentrations below 1 MAC, $Paco_2$ reactivity remains intact, permitting control of vasodilation by hypocapnia.[22,25,35] (However, the presence of a pathologic brain condition or use of a high-MAC volatile anesthetic may impair or even abolish $Paco_2$ reactivity and autoregulation.)[36,37]

NITROUS OXIDE

Nitrous oxide is cerebrostimulatory, increasing CBF, CMR, and sometimes ICP. Its effect is not uniform throughout the brain but is limited to selected brain regions (basal ganglia, thalamus, insula), changing the regional distribution of CBF.[38,39] If substituted for an equipotent concentration of a volatile anesthetic agent, nitrous oxide increases CBF.[40-43] For the normal brain, the resulting cerebral vasodilation can be controlled by hypocapnia or the addition of an intravenous anesthetic. However, volatile agents have no such attenuating effect[44]; CMR and CBF are higher during 1 MAC anesthesia produced by a nitrous oxide–volatile anesthetic combination than that produced only by a volatile anesthetic.[43,44] This effect is especially deleterious in the actual or potential presence of brain ischemia. Particularly for repeat craniotomy, the potential of nitrous oxide, which is poorly soluble, to diffuse into and hence expand hollow spaces must be remembered as it could cause tension pneumocephalus in patients with intracranial air (repeat neurosurgery or head trauma).[45-47]

OPIOIDS

Opioids have been associated with short-term increases in ICP,[48-52] particularly sufentanil or alfentanil. Reflex cerebral vasodilation after decreases in MAP and hence in CPP is the underlying mechanism for the transient increases in ICP,[44,53-56] although a direct modest cerebral vasodilator effect has been demonstrated.[50] This effect demonstrates the sensitivity of intracerebral drug effects to the intracranial and extracranial environment and the importance of maintaining normovolemia for ICP stability. Generally, opioids modestly reduce CMR and do not affect flow-metabolism coupling, autoregulation, or the carbon dioxide sensitivity of the cerebral vessels. Remifentanil has been extensively studied. Its cerebral effects are comparable to those of other opioids, and its use in neuroanesthesia has been validated in clinical trials.[11,57-60]

OTHER DRUGS

Vasodilating antihypertensive agents such as nitroglycerine, nitroprusside, and nicardipine increase ICP and should be avoided.[61,62] Cerebral vasodilation may result from a normal autoregulation response or direct arterial vasodilation. For example, sodium nitroprusside increases ICP[63] but intracarotid injection of nitroprusside does not change CBF.[64] Conversely, verapamil decreases cerebrovascular resistance in humans by inducing direct cerebral vasodilation.[65] Theophylline constricts cerebral vessels but increases CSF production and is a potent central nervous system (CNS) stimulant, raising the risk of convulsions. Most β-adrenergic blockers, especially esmolol, do not interfere with cerebral blood flow or metabolism.[66]

Reducing ICP, Brain Bulk, and Tension

The anesthesiologist possesses a number of instruments to achieve ICP reduction and brain relaxation (Box 11-2), and thus to improve the quality of surgical exposure and to reduce retractor pressure. The effectiveness of these instruments depends on intact intracerebral homeostatic mechanisms.

BOX 11–2 *Management of Intracranial Hypertension and Brain Bulging*

Prevention

Euvolemia
Sedation, analgesia, anxiolysis
No noxious stimulus applied without sedation and local anesthesia
Head-up position, no compression of the jugular veins, head straight
Osmotic agents: mannitol, hypertonic saline
β-Blockers or clonidine or lidocaine
Steroids, if a tumor is present
Adequate hemodynamics: mean arterial blood pressure, central venous pressure, pulmonary capillary wedge pressure, heart rate
Adequate ventilation: Pao_2 >100 mm Hg, $Paco_2$ 35 mm Hg
Intrathoracic pressure as low as possible
Hyperventilation on demand before induction
Use of intravenous anesthetic agents for induction and maintenance in case of tensed brain

Treatment

Cerebrospinal fluid drainage if ventricular or lumbar catheter in situ
Osmotic agents
Hyperventilation
Augmentation of anesthesia with intravenous anesthetic agents: propofol, thiopentone, etomidate
Muscle relaxants
Venous drainage: head up, no positive end-expiratory pressure, reduction of inspiratory time
Mild controlled hypertension if autoregulation present

INTRAVENOUS ANESTHETICS

Intravenous anesthetics reduce CMR, CBF, and hence CBV and ICP, leading to a diminution of brain bulk, as discussed previously. Cerebral vasoconstriction depends on intact flow-metabolism coupling (Figs. 11-4 and 11-5) and is dose related up to neuronal electrical silence (EEG burst suppression). Like autoregulation, flow-metabolism coupling is impaired by brain contusion and other intracerebral pathologic conditions.

HYPERVENTILATION

Hyperventilation results in hypocapnia and subsequent cerebral vasoconstriction. In the context of intact autoregulation, CBF is roughly linearly related to $Paco_2$ between 20 and 70 mm Hg.[12] However, the carbon dioxide reactivity of cerebral vessels may be impaired or abolished in the presence of head injury or other intracerebral pathologic conditions, by high inspired concentrations of volatile anesthetics, or, particularly if the vessels are already dilated, by nitrous oxide. The CBF-, CBV-, and ICP-reducing effects of hypocapnia are acute and apparent for less than 24 hours.[67] A typical value to aim for is a $Paco_2$ of 30 to 35 mm Hg; arterial blood gas analysis rather than end-tidal CO_2 ($ETCO_2$) should be used as a controlling variable because of the possibility of large arterioalveolar CO_2 gradients in neurosurgical patients. The effectiveness of hyperventilation ($Paco_2$ at 25 ± 2 mm Hg) for controlling brain bulk in the patient under either isoflurane or propofol anesthesia has been demonstrated.[68]

The main complication associated with hyperventilation is reduction of CBF, which gives rise to cerebral ischemia.[69] Thus, the anesthesiologist must balance the benefit of brain relaxation against the risk of cerebral hypoperfusion. Other side effects are linear reduction in coronary artery flow,

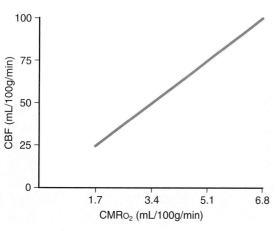

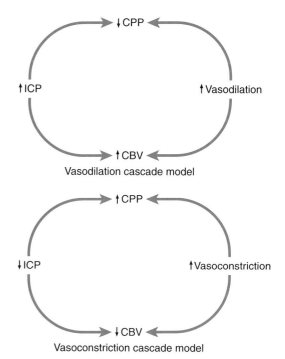

Figure 11–5 Coupling between cerebral blood flow (CBF) and cerebral metabolic rate of O2 production (CMR_{O_2}) coupling (flow-metabolism coupling). Normally, a CMR_{O_2} of 4 mL/100 g/min is coupled to a CBF of 50 mL/100 g/min.

Figure 11–6 Vasodilatory cascade model proposes that a decrease (↓) in cerebral perfusion pressure (CPP) can lead to cerebral vasodilation with subsequent increases (↑) in cerebral blood volume (CBV) and intracranial pressure (ICP). In contrast, the vasoconstriction cascade model suggests that an increase in CPP can reduce CBV and thus ICP. *(Modified from Rosner MJ, Daughton S: Cerebral perfusion pressure management in head injury. J Trauma 1990;30:933-940.).*

reduced cardiac venous return, hypokalemia, and potentiation of the brain's response to opioids.[70]

DIURETICS

Osmotic diuretics such as mannitol and hyperosmotic saline increase blood osmolality acutely, thus reducing brain water content (mainly in healthy brain tissue with an intact blood-brain barrier) and hence brain bulk and ICP.[71] This response improves brain deformability and thereby facilitates surgical exposure. A further beneficial effect is improvement in blood rheology[72] as a result of the reduction in edema of vascular endothelium and erythrocytes (increasing erythrocyte deformability)—the basis of mannitol's classic "antisludge" effect.[73] A typical regimen is to give 0.5 to 1 g/kg mannitol (150–400 mL 20% Mannitol) intravenously, split between a more rapid pre-craniotomy dose and a slower infusion, until brain dissection is complete. The ICP effect is prompt,[74] removes about 90 mL of brain water at peak effect,[75] and lasts for 2 to 3 hours. Normally the aim is to keep osmolality at less than 320 mOsm/kg. Problems with the use of osmotic diuretics include hypernatremia, hypokalemia, and acute hypervolemia, which could be deleterious in patients with congestive heart failure. There is no additional benefit to using loop diuretics such as furosemide, which induces hypovolemia and does not reduce brain water content.[76] On the contrary, serum saline should be infused to replace urinary losses in order to avoid hypovolemia and maintain blood pressure.

CEREBROSPINAL FLUID DRAINAGE

CSF drainage is achieved either by intraoperative direct puncture of the lateral ventricle or through a lumbar spinal catheter placed preoperatively. The latter is effective only if there is no caudal block to CSF outflow. Because of the risk of causing acute brain herniation, lumbar CSF drainage should be used cautiously and only when the dura is open. The patient should receive at least mild hyperventilation when CSF is drained. Normally removal of 10 to 20 mL of CSF is very effective in reducing brain tension. Up to 50 mL can be drained if necessary.

OTHER FACTORS

Other factors causing cerebral vasodilation and that can be corrected by the anesthesiologist include hypovolemia and hypoxia. The position of the patient (head down, extreme turning of the neck) also influences brain volume because of impaired venous drainage of the brain.[77] This should be kept in mind when brain swelling is observed without any obvious reason after the dura is opened. Repositioning of the head to avoid excessive rotation and compression of the jugular vein may be the solution.

VASOCONSTRICTIVE CASCADE

Finally, the anesthesiologist can use the vasoconstrictive cascade[78] by mildly increasing MAP, thus increasing CPP and decreasing CBV and ICP (Fig. 11-6).

General Anesthetic Management

Preoperative Assessment

Determination of anesthetic strategy for a given neurosurgical intervention depends on thorough knowledge of the neurologic and general state of the patient, the planned intervention, and holistic integration of these factors. The patient and the planned intervention should be discussed with the neurosurgeon involved.

NEUROLOGIC STATE OF PATIENT

A major aim in evaluating neurologic status is to estimate how much ICP is raised, the extent of impairment of intracranial compliance and autoregulation, and how much homeostatic reserve for ICP and CBF remains before brain ischemia and neurologic impairment occur. The goal is also to assess how much permanent and reversible neurologic damage is already present. Typical pointers to these elements in the patient history, physical examination, and technical examinations are listed in Box 11-3. The minimum examination should involve

BOX 11–3 *Preoperative Neurologic Evaluation*

History

Seizure (type, frequency, treatment)
Increased intracranial pressure (ICP): headache, nausea, vomiting, blurred vision
Decreased level of consciousness, somnolence
Focal neurologic signs: hemiparesis, sensory deficits, cranial nerve deficits, etc.
Paraneoplastic syndromes, including presence of thrombosis

Physical Evaluation

Mental status
Papilledema (increased ICP)
Signs of Cushing's response: hypertensive bradycardia
Pupil size, speech deficit, Glasgow Coma Scale score, focal signs

Medication

Steroids
Antiepileptic drugs

Technical Examination (Computed Tomography or Magnetic Resonance Imaging)

Size and location of the tumor: silent or eloquent area, near a major vessel, etc.
Intracranial mass effect: midline shift, decreased size of the ventricles, temporal lobe hernia
Intracranial mass effect: hydrocephalus, cerebrospinal fluid space around brainstem
Others: edema, brainstem involvement, pneumocephalus (repeat craniotomy)

Evaluation of Hydration Status

Fever; infection
Duration of bed rest
Fluid intake
Diuretics
Inappropriate secretion of antidiuretic hormone

Neurologic Working Diagnosis

Tissue type of tumor

---

a neurologic mini-mental status assessment, comprising the patient's ability to follow commands, the patient's degree of orientation, the presence or absence of speech deficit, and the Glasgow Coma Scale score. Elucidating what medication the patient is receiving and for how long is important because this medication may also affect intracranial compliance, perfusion, and reserves, as well as modify the pharmacokinetics and dynamics of anesthetic drugs.

The patient's CT scan or magnetic resonance image should be examined for the size and localization of the tumor and for signs of increased ICP. The latter include effacement of the lateral ventricle by tumor mass, lateral ventricle extension resulting from obstructive hydrocephalus, and midline shift (midline shift > 5 mm).[79,80] The presence of such signs warns that the ICP-volume curve is close to decompensation (the "knee" of the hyperbolic ICP-volume curve; see Fig. 11-1), with small increases in intracranial volume leading to disproportionate ICP increases and brain swelling. The preoperative treatment of brain edema with steroids should not mislead the neuroanesthetist into thinking that the patient is no longer at risk for perioperative intracranial hypertension. If the patient has presented with symptoms and signs of elevated ICP, the patient should be regarded as being at risk for perioperative

intracranial hypertension even if the presenting clinical tableau is no longer present.

GENERAL STATE OF PATIENT

Cardiovascular and respiratory functions are important because brain perfusion and oxygenation ultimately depend on them; their function should therefore be optimized preoperatively. Some intracranial pathologic conditions alter cardiovascular function (e.g., effects of raised ICP on cardiac conduction). Supratentorial surgery (particularly for meningiomas, metastasis) can be associated with significant blood loss, and hypovolemia and hypotension have detrimental effects in the neurosurgical context. The neuroanesthetist should note that both hyperventilation—often used to control ICP, CBF, CBV, and brain tension—and the head-up or sitting position make additional demands on the respiratory and cardiovascular systems. Finally, especially in neurosurgery for metastases, the primary tumor can itself impair cardiorespiratory function (e.g., 40% of brain metastases originate from the lung[81]) as can anticancer chemotherapy or radiotherapy. Examples are cardiomyopathy and doxorubicin (Adriamycin) or cyclophosphamide (Cytoxan) therapy and inhibition of plasma cholinesterase activity.[82]

Further problems associated with malignant tumors include coagulation disorders, which are associated with an increased risk of thromboembolism, as high as 21% in the first year after surgery.[83] Thus, despite the risk of bleeding, low-molecular-weight heparin may be indicated after craniotomy to prevent venous thromboembolism.[84]

Other systems interacting with neuroanesthesia are the renal system (e.g., diuretics and subsequent changes in plasma electrolytes, diabetes insipidus, decreased fluid intake), the endocrine system (altered by the intracranial disease process, such as pituitary adenoma, or by therapeutic drugs, such as the effect of glucocorticosteroids on hyperglycemia and cerebral ischemia), and the gastrointestinal tract (e.g., mucosal effects of steroids, motility effects of raised ICP). Hypercalcemia should be ruled out when brain tumors are associated with bone metastasis. A thorough history, supplemented by appropriate physical and technical examinations, is important for the elucidation and definition of these problems. It is important to remember that elderly patients (especially those with impaired cardiac and pulmonary function) pose particular challenges for anesthetic and perioperative management in this context.

PLANNED OPERATIVE INTERVENTION

For a planned operative intervention, the important points to clarify include the size and position of the tumor, the tissue diagnosis, the surgical approach, the structures in proximity and the likelihood of their involvement by surgery, and whether the tumor is to be removed radically. Knowing whether the mass to be resected is a tumor, a hematoma (acute or chronic), an abscess, a metastasis, or something else is useful information. The surgical approach determines the positioning of the patient; common approaches to supratentorial masses are either pterional or temporal and frontal craniotomies. In a bifrontal approach, the sagittal venous sinus is traversed, thereby raising the risk of bleeding and venous air embolism.[85]

When the tissue diagnosis is meningioma, the anesthesiologist should anticipate an operation with the goal of complete excision, which is generally curative.[86] Meningiomas can grow quite large, particularly in neurologically silent areas such as the frontal region, because they often grow slowly. They are often in difficult locations because of either surrounding structures or problematic access (e.g., sagittal sinus, optic nerve sheath, clivus, tentorial notch, ventricles, bone invasion). The combination of large size, difficult location, and the desire for radical excision makes for long and technically demanding operations. Such procedures are often accompanied by significant bleeding (from surrounding structures and because meningiomas are often highly vascular) and require maximal reduction of brain tension to facilitate surgical access. Preoperative embolization may reduce intraoperative bleeding during meningioma resection. Intraoperative blood salvage and autotransfusion may limit homologous transfusion in about 15% of patients.[87] In contrast, glioma resections are often easy debulking operations, of simple surgical access and low propensity to stimulate bleeding.

Colloid cysts of the third ventricle and epidermoid tumors arising in the basal cisterns are the most common nonpituitary supratentorial lesions. Colloid cysts of the third ventricle may be accompanied by obstructive hydrocephalus and thus high ICP at anesthesia induction. The relatively deep location of colloid cysts, epidermoid tumors of the basal cisterns, and pituitary tumors (if operated transcranially) make the provision of excellent brain relaxation for their exposure at the skull base the major anesthesiologic challenge during resection. Transsphenoidal resection of a pituitary adenoma is an essentially extracranial operation.

DETERMINATION OF ANESTHETIC STRATEGY

After consideration of the preceding factors, the following issues are addressed:

Vascular access: Consider risk of bleeding and venous air embolism, need for hemodynamic and metabolic monitoring, and requirements for infusion of vasoactive and other substances.

Fluid therapy: Aim for normovolemia and normotension, avoid hypo-osmolar fluids (lactated Ringer's solution), and avoid glucose-containing solutions in order to prevent hyperglycemia, which exacerbates ischemic brain injury.

Anesthetic regimen: Use (1) volatile agent–based anesthesia for "simple" procedures with low risk of ICP problems, ischemia, and need for brain relaxation and (2) total intravenous anesthesia for more complex procedures with anticipation of ICP problems, significant risk of cerebral ischemia, and need for excellent brain relaxation.

Ventilatory regimen: Aim for mild hypocapnia, mild hyperoxia, and low intrathoracic pressures (to improve cerebral venous return).

Extracranial monitoring: Assess cardiovascular and renal function (anticipate the management of venous air embolism).

Intracranial monitoring: Check general intracranial environment versus specific functions or pathways, for example, neurophysiologic (EEG, evoked potentials), metabolic (jugular venous bulb oxygenation, transcranial oximetry), and functional (transcranial Doppler ultrasonography).

Special techniques: Take into account surgical needs that may modify anesthetic management (brain stimulation and use of muscle relaxants, for example).

Preoperative Preparation

PREMEDICATION

Sedation carries the risk of hypercapnia, hypoxemia, and partial upper airway obstruction, all of which are detrimental in the context of increased ICP. However, avoiding stress (increased CMR, CBF) and hypertension (increased CBF, possibly vasogenic edema with impaired autoregulation) is also desirable.[88] Thus analgesia and sedation (e.g., midazolam 0.5 to 2 mg and/or fentanyl 25 to 100 μg or sufentanil 5 to 20 μg) may be provided during the placement of preoperative vascular access and monitoring devices by small, titrated, and intravenous increments under the direct and continuing control and observation of the anesthesiologist. The patient must never be left unsupervised in this context; respiratory support should be provided as necessary. However, in patients with tumors with no clinical or other signs of increased ICP (no shift, etc.), a small dose of benzodiazepine can help decrease the level of anxiety. Small doses of benzodiazepines or narcotics can unmask or worsen a preexisting compensated neurologic deficit.[89,90] This event may be difficult to distinguish from rapid worsening of mass effect and intracranial hypertension.

Steroids should be continued on the morning of the operation (methylprednisolone or dexamethasone). Histamine (H_2) blockers and gastric prokinetic agents should be considered to counteract the reduced gastric emptying and greater acid secretion associated with increased ICP and steroid therapy, particularly in patients with cranial nerve (IX, X) palsies (impairment or absence of gag reflexes). Other regular medication, particularly anticonvulsants,[91-93] as well as antihypertensive and other cardiac medications, should be continued, although drug interactions may occur with phenytoin. Consideration should be given to starting anticonvulsant therapy if it was not already initiated (e.g., a loading dose of 15 mg/kg phenytoin over 30 minutes during the procedure; this also helps hemodynamic control at the end of the operation). Perioperative fluctuations in antiepileptic medications may occur, contributing to perioperative development of seizures.[92,93] Monitoring of plasma levels or temporary augmentation of dosage of such medications may be necessary.

VASCULAR ACCESS

Two large-bore peripheral intravenous lines are usually placed for a full craniotomy; one line should suffice for stereotactic biopsy. Central venous access is indicated if a clinically significant risk of venous air embolism exists,[85] if substantial bleeding is anticipated (e.g., a large vascular tumor, proximity to major arteries or venous sinuses, or extensive bone resection), if major cardiovascular compromise is evident (with severely restricted myocardial function, pulmonary artery catheterization or transesophageal echocardiography should be considered), and if vasoactive drugs are to be infused continuously. We recommend the internal jugular approach with a meticulous cannulation technique and minimization of head-down positioning and neck rotation. Such positioning and neck rotation, together with the inevitable element of patient discomfort, can increase ICP. Thus in a stable patient, consideration can be given to putting these lines in once the patient is asleep. If the central line is placed for the management of venous air embolism, its position must be carefully controlled radiographically (tip at transition between vena cava and right atrium) or with the use of an electrocardiography lead.

Modern neuroanesthesia for full craniotomy with arterial cannulation is recommended, because of the need for very tight monitoring and control of CPP (obtainable by transducing arterial pressure at the mid-ear level of the circle of Willis and using the formula CPP = MAP − ICP). After the dura is opened, ICP equals the atmospheric pressure, so CPP equals MAP. In addition, frequent blood sampling is necessary for

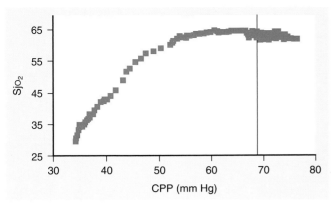

Figure 11–7 Jugular venous bulb oxygen saturation (Sjo_2) versus cerebral perfusion pressure (CPP) during administration of a methoxamine bolus for hypotension. Sjo_2 starts to decline. *(Courtesy Andrews PJD, Wang FC, Miller JD, unpublished data.)*

measurements of $Paco_2$, particularly if the patient is hyperventilated, is elderly, or has chronic obstructive pulmonary disease,[94,95] and for plasma glucose, potassium, osmolality, and other measurements. Monitoring of $ETCO_2$ is no substitute for $Paco_2$ measurement because the two often correlate poorly, especially with impaired ventilation-perfusion matching as occurs in chronic obstructive pulmonary disease, in elderly patients, or with long procedures.

Monitoring of jugular venous bulb oxygen saturation via a catheter placed by retrograde cannulation of the internal jugular vein permits continuous monitoring of cerebral oxygen extraction and hemoglobin oxygen saturation in jugular venous bulb blood ($Sjvo_2$). Under the assumption that CMR is constant, or through observation of its alteration by EEG monitoring, conclusions can be drawn about the global adequacy of cerebral perfusion (Fig. 11-7).[96]

Monitoring

As already noted, close hemodynamic monitoring is fundamental during neurosurgery. This includes beat-to-beat monitoring of arterial blood pressure and the electrocardiogram for the diagnosis of myocardial ischemia and arrhythmias. Pulse oximetry (for the detection of systemic hypoxia), $ETCO_2$ (as a *trend* monitor for $Paco_2$ and to help in the detection of venous air metabolism), and temperature monitoring (e.g., esophageal or urinary bladder) represent standard monitoring. A urinary catheter is placed to monitor urine output.

The occurrence of air embolism[85] is best detected by precordial Doppler ultrasonography, the most sensitive monitor (together with transesophageal echocardiography) for air bubbles in the venous circulation. If myorelaxants are used during the operation, neuromuscular block should be monitored. However, neuromuscular transmission should not be monitored on hemiplegic extremities because the greater acetylcholine receptor density of lower motor neuron units innervated by dysfunctional or nonfunctional upper motor neurons leads to resistance to nondepolarizing myorelaxants. If myorelaxant dosing is based on peripheral nerve stimulation of a hemiplegic extremity, overdosing of normal neuromuscular units will result.[97,98] In this context hemiparesis is probably not associated with hyperkalemia as appears in paraplegic or burn patients, and the use of succinylcholine is therefore not contraindicated from this point of view.[99] Because general anesthesia and steroid therapy both raise blood glucose levels

and because brain retraction is often associated with at least some focal cerebral ischemia,[100] blood glucose levels should be monitored regularly; hyperglycemia worsens neuronal damage during ischemia.[101-104] In this context, monitoring plasma electrolytes (particularly potassium) and osmolality (particularly if mannitol is used) would also appear to be prudent, as would hemoglobin and hematocrit determinations in the context of bleeding.

Monitoring of the intracranial environment or cerebral function is increasingly practiced during neurosurgery. As stated, $Sjvo_2$ monitoring provides useful global information on the adequacy of cerebral perfusion and oxygenation, and EEG monitoring can inform the anesthesiologist about CMR, cerebral ischemia, and depth of anesthesia. For some operations, monitoring of evoked potentials is helpful in observing the intactness of specific central nervous pathways. The surgical treatment of tumors located near eloquent brain areas carries a high risk of worsening neurologic deficits. Intraoperative electrostimulation (IES) has been developed to optimize the benefit-risk ratio of surgery. Motor mapping with the patient under general anesthesia or conscious sedation is being increasingly used to localize motor cortex adequately and improve the quality of surgical tumor removal. Compared with general anesthesia, conscious sedation improved the chance of achieving successful stimulation.[105] For patients who do not tolerate awake surgery, close cooperation of the anesthesiologist with the neurosurgeon is mandatory to obtain good results (avoid muscle relaxants, decrease the dosage of anesthetics as low as possible, maintain normothermia).

Preoperative ICP monitoring for elective supratentorial tumor surgery is rarely used today because of the impact of corticosteroids on preoperative ICP reduction and the ability of modern anesthetic techniques to control ICP during induction. Intraoperatively, once the dura is open, ICP is 0 (and MAP = CPP), making ICP monitoring of little use. These caveats do not, of course, apply to neurotraumatology, in which ICP monitoring is vital for therapy from the patient's entry in the emergency department onward. With the advent of relatively safe and simple-to-use catheter-tip ICP monitoring, there is, however, a trend toward more use of postoperative ICP monitoring, particularly for patients at risk (especially for removal of large tumors with extensive surrounding edema or for emergency surgery in patients with intracranial hypertension and altered consciousness). Intracranial hypertension develops in up to 20% of patients in the immediate postoperative period from brain swelling or hematoma formation, and such patients benefit from prompt therapeutic intervention.[106] Postoperative ICP monitoring may also help with the differential diagnosis in patients who do not emerge from anesthesia after operation. For all of these uses, looking at the shape of the ICP curve is important to ensure that the pressures displayed are reliable.

If lumbar CSF drainage is used, it can provide a reflection of ICP as long as the CSF pathways are not blocked. This approach can be tested by determining whether compression of the jugular veins increases lumbar CSF pressure (Queckenstedt maneuver). The lumbar CSF pressure can then be used to provide information to the surgeon and anesthesiologist about the influence of positioning, anesthesia, and surgery on potential brain perfusion pressure.

Transcranial Doppler ultrasonography (TCD) is being increasingly used in anesthesia and intensive care for monitoring blood flow velocity (FV). The middle cerebral artery is most commonly insonated because it carries about 60% of

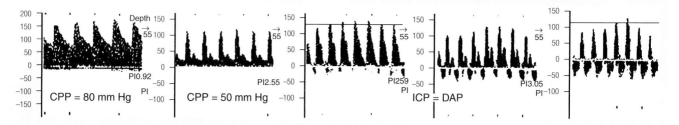

Figure 11–8 Changes seen on transcranial Doppler ultrasonography with decreasing cerebral perfusion pressure (CPP). Cerebral diastolic velocities decrease to zero when intracranial pressure (ICP) reaches diastolic arterial pressure (DAP). Ultimately, a reverse flow pattern with upward flow during systole and downward flow during diastole indicates cerebral circulatory arrest. PI, xx.

ipsilateral carotid artery blood flow and access through the temporal window is easy. TCD allows estimation of pressure autoregulation and CO_2 reactivity.[107] Autoregulation may be disturbed even after mild brain injury. After induction of anesthesia, MAP levels that are adequate in the vast majority of patients may be too low for neurosurgical patients. TCD measurement may help determine the adequacy of cerebral perfusion and change the hemodynamic management of a patient.[37] In addition, TCD is the only convenient noninvasive method both to detect intracranial complications that lead to increased ICP and to assess cerebral perfusion in anesthetized patients (Fig. 11-8).[108] During emergence from anesthesia, FV monitoring can detect cerebral hyperemia.[109] Although the implications of this physiologic change are not clear, cerebral hemorrhage after severe cerebral hyperemia has been reported.[110] Intraoperative Doppler monitoring in the surgical field, by means of a microvascular ultrasonic flow probe, has been used mostly in aneurysm surgery.[111] It may be used in tumor surgery to assess vessel patency during difficult dissection from the tumor.

Induction of Anesthesia
GOALS AND DRUGS

The major factors to be considered for anesthesia induction for elective supratentorial neurosurgery are ventilatory control (avoidance of hypercapnia and hypoxemia, early establishment of mild hyperventilation), sympathetic and thus blood pressure control (i.e., adequate depth of anesthesia and antinociception to prevent CNS arousal), and prevention of cranial venous outflow obstruction (head positioning). Attention to these details improves the patient's intracranial pressure-volume curve status, ensures the adequacy of cerebral perfusion, helps prevent untoward increases in ICP, and decreases brain perfusion pressure. A typical scheme for achieving these goals is detailed in Box 11-4, with thiopental or propofol given as a "starter," and an opioid, together with gentle hyperventilation, administered before intubation.

The use of propofol infusion permits the safer use of nitrous oxide by suppressing the latter's undesirable cerebrostimulatory effects. For induction in more frail or elderly patients, etomidate (0.2 to 0.4 mg/kg) may be used instead of propofol.

Fentanyl may be replaced by alfentanil (5 to 10 µg/kg followed by infusion at 5 to 10 µg/kg/hr), by sufentanil (0.5 to 1.5 µg/kg followed by infusion at 0.1 to 0.3 µg/kg/hr) for smoother hemodynamic control, or by remifentanil (0.5 to 1 µg/kg followed by infusion at 0.1 to 0.2 µg/kg/hr) for rapid awakening

---

BOX 11–4 *Suggested Anesthesia Induction Sequence for Intracranial Surgery*

1. Adequate anxiolysis in the anesthetic room. Adequate fluid loading (5 to 7 mL/kg of NaCl 0.9%). Electrocardiogram leads in place; capnometer, pulse oximeter, and noninvasive blood pressure monitors. Insertion of intravenous and arterial lines under local anesthesia.
2. Induction of general anesthesia. Fentanyl 1 to 2 µg/kg or sufentanil or remifentanil. Preoxygenation and voluntary hyperventilation Propofol 1.25 to 2.5 mg/kg or thiopentone 3 to 6 mg/kg for induction. Nondepolarizing muscle relaxant: vecuronium, rocuronium, or cisatracurium. Controlled ventilation at $PaCO_2$ of 35 mm Hg. Propofol 50 to 150 µg/kg/min or isoflurane 0.5% to 1.5% (or sevoflurane or desflurane) for maintenance and fentanyl (or alfentanil, sufentanil, or remifentanil) 1 to 2 µg/kg/hr (or bolus) for analgesia.
3. Intubation.
4. Local anesthesia or intravenous remifentanil 0.5 to 1 µg/kg for skull-pin head-holder placement and skin incision.
5. Adequate head-up positioning; no compression of the jugular veins.
6. Brain relaxation. Mannitol 0.5 to 0.75 g/kg if needed. Insertion of a lumbar drain if needed. Normovolemia with the use of NaCl 0.9% or starch 6%—no lactated Ringer's solution.

---

and early neurologic assessment independent of the duration of anesthesia.[60,112,113]

MUSCLE RELAXANTS

Modern nondepolarizing myorelaxants have minimal effects on intracerebral hemodynamics. It is thought that the use of succinylcholine should be reserved for patients with possible intubation difficulties or when rapid-sequence induction is absolutely unavoidable. Succinylcholine can cause transient increases in CMR, CBF, and ICP, although such increases usually can be controlled by hyperventilation or deepened anesthesia and are of consequence mainly in patients who have precariously elevated ICP.

We strongly recommend avoiding longer-acting myorelaxants, such as pancuronium, and prefer the use of middle- to short-acting myorelaxants, such as vecuronium, cisatracurium, mivacurium, and rocuronium. Our recommendation is based on the fact that neurosurgical patients are particularly susceptible to the effects of myorelaxant hangover (difficult to detect with manual assessment of peripheral nerve stimulation). In this context, the interaction (need for up to 50% to 60% higher doses) between long-term phenytoin[91,114] or carbamazepine treatment[115] (>7 days) and pancuronium, vecuronium, atracurium, or cisatracurium[116,117] should be noted, as should the need to monitor neuromuscular transmission on nonhemiplegic extremities (as discussed previously). The anesthesiologist should keep in mind, however, that immobility of the patient must be guaranteed during the procedure.

PATIENT POSITIONING

Pin holder application is a maximal nociceptive stimulus. It must be adequately blocked by deepening of analgesia (bolus of remifentanil 0.25 to 1 µg/kg, fentanyl 1 to 3 µg/kg or alfentanil 10 to 20 µg/kg) or anesthesia (e.g., intravenous bolus of thiopental 1 mg/kg or propofol 0.5 mg/kg), preferably in conjunction with local anesthetic infiltration of the pin site to prevent undesirable CNS arousal and hemodynamic activation.[118] Alternatively, hemodynamic control can be achieved with antihypertensive agents such as esmolol (1 mg/kg) and labetalol (0.5 to 1 mg/kg). *Pin insertion can be associated with venous air embolism.*

Patient positioning must be closely surveyed by both the anesthesiologist and the surgeon, with extreme positioning being avoided. Careful attention should be paid to padding or fixing of regions susceptible to injury by pressure, abrasion, or movement, such as falling extremities. A mild head-up position helps venous drainage. Severe lateral extension or flexion of the head on the neck should be prevented (there should be at least two fingers' space between chin and nearest bone) to avoid endotracheal tube kinking, postoperative airway swelling and compromise, and impairment of cerebral venous drainage (brain swelling). The knees should be mildly flexed to avoid lumbosacral injury. If the head is turned laterally (e.g., for pterional or frontotemporal craniotomy), the contralateral shoulder should be elevated (with a wedge or roll) to prevent brachial plexus stretch injury. The lateral and sitting positions have their own specific positioning precautions. The endotracheal tube must be fixed and packed securely to prevent accidental extubation or abrasions resulting from movement and must be accessible intraoperatively (note: there is increased dead space if extension tubing is used distal to the Y-piece). Finally, the eyes should be taped closed to prevent corneal damage from exposure or irrigation with antiseptic or other fluids.

Maintenance of Anesthesia
GOALS

The main anesthetic aims during supratentorial surgery are (1) control of brain tension via control of CBF and CMR (the so-called chemical brain retractor concept [Box 11-5]) and (2) neuroprotection through maintenance of an optimal intracranial environment. The first goal depends on the prevention of CNS arousal; it is achieved through good depth of anesthesia and antinociception (Fig. 11-9), antiepileptic prophylaxis,[119,120] as well as control of the consequences of CNS arousal should it occur (with antihypertensives, sympatholytics). The second goal depends on maintaining a good match between cerebral substrate demand and supply, as well as attempts at specific neuroprotection if mismatch occurs (note: ischemia occurs under the retractor in 5% to 10% of patients).[100] Many anesthesiologists use modest passive hypothermia (35° C) to provide neuroprotection, on the

---

BOX 11–5 *Chemical Brain Retractor Concept*

Mild hyperosmolality (use NaCl 0.9% [304 mOsm/kg] as baseline infusion; give 20% mannitol [1245 mOsm/kg] 0.5 to 0.75 g/kg or hypertonic saline [7.5%, 2498 mOsm/kg] 2 to 4 mL/kg before bone flap removal)

Intravenous anesthetic agent (propofol), adequate depth of anesthesia

Mild hyperventilation, mild hyperoxygenation

Mild controlled hypertension: mean arterial blood pressure maintained around 100 mm Hg in order to decrease cerebral blood volume and intracranial pressure

Normovolemia; no vasodilators

Mild hyperoxia

Together with:
- Head-up positioning with unimpeded cerebral venous drainage; no compression of the jugular veins
- Minimal positive end-expiratory pressure
- Adequate anesthetic depth or muscle relaxant to prevent bucking on ventilator
- Lumbar drainage
- Avoidance of brain retractors

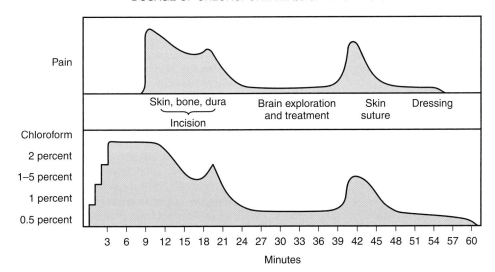

Figure 11–9 Nociception and depth of anesthesia as illustrated by this graph of chloroform requirements during various levels of operative nociception. *(From Horsley V: On the technique of operations on the central nervous system: Address in surgery. Lancet 1906; ii; 484.)*

DOSAGE OF CHLOROFORM REQUISITE DURING OPERATION

basis of the abundant experimental literature demonstrating its efficacy after brain injury. However, clinical studies have not demonstrated any beneficial effect of hypothermia in neurosurgical patients.[121] In addition, hypothermia impairs platelet function and the coagulation cascade. Consequently, even mild hypothermia ($<1°$ C) may increase blood loss and the risk for transfusion.[122] Although a higher risk of cerebral bleeding due to hypothermia has not been demonstrated during neurosurgery, this theoretical effect should be considered in the risk-benefit analysis of inducing hypothermia. Other complications of hypothermia are surgical wound infection,[123] adverse myocardial outcomes,[124] prolonged recovery, and shivering.[125] Thus, normothermia should be a major goal of neuroanesthetic management. Hypothermia should be considered only in cases with a major risk of cerebral ischemic injury.

CHOICE OF TECHNIQUE

There has been a long-standing controversy surrounding the use of intravenous versus volatile anesthetics for intracranial procedures. So far, no study comparing intravenous with volatile agent–based neuroanesthesia has been able to demonstrate major outcome differences.[80,126]

At present, the major argument for the still extensive and successful use of volatile agent–based techniques remains controllability, predictability, and the attainability of early awakening.[127] However, volatile anesthetics are otherwise far from ideal agents for neuroanesthesia because of their ability to increase CBF, ICP, and brain bulk.[15,16,92] In a prospective randomized study comparing propofol-fentanyl, isoflurane-fentanyl, and sevoflurane-fentanyl anesthesia in normocapnic patients, the rate of ICP and cerebral swelling was lower in the propofol-fentanyl group.[126] However, in patients with no evidence of midline shift on preoperative CT scan, neither isoflurane nor desflurane induced any significant variation in ICP.[128] Similarly, there was no difference in surgeon's assessment of brain swelling between patients anesthetized with isoflurane and those anesthetized with propofol.[68] Thus, despite evidence that ICP is lower with total intravenous techniques, the clinical impact of this technique in patients with elevated ICP has yet to be evaluated.[129] Although intravenous agents offer good control of CBF, ICP, and brain bulk,[15,126,129] prolonged or unpredictable awakening remains the main concern with intravenous techniques, with possible resulting difficulties in the differential diagnosis of delayed awakening and the need for emergency CT to rule out surgical complications. This problem is increasingly mitigated by the use of computer-controlled infusion schemes (target-controlled infusion pumps) and the availability of short-acting or infusion duration–insensitive drugs, such as propofol and remifentanil.

At this time, we would consider intravenous techniques to be most clearly indicated for the problem neurosurgical patient (high risk of ICP problems and brain swelling), whereas volatile techniques are best used for the uncomplicated neurosurgical case.[127] In this context, nitrous oxide may be used as a rapid-acting analgesic supplement while the dura is open and the brain is slack. However, as evidenced, the concurrent use of nitrous oxide and volatile anesthetics is best avoided in the problem patient because of their synergistic effects in increasing cerebral metabolism and blood flow, as discussed previously.[16,22,40,42,43,130,131] Clearly, if measures to control brain bulk (hyperventilation, osmotic diuretics, blood pressure control, positioning, lumbar drainage) are unsuccessful during anesthesia with volatile agents, consideration

should be given to converting to a total intravenous anesthetic technique (see Box11-2).

If undesirable CNS arousal and hemodynamic activation occur despite an adequate depth of anesthesia and analgesia, these problems may be controlled by an antisympathetic drug such as esmolol (initial dose of 1 mg/kg), labetalol (initial dose of 0.5 to 1 mg/kg), or clonidine (initial dose of 0.5 to 1 µg/kg).

MANAGEMENT OF INCREASES IN INTRACRANIAL PRESSURE AND BRAIN BULK

Details of prevention and treatment of increases in ICP and brain bulk are shown in Box 11-2. The occurrence of brain protrusion requires *immediate* intervention, which should include deepening anesthesia with intravenous agents (the capnogram curve should be checked to rule out "fighting" against the ventilator), increasing hyperventilation, performing CSF drainage, and changing to head-up positioning without delay.

FLUID THERAPY

The practice of maintaining normovolemia and normotension during intracranial surgery is now well-established. Hyperglycemia, which worsens the consequences of cerebral ischemia,[101,103,132] and hypo-osmolality (target osmolality, 290 to 320 mOsm/kg), which can increase brain edema, should be avoided. Colloid oncotic pressure plays an unclear role in brain edema. Glucose-containing or hypo-osmolar solutions (e.g., lactated Ringer's solution, 254 mOsm/kg) should be avoided. Suitable choices for infusion liquids during intracranial surgery include 0.9% NaCl and modern 6% hydroxyethyl starch 130/0.4 solutions (304 mOsm/kg) with no deleterious effect on coagulation. The hematocrit should be kept above 28%. Fluids should be warmed at the end of the procedure to ensure normothermia for emergence from anesthesia.

Emergence from Anesthesia

Emergence from anesthesia has respiratory, cardiovascular, metabolic-endocrine, and neurologic consequences.[133,134] In the early postoperative period after elective craniotomy, autoregulation is often impaired, with 20% of patients demonstrating raised ICP.[106] Particularly in the neurosurgical context, extubation criteria must be strictly observed: Respiratory drive and airway protection are likely to be impaired after brain surgery, and both hypercapnia and hypoxia carry the risk of causing additional systemic secondary brain damage (see Box 11-1). Awakening and extubation after anesthesia are associated with hemodynamic arousal lasting 10 to 25 minutes[133] and only weakly correlating to rises in oxygen consumption (Fig. 11-10).[133] This activation is partially mediated by elevations in catecholamine levels and partially by nociceptive stimuli. A link between perioperative hypertension and intracranial hemorrhage after craniotomy has been demonstrated.[135] In the study, patients with postoperative intracranial hemorrhage were 3.6 times more likely to be hypertensive than their matched controls. The very strong association of intracranial hemorrhage with the pattern of blood pressure remaining in the normal range intraoperatively but hypertension occurring during emergence from anesthesia suggested that loose surgical hemostasis achieved at a low blood pressure may result in bleeding at a higher one. Changes in the cerebral circulation may also contribute to postoperative cerebral complications (hemorrhage or edema). Tracheal extubation is associated with a 60% to 80% increase in cerebral blood flow

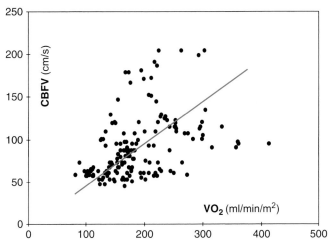

Figure 11–10 Relationship between body oxygen consumption and cerebral hemodynamic activation assessed by transcranial cerebral blood flow velocity (CBFV) at extubation (N Bruder, P Ravussin, unpublished data).

velocity from preinduction baseline value with an increase in $SjvO_2$.[109] It seems clear that the association of arterial hypertension and postoperative cerebral hyperemia may be dangerous for the patients. Analgesia, prevention of hypothermia and shivering, and timely tracheal extubation to avoid fighting of the patient against the tube are required to limit catecholamine release and hemodynamic changes. β-Adrenergic blocking agents improve hemodynamic stability during emergence and mitigate CBF changes.[136] Esmolol, a short-acting beta-blocker (half-life 9 minutes), may be used as a bolus (1 mg/kg) followed by a continuous infusion (100 to 300 μg/kg/min) for 15 to 30 minutes after tracheal extubation.

Aims of Emergence After Neurosurgery

The main aim during emergence from anesthesia after neurosurgery is maintenance of intracranial and extracranial homeostasis, particularly of the following parameters: MAP, CBF, ICP, $PaCO_2$, PaO_2, CMR, and temperature (Box 11-6). Factors likely to cause intracranial bleeding or to affect CBF or ICP, such as coughing, fighting against the ventilator, hypertension,[135] and airway overpressure, should be avoided. The patient should be responsive to verbal commands, calm, and cooperative soon after emergence. The most common signs of deterioration after intracranial surgery are a decrease in the level of consciousness and clinical signs of focal neurologic deficit. The most feared postoperative complication, cerebral hemorrhage, occurs most often in the first 6 hours after surgery, justifying close clinical monitoring in the first postoperative hours.[137] In a retrospective analysis, factors associated with postoperative complications were tumor severity score (combining tumor location, mass effect, and midline shift), estimated blood loss and intraoperative fluids volume, duration of surgery more than 7 hours, and postoperative ventilation. The shortage in intensive care unit resources may justify a prolonged stay in a post-anesthesia care unit and return to the neurosurgical ward by bypassing the intensive care unit only for patients at low risk of cerebral complications. But one postoperative catastrophe may far outweigh the potential cost saving needing to establish clear postoperative protocols in case of neurologic worsening.[138]

Neurosurgical awakening should provide: optimal conditions for neurologic examination.

Early versus Late Emergence

Ideally, patients recovering from neurosurgery should emerge rapidly from anesthesia to permit immediate assessment of the results of surgery and to provide a baseline for continuing postoperative neurologic follow-up.[133] However, there are still some categories of patients in which early emergence is not appropriate. Advantages and disadvantages of early versus late emergence are summarized in Table 11-1.

Indications for Late Emergence

If the patient had obtunded consciousness or inadequate airway control preoperatively, the problem is not likely to improve postoperatively, making successful early extubation unlikely. If there is a high postoperative risk of brain edema, raised ICP, or deranged intracerebral hemostasis or homeostasis, early awakening is not appropriate. Such a risk is increased after long (>6 hours) and extensive surgery (particularly if associated with bleeding), repeat surgery, major glioblastoma surgery, surgery involving or close to vital brain areas, and surgery associated with significant brain ischemia (e.g., long vascular clipping times, extensive retractor pressure). If delayed emergence is chosen, adequate sedation and analgesia should be ensured, preferably with short-acting drugs.

Preconditions for Early Emergence

Early emergence from anesthesia necessitates planning. It entails an anesthetic technique pharmacologically adequate to permit early awakening and requires meticulous attention to the detail of intraoperative systemic and brain homeostasis (preservation of normal oxygenation, temperature, intravascular volume, blood pressure, cardiovascular function, and CNS metabolism) (Box 11-7). To avoid the trauma of mechanical brain retraction, ICP and brain bulk should be controlled pharmacologically during the operation (see Box 11-5). The neurosurgeon contributes by minimizing blood loss via obsessive hemostasis and reduction of surgical invasiveness with the use of microsurgery and small operative fields. If these conditions are fulfilled, early emergence can be associated with less metabolic, hemodynamic, and endocrine activation than delayed emergence (Fig. 11-11).[133]

Conduct of Early Emergence

The essentials of conducting a patient's early emergence from anesthesia are listed in Box 11-8. The cardinal prerequisite for a "soft landing" is careful titration of anesthetics and analgesics at the end of the procedure. This goal is achieved with the use of small "top-up" doses of intravenous anesthetics or

Table 11–1 **Pros and Cons: Early versus Delayed Awakening**

	Early Awakening	Delayed Awakening
Advantages	Earlier neurologic examination and reintervention if necessary Easier transfer to intensive care unit (ICU) Earlier indications for further investigations Setting of neurologic scene for following hours (baseline for further clinical assessment) Less hypertension, less catecholamine burst Performed by anesthetist who knows patient: brain tightness, bleeding, surgery, etc. Potential lower costs	Less risk of hypoxemia or hypercapnia Better late hemostasis Stabilization period in same position as during surgery
Disadvantage(s)	Greater risk of hypoxemia, hypercapnia Larger hemodynamic changes Difficult respiratory monitoring during transfer to ICU	Less neurologic monitoring

BOX 11–7 *Preconditions for Early Emergence from Anesthesia: Homeostasis*

Systemic Homeostasis

Normovolemia, normothermia
Normotension (mean arterial blood pressure 80 mm Hg)
Mild hypocapnia ($Paco_2$ 35 mm Hg)
Normoglycemia (serum glucose 4 to 6 mmol/L)
Mild hyperosmolality (285 ± 5 mOsm/kg)
Hematocrit approximately 30%

Brain Homeostasis

Normal cerebral metabolic rate, cerebral blood flow, and intracranial pressure
Antiepileptic prophylaxis
Adequate head-up position

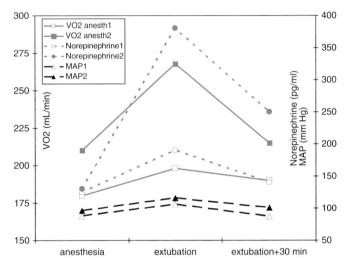

Figure 11–11 Early versus delayed recovery after neurosurgery: differences in body oxygen consumption (VO2, squares left axis), norepinephrine blood concentration (circles right axis), and mean arterial pressure (MAP, triangles right axis). The measures were recorded during anesthesia, at extubation and 30 minutes after extubation (x-axis). In this study, patients were divided into two groups, those extubated in the operating room (group 1) and those extubated more than 2 hours later in the intensive care unit (group 2). Despite similar changes in blood pressure, patients in group 2 had higher VO2 and catecholamine blood level at extubation. *(modified from Bruder N, Stordeur JM, Ravussin P: Metabolic and hemodynamic changes during recovery and tracheal extubation in neurosurgical patients: immediate versus delayed recovery. Anesth Analg 1999; 89:674-8)*

analgesics (opioids, lidocaine) or, alternatively, a short burst of volatile agents, or both. The judicious use of sympatholytic agents may be indicated. Prevention of postoperative pain is mandatory, especially after remifentanil analgesia. The infusion of a single nonnarcotic analgesic does not provide adequate analgesia in all patients. A combination of 2 nonnarcotic analgesics, associated with small doses of morphine after extubation as needed, is mandatory.[139] A scalp nerve block or bupivacaine infiltration of the wound provides adequate analgesia in the early postoperative period and should be considered.[140] Adequate antiepileptic prophylaxis relies mostly on a phenytoin (or fosphenytoin) loading dose during surgery, but other intravenous antiepileptic agents (valproate, levetiracetam, etc.) may be used. Prospective trials comparing various antiepileptic agents for early postoperative prophylaxis are lacking.

DIFFERENTIAL DIAGNOSIS OF UNPLANNED DELAYED EMERGENCE

If the patient is not awake enough to obey simple verbal commands 20 to 30 minutes after pharmacologically adequate cessation of anesthesia, nonanesthetic causes of delayed emergence must be considered and ruled out (with CT or magnetic resonance imaging) or treated. The differential diagnosis includes seizure, cerebral edema, intracranial hematoma, pneumocephalus, vessel occlusion, and ischemia as well as metabolic or electrolyte disturbances. If opioid overdose is suspected, it is not unreasonable to try carefully titrated antagonization with small doses of naloxone or naltrexone.

Specific Anesthetic Management

Difficult Airway

The avoidance of hypoxia is more important than the prevention of ICP increases. With the advances in fiberoptic intubation techniques, awake intubation in the electively prepared, cooperative patient with a difficult airway is the method of choice before supratentorial tumor surgery. Fiberoptic intubation must be carefully prepared. It begins with a good explanation of the procedure to the patient, continues with meticulous local anesthesia of the nasopharynx and airways, and is supplemented by judicious use of small doses of sedatives (e.g., 0.5- to 1-mg bolus of midazolam, 25- to 50-μg bolus of fentanyl, or the use of a low-dose infusion of propofol at 1 to 2 mg/kg/hr). The cerebral consequences of deep sedation and hypercapnia should be kept in mind during this procedure.

BOX 11–8 *Conduct of Early Emergence from Anesthesia after Intracranial Surgery*

Checklist before Attempting an Early "Landing"

Adequate preoperative state of consciousness

Limited brain surgery, no major brain laceration

No extensive posterior fossa surgery involving cranial nerves IX to XII

No major arteriovenous malformation resection, which may give rise to malignant postoperative edema

Normal body temperature and oxygenation; cardiovascular stability

Suggested Awakening Sequence

1. Discontinue long-lasting opioids (fentanyl or sufentanil) approximately 60 minutes before planned emergence or remifentanil at the end of skin closure.
2. Allow progressive rise of $PaCO_2$ to normoventilation.
3. Let neuromuscular block decrease to two twitches (TOF) if myorelaxation is used.
4. Treat blood pressure bursts resulting from nociception with boluses of intravenous agents or high-concentration volatile bursts; if hypertension persists, consider sympatholytics.
5. Stop anesthetic administration during skin closure (syringe of intravenous agent ready or hand on vaporizer).
6. Remove head pins as early as possible—esmolol or lidocaine 1.5 mg/kg for short-term hemodynamic control.
7. Stop nitrous oxide if used (antagonize myorelaxants if necessary—should be avoided if possible).
8. Try for spontaneous ventilation as soon as possible. Remove packing, perform adequate suctioning before extubation.
9. Keep blood pressure in the preoperative range by quickly treating arterial hypertension.
10. Perform brief, targeted neurologic status examination.

Transfer patient to postanesthetic care unit or intensive care unit.

Hemodynamic activation should be treated promptly by antihypertensive agents (e.g., labetalol or esmolol).

Infectious Tumors (Abscess)

Brain abscesses form part of the differential diagnosis of supratentorial mass lesions, and their effects on the brain and ICP pressure are similar. Risk factors include contiguous infections (sinus, ear), right-to-left cardiac shunt, immunosuppression (extraneous or intrinsic), and intravenous drug abuse.[141] Brain abscess is often accompanied by a low-grade fever. If its presence is suspected, initial treatment includes antibiotics to control the infection and corticosteroids to try to control brain edema—sometimes in conjunction with diuretics. Definitive diagnosis and treatment are achieved with craniotomy or stereotaxy and aspiration of the abscess. The surgical and anesthetic management is similar to that for supratentorial neoplasms. If the patient is immunocompromised (e.g., acquired immunodeficiency syndrome [AIDS]), sterile technique and aseptic precautions must be adhered to with particular vigor. It is notable that human immunodeficiency virus (HIV) infection is associated with non-Hodgkin's lymphoma of the brain.

Craniofacial and Skull Base Surgery

Craniofacial and skull base surgery is an approach that is increasingly used for tumors near the posterior wall of the nasal sinuses, the orbits, and so on. These are complex operations requiring a multidisciplinary surgical approach and often involving sensory and motor neurophysiologic monitoring of cranial nerves. Because of the transfacial surgical approach, oral intubation or tracheostomy is often required. The extensive bony involvement of the procedure carries the potential for significant blood loss, hemorrhagic diathesis, and venous air embolism, particularly if the head is elevated. If cranial nerve monitoring (particularly of motor nerves) is performed, neuromuscular blockade should be avoided. For a second procedure of this type, skull base exposures involve extensive temporalis muscle mobilization and often result in mandibular pseudoankylosis with subsequent limitation of mouth opening and difficult intubation.[142-144]

Awake Craniotomy or Stereotactic Procedures

The most common indications for awake neurosurgery are stereotactic biopsies or procedures and the surgery of small lesions in close proximity to speech or motor areas (including epilepsy surgery). Retrospective studies have shown that intraoperative electrical stimulation reduced by approximately twofold the incidence of severe permanent neurologic deficits and markedly improved the completeness of surgical resection.[145] Motor mapping may be performed in a patient under general anesthesia, although the results of stimulation are better in conscious patients.[105] However, surgery of a tumor involving speech areas needs the intraoperative cooperation of a fully awake patient. The main prerequisites for awake neurosurgical procedures are a motivated and understanding neurosurgeon and a patient who is cooperative, fully conscious (to test neurologic function during the operation), and willing to put up with the discomfort of an awake procedure, which is often long and tedious for all involved. Most often, the patient is not awake during the entire procedure but only during the period of tumor removal, thus achieving an asleep-awake-asleep technique. Equally important is ensuring safety by monitoring the patient's vital functions and providing emergency treatment if sudden neurologic (or other) deterioration occurs (e.g., bleeding, intracranial hypertension, vasospasm, seizure, respiratory or cardiac arrest). Thus the attending anesthesiologists should always be prepared and equipped to deal with emergencies involving the patient's airway or intravascular volume status. They should also be familiar with the procedure for rapidly removing the stereotactic frame (halo cast) in an emergency.

If full cooperation of the patient is needed during the procedure, the patient should not receive any kind of sedation, including sedative premedication. Common complications of the procedure are nausea and vomiting, epileptic fits, and wound pain. Nausea is treated with ondansetron or droperidol (< 1 mg to avoid sedation). Epilepsy is treated first by spreading of cold fluids over the cortical surface and then with antiepileptic agents. Pain is treated with application of supplemental local anesthesia in the surgical wound and infusion of nonnarcotic, nonsedative analgesics. Low-doses narcotic may be used only as second-line agents in order to avoid sedation. Motor stimulation allows conscious sedation. The aim of sedation is to have a patient able to respond to verbal commands while being sufficiently analgesic and anxiolytic to tolerate the discomfort of an often long procedure. This goal is generally achieved with careful and meticulous titration to effect a combination of a hypnotic drug and an opioid drug at small doses. Typical hypnotics are propofol (often as an infusion), midazolam, and droperidol; typical opioids are remifentanil, fentanyl, alfentanil, and sufentanil. The most common complication of such sedation is respiratory depression; this problem must be guarded against by mask oxygen supplementation and close respiratory monitoring, including clinical observation, pulse oximetry, and capnography (via a small catheter in the nares under the oxygen mask). The drugs (e.g., opioid antagonists) and equipment necessary to treat respiratory depression must be close at hand. The problems of respiratory depression are compounded by the presence of the halo cast necessary for stereotactic procedures. Most halo casts make mask ventilation impossible and endotracheal intubation difficult.

In elective cases, if stereotaxy is to precede surgery, the policy regarding intubation must be carefully planned: Either stereotaxy and surgery are carried out with the patient under general anesthesia, and intubation takes place before application of the halo, or, if stereotaxy must be performed while the patient is awake, the surgeon must pay attention to placement of the stereotactic frame in order to allow tracheal intubation. Fiberoptic intubation with use of local anesthesia is another option before induction of general anesthesia. In emergencies, the anesthesiologist should have no hesitation about removing the halo cast.

ANESTHESIA FOR INTRACRANIAL HEMATOMAS

General Considerations

Even more than with supratentorial tumors, the effects of intracranial hematomas on neurologic status and ICP depend on the speed with which they arise. At one end of the time spectrum, patients with chronic subdural hematomas show only subtle neurologic signs with small increases in ICP and can thus be anesthetized with a technique similar to that for supratentorial tumors. At the other extreme, acute epidural or subdural hematomas arise much more rapidly than tumors, with massive neurologic impairment and potentially acutely life-threatening ICP elevations.[146,147] In these patients, anesthetic management must entail aggressive reduction of ICP together with measures to preserve brain oxygenation and perfusion, followed by urgent surgical decompression.

Anesthetic Management of Acute Intracranial Hematoma

Induction

Ensuring oxygenation is paramount during induction of the patient with acute intracranial hematoma. It begins with securing of the airway and is followed by mild hyperventilation with 100% oxygen. In the context of head trauma, cervical spine fracture should be ruled out with preoperative CT if the patient's ventilatory state permits it. Intubation following hyperventilation by mask ideally should be swift, atraumatic, and associated with minimal ICP rise. Anesthesia must be deep enough to avoid coughing or arterial hypertension. However, compromises as to the depth of anesthesia are inevitable in the polytraumatized, hypovolemic, and possibly comatose patient with a full stomach (rapid-sequence induction with cricoid pressure). In a deeply unconscious patient, one might tend to intubate without any further use of drugs. In case of severe arterial hypertension due to intracranial hypertension (Cushing's response), thiopental 3 to 5 mg/kg is probably a good choice to decrease both arterial pressure and ICP, thus maintaining CPP before intubation. Judicious use of a sedative

(e.g., etomidate 0.2 to 0.5 mg/kg, propofol 0.5 to 1 mg/kg) together with a myorelaxant is necessary for a semiconscious, struggling patient. The decision regarding which myorelaxant procedure to use to achieve rapid-sequence induction in this context is still controversial. Options include succinylcholine alone, a small dose of nondepolarizing myorelaxant (e.g., 1 mg vecuronium) followed by an increased (1.5 mg/kg) dose of succinylcholine,[99] a priming dose of a nondepolarizing myorelaxant followed 3 minutes later by a full dose of the same myorelaxant,[148] and large doses of rocuronium,[149] which permit intubation 1 minute later. Large doses of non depolarizing myorelaxant is *not* recommended for difficult airways and carries the risk of creating a "cannot intubate, cannot ventilate" situation. These important limitations may change with the availability of suggamadex, a nondepolarizing myorelaxant antagonist.[150] In all of these cases, consideration should be given to aspiration prophylaxis in conscious patients (e.g., 50 mg ranitidine IV, if possible, 20 minutes before induction or, if the patient is cooperative, sodium citrate PO).

Once ventilation and the airway are controlled, thought should be given to early and continuing control of ICP and brain swelling. Typically, osmotic diuretics such as mannitol are given at this stage. Corticosteroids have not been shown to be effective for improving outcome for intracranial hematomas, either traumatic or primary, and they raise mortality risk in head-injured patients.[151,152] The use of myorelaxants is indicated even in comatose patients because increased muscle tone and shivering increase CO_2 production, complicating ICP control through hyperventilation.

Anesthesia Maintenance

The main aim of anesthesia for acute intracranial hematoma is to control ICP and brain swelling while maintaining adequate cerebral perfusion and oxygenation (i.e., matching CMR and CBF). Particular attention is required upon hematoma evacuation, which may result in rapid and severe hypotension (loss of Cushing's response). Vasopressors should be ready to use at this time. An epinephrine bolus (0.1 mg) may be necessary in some patients.

Monitoring

Patients with acute intracranial hematoma are often hemodynamically unstable (hypertension, hypovolemia). Invasive arterial pressure monitoring is used to permit close hemodynamic control and for repeated laboratory determinations (blood gas analysis, hematocrit, etc.). Arterial cannulation is commenced, preferably before induction, particularly in polytraumatized patients, except in case of impending brain herniation, when every minute counts. If a hematoma is to be evacuated, ICP monitoring is generally installed once evacuation has been performed. Electrocardiographic monitoring is particularly important in patients with multiple trauma because electrocardiogram changes can result from cerebral (e.g., blood in the CSF causing T-wave inversion) and cardiac (e.g., ST-segment change in cardiac contusion) causes. Blood gas analysis forms the basis for various interventions in acid-base balance, ventilation, and so on. Blood glucose levels should be followed closely, and any hyperglycemia should corrected because it has been shown to worsen the effects of brain ischemia.[101,103,132] Also of note is that brain tissue damage releases large quantities of thromboplastin into the circulation, adversely affecting blood coagulation, which should be checked regularly (coagulation status, activated partial thromboplastin time). If osmotic diuretics have been started (mannitol), their further use should be guided by determinations of blood osmolality (maximum, 320 mOsm/kg). More detail on the management and monitoring of head injury patients is given in Chapters, 10, 18 and 22.

ANESTHETIC TECHNIQUE

Intravenous anesthetics that increase CVR, decrease CBF and CBV (brain relaxation), and reduce CMR[129] are the mainstays of anesthesia for acute intracranial hematoma. The use of volatile anesthetics is not recommended because they can cause unacceptable rises in ICP and brain tension to the point of acute transtentorial or transcraniotomy herniation, even in the context of preexisting hypocapnia.

Arterial hypotension subsequent to use of intravenous anesthetics or opioids must be avoided to prevent cerebral ischemia and because reductions in CPP can cause reflex cerebral vasodilation and consequent ICP increases not controlled by hypocapnia (see earlier). The management of controlled arterial hypertension in the context of acute intracranial hematoma is controversial and must carefully balance the maintenance of adequate CPP to areas of the brain ischemia caused by hematoma compression against the risks of producing more vasogenic brain edema and resuming hemorrhage. TCD just before or just after induction of anesthesia may help assess cerebral perfusion and determine the optimal blood pressure level. $SjvO_2$ monitoring may help in providing a global assessment of the adequacy of CPP[153]; however, globally adequate CPP does not rule out regional CPP inadequacies and thus regional brain ischemia. If a reduction in arterial hypertension is indicated, the first line of management should be improved analgesia (i.e., opioids) followed by an increased depth of anesthesia (propofol, barbiturates, etomidate). Only then should specific antihypertensive measures be considered, generally with antisympathetic drugs (e.g., esmolol, labetalol, clonidine). Vasodilating antihypertensive agents (nitroprusside, nitroglycerine, hydralazine, nicardipine) should be avoided because they risk the perverse effect of raising ICP via cerebral vasodilation at the same time as decreasing MAP and hence CPP.[154]

However, it may be difficult to differentiate direct cerebral vasodilating effects and vasodilation secondary to autoregulation due to systemic hypotension. For example, intracarotid nitroprusside does not augment CBF, but verapamil decreases cerebrovascular resistance in humans.[64,65]

EMERGENCE FROM ANESTHESIA

In general, patients suffering from acute cerebral hematomas have suffered significant brain injury with significant actual and potential brain swelling. They should thus undergo slow weaning and delayed extubation in a neurointensive care unit (see Chapter 22) with all of the monitoring and therapeutic facilities it provides. Patients with chronic subdural hematomas often have minimal neurologic signs and impairment of consciousness preoperatively and can therefore usually be extubated immediately after surgery.

SUMMARY

The basis of neuroanesthesia for surgery of supratentorial masses is an understanding of the following:

- Pathophysiology of raised ICP
- Regulation and maintenance of cerebral perfusion
- Effects of anesthesia and surgery on ICP, cerebral perfusion, and intracerebral homeostasis
- Differences between the pathophysiology and management of rapidly expanding masses, such as acute hematomas, and slowly growing masses, such as brain tumors

The main objectives of anesthesia for excision of a cerebral tumor are as follows:

1. The preservation during the procedure of the uninjured cerebral territories by global maintenance of cerebral homeostasis and protection by:
   - Normovolemia and normotension
   - Normoglycemia
   - Mild hyperoxia and hypocapnia
   - Mild hyperosmolality
2. The preservation of CBF autoregulation versus MAP, as well as cerebral vasoreactivity to $PaCO_2$.
3. The minimization of the need for surgical retraction through the use of "chemical brain retraction," which consists of:
   - The control of $CMRO_2$, CBF, and CBV
   - Moderate hyperventilation
   - Strict maintenance of CPP
   - Osmotherapy
   - CSF drainage
   - Use of intravenous anesthetics for tight brain
4. The provision of early neurosurgical awakening, thus permitting:
   - Adequate immediate postoperative neurologic assessment
   - Continuing further postoperative evaluation
   - Diagnosis of complications by the neurologic team without delay
   - Immediate CT scanning or surgery if necessary
5. Management of anesthesia and surgical recovery consists of:
   - Adequate pain relief
   - Prevention of postoperative nausea and vomiting
   - Hemodynamic control

The main objectives of anesthesia for acute cerebral hematoma are as follows:

- Aggressive control of ICP and brain swelling
- Adequate blood pressure to maintain CPP and limit cerebral hemorrhage or edema
- Time management in the context of impending brain herniation

REFERENCES

1. Central Brain Tumor Registry of the United States. Available at http://www.cbtrus.org. http://www.cbtrus.org/reports//2007-2008/2007report.pdf, last consulted Sept 14th, 2009
2. Hoffman S, Propp JM, McCarthy BJ: Temporal trends in incidence of primary brain tumors in the United States, 1985-1999, Neuro Oncol 8:27–37, 2006.
3. Gavrilovic IT, Posner JB: Brain metastases: Epidemiology and pathophysiology, J Neurooncol 75:5–14, 2005.
4. Carrel M, Moeschler O, Ravussin P, et al: Prehospital air ambulance and systemic secondary cerebral damage in severe craniocerebral injuries [in French], Ann Fr Anesth Reanim 13:326–335, 1994.
5. Chesnut RM, Marshall SB, Piek J, et al: Early and late systemic hypotension as a frequent and fundamental source of cerebral ischemia following severe brain injury in the Traumatic Coma Data Bank, Acta Neurochir 59(Suppl):121–125, 1993.
6. Langfitt TW, Weinstein JD, Kassell NF: Cerebral vasomotor paralysis produced by intracranial hypertension, Neurology 15:622–641, 1965.

7. Bell BA, Smith MA, Kean DM, et al: Brain water measured by magnetic resonance imaging, *Lancet* 1(8524):66–69, 1987.

8. Bruce JN, Crisculo GR, Merrill MJ, et al: Vascular permeability induced by protein product of malignant brain tumors: Inhibition by dexamethasone, *J Neurosurg* 67:880–884, 1987.

9. Tatagiba M, Mirzai S, Samii M: Peritumoral blood flow in intracranial meningiomas, *Neurosurgery* 28:400–404, 1991.

10. Neuwelt E, Abbott NJ, Abrey L, et al: Strategies to advance translational research into brain barriers, *Lancet Neurol* 7:84–96, 2008.

11. Baker KZ, Ostapkovich N, Sisti MB, et al: Intact cerebral blood flow reactivity during remifentanil/nitrous oxide anesthesia, *J Neurosurg Anesthesiol* 9:134–140, 1997.

12. Grubb RL, Raichle ME, Eichling JO, et al: The effects of changes in $PaCO_2$ on cerebral blood volume, blood flow, and vascular mean transit time, *Stroke* 5:630–639, 1974.

13. Chaudhri S, White M, Kenny GNC: Induction of anaesthesia with propofol using a target-controlled infusion system, *Anaesthesia* 47:551–553, 1992.

14. Bekker AY, Mistry A, Ritter AA, et al: Computer simulation of intracranial pressure changes during induction of anesthesia: Comparison of thiopental, propofol, and etomidate, *J Neurosurg Anesthesiol* 11:69–80, 1999.

15. Kaisti KK, Metsahonkala L, Teras M, et al: Effects of surgical levels of propofol and sevoflurane anesthesia on cerebral blood flow in healthy subjects studied with positron emission tomography, *Anesthesiology* 96:1358–1370, 2002.

16. Kaisti KK, Langsjo JW, Aalto S, et al: Effects of sevoflurane, propofol, and adjunct nitrous oxide on regional cerebral blood flow, oxygen consumption, and blood volume in humans, *Anesthesiology* 99:603–613, 2003.

17. Renou AM, Vernhiet J, Macrez P, et al: Cerebral blood flow and metabolism during etomidate anaesthesia in man, *Br J Anaesth* 50:1047–1051, 1978.

18. Robertson SC, Brown P 3rd, Loftus CM: Effects of etomidate administration on cerebral collateral flow, *Neurosurgery* 43:317–323, 1998.

19. Todd MM, Weeks J: Comparative effects of propofol, pentobarbital, and isoflurane on cerebral blood flow and blood volume, *J Neurosurg Anesthesiol* 8:296–303, 1996.

20. Langsjo JW, Maksimow A, Salmi E, et al: S-Ketamine anesthesia increases cerebral blood flow in excess of the metabolic needs in humans, *Anesthesiology* 103:258–268, 2005.

21. Langsjo JW, Salmi E, Kaisti KK, et al: Effects of subanesthetic ketamine on regional cerebral glucose metabolism in humans, *Anesthesiology* 100:1065–1071, 2004.

22. Eng C, Lam AM, Mayberg T, et al: The influence of propofol with and without nitrous oxide on cerebral blood flow velocity and CO2 reactivity in humans, *Anesthesiology* 77:872–879, 1992.

23. Fox J, Gelb AW, Enns J, et al: The responsiveness of cerebral blood flow to changes in arterial carbon dioxide is maintained during propofol nitrous oxide anesthesia in humans, *Anesthesiology* 77:453–456, 1992.

24. Johnston AJ, Steiner LA, Chatfield DA, et al: Effects of propofol on cerebral oxygenation and metabolism after head injury, *Br J Anaesth* 91:781–786, 2003.

25. Strebel S, Kaufmann M, Guardiola PM, Schaefer HG: Cerebral vasomotor responsiveness to carbon dioxide is preserved during propofol and midazolam anesthesia in humans, *Anesth Analg* 78:884–888, 1994.

26. Veselis RA, Feshchenko VA, Reinsel RA, et al: Propofol and thiopental do not interfere with regional cerebral blood flow response at sedative concentrations, *Anesthesiology* 102:26–34, 2005.

27. Vinclair M, Broux C, Faure P, et al: Duration of adrenal inhibition following a single dose of etomidate in critically ill patients, *Intensive Care Med* 34:714–719, 2008.

28. Adams RW, Cucchiara RF, Gronert GA, et al: Isoflurane and cerebrospinal fluid pressure in neurosurgical patients, *Anesthesiology* 54:97–99, 1981.

29. Matta BF, Mayberg TS, Lam AM: Direct cerebrovasodilatory effects of halothane, isoflurane, and desflurane during propofol-induced isoelectric electroencephalogram in humans, *Anesthesiology* 83:980–985, 1995.

30. Stullken EH Jr, Milde JH, Michenfelder JD, Tinker JH: The nonlinear responses of cerebral metabolism to low concentrations of halothane, enflurane, isoflurane, and thiopental, *Anesthesiology* 46:28–34, 1977.

31. Alkire MT: Quantitative EEG correlations with brain glucose metabolic rate during anesthesia in volunteers, *Anesthesiology* 89:323–333, 1998.

32. Bedforth NM, Hardman JG, Nathanson MH: Cerebral hemodynamic response to the introduction of desflurane: A comparison with sevoflurane, *Anesth Analg* 91:152–155, 2000.

33. Holmstrom A, Akeson J: Cerebral blood flow at 0.5 and 1.0 minimal alveolar concentrations of desflurane or sevoflurane compared with isoflurane in normoventilated pigs, *J Neurosurg Anesthesiol* 15:90–97, 2003.

34. Laitio RM, Kaisti KK, Langsjo JW, et al: Effects of xenon anesthesia on cerebral blood flow in humans: A positron emission tomography study, *Anesthesiology* 106:1128–1133, 2007.

35. Young WL, Prohovnik I, Correl JW, et al: A comparison of cerebral blood flow reactivity to CO2 during halothane versus isoflurane anesthesia for carotid endarterectomy, *Anesth Analg* 73:416–421, 1991.

36. Ringaert KRA, Mutch WAC, Malo LA: Regional cerebral blood flow and response to carbon dioxide during controlled hypotension with isoflurane anesthesia in the rat, *Anesth Analg* 67:383–388, 1988.

37. Strebel S, Lam AM, Matta BF, Newell DW: Impaired cerebral autoregulation after mild brain injury, *Surg Neurol* 47:128–131, 1997.

38. Reinstrup P, Ryding E, Algotsson L, et al: Effects of nitrous oxide on human regional cerebral blood flow and isolated pial arteries, *Anesthesiology* 81:396–402, 1994.

39. Reinstrup P, Ryding E, Ohlsson T, et al: Regional cerebral metabolic rate (positron emission tomography) during inhalation of nitrous oxide 50% in humans, *Br J Anaesth* 100:66–71, 2008.

40. Drummond JC, Sheller MS, Todd MM: The effect of nitrous oxide on cortical blood flow during anaesthesia with halothane and isoflurane, with and without morphine, in the rabbit, *Anesth Analg* 66:1083–1089, 1987.

41. Drummond JC, Todd MM: The response of the feline cerebral circulation to Paco2 during anesthesia with isoflurane and halothane and during sedation with nitrous oxide, *Anesthesiology* 62:268–273, 1985.

42. Hoffman WE, Charbel FT, Edelman G, et al: Nitrous oxide added to isoflurane increases brain artery blood flow and low frequency brain electrical activity, *J Neurosurg Anesthesiol* 7:82–88, 1997.

43. Lam AM, Mayberg TS, Eng CC, et al: Nitrous oxide-isoflurane anesthesia causes more cerebral vasodilatation than an equipotent dose of isoflurane in humans, *Anesth Analg* 74:462–468, 1994.

44. Jung R, Reinsel R, Marx W, et al: Isoflurane and nitrous oxide: Comparative impact on cerebrospinal fluid pressure in patients with brain tumors, *Anesth Analg* 75:724–728, 1992.

45. Artru AA: Nitrous oxide plays a direct role in the development of tension pneumocephalus intraoperatively, *Anesthesiology* 57:59–61, 1982.

46. Goodie D, Traill R: Intraoperative subdural tension pneumocephalus arising after opening of the dura, *Anesthesiology* 74:193–195, 1991.

47. Yates H, Hamill M, Borel CO, et al: Incidence and perioperative management of tension pneumoencephalus following craniofacial resection, *J Neurosurg Anesthesiol* 6:15–20, 1994.

48. Albanese J, Durbec O, Viviand X, et al: Sufentanil increases intracranial pressure in patients with head trauma, *Anesthesiology* 79:493–497, 1993.

49. Albanese J, Viviand X, Potie F, et al: Sufentanil, fentanyl, and alfentanil in head trauma patients: A study on cerebral hemodynamics, *Crit Care Med* 27:407–411, 1999.

50. de Nadal M, Munar F, Poca MA, et al: Cerebral hemodynamic effects of morphine and fentanyl in patients with severe head injury: Absence of correlation to cerebral autoregulation, *Anesthesiology* 92:11–19, 2000.

51. Engelhard K, Reeker W, Kochs E, Werner C: Effect of remifentanil on intracranial pressure and cerebral blood flow velocity in patients with head trauma, *Acta Anaesthesiol Scand* 48:396–399, 2004.

52. Jamali S, Ravussin P, Archer DP, et al: The effects of bolus administration of opioids on cerebrospinal fluid pressure in patients with supratentorial lesions, *Anesth Analg* 82:600–606, 1996.

53. From RP, Warner DS, Todd MM, et al: Anesthesia for craniotomy: A double blind comparison of alfentanil, fentanyl, and sufentanil, *Anesthesiology* 73:896–904, 1990.

54. Hormann C, Langmayr J, Schalow S, et al: Low-dose sufentanil increases cerebrospinal fluid pressure in human volunteers, *J Neurosurg Anesthesiol* 7:7–13, 1995.

55. Marx W, Shah N, Long C, et al: Sufentanil, alfentanil and fentanyl: Impact on cerebral spinal fluid pressure in patients with brain tumors, *J Neurosurg Anesthesiol* 1:3–7, 1989.

56. Mayer N, Weistahl C, Podreka L, et al: Sufentanil does not increase cerebral blood flow in healthy human volunteers, *Anesthesiology* 73:240–243, 1990.

57. Coles JP, Leary TS, Monteiro JN, et al: Propofol anesthesia for craniotomy: A double-blind comparison of remifentanil, alfentanil, and fentanyl, *J Neurosurg Anesthesiol* 12:15–20, 2000.

58. Ostapkovich ND, Baker KZ, Fogarty-Mack P, et al: Cerebral blood flow and CO2 reactivity is similar during remifentanil/N2O and fentanyl/N2O anesthesia, *Anesthesiology* 89:358–363, 1998.

59. Sneyd JR, Whaley A, Dimpel HL, Andrews CJ: An open, randomized comparison of alfentanil, remifentanil and alfentanil followed by remifentanil in anaesthesia for craniotomy, *Br J Anaesth* 81:361–364, 1998.

60. Warner DS: Experience with remifentanil in neurosurgical patients, *Anesth Analg* 89:S33–S39, 1999.

61. Nishikawa T, Omote K, Namiki A, Takahashi T: The effects of nicardipine on cerebrospinal fluid pressure in humans, *Anesth Analg* 65:507–510, 1986.

62. Pinaud M, Souron R, Lelausque JN, et al: Cerebral blood flow and cerebral oxygen consumption during nitroprusside-induced hypotension to less than 50 mmHg, *Anesthesiology* 70:255–260, 1989.

63. Griswold WR, Reznik V, Mendoza SA: Nitroprusside-induced intracranial hypertension, *JAMA* 246:2679–2680, 1981.

64. Joshi S, Young WL, Duong H, et al: Intracarotid nitroprusside does not augment cerebral blood flow in human subjects, *Anesthesiology* 96:60–66, 2002.

65. Joshi S, Meyers PM, Pile-Spellman J, et al: Intracarotid verapamil decreases both proximal and distal human cerebrovascular resistance, *Anesthesiology* 100:774–781, 2004.

66. Heinke W, Zysset S, Hund-Georgiadis M, et al: The effect of esmolol on cerebral blood flow, cerebral vasoreactivity, and cognitive performance: A functional magnetic resonance imaging study, *Anesthesiology* 102:41–50, 2005.

67. Albrecht RF, Miletich DJ, Ruttle M: Cerebral effects of extended hyperventilation in unanesthetized goats, *Stroke* 18:649–655, 1987.

68. Gelb AW, Craen RA, Rao GS, et al: Does hyperventilation improve operating condition during supratentorial craniotomy? A multicenter randomized crossover trial, *Anesth Analg* 106:585–594, 2008.

69. Coles JP, Fryer TD, Coleman MR, et al: Hyperventilation following head injury: Effect on ischemic burden and cerebral oxidative metabolism, *Crit Care Med* 35:568–578, 2007.

70. Matteo RS, Ornstein E, Schwartz AE, et al: Effects of hypocarbia on the pharmacodynamics of sufentanil in humans, *Anesth Analg* 75:186–192, 1992.

71. Muizelaar JP, Lutz HA 3rd, Becker DP: Effect of mannitol on ICP and CBF and correlation with pressure autoregulation in severely head-injured patients, *J Neurosurg* 61:700–706, 1984.

72. Muizelaar JP, Wei EP, Kontos HA, Becker DP: Mannitol causes compensatory cerebral vasoconstriction and vasodilation in response to blood viscosity changes, *J Neurosurg* 59:822–828, 1983.

73. Burke AM, Quest DO, Chien S, et al: The effect of mannitol on blood viscosity, *J Neurosurg* 55:550–553, 1981.

74. Ravussin P, Abou-Madi M, Archer D, et al: Changes in CSF pressure after mannitol in patients with and without elevated CSF pressure, *J Neurosurg* 69:869–876, 1988.

75. Cascino T, Baglivo J, Conti J, et al: Quantitative CT assessment of furosemide- and mannitol-induced changes in brain water content, *Neurology* 33:898–903, 1983.

76. Todd MM, Cutkomp J, Brian JE: Influence of mannitol and furosemide, alone and in combination, on brain water content after fluid percussion injury, *Anesthesiology* 105:1176–1181, 2006.

77. Mavrocordatos P, Bissonnette B, Ravussin P: Effects of neck position and head elevation on intracranial pressure in anaesthetized neurosurgical patients: Preliminary results, *J Neurosurg Anesthesiol* 12:10–14, 2000.

78. Rosner MJ, Daughton S: Cerebral perfusion pressure management in head injury, *J Trauma* 30:933–940, 1990.

79. Bedford RF, Morris L, Jane JA: Intracranial hypertension during surgery for supratentorial tumor: Correlation with preoperative computed tomography scans, *Anesth Analg* 61:430–433, 1982.

80. Todd MM, Warner DS, Sokol MD, et al: A prospective comparative trial of three anesthetics for elective supratentorial craniotomy: Propofol/fentanyl, isoflurane/nitrous oxide, and fentanyl/nitrous oxide, *Anesthesiology* 78:1005–1020, 1993.

81. Black PM: Brain tumors: Part 1, *N Engl J Med* 324:1471–1476, 1991.

82. Pai VB, Nahata MC: Cardiotoxicity of chemotherapeutic agents: incidence, treatment and prevention, *Drug Saf* 22:263–302, 2000.

83. Brandes AA, Scelzi E, Salmistraro G, et al: Incidence of risk of thromboembolism during treatment high-grade gliomas: A prospective study, *Eur J Cancer* 10:1592–1596, 1997.

84. Agnelli G, Piovella F, Buoncristiani P, et al: Enoxaparin plus compression stockings compared with compression stockings alone in the prevention of venous thromboembolism after elective neurosurgery, *N Engl J Med* 339:80–85, 1998.

85. Albin MS, Carroll RG, Maroon JC: Clinical considerations concerning detection of venous air embolism, *Neurosurgery* 3:380–384, 1978.

86. Ayerbe J, Lobato RD, de la Cruz J, et al: Risk factors predicting recurrence in patients operated on for intracranial meningioma: A multivariate analysis, *Acta Neurochir (Wien)* 141:921–932, 1999.

87. Cataldi S, Bruder N, Dufour H, et al: Intraoperative autologous blood transfusion in intracranial surgery, *Neurosurgery* 40:765–771, 1997.

88. Lunn JK, Stanley TH, Webster LR, et al: Arterial blood pressure and pulse rate responses to pulmonary and radial arterial catheterization prior to cardiac and major vascular operations, *Anesthesiology* 51:265–269, 1979.

89. Lazar RM, Fitzsimmons BF, Marshall RS, et al: Reemergence of stroke deficits with midazolam challenge, *Stroke* 33:283–285, 2002.

90. Thal GD, Szabo MD, Lopez-Bresnahan M, Crosby G: Exacerbation or unmasking of focal neurologic deficits by sedatives, *Anesthesiology* 85:21–51, 1996.

91. Ornstein E, Matteo RS, Schwartz AE, et al: The effect of phenytoin on the magnitude and duration of neuromuscular block following atracurium and vecuronium, *Anesthesiology* 67:191–196, 1987.

92. Paul F, Veauthier C, Fritz G, et al: Perioperative fluctuations of lamotrigine serum levels in patients undergoing epilepsy surgery, *Seizure* 16:479–484, 2007.

93. Yeh JS, Dhir JS, Green AL, et al: Changes in plasma phenytoin level following craniotomy, *Br J Neurosurg* 20:403–406, 2006.

94. Grenier B, Verchere E, Mesli A, et al: Capnography monitoring during neurosurgery: Reliability in relation to various intraoperative positions, *Anesth Analg* 88:43–48, 1999.

95. Whitesell R, Asiddao C, Gullman D, et al: Relationship between arterial and peak expired carbon dioxide pressure during anesthesia and factors influencing the difference, *Anesth Analg* 60:508–512, 1981.

96. Valadka AB, Furuya Y, Hlatky R, Robertson CS: Global and regional techniques for monitoring cerebral oxidative metabolism after severe traumatic brain injury, *Neurosurg Focus* 92000:e3.

97. Graham DH: Monitoring neuromuscular block may be unreliable in patients with upper motor neuron lesions, *Anesthesiology* 52:74–75, 1980.

98. Shayevitz JR, Matteo RS: Decreased sensitivity to metocurine in patients with upper motoneuron disease, *Anesth Analg* 64:767–772, 1985.

99. Minton MD, Grosslight K, Stirt JA, et al: Increases in ICP from succinylcholine: Prevention by prior nondepolarizing blockade, *Anesthesiology* 65:165–169, 1986.

100. Andrews RJ, Bringas JR: A review of brain retraction and recommendations for minimizing intra-operative brain injury, *Neurosurgery* 33:1052–1063, 1993.

101. Kimura K, Iguchi Y, Inoue T, et al: Hyperglycemia independently increases the risk of early death in acute spontaneous intracerebral hemorrhage, *J Neurol Sci* 255:90–94, 2007.

102. Lanier WL, Stangland KJ, Scheithauer BW, et al: The effects of dextrose infusion and head position on neurologic outcome after complete cerebral ischemia in primates: Examination of a model, *Anesthesiology* 66:39–48, 1987.

103. McGirt MJ, Woodworth GF, Brooke BS, et al: Hyperglycemia independently increases the risk of perioperative stroke, myocardial infarction, and death after carotid endarterectomy, *Neurosurgery* 58:1066–1073, 2006.

104. Ribo M, Molina CA, Delgado P, et al: Hyperglycemia during ischemia rapidly accelerates brain damage in stroke patients treated with tPA, *J Cereb Blood Flow Metab* 27:1616–1622, 2007.

105. Vitaz TW, Marx W, Victor JD, Gutin PH: Comparison of conscious sedation and general anesthesia for motor mapping and resection of tumors located near motor cortex, *Neurosurg Focus* 15:E8, 2003.

106. Constantini S, Cotev S, Rappaport ZH, et al: Intracranial pressure monitoring after elective intracranial surgery: A retrospective study of 514 consecutive patients, *J Neurosurg* 69:540–544, 1988.

107. Moppett IK, Mahajan RP: Transcranial Doppler ultrasonography in anaesthesia and intensive care, *Br J Anaesth* 93:710–724, 2004.

108. Eng CC, Lam AM, Byrd S, Newell DW: The diagnosis and management of a perianesthetic cerebral aneurysmal rupture aided with transcranial Doppler ultrasonography, *Anesthesiology* 78:191–194, 1993.

109. Bruder N, Pellissier D, Grillo P, Gouin F: Cerebral hyperemia during recovery from general anesthesia in neurosurgical patients, *Anesth Analg* 94:650–654, 2002.

110. Meyers PM, Higashida RT, Phatouros CC, et al: Cerebral hyperperfusion syndrome after percutaneous transluminal stenting of the craniocervical arteries, *Neurosurgery* 47:335–343, 2000.

111. Amin-Hanjani S, Meglio G, Gatto R, et al: The utility of intraoperative blood flow measurement during aneurysm surgery using an ultrasonic perivascular flow probe, *Neurosurgery* 58(Suppl 2)2006:ONS-305-ONS-312.

112. Shafer SL, Stanski DR: Improving the clinical utility of anesthetic drug pharmacokinetics, *Anesthesiology* 76:327–330, 1992.

113. Shafer SL, Varvel JR: Pharmacokinetics, pharmacodynamics and rational opioid selection, *Anesthesiology* 74:53–63, 1991.

114. Wright PM, McCarthy G, Szenohradszky J, et al: Influence of chronic phenytoin administration on the pharmacokinetics and pharmacodynamics of vecuronium, *Anesthesiology* 100:626–633, 2004.

115. Spacek A, Neiger FX, Krenn CG, et al: Rocuronium-induced neuromuscular block is affected by chronic carbamazepine therapy, *Anesthesiology* 90:109–112, 1999.

116. Richard A, Girard F, Girard DC, et al: Cisatracurium-induced neuromuscular blockade is affected by chronic phenytoin or carbamazepine treatment in neurosurgical patients, *Anesth Analg* 100:538–544, 2005.

117. Tempelhoff R, Modica PA, Jellish WS, Spitznagel EL: Resistance to atracurium-induced neuromuscular blockade in patients with intractable seizure disorders treated with anticonvulsants, *Anesth Analg* 71:665–669, 1990.

118. Bayer-Berger M, Ravussin P, Fankhauser H, et al: Effect of 3 pretreatment techniques on hemodynamic and CSFP responses to skullpin head-holder application during thiopental-isoflurane or propofol anesthesia, *J Neurosurg Anesthesiol* 1:227–232, 1987.

119. Beenen LF, Lindeboom J, Kasteleijn-Nolst Trenite DG, et al: Comparative double blind clinical trial of phenytoin and sodium valproate as anticonvulsant prophylaxis after craniotomy: Efficacy, tolerability, and cognitive effects, *J Neurol Neurosurg Psychiatry* 67:474–480, 1999.

120. North JB, Penhall RR, Haneih A, et al: Phenytoin and postoperative epilepsy: A double-blind trial, *J Neurosurg* 58:672–677, 1983.

121. Todd MM, Hindman BJ, Clarke WR, Torner JC: Mild intraoperative hypothermia during surgery for intracranial aneurysm, *N Engl J Med* 352:135–145, 2005.

122. Rajagopalan S, Mascha E, Na J, Sessler DI: The effects of mild perioperative hypothermia on blood loss and transfusion requirement, *Anesthesiology* 108:71–77, 2008.

123. Kurz A, Sessler DI, Lenhardt R: Perioperative normothermia to reduce the incidence of surgical-wound infection and shorten hospitalization. Study of Wound Infection and Temperature Group, *N Engl J Med* 334:1209–1215, 1996.

124. Frank SM, Beattie C, Christopherson R, et al: Unintentional hypothermia is associated with postoperative myocardial ischemia. The Perioperative Ischemia Randomized Anesthesia Trial Study Group, *Anesthesiology* 78:468–476, 1993.

125. Lenhardt R, Marker E, Goll V, et al: Mild intraoperative hypothermia prolongs postanesthetic recovery, *Anesthesiology* 87:1318–1323, 1997.

126. Petersen KD, Landsfeldt U, Cold GE, et al: Intracranial pressure and cerebral hemodynamic in patients with cerebral tumors: A randomized prospective study of patients subjected to craniotomy in propofol-fentanyl, isoflurane-fentanyl, or sevoflurane-fentanyl anesthesia, *Anesthesiology* 98:329–336, 2003.

127. Ravussin P, de Tribolet N, Wilder-Smith OHG: Total intravenous anesthesia is best for neurological surgery, *J Neurosurg Anesthesiol* 6:285–289, 1994.

128. Fraga M, Rama-Maceiras P, Rodino S, et al: The effects of isoflurane and desflurane on intracranial pressure, cerebral perfusion pressure, and cerebral arteriovenous oxygen content difference in normocapnic patients with supratentorial brain tumors, *Anesthesiology* 98:1085–1090, 2003.

129. Cole CD, Gottfried ON, Gupta DK, Couldwell WT: Total intravenous anesthesia: Advantages for intracranial surgery, *Neurosurgery* 61:369–377, 2007.

130. Hansen TD, Warner DS, Todd MM, et al: Effects of nitrous oxide and volatile anaesthetics on cerebral blood flow, *Br J Anaesth* 63:290–295, 1989.

131. Jung R, Reinsel R, Marx W, et al: Isoflurane and nitrous oxide: Comparative impact on cerebrospinal fluid pressure in patients with brain tumors, *Anesth Analg* 75:724–728, 1992.

132. Rovlias A, Kotsou S: The influence of hyperglycemia on neurological outcome in patients with severe head injury, *Neurosurgery* 46:335–342, 2000.

133. Bruder N, Ravussin P: Recovery from anesthesia and postoperative extubation of neurosurgical patients: A review, *J Neurosurg Anesthesiol* 11:282–293, 1999.

134. Muzzi DA, Black S, Losasso T, et al: Labetalol and esmolol in the control of hypertension after intracranial surgery, *Anesth Analg* 70:68–71, 1990.

135. Basali A, Mascha E, Kalfas I, Schubert A: Relation between perioperative hypertension and intracranial hemorrhage after craniotomy, *Anesthesiology* 93:48–54, 2000.

136. Grillo P, Bruder N, Auquier P, et al: Esmolol blunts the cerebral blood flow velocity increase during emergence from anesthesia in neurosurgical patients, *Anesth Analg* 96:1145–1149, 2003.

137. Fabregas N, Bruder N: Recovery and neurological evaluation, *Best Pract Res Clin Anaesthesiol* 21:431–447, 2007.

138. Ziai WC, Varelas PN, Zeger SL, et al: Neurologic intensive care resource use after brain tumor surgery: An analysis of indications and alternative strategies, *Crit Care Med* 31:2782–2787, 2003.

139. Verchere E, Grenier B, Mesli A, et al: Postoperative pain management after supratentorial craniotomy, *J Neurosurg Anesthesiol* 14:96–101, 2002.

140. Ayoub C, Girard F, Boudreault D, et al: A comparison between scalp nerve block and morphine for transitional analgesia after remifentanil-based anesthesia in neurosurgery, *Anesth Analg* 103:1237–1240, 2006.

141. Mathisen GE, Johnson JP: Brain abscess, *Clin Infect Dis* 25:763–779, 1997.

142. Coonan TJ, Hope CE, Howes WJ, et al: Ankylosis of the temporomandibular joint after temporal craniotomy: A cause of difficult intubation, *Can Anaesth Soc J* 32:158–160, 1985.

143. Kawaguchi M, Sakamoto T, Ohnishi H, et al: Do recently developed techniques for skull base surgery increase the risk of difficult airway management? Assessment of pseudoankylosis of the mandible following surgical manipulation of the temporalis muscle, *J Neurosurg Anesthesiol* 7:183–186, 1995.

144. Nitzan DW, Azaz B, Constantini S: Severe limitation in mouth opening following transtemporal neurosurgical procedures: Diagnosis, treatment, and prevention, *J Neurosurg* 76:623–625, 1992.

145. Duffau H, Lopes M, Arthuis F, et al: Contribution of intraoperative electrical stimulations in surgery of low grade gliomas: A comparative study between two series without (1985-96) and with (1996-2003) functional mapping in the same institution, *J Neurol Neurosurg Psychiatry* 76:845–851, 2005.

146. Ropper AH: Lateral displacement of the brain and level of consciousness in patients with an acute hemispheral mass, *N Engl J Med* 314:953–958, 1986.

147. Ross DA, Olsen WL, Ross AM, et al: Brain shift, level of consciousness and restoration of consciousness in patients with acute intracranial hematoma, *J Neurosurg* 71:498–502, 1989.

148. Mehta MP, Choi WW, Gergis SD, et al: Facilitation of rapid endotracheal intubations with divided doses of nondepolarizing neuromuscular blocking drugs, *Anesthesiology* 62:392–395, 1985.

149. Pühringer FK, Khuenl-Brady KS, Koller J, et al: Evaluation of the endotracheal intubating conditions of rocuronium (ORG 9426) and succinylcholine in outpatient surgery, *Anesth Analg* 75:37–40, 1992.

150. de Boer HD, Driessen JJ, Marcus MA, et al: Reversal of rocuronium-induced (1.2 mg/kg) profound neuromuscular block by sugammadex: A multicenter, dose-finding and safety study, *Anesthesiology* 107:239–244, 2007.

151. Edwards P, Arango M, Balica L, et al: Final results of MRC CRASH, a randomised placebo-controlled trial of intravenous corticosteroid in adults with head injury-outcomes at 6 months, *Lancet* 365:1957–1959, 2005.

152. Roberts I, Yates D, Sandercock P, et al: Effect of intravenous corticosteroids on death within 14 days in 10008 adults with clinically significant head injury (MRC CRASH trial): Randomised placebo-controlled trial, *Lancet* 364:1321–1328, 2004.

153. Gopinath SP, Cormio M, Ziegler J, et al: Intraoperative jugular desaturation during surgery for traumatic intracranial hematomas, *Anesth Analg* 83:1014–1021, 1996.

154. Marsh ML, Shapiro HM, Smith RW, et al: Changes in neurologic status and intracranial pressure associated with sodium nitroprusside administration, *Anesthesiology* 51:336–338, 1979.

Chapter 12

ANESTHETIC MANAGEMENT FOR POSTERIOR FOSSA SURGERY

David S. Smith

The confines of the posterior fossa and the myriad of neuronal and vascular structures that traverse it create a challenge for the anesthesiologist, whose intraoperative goals are to facilitate surgical access, minimize nervous tissue trauma, and maintain respiratory and cardiovascular stability. This discussion focuses on the anesthetic considerations for posterior fossa surgery in adult patients; preoperative evaluation, preparation, and premedication; general monitoring considerations; choice of position for surgery; anesthetic considerations, risks, prevention, detection, treatment, and complications of air embolism; and special monitoring issues.

PREOPERATIVE EVALUATION AND PREPARATION

Patient physical status, particularly in reference to cardiovascular and pulmonary stability and airway manageability, is a determinant of the choice of patient position for posterior fossa surgery. The efforts to obtain optimal operating conditions and maintain a stable perioperative course may sometimes be at cross-purposes. For example, patients with previous cerebrospinal fluid shunting procedures may be at greater risk for subdural pneumocephalus with surgery in the head-up position. Thus a thorough evaluation of previous operations and cardiopulmonary problems, current cardiac and respiratory status, evidence of cerebrovascular compromise, and suitability of vascular access for right atrial catheter placement are of particular importance in the patient undergoing posterior fossa surgery.

In patients with altered limits of cerebral autoregulation, impaired cerebral perfusion, or abnormal baroreceptor function resulting from hypertension, cardiovascular disease, cerebrovascular insufficiency, or prior carotid endarterectomy, the occurrence of hypotension during anesthesia in the head-up position may be especially detrimental.

Intravascular volume depletion may result from decreased oral intake, supine diuresis, vomiting, and administration of intravenous contrast agents for diagnostic studies. Incremental administration of intravenous fluids before induction may help limit hypotension during anesthesia induction and positioning. Application of thigh-high compression stockings to the legs limits venous pooling in the lower extremities.

Assessment of vascular access for right atrial catheter placement helps determine the most promising route. Patients who are obese, have poor vasculature due to disease or chronic intravenous cannulation, or have short, thick necks should be identified early so that necessary time may be allotted for

catheter placement. Some authorities have advocated echocardiography to detect patent foramen ovale (PFO) in patients scheduled for surgery in the head-up position; the use of an alternative position for those who have PFO might reduce the occurrence of paradoxical air embolism (PAE).[1,2] A detection rate of 10% to 30% with use of echocardiography is comparable with the 20% to 30% incidence reported in autopsy findings.[3] The noninvasive nature of echocardiography makes it attractive for screening purposes; its specificity is reported to be 64% to 100%.[4-6] However, preoperative screening echocardiography lacks sensitivity (i.e., nondetection of PFO does not guarantee its absence).[7,8] Transesophageal echocardiography (TEE) is used after induction of anesthesia in some institutions,[9] but it is not 100% sensitive for detection of PFO.[10] More recently Kwapisz and associates[11] described their experience in 35 patients scheduled for posterior fossa surgery in the sitting position. After induction of anesthesia, contrast-enhanced transesophageal echocardiography was performed to check for PFO. Three of the 35 patients were shown to have PFO, and the planned surgical position was altered.

GENERAL MONITORING ISSUES

The goals of monitoring are to ensure adequate central nervous system perfusion, maintain cardiorespiratory stability, and detect and treat air embolism. Box 12-1 lists the monitors used regardless of patient position; monitors that are not in

---

BOX 12–1 *Monitors for Posterior Fossa Surgery*

Preinduction and Induction

Five-lead electrocardiogram
Blood pressure monitoring
Pulse oximetry
Precordial stethoscope
$ETCO_2$ monitoring
Electrophysiologic monitoring*

Postinduction

Central venous (right atrial, pulmonary artery) catheter
Precordial Doppler ultrasound probe
Esophageal stethoscope
Esophageal or nasopharyngeal temperature probe
$ETCO_2$, ETN_2 monitoring
Transesophageal echocardiogram*

---

*Not routine but provide specialized information during certain procedures.

routine use but that provide specialized information during certain procedures are listed with an asterisk. Not every "routine" monitor listed in the box is always used for every posterior fossa procedure.

For surgery on the head or neck, many clinicians prefer placement of central venous catheters in the forearm or the antecubital fossa, preferably via the basilic vein after induction of anesthesia. In patients with small veins, a modified Seldinger technique can be used for specialized right atrial catheters or pulmonary angiography catheters. Prolonged head-down position and head rotation for jugular vein catheter placement should be minimized because these maneuvers may reduce cerebral blood perfusion. A specialized Doppler ultrasound device can be used to localize the jugular or subclavian vein before needle insertion.[12] Whenever catheters are placed via the neck or subclavian routes, the insertion sites should be sealed with bacteriostatic ointment and dressing to minimize air entrainment, especially for patients in head-up positions. Another precaution is to place and remove these central lines while the patient is flat or has the head down, never in the head-up position, because air embolism has been reported in patients in the head-up position.

CHOICE OF PATIENT POSITION

Surgical access to the posterior fossa can be obtained through various patient positions, such as the sitting position and variants of the horizontal position, which include supine, prone, three-quarter prone, and lateral positions.

Sitting Position

To establish the sitting position, the patient's skull should be secured in a three-pin head holder; infiltration of the scalp and periosteum at the pin sites reduces the hypertensive response to insertion of pins into the outer table of the skull.[13] The arterial pressure transducer is zeroed at the skull base during positioning and throughout the procedure to make maintenance of adequate cerebral perfusion pressure (CPP) easier. Bony prominences should be well padded, the legs placed in thigh-high compression stockings to limit pooling of blood, elbows supported by pillows or pads to avoid contact with the table or stretch on the brachial plexus, and the legs freed of pressure at the level of the common peroneal nerve just distal and lateral to the head of the fibula. Efforts to prevent cervical cord stretching and obstruction of venous drainage from the face and tongue include maintenance of at least a 1-inch space between chin and chest, avoidance of large airways and bite blocks in the pharynx, and avoidance of excessive neck rotation, especially in elderly patients. Abdominal compression, lower extremity ischemia, and sciatic nerve injury are prevented by avoidance of excessive flexion of the knees toward the chest. Compression stockings should be applied carefully to avoid a tourniquet effect and ischemic injury to the leg.

A "lounge chair" modification of the sitting position, with the thoracic cage raised 30 to 45 degrees, may be used for lateral lesions. Access to more midline structures may be impeded by the degree of neck flexion required. Another modification, the lateral sitting position, allows rapid head lowering to the left lateral decubitus position and continuation of the operation in the event of hypotension or persistent venous air embolism (VAE).

For the anesthesiologist, advantages of the sitting position include lower airway pressures and ease of diaphragmatic excursion, improved ability for hyperventilation, better access to the endotracheal tube and thorax for monitoring, access to the extremities for monitoring, fluid or blood administration and blood sampling, and visualization of the face for observation of motor responses during cranial nerve stimulation.

Improved postoperative cranial nerve function has been reported in patients undergoing acoustic neuroma resection in the sitting position than in those operated on in horizontal positions.[14] Relative contraindications to the sitting position are known intracardiac defects, known pulmonary arteriovenous malformations, severe hypovolemia or cachexia, severe hydrocephalus, and lesion vascularity.

Physiologic Changes in the Sitting Position

Head elevation above the right atrium reduces dural sinus pressure, which decreases venous bleeding, and raises the risk of VAE. Head elevation to the 90-degree sitting position produces decreases in dural sinus pressure of up to 10 mm Hg. Jugular bulb venous pressure is not a reliable indicator of dural sinus pressure.

Cardiovascular effects include increases in pulmonary and systemic vascular resistance and decreases in cardiac output, venous return, and CPP.[15,16] For each 1.25-cm movement of the head above the level of the heart, local arterial pressure is reduced by approximately 1 mm Hg.[17] Dysrhythmias, such as bradycardia, tachycardia, premature ventricular contractions, and asystole, may result from manipulation or retraction of cranial nerves or the brainstem regardless of patient position.[18-20] Their negative effects on cardiac output may be more pronounced for patients in the sitting position than in a horizontal position. These factors should be considered in the assessment of an elderly patient or a patient with impaired cardiac function for possible placement in the sitting position.

Pulmonary vital capacity and functional residual capacity are improved in the sitting position, but hypovolemia may decrease perfusion of the upper lung, leading to ventilation or perfusion abnormalities and hypoxemia. Inhalational anesthetics may increase the likelihood of transpulmonary passage of air in a dose-dependent manner,[21-23] a feature that influences the choice of anesthetic in the sitting position.

The use of N_2O in the sitting position continues to be controversial. It increases the size of intravascular air bubbles if air embolism occurs.[24] However, N_2O has not been determined to be a factor in perioperative morbidity in several series of patients undergoing posterior fossa surgery at different institutions, regardless of patient position and occurrence of VAE.[25,26]

Because N_2O raises pressure in a closed air space, some clinicians recommend discontinuation of its use before the dura is completely closed to prevent the buildup of gas pressure and possible neurologic deficit from tension pneumocephalus.[27,28] Others have demonstrated that continued use of N_2O until the end of the procedure actually promotes removal of the gas after the N_2O is discontinued, because of the gradient created between the gas space and blood, provided that circulation to that area is intact.[29] Discontinuation of N_2O has not been effective in preventing pneumocephalus.[30]

The incidence of pneumocephalus was reported to be 100% for intracranial procedures performed with patients in the sitting position, 72% for those in the "park-bench" (semiprone lateral) position, and 57% for those in the prone position.[31,32] Pneumocephalus is usually asymptomatic and resolves spontaneously. However, tension pneumocephalus may produce postoperative neurologic deficits.[33-35] It may be diagnosed intraoperatively from decreases in somatosensory evoked potentials (SSEPs) (if monitored)[36,37] and postoperatively on computed tomography. Treatment is supportive, consisting of 100% O_2 administration and, in severe cases, removal of gas by aspiration or reopening of the dura.

Prone Position

The prone position is associated with a lower incidence of VAE.[14,25] However, the patient's head is usually elevated above the heart to decrease venous bleeding, so the risk of VAE is not eliminated. Access to superior posterior fossa structures and ease of head manipulation are not as favorable as in the sitting position; the sitting position may also offer better operating conditions for high cervical decompression, in which neck flexion and weight-bearing on the head are detrimental.[38]

When the patient is in the head-elevated position, placement of the shoulders at or above the edge of the operating table back prevents the face from becoming compressed against the cephalad edge of the table when it is inclined. Eye compression can produce blindness from retinal artery thrombosis; this risk is greater for prone and lateral patient positions, particularly when a padded facial headrest is used. Conjunctival edema is a benign consequence of the prone position that resolves quickly. Visual loss from a variety of mechanisms, usually perioperative ischemic optic neuropathy, is a rare but catastrophic outcome of operative intervention and may be of particular relevance in spinal fusion procedures.

Venous pooling sufficient to impair venous return can occur in the lower extremities when they lie below the right atrium. Elderly, debilitated patients may not tolerate even a brief discontinuation of monitoring during the turn to the prone position without suffering severe hypotension. In these patients, monitoring cables and transducers should be oriented to allow uninterrupted electrocardiogram (ECG) and arterial blood pressure monitoring throughout the turn to the prone position and positioning adjustments.

Lateral, Three-Quarter Prone, and Park-Bench Positions

The lateral position is used for unilateral neurosurgical procedures in the upper posterior fossa. The three-quarter prone position, a modification of the prone and lateral positions, and the park-bench position are used for similar procedures to permit greater head rotation and access to more axial structures.

Risk-Benefit Analysis of Sitting Position Compared with Other Positions

The usefulness or appropriateness of the sitting surgical position for access to the posterior fossa continues to spark debate among neurosurgeons and neuroanesthesiologists, because alternative positions can be used for posterior fossa access and the occurrence of VAE is more common and severe in posterior fossa procedures performed in the sitting position than in alternative positions. Investigators from different institutions have reported their experience with the sitting position, with particular emphasis placed on complications and outcome (Table 12-1).[18,26] Some of the reported complications might

have been prevented or reduced if the sitting position had not been used (Table 12-2).

ANESTHETIC CONSIDERATIONS

The clinical significance of theoretic considerations regarding the choice of anesthetic drugs for patients who undergo posterior fossa exploration remains to be determined. First is the question of the effects of inhalational versus intravenous anesthetic drugs on the lungs' ability to retain air that enters the venous circulation, preventing its passage to the arterial circulation. Transpulmonary air passage occurs in humans and is supported by reports of cerebral air emboli in the absence of an intracardiac defect,[39] as well as detection of left-sided heart air on echocardiogram without demonstration of an intracardiac defect.[5] The intravenous anesthetics pentobarbital, fentanyl, and ketamine maintain a higher threshold for trapping air bubbles in the pulmonary circulation than halothane.[21-23] Thus such agents may decrease the risk and severity of air emboli if they occur.

A second consideration is the maintenance of adequate CPP. Before surgical incision, administration of intravenous anesthetic drugs has been demonstrated to have less effect on cardiovascular function than inhalational anesthetics in patients placed in the sitting position.[40] Whether the relationship continues after the start of surgery has not been investigated.

A third issue is the potential benefit of preserving cardiovascular responsiveness to surgical manipulation of brainstem structures. In such instances, the avoidance of anticholinergic drugs or long-acting β-adrenergic blockers that would mask cardiovascular response may provide useful information to the surgeon and anesthesiologist.

An additional consideration surrounds the use of N_2O in cases in which the risk of VAE is increased. A prospective, randomized study of patients requiring posterior fossa exploration or cervical spine surgery demonstrated that 50% N_2O had no significant effect on the incidence or severity of VAE if the N_2O was discontinued when air was detected by Doppler ultrasonography. Its analgesic effect, rapid elimination and emergence characteristics, and facilitation of the postoperative neurologic assessment continue to make it a popular adjunct. However, fentanyl-based anesthesia with supplemental isoflurane has been administered with no difference in time to emergence from anesthesia between patients who received 50% N_2O and those who did not.[9]

Premedication

Administration of surgical premedication is individualized by patient physical status, evidence of increased intracranial pressure (ICP), and level of patient anxiety. Long-term antihypertensive therapy is continued; perioperative corticosteroids and antibiotics are routinely ordered by the neurosurgeon. Narcotic premedication is avoided in patients with space-occupying lesions or hydrocephalus from fourth ventricle occlusion because the resultant hypoventilation and CO_2 retention may raise ICP. Oral benzodiazepines given 60 to 90 minutes before the patient's arrival in the operating room are effective in reducing anxiety and do not have significant effects on ICP. Often, however, now that most patients come to the hospital on the day of surgery, no premedication is given until arrival in the operating room. Often it is not given at all.

Table 12–1 Complications Associated with Surgical Position in Posterior Fossa Surgery

Complication(s)	Sitting Position	Prone Position	Lateral, Three-Quarter Prone Position	Park-Bench, "Lounge" Position
Nervous System				
Cerebral ischemia	++	+	0	+
Cervical spine ischemia	++	+	0	+
Palsies:				
Cranial nerve	+	++	++	
Brachial plexus	+		++	++
Sciatic nerve	+	0	0	0
Peroneal nerve	+	0	?	
Airway				
Edema of face, tongue, neck (postoperative obstruction)	++	++	+	0
Endotrachael tube migration	++	++	+	+
Pulmonary				
Ventilation/perfusion abnormalities	+	+	+	+
Increased airway pressures	0	++	0-+	0
Tension pneumocephalus	+	+	0	0
Cardiovascular				
Hypotension	++	++	0	+
Dysrhythmias	++	++	±	++
Need for blood transfusion	+	++	±	+
Miscellaneous				
Eye compression	0	+++	++	+
"Compartment syndrome"	+	0	0	0
Venous air embolism	+++	++	+	++
Paradoxical air embolism	++	+	?	?

0, +, ++, ++ indicate relative probability from no risk to high risk.

Table 12–2 Posterior Fossa Craniotomy: Intraoperative Surgical Problems by Patient Position

Problem	Sitting Position*	Horizontal Position*
Total number of patients	333	246
Hypotension:		
With positioning	63 (19%)	60 (24%)
During procedure	86 (26%)	54 (22%)
Entire anesthetic	121 (36%)	94 (38%)
Without cardiac disease	101/297 (34%)	130/197 (34%)
With cardiac disease	30/36 (56%)	27/49 (55%)
Transfusion of > 2 units of blood	3%	13%[†]
Average blood replacement	359 mL	507 mL[‡]
Postoperative cranial nerve function:		
Improved	41 (12)	50 (20)[§]
Unchanged	218 (65)	112 (45)
Deteriorated	74 (22)	84 (34)

*Unless otherwise indicated, first number is number of patients affected, and number in parentheses is percentage of total patients.
[†]$P < .01$ (chi-square test).
[‡]$P < .05$ (Student t test).
[§]26% of patients in horizontal position had decompression for tic douloureux.
Adapted from Black S, Ockert DB, Oliver WC, et al: Outcome following posterior fossa craniotomy in patients in the sitting or horizontal positions. Anesthesiology 1988;69:49-56.

Induction of Anesthesia

Direct arterial blood pressure monitoring established before induction of anesthesia allows tighter control of blood pressure and CPP during induction and intubation, especially in patients at risk for increased ICP. The use of a low-dose (4 to 6 μg/kg fentanyl), narcotic-based, muscle relaxant technique with 0.5 to 1.0 MAC volatile inhalational anesthetic after intravenous induction with thiopental or propofol affords adequate analgesia and amnesia, preservation of autonomic nervous system activity, and rapid awakening after discontinuation of the inhalational anesthetics; thus an early postoperative neurologic examination is facilitated if desired. Some anesthesiologists continue to use nitrous oxide in oxygen (typically 50%) unless air embolism occurs, but with desflurane there appears to be little advantage to nitrous oxide. A propofol infusion (50-100 μg/kg/min) often provides better surgical access than inhalational anesthetic alone. β-Adrenergic blocking drugs and direct-acting vasodilators may be used alone or in combination to treat increases in blood pressure. Use of long-acting antihypertensive drugs is avoided until the patient has been placed in the operating position. The need for vasopressor administration may arise after induction of anesthesia or positioning, especially in chronically hypertensive or debilitated patients. Short-acting drugs, such as small boluses of ephedrine or phenylephrine, are usually effective. Rarely, after all correctable derangements such as hypovolemia have been ruled out, inotrope infusions may be required throughout the surgical procedure, but a cause for an underlying mechanism should be sought.

Verification of appropriate placement of the endotracheal tube after final positioning, but before surgical incision, is of utmost importance, regardless of the position employed. Intraoperative access to the airway is limited by virtue of the proximity of the operative site, and neck flexion or extension can produce caudad or cephalad displacement of the endotracheal tube, respectively, by as much as 2 cm. Palpation of the endotracheal tube cuff above the sternal notch is a useful maneuver to ensure that the tip of the endotracheal tube rises above the carina.

Maintenance of Anesthesia

Controlled positive-pressure ventilation with paralysis has the following advantages:

- Maintenance of lighter levels of anesthesia
- Hyperventilation, which diminishes $Paco_2$, thereby decreasing both sympathetic stimulation and blood pressure at any given depth of anesthesia
- Cerebral vasoconstriction
- Less bleeding
- Lower ICP
- Less cardiovascular depression because of decreased anesthetic depth
- Less likelihood of patient movement

The MAC for desflurane (and presumably other anesthetic drugs) is not altered by the sitting position.[41] Excessive decreases in inhaled agent concentration as a strategy to combat hypotension may allow awareness. Intraoperative hypothermia should be avoided.

More liberal administration of intravenous fluids may be required during head-elevated prone procedures because of relaxation of the lower extremity capacitance vessels and resultant venous pooling. This pooling may be offset by preoperative application of compression stockings, but some loss of intravascular fluid to the extravascular space will occur over time. If large volumes of fluid are administered during surgery, a small prophylactic dose (5 to 10 mg) of furosemide will promote postoperative diuresis of excess fluids reabsorbed from the extravascular space. Glucose-containing solutions are not used because of the possible detrimental effects of hyperglycemia on areas of the brain at risk for cerebral ischemia.[42]

The administration of osmotic and loop diuretics for tumor resection and vascular procedures may predispose sitting patients to electrolyte disturbances or cardiovascular instability caused by hypovolemia.[43] Also, the size of the pneumocephalus may be increased.[32] Simultaneous administration of intravenous colloid is appropriate to maintain CPP and should probably have minimal effect on the cerebral dehydrating action of the diuretic.

Emergence from Anesthesia

The anesthetic goals during emergence from anesthesia are to prevent abrupt rises in blood pressure, effect rapid awakening, return motor strength, and minimize coughing and straining on the endotracheal tube. The feasibility of immediate postoperative extubation is determined by the nature and extent of surgery (e.g., extensive brainstem manipulation with a greater likelihood of postoperative brainstem edema or brainstem injury caused by a difficult tumor resection).[44,45] If extensive manipulation of the medullary structures or significant edema is a factor, a secured airway should be maintained until the patient is awake, following commands, and demonstrating return of protective airway reflexes. Additional sedation may be required until this point of recovery is reached. Persistent postoperative hypertension in a previously normotensive patient should alert the anesthesiologist to possible brainstem compression, ischemia, or hematoma.

VENOUS AIR EMBOLISM

Documentation of venous air embolism has existed for more than 100 years (Table 12-3). VAE is associated most often with posterior fossa procedures in the sitting position because of facilitation of air entry by subatmospheric pressure in an opened vein and the presence of noncollapsible venous channels, such as diploic veins and dural sinuses. Cases in which air entered the venous circulation via burr holes or wounds from the skull head holder have also been reported, particularly when the head was elevated.[26,46,47] Often unappreciated is the potential for venous air embolism originating from the sites of central venous access. Air can be entrained around the site of catheter entry. Air embolism may also occur when central catheters are removed with the patient's head up.

VAE in neurosurgery is a subset of the larger problem of VAE in the medical population. Several reviews addressing this issue have been published.[48, 49]

Pathophysiology

Review of the pathophysiologic effects of gas bubbles on the vascular endothelium suggests that a form of ischemia/reperfusion injury occurs that is common to all organs involved. During slow, continuous air entrainment, air is dissipated into the peripheral pulmonary circulation. The mechanical obstruction

Table 12-3 Early Historical Perspective on Air Embolism

Year(s)	Finding	Discoverer
1667	Death in animals when air enters vein	Redi
1681	Characteristic noise of air entrainment	Hardner
1683-1686	Right-heart dilation from air insufflation; mortality is rate- and dose-dependent	Camerarius, de Heyde
1800	First recorded case of air embolism during excision of a neck tumor (not realized until 30 years later)	Barlow
1811	Small air dose well tolerated; right ventricular distention is cause of death	Nysten
1818	Sudden death associated with hissing noise in young patient having clavicular tumor resection in sitting position	Bauchene
1821	Development of experimental surgery to investigate clinical findings	Magendie
1823	Treatment of air embolism during tumor resection by closing vein wound when hissing noise occurred	Wattmann
1832	Treatment for traumatic air embolism published (but overlooked)	Wattmann
1839	Establishment of conditions, treatment for venous air embolism in humans, including air aspiration	Amussat
1843	Approximately 40 cases of air embolism described	Various scientists
1845	Wattmann's work recognized	
1846	Concept and term "embolism" created	Virchow
1877	Paradoxical embolism associated with patent foramen ovale	Cohnheim
1885	Importance of head position in air entrainment	Senn

or local hypoxemia produced creates sympathetic reflex vasoconstriction. Microvascular bubbles can activate the endothelium, resulting in complement production, cytokine release, and production of reactive O_2 molecules. Pulmonary manifestations include pulmonary hypertension, impairment of gas exchange and hypoxemia,[50] CO_2 retention, increased pulmonary dead space, and decreased end-tidal CO_2 (ETCO$_2$). Bronchoconstriction results in increased airway pressures. Reduced venous return leads to decreases in cardiac output and systemic arterial blood pressure.[51] Myocardial and cerebral ischemia may result from severe, persistent hypoxemia or hypotension.

A rapidly entrained air bolus may result in an air lock within the right side of the heart or a cumulative gas volume that exceeds pulmonary arterial capacity (estimated to be 5 mL/kg), blockage of the right ventricular outflow tract, air or blood layer formation with obstructed venous return, decreased cardiac output, acute right ventricular dilation and failure, myocardial and cerebral ischemia, dysrhythmias, and cardiovascular collapse.[51,52]

Morbidity and mortality are directly related to the amount and rate of air entry. The "symptomatic dose" of venous air is not well documented in humans, but in a review of the clinical manifestations of VAE,[53] more than 50 mL have been retrieved in patients manifesting clinical changes such as decreases in blood pressure, dysrhythmia, and ECG changes. This same review summarized a collection of 93 early case reports in which 37 of 40 (93%) untreated patients died, and the lethal dose of intravascular air in humans has been estimated to be greater than 300 mL. Early investigations in dogs reported tolerance of as much as 1000 mL of air infused over 50 to 100 minutes, but fatality with a 100-mL bolus.[52]

Factors contributing to the occurrence and severity of VAE include the surgical site, such as the posterior fossa, where venous channels are stented open by surrounding structures, and the extent of head elevation and negative pressure

between the right atrium and the surgical site. VAE is more common and severe in posterior fossa craniotomies than in laminectomies.[26,54,55] Children experience greater hemodynamic derangements from VAE than adults.[26,54] In addition, air entrainment in children is more difficult to treat. The incidence is decreased by careful surgical dissection, hemostasis, and liberal use of bone wax. Hypovolemia lowers central venous pressure and increases the negative pressure gradient between the elevated head and the right side of the heart.

Incidence

A 1988 study reported the incidence of VAE to range from as low as 25% to as high as 60% in patients when the head is higher than the heart (Table 12-4).[56] Several later series have not changed this incidence but suggest that a higher incidence is detected with Doppler monitoring is used (43%) than with ETCO$_2$ monitoring (9%-28%).[57-60]

Risks of Air Embolism

The greater the pressure gradient between cerebral veins and the right atrium and the lower the central venous pressures, the greater is the tendency for air to enter venous openings at the craniotomy site. The risk of catastrophic air embolism has been reduced dramatically by improved detection and prompt treatment of VAE.[61-63] More attention has been directed toward recognition and treatment of paradoxical air embolism (PAE).

Risks of Paradoxical Air Embolism

Clinical evidence of PAE in the perioperative period is less frequent than calculated estimates based on the incidence of VAE and the prevalence of PFO.[64] However, complications,

Table 12–4	Incidence of Venous Air Embolism (VAE) in Posterior Fossa Surgery				
Investigator(s)	Year Reported	Surgical Position	Incidence	Percentage of Patients with VAE	Method of Detection
Michenfelder et al.[63]	1969	Sitting	37/751	5	Right-atrial catheter, aspiration
Michenfelder et al.[78]	1972	Sitting	26/69	42	Right-atrial catheter, Doppler
Albin et al.[25]	1987	Sitting	100/400	25	Right-atrial catheter, Doppler
		Horizontal	13/118	11	Right-atrial catheter, Doppler
Marshall & Bedford[131]	1980	Sitting	20/52	38	Doppler only
			13/52	25	Doppler, ↑PAP, ↓ETCO$_2$
Voorhies et al.[130]	1983	Sitting	41/81	50	Doppler, PEEP (no right-atrial catheter)
Standefer et al.[126]	1984	Sitting	22/382	6	Right-atrial catheter, Doppler
Matjasko et al.[54]	1985	Sitting	130/554	23.5	Right-atrial catheter, Doppler (ETCO$_2$ in 94 pts)
Young et al.[55]	1986	Sitting	70/255	30	Right-atrial catheter, Doppler
Black et al.[14]*	1988	Sitting	150/333	45	Right-atrial catheter, Doppler
		Horizontal	30/246	12	Right-atrial catheter (33%), Doppler (30%)
Von Gösseln et al.[127]	1991	30- to 45-degree head elevation	46/704	6.5	Right-atrial catheter, Doppler, ETCO$_2$

*Mass spectroscopy after 1982.
Doppler, precordial Doppler ultrasonography; PAP, Pulmonary artery pressure; PEEP, positive end-expiratory pressure; ↑, increase; ↓, decrease.

such as myocardial or cerebral ischemia resulting from PAE, may be devastating. Improvement in detection and prevention of the occurrence of PAE constitute areas of active clinical investigation.

The most likely mechanism of PAE in humans is right-to-left shunting through an intracardiac defect. A PFO is reported to exist in 20% to 30% of the population.[3] The likelihood of right-to-left shunt may be increased if the right atrial pressure exceeds left atrial pressure, and up to 50% of patients may experience reversal of an existing left-to-right atrial pressure gradient with the potential for PAE after 1 hour in the sitting position.

The calculated risk of PAE is 5% to 10%, but not all patients with a PFO will have PAE. Two-dimensional echocardiography during Valsalva maneuver in healthy volunteers revealed an 18% incidence of right-to-left shunting at the atrial level.[6]

The conditions under which PAE can occur through the pulmonary vascular bed in humans have not been well defined. Echocardiographic studies and numerous case reports describe its occurrence.[44,65,66] Findings regarding the occurrence and threshold for transpulmonary air passage differ in awake and anesthetized animal models, and the type of anesthetic appears to influence the threshold.[22,23] Although the true incidence of PAE is unknown, it may occur without postoperative sequelae, depending on both the volume and ultimate destination of the air that enters the arterial circulation. PAE to the cerebral circulation should be suspected in any patient who manifests an unexpected neurologic deficit after a surgical procedure known to be associated with a risk of air embolism, regardless of the intraoperative patient position.

Hypovolemia has been proposed as a predisposing factor to the occurrence of PAE as well as of VAE.[67] Intravenous fluid loading has been recommended to decrease the likelihood of right-to-left shunting and PAE in patients undergoing surgery in the sitting position.[68]

Use of Positive End-Expiratory Pressure

VAE and positive end-expiratory pressure (PEEP) may both increase right atrial pressure, and PEEP may raise cerebral venous pressure. PEEP has been proposed as a prophylactic measure against VAE.[69] However, it may impair surgical conditions, decrease venous return, and increase the chance that right atrial pressure will exceed left atrial pressure, thus predisposing an at-risk patient to PAE. Giebler and colleagues[70] found no reduction in the incidence of air embolism when they compared 10 cm PEEP with no PEEP in a prospective randomized study of patients operated on in the sitting position; these researchers suggested that the use of PEEP in sitting cases be abandoned. Jugular venous compression has been demonstrated to be effective in reducing air entry.[71,72]

Monitoring for Venous Air Embolism

Table 12-5 summarizes the monitors that may be used to detect VAE.

Doppler Ultrasound Transducer

The precordial Doppler ultrasound transducer is the most sensitive device commonly available for the detection of air in the right atrium.[73-75] Patient position influences air detection and retrieval.[76] Correct positioning of the Doppler probe over the right side of the heart may be difficult.

The Doppler probe generates a 2.5-MHz continuous ultrasonic signal that is reflected by moving blood and cardiac structures,[77,78] and the frequency change between transmitted and reflected signal is electronically converted into a readily detectable audible sound. Small volumes of air are detected

Table 12–5 Monitors for Detection of Venous Air Embolism

Monitor	Advantages	Disadvantages
Doppler	Most sensitive noninvasive monitor Earliest detector (before air enters pulmonary circulation)	Not quantitative May be difficult to place in obese patients, patients with chest wall deformity, or those in the prone/lateral positions False-negative result if air does not pass beneath ultrasonic beam (about 10% of cases); useless during electrocautery IV mannitol may mimic intravascular air
PA catheter	Quantitative, slightly more sensitive than $ETCO_2$ Widely available Placed with minimal difficulty in experienced hands Can detect right-atrial pressure greater than pulmonary capillary wedge pressure	Small lumen, less air aspirated than with right-atrial catheter Placement for optimal air aspiration may not allow pulmonary capillary wedge pressure measurement Nonspecific for air
$ETCO_2$	Noninvasive Sensitive Quantitative Widely available	Nonspecific for air Less sensitive than Doppler ultra, PA catheter Accuracy affected by tachypnea, low cardiac output, chronic obstructive pulmonary disease
ETN_2	Specific for air Detects air earlier than $ETCO_2$	May not detect subclinical air embolism May indicate air clearance from pulmonary circulation prematurely Accuracy affected by hypotension
TEE	Most sensitive detector of air Can detect air in left heart, aorta	Invasive, cumbersome Expensive Must be observed continuously Not quantitative May interfere with Doppler ultrasonography

Doppler, precordial Doppler ultrasonography; PA, pulmonary artery; TEE, transesophageal echocardiography.

easily with the probe because air is a good acoustic reflector. The precordial probe is placed just to the right of the sternum and a few inches above the xiphoid, where maximal signal is detected. Position of the probe is confirmed by injection of 0.25 to 0.5 mL CO_2 or 5 mL saline[77,79] through a right atrial catheter and listening for the characteristic change in the Doppler tones.

Right Atrial Catheter

The right atrial catheter (RAC) is used to aspirate air entering the right side of the heart; air aspiration is therapeutic during episodes of VAE. This procedure is useful in confirming the diagnosis of air embolism, particularly during electrocautery use, when the Doppler signal is obscured.[51,80] Optimal catheter placement requires that the orifice(s) be placed in or near the air-blood interface.[76,81,82]

The RAC is placed with a minimum of difficulty. Large-diameter catheters can retrieve large quantities of air, and aspiration of air has been demonstrated to be therapeutic when larger quantities have been entrained.[83] Disadvantages are that the catheter's position can change (especially after patient repositioning)[84] and that it may not retrieve all intravascular air. Multiple-orifice RACs are more effective than single-orifice catheters in aspirating air from the circulation.[25] There is greater air recovery with the tip at or 2 cm below the sinoatrial node. On the basis of modeling studies, with the RAC at an 80-degree atrial tilt, the proximal port should be located 1 to 3 cm above the sinoatrial node.[76]

Factors that influence air retrieval include catheter length and diameter, extent of patient inclination (retrieval is most efficient at 80%; retrieval at 60% is equal to that at 90%), number and size of orifices, and distance between orifices (Table 12-6).[85-87] A sheath (9 Fr diameter) allows air aspiration through the multiple-orifice end and simultaneous placement

of a pulmonary artery (PA) catheter. RAC positioning for optimal air aspiration can be accomplished with intravascular electrocardiography.[65,85] A method for ECG-guided catheter placement is performed as follows:

1. For the arm or neck, perform a venipuncture aseptically using a modified Seldinger technique.
2. Advance the catheter at least 20 cm via the arm or 15 cm via the neck.
3. Place a specially adapted conductive connector for ECG attachment (Arrow-Johans ECG adapter, Arrow International, Inc., Reading, PA) in the right atrial line next to the standard stopcock. Flushing the catheter with $NaHCO_3$ will reduce electrical impedance and improve the signal.
4. Set the ECG monitor for lead II and attach the right arm lead to the conductive connector. Some centers use lead V, which results in deflection of the P wave in the opposite direction.
5. Observe the ECG trace and pressure waveform on the monitor, and manipulate the catheter until the tip is in the right ventricle, and then withdraw it into the mid-right atrium to detect a biphasic P wave.
6. Withdraw the catheter until the P wave is approximately the height of the QRS complex (Fig. 12-1). Withdraw an additional centimeter, at which point the P wave should be slightly smaller than the QRS complex, and then secure the catheter.

The intracardiac ECG should be rechecked after the patient has been placed in the final position because sitting, as well as movement of the neck or the catheterized arm, may move the catheter.[84,85] Although a high incidence of catheter migration has been reported, the conductive connector should be removed after the patient is sitting and the catheter position has been reconfirmed in order to eliminate its electrical microshock hazard. The catheter tip should be withdrawn

Table 12–6   Characteristics of Catheters Used for Venous Air Aspiration

Catheter (Manufacturer)	Length (cm)	Diameter (Fr)	Distance from Proximal to Distal Orifice (cm)
Multiple-Orifice			
Bunegin-Albin multiorifice (Cook Medical, Inc., Bloomington, IN)	80 (arm)	5.8	4.2
	30 (neck)	5.8	
Flow-directed angiography (Baxter Healthcare, Deerfield, IL)	110	7	1.0
8 Fr multiorifice angiography (Edwards Medical Supply, Bolingbroke, IL)	110	8	4.9
PAC multiorifice sheath (Cook Medical)	25	9	4.2
Single-Orifice			
Swan-Ganz thermodilution (Baxter Healthcare) (single distal orifice and CVP port)	110	7	NA
Swan-Ganz pulmonary artery (Edwards Medical Supply) (single distal orifice and CVP port)	110	I7	NA
Single orifice CVP (Sorenson Medical Products, Inc., West Jordan, UT)	23.5	I5.5	NA
Single orifice drum cartridge (Abbott Laboratories, Abbott, IL)	71	5	NA

CVP, central venous pressure.

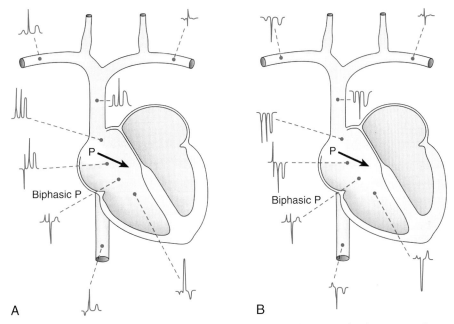

Figure 12–1 Positioning a right atrial catheter. **A,** P wave changes seen with lead II as the sensing lead. **B,** P wave changes seen with lead V as the sensing lead. P represents the origin of the P wave vector at the sinoatrial node.

from the right atrium at the end of surgery to prevent atrial perforation.

Observation of the ECG configuration to confirm proper catheter placement in the right atrium is more precise than chest radiography. However, changes in the venous pressure waveform during pressure-wave transduction for catheter placement are reportedly as accurate as changes in the ECG waveform.[88] Pressure wave forms may be of greatest benefit in rechecking catheter position periodically throughout surgery. Schummer and colleagues[89] have questioned the accuracy of ECG configuration changes as a guide to central line placement when a the left internal jugular vein is used and suggested that the transesophageal echocardiograph or chest radiograph should be the final determinant of placement.[89]

Pulmonary Artery Catheter

The PA catheter detects the pulmonary hypertension resulting from mechanical obstruction and reflex vasoconstriction from local hypoxemia caused by transpulmonary air.[90] PA pressure measurement is slightly more sensitive than capnography for detection of VAE; however, it is more invasive, and the PA catheter's lumen makes air aspiration more difficult than with larger catheters. In addition, the fixed distance between the PA catheter tip and the right atrial port makes simultaneous optimal positioning for pulmonary capillary wedge pressure measurements and air aspiration difficult. Use of pulmonary capillary wedge pressure to determine when left atrial pressure exceeds right atrial pressure has been advocated, but pulmonary capillary wedge pressure may not be a reliable estimate of left atrial pressure at higher pulmonary pressures.[70]

Figure 12–2 Visualization of intracardiac air by transesophageal echocardiography. Long-axis view of heart at the level of the left atrium and left ventricle; the left-ventricular outflow tract is shown. Microbubbles represented by high-intensity echoes are noted in all three structures. LA, Left atrium; LV, left ventricle; LVOT, left ventricular outflow tract.

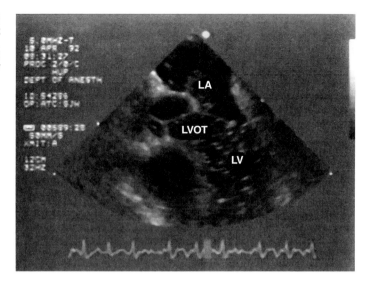

Exhaled Gas Analysis

Exhaled gas monitoring can be performed in the operating room with the use of infrared analysis, mass spectroscopy, or Raman light-scattering spectroscopy. However, in the United States, infrared spectroscopy has become the virtually exclusive measurement device. It can measure concentrations of volatile inhalational anesthetics in addition to O_2, N_2O, and CO_2 but not N_2. For many years my colleagues and I had access to Raman spectroscopy and could use exhaled nitrogen as one of the indicators of air embolism; however, at my institution, we can do longer do so, having changed to infrared technology.

Capnography

Capnography ($ETCO_2$ monitoring) has a specific role for air embolism location in enabling detection of the increased arterial–to–end-tidal CO_2 gradient associated with its occurrence. Factors that may influence the capnograph's accuracy include rapid respiratory rate, low cardiac output, and chronic obstructive pulmonary disease.

End-Tidal Nitrogen (ETN_2) Monitoring

Advantages of ETN_2 monitoring over capnography are its specificity for air and earlier detection than $ETCO_2$ when air enters the pulmonary circulation.[91] However, the sensitivity of current N_2 monitoring technology available for clinical use may not be sufficient to detect subclinical VAE. In addition, ETN_2 decreases with hypotension, and it may indicate prematurely that N_2 has been eliminated from the pulmonary circulation.[92] As noted previously, the capability for ETN_2 measurement is rapidly being lost as the clinical respiratory gas monitors that do this are no longer being manufactured.

Transesophageal Echocardiography

TEE detects air bubbles with a 3.5- to 5-MHz echocardiographic probe placed behind the heart; a visual image is produced with two-dimensional TEE[93,94] (Fig. 12-2) and, like Doppler ultrasonography, TEE detects air when it is still in the right side of the heart. A major advantage of TEE over other monitors currently available is that it can detect air in the left side of the heart and in the aorta. However, its detection of air bubbles is qualitative, not quantitative; thus microbubbles can generate a dramatic image. The use of TEE in screening of anesthetized sitting patients for PFOs has been described.[10,95]

Other Monitoring Methods

Doppler Monitoring of Carotid and Middle Cerebral Arteries

Doppler ultrasonographic monitoring of the cerebral circulation uses the same technology currently in use for VAE detection. Routine carotid Doppler monitoring may not be specific for PAE, because any air in the adjacent internal jugular veins would also be detected by the probe. Transcranial Doppler ultrasonographic monitoring of the middle cerebral artery has become increasingly useful in the perioperative setting. Efforts continue to enable quantification of embolic air and to make the equipment less cumbersome.

Brain Electrical Activity

Charzot and colleagues[96] and Kin and associates[97] reported acute decrements in the bispectral index as a consequence of air embolism. However these changes are not specific for air entrainment and may occur for many other reasons, including an increase in anesthetic concentration.

Complications Resulting from Venous Air Embolism

Table 12-7 summarizes the complications of venous air embolism in posterior fossa surgery.

Intraoperative Complications

Cardiovascular instability due to VAE may manifest in a number of ways. The most common dysrhythmia is premature ventricular contraction, but murmurs, tachycardia, bradycardia, and ventricular tachycardia may occur.[51,63,80] Hypertension and tachycardia may occur initially in response to air entry into the pulmonary microcirculation. Marked alterations in blood pressure and the characteristic changes in heart sounds usually do not appear until large emboli are present. Hypotension is most likely due to decreases in cardiac output associated with larger volumes of intravascular air.[51] However, the duration of changes in heart tones[98] may be brief (i.e., < 5 minutes), although air is still present. ECG changes are generally too late to be useful diagnostically; however, evidence of transmural myocardial ischemia may indicate airflow into the coronary arteries.[99] Right ventricular failure results from acute dilation and pulmonary outflow obstruction.[51] Rapid

Table 12–7   Complications of Venous Air Embolism

Location	Intraoperative Complications	Postoperative Complications
Cardiovascular	Dysrhythmias	Myocardial ischemia
	Hypotension/hypertension	Right-ventricular failure
	Changes in heart sounds, murmurs	
	Electrocardiographic evidence of ischemia	
	Acute right-ventricular failure	
	Cardiac arrest	
Pulmonary	Hypercarbia	Perfusion defects
	Hypoxemia	
	Pulmonary hypertension	
	Pulmonary edema	
Central nervous system	Hyperemia	Neurologic deficits, stroke, coma
	Brain swelling	

accumulation of large volumes of air may overwhelm the pulmonary circulation or produce air lock in the right-sided heart chambers, leading to cardiac arrest.

Animal studies of intracoronary air have reported ECG changes resulting from as little as 0.025 mL air injected into the anterior descending coronary artery of the dog, and 0.05 mL in the same model has resulted in death. In studies of the effects of intracerebral air embolism, acute hypertension and severe cardiac dysrhythmias have been described after infusion of 2 mL/kg of air into the vertebral arteries of cats. Similar findings have been reported in dogs with carotid injections of air.

A "gasp" has been described as a classic clinical finding when air embolism occurs.[51,100] The likelihood of this occurrence is greater in a patient who has not undergone respiratory paralysis. The extent of pulmonary dysfunction depends on the amount of air that reaches the pulmonary circulation. Hypercapnia, hypoxemia, and pulmonary hypertension may be mild, moderate, or severe.

Pulmonary edema may follow both small and large air emboli. Its development is believed to involve mechanisms similar to those of clot emboli rather than neurogenic pulmonary edema. The association of pulmonary edema with elevations in pulmonary capillary wedge pressure can be used to distinguish it from neurogenic pulmonary edema, which after the acute sympathetic response is associated with a normal wedge pressure.[101,102] Damage to the pulmonary vascular endothelium may result from repeated bouts of pulmonary hypertension.[103] Perfusion defects similar to those found in instances of pulmonary clot emboli have been described after pulmonary air embolism.[104] Their distinguishing feature is the more rapid resolution of the defect.

Postoperative Complications

Complications arising from air embolism primarily involve the central nervous, cardiovascular, and pulmonary systems. Neurologic deficits, stroke, and coma may result from surgical manipulation, hypoxic or ischemic injury, or cerebral air embolism. Dose and rate of air entrainment appear to influence the clinical findings. Increases in ICP appear to be associated with more severe injury.

Available studies in humans have been unable to correlate morbidity and mortality with the volume of cerebral arterial air introduced. However, clear laboratory findings and clinical evidence have shown that cerebral air can produce brain injury.[105,106] Other studies have reported altered sensorium, convulsions, hemiplegia, monoplegia, hemianesthesia, hemianopsia, nystagmus, strabismus, and respiratory disturbances. A case report described suspected arterial air embolism from an indeterminate volume of air flushed retrograde through a radial artery catheter.[107]

Potential postoperative cardiovascular complications resulting from VAE include right ventricular failure (from pulmonary hypertension) and myocardial ischemia (from coronary air embolism or right-sided heart strain). Postoperative pulmonary edema may produce chest radiograph abnormalities and perfusion defects, but it is usually self-limited and responsive to conservative therapy, such as supplemental O_2 or small doses of furosemide.[104,108]

Prevention of Air Embolism

No maneuver is 100% effective in preventing the occurrence of VAE if a gradient exists between the operative site and the right atrium, regardless of patient position. However, the incidence and severity can be decreased by the use of controlled positive-pressure ventilation, adequate hydration, proper wrapping of the lower extremities, positioning so that head elevation is the lowest possible while still providing good surgical exposure, meticulous surgical technique with careful dissection and liberal use of bone wax, avoidance of N_2O in patients with known intracardiac defects, and avoidance of drugs that may increase venous capacitance (e.g., nitroglycerin).

Treatment of Venous Air Embolism

Box 12-2 summarizes the treatment of VAE.

Intraoperative Period

The intraoperative goals in the treatment of VAE are to stop further air entry, remove air already present, and correct hypotension, hypoxemia, and hypercapnia. If Doppler ultrasonography changes occur or ETCO$_2$ decreases more than 2 mm Hg, the surgeon should be informed immediately.

Jugular compression has been shown to be effective in raising dural sinus pressure in patients in both the supine and

BOX 12–2 *Treatment of Venous Air Embolism*

Intraoperative Goals

1. Inform surgeon immediately.
2. Discontinue N_2O, increase O_2 flows.
3. Modify the anesthetic.
4. Have the surgeon flood the surgical field with fluids.
5. Provide jugular vein compression.
6. Aspirate the right atrial catheter.
7. Provide cardiovascular support.
8. Change the patient's position.

Postoperative Goals

1. Provide supplemental O_2.
2. Perform electrocardiography, chest radiographs.
3. Measure serial arterial blood gas levels.
4. If arterial air emboli are suspected, provide hyperbaric oxygen compression if available.

sitting positions.[71] However, there is concern that the technique of jugular venous compression may cause the following:

- Cerebral venous outflow obstruction with a resulting decrease in cerebral blood flow.
- Carotid artery compression or dislodgment of atherosclerotic plaques.
- Venous engorgement, leading to brain swelling and cerebral edema.
- Carotid sinus compression and bradycardia. Maintenance of CPP greater than 50 mm Hg in normotensive patients should minimize the risk of cerebral hypoperfusion. Higher perfusion pressures should be maintained in patients with chronic hypertension.

Aspiration of the RAC should be initiated as quickly as possible after Doppler ultrasonography or TEE detection of intravascular air. This maneuver has been demonstrated as effective in reducing morbidity from VAE.[51,63,80,83]

Patient position should be changed to lower the head to heart level when feasible. Other measures are greater intravenous fluid administration, vasopressors if hypotension occurs, antidysrhythmics, and modification of the anesthetic technique in the absence of N_2O with more anesthetic drugs. External cardiac massage has been shown to be effective in disrupting a large air lock in the event of cardiovascular collapse.[109] Changing the patient's position to left lateral decubitus to limit airflow through the pulmonary outflow tract is of limited benefit in the presence of a continuous stream of air. PEEP or Valsalva maneuver may increase the likelihood of PAE after VAE has occurred and should therefore be avoided.[1,5,6,70] On the basis of data from a porcine model of cerebral air embolism, hyperventilation is not helpful.[110,111]

Postoperative Period

Postoperative goals in the treatment of VAE include prevention of hypoxemia or other respiratory compromise, detection and treatment of myocardial ischemia, and treatment of clinical evidence of PAE. Useful diagnostic studies include arterial blood gas measurements, ECG, and electrophysiologic monitoring. Air bubbles in the retinal vessels, seen through funduscopic examination, have been described as a diagnostic sign for cerebral air embolism. In patients with suspected cerebral air embolism, a CT scan may aid in the diagnosis. However, radiographic evidence of cerebral air may vary among patients, initial CT scans may be normal, and the findings may change over time.[112,113] The role of magnetic resonance imaging in the diagnosis of air embolism remains to be determined. Although magnetic resonance imaging has been described as more sensitive than CT in detecting ischemic cerebral and diving-related spinal injuries,[114] technical constraints may limit its use in critically ill patients.

Annane and coworkers[115] demonstrated that experimental cerebral air embolism in beagles is cleared faster when the animals undergo mechanical ventilation with 100% oxygen than for spontaneous ventilation on room air.[115] Because patients undergoing posterior fossa surgery are already intubated, this finding would not change practice; however, patients with suspected, neurologically significant cerebral air detected after extubation might benefit from reintubation.

Hyperbaric oxygen (HBO) therapy for the treatment of suspected cerebral air embolism is used when appropriate equipment is available. Rapid application of very high pressure reduces air bubble volume, which should speed elimination of dissolved gas and reduce cerebral edema.[116] Numerous reports, some dramatic, describe the benefits of HBO therapy for decompression sickness and arterial gas embolism.[117] In a review of 86 patients treated for iatrogenic air embolism between 1980 and 1999, Blanc and colleagues[118] found better neurologic outcome when therapy was started less than 6 hours from the time of insult. Thus if HBO is to be used, treatment should be started as soon as possible.

Electrophysiologic Monitoring

Various forms of monitoring, such as raw or processed electroencephalogram (EEG), brainstem auditory evoked potentials (BAEPs), and somatosensory and motor nerve stimulation, are being used with increasing frequency to determine the integrity of cerebral function during posterior fossa surgery. Such monitoring is used in selected intracranial, spinal, and cerebrovascular procedures and is generally handled by experienced electrophysiologists. Bimodal or multimodal measurements of EEG, BAEPs, and SSEPs have been advocated as a more effective means of monitoring central nervous system function for posterior fossa surgery than single-modality monitoring.[119]

Brainstem Auditory Evoked Potentials

BAEPs are robust signals that are minimally influenced by the type or depth of anesthesia. Cranial nerve VIII monitoring during acoustic neuroma resection or microvascular decompression has been advocated to help preserve nerve VIII function.[120-122] Bilateral changes in BAEPs are indicative of brainstem compromise.[123,124] Normalization of BAEPs during emergency posterior fossa decompression has been used to guide postoperative management and timing of extubation.

Somatosensory Evoked Potentials

SSEPs may be of use in detecting morbidity from cerebral air embolism,[125] spinal cord ischemia caused by hypotension, or stretch of the cord due to excessive neck flexion. Monitoring of short-latency SSEPs, which monitor subcortical components of central sensory pathways, has been advocated for surgery on the cervical cord and posterior fossa.[124] Long-latency components of SSEPs may be difficult to evaluate because of greater variability in both latency and amplitude.

Electroencephalogram

EEG signals provide information regarding depth of anesthesia because they are sensitive to both inhalational and intravenous anesthetics. Intraoperative EEG monitoring during posterior fossa surgery can detect decreased cortical responses resulting from deep anesthesia or ischemia. The information from the cortical components of SSEPs is similar to that from EEG signals.

Facial Nerve Monitoring

Monitoring of facial nerve (VII) function may help reduce complications of surgical dissection and manipulation for resection of acoustic neuromas and microvascular decompression.[120] Muscle paralysis, which can interfere with the signal, should be significantly reduced or avoided when muscle stimulation is required.

SUMMARY

The patient undergoing posterior fossa surgery poses challenges to the anesthesiologist in terms of preoperative evaluation, positioning, choice of anesthetic agents, and monitoring, particularly for prevention of air embolism and preservation of neurologic function. The goals of monitoring are maintenance of hemodynamic stability and early detection of air embolism. Active clinical and basic science investigations continue to improve the means by which these challenges may be met in optimal fashion.

REFERENCES

1. Cucchiara RF, Seward JB, Nishimura RA, et al: Identification of patent foramen ovale during sitting position craniotomy by transesophageal echocardiography with positive airway pressure, Anesthesiology 63:107–109, 1985.
2. Guggiari M, Ph Lechat, Garen-Colonne C, et al: Early detection of patent foramen ovale by two-dimensional contrast echocardiography for prevention of paradoxical air embolism during sitting position, Anesth Analg 67:192–194, 1988.
3. Hagen PT, Scholz DG, Edwards WD: Incidence and size of patent foramen ovale during the first 10 decades of life: An autopsy study of 965 normal hearts, Mayo Clin Proc 59:17–23, 1984.
4. Banas JS, Meister SG, Gazzaniga AB, et al: A simple technique for detecting small defects in the atrial septum, Am J Cardiol 28:467–471, 1971.
5. Kronik G, Mosslacher H: Positive contrast echocardiography in patients with patent foramen ovale and normal right heart hemodynamics, Am J Cardiol 49:1806–1809, 1982.
6. Lynch JJ, Schuchard GH, Gross CM, et al: Prevalence of right-to-left atrial shunting in a healthy population: Detection by Valsalva maneuver contrast echocardiography, Am J Cardiol 53:1478–1480, 1984.
7. Black S, Muzzi DA, Nishimura RA, et al: Preoperative and intraoperative echocardiography to detect right-to-left shunt in patients undergoing neurosurgical procedures in the sitting position, Anesthesiology 72:436–438, 1990.
8. Cucchiara RF, Nishimura RA, Black S: Failure of preoperative echo testing to prevent paradoxical air embolism: Report of two cases, Anesthesiology 71:604–607, 1989.
9. Losasso TJ, Muzzi DA, Dietz NM, et al: Fifty percent nitrous oxide does not increase the risk of venous air embolism in neurosurgical patients operated upon in the sitting position, Anesthesiology 77:21–30, 1992.
10. Papadopoulos G, Kuhly P, Brock M, et al: Venous and paradoxical air embolism in the sitting position: A prospective study with transesophageal echocardiography, Acta Neurochir 126:140–143, 1994.
11. Kwapisz MM, Deinsberger W, Muller M, et al: Transesophageal echocardiography as a guide for patient positioning before neurosurgical procedures in semi-sitting position, J Neurosurg Anesthesiol 16:277–281, 2004.
12. Troianos CA, Jobes DR, Ellison N: Ultrasound-guided cannulation of the internal jugular vein: A prospective, randomized study, Anesth Analg 72:823–826, 1991.
13. Colley PS, Dunn R: Prevention of blood pressure response to skull-pin head holder by local anesthesia, Anesth Analg 58:241–243, 1979.
14. Black S, Ockert DB, Oliver WC, et al: Outcome following posterior fossa craniotomy in patients in the sitting or horizontal positions, Anesthesiology 69:49–56, 1988.
15. Coonan TJ, Hope CE: Cardio-respiratory effects of change of body position, Can Anaesth Soc J 30:424–437, 1983.
16. Darymple DG, MacGowan SW, MacLeod GF: Cardiorespiratory effects of the sitting position in neurosurgery, Br J Anaesth 51:1079–1081, 1979.
17. Enderby GEH: Postural ischaemia and blood pressure, Lancet 266:185–187, 1954.
18. Albin MS, Babinski M, Maroon JC, et al: Anesthetic management of posterior fossa surgery in the sitting position, Acta Anaesthesiol Scand 20:117–128, 1976.
19. Millar RA: Neuroanesthesia in the sitting position, Br J Anaesth 44:495, 1972.
20. Whitby JD: Electrocardiography during posterior fossa operations, Br J Anaesth 35:624–630, 1963.
21. Butler BD, Leiman BC, Katz J: Arterial air embolism of venous origin in dogs: Effect of nitrous oxide in combination with halothane and pentobarbitone, Can J Anaesth 34:570–576, 1987.
22. Yahagi N, Furuya H: The effects of halothane and pentobarbital on the threshold of transpulmonary passage of venous air emboli in dogs, Anesthesiology 67:905–909, 1987.
23. Yahagi N, Furuya H, Yoshikazu S, et al: Effect of halothane, fentanyl, and ketamine on the threshold for transpulmonary passage of venous air emboli in dogs, Anesth Analg 75:720–723, 1992.
24. Munson ES, Merrick HC: Effects of nitrous-oxide on venous air embolism, Anesthesiology 27:783–787, 1986.
25. Albin MS, Carroll RG, Maroon JC: Clinical considerations concerning detection of venous air embolism, Neurosurgery 3:380–384, 1978.
26. Cabezudo JM, Gilsanz F, Vaquero J, et al: Air embolism from wounds from a pin-type head-holder as a complication of posterior fossa surgery in the sitting position, J Neurosurg 55:147–148, 1981.
27. Artru AA: Nitrous oxide plays a direct role in the development of tension pneumocephalus intraoperatively, Anesthesiology 57:59–61, 1982.
28. Artru AA: Breathing nitrous oxide during closure of the dura and cranium is not indicated, Anesthesiology 66:719, 1987.
29. Skahen S, Shapiro HM, Drummond JC, et al: Nitrous oxide withdrawal reduces intracranial pressure in the presence of pneumocephalus, Anesthesiology 65:192–196, 1986.
30. Friedman GA, Norfleet EA, Bedford RF: Discontinuance of nitrous oxide does not prevent pneumocephalus, Anesth Analg 60:57–58, 1981.
31. Di Lorenzo N, Caruso R, Floris R, et al: Pneumocephalus and tension pneumocephalus after posterior fossa surgery in the sitting position: A prospective study, Acta Neurochir (Wien) 83:112–115, 1986.
32. Toung TJK, McPherson RW, Ahn H, et al: Pneumocephalus: Effects of patient position on the incidence and location of aerocele after posterior fossa and upper cervical cord surgery, Anesth Analg 65:65–70, 1986.
33. Kishan A, Naidu MR, Muralidhar K: Tension pneumocephalus following posterior fossa surgery in sitting position: A report of 2 cases, Clin Neurol Neurosurg 92:245–248, 1990.
34. Kitahata LM, Katz JD: Tension pneumocephalus after posterior fossa craniotomy: A complication of the sitting position, Anesthesiology 45:578, 1976.
35. MacGillivray RG: Pneumocephalus as a complication of posterior fossa surgery in the sitting position, Anaesthesia 37:722–725, 1982.
36. McPherson RW, Toung TJK, Johnson RM, et al: Intracranial subdural gas: A cause of false-positive change of intraoperative somatosensory evoked potential, Anesthesiology 62:816–819, 1985.
37. Schubert A, Zornow MH, Drummond JC, et al: Loss of cortical evoked responses due to intracranial gas during posterior fossa craniectomy in the seated position, Anesth Analg 65:203–206, 1986.
38. Rayport M: The head-elevated positions: Neurosurgical aspects: Approaches to the occiput and cervical spine. In Martin JT, editor: Positioning in Anesthesia and Surgery, ed 2, Philadelphia, 1987, WB Saunders.
39. Black M, Calvin J, Chan KL, et al: Paradoxic air embolism in the absence of an intracardiac defect, Chest 99:754–755, 1991.
40. Marshall WK, Bedford RF, Miller ED: Cardiovascular responses in the seated position: Impact of four anesthetic techniques, Anesth Analg 62:648–653, 1983.
41. Lin C-M, Wu C-T, Lee S-T, et al: Sitting position does not alter minimum alveolar concentration for desflurane, Can J Anaesth 54:523–530, 2007.

42. Sieber FE, Smith DS, Traystman RJ, et al: Glucose: A reevaluation of its intraoperative use, *Anesthesiology* 67:72–81, 1987.

43. Cottrell JE, Robustelli A, Post K, et al: Furosemide and mannitol-induced changes in intracranial pressure and serum osmolarity and electrolytes, *Anesthesiology* 47:28–30, 1977.

44. Artru AA, Cucchiara RF, Messick JM: Cardiorespiratory and cranial nerve sequelae of surgical procedures involving the posterior fossa, *Anesthesiology* 52:83–86, 1980.

45. Howard R, Mahoney A, Thurlow AC: Respiratory obstruction after posterior fossa surgery, *Anaesthesia* 45:222–224, 1990.

46. Edelman JD, Wingard DW: Air embolism arising from burrholes, *Anesthesiology* 53:167–168, 1980.

47. Wilkins RH, Albin MS: An unusual entrance site of venous air embolism during operation in the sitting position, *Surg Neurol* 7:71, 1977.

48. Mirski MA, Lele AV, Fitzsimmons L, et al: Diagnosis and treatment of vascular air embolism, *Anesthesiology* 106:164–177, 2007.

49. Muth CM, Shank ES: Gas embolism, *N Engl J Med* 342:476–482, 2000.

50. Pfitzner J, Petito SP, McLean AG: Hypoxaemia following sustained low-volume venous air embolism in sheep, *Anaesth Intensive Care* 16:164–170, 1988.

51. Adornato DC, Gildenberg PL, Ferrario CM, et al: Pathophysiology of intra venous air embolism in dogs, *Anesthesiology* 49:120–127, 1978.

52. Durant TM, Long J, Oppenheimer MJ: Pulmonary (venous) air embolism, *Am Heart J* 33:269–281, 1947.

53. Gottlieb JD, Ericsson JA, Sweet RB: Venous air embolism: A review, *Anesth Analg* 44:773–778, 1963.

54. Matjasko J, Petrozza P, Cohen M, et al: Anesthesia and surgery in the seated position: Analysis of 554 cases, *Neurosurgery* 17:695–702, 1985.

55. Young ML, Smith DS, Murtagh F, et al: Comparison of surgical and anesthetic complications in neurosurgical patients experiencing venous air embolism in the sitting position, *Neurosurgery* 18:157–161, 1986.

56. Gottdiener JS, Papademetriou V, Notargiacomo A, et al: Incidence and cardiac effects of systemic venous air embolism: Echocardiographic evidence of arterial embolization via noncardiac shunt, *Arch Intern Med* 148:795–800, 1988.

57. Domaingue CM: Neurosurgery in the sitting position: A case series, *Anaesth Intensive Care* 33:332–335, 2005.

58. Bithal PK, Pandia MP, Dash HH, et al: Comparative incidence of venous air embolism and associated hypotension in adults and children operated for neurosurgery in the sitting position, *Eur J Anaesthesiol* 21:517–522, 2004.

59. Rath GP, Bithal PK, Chaturvedi A, et al: Complications related to positioning in posterior fossa craniectomy, *J Clin Neurosci* 14:520–525, 2007.

60. Leslie K, Hui R, Kaye AH: Venous air embolism and the sitting position: A case series, *J Clin Neurosci* 13:419–422, 2006.

61. Bedford RF: Perioperative venous air embolism, *Semin Anesth* 6:163–170, 1987.

62. Michenfelder JD: The 27th Rovenstine Lecture: Neuroanesthesia and the achievement of professional respect, *Anesthesiology* 70:695–701, 1989.

63. Michenfelder JD, Martin JT, Altenburg BM, et al: Air embolism during neurosurgery: An evaluation of right atrial catheters for diagnosis and treatment, *JAMA* 208:1353–1358, 1969.

64. Black S, Muzzi DA, Nishimura RA, et al: Preoperative and intraoperative echocardiography to detect right-to-left shunt in patients undergoing neurosurgical procedures in the sitting position. *Anesthesiology* 72:436–8, 1990.

65. Bowdle TA, Artru AA: Positioning the air aspiration pulmonary artery catheter introducer sheath by intravascular electrocardiography, *Anesthesiology* 69:276–279, 1988.

66. Marquez J, Sladen A, Gendell H, et al: Paradoxical cerebral air embolism without an intracardiac septal defect, *J Neurosurg* 55:997–999, 1981.

67. Pfitzner J, McLean AG: Venous air embolism and active lung inflation at high and low CVP: A study in upright anesthetized sheep, *Anesth Analg* 66:1127–1134, 1987.

68. Colohan ART, Perkins NAK, Bedford RF, et al: Intravenous fluid loading as prophylaxis for paradoxical air embolism, *J Neurosurg* 62:839–842, 1985.

69. Perkins NAK, Bedford RF: Hemodynamic consequences of PEEP in seated neurosurgical patients: Implications for paradoxical air embolism, *Anesth Analg* 63:429–432, 1984.

70. Giebler R, Kollenberg B, Pohlen G, et al: Effect of positive end-expiratory pressure on the incidence of venous air embolism and on the cardiovascular response to the sitting position during neurosurgery, *B J Anaesthesiol* 80:30–35, 1998.

71. Grady MS, Bedford RF, Park TS: Changes in superior sagittal sinus pressure in children with head elevation, jugular venous compression and PEEP, *J Neurosurg* 65:199–202, 1986.

72. Toung TJK, Miyabe M, McShane AJ, et al: Effect of PEEP and jugular venous compression on canine cerebral blood flow and oxygen consumption in the head elevated position, *Anesthesiology* 68:53–58, 1988.

73. Edmonds-Seal J, Maroon JC: Air embolism diagnosed with ultrasound, *Anaesthesia* 24:438–440, 1969.

74. Edmonds-Seal J, Prys-Roberts C, Adams AP: Air embolism: A comparison of various methods of detection, *Anaesthesia* 26:202–208, 1971.

75. Gildenberg PL, O'Brien RP, Britt WJ, et al: The efficacy of Doppler monitoring for the detection of venous air embolism, *J Neurosurg* 54:75–78, 1981.

76. Bunegin L, Albin MS, Helsel PE, et al: Positioning the right atrial catheter: A model for reappraisal, *Anesthesiology* 55:343–348, 1981.

77. Maroon JC, Albin MS: Air embolism diagnosed by Doppler ultrasound, *Anesth Analg* 53:399–402, 1974.

78. Michenfelder JD, Miller RH, Gronert GA: Evaluation of an ultrasonic device (Doppler) for the diagnosis of venous air embolism, *Anesthesiology* 36:164–168, 1972.

79. Tinker JH, Gronert GA, Messick JM, et al: Detection of air embolism: A test for positioning of right atrial catheter and Doppler probe, *Anesthesiology* 43:104–105, 1975.

80. Alvaran SB, Toung JK, Graff TE, et al: Venous air embolism: Comparative merits of external cardiac massage, intracardiac aspiration, and left lateral decubitus position, *Anesth Analg* 57:166–170, 1978.

81. Bunegin L, Albin MS: Balloon catheter increases air capture, *Anesthesiology* 57:66–67, 1982.

82. Diaz PM: Balloon catheter should increase recovery of embolized air, *Anesthesiology* 57:66, 1982.

83. Colley PS, Artru AA: Bunegin-Albin catheter improves air retrieval and resuscitation from lethal venous air embolism in upright dogs, *Anesth Analg* 68:298–301, 1989.

84. Lee DS, Kuhn J, Shaffer MJ, et al: Migration of tips of central venous catheters in seated patients, *Anesth Analg* 63:949–952, 1984.

85. Colley PS, Artru AA: ECG-guided placement of Sorenson CVP catheters via arm veins, *Anesth Analg* 63:953–956, 1984.

86. Johans TG: Multi-orificed catheter placement with an intravascular electrocardiographic technique, *Anesthesiology* 64:411–413, 1986.

87. Warner DO, Cucchiara RF: Position of proximal orifice determines electrocardiogram recorded from multiorificed catheter, *Anesthesiology* 65:235–236, 1986.

88. Mongan P, Peterson RE, Culling RD: Pressure monitoring can accurately position catheters for air embolism aspiration, *J Clin Monit* 8:121–125, 1992.

89. Schummer W, Herrmann S, Schummer C, et al: Intra-atrial ECG is not a reliable method for positioning left internal jugular vein catheters, *B J Anaesth* 91:481–486, 2003.

90. Munson ES, Paul WC, Perry JC, et al: Early detection of venous air embolism using a Swan-Ganz catheter, *Anesthesiology* 42:223–226, 1975.

91. Matjasko MJ, Hellman J, Mackenzie CF: Venous air embolism, hypotension and end-tidal nitrogen, *Neurosurgery* 21:378–382, 1987.

92. Drummond JC, Prutow RJ, Scheller MS: A comparison of the sensitivity of pulmonary artery pressure, end-tidal carbon dioxide, and end-tidal nitrogen in the detection of venous air embolism in the dog, *Anesth Analg* 64:688–692, 1985.

93. Glenski JA, Cucchiara RF, Michenfelder JD: Transesophageal echocardiography and transcutaneous O_2 and CO_2 monitoring for detection of venous air embolism, *Anesthesiology* 64:541–545, 1986.

94. Sato S, Toya S, Ohira T, et al: Echocardiographic detection and treatment of intraoperative air embolism, *J Neurosurg* 64:440–444, 1986.

95. Mammoto T, Hayashi Y, Osnishi Y, et al: Incidence of venous and paradoxical air embolism in neurosurgical patients in the sitting position: Detection by transesophageal echocardiography, *Acta Anaesthesiol Scand* 42:643–647, 1998.

96. Chazot T, Liu N, Tremelot L, et al: Detection of gas embolism by bispectral index and Entropy monitoring in two cases, *Anesthesiology* 101:1053–1054, 2004.

97. Kin N, Konstadt SN, Sato K, et al: Reduction of bispectral index value associated with clinically significant air embolism, *J Cardiothor Vasc Anesth* 18:82–84, 2004.

98. Whitby JD: Early cases of air embolism, *Anaesthesia* 19:579–584, 1964.

99. Durant TM, Oppenheimer MJ, Webster MR, et al: Arterial air embolism, *Am Heart J* 38:481–500, 1949.

100. Lesky E: Notes on the history of air embolism, *German Med Monthly* 6:159–161, 1961.

101. Chandler WF, Dimsheff DG, Taren JA: Acute pulmonary edema following venous air embolism during a neurosurgical procedure, *J Neurosurg* 40:400–404, 1974.

102. Peterson BT, Petrini MF, Hyde RW, et al: Pulmonary tissue volume in dogs during pulmonary edema, *J Appl Physiol* 44:782–795, 1978.

103. Ohkuda K, Nakahara K, Binder A, et al: Venous air emboli in sheep: reversible increase in lung microvascular permeability, *J Appl Physiol* 51:887–894, 1981.

104. Sessler CN, Kiser PE, Raval V: Transient pulmonary perfusion scintigraphic abnormalities in pulmonary air embolism, *Chest* 95:910–912, 1989.

105. Gronert GA, Messick JM, Cucchiara RF, et al: Paradoxical air embolism from a patent foramen ovale, *Anesthesiology* 50:548–549, 1979.

106. Mills NL, Ochsner JL: Massive air embolism during cardiopulmonary bypass: Causes, prevention, and management, *J Thorac Cardiovasc Surg* 80:708–717, 1980.

107. Chang C, Dughi J, Shitabata P, et al: Air embolism and the radial arterial line, *Crit Care Med* 16:141–143, 1988.

108. Perschau RA, Munson ES, Chapin JC: Pulmonary interstitial edema after multiple venous air emboli, *Anesthesiology* 45:364–366, 1976.

109. Ericsson JA, Gottlieb JD, Sweet RB: Closed-chest cardiac massage in the treatment of venous air embolism, *N Engl J Med* 270:1353–1354, 1964.

110. Hirabuki N, Miura T, Mitomo M, et al: Changes of cerebral air embolism shown by computed tomography, *Br J Radiol* 61:252–255, 1988.

111. Muth C-M, Shank ES: Cerebral arterial gas embolism: Should we hyperventilate these patients? *Intensive Care Med* 30:742–743, 2004.

112. van Hulst RA, Haitsma JJ, Lameris TW, et al: Hyperventilation impairs brain function in acute cerebral air embolism in pigs, *Intensive Care Med* 30:944–950, 2004.

113. Jensen ME, Lipper MH: CT in iatrogenic cerebral air embolism, *AJNR Am J Neuroradiol* 7:823–827, 1986.

114. Warren LP Jr, Djang WT, Moon RE, et al: Neuroimaging of scuba diving injuries to the CNS, *Am J Roentgenol* 151:1003–1008, 1988.

115. Annane D, Troche G, Delisle F, et al: Effects of mechanical ventilation with normobaric oxygen therapy on the rate of air removal from cerebral arteries, *Crit Care Med* 22:851–857, 1994.

116. Dutka AJ: A review of the pathophysiology and potential application of experimental therapies for cerebral ischemia to the treatment of cerebral arterial gas embolism, *Undersea Biomed Res* 12:403–421, 1985.

117. Dutka AJ: Air or gas embolism. In Camporesi EM, Barker AC, editors: *Hyperbaric Oxygen Therapy: A Critical Review*, Bethesda, 1991, Undersea and Hyperbaric Medical Society, pp 1–10.

118. Blanc P, Boussuges A, Henriette K, et al: Iatrogenic cerebral air embolism: Importance of an early hyperbaric oxygenation, *Intensive Care Med* 28:559–563, 2002.

119. Schramm J, Watanabe E, Strauss C, et al: Neurophysiologic monitoring in posterior fossa surgery. I: Technical principles, applicability and limitations, *Acta Neurochir (Wien)* 98:9–18, 1989.

120. Linden RD, Tator CH, Benedict D, et al: Electrophysiological monitoring during acoustic neuroma and other posterior fossa surgery, *Can J Neurol Sci* 15:73–81, 1988.

121. Radtke RA, Erwin CW, Wilkins RH: Intraoperative brainstem auditory evoked potentials: Significant decrease in postoperative morbidity, *Neurology* 39:187–191, 1989.

122. Watanabe E, Schramm J, Strauss C, et al: Neurophysiologic monitoring in posterior fossa surgery. II: BAEP waves I and V and preservation of hearing, *Acta Neurochir (Wien)* 98:118–128, 1989.

123. Grundy BL, Linda A, Procopio PT, et al: Reversible evoked potential changes with retraction of the eighth cranial nerve, *Anesth Analg* 60:835–838, 1981.

124. Radtke RA, Erwin CW: Intraoperative monitoring of auditory and brain-stem function, *Neurol Clin* 6:899–915, 1988.

125. Reasoner DK, Dexter F, Hindman BJ, et al: Somatosensory evoked potentials correlate with neurological outcome in rabbits undergoing cerebral air embolism, *Stroke* 27:1859–1864, 1996.

126. Standefer M, Bay JW, Trusso R: The sitting position in neurosurgery: a retrospective analysis of 488 cases, *Neurosurgery* 14:649–659, 1984.

127. Von Gösseln H, Samii M, Suhr D, et al: The lounging position for posterior fossa surgery: anesthesiological considerations regarding air embolism, *Childs Nerv Syst* 7:568–574, 1991.

128. Bedford RF: Venous air embolism: a historical prospective, *Semin Anesth* 11:169–176, 1983.

129. Senn N: An experimental and clinical study of air embolism, *Ann Surg* 2:129–147, 1885.

130. Voorhies RM, Fraser RA, Van Poznak A: Prevention of air embolism with positive end expiratory pressure, *Neurosurgery* 12:503–506, 1983.

131. Marshall MK, Bedford RF: Use of a pulmonary – artery catheter for detection and treatment of venous air embolism: a prospective study in man, *Anesthesiology* 52:131-134, 1980.

Chapter 13

ANESTHETIC MANAGEMENT OF CEREBRAL ANEURYSM SURGERY

Ryan P. Pong • Arthur M. Lam

Although it is simplistic, the statement by the British neurosurgeon J. Gillingham that "in the early years anaesthetists spent their time pushing the brain out of the skull while in recent times they have been sucking it back in"[1] underscores the importance and contribution of neuroanesthesia to the improved results of the surgical treatment of cerebral aneurysms. Other advances are the improvements in microsurgical instrumentation such as the operating microscope, neuroradiology, and the development of specialized centers with surgeons and anesthesiologists dedicated to the treatment of patients with cerebral aneurysms. However, data published from The International Cooperative Study on the Timing of Aneurysm Surgery (Cooperative Study) in 1990 indicated that overall surgical mortality was high, at approximately 20%.[2,3] To a certain extent these results might have been biased because of the trend toward early operative intervention in high-risk patients who were previously considered unsuitable for surgery. Nonetheless, even patients admitted in good condition with a level of consciousness score equivalent to Hunt and Hess grades I and II (see later discussion) have a "good" recovery rate of only 58% and a mortality rate of 26%.[2] Thus much room exists for improvement in all aspects of cerebral aneurysm treatment. Considerable variations in mortality and morbidity exist among centers of the Cooperative Study, the reasons for which are not apparent. The leading causes of death and disability were, in descending order, vasospasm, the direct effects of the initial bleed (massive subarachnoid, subdural, or intracerebral hematoma, permanent ischemic effects of increased intracranial pressure [ICP]), rebleeding, and surgical complications.[2] Successful anesthetic management of patients with cerebral aneurysms requires a thorough understanding of the natural history, pathophysiology, and surgical requirements of the procedures.

Endovascular treatment using thrombogenic coils is an alternative to surgical treatment. The results of the International Subarachnoid Trial (ISAT) showed that when an aneurysm is amenable to either endovascular coiling or surgical clipping, outcomes favor the coiling.[4,5] Subsequent follow-up studies have questioned this result and have raised questions as to which modality is superior,[6] and there is interest in establishing in which cohort one treatment is favored over the other. Multiple factors must be evaluated, including aneurysm factors such as location and anatomy and patient factors such as age, comorbidities, and patient wishes.[6]

PREOPERATIVE CONSIDERATIONS

The main steps in preoperative evaluation are as follows:
1. Assessment of the patient's neurologic condition and clinical grading of the subarachnoid hemorrhage (SAH).
2. A review of the patient's intracranial pathologic condition, including the performing of computed tomography (CT) and angiograms.
3. Monitoring of ICP and transcranial Doppler ultrasonography (TCD) if available.
4. Evaluation of other systemic functions, premorbid as well as current condition, with emphasis on systems known to be affected by SAH.
5. Communication with the neurosurgeon regarding positioning and special monitoring requirements.
6. Optimization of the patient's condition by correcting any existing biochemical and physiologic disturbances.

The preoperative assessment allows appropriate planning of an anesthetic regimen with consideration of the pathophysiology of all organ systems as well as the surgical and monitoring requirements. This approach facilitates the goals of smooth anesthesia for an uncomplicated aneurysm and ensures a heightened level of preparedness for a complicated one.

The Central Nervous System

To allow better assessment of surgical risk and prognosis, Botterell and colleagues[7] in 1956 first proposed the grading of subarachnoid hemorrhage (Table 13-1),[7] which was later modified by Hunt and Hess (Table 13-2).[8] In the 1980s a grading scale based on the Glasgow Coma Scale was introduced by the World Federation of Neurological Surgeons (Table 13-3).[9] In the World Federation classification, the most important correlate with outcome is the preoperative level of consciousness.[2] These clinical grading schemes allow evaluation of operative risk, communication among physicians about a patient's condition, and conduct of comparative studies of therapy on outcome. The modified Hunt and Hess grading scale is still the most commonly used, because of both familiarity and ease of application.

Despite successful surgical treatment, delayed ischemic neurologic deficits resulting in permanent neurologic injury or death can occur in patients in whom the complication vasospasm develops. Because the incidence and severity of vasospasm is related to the amount of subarachnoid blood present, Computed Tomography (CT) findings are often graded according to the Fisher's grading system (Table 13-4).[10] Despite criticisms of Fisher grading[11] and proposed modifications,[12] it remains the primary method of describing the CT findings with regard to clot burden and the risk of vasospasm in aneurysmal SAH.

Although the surgical mortality and morbidity vary with different institutions, patients in good preoperative condition (assigned to clinical grades I and II) can be expected to do well; patients with grade V status have a high mortality and

Table 13–1 Botterell's Clinical Grades for Patients with Subarachnoid Hemorrhage

Grade	Criteria
I	Conscious with or without meningeal signs
II	Drowsy without significant neurologic deficit
III	Drowsy with neurologic deficit and probable cerebral clot
IV	Major neurologic deficits present
V	Moribund with failing vital centers and extensor rigidity

Data from Botterell EH, Lougheed WM, Scott JW, Vandewater SL: Hypothermia, and interruption of carotid, or carotid and vertebral circulation, in the surgical management of intracranial aneurysms. J Neurosurg 1956;13:1-42.

Table 13–3 World Federation of Neurological Surgeons' Grades for Patients with Subarachnoid Hemorrhage

Grade	Glasgow Coma Scale Score	Motor Deficit
I	15	Absent
II	14-13	Absent
III	14-13	Present
IV	12-7	Present or absent
V	6-3	Present or absent

Data from Report of World Federation of Neurological Surgeons Committee on a Universal Subarachnoid Hemorrhage Grading Scale. J Neurosurg 1988;68:985-986.

Table 13–2 Modified Hunt and Hess Clinical Grades for Patients with Subarachnoid Hemorrhage*

Grades	Criteria
0	Unruptured aneurysm
I	Asymptomatic or minimal headache and slight nuchal rigidity
II	Moderate to severe headache, nuchal rigidity, but no neurologic deficit other than cranial nerve palsy
III	Drowsiness, confusion, or mild focal deficit
IV	Stupor, mild or severe hemiparesis, possible early decerebrate rigidity, vegetative disturbance
V	Deep coma, decerebrate rigidity, moribund appearance

*Serious systemic disease such as hypertension, diabetes, severe arteriosclerosis, chronic pulmonary disease, and severe vasospasm seen on arteriography result in assignment of the patient to the next less favorable category.

Table 13–4 Fisher Grades for Computed Tomography (CT) Findings in Subarachnoid Hemorrhage

Grade	CT Finding(s)
1	No blood detected
2	Diffuse thin layer of subarachnoid blood (vertical layers < 1 mm thick)
3	Localized clot or thick layer of subarachnoid blood (vertical layers ≥ 1 mm thick)
4	Intracerebral or intraventricular blood with diffuse or no subarachnoid blood

Data from Fisher CM, Kistler JP, Davis JM: Relation of cerebral vasospasm to subarachnoid hemorrhage visualized by computerized tomographic scanning. Neurosurgery 1980;6:1-9.

Table 13–5 Surgical Mortality and Major Morbidity of Subarachnoid Hemorrhage According to Clinical Grades*

Grade (Hunt and Hess)	Mortality (%)	Morbidity (%)
0	0-2	0-2
I	2-5	0-2
II	5-10	7
III	5-10	25
IV	20-30	25
V	30-40	35-40

*Pooled from the literature and experience in the author's (A.M.L.) institution.

morbidity, but aggressive management has resulted in substantial improvement (Table 13-5).[13] The clinical grade also indicates the severity of associated cerebral pathophysiology. The higher the clinical grade, the more likely the occurrence of vasospasm, elevated ICP,[14,15] impairment of cerebral autoregulation,[16,17] and a disordered cerebrovascular response to hypocapnia.[17] A worse clinical grade is also associated with a higher incidence of cardiac arrhythmia and myocardial dysfunction.[18,19]

Patients with worse clinical grades have a tendency to become hypovolemic and hyponatremic.[20,21] Thus, understanding the grading scale allows the anesthesiologist to communicate effectively with other physicians and facilitates assessment of pathophysiologic derangements and the planning of perioperative anesthetic management.

Intracranial Pressure

ICP increases rapidly after an SAH and may approach the levels of the systemic blood pressure. This phase lasts minutes and is thought to limit the amount of blood leakage through the ruptured aneurysm. With recurrent rupture of the aneurysm, ICP increases further from mass effect (clot), cerebral edema, or hydrocephalus due to a blocked aqueduct. A communicating hydrocephalus may later develop because of arachnoidal adhesions from the extravascular blood that interferes with reabsorption of cerebrospinal fluid (CSF). In several large studies the incidence of hydrocephalus ranged from 15%[2] to 41%.[22] Elevated ICP with hypovolemia may increase the likelihood of delayed cerebral ischemia and infarction.[21] Patients with SAH generally have decreased cerebral blood flow (CBF) and cerebral metabolic rate.[23,24] The development of vasospasm can also exacerbate a rise in ICP because the reduction in CBF resulting from vasoconstriction of large conductance vessels is accompanied by vasodilation in the distal vessels, leading to an increase in cerebral blood volume (CBV) and a subsequent rise in ICP. Another factor that would contribute to increases in ICP is an intracerebral (17%) or intraventricular (17%) hematoma.[2] Clinically, hydrocephalus is characterized by progressive obtundation and nonreactive small pupils. The clinical features are present in only about 50% of cases, and therefore radiologic diagnosis is essential. However, the causal relation between acute hydrocephalus and delayed cerebral ischemia remains in question.[25]

ICP correlates well with clinical grade. It is generally normal in patients with grade I and II status but is elevated in those with grade IV and V status (Fig. 13-1). However, a normal ICP does not necessarily imply normal intracranial compliance (elastance). It is important not to normalize the ICP too rapidly, because doing so may increase the transmural pressure (TMP) gradient across the aneurysm wall and cause further hemorrhage. A cerebral perfusion pressure (CPP) value of 60 to 80 mm Hg is a reasonable goal.[26]

Impairment of Autoregulation and Carbon Dioxide Reactivity

Patients with SAH have both an impairment in autoregulatory capacity[27] and a rightward shift in the lower limit of autoregulation. The severity of autoregulatory impairment correlates directly with the clinical grade.[16,17,27] Nornes and colleagues[28] observed that the lower limit of autoregulation was significantly higher in patients with clinical grade III than in those with clinical grade I and II during intracranial surgery. The development of impaired autoregulation closely correlates with the occurrence of vasospasm.[29] This impaired autoregulation in the presence of vasospasm may result in delayed ischemic deficits.[30,31]

If neurologic deterioration occurs, it is vital to review the hemodynamic measurements for any associated relationship. Many well-documented cases describe patients with SAH in whom a new neurologic deficit developed in association with a decrease in blood pressure and a subsequent reversal of the deficit with a pharmacologically induced increase in blood pressure.[32] Thus, the anesthesiologist must not allow

the perfusion pressure to decrease below this lower limit perioperatively. This situation represents a relative contraindication to induced hypotension during surgery, as discussed later. One study looked at outcome in relation to the incidence and magnitude of decrease in blood pressure and failed to find any difference in poor outcomes.[33] While seemingly tolerated, induced hypotension may predispose to inadequate CPP values as well as exacerbate elevated ICP and so is best avoided.

The cerebrovascular response to hyperventilation is generally preserved after SAH.[16,17] Although impairment of autoregulation may occur in patients assigned relatively good clinical grades, a decline in CO_2 reactivity does not occur until there is severe damage.[17] Thus hyperventilation remains effective in reducing CBF and CBV during perioperative management for most patients and potentially could improve autoregulation in those compromised by the SAH.[34]

Systemic Effects

Intravascular Volume Status and Hyponatremia

The intravascular volume status has been found to be abnormally low in 36% to 100% of patients with SAH, and the level of hypovolemia correlates with the clinical grade.[21,35] Moreover, patients with signs of increased ICP on CT scan have a greater likelihood of systemic hypovolemia.[21] The reasons are multifactorial and probably include bed rest, supine diuresis, negative nitrogen balance, decreased erythropoiesis, and iatrogenic blood loss. Hypovolemia may exacerbate vasospasm and is associated with cerebral ischemia and infarction.[21,35,36]

Paradoxically, hypovolemia has often been observed to be associated with hyponatremia, which is observed in approximately 30% to 57%[37,38] of cases of SAH. The etiology of hyponatremia is still a matter of debate. The syndrome of inappropriate antidiuretic hormone secretion has been implicated,[38] treatment for which consists of fluid restriction. However, the preponderance of data now suggests that the hyponatremia is related to release of natriuretic peptides—which has been referred to as *cerebral salt wasting syndrome*.[39] Whether the peptides are released from the hypothalamus in response to hydrocephalus that causes distention of the cerebral ventricles[8,24] or released from the walls of the myocardium[40] is unknown. The release of brain natriuretic peptide has been correlated with cerebral vasospasm and hyponatremia.[41,42]

Other significant electrolyte abnormalities are hypokalemia and hypocalcemia. In a series of 406 patients with SAH, both hypokalemia (serum K^+ value < 3.4 mmol/L) and hypocalcemia (serum Ca^{2+} value 2.2 mmol/L) were noted (in 41% and 74% of cases, respectively).[43]

Cardiac Effects

The effects of SAH on the myocardium can range from alterations in the electrocardiogram, to leakage of cardiac troponins to wall motion abnormalities evident on echocardiography. Preexisting coronary artery disease in the setting of the profound stress induced by SAH may result in myocardial ischemia. However, the majority of patients with cardiac dysfunction secondary to SAH has normal coronary artery anatomy and suffers from a neurogenic stressed myocardium.[44]

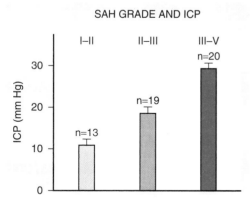

SAH GRADE AND ICP

Figure 13–1 The relationship between grade of subarachnoid hemorrhage (SAH) (Hunt and Hess) and intracranial pressure (ICP). *(Data From Voldby B, Enevoldsen EM: Intracranial pressure changes following aneurysm rupture. Part 1: Clinical and angiographic correlations. J Neurosurg 1982;56:186-196.)*

Electrocardiographic Changes

Electrocardiographic (ECG) abnormalities occur in 40% to 100% of patients with SAH.[45,46] These abnormalities include sinus bradycardia, sinus tachycardia, atrioventricular dissociation, and bradycardia-tachycardia to more serious and potentially life-threatening rhythms such as ventricular tachycardia and fibrillation. Morphologic changes in the ECG tracing include T-wave inversion, depression of the ST segment, the appearance of U waves, prolonged QT interval, and, rarely, Q waves. A prolonged QT interval may occur in 20% to 41% of patients predisposing them to dangerous ventricular arrhythmias. Atrial arrhythmias including fibrillation and flutter occur in 4% of patients and have been found to be associated with a higher risk of severe disability and death.[47] The incidence of ECG changes correlates with the amount of intracranial blood, patients with Fisher grades 3 and 4 CT findings having more abnormalities.[46] Potassium and calcium abnormalities may contribute to the ECG changes.

Myocardial Function

After SAH, damage to the myocardium can be indicated by an increase in circulating levels of cardiac Troponin I (cTi) found in 17% to 68% of patients.[48,49] This cTi elevation following SAH-induced myocardial insult is much less than that related to myocardial infarction.[50] Elevation of cTi has been found to be associated with regional wall motion abnormalities and left ventricular dysfunction[49] as well as hypotension, delayed cerebral ischemia from vasospasm, and death and disability at 90 days.[49,51]

Echocardiography of patients with SAH has shown depressed left ventricular function and regional wall motion abnormalities in 13% to 18% of cases.[19,52] Predictors of ventricular dysfunction include elevated cTi,[19,49,50] poor clinical grade (Hunt and Hess III to V),[19,52] and female gender.[52]

The mechanism of myocardial dysfunction has garnered much attention lately, leading to the proposal of several mechanisms.[44] The arterial supply to the heart has been implicated. Multivessel coronary artery spasm seems unlikely, given that the available coronary angiographic studies demonstrate normal coronary structure even in the presence of ongoing ECG and echocardiographic evidence of myocardial dysfunction.[53,54] Currently the favored mechanism is increased release of localized catecholamines in the myocardium. This intense stimulation leads to contraction band necrosis and subsequent myocardial dysfunction. The fact that regional wall motion abnormalities span the myocardium in a pattern outside the territories of known coronary artery distributions lends credence to this theory.[55]

Takotsubo cardiomyopathy has been reported in aneurysmal subarachnoid hemorrhage.[56] and typically, ventricular dysfunction secondary to SAH is associated with apical sparing.[55] The prognosis of SAH-induced ventricular dysfunction is good and generally reversible.[57]

Anesthetic Implications

Patients with prolonged QT interval, T-wave abnormalities, and Q waves should undergo prompt correction of electrolyte disturbances. Experimentally, pharmacologic or surgical blockade of the sympathetic nervous system prevents or abolishes these ECG changes. However, no evidence exists that the prophylactic administration of a β-adrenergic or other autonomic antagonist significantly alters the outcome in such patients, and the use of these agents for this purpose is probably not warranted.[58]

Q waves and other ECG evidence of ischemia are always worrisome and, when observed in a patient with SAH, pose a diagnostic dilemma. Although most ECG abnormalities after SAH appear to be neurogenic rather than cardiogenic in nature, diagnostic difficulty has on occasion led to a delay in surgery. Moreover, microscopic hemorrhages and myocytolysis have been observed in a postmortem study, although other studies have reported no signs of myocardial damage.

The three possibilities for ECG abnormalities consistent with infarction are: (1) coincidental acute myocardial infarction, (2) SAH-induced myocardial infarction, and (3) ECG changes without infarction. Cardiac enzyme measurements and echocardiography should be obtained in suspicious cases. As with any surgical procedure, the decision to proceed with surgery should be based on a risk-benefit analysis and therefore depends on the urgency of the situation. Because of the risk of rebleeding, surgical therapy of a ruptured aneurysm is almost always considered urgent.

In summary, ECG changes are prevalent after SAH and likely represent hyperactivity of the sympathetic system with increased levels of norepinephrine. Although in some patients there is no myocardial pathologic condition, in others there may be ventricular dysfunction, and in rare cases necrosis and other myopathology can occur. In suspicious cases, serial cTi measurements should be obtained. Because the electrocardiographic changes reflect the severity of neurologic damage and have not been shown to materially contribute to perioperative mortality or morbidity,[59] the decision to operate should not be influenced by these ECG changes. These considerations, however, may influence the decision about the choice of invasive monitoring. The various ECG changes and their potential correlation with ventricular dysfunction and pathology are summarized in Table 13-6.

Respiratory System

Pulmonary edema has been observed to accompany SAH in 8% to 28% of cases,[60,61] and in addition to a sympathetic mechanism, an inflammatory component has been implicated.[62] Parallel to myocardial dysfunction, the incidence of pulmonary edema is correlated closely with clinical grade.[60] Aspiration and hydrostatic pneumonia are other potential complications.

Table 13–6 Electrocardiography and Myocardial Dysfunctions seen in Subarachnoid Hemorrhage*

Benign changes	Sinus bradycardia
	Sinus tachycardia
	Atrioventricular dissociation
	Premature ventricular contractions
	Nonspecific ST segment depression
	T wave inversion
	U wave
Possible and actual wall motion abnormalities	Symmetrical T wave inversion[217,218]
	Prolonged QT interval > 500 msec[218]
	ST segment elevation[219]
	Left ventricular dysfunction with apical sparing[49]
	Regional wall motion abnormalities[19]
Possible and actual myocardial injury	Q wave
	ST segment elevation
	Elevated myocardial enzyme values
	Elevated troponin I value

*Superscript numbers are chapter references.

Other Major Medical Problems

On the basis of the findings of the Cooperative Study, other major medical problems associated with SAH are systemic hypertension (21%), heart disease (3%), and diabetes mellitus (2%).[2]

Concurrent Medical Treatments

Patients receiving diuretic therapy for chronic hypertension may have preexisting fluid and electrolyte problems before SAH.

Anticonvulsant medications such as phenytoin and carbamazepine antagonize the actions of nondepolarizing agents such as pancuronium and vecuronium, leading to higher dose requirements and shortened duration of action for muscle relaxants. Acute anticonvulsant therapy of less than 7 days' duration probably has little effect. The mechanism is unclear but is probably pharmacodynamic rather than pharmacokinetic in origin. Although the results are not consistent, atracurium appears to be less affected than other nondepolarizing agents. One report suggests that anticonvulsant therapy also increases fentanyl requirements. The effect of the newer anticonvulsants lamotrigine and levetiracetam on nondepolarizing agents has not been rigorously studied. However, preliminary data indicate that higher doses are not needed and shortened duration of neuromuscular blockade does not occur.[63]

Some hospitals continue to use antifibrinolytic agents such as ε-aminocaproic acid and tranexamic acid to prevent rebleeding while the patient is waiting for surgery. Although these agents have been found to decrease the risk of rebleeding, they are associated with a risk of cerebral ischemia, and no overall benefit has been shown for their use.[64] The anesthesiologist should be aware that patients on antifibrinlytics may have a greater incidence of vasospasm and hydrocephalus. They also have a higher incidence of venous thrombosis and pulmonary embolism. Use of recombinant factor VII (rFVIIIa) to decrease the incidence of rebleeding has been deterred by critical thrombosis in an early trial.[65]

Calcium channel antagonists (usually oral nimodipine) are now routinely administered for vasospasm prophylaxis. This therapy has specific anesthetic implications that are discussed later.

Timing of Surgery

The two major complications contributing to significant morbidity and mortality after SAH are rebleeding and vasospasm, with each accounting for about 7% of mortality.[2] Because the brain is acutely swollen with fresh clots following SAH, it was generally believed that early operation increases the incidence of postoperative vasospasm. The Cooperative Study data influenced most surgeons to wait 7 to 10 days for the acute inflammatory process to subside before any operative intervention. Indeed, results from the Cooperative Study indicate that the brain was considered "tight" in 50% of cases with early surgery (same day as SAH), but in only 20% of cases undergoing operation after 10 days (Fig. 13-2).[3] Although delaying surgery does allow brain swelling to decrease, both rebleeding and vasospasm can occur during this waiting period. When surgery was delayed, antifibrinolytic agents were usually given to prevent lysis of the clot and rebleeding from the rent of the aneurysm. However, randomized clinical trials showed that

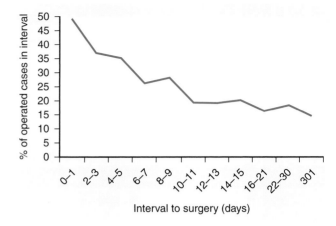

Figure 13–2 The percentage of patients with a "tight" brain during surgical exposure correlated with the number of day(s) after subarachnoid hemorrhage that the operation was performed. *(From Kassell NF, Torner JC, Haley EC Jr, et al: The International Cooperative Study on the Timing of Aneurysm Surgery. Part 1: Overall management results. J Neurosurg 1990;73:18-36.)*

although these agents are effective in reducing the incidence of rebleeding, the incidence of vasospasm increases, leaving the overall morbidity and mortality unchanged.

In an attempt to improve the overall outcome, there is a growing trend toward early operation, so that the risk of rebleeding can be eliminated and any vasospasm more aggressively treated. However, the results from the Cooperative Study showed that the overall management results for early (3 days or sooner) and late (after 10 days) surgery are not significantly different, although the results were the worst when surgery was performed between 7 and 10 days.[2] A subsequent analysis of data derived from only North American centers varied from the overall findings and indicated that the best results were achieved when surgery was planned within 3 days of SAH, therefore arguing strongly in favor of early surgery.[66] Although they should never be the primary consideration, substantial economic savings are also realized with early surgery. The trend toward early operation will probably continue, and patients in less-than-ideal condition for surgery will be coming to the operating room.

Rebleeding

Previous studies suggest that rebleeding following the initial SAH peaks at the end of the first week. The Cooperative Study data indicate that rebleeding peaks at 4% during the first 24 hours and then levels off at 1.5% per day on subsequent days. The overall incidence is 11%,[66] which accounts for 8% of the mortality and disability.[2] The incidence is lower in patients receiving antifibrinolytic agents.[2] Rebleeding remains a major threat in hospitals where delayed surgery is the standard practice. With the trend toward early operation, the risk of rebleeding is reduced but not eliminated. A combination of antifibrinolytic therapy for rebleeding and a calcium channel blocker for vasospasm has been suggested as a possible remedy.[67]

Vasospasm

INCIDENCE

In patients who initially survive a SAH, cerebral vasospasm causing ischemia or infarction remains an important cause of morbidity and mortality. In the Cooperative Study, vasospasm accounted for 13.5% of the overall mortality and major morbidity.[2] Not all patients with SAH have vasospasm, and the severity, time course, and prognosis of vasospasm are largely unpredictable. The incidence and severity of delayed cerebral vasospasm have been shown to correlate with the amount and location of blood in the basal cisterns. The frequency of occurrence as determined by angiography is estimated to be 40% to 60%. However, clinically significant and symptomatic vasospasm occurs at a lower frequency (20% to 30%). The difference may be explained by the varying severity of vasospasm. It has been established that the lower limit of CBF compatible with normal brain function is approximately 15 to 20 mL/100 g/min. Thus considerable reduction in CBF can occur from vasospasm without clinical symptoms. Of patients in whom symptomatic vasospasm develops, approximately 50% die or are left with a serious residual neurologic deficit. Typically, angiographically detectable vasospasm is not seen until 72 hours after SAH, the incidence peaks 7 days after SAH, and the problem is seldom seen after 2 weeks. Endovascular aneurysm therapy and surgical clipping of the aneurysm appear to have the same incidences of vasospasm.[68]

Pathogenesis. The vasospastic artery has structural and pathologic changes within the vessel wall, such as swelling and necrosis of the smooth muscle cells. Although the exact mechanism and cause of spasm have not been completely elucidated, a reasonable hypothesis is that one or more vasoactive substances contained in the blood in the basal cisterns induce changes in the cerebral arteries to cause severe constriction. The component in the blood implicated in the pathogenesis of vasospasm is currently thought to be oxyhemoglobin.[69] The normal cerebrovascular tone is regulated by a balance between vasodilating and vasoconstricting factors. The suppressive interaction of oxyhemoglobin with endothelium-derived relaxing factor or nitric oxide (potent vasodilator) coupled with stimulated production of endothelin (potent vasoconstrictor) is the postulated cause of cerebral vasospasm. In experimental vasospasm, the rises in perivascular concentrations of oxyhemoglobin and deoxyhemoglobin parallel the time course of vasospasm.[70] In support of this hypothesis, early intracranial operation (within 48 hours) to remove extravasated subarachnoid blood has been shown to be effective in reducing the occurrence of vasospasm and associated neurologic deterioration. Delayed cerebral ischemia occurred only in patients in whom the subarachnoid blood clot remained in the cisterns. Because subarachnoid blood may be widely dispersed from a ruptured aneurysm, the removal of blood must be aggressive and extensive, including from tissue beyond the vicinity of the aneurysm and the adjacent cisterns. Instillation of human recombinant tissue plasminogen activator into the subarachnoid space is effective in lysing the clot and also reduces the severity of vasospasm.[71,72]

CLINICAL MANIFESTATIONS

Delayed cerebral ischemia from vasospasm after SAH is a multivascular or diffuse process in most patients. The clinical manifestations of vasospasm include a decrease in the level of consciousness, new onset of focal signs, and mutism. In a prospective study, Hijdra and associates[73] found that the majority of patients with delayed cerebral ischemia from vasospasm had decrease in level of consciousness that was sometimes accompanied by but never preceded by focal signs. Clinical manifestations most commonly appear gradually but may also occur abruptly.

DIAGNOSIS

After the appearance of new focal signs or a decrease in level of consciousness, the diagnosis of cerebral vasospasm is confirmed by angiography. A CT scan may show hypodense lesions in brain areas that are consistent with the clinical signs. The diagnosis of vasospasm may also be predicted or anticipated before the onset of clinical vasospasm with the use of TCD. With vasospasm, cerebral artery flow velocities increase,[74] although confirmation with angiography is necessary. The noninvasive technology of TCD also allows continual evaluation of the patient in vasospasm without resorting to frequent angiographic investigations. However, in patients treated with hypertensive therapy, increase in flow velocity may represent increase in local cerebral blood flow instead of worsening vasospasm.[75,76] Radiologic confirmation with angiography, single-photon emission computerized tomography (SPECT), or xenon CT cerebral blood flow studies may be necessary.

TREATMENT

Pharmacologic. Numerous drugs have been investigated for prevention or treatment of vasospasm, but most are ineffective. Calcium channel blockers, of which nimodipine has been most extensively studied, are the only class of drugs that have been shown to consistently reduce the morbidity and mortality from vasospasm. Depending on the study, the incidence of poor outcome is reduced by 40% to 70%.[77] Interestingly, none of these studies with favorable results for calcium channel blocker prophylaxis was able to demonstrate any significant change in the incidence or severity of vasospasm, suggesting that the beneficial effects of nimodipine may be occurring at either a distal vessel site or a cellular level. The only study that demonstrated a significant improvement in angiographic vasospasm with a calcium channel blocker used the experimental agent fasudil hydrochloride (AT877). Its use has yielded clinical outcomes similar to those for nimodipine.[78] High-dose intravenous nicardipine has been investigated for prevention of vasospasm. Although the incidence of symptomatic vasospasm was reduced from 38% to 25%, there was no difference in outcome at 3 months, presumably because hypervolemic hypertensive therapy is effective in ameliorating the ischemic deficits from vasospasm.[79]

Because cerebral vasospasm is frequently the cause of poor outcomes after successful surgical or endovascular treatment, there are many investigations looking for new pharmacologic therapies. Magnesium sulfate is thought to be a cerebral vasodilator by way of blocking voltage-dependent calcium channels. This property, paired with its ability to antagonize *N*-methyl-D-aspartate receptors, thereby limiting the damaging excitatory glutamate stimulation, has led to many preliminary studies. So far, magnesium sulfate has shown a similar efficacy in replacing nimodipine,[80] and when use of these two agents in conjunction has led to positive results in decreasing vasospasm and improving outcome.[81] The enthusiasm, however, must be tempered with the concern for hypotension and hypocalcemia that accompany its use.[82] Endothelin receptor antagonists, in early and small trials, have shown ability to prevent[83] as well as treat established vasospasm.[84] The evolution in the uses of statins has reached the realm of cerebral vasospasm, via the anti-inflammatory and modulating effect on the cerebral vasculature. Initially, in two small prospective studies, statins reduced the incidence of vasospasm significantly.[85-87] However, a larger follow-up retrospective study by

Kramer and associates[88] casts doubt on the efficacy of statins because they were unable to show any benefit from its use. Large-scale randomized and blinded studies are needed before use of any of these therapies becomes routine.

Several other medications have shown early promise but since have failed to materialize into clinical use. Of these, tirilazad, a potent lipid peroxidation inhibitor that was reported to have positive results in a European trial,[89] failed to demonstrate any improvement over placebo in North American trials.[90] Nicaraven, a hydroxyl radical scavenger, afforded a 35% reduction in the incidence of delayed ischemic deficits at 1 month. However, the results were no longer favorable at 3 months.[91]

Nonpharmacologic

Surgical. The presence of subarachnoid blood is related to the occurrence of vasospasm both qualitatively and quantitatively. By operating on patients with SAH within 48 hours of hemorrhage, Taneda[92] reduced the incidence of delayed ischemic deficits from 25% (11 of 44 patients who underwent surgery 10 days or more after the hemorrhage) to 11% (11 of 101 patients). Thus early operation with extensive irrigation of the cisterns may have lowered the incidence or severity of vasospasm.

Reduction of ICP. If the patient has elevated ICP, cerebral perfusion may be improved by lowering of the ICP. Improvement in neurologic status with this treatment alone has been reported.

Hypervolemic, Hypertensive, and Hemodilution Therapy. The most consistently effective regimen now available to prevent and treat ischemic neurologic deficits due to cerebral vasospasm uses hypervolemia, hypertension, and hemodilution (triple-H therapy). The rationale behind induced hypervolemia and hypertension is that in SAH the ischemic areas of the brain have impaired autoregulation and thus CBF depends on perfusion pressure, which partly depends on the intravascular volume and mean arterial blood pressure.[93,94]

This therapy is most successful if instituted early, when the neurologic deficits are mild and before the onset of infarction.[32] However, prophylactic treatment initiated before aneurysm clipping is associated with a significant risk of rebleeding (19% in one series). Other concerns are worsening of cerebral edema, increasing ICP, and causing hemorrhage into an infarcted area. With early surgery there is less likelihood of rebleeding from the hypervolemic, hypertensive therapy.[95] Other systemic complications are pulmonary edema (7%-17%), myocardial infarction (2%), dilutional hyponatremia (3%-35%), and coagulopathy (3%).[32]

To optimize therapy and minimize the potential cardiovascular and pulmonary complications, the use of invasive monitors, including arterial blood pressure and either central venous pressure (CVP) or pulmonary artery catheter (PAC), is essential. Sufficient intravenous fluids are infused to raise the CVP to 10 mm Hg or the pulmonary artery wedge pressure (PAWP) to 12 to 20 mm Hg.[32,94,95] In a study in which a Starling curve was constructed in nine patients with ruptured intracranial aneurysm, Levy and Giannotta[94] observed that raising the PAWP from 8 to 14 mm Hg correlated with significant increases in left ventricular stroke work index, stroke volume index, and cardiac index. However, further volume expansion to raise PAWP to above 14 mm Hg resulted in a decline in the cardiac index. No correlation existed between changes in CVP and changes in PAWP during volume expansion. They recommend that PAWP should be the variable to observe during hypervolemic therapy.[94] Because a growing

number of studies have implicated PACs as increasing complication rates with no improvement in outcome,[96] it is our practice not to routinely place a PAC to guide triple-H therapy. Select cases where neurogenic cardiac stunning may complicate triple-H therapy may warrant the addition of a PAC to guide fluid therapy.

Hypervolemia is generally achieved with infusions of colloids (e.g., 5% albumin) as well as crystalloids. Hetastarch and dextran solutions should be used sparingly or not at all because of the potential complication of coagulopathy through interference with platelets and factor VIII.[97,98] Trumble and colleagues[99] examined the use of hetastarch for hypervolemic treatment of vasospasm and reported the occurrence of coagulation abnormalities in all patients. Thus they were unable to formulate any dose guideline for its safe use. The lower-molecular-weight dextran (pentastarch) appears to be associated with fewer coagulation problems.[100] Although intravenous fluid loading alone is often effective,[32] it is at times insufficient to raise the blood pressure or reverse ischemic symptoms; vasopressors are then initiated to induce hypertension. The most widely used vasopressors are dopamine, dobutamine, and phenylephrine. The hypertensive, hypervolemic therapy may induce a vagal response as well as a profound diuresis, requiring administration of large amounts of intravenous fluids. Atropine (1 mg intramuscularly every 3 to 4 hours) may be given to maintain the heart rate between 80 and 120 beats/min, and aqueous vasopressin (Pitressin) (5 units intramuscularly) may be administered to maintain the urine output at less than 200 mL/hr. With this regimen, often only small amounts of vasopressor drugs are required.[32] The blood pressure is titrated to a level necessary to reverse the signs and symptoms of vasospasm or to a maximum of 160 to 200 mm Hg systolic in the patient whose aneurysm has been clipped.[32] If the aneurysm has not been clipped, the systolic blood pressure is increased to only 120 to 150 mm Hg. The elevated blood pressure must be maintained until the vasospasm resolves, usually in 3 to 7 days. Response to therapy can now be monitored noninvasively with TCD. Improvement in vasospasm may be associated with a decrease in flow velocity, however, so angiography may be necessary.

Hemodilution, the last component of the triple-H therapy, is based on the correlation of hematocrit and whole blood viscosity. As the hematocrit and viscosity diminish, the cerebrovascular resistance correspondingly decreases and CBF increases. One argument against hemodilution is that oxygen-carrying capacity is also reduced. Experimental studies have suggested that a hematocrit of 33% provides an optimal balance between viscosity and oxygen-carrying capacity, and this value has been applied clinically. With the growing concern about greater morbidity and mortality with blood transfusion, this value is now often revised downwards to between 27% and 30%.

Transluminal Angioplasty. In all major vessels that are accessible, transluminal angioplasty has been used in patients with vasospasm refractory to conventional treatment, reversal of deficits being achieved in 65% of the patients treated.[101] The time frame for institution of angioplastic therapy, or even its prophylactic use, has not yet been established. In distal vessels that are not accessible for angioplasty, the administration of vasodilators (papaverine, verapamil, milrinone) via superselective intra-arterial infusion has been shown to be effective. Improvement in cerebral venous oxygen saturation and metabolic profile with this treatment has been demonstrated.[102]

For vessels that are accessible, however, transluminal balloon angioplasty appears to be superior to papaverine treatment.[103] Although rare, complications from intra-arterial papaverine infusion include severe thrombocytopenia,[104] increase in ICP,[105] and transient brainstem dysfunction (when infused into the posterior circulation).[106] Intraoperative cisternal injection of papaverine to reduce the risk of vasospasm has also been reported to cause transient pupillary dysfunction, which may interfere with neurologic assessment.[107] The newer vasodilators used for intra-arterial injection seem to decrease these side effects, although their efficacy and safety have not been fully evaluated.[108,109] Intrathecal use of nicardipine[110] and nimodipine[111] in initial studies has shown some benefit in the treatment of vasospasm. Intraventricular administration of sodium nitroprusside has also been reported to reverse vasospasm refractory to conventional triple-H therapy.[112]

ANESTHETIC CONSIDERATIONS

Hypertensive Therapy. The anesthetic management of patients who have or are at risk for vasospasm requires an understanding of the natural course of vasospasm, concurrent therapy, the importance of intravascular volume status, the changes in electrolyte concentration that occur with the treatment of vasospasm, and which hemodynamic variables are associated with vasospasm. Although it is generally believed that early surgery raises the risk of vasospasm, there are no substantiating data, and some data suggest otherwise.[2,95] Further investigations indicate that the interplay of vasospasm and surgical timing must account for the severity of the bleeding.[113]

Asymptomatic patients at risk for vasospasm include all patients who undergo surgery before the onset of vasospasm. Although it is not possible to predict the occurrence of postoperative vasospasm, patients with good SAH grades and low Fisher grade tend to have a lower incidence. These patients should be kept in a normovolemic state, with volume loading initiated toward the end of the operation, after the aneurysm has been clipped. Intraoperatively, controlled hypotension can be provided safely, if so requested by the surgeon.[114] Treatment of postoperative hypertension should not be too aggressive.

Some physicians consider patients who are symptomatic from vasospasm as being at high risk and not eligible for surgery. Many other surgeons, however, believe the most effective treatment of vasospasm is immediate clipping of the aneurysm so that aggressive hypertensive and hypervolemic therapy can be implemented. Symptomatic patients presenting for emergency clipping of aneurysms should be treated aggressively, and hypervolemia should be maintained and guided with invasive monitoring. For patients who have already been treated with hypertensive therapy, the threshold blood pressure below which the patient becomes symptomatic must be noted, and the blood pressure should not be allowed to fall below this value. Buckland and coworkers[115] have advocated intraoperative induced hypertension as a prophylactic measure. This approach, however, must be balanced against the risk of rerupture of the aneurysm as well as increased brain swelling and difficulty with intraoperative brain retraction. Because the main aim must be to maintain adequate CPP, induced hypotension is contraindicated in these patients.

With respect to asymptomatic patients who undergo operation on a delayed basis, vasospasm seldom occurs more than 12 days after SAH. Therefore patients who have surgery later than 10 to 12 days after SAH have a low risk of vasospasm and can be managed in a normal fashion.

Calcium Channel Antagonists. Calcium channel antagonists have a proven efficacy in reducing the neurologic complications of vasospasm. In most institutions, all patients with SAH are prophylactically treated with nimodipine. Clinical experience suggests that these drugs do not present any difficulty for anesthetic management, although 5% of the patients who receive nimodipine and 23% of the patients who receive intravenous nicardipine demonstrate mild hypotension as a result of systemic vasodilation. A similar tendency toward lower systemic blood pressure was also observed intraoperatively, and there was a reduced demand for hypotensive agents when controlled hypotension was used.

Premedication

To allow accurate assessment of the patient's immediate preoperative neurologic condition and clinical grade, preoperative medications are best omitted. A proper preoperative visit by the anesthesiologist with a thorough explanation usually obviates any need for preoperative medication. However, an anxious patient may become hypertensive, with greater risk of rebleeding. On the other hand, premedications such as barbiturates and narcotics may cause respiratory depression, resulting in an increase in CBF and CBV; therefore such medication must be used judiciously in patients with elevated ICP. Premedication should be individualized. Patients with a good clinical grade may receive morphine, 1 to 5 mg, and/or midazolam, 1 to 5 mg, intravenously for sedation. Best results are achieved when administration is titrated in 1-mg increments. Patients already treated with mechanical ventilation may receive higher doses (morphine, 10 to 20 mg; midazolam, 5 to 10 mg) if hemodynamic stability is maintained. Muscle relaxants may also be required for transport of intubated patients. Patients should continue to receive their regular doses of nimodipine and dexamethasone.

INTRAOPERATIVE CONSIDERATIONS AND INDUCTION OF ANESTHESIA

The incidence of aneurysm rupture during induction of anesthesia, although rare (reported to be 2% in one series but probably less than 1% with modern anesthetic techniques), is usually precipitated by a sudden rise in blood pressure during tracheal intubation and is associated with a high mortality. Therefore the goal during induction of anesthesia for aneurysm surgery is to reduce the risk of aneurysm rupture by minimizing the TMP while simultaneously maintaining an adequate CPP. As illustrated in Figure 13-3, both TMP and CPP are determined by the same equation, mean arterial blood pressure (MAP) minus ICP (MAP − ICP). Therefore these goals represent opposite objectives. Ideally the TMP or CPP should be kept at the preoperative value throughout the induction period, particularly in patients with good SAH grades, however, this is not always possible.

As a general principle, the patient's blood pressure should be reduced to 20% to 25% below the baseline value, and prophylaxis for the normal hypertensive response to intubation should be instituted before tracheal intubation is attempted. Another useful approach is to balance the risk of ischemia from a reduction in CPP against the benefit of a reduced chance of aneurysmal rupture from a decrease in TMP, taking into consideration the patient's clinical grade. Patients with SAH grades 0, I, and II generally have normal

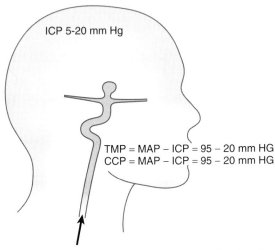

ICP 5-20 mm Hg

TMP = MAP – ICP = 95 – 20 mm HG
CCP = MAP – ICP = 95 – 20 mm HG

Figure 13–3 Determinants of transmural pressure (TMP) and cerebral perfusion pressure (CPP). Both are determined by the difference between mean arterial pressure (MAP) and intracranial pressure (ICP) and are therefore numerically identical.

ICP and are not experiencing acute ischemia.[29] Therefore these patients will tolerate a bigger transient decrease in blood pressure (30% to 35%, or systolic blood pressure at about 100 mm Hg). In contrast, patients with poor clinical grades frequently have increased ICP,[29] low CPP, and ischemia. The elevated ICP decreases the TMP and partially protects the aneurysm from rerupture. These patients may not tolerate transient hypotension as well, and the duration and magnitude of blood pressure decrease should be moderated. The same consideration applies to the use of hyperventilation. Patients with a good clinical grade should not be hyperventilated, because the reduction in CBF will lead to a reduction in ICP and, consequently, an increase in TMP. Conversely, patients with poor clinical grades should be managed with moderate hyperventilation to improve cerebral perfusion. To reduce the risk of aneurysm rupture or ischemia, the change in TMP or CPP should always be gradual, not abrupt.

If these principles and objectives are adhered to, a variety of anesthetic agents and techniques can be used successfully. Irrespective of the technique used, vigilant monitoring of blood pressure is required, which may be achieved by direct intra-arterial blood pressure monitoring.

Conceptually, it is convenient to think of the induction phase as consisting of two parts, (1) induction to achieve loss of consciousness and (2) prophylaxis to prevent a rise in blood pressure in response to laryngoscopy and intubation.

Induction

Achieve Loss of Consciousness

Propofol (1.5 to 2 mg/kg), or thiopental (3 to 5 mg/kg) in combination with fentanyl (3 to 5 μg/kg) or sufentanil (0.3 to 0.5 μg/kg) is suitable. Propofol has superseded thiopental, and remifentanil or fentanyl are the preferred narcotics. Other alternatives are etomidate (0.3 to 0.4 mg/kg) and midazolam (0.1 to 0.2 mg/kg). Propofol is similar in action to thiopental. It reduces CBF and metabolic rate,[116] and with careful titration (1.5 to 2.5 mg/kg) it can be used without compromising cerebral perfusion.

Regarding the use of narcotics, Marx and associates[117] observed that sufentanil may cause an increase in ICP in patients with supratentorial tumors and suggested that this increase may be secondary to cerebral vasodilation. However, both fentanyl and sufentanil have been shown to raise ICP in patients with head trauma,[118] and Trindle and colleagues[119] reported that both agents increase CBF velocity. Other investigators, however, were unable to document either an increase in flow or a change in ICP with sufentanil.[120,121] Similarly, Mayberg and coworkers[122] did not observe an increase in flow velocity or ICP with alfentanil.[122] In view of these studies, the mechanism of the rise in ICP remains unclear and may be related to the simultaneous decrease in systemic blood pressure resulting in autoregulation-mediated compensatory vasodilation. The study by Werner and associates[123] in patients with head injury supports this possibility; they observed an increase in ICP only in the patient group in whom systemic hypotension developed after sufentanil administration. This mechanism has been questioned by de Nadal and colleagues,[124] who found that autoregulatory status was not predictive of ICP changes induced with opioids in head-injured patients.

These studies leave the mechanism of ICP change with opioids in question, although the importance of maintaining normotension with administration of synthetic narcotics cannot be neglected. When used in combination with a vasoconstrictive agent such as thiopental or propofol, these narcotics should be safe for use in patients with SAH, although mild hyperventilation should be instituted in patients with elevated ICP. The action of the most recently introduced narcotic remifentanil appears to be similar to that of fentanyl,[125-127] with the exception that the context-sensitive half-life is very short at 3 minutes after a 3-hour infusion.[128] This ultra–short-acting narcotic facilitates the emergence of the patient from anesthesia and allows immediate assessment of neurologic function. It is often used in combination with propofol infusion as part of total intravenous anesthesia regimen.

Intubation

Prophylaxis against a Rise in Blood Pressure during Laryngoscopy

The aforementioned regimen deals only with induction of unconsciousness, and other agents are required before tracheal intubation is attempted. Many anesthetic adjuncts have been used successfully to prevent the rise in blood pressure that occurs with laryngoscopy and tracheal intubation. They include the use of high-dose narcotics (e.g., fentanyl, 5 to 10 μg/kg, or sufentanil, 0.5 to 1.0 μg/kg), β-adrenergic antagonists (e.g., esmolol, 0.5 mg/kg), labetalol (10 to 20 mg), intravenous or topical lidocaine (1.5 to 2.0 mg/kg), a second dose of propofol (0.5 to 1 mg/kg) or thiopental (1 to 2 mg/kg), or a deep level of an inhalation anesthetic such as isoflurane or sevoflurane. Intravenous adjuncts are preferred in patients with poor SAH grade, whereas deep inhalation anesthetics are appropriate for patients with good SAH grades but should be avoided in patients with increased ICP. We routinely administer intravenous lidocaine, 1.5 mg/kg 2 to 3 minutes before intubation.

Choice of Muscle Relaxant

Although succinylcholine has been reported to increase ICP,[129] it has been used successfully in many aneurysm patients with no known sequelae. Moreover, this increase in ICP is not seen when the patients are deeply anesthetized[130] or when succinylcholine is preceded by a defasciculating dose of a nondepolarizing agent. Another potential concern with succinylcholine is the possibility of potassium release. An early study reported potassium release to be a significant complication, but this observation was not confirmed by a later investigation.[131] In all likelihood, succinylcholine is probably safe to use in the patient with acute SAH but should be avoided in patients with motor deficits in the subacute stages.

In view of these potential complications, many anesthesiologists prefer to use a nondepolarizing agent. Atracurium, which may be associated with histamine-mediated hypotension, is devoid of this side effect in its pure isomer, cisatracurium. Pancuronium, on the other hand, may cause tachycardia and hypertension, although this effect is attenuated by the simultaneous administration of synthetic narcotics such as fentanyl or sufentanil. Vecuronium is associated with hemodynamic stability. Rocuronium, given at 1.2 mg/kg, is similar in onset time to succinylcholine and may be the nondepolarizing muscle relaxant of choice in neurosurgical anesthesia. Overall, the choice of muscle relaxant depends on the anesthesiologist's preference as well as the nature of other drugs being administered at the time of induction. For subsequent neuromuscular blockade, any of the nondepolarizing agents can be used. If neurophysiologic monitoring (specifically motor evoked potential [MEP] monitoring) is employed, subsequent doses of muscle relaxants may impede adequate monitoring.[132]

To avoid coughing, the neuromuscular junction should be monitored, and tracheal intubation should be attempted only when muscle paralysis is complete. The blood pressure should also be watched closely during laryngoscopy. If the blood pressure begins to rise unexpectedly (above the preinduction value), the intubation attempt must cease, and additional anesthetic agents or adjuncts should be given.

The Patient with a Full Stomach

If the patient has a full stomach, the anesthesiologist must balance the risk of aneurysm rupture against the risk of aspiration. One approach is to treat the patient like any patient at risk of regurgitation and aspiration, using a rapid-sequence induction with cricoid pressure. To obtund the hypertensive response to tracheal intubation, fentanyl 5-10 µg/kg or sufentanil 0.1 µg/kg, should be used in combination with propofol or thiopental. Either succinylcholine (1.5 to 2.0 mg/kg, preceded by defasciculation) or rocuronium (1.0 to 1.2 mg/kg) can be used for muscle relaxation. Without the ability to titrate the drugs to response, this technique is associated with a risk of systemic hypotension. An alternative approach is to accept the small risk of regurgitation and to titrate in the appropriate amount of narcotics and hypnotics as indicated by the blood pressure response while maintaining oxygenation and ventilation with mask and cricoid pressure. With either approach, if the blood pressure starts to rise with laryngeal stimulation, the anesthesiologist should abort the laryngoscopy, maintain ventilation with cricoid pressure, and increase the depth of anesthesia before another attempt at tracheal intubation. Esmolol (0.5 mg/kg) given intravenously may be a useful adjunct in this situation. Labetalol, 10 to 30 mg in 5-mg increments, is also effective.

The Patient with a Potentially Difficult Airway

The potential risk of aneurysm rupture is increased in patients with a difficult airway.

When a difficult airway is anticipated, fiberoptic intubation is the method of choice. Because translaryngeal injection may cause coughing and hypertension, it is preferable in the patient with a difficult airway to provide topical anesthesia by inhalation of nebulized lidocaine (4%). Sufficient time (20 to 30 minutes), however, must be allowed for this method to be effective. Intravenous fentanyl and midazolam in 50-µg and 1-mg increments, respectively, may be administered judiciously, provided that the patient does not have elevated ICP. Alternatively, after appropriate sedation as outlined previously, translaryngeal injection through the cricothyroid membrane of lidocaine (2.5 to 3.0 mL of 4% lidocaine) can be performed. After obtundation of the cough reflex with intravenous narcotics, the cough response to the translaryngeal injection should be brief and attenuated. To anesthetize the upper pharynx and laryngopharynx, topical benzocaine spray can be used. Other authorities advocate supplementation with bilateral superior laryngeal nerve block by injecting 0.75 mL lidocaine (2%) subcutaneously on either side of the hyoid arch. We have found the combination of topical spray and translaryngeal injection satisfactory.

If there is an unexpectedly difficult airway but ventilation is adequate and tracheal intubation is impossible, the patient should be kept anesthetized with either intravenous or inhalation agents. The usual approach to a difficult intubation with adequate mask ventilation should be employed, utilizing adjunctive measures such as a fiberoptic bronchoscope or intubating laryngeal mask airway. Attention must simultaneously be directed to control of systemic blood pressure. If neither ventilation nor intubation is possible, transtracheal jet ventilation should be implemented and oxygenation maintained while fiberoptic intubation is attempted. Cricothyroidotomy or tracheostomy may be necessary. The availability of the laryngeal mask airway has improved safety under these conditions.

After Intubation

Monitoring Requirements

Following induction of anesthesia and tracheal intubation, additional monitors and catheters are placed. In addition to ECG tracings, a neuromuscular blockade monitor, noninvasive blood pressure monitor, pulse oximetry, end-tidal capnography monitor, urinary catheter, and temperature monitor should be used. Monitoring for aneurysm surgery should also include direct intra-arterial blood pressure measurement, preferably instituted before laryngoscopy or induction of anesthesia. Adequate intravenous access is important, and at least one 16-gauge or 14-gauge peripheral catheter should be inserted in addition to the central venous catheter or PAC. To accurately reflect the CPP, the arterial transducer should be placed at the level of the base of the skull and adjusted with any change in the patient's position. Intermittent blood sampling for determination of hematocrit, blood gas, glucose, osmolarity, and electrolyte values is also important. Osmolarity measurement helps determine the efficacy of additional mannitol when the brain is judged "tight"; if serum osmolarity exceeds 320 mOsm, additional mannitol may cause renal dysfunction. Patients placed in the seated position have other requirements, which are discussed in other chapters.

It has been well shown that hyperglycemia can exacerbate cellular injury during cerebral ischemia.[133,134] There has now been a movement toward tight glycemic control utilizing intensive insulin therapy to achieve this goal. Although avoiding very high levels of glucose is important, the rigidity with which such control is achieved may lead to hypoglycemic events and equally devastating neurologic injury.[135] Blood glucose values exceeding 200 mg/dL should be judiciously treated with insulin.

The patient is then positioned for surgery. Insertion of the pins for the Mayfield or other pin fixation device represents a very noxious stimulus and can raise the blood pressure dramatically if the patient is not pretreated. Infiltration with local anesthesia[136] and administration of additional propofol, thiopental, or narcotics is an effective regimen. Alternatively, esmolol (0.5 mg/kg) or labetalol (10 to 20 mg) can be used.

CENTRAL VENOUS PRESSURE CATHETER VERSUS PULMONARY ARTERY CATHETER

A CVP catheter should be placed in all patients undergoing craniotomy for aneurysm surgery, for the following reasons: (1) the prevalence of preexisting hypovolemia, (2) the large intraoperative fluid shift with the use of osmotic and loop diuretics, (3) the potential risk of aneurysm rupture, necessitating blood and fluid resuscitation, and (4) the possible presence of myocardial dysfunction. Many anesthesiologists insert a PAC when the patient (1) has known coronary artery disease or ventricular dysfunction, (2) has symptomatic vasospasm necessitating preoperative hypertensive therapy, or (3) has a poor clinical grade and is at high risk of postoperative vasospasm, and intravascular volume expansion is planned.

SITE OF CENTRAL VENOUS CATHETER AND PULMONARY ARTERY CATHETER PLACEMENT

Central venous access can be established via the internal jugular vein, the subclavian vein, or the antecubital vein. Each route has advantages and disadvantages. The internal jugular vein is readily accessible and easy to locate, but some neurosurgeons are concerned about potential venous obstruction. We have not found this possibility to be a problem, and it is our method of choice. For subtemporal incisions, as well as in procedures in which the extracranial internal carotid artery may be temporarily occluded, we place the catheter on the contralateral side to avoid interference with the surgical field.

The subclavian route does not interfere with cerebral venous drainage but is associated with a significant risk of pneumothorax. The antecubital approach is least invasive but has a lower success rate, which, however, can be improved with ECG guidance.

Although it is customary to place the patient in Trendelenburg position to facilitate placement of the central venous catheter, this practice is potentially dangerous in patients with elevated ICP. We generally do not use more than a 5% to 10% tilt, and for patients with known elevated ICP, we prefer to attempt placement in the neutral supine position.

Because of the potential risk of intraoperative aneurysm rupture, at least 4 to 6 units of blood should have been typed and crossmatched for the patient and should be available at the time of surgical incision.

OTHER MONITORING

Other monitoring includes jugular bulb oxygen saturation, noninvasive cerebral oximetry, and TCD.

Placement of a catheter (continuous fiberoptic oximetry or intermittent sampling) in the jugular bulb allows monitoring of the cerebral venous oxygen saturation ($SjvO_2$). Because the cerebral metabolic rate for oxygen is equal to the product of CBF and arteriovenous oxygen content difference—assuming 100% arterial oxygen saturation—$SjvO_2$ reflects the balance between cerebral metabolic supply and demand. This approach is analogous to monitoring of mixed venous oxygen saturation as an index of the balance between systemic metabolic requirement and cardiac output. The use of jugular venous oximetry in the intensive care of head-injured patients is relatively well established. Its use in the intraoperative management of patients undergoing cerebral aneurysm surgery, however, remains investigative rather than routine. Matta and colleagues[137] reported on the feasibility and safety of the use of retrograde catheters in a variety of neurosurgical procedures. Although outcome is not addressed in their report, they observed that venous oximetry monitoring in patients undergoing aneurysm surgery allows optimization of ventilation with fine-tuning of $PaCO_2$ to avoid potential cerebral ischemia. Moss and colleagues[138] determined that jugular venous oximetry may facilitate intraoperative blood pressure management, whereas Clavier and associates[139] observed that it can be used to diagnose hyperemia or luxury perfusion. Acute decrease in jugular venous oxygen saturation during intraoperative aneurysm rupture has also been described.[140]

Regional cerebral oximetry uses optical spectroscopy to measure brain vascular hemoglobin saturation in a noninvasive manner to provide similar information. At present, however, it is not reliable enough to be used clinically. Continuous TCD monitoring may improve the safety of induced hypotension by correlating the blood velocity change with the decline in blood pressure. It has also been used perioperatively to confirm the diagnosis of aneurysmal rupture,[141] but its routine use in this regard is impractical.

Positioning of the Patient

The location and the size of the aneurysm generally determine the position of the patient for the surgical procedure. Preoperative review of the angiogram and CT scan will facilitate proper positioning of the patient. Anterior circulation aneurysms are usually approached through a frontal temporal incision with the patient in the supine position. Basilar tip aneurysms are approached through a subtemporal incision with the patient in the lateral position or an incision allowing the patient to remain supine. Vertebral and basilar trunk aneurysms are often approached through a suboccipital incision, with the patient either in the seated position or the "park-bench" (semiprone lateral) position. The risk of air embolism is always present, although it is significantly higher in the seated position than in the supine position. As a general principle, because of the duration of these surgical procedures, all bony prominences must be well padded and all extremities well supported before the surgical procedure begins. Equally important before draping is a final inspection of the head and neck position in relationship to the body and palpation of the neck to ensure that jugular venous obstruction does not occur. Failure to make this inspection is a common cause of unexplained intraoperative cerebral swelling. Therefore it is generally advisable to secure the tracheal tube with tapes rather than a tie around the neck because a tie may slip and tighten around the neck. Although not proven, partial venous obstruction may contribute to reported postoperative tongue swelling and airway obstruction in posterior fossa procedures.[142,143] For this reason a soft bite block is preferable to an oropharyngeal airway.

After final positioning, the lung fields should be auscultated to rule out bronchial intubation. Flexion of the head tends to advance of the endotracheal tube, whereas extension of the head has the opposite effect. Careful initial placement of the endotracheal tube, ensuring that it measures between 20 and 24 cm at the teeth (in the average-sized adult), will diminish but not eliminate the possibility of bronchial intubation with flexing of the patient's head.

Maintenance of Anesthesia

The goals during maintenance of anesthesia are to (1) provide a relaxed or "slack" brain that will allow minimal retraction pressure, (2) maintain perfusion to the brain, (3) reduce TMP if necessary during dissection of the aneurysm and final clipping, and (4) allow prompt awakening and assessment of patients with good SAH grades.

With the trend toward early surgery, the anesthesiologist can expect to see more difficult conditions in which maximal brain "relaxation" therapy is required. Because no data exist about the influence of anesthetic drugs on the outcome of aneurysm surgery, the choice should be based on both the brain condition and the overall management plan, with the patient's preoperative clinical grade taken into consideration. In general, a patient with SAH grades I, II, or III undergoing an uneventful aneurysm clipping should be allowed to awaken and should be extubated in the operating room. Either an intravenous or inhalation anesthetic or a combination of both can be used to provide such conditions.

Nitrous oxide is a cerebral vasodilator when used in combination with a potent inhaled anesthetic.[144,145] It has also been reported to cause cerebral stimulation with an increase in cerebral metabolic rate.[145] Although no outcome studies suggest that nitrous oxide may have a detrimental effect, there is little or no advantage in using it with a potent inhaled anesthetic. On the other hand, the vasodilatory properties of nitrous oxide are attenuated when it is used in combination with an intravenous anesthetic agent.[116] Generally, nitrous oxide is omitted when isoflurane is used but may be combined with propofol and fentanyl infusion.

With regard to narcotic agents, fentanyl and sufentanil, given either in bolus (50 to 100 μg and 5 to 10 μg, respectively) in response to hemodynamic changes or in continuous infusion (1 to 2 μg/kg/hr or 0.1 to 0.2 μg/kg/hr, respectively), when combined with isoflurane (0.5% to 1.0%) provide satisfactory conditions for most patients in good condition. Desflurane (4% to 6%), which appears to be similar in cerebrovascular effects to those of isoflurane, could be used as an alternative. Its low blood gas solubility is a theoretical advantage. However, in high concentration it can cause sympathetic stimulation. Sevoflurane has a similar blood gas solubility. Although its cardiovascular and cerebrovascular properties appear to be similar to those of other inhaled anesthetics,[146,147] it is unique in that autoregulation appears to be preserved at all concentrations of sevoflurane, whereas other inhaled anesthetics impair the autoregulatory capacity in a dose-related manner.[148,149]

Fentanyl and sufentanil infusions should be discontinued approximately 1 hour before the surgical dressing is applied. The ultra–short-acting remifentanil, used at a rate of 0.125 to 0.25 μg/kg/min, can be infused until about 5 minutes before the end of dressing application. Systemic hypotension is a potential complication with remifentanil. For the other narcotics, the total dosage should not exceed 10 μg/kg for fentanyl and 2 μg/kg for sufentanil, to allow awakening and immediate neurologic assessment.

No differences among the narcotic drugs have been found with respect to observed brain "tightness"[150] or the amount of retractor pressure required for intraoperative brain retraction. Fentanyl and alfentanil exhibit no significant clinical differences with respect to emergence from anesthesia.[151] Total intravenous anesthesia with propofol and alfentanil infusion has also been used successfully. High-dose narcotics (fentanyl 20 to 50 μg/kg; sufentanil 2 to 5 μg/kg), however, will prolong recovery and are unsuitable if rapid awakening and assessment are desired. For patients with poor preoperative SAH grades, extubation of the trachea at the end of the surgical procedure is not planned, and an intravenous anesthetic–based technique is more appropriate (fentanyl or sufentanil with propofol). In difficult cases in which the brain remains tight, continuous thiopental infusion at 5 to 6 mg/kg/hr should be considered. Alternatively, etomidate (0.2 to 0.3 mg/kg/hr) or propofol (150 to 200 μg/kg/hr) infusion can be used. These latter two agents may have the added advantage of a shorter recovery time if extubation of the trachea is contemplated at the end of the procedure.

Irrespective of the anesthetic technique used, an important factor to recognize is that the surgical stimulus during cerebral aneurysm surgery varies at different times. Noxious stimuli begin with insertion of the pin head holder and intensify with the raising of the bone flap; once the dura is open there is little or no surgical stimulation. The anesthetic plan must therefore take this process into consideration to avoid wide fluctuations in CPP or dangerous increases in blood pressure. Of note is the fact that retraction of cranial nerves and the brainstem (posterior fossa aneurysms) may be associated with sudden increases in blood pressure or heart rate. Thus a deeper level of anesthesia must be maintained with these circumstances.

Brain Relaxation

Various maneuvers and adjuncts are used to relax the brain. Although the details of practice vary, they are all directed at the components of the intracranial vault: brain tissue volume, CSF volume, and blood volume.

Patient position can have a profound impact on ICP and brain relaxation. Tankisi and associates[152] found that 10 degrees of reverse Trendelenburg positioning had a favorable effect on ICP while maintaining CPP.

To reduce brain tissue volume, 20% mannitol (0.5 to 2 g/kg) is usually given over 30 minutes to effect osmotic diuresis. The usual dose is 1 g/kg; an additional dose is given when indicated by the brain conditions. A total dose of 2 g/kg is frequently given when temporary artery occlusion is planned (also see the section on temporary occlusion). Mannitol's action begins within 4 to 5 minutes and peaks in about 30 to 45 minutes. Although the classic mechanism is believed to be movement of intracellular water into the intravascular volume along the osmotic gradient (the osmolarity of 20% mannitol is 1098 mOsm/L), some evidence exists that the rapid action of mannitol can be mediated by decreased production of CSF.[153] The cardiovascular and cerebrovascular actions of mannitol can be considered to be triphasic: transient, delayed, and late. Because of mannitol's high osmolarity, it transiently increases CBF, CBV, and ICP, which are followed by decreases in CBV and ICP.[154] Systemically, an acute decrease in peripheral vascular resistance occurs, particularly when mannitol is given quickly (<10 minutes). This may result in transient hypotension, followed by a marked rise in CVP, PAWP, and cardiac output. Therefore the full dose of mannitol should be given over 30 minutes. It also transiently reduces hematocrit, increases serum osmolarity, and causes hyponatremia, hypochloremia, and hyperkalemia.[155] Potential complications from the delayed effects therefore include fluid overload and pulmonary edema in patients with poor cardiac function. Within 45 minutes the cardiovascular effects have dissipated, and with the onset of full diuresis the intravascular volume may start to contract. Theoretically mannitol should not be given before the dura is open to minimize fluctuation in ICP. Shrinkage of the brain may also cause tearing of the bridging veins. In clinical practice, slow mannitol infusion (100 to 200 mL/hr) is frequently begun after final positioning of the patient, and the infusion rate increased after the bone flap has been raised (400 to 500 mL/hr). Some practitioners routinely use furosemide (0.1 to 0.5 mg/kg) to augment the action of mannitol. Additional mannitol, to a total of 2 g/kg, because of its potential brain-protective effect, is often administered before temporary occlusion of major feeding arteries.[155]

Hypertonic saline is a reasonable alternative to mannitol for brain relaxation. An investigation comparing 20% mannitol with 3% hypertonic saline found no difference between them in the extent of brain relaxation.[156] Volume shift and fluid requirement were lower in the hypertonic saline group.

Reducing the volume of the CSF compartment by drainage of CSF with a lumbar subarachnoid drain facilitates surgical exposure, because the average adult has approximately 150 mL of CSF. Extreme care should be exercised during insertion of the drain to minimize CSF loss and a sudden decrease in ICP, so as to avoid an abrupt increase in TMP and a rebleed. Because of the risk of brainstem herniation, lumbar drainage of CSF is contraindicated in patients with intracerebral hematoma. In theory, free drainage should be allowed only after the dura is open to minimize the risk of rebleeding; in practice, however, 20 to 30 mL of CSF is usually drained just before dural opening to facilitate dural incision. Rapid drainage can cause sudden reflex hypertension, presumably from stimulation of the brainstem. Barker[157] has suggested that the drainage rate should not exceed 5 mL/min. The drain is usually left open during the procedure, until the aneurysm is clipped or until the beginning of dural closure.

The equipment used for subarachnoid lumbar drainage varies among different hospitals, and some neurosurgeons prefer not to use CSF drainage, relying on mannitol and hyperventilation instead. We use a standard commercially available kit (Lumbar Catheter Accessory Kit, Cordis Corporation, Miami, FL), which essentially consists of a 14-gauge Touhy needle and a soft flexible catheter having multiple orifices at the end. In essence the subarachnoid drain differs from a subarachnoid catheter inserted for continuous spinal analgesia only in size. Regular lumbar epidural kits designed for epidural anesthesia are generally not satisfactory because the size of the catheter is too small, and in patients with acute SAH, blood clots frequently block the drainage. Pediatric feeding catheters have also been used with success, but the stiffness of these catheters increases the risk of potential spinal cord damage. On the other hand, caution must be exercised with the insertion and removal of the soft, flexible catheters. Withdrawal of the catheter through the needle and the use of guidewires increase the risk of catheter shearing.[158] Because the catheter is placed with the patient in the flexed position but often is removed with the patient in the extended or neutral position, the catheter has been known to break off at the site of compression between the vertebral bodies.[158] The patient should therefore be placed in the flexed position whenever difficulty

with catheter removal is encountered. To avoid the difficulty with insertion and removal of these catheters, some hospitals use malleable spinal needles and simply bend the needle to the patient's contour after placement. This approach is most suited to patients who have been placed in the lateral position for surgery.

CBV can be reduced. Within the physiologic range of $Paco_2$ (20 to 70 mm Hg), CBF bears an almost linear relationship to arterial $Paco_2$, changing 2% to 3% for each 1–mm Hg change in $Paco_2$. Controlled hyperventilation therefore can be used to decrease the CBV, which probably changes by about 1% for each 1–mm Hg change in $Paco_2$. Although anesthetic agents may influence the response to CO_2, the changes are small and CO_2 reactivity is generally well preserved. CO_2 reactivity is normal in patients with good SAH grades but may be impaired in those with poor SAH grades. Although it is generally safe to maintain $Paco_2$ in the range of 25 to 35 mm Hg, it should be individualized according to the operating conditions. A reasonable approach is to institute mild hypocapnia (30 to 35 mm Hg) before the dura is open, moderate hypocapnia (25 to 30 mm Hg) after the dura is open, and relative normocapnia during induced hypotension and after the aneurysm is clipped. The advantages of extreme hypocapnia in reducing CBV should always be balanced against the risk of potential cerebral ischemia. Because the objective is to relax the brain without causing ischemia, the efficacy of hyperventilation should be continuously assessed by observing the intraoperative brain relaxation in order to achieve the optimal $Paco_2$.

In difficult situations, brain relaxation may remain unsatisfactory and refractory to the regimen just described. If this occurs, the anesthesiologist should:

1. Make sure that there is no hypoxemia or systemic hypertension.
2. Check the patient's neck to rule out venous obstruction.
3. Inspect the subarachnoid drain to ensure patency and proper drainage of CSF.
4. Since nitrous oxide is a cerebral vasodilator when used in conjunction with an inhaled anesthetic,[144] discontinue nitrous oxide.
5. After communication with the surgeon, implement a head-up tilt to facilitate venous blood and CSF drainage.[152]
6. Finally, give a test dose of thiopental (150 to 200 mg) and, if brain relaxation improves, start a continuous infusion (4 to 5 mg/kg/hr). This will usually, but not always, produce a prolonged recovery from anesthesia.

Occasionally, uncontrolled intraoperative swelling may be due to an intracerebral hematoma.

Fluid and Electrolyte Balance

Fluid should be administered according to the patient's need and guided by intraoperative blood loss, urine output, and CVP or PAWP value. Intravenous fluid should not be withheld if induced hypotension is planned, because hypovolemic hypotension is detrimental to organ perfusion. The aim is to maintain normovolemia before aneurysm clipping and slight hypervolemia after clipping. Electrolytes should be replaced as needed. Glucose-containing solutions should not be given, because evidence exists that hyperglycemia may aggravate both focal and global transient cerebral ischemia.[133,134] Because lactated Ringer's solution is relatively hypo-osmolar, a more physiologic solution, such as Plasma-Lyte, Normosol, or normal saline, is preferred. Some practitioners use 5% albumin after clipping of the aneurysm, but the advantages of this protocol have not been documented. On the other hand, hetastarch probably should not be used or should be used in small amounts (less than 500 mL) because of the risk of intracranial bleeding.[97,98]

Other Considerations

Controlled Hypotension versus Temporary Occlusion

Because of the enlargement of the aneurysmal sac, the wall stress increases proportionately to increases in blood pressure, as dictated by the law of Laplace, as follows:

$$T = R \times P/2$$

where T is wall tension, P is mean blood pressure, and R is the radius of the aneurysm (Fig. 13-4); hence, large aneurysms are more likely to rupture than small ones. Therefore, the blood pressure is traditionally lowered during microscopic dissection of the aneurysm, particularly during clip placement, to reduce

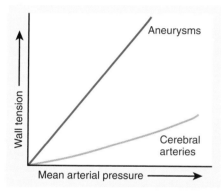

Figure 13–4 The relationship between wall tension and mean arterial pressure (intracranial pressure is 0 when the dura is open). For any given pressure, wall stress and therefore the tendency to rupture are higher in an aneurysmal sac than in a normal cerebral artery. *(From Ferguson GG: The rationale for controlled hypotension. In Varkey GP [ed]: Anesthetic Considerations in the Surgical Repair of Intracranial Aneurysms. Boston, Little, Brown, 1982.)*

the risk of rupture. Hypotension also reduces bleeding, allowing better visualization of the anatomy of the aneurysm and the perforating vessels. Although the risk of hypotension-induced global cerebral ischemia always exists, deliberate hypotension has been used successfully for many years without apparent ill effects. However, the demonstration of impairment of autoregulatory capacity after SAH,[16,17] the unpredictable cerebrovascular response to induced hypotension, increased risk of vasospasm,[114] and poorer outcomes[114,159] have led to the rare use of routine deliberate hypotension. Patients with vasospasm, as evidenced by angiography or symptoms, are particularly at risk of ischemia during hypotension.

To reduce the risk of aneurysm rupture without using hypotension, many surgeons are now using temporary occlusion of the major feeding artery[160-162] (Fig. 13-5; modified from 161). The potential risks of temporary occlusion include focal cerebral ischemia and subsequent infarction as well as damage to the feeding artery from the occlusion. With improved design of temporary clips, the latter complication is now of less concern. The risk of cerebral infarction remains, however, and depends on the duration of the temporary occlusion as well as the state of the collateral circulation.

The anesthetic management of patients during induced hypotension clearly differs from their management during temporary occlusion. The major differences are summarized in Table 13-7.

CONTROLLED HYPOTENSION

The major concerns with controlled hypotension are avoidance of cerebral ischemia and maintenance of organ perfusion. No ideal hypotensive agent exists, but many hypotensive drugs and techniques have been used successfully and are discussed in detail elsewhere in this book.

TEMPORARY OCCLUSION

Because the tolerable duration of temporary occlusion varies with different arteries as well as among individuals, it is difficult to predict the upper time limit in any given situation. Five to 7 minutes of occlusion with prompt reperfusion is usually well tolerated, but this time period is generally insufficient for

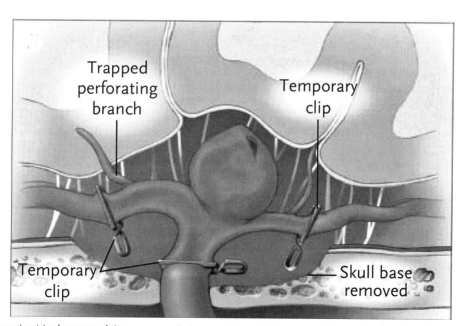

Figure 13–5 To reduce the risk of rupture of the aneurysm during surgical repair, temporary clips can be placed on the proximal artery as well as on the distal arteries to reduce the pressure inside the aneurysmal sac.

Table 13–7 Temporary Arterial Occlusion versus Controlled Hypotension during Cerebral Aneurysm Surgery

Temporary Occlusion	Controlled Hypotension
Normotension or hypertension	Systemic hypotension
Temporary cessation of flow	Uninterrupted flow
Regional ischemia	Global ischemia
Short duration (10-20 min)	Longer duration
Dependent on collateral vessels	Independent of collateral vessels
Potential vessel damage	No vessel damage
Possibly complete control	Lack of complete control

clipping difficult or giant aneurysms. Although no randomized clinical trials have been conducted, a number of regimens have been used to extend the occlusion duration. Suzuki[164] introduced the technique of high-dose mannitol (2 g/kg) for temporary arterial occlusion, and experimental studies have supported a brain-protective role for mannitol. Because neuronal damage may be mediated by the production of free radicals, Suzuki[164] advocates a combination of mannitol (500 mL of a 20% solution, or 100 g), vitamin E (500 mg), and dexamethasone (50 mg), often referred to as the "Sendai cocktail," for temporary arterial occlusion. Up to 60 minutes of temporary arterial occlusion has been obtained with use of this regimen without apparent postoperative neurologic deficits. In general, however, 15 to 20 minutes is considered to be the upper limit of safety.[165]

Other surgeons use pharmacologic metabolic suppression, theorizing that, decreasing cerebral metabolic rate enables the tissues distal to the occlusion to tolerate a longer period of ischemia. Thiopental, etomidate, and propofol have been used for this purpose.[166] Administration of any of these agents prior to temporary clipping usually achieves the endpoint of burst suppression, as indicated by EEG monitoring, in 2 to 3 minutes. Additional doses may be given as indicated by EEG. However, the additional doses may not be effective if collateral circulation is inadequate for delivery of the agent. On the other hand, in this situation the agent that has been given would also stay in the ischemic area longer because of the diminished blood flow for washout. Although there have been no controlled clinical studies, good results have been reported whether thiopental,[167] etomidate,[166] or mannitol[165] was used for cerebral protection. Theoretically, because there is less associated systemic hypotension, etomidate may be preferable to thiopental. However, some studies suggest that etomidate, despite reducing global cerebral metabolic rate, may cause cerebral tissue hypoxia during temporary occlusion, as determined with intracerebral oxygen tension measurements.[168] On the other hand, Lavine and associates[166] reported their results comparing patients who received intravenous brain-protective therapy (barbiturates or etomidate) with those who did not (inhalation anesthetics only) during temporary occlusion; they concluded that brain protective therapy can extend the occlusion duration from 12 minutes to 19 minutes without cerebral infarction.

In general, if the temporary occlusion time is kept below 10 minutes, the risk of infarction is low irrespective of anesthetic agents used. In an earlier series, Samson and colleagues[169] reported that patients older than 61 years and

in poor condition (Hunt and Hess grades III to V) did not tolerate temporary occlusion as well as patients who were younger and in better neurologic condition. In this series all patients in whom occlusion time exceed 31 minutes had cerebral infarction. Traditionally, to use pharmacologic protection efficiently, it is necessary to monitor the EEG to define the endpoint, because no further metabolic benefits can be derived with doses greater than those needed to produce burst suppression or electrical silence. Warner and coworkers[170] observed in experimental ischemia that maximal protection with barbiturates need not occur at burst suppression, and such findings have raised questions about this practice. In the absence of clinical data to support this observation, it remains prudent to use burst suppression as the endpoint.

Cardiac Standstill Using Adenosine (Transient Cardiac Pause)

To facilitate clipping of a large aneurysm with a broad neck and reduce the risk of rupture, transient cardiac arrest can be induced with a bolus of adenosine. This technique has been reported with embolization of arteriovenous malformations (AVMs)[171] and has been used by some surgeons for clipping of posterior fossa aneurysms, although there are few reports in the literature.[172] After a dose response has been established with the use of two to three incremental doses of adenosine between 6 and 18 mg, a duration of approximately 30 seconds of asystole can be induced with an average dose of 30 to 36 mg of adenosine. Recovery of cardiac rhythm is spontaneous and may be followed by rebound tachycardia and hypertension. This technique is contraindicated in patients with preexisting cardiac conduction abnormalities or severe asthma.

Electrophysiologic monitoring can also be used to determine the upper limit of occlusion duration, thus allowing the surgeon to proceed without haste as long as the monitoring suggests normal function. This approach allows the anesthesiologist to recognize the need for brief periods of reperfusion when the monitoring indicates deterioration. EEG or evoked potentials, including MEPs and SSEPs, are increasingly being used for such purposes. It is important to realize the limitations of these modalities: The deep levels of anesthesia given to obtain burst suppression can affect signal quality for the monitoring modalities. Some surgeons use mild hypotension during dissection and then apply temporary arterial occlusion during actual placement of the clip. It is important to restore the blood pressure to normal before the placement of the temporary clips to maximize collateral blood flow.

Moderate Hypothermia and Neuroprotection

Moderate hypothermia (28° to 32° C) has also been used in the past to extend the duration of tolerable occlusion.[164] Because experimental studies in cerebral ischemia have demonstrated that even mild hypothermia can exert significant cerebroprotective effects by suppressing release of excitotoxic amino acids,[173,174] the practice of maintaining the body temperature between 33° and 35° C during the periods when the patient is considered to be at risk for cerebral ischemia was quite routine. Although it is clear that metabolic suppression is achieved, potential complications include ventricular arrhythmia, myocardial depression, coagulopathy, and postoperative shivering. The Intraoperative Hypothermia for Aneurysm Surgery Trial (IHAST) evaluated the effects of mild hypothermia (33.5° C) and found no effect on neurologic outcome in patients with favorable clinical grade aneurysms.[22] No significant complications were noted in the hypothermia group, and specifically, no

---

BOX 13–1   *Protocol for Circulatory Arrest*

1. Place intra-arterial and large-bore intravenous catheters before induction of anesthesia. The usual precautions for induction of anesthesia in patients with a cerebral aneurysm apply.
2. Once anesthesia is induced and the trachea intubated, place the following devices:
   - Either a central venous line or PAC.
   - A second intra-arterial catheter to allow phlebotomy.
   - A lumbar subarachnoid drain
   - Electrophysiologic monitors (EEG and/or somatosensory evoked potentials)
   - Both nasopharyngeal and esophageal temperature probes
   Anticipate periods of stimulation, such as during tracheal intubation, head pinning, and periosteal retraction, which can cause hypertension.
3. Begin surface cooling by using a cooling blanket and lowering the room temperature. The rate of decrease should proceed at approximately 0.2° C/min.
4. If barbiturates are to be used, administer a 3 to 5 mg/kg bolus of thiopental to induce either a burst suppression pattern at a 1:5 ratio (i.e., time period in burst relative to electrical silence, or a burst suppression ratio of 80%) or an isoelectric EEG. This can be followed by a continuous infusion of thiopental at 0.1 to 0.5 mg/kg/min. Once cooling begins, continue the infusion at this rate for the entire period of cardiopulmonary bypass.
5. Perform hemodilution to a hematocrit of 28% to 30% by collecting blood into an anticoagulant solution kept at room temperature. Maintain intravascular volume with up to 4 L of cold intravenous saline containing potassium chloride (4 to 6 mEq/L).
6. After the aneurysm is dissected and hemostasis obtained, begin extracorporeal circulation via femoral artery–femoral vein bypass when the patient's temperature reaches 34° C. Just before initiation of bypass, ensure surgical hemostasis and then give heparin, 300 to 400 IU/kg, to maintain the ACT between 450 and 480 seconds.
7. Cool the patient to between 15° and 18° C. Be aware of electrocardiographic changes; at 28° C, the myocardium is extremely irritable and may fibrillate continuously. Fibrillation should be stopped with 40 to 80 mEq of potassium chloride, but if fibrillation is persistent, defibrillator should be used at 100 to 250 watts/sec. Administer additional doses of potassium chloride as needed.
8. Circulatory arrest occurs between 15° and 18° C and should be limited to the period of clip application. The EEG should be isoelectric before arrest. If barbiturates were not used earlier, they may be added at this point to achieve a silent EEG. Elevate the patient's head slightly to facilitate venous drainage, keeping in mind that this position increases the potential risk of air embolism and no-reflow phenomenon in small vessels.
9. The circulatory arrest time should be limited to less than 60 minutes for optimal results. This arrest time can be further minimized with intermittent perfusion with or dissection under low flow until the clip is ready to be placed.
10. Once the aneurysm is clipped, bypass is reestablished and the patient is rewarmed at a rate of 0.2° to 0.5° C/min. Too-rapid rewarming can cause tissue acidosis and hypoxia. Sodium nitroprusside may be used to allow a more homogeneous rewarming.
11. With rewarming, the heart will fibrillate. Perform cardioversion with 200 to 400 joules through external defibrillating pads. Antiarrhythmic drugs may be required to restore a normal sinus rhythm. In addition, the patient may require inotropic support.
12. Discontinue extracorporeal circulation when the patient's temperature is 34° C and the heart can maintain a normal cardiac output and sinus rhythm. An after-drop in temperature can be expected, and it is important to use other ancillary devices, such as forced warm air, to keep the patient warm.
13. Correct the ACT to 100 and 150 seconds with protamine sulfate. Transfuse the autologous blood containing platelet-rich plasma. Other blood products may be necessary to restore hemostasis.

ACT, activated clotting time; EEG, electroencephalogram.

---

coagulopathy was observed. The protective effects of moderate hypothermia in patients with poor clinical grade and those with prolonged temporary occlusion, however, have not been studied. Consequently, considering that the cerebroprotective effect of moderate hypothermia following global ischemia has been documented with respect to ventricular fibrillation,[175,176] the intraoperative use of this maneuver for aneurysm surgery in patients at high risk for infarction due to prolonged temporary occlusion needs further evaluation.

Improvements in cardiopulmonary bypass technology and coagulation management have led to a revival of interest in the use of profound hypothermia and circulatory arrest for complex or giant aneurysms (Box 13-1).[177]

In corollary to hypothermia, any increase in body temperature above normal must be vigorously treated. The site of temperature monitoring should reflect the temperature in the brain. Clearly, the temperatures at the surface and deeper part of the brain may be different,[178] but in general, nasopharyngeal and tympanic membrane temperature closely approximates that of the deep brain structures.[179]

Pharmacologic metabolic suppression or use of mannitol appears to provide some brain protection without the complications of hypothermia. In some centers the routine practice is to use additional mannitol to a total of 2 g/kg just before the proximal vessel occlusion. In patients in whom the collateral circulation has been demonstrated to be poor or nonexistent angiographically and yet temporary occlusion is deemed necessary, we would induce burst suppression with thiopental or propofol in addition to the use of mannitol. Prior communication between the neurosurgeon and the anesthesiologist is clearly needed for the successful management of these patients. The placement of EEG electrodes must not interfere with the surgical field and the electrodes must be well shielded and protected from both preparation solution and blood to allow proper intraoperative monitoring of EEG. Fortunately, a simple bihemispheric fronto-occipital montage suffices. It can be accomplished by placing surface gel electrodes with appropriate occlusive dressing or needle electrodes over the forehead just above the eyes, which are then referenced to the respective electrodes placed over the ipsilateral mastoid processes.

Electrophysiologic Monitoring

Electrophysiologic monitoring such as EEG and evoked potentials may allow intraoperative detection of cerebral ischemia, leading to a change in surgical technique that improves perfusion. Although there are no randomized clinical trials on the efficacy of evoked potential monitoring, this technique is increasingly used as routine monitoring during aneurysm surgery. Optimal monitoring of SSEPs and MEPs usually necessitates the use of total intravenous anesthesia and the omission of muscle relaxants.

EEG has been used to determine the lowest blood pressure tolerable during induced hypotension, but the results are not consistent. This is not surprising because a significant decrease in EEG activity can be compatible with normal neurologic recovery. A report described the use of intraoperative bihemispheric computer-processed EEG and found that changes correspond to postoperative outcome. However, the series is too small for any conclusions to be drawn about the utility of routine EEG monitoring. In contrast, EEG monitoring may be indicated when temporary occlusion is planned, either to determine the duration of tolerance or for titration of anesthetic agents when pharmacologic metabolic suppression is desired.

SSEP monitoring has been investigated for use during procedures on both anterior and posterior circulation aneurysms, whereas brainstem auditory evoked potential (BAEP) monitoring has been investigated primarily for use during procedures on vertebrobasilar aneurysms. Both monitors are probably most useful when temporary or permanent vessel occlusion is planned. Evoked potentials can be recorded even when the EEG signal is suppressed with high-dose barbiturates and therefore represent the only electrophysiologic monitoring technique available when maximal pharmacologic metabolic suppression is used. Like all types of electrophysiologic monitoring, even during temporary occlusion, SSEP monitoring lacks specificity, and a high false-alarm rate can be expected. The false-negative rate (SSEP unchanged but neurologic deficit occurs) is lower but remains significant in most series. Table 13-8 summarizes the reported series on the use of SSEPs during temporary arterial occlusion as well as later series on MEPs. Most studies report a high false-positive rate as well as a considerable false-negative rate. Despite these results, routine use of evoked potential monitoring is growing.

In selected cases for which permanent occlusion of a major vessel is anticipated, SSEP or BAEP monitoring may be useful. In a series examining the use of both SSEPs and BAEPs in posterior circulation aneurysms, neither modality was superior in predicting neurologic deficits, but the combination reduced the false-positive and false-negative rates to 13% and 20%, respectively.[180] These results are better than reported by most other studies.

Spontaneous breathing has been used in the past as an indicator of brainstem function, particularly when extreme hypotension is used. It is seldom used today, because optimal brain relaxation is difficult to achieve and extreme hypotension is no longer used. However, with aneurysms involving the low basilar artery and the vertebral arteries, where temporary or permanent occlusion of the feeding vessel is contemplated, spontaneous breathing may provide additional and more specific information than cardiovascular monitoring. Disturbances ranging from tachypnea to apnea have been observed.[180] Spontaneous ventilation has been compared with BAEP as a monitor of brainstem function during vertebrobasilar aneurysm surgery, and its complementary efficacy demonstrated.[181] Fortunately these situations are extremely rare.

Monitoring of MEPs has now been added to multimodality monitoring during intracranial aneurysmal surgery. With the significant false-negative rate for SSEP monitoring, the addition of MEPs was sought to improve both the sensitivity and specificity for ischemia resulting in postoperative deficit, particularly that secondary to ischemia of subcortical structures.[182] Several case series have shown promising results with better sensitivity than SSEP in both anterior[183] and posterior circulation aneurysms.[184] The proliferation of MEP monitoring for aneurysm surgery may dictate a change in anesthetic plan with regard to the use of inhaled anesthetics as well as neuromuscular blocking agents, both of which have been shown to preclude adequate MEP recording.[185] One must also consider the profound depressive effects that pharmacologic burst suppression has on MEP signal quality. The effect can be so pronounced that MEP signal may be lost completely (Authors' unpublished data 2009).

Table 13–8 Monitoring of SSEPs and MEPs in Temporary Arterial Occlusion for Cerebral Aneurysm Surgery

Study*	No. of Patients	Temporary Occlusion	False-Positive Results	False-Negative Results
MEP monitoring:				
Szelenyi et al (2006)[220]	119	71	4	7
Horiuchi et al (2005)[183]	53	?	6	0
SSEP monitoring:				
Manninen et al (1994)[180]	70	52	11	47
Mizoi et al (1993)[221]	124	97	57	25
Schramm et al (1990)[222]	113	34	40%	34%
Manninen et al (1990)[223]	157	97	43%	14%
Mooij et al (1987)[162]	5	5	?	0%
Momma et al (1987)[161]	40	40	60%	5%
Kidooka et al (1987)[224]	31	15	38%	22%
Symon et al (1984)[225]	34	15	40%	7%

MEP, motor evoked potential; SSEP, somatosensory evoked potential.
*Superscript numbers indicate chapter references.

Intraoperative Aneurysm Rupture

The incidence of aneurysm rupture varies with the size and the anatomic location of the aneurysm, larger arteries, posteroinferior cerebellar arteries, and anterior and posterior communicating arteries being more likely to rupture.[186] There also appear to be differences between institutions. In the Cooperative Study, an intraoperative aneurysm leak occurred in about 6% of patients, whereas frank rupture occurred in 13%,[4] for a combined incidence of 19%. In a later series, the rate of rupture was down to 3.8% for frank rupture and 7.9% for all ruptures, including leaks.[186] These findings are similar to those reported by Bater and Samson.[187] In approximately 8% of the cases reported by the Cooperative Study, the rupture resulted in frank hemorrhagic shock.[4] In Batjer and Samson's series,[187] 7% of the ruptures occurred before dissection of the aneurysm, 48% during dissection, and 45% during clip application. Mortality and morbidity are higher with intraoperative aneurysm rupture. A multicenter study examining intraprocedure rupture of aneurysms similarly reported an incidence of 19% with clipping, and 31% of these cases were associated with death or disability.[188]

Management of aneurysm rupture during surgery partially depends on the ability to maintain the blood volume during the rupture. If the leak is small and dissection is complete, the surgeon can gain control with suction and then apply the permanent clip to the neck of the aneurysm. Alternatively, temporary clips can be applied proximally and distally to the aneurysm to gain control. The keys to anesthetic management are good communication with the surgeon and close monitoring of the patient's vital signs as well as the surgical conditions. Video monitors allowing the anesthesiologist to view the surgical field greatly facilitate patient care during this acute, rapidly changing situation. If temporary occlusion is not planned or not possible and blood loss is not significant, the MAP should be decreased transiently to 50 mm Hg or even lower to facilitate surgical control. Proximal and distal temporary occlusion, however, is the preferred method. Thiopental, propofol, or etomidate may be given to provide some protection before placement of the temporary clip. The last agent is preferable if the status of the patient's blood volume is uncertain. If frank hemorrhage occurs, aggressive fluid resuscitation and blood transfusion must begin immediately. Administration of a cerebroprotective agent may not be possible because of its associated hemodynamic effects. Induced hypotension under these circumstances may not be possible, because the intravascular volume must be restored first. During temporary occlusion, normotension must be maintained to maximize collateral perfusion. Excellent results have been achieved by Batjer and Samson[187] with the use of temporary occlusion for intraoperative aneurysm rupture.

Intraoperative Catheter Angiography and Indocyanine Green Videoangiography

Many surgeons routinely perform intraoperative contrast angiography to confirm the proper placement of the clip and patency of the vessels. This practice requires the use of special radiolucent operating room table attachments and the prior placement of intra-arterial sheath for catheter angiography. Near-infrared indocyanine green (ICG) videoangiography has now been introduced.[189] Injection of 25 mg of ICG and use of a specially equipped camera allows the anatomy of the aneurysm and the associated arteries to be visualized. Whether this method would replace intraoperative catheter angiography remains to be seen.[190]

Emergence and Recovery

Communication between the surgeon and the anesthesiologist is again essential for optimal management of the patient's emergence from anesthesia. If the surgical procedure is uneventful, patients with preoperative SAH grade I or II should be allowed to awaken, and their tracheas may be extubated in the operating room. To minimize coughing, particularly during movement of the head when the surgical dressing is applied, intravenous lidocaine, 1.5 mg/kg, is effective, but its duration of action is only about 3 to 5 minutes. It can be safely repeated if necessary. Because hypertensive therapy is effective in reversing delayed cerebral ischemia from vasospasm, modest levels of postoperative hypertension (<180 mm Hg systolic) are not aggressively treated. Nonetheless, severe hypertension (>200 mm Hg systolic) may cause increased swelling or cerebral hemorrhage. Labetalol and esmolol are both effective in controlling emergence hypertension. Labetalol is usually given in 5- to 10-mg increments, and esmolol in 0.1- to 0.5–mg/kg increments, until blood pressure is controlled. Other hypotensive drugs, including sodium nitroprusside, nitroglycerin, hydralazine, and nicardipine, can also be used. However, these drugs may cause cerebral vasodilation and increase ICP. In institutions where ICP monitors are placed routinely at the end of the surgical procedure and ICP is monitored postoperatively, it is safe to use these vasodilators for control of blood pressure. They are equally safe in patients who are awake and whose neurologic signs are being monitored continually.

Depending on preoperative ventilatory status and the duration and difficulty of the surgical procedure, the patient with preoperative SAH grade III may or may not undergo tracheal extubation in the operating room. In general, one should err on the side of caution. Only when the surgical procedure is uneventful, brain relaxation has not been a problem, and the patient can maintain adequate ventilation with intact laryngeal reflexes should extubation of the trachea be considered. Patients with preoperative SAH grade IV or V usually require postoperative ventilatory support and continuous neurointensive care. In patients with multiple aneurysms, systemic blood pressure must continue under strict control (within 20% of their normal blood pressure) to prevent rupture of unclipped aneurysms during emergence and recovery from anesthesia.

Patients who have experienced intraoperative aneurysm rupture and patients with vertebrobasilar aneurysms must be considered individually irrespective of their preoperative clinical SAH grade. In both groups the recovery may be slow, and immediate tracheal extubation may not be possible. In the former group, intraoperative cerebral ischemia may have occurred, and in the latter, transient or permanent cranial nerve dysfunction may have resulted from perforator vessel occlusion or brainstem retraction.

POSTOPERATIVE CONSIDERATIONS

In the immediate postoperative period, the anesthesiologist should assess the patient who has undergone subarachnoid aneurysm surgery to ensure that the recovery is satisfactory and consistent with the anesthetic given. The time of recovery clearly depends on the type and dose of anesthetic given as well as the patient's sensitivity to drugs given. There is no hard-and-fast rule to discriminate between anesthetic effects and surgical complications. Nevertheless, distinguishing residual anesthesia from surgical complications, such as development of subdural or epidural hematomas, is important. The following general guidelines are useful:

1. Anesthesia causes global depression, and any new focal neurologic deficit should be assumed to a surgical cause, although sedatives and analgesics have been reported to exacerbate or unmask focal neurologic findings in patients with previous strokes.[191]
2. The effect of potent inhaled anesthetics should have largely dissipated after 30 to 60 minutes.
3. Patients whose pupils are mid-sized and reactive to light and whose respiration is not depressed are unlikely to be experiencing narcotic overdose.
4. The postoperative presence of unequal pupils in a patient without this sign before operation always suggests a surgical event.
5. The patient's neurologic status should be assessed every 15 minutes in the recovery room or intensive care unit, and in some patients an immediate CT scan or angiogram may be necessary.

SUBARACHNOD HEMORRHAGE AND PREGNANCY

Intracranial hemorrhage from either a cerebral aneurysm or AVM is seen in 0.01% to 0.05% of all pregnant women,[192,193] a rate no different from its occurrence in the general population. Thus pregnancy does not predispose the patient to the development of SAH, and the occurrence of SAH, once thought to be not related to parity,[193] may actually be decreased in those with higher parity.[194] Most intracranial hemorrhages in pregnancy are caused by aneurysmal rupture (77%) rather than by AVM rupture (23%).[192] The mean age for patients with aneurysmal hemorrhage has been reported to be 28 to 30 years.[192,193]

Time Course of Bleeding

Most studies have found that aneurysms bleed more frequently during the third trimester, although bleeding has occurred as early as 6 weeks of gestation.[192,193] The tendency to bleed as pregnancy progresses may be due to cardiovascular changes. Cardiac output increases with pregnancy, with peak periods at 28 to 32 weeks, during labor and delivery, and in the initial postpartum period. Maternal blood volume, systolic blood pressure, stroke volume, and heart rate increase continually throughout pregnancy and reach maximum at term. During labor and delivery the cardiac output and blood pressure both increase in short bursts with uterine contractions secondary to pain and autotransfusion. The importance of these short bursts in facilitating aneurysmal rupture is uncertain. One school of thought is that labor is not a precipitating factor and that aneurysmal rupture during labor is a rare event. Of note, these cardiovascular changes associated with contractions can be blunted with epidural anesthesia.

Maternal and Fetal Outcome

The reported maternal mortality from aneurysmal SAH has been reported to be 35%, similar to that in the nongravid population, and the fetal mortality to be 17%.[192] The maternal mortality varied directly with Hunt and Hess clinical

grade.[192] Both maternal mortality (11% vs. 63%, respectively) and fetal mortality (5% vs. 27%, respectively) are significantly better with surgical treatment than with conservative management.[192]

Diagnosis

The clinical features of SAH in pregnant patients are similar to those in the general population. However, other disorders associated with pregnancy may mimic SAH and must be ruled out. They include pituitary apoplexy, cerebral sinus thrombosis, intracranial arterial occlusion, migraine headaches, post–dural puncture headaches, and preeclampsia. Other disorders causing neurologic symptoms suggestive of elevated ICP that may be confused with SAH are intracranial tumor or other mass lesion, meningitis, encephalitis, and demyelinating disease. A high index of suspicion is necessary to make the diagnosis of SAH in a pregnant patient. Preeclampsia—defined as hypertension, proteinuria, and peripheral edema—is another common cause of intracranial hemorrhage during the third trimester of pregnancy. The diagnosis of SAH is confirmed by CT scan or lumbar dural puncture followed by angiography. With proper shielding of the uterus, radiation exposure of the fetus is minimal. Iodinated contrast agents do not cross the placental barrier and pose little risk to the fetus. However, because of their osmotic effect, fetal dehydration may occur. Consequently, the mother should have adequate intravenous hydration during and after administration of the contrast agent, and her serum osmolarity and urine output should be monitored to avoid fetal dehydration.

Obstetric Management of Subarachnoid Hemorrhage in Pregnancy

Until recently, the treatment of choice for SAH during pregnancy was clearly surgical,[193] but the use of coils to occlude the aneurysm has arisen as an alternative treatment option.[195] Management depends on the gestational age of the fetus as well as the clinical status of the mother. Before fetal viability and in patients with good SAH grades, surgical clipping or coiling should be performed as soon as possible to prevent rebleeding.[193] Approximately 80% of aneurysm ruptures occur before 36 weeks of gestation, and in these patients, aneurysm clipping followed by delivery at full term generally results in a satisfactory outcome for both mother and infant. During craniotomy, continuous fetal heart rate monitoring should be used with an obstetric team available. If fetal distress develops, cesarean delivery may be considered. If labor begins and delivery appears imminent, the craniotomy should be temporarily halted and the fetus delivered by cesarean section.[192] If the fetus is near term or signs of fetal distress are apparent, the fetus should be delivered by cesarean section first and then the aneurysm should be clipped or coiled.[192] Oxytocic drugs have been used to decrease uterine atony and bleeding after delivery without deleterious neurologic effects, although these agents have not been studied extensively in this setting.[196] The most common hemodynamic alteration with oxytocin is hypotension, whereas hypertension is associated with methylergonovine maleate (Methergine) and prostaglandins (Hemabate).

In the gravid patient with a surgically inaccessible or undetermined aneurysm and in whom delivery is scheduled, obstetric management is controversial. The risk of bleeding during vaginal delivery is not significantly different from that during cesarean delivery. Although some authorities contend that all such patients should have cesarean deliveries to avoid the strain induced by labor, there are no significant differences in maternal and fetal mortality rates between vaginal delivery and cesarean delivery in patients with untreated aneurysms.[192]

One unusual circumstance in which emergency cesarean delivery is indicated is a patient in her third trimester whose aneurysm has bled, who is now moribund, and who is undergoing neuroresuscitation.[196]

Physiologic Changes in Pregnancy

Pregnancy is accompanied by a progressive increase in minute ventilation and a decrease in functional residual capacity. These changes make pregnant women prone to development of hypoxemia. The minimum alveolar concentration for inhaled anesthetics decreases. The greater minute ventilation that occurs with pregnancy lowers the $Paco_2$ to approximately 32 mm Hg and changes the set point for the cerebrovascular response to hyperventilation. Attempts to lower ICP therefore necessitate lowering $Paco_2$ to 25 mm Hg or less. Further decreases in $Paco_2$, however, may cause fetal hypoxia and acidosis through a decrease in uterine blood flow and reduced release of oxygen secondary to a shift of the oxygen-hemoglobin dissociation curve to the left. For these reasons, maternal $Paco_2$ should be maintained at approximately 30 mm Hg.

Uterine Blood Flow

Uterine blood flow is not autoregulated. It varies directly with systemic maternal blood pressure and is inversely proportional to uterine vascular resistance. A maternal systolic blood pressure of less than 100 mm Hg may produce uterine hypoperfusion and fetal bradycardia. Hypotension during aneurysm clipping may occur as a result of hypovolemia, administration of anesthetic agents, excessive positive-pressure ventilation, hemorrhage, or the use of nimodipine. Whatever the cause, maternal hypotension must be treated vigorously. Although induced hypotension may have adverse effects on the fetus, it has been used successfully to facilitate aneurysm clipping.[197,198] Positioning of the patient in her third trimester also affects uterine blood flow; a supine or right lateral position may cause the aorta–vena caval syndrome, resulting in maternal hypotension. Therefore left uterine displacement must be maintained with a roll or wedge under the right hip. Uterine blood flow may decrease during controlled ventilation secondary to the effect of hypocapnia on the uterine blood vessels or the mechanical effect of positive-pressure ventilation on cardiac output.

Anesthetic Management

Because cerebral aneurysms manifest primarily in the third trimester of pregnancy, the anesthesiologist must face the possible complications associated with pregnancy as well as the special considerations for aneurysm clipping. The anesthetic management also depends on the gestational age and obstetric plan—that is, whether delivery of the fetus will precede the neurosurgical procedure or whether aneurysm clipping will be followed by normal maturation of the fetus and subsequent delivery at term. Benefits of anesthetic drugs and technique used for the mother must always be balanced against potential risks to the fetus.

General Principles

The goals of anesthesia during pregnancy are to ensure recovery of the mother and normal continuation of the pregnancy without damage to the fetus. The anesthetic management should be the same as for the nonpregnant patient with an aneurysm, except that a pregnant patient is actually two patients. Pregnant patients have special needs because of the physiologic changes that occur during pregnancy, including: (1) consideration for the decrease in minimum alveolar concentration (MAC); (2) a greater potential for aspiration and a difficult airway; (3) special positioning; (4) the influence of anesthetic-induced depression on maternal blood pressure; and (5) the risk of inducing premature labor. Special needs with respect to the fetus are (1) adequate fetal-maternal oxygen exchange, which depends on adequate maternal blood pressure; (2) potential for the teratogenic effects of anesthetic drugs; and (3) perioperative monitoring of the fetus.[192]

Measures should be taken to prevent aspiration of gastric contents, because all pregnant patients are considered to have full stomachs, and to prevent the hypertensive response to intubation that may increase the potential of cerebral aneurysm rupture.[197] Pregnant patients should fast overnight, should receive a histamine H_2 receptor antagonist such as ranitidine, and should be given metoclopramide preoperatively to reduce the volume of gastric contents. The induction technique is essentially the same as already described for a nonpregnant patient with a full stomach.

In positioning of the patient in the third trimester of pregnancy, it is important to prevent aortocaval compression by using left uterine displacement. Immediately after positioning, the fetal heart rate should be monitored, the only practical way of monitoring fetal well-being during anesthesia.

Loss of beat-to-beat variation in fetal heart rate may be an early sign of fetal hypoxia during awake conditions but is normal for the anesthetized fetus. Interpretation of the intraoperative fetal heart rate should be made through comparison of a preinduction recording with the various changes during the course of anesthesia and surgery. If the fetus demonstrates tachycardia or bradycardia during maternal hypotension, the surgeon should be immediately informed, the blood pressure increased, and an obstetrician consulted.

Use of Induced Hypotension

Induced hypotension has been employed with success to facilitate aneurysm clipping during pregnancy.[193,196] Hypotensive agents that have been used include sodium nitroprusside,[198] trimethaphan, and high concentrations of isoflurane.[197] Sodium nitroprusside acts directly on the smooth muscle of the blood vessel and is freely permeable to the placenta, although this property is probably species dependent.[198] It may decrease uterine blood flow[198] as well as cause fetal cyanide toxicity. Although trimethaphan has been used for hypotension during pregnancy, it causes reductions in both cardiac output and CBF and therefore may be unsuitable for this purpose. Isoflurane is an alternative, because it has little effect on cardiac output[199] and CBF.[200] In the pregnant ewe at 1.5 MAC, uteroplacental blood flow was maintained and did not cause fetal hypoxemia or metabolic acidosis.[201] The use of hypotension, however, remains controversial, and several writers have suggested that the technique be avoided in pregnant patients. With the trend toward temporary arterial occlusion, there should be no need for induced hypotension during pregnancy. If hypotension is to be used, the fetal heart rate must be monitored closely, and the blood pressure raised if fetal bradycardia or tachycardia occurs.

Other Considerations

Mannitol has been shown to cross the placenta, so it may accumulate in the fetus and lead to changes in fetal osmolality, volume, and the concentrations of various electrolytes. Mannitol infusions of 12.5 g/kg in pregnant rabbits shift free water from the fetus to the mother, which increases fetal osmolality by 22%, raising plasma sodium concentration to 162 mEq/L and decreasing plasma volume by 50%.[202] In a human study the administration of 200 g of mannitol to the mother before delivery altered the volume, osmolality, and concentration of solutes in the fetus.[203] However, in dosages used clinically in aneurysm clipping (0.5 to 1.0 g/kg), mannitol is unlikely to cause severe fluid or electrolyte abnormalities in the fetus. Mannitol is also not always essential for brain relaxation; however, if it is required, moderate doses should be used.[197]

β-Adrenergic antagonists have been reported to cause intrauterine growth retardation, premature labor, worsening of preexisting fetal distress, neonatal acidosis, bradycardia, hypoglycemia, apnea, and diminished response to hypoxia and acidosis.[196,198] To what extent these theoretic considerations should influence clinical decisions regarding the use of β-blockers is not clear. A rational approach would be to limit the use of these agents to clear indications and to always be aware of their potential adverse effects. Table 13-9 contains a summary of the effects of some drugs on the uterus and placenta.

Table 13–9   Adverse Uteroplacental Effects of Various Drugs

Drug	Adverse Effect(s)
Phenytoin	Minimal
Thiopental	Neonatal depression (> 8 mg/kg in humans); worsening of preexisting fetal distress caused by maternal hemodynamics effects
Lidocaine	Uterine hypertonus and vasoconstriction with fetal distress (toxic doses in sheep); worsening of preexisting fetal distress
Mannitol	Oligohydramnios with fetal hyperosmolarity, hypernatremia, dehydration, cyanosis, bradycardia (at 12.5 g/kg in rabbits); fetal hyperosmolarity in humans 1 hr after 200 g IV
Furosemide	Possible dilation of ductus arteriosus; electrolyte abnormalities
Nitroprusside	Decreased uterine vascular resistance; electrolyte abnormalities
Nitroprusside	Decreased uterine vascular resistance; lethal fetal cyanide levels with onset of maternal tachyphylaxis in sheep
Nitroglycerin	Decreased uterine vascular resistance
Hydralazine	Decreased uterine vascular resistance
Propranolol	Decreased umbilical blood flow in sheep; premature labor, worsening of preexisting fetal distress, neonatal acidosis, bradycardia, hypoglycemia, apnea, diminished response to hypoxia and acidosis

Preterm Clipping of Aneurysm with Normal Delivery at Term

When the pregnant patient is to undergo aneurysm clipping followed by continuation of pregnancy to term, the emphasis during the surgical procedure is to treat the patient as any patient with SAH while being cognizant of the effects of anesthetic drugs and techniques on fetal well-being. Because delivery is not immediate, neonatal depression is not a significant concern. Perioperative and postoperative fetal heart rate monitoring is mandatory. Patients who have undergone successful clipping of their aneurysms during pregnancy do not require specialized management of labor or delivery and may receive an oxytocic agent for induction of labor for vaginal delivery unless there are obstetric indications for abdominal delivery.[193]

Cesarean Delivery Followed by Aneurysm Clipping

In a patient undergoing cesarean delivery before aneurysm clipping, the aim is to prevent rupture of the aneurysm while the cesarean delivery is being performed. A light anesthetic, although normally appropriate to minimize neonatal depression, may allow for maternal hypertension and rupture of the aneurysm. Both intravenous and inhaled anesthetic agents, however, will cross the placental barrier, resulting in neonatal depression. On balance, the anesthesiologist should anesthetize the patient to an adequate depth of anesthesia with the aim of preventing aneurysmal rupture during induction as well as during maintenance and accept the price of neonatal depression. Equipment and personnel for neonatal resuscitation should be at hand when delivery occurs.

GIANT ANEURYSMS

Giant cerebral aneurysms are defined as those greater than 2.5 cm in diameter, representing a subset of cerebral aneurysms that may present technical difficulty because of their size or lack of an anatomic neck. They often have perforating vessels originating in, or probably more typically, adherent to the wall of the aneurysm, as well as a high likelihood of atheromatous changes. The incidence of giant aneurysm is 2% of all patients in the Cooperative Study.[2] Most giant aneurysms manifest as symptoms of a mass lesion, such as headache, visual disturbance, and cranial nerve palsies.

The surgical treatment of these aneurysms is associated with significant perioperative morbidity and mortality. In a series of 174 patients with giant aneurysms who underwent standard surgical treatment, Drake[204] reported that 71.5% of the patients had good outcomes, 13% were severely disabled, and 15.5% died. The series of 174 included 73 patients with giant basilar aneurysms that were associated with a complication rate of near 50% (23% had poor outcome and 25% died). Surgery for giant aneurysm remains a formidable challenge, and some neurosurgeons advise their patients against operative intervention unless immediate life-threatening risks are present.[205] Two surgical techniques are used for the management of giant aneurysms considered otherwise inoperable: (1) the use of proximal and distal temporary occlusion to collapse the aneurysm and (2) the use of circulatory arrest with profound hypothermia.[206] Although the former approach has been advocated by some surgeons,[207] it is not considered uniformly applicable. The latter approach had been used as a general approach for all cerebral aneurysms but fell into disfavor as improvements in microsurgical technique and neuroanesthesia allowed conventional approaches to achieve better results. However, interest in using hypothermic circulatory arrest for giant aneurysms has been revived, with several groups reporting good results and a mortality ranging from 0% to 25%. The main advantages of hypothermic circulatory arrest for giant aneurysm are (1) decompression of the aneurysmal sac, (2) better visualization of the anatomy, (3) a totally bloodless field, and (4) greater ease in placement of the clip across a large or anatomically complicated aneurysm neck. Circulatory arrest can be performed with use of closed-chest femoral vein-femoral artery bypass or through an open chest with median sternotomy and ventricular venting. The closed-chest method is associated with lower morbidity and is preferred.

The anesthetic management of temporary occlusion has already been described; therefore only circulatory arrest under profound hypothermia is discussed here. The major issues concern brain protection and the complications of cardiopulmonary bypass. For details on physiology and management of cardiopulmonary bypass, the reader should consult a standard textbook on cardiovascular anesthesia.

Brain Protection in Circulatory Arrest

Cerebral hypoxia and ischemia are the factors that limit the duration of the circulatory arrest. The metabolic oxygen consumption of the brain may be divided into an active component, which can be regarded as any neuronal activity, and a basal component, which is related to maintenance of cellular integrity. Pharmacologic and nonpharmacologic methods that reduce metabolic oxygen consumption increase the duration of arrest tolerated. At present, these include the use of barbiturates or propofol and profound hypothermia. A number of investigators have reported good results with giant aneurysm surgery utilizing the combination of barbiturate therapy and profound hypothermia during circulatory arrest.[205,208-211] High-dose propofol has also been used to achieve a similar purpose. However, similar results have also been obtained with profound hypothermia alone.[212]

Barbiturates

Barbiturates can reduce the cerebral metabolic rate for oxygen ($CMRo_2$) attributed to the active component to zero and, therefore, reduce the overall $CMRo_2$ to a maximum of 50%. Additional barbiturate administration beyond what is required to cause electrical silence in the EEG will not decrease the metabolic rate further. However, barbiturates may have other actions, including free radical scavenging and membrane stabilization.[209] Therefore barbiturates may provide additional cerebral protection even during profound hypothermia, although this notion remains controversial. Barbiturate therapy is most effective in preventing cerebral injury secondary to temporary focal ischemia. It is less well established in the situation of temporary global ischemia.

Two modes of administering barbiturates (primarily, sodium thiopental) before cooling and arrest are used, a single bolus and a continuous infusion. In studies in which a single dose of thiopental was given, the amount ranged from 30 to 40 mg/kg administered over 30 minutes.[208,210,213] In most of the reported studies, however, EEG monitoring was not used to determine the endpoint. Monitoring the EEG allows the anesthesiologist to titrate the loading dose and the maintenance

infusion to achieve EEG burst suppression throughout the procedure.[209,211] A simple bihemispheric two-channel EEG device will suffice. Burst suppression may be accomplished with an initial loading dose of thiopental, 3 to 5 mg/kg, followed by a continuous infusion varying from 0.1 to 0.5 mg/kg/min for the entire period of cardiopulmonary bypass. With profound hypothermia at temperatures below 18° C, the EEG is rendered isoelectric even without pharmacologic suppression (in contrast, evoked responses are abolished between 15° and 18° C). It is recommended that the thiopental infusion rate established during normothermia be maintained during circulatory arrest.[209] In patients with heart disease, thiopental loading may lead to severe myocardial dysfunction, preventing separation of the patient from cardiopulmonary bypass after the aneurysm is clipped. Several small studies examining the cardiac performance in patients undergoing profound hypothermia for cerebral aneurysm surgery demonstrated that cardiac function was only minimally impaired. Similar observations were made with the use of high-dose propofol.[214]

Hypothermia

Hypothermia (Table 13-10), a nonpharmacologic method of reducing the $CMRo_2$, is different from barbiturates in that it reduces not only the active component but also the basal component of the $CMRo_2$. Hypothermia causes a significant reduction in cerebral oxygen consumption and has been demonstrated to protect the brain during anoxic conditions. The period of circulatory arrest tolerated at normothermia is only 4 to 5 minutes, but it doubles for every 8° C in temperature reduction. Thus the $CMRo_2$ value drops to 50% of normal with hypothermia at 30° C, to 25% of normal at 25° C, 15% of normal at 20°C, and to 10% of normal at 15°C. At 15° C, continuous circulatory arrest can be tolerated for 32 to 40 minutes. The maximum time of deep hypothermic arrest has not been definitively established, but in clinical practice the maneuver has been safely used for up to 60 minutes.[212]

Because substantial gradients in temperature can develop between the brain and the periphery during cooling and rewarming, it is important to monitor the brain temperature accurately before circulatory arrest. Williams and associates[212] reported close correlation of brain temperatures measured with esophageal, tympanic membrane, and nasopharyngeal sensors. In contrast, rectal temperatures were unreliable and bladder temperature reliability varied among studies.[215] Direct brain temperature monitoring has also been advocated.[178] To improve safety, at least two temperature monitoring sites should be used.

The depth of hypothermia and the duration of circulatory arrest reported in various studies for treatment of giant

Table 13–10 Hypothermia for Treatment of Giant Cerebral Aneurysms

Body Temperature (° C)	Percentage of Normal Cerebral Metabolic Rate	Period of Tolerated Circulatory Arrest (min)
38	100	4-5
30	50	8-10
25	25	16-20
20	15	32-40
10	10	64-80

Table 13–11 Reports of Circulatory Arrest for Treatment of Giant Cerebral Aneurysms

Study*	No. of Cases	Body Temperature (° C)	Duration of Arrest (min)		Rate of Major Morbidity (%)	Rate of Mortality (%)
			Median	Range		
Spetzler et al (2008)[226][†]	105	?	?	?	?	13.3
Mack et al (2007)[177]	66	17.6	26.2	6-77	31	12
Levati et al (2007)[211][‡]	12	14.1	26.5	9-54	25	0
Lawton et al (1998)[227][§]	60	9-19	23	2-72	13.3	8.3
Greene et al (1994)[228][¶¶]	2	15-18	40,70	40-70	0	0
Ausman et al (1993)[229]	9	17-18	20	12-37	22	33
Williams et al (1991)[212]	10[¶]	8.4-13.7	25	1.25-60	20	10
Solomon et al (1991)[205][‡]	14	15-22.5	22	8-51	50	0
Thomas et al (1990)[210][‡]	1	15.4	35	—	0	0
Spetzler et al (1988)[209][‡]	7	17.5-21	11	7-53	29	14
Gonski et al (1986)[230][‡]	40	25	10	0-35	23	25
Baumgartner et al (1983)[208][‡]	15**	16-21.5	19	0-51	20	0
McMurtry et al (1974)[231]	12[††]	28-29	9	1-28	50	8
Sundt et al (1972)[232]	1	13	30	—	100	0
Drake et al (1964)[206]	10	13-17	14	2-18	40	30
Michenfelder et al (1964)[233]	15	13-16	17	0-39	40	20
Patterson & Ray (1962)[216]	7	14-17	25	9-43	0	30
Woodhall et al (1960)[234]	1[‡‡]	12	30	—	100	0

?, means unknown (not reported); —, information not available from the reference.
*Superscript numbers indicate chapter references.
[†]Citing unpublished data.
[‡]Barbiturate therapy was also used.
[§]Includes patients from previously published series
[¶¶]Pediatric cases.
[¶]Only 4 out of 10 are giant aneurysms. The patient who died had an AVM; the patients with morbidity included 1 with AVM and 1 with aneurysm.
**Two of 15 are patients with medullary hemangioblastoma.
[††]One of 12 with AVM.
[‡‡]Patient with metastatic bronchogenic carcinoma.

aneurysms are summarized in Table 13-11. Note that the amount of time necessary for the clipping is usually less than the tolerable safe limit at the temperature used. Compared to early experience, the mortality and morbidity have declined substantially. The more recent series suggest that temperature should be decreased to 15° to 18°C, since the series with the highest mortality (25%) was associated with circulatory arrest at 25°C.[216]

CARDIOVASCULAR EFFECTS OF PROFOUND HYPOTHERMIA

Hypothermia induces characteristic cardiovascular changes. As temperature decreases, systemic vascular resistance increases while cardiac output decreases. To allow high pump flow to facilitate rapid cooling and subsequent rewarming, use of vasodilators such as sodium nitroprusside may be necessary. Progressive bradycardia occurs as the temperature approaches 30° C, and the atrium frequently begins to develop flutter or fibrillation below 30° C. The ventricles usually fibrillate below 28° C. Because continuous ventricular fibrillation may cause ischemic injury to the heart, electrical activity should be terminated with administration of 40 to 80 mEq of potassium chloride to the pump or with cardioversion (100 to 250 watts/sec).

HEMATOLOGIC EFFECTS OF PROFOUND HYPOTHERMIA

The coagulation system is severely perturbed by hypothermia, and the problem is compounded by inadequate surgical hemostasis or incomplete reversal of heparin with protamine.[208,209,212] Hypothermia-induced coagulopathy is caused by a multitude of factors, including (1) reduction of the platelet count, probably from splenic sequestration, (2) a reversible platelet dysfunction through a decrease in adhesiveness, (3) slowing down of the enzyme-mediated steps in the coagulation cascade, and (4) decrease in the metabolism of heparin. The dilutional effect of priming solutions with cardiopulmonary bypass on coagulation factors I, II, V, VII, and XIII also contributes to difficulty with hemostasis.

Hypothermia also causes an increase in viscosity, leading to sludging of the red blood cells. However, this problem can be effectively treated through a deliberate lowering of the hematocrit with phlebotomy and simultaneously replacement of the blood volume with a crystalloid solution. The phlebotomy not only decreases the hematocrit but also preserves platelet-rich autologous blood for subsequent transfusion during the rewarming phase. The lower hematocrit reduces oxygen-carrying capacity, but this effect is partially compensated for by the greater amount of dissolved oxygen, which results from the higher oxygen solubility that occurs with hypothermia. The hemoglobin-oxygen dissociation curve, however, is also shifted to the left and may reduce unloading of oxygen in ischemic tissue.

HYPERGLYCEMIA

Hypothermia prevents proper utilization and metabolism of glucose and may cause hyperglycemia. As mentioned previously, hyperglycemia may exacerbate neuronal damage during ischemia[133,134] and therefore should be treated with insulin. Frequent monitoring of serum glucose and electrolyte concentrations in addition to acid-base balance is therefore essential.

ANESTHETIC CONSIDERATIONS

In addition to the normal evaluation of the patient with SAH, preoperative consideration of patients scheduled for hypothermic circulatory arrest must include special emphasis on coexisting cardiac, pulmonary, hematologic, or neurologic disorders that may require modification of this form of therapy or exclude the patient from undergoing it. For example, patients with aortic valve insufficiency may require the open-chest method of cardiopulmonary bypass to prevent ventricular distention. On the other hand, patients with poor ventricular function, existing coagulopathy, or significant carotid artery disease may be considered unsuitable for the procedure.

Although induction of anesthesia is similar to what has been covered previously regarding monitors, blood pressure control, and intubation, several additional monitors should be considered. These include EEG, SSEP and BAEP monitoring, transesophageal echocardiography, and TCD. The EEG monitors cortical activity and is necessary as an endpoint for barbiturate-induced burst suppression when barbiturates are used for added protection. SSEP monitoring, on the other hand, is a measure of the sensory conduction to the cortex and can be recorded even during a barbiturate-induced silent EEG. The BAEP reflects the function of the auditory pathway through the brainstem and so its monitoring may be useful during procedures on vertebrobasilar aneurysms.[209] During profound hypothermia at 15° to 18° C, all electrophysiologic activity is abolished; nevertheless, SSEP monitoring may allow assessment of neurologic function during cooling as well as rewarming and may have prognostic value. Transesophageal echocardiography allows visualization of the cardiac chambers and assessment of ventricular function and is useful in management of patients with cardiac disease.[205] In addition, TCD has been used during these procedures,[205] presumably to monitor CBF velocity and emboli, although its value has not been established.

The overall management necessitates a team effort requiring effective communication from all participants. To administer anesthesia safely for hypothermic circulatory arrest, a thorough understanding of the cardiovascular and hematologic perturbations in response to hypothermia must be appreciated. The technique also demands knowledge of the use of the various electrophysiologic monitors that guide efforts to provide cerebral protection. Although the actual practice varies among different institutions, a suggested protocol is appended.

The major and most feared postoperative complication associated with hypothermic cardiac arrest for aneurysm surgery is coagulopathy leading to cerebral hemorrhage. A small leak at the operative site can be disastrous. To reduce this risk, the surgeon should complete the dissection of the aneurysm and verify absolute hemostasis before initiating hypothermic circulatory arrest. Heparinization should be evaluated and followed with the activated clotting time, which should be maintained within 400 to 450 seconds. Once rewarming has occurred and the patient no longer requires bypass, protamine sulfate is titrated to reverse the effect of heparin until the activated clotting time is between 100 and 150 seconds. The phlebotomized blood removed earlier is transfused back, and additional blood products, such as fresh frozen plasma, cryoprecipitate, and platelets, are often required. Meticulous achievement of surgical hemostasis is again necessary before dural closure begins.

The anesthesiologist must also watch for any cardiovascular complications associated with cardiopulmonary bypass, including hypotension, low cardiac output, and hypertension, and must correct any rhythm abnormalities during the cooling or rewarming phase. The patient may also require inotropic support during warming and the immediate postoperative course. With or without additional barbiturate protection, the patient is generally transferred directly to the intensive care unit for continued care. Extubation of the trachea and assessment of neurologic function can usually be accomplished within 12 to 24 hours postoperatively.

SUMMARY

Because of the associated systemic effects and the surgical requirements, patients with cerebral aneurysms present a unique challenge to the anesthesiologist. This chapter has highlighted the major considerations and suggested rational approaches. The important steps are:

1. A thorough understanding of the patient's pathophysiology in relation to the subarachnoid hemorrhage as well as other related systemic effects
2. Communication with the neurosurgeon to clarify the surgical approach and the necessity for any specific monitoring
3. Outline of the anesthetic objectives
4. Formulation of anesthetic plan to meet the objectives, taking into consideration one's knowledge of anesthetic drugs and clinical experience (this should also include planning for untoward events intraoperatively such as rupture of the aneurysm)
5. Implementation of the plan.

There will always be patients who, despite our best efforts, fail to benefit from the surgical procedure. It is hoped, however, that with proper planning, optimal results can be achieved.

REFERENCES

1. Drake CG: Aneurysm surgery: past, present, and future. In Varkey GP [ed]: Anesthetic Considerations in the Surgical Repair of Intracranial Aneurysms. Boston, Little, Brown, 1982.
2. Kassell NF, Torner JC, Haley EC Jr, et al: The International Cooperative Study on the Timing of Aneurysm Surgery. Part 1: Overall management results, J Neurosurg 73:18–36, 1990.
3. Kassell NF, Torner JC, Jane JA, et al: The International Cooperative Study on the Timing of Aneurysm Surgery. Part 2: Surgical results, J Neurosurg 73:37–47, 1990.
4. Molyneux A, Kerr R, Stratton I, et al: International Subarachnoid Aneurysm Trial (ISAT) of neurosurgical clipping versus endovascular coiling in 2143 patients with ruptured intracranial aneurysms: A randomised trial, Lancet 360:1267–1274, 2002.
5. Molyneux AJ, Kerr RS, Yu LM, et al: International Subarachnoid Aneurysm Trial (ISAT) of neurosurgical clipping versus endovascular coiling in 2143 patients with ruptured intracranial aneurysms: A randomised comparison of effects on survival, dependency, seizures, rebleeding, subgroups, and aneurysm occlusion, Lancet 366:809–817, 2005.

6. Campi A, Ramzi N, Molyneux AJ, et al: Retreatment of ruptured cerebral aneurysms in patients randomized by coiling or clipping in the International Subarachnoid Aneurysm Trial (ISAT), *Stroke* 38:1538–1544, 2007.

7. Botterell EH, Lougheed WM, Scott JW, Vandewater SL: Hypothermia, and interruption of carotid, or carotid and vertebral circulation, in the surgical management of intracranial aneurysms, *J Neurosurg* 13:1–42, 1956.

8. Hunt WE, Hess RM: Surgical risk as related to time of intervention in the repair of intracranial aneurysms, *J Neurosurg* 28:14–20, 1968.

9. Report of World Federation of Neurological Surgeons Committee on a Universal Subarachnoid Hemorrhage Grading Scale, *J Neurosurg* 68:985–986, 1988.

10. Fisher CM, Kistler JP, Davis JM: Relation of cerebral vasospasm to subarachnoid hemorrhage visualized by computerized tomographic scanning, *Neurosurgery* 6:1–9, 1980.

11. Smith ML, Abrahams JM, Chandela S, et al: Subarachnoid hemorrhage on computed tomography scanning and the development of cerebral vasospasm: The Fisher grade revisited, *Surg Neurol* 63:229–234, 2005:discussion 234–235.

12. Frontera JA, Claassen J, Schmidt JM, et al: Prediction of symptomatic vasospasm after subarachnoid hemorrhage: The modified Fisher scale, *Neurosurgery* 59:21–27, 2006.

13. Le Roux PD, Elliott JP, Newell DW, et al: Predicting outcome in poor-grade patients with subarachnoid hemorrhage: A retrospective review of 159 aggressively managed cases [see comments], *J Neurosurg* 85:39–49, 1996.

14. Voldby B, Enevoldsen EM: Intracranial pressure changes following aneurysm rupture. Part 1: Clinical and angiographic correlations, *J Neurosurg* 56:186–196, 1982.

15. Heuer GG, Smith MJ, Elliott JP, et al: Relationship between intracranial pressure and other clinical variables in patients with aneurysmal subarachnoid hemorrhage, *J Neurosurg* 101:408–416, 2004.

16. Dernbach PD, Little JR, Jones SC, Ebrahim ZY: Altered cerebral autoregulation and CO_2 reactivity after aneurysmal subarachnoid hemorrhage, *Neurosurgery* 22:822–826, 1988.

17. Tenjin H, Hirakawa K, Mizukawa N, et al: Dysautoregulation in patients with ruptured aneurysms: Cerebral blood flow measurements obtained during surgery by a temperature-controlled thermoelectrical method, *Neurosurgery* 23:705–709, 1988.

18. Davies KR, Gelb AW, Manninen PH, et al: Cardiac function in aneurysmal subarachnoid haemorrhage: A study of electrocardiographic and echocardiographic abnormalities, *Br J Anaesth* 67:58–63, 1991.

19. Kothavale A, Banki NM, Kopelnik A, et al: Predictors of left ventricular regional wall motion abnormalities after subarachnoid hemorrhage, *Neurocrit Care* 4:199–205, 2006.

20. Diringer MN, Lim JS, Kirsch JR, Hanley DF: Suprasellar and intraventricular blood predict elevated plasma atrial natriuretic factor in subarachnoid hemorrhage, *Stroke* 22:577–581, 1991.

21. Nelson RJ, Roberts J, Rubin C, et al: Association of hypovolemia after subarachnoid hemorrhage with computed tomographic scan evidence of raised intracranial pressure, *Neurosurgery* 29:178–182, 1991.

22. Todd MM, Hindman BJ, Clarke WR, Torner JC: Mild intraoperative hypothermia during surgery for intracranial aneurysm, *N Engl J Med* 352:135–145, 2005.

23. Carpenter DA, Grubb RL Jr, Tempel LW, Powers WJ: Cerebral oxygen metabolism after aneurysmal subarachnoid hemorrhage, *J Cereb Blood Flow Metab* 11:837–844, 1991.

24. Jakobsen M, Enevoldsen E, Bjerre P: Cerebral blood flow and metabolism following subarachnoid haemorrhage: Cerebral oxygen uptake and global blood flow during the acute period in patients with SAH, *Acta Neurol Scand* 82:174–182, 1990.

25. Bakker AM, Dorhout Mees SM, Algra A: Rinkel GJ: Extent of acute hydrocephalus after aneurysmal subarachnoid hemorrhage as a risk factor for delayed cerebral infarction, *Stroke* 38:2496–2499, 2007.

26. Shapiro HM: Intracranial hypertension: Therapeutic and anesthetic considerations, *Anesthesiology* 43:445–471, 1975.

27. Schmieder K, Moller F, Engelhardt M, et al: Dynamic cerebral autoregulation in patients with ruptured and unruptured aneurysms after induction of general anesthesia, *Zentralbl Neurochir* 67:81–87, 2006.

28. Nornes H, Knutzen HB, Wikeby P: Cerebral arterial blood flow and aneurysm surgery. Part 2: Induced hypotension and autoregulatory capacity, *J Neurosurg* 47:819–827, 1977.

29. Voldby B, Enevoldsen EM, Jensen FT: Cerebrovascular reactivity in patients with ruptured intracranial aneurysms, *J Neurosurg* 62:59–67, 1985.

30. Lam JM, Smielewski P, Czosnyka M, et al: Predicting delayed ischemic deficits after aneurysmal subarachnoid hemorrhage using a transient hyperemic response test of cerebral autoregulation, *Neurosurgery* 47:819–825, 2000:discussion 825–826.

31. Jaeger M, Schuhmann MU, Soehle M, et al: Continuous monitoring of cerebrovascular autoregulation after subarachnoid hemorrhage by brain tissue oxygen pressure reactivity and its relation to delayed cerebral infarction, *Stroke* 38:981–986, 2007.

32. Kassell NF, Peerless SJ, Durward QJ, et al: Treatment of ischemic deficits from vasospasm with intravascular volume expansion and induced arterial hypertension, *Neurosurgery* 11:337–343, 1982.

33. Hoff RG, Vand GW, Mettes S, et al: Hypotension in anaesthetized patients during aneurysm clipping: Not as bad as expected? *Acta Anaesthesiol Scand* 52:1006–1011, 2008.

34. Ma X, Willumsen L, Hauerberg J, et al: Effects of graded hyperventilation on cerebral blood flow autoregulation in experimental subarachnoid hemorrhage, *J Cereb Blood Flow Metab* 20:718–725, 2000.

35. Wijdicks EF, Vermeulen M, Hijdra A, van Gijn J: Hyponatremia and cerebral infarction in patients with ruptured intracranial aneurysms: Is fluid restriction harmful? *Ann Neurol* 17:137–140, 1985.

36. Hasan D, Wijdicks EF, Vermeulen M: Hyponatremia is associated with cerebral ischemia in patients with aneurysmal subarachnoid hemorrhage, *Ann Neurol* 27:106–108, 1990.

37. Betjes MG: Hyponatremia in acute brain disease: The cerebral salt wasting syndrome, *Eur J Intern Med* 13:9–14, 2002.

38. Sherlock M, O'Sullivan E, Agha A, et al: The incidence and pathophysiology of hyponatraemia after subarachnoid haemorrhage, *Clin Endocrinol (Oxf)* 64:250–254, 2006.

39. Harrigan MR: Cerebral salt wasting syndrome: A review, *Neurosurgery* 38:152–160, 1996.

40. Tung PP, Olmsted E, Kopelnik A, et al: Plasma B-type natriuretic peptide levels are associated with early cardiac dysfunction after subarachnoid hemorrhage, *Stroke* 36:1567–1569, 2005.

41. Sviri GE, Shik V, Raz B, Soustiel JF: Role of brain natriuretic peptide in cerebral vasospasm, *Acta Neurochir (Wien)* 145:851–860, 2003:discussion 860.

42. McGirt MJ, Blessing R, Nimjee SM, et al: Correlation of serum brain natriuretic peptide with hyponatremia and delayed ischemic neurological deficits after subarachnoid hemorrhage, *Neurosurgery* 54:1369–1373, 2004:discussion 1373–1374.

43. Rudehill A, Gordon E, Sundqvist K, et al: A study of ECG abnormalities and myocardial specific enzymes in patients with subarachnoid haemorrhage, *Acta Anaesthesiol Scand* 26:344–350, 1982.

44. Lee VH, Oh JK, Mulvagh SL, Wijdicks EF: Mechanisms in neurogenic stress cardiomyopathy after aneurysmal subarachnoid hemorrhage, *Neurocrit Care* 5:243–249, 2006.

45. Lanzino G, Kongable GL, Kassell NF: Electrocardiographic abnormalities after nontraumatic subarachnoid hemorrhage, *J Neurosurg Anesthesiol* 6:156–162, 1994.

46. Manninen PH, Ayra B, Gelb AW, Pelz D: Association between electrocardiographic abnormalities and intracranial blood in patients following acute subarachnoid hemorrhage, *J Neurosurg Anesthesiol* 7:12–16, 1995.

47. Frontera JA, Parra A, Shimbo D, et al: Cardiac arrhythmias after subarachnoid hemorrhage: Risk factors and impact on outcome, *Cerebrovasc Dis* 26:71–78, 2008.

48. Horowitz MB, Willet D, Keffer J: The use of cardiac troponin-I (cTnI) to determine the incidence of myocardial ischemia and injury in patients with aneurysmal and presumed aneurysmal subarachnoid hemorrhage, *Acta Neurochir* 140:87–93, 1998.

49. Naidech AM, Kreiter KT, Janjua N, et al: Cardiac troponin elevation, cardiovascular morbidity, and outcome after subarachnoid hemorrhage, *Circulation* 112:2851–2856, 2005.

50. Bulsara KR, McGirt MJ, Liao L, et al: Use of the peak troponin value to differentiate myocardial infarction from reversible neurogenic left ventricular dysfunction associated with aneurysmal subarachnoid hemorrhage, *J Neurosurg* 98:524–528, 2003.

51. Yarlagadda S, Rajendran P, Miss JC, et al: Cardiovascular predictors of in-patient mortality after subarachnoid hemorrhage, *Neurocrit Care* 5:102–107, 2006.

52. Mayer SA, Lin J, Homma S, et al: Myocardial injury and left ventricular performance after subarachnoid hemorrhage, *Stroke* 30:780–786, 1999.

53. Zaroff JG, Rordorf GA, Titus JS, et al: Regional myocardial perfusion after experimental subarachnoid hemorrhage, *Stroke* 31:1136–1143, 2000.

54. de Chazal I, Parham WM 3rd, Liopyris P, Wijdicks EF: Delayed cardiogenic shock and acute lung injury after aneurysmal subarachnoid hemorrhage, *Anesth Analg* 100:1147–1149, 2005.

55. Zaroff JG, Rordorf GA, Ogilvy CS, Picard MH: Regional patterns of left ventricular systolic dysfunction after subarachnoid hemorrhage: Evidence for neurally mediated cardiac injury, *J Am Soc Echocardiogr* 13:774–779, 2000.

56. Lee VH, Connolly HM, Fulgham JR, et al: Tako-tsubo cardiomyopathy in aneurysmal subarachnoid hemorrhage: An underappreciated ventricular dysfunction, *J Neurosurg* 105:264–270, 2006.

57. Banki N, Kopelnik A, Tung P, et al: Prospective analysis of prevalence, distribution, and rate of recovery of left ventricular systolic dysfunction in patients with subarachnoid hemorrhage, *J Neurosurg* 105:15–20, 2006.

58. Grad A, Kiauta T, Osredkar J: Effect of elevated plasma norepinephrine on electrocardiographic changes in subarachnoid hemorrhage, *Stroke* 22:746–749, 1991.

59. Zaroff JG, Rordorf GA, Newell JB, et al: Cardiac outcome in patients with subarachnoid hemorrhage and electrocardiographic abnormalities, *Neurosurgery* 44:34–39, 1999:discussion 39–40.

60. Muroi C, Keller M, Pangalu A, et al: Neurogenic pulmonary edema in patients with subarachnoid hemorrhage, *J Neurosurg Anesthesiol* 20:188–192, 2008.

61. McLaughlin N, Bojanowski MW, Girard F, Denault A: Pulmonary edema and cardiac dysfunction following subarachnoid hemorrhage, *Can J Neurol Sci* 32:178–185, 2005.

62. Baumann A, Audibert G, McDonnell J, Mertes PM: Neurogenic pulmonary edema, *Acta Anaesthesiol Scand* 51:447–455, 2007.

63. Audu P, Kim LI, Mehta MY, Kim J: Newer anti-epileptic drugs do not cause resistance to non-depolarizing neuromuscular blockade, *Anesthesiology* 105:A115, 2006.

64. Roos YB, Rinkel GJ, Vermeulen M et al: Antifibrinolytic therapy for aneurysmal subarachnoid haemorrhage, *Cochrane Database Syst Rev* (2)2003:CD001245.

65. Pickard JD, Kirkpatrick PJ, Melsen T, et al: Potential role of NovoSeven in the prevention of rebleeding following aneurysmal subarachnoid haemorrhage, *Blood Coagul Fibrinolysis* 11(Suppl 1):S117–S120, 2000.

66. Haley EC Jr, Kassell NF, Torner JC: The International Cooperative Study on the Timing of Aneurysm Surgery: The North American experience, *Stroke* 23:205–214, 1992.

67. Chwajol M, Starke RM, Kim GH, et al: Antifibrinolytic therapy to prevent early rebleeding after subarachnoid hemorrhage, *Neurocrit Care* 8:418–426, 2008.

68. de Oliveira JG, Beck J, Ulrich C, et al: Comparison between clipping and coiling on the incidence of cerebral vasospasm after aneurysmal subarachnoid hemorrhage: A systematic review and meta-analysis, *Neurosurg Rev* 30:22–30, 2007:discussion 30–31.

69. Macdonald RL, Weir BK: A review of hemoglobin and the pathogenesis of cerebral vasospasm, *Stroke* 22:971–982, 1991.

70. Pluta RM, Afshar JK, Boock RJ, Oldfield EH: Temporal changes in perivascular concentrations of oxyhemoglobin, deoxyhemoglobin, and methemoglobin after subarachnoid hemorrhage, *J Neurosurg* 88:557–561, 1998.

71. Findlay JM, Kassell NF, Weir BK, et al: A randomized trial of intraoperative, intracisternal tissue plasminogen activator for the prevention of vasospasm, *Neurosurgery* 37:168–176, 1995:discussion 177–178.

72. Zabramski JM, Spetzler RF, Lee KS, et al: Phase I trial of tissue plasminogen activator for the prevention of vasospasm in patients with aneurysmal subarachnoid hemorrhage, *J Neurosurg* 75:189–196, 1991.

73. Hijdra A, Van Gijn J, Stefanko S, et al: Delayed cerebral ischemia after aneurysmal subarachnoid hemorrhage: Clinicoanatomic correlations, *Neurology* 36:329–333, 1986.

74. Seiler RW, Grolimund P, Aaslid R, et al: Cerebral vasospasm evaluated by transcranial ultrasound correlated with clinical grade and CT-visualized subarachnoid hemorrhage, *J Neurosurg* 64:594–600, 1986.

75. Clyde BL, Resnick DK, Yonas H, et al: The relationship of blood velocity as measured by transcranial Doppler ultrasonography to cerebral blood flow as determined by stable xenon computed tomographic studies after aneurysmal subarachnoid hemorrhage, *Neurosurgery* 38:896–904, 1996:discussion 904–905.

76. Manno EM, Gress DR, Schwamm LH, et al: Effects of induced hypertension on transcranial Doppler ultrasound velocities in patients after subarachnoid hemorrhage, *Stroke* 29:422–428, 1998.

77. Dorhout Mees SM, Rinkel GJ, et al: Calcium antagonists for aneurysmal subarachnoid haemorrhage, *Cochrane Database Syst Rev* (3)2007:CD000277.

78. Zhao J, Zhou D, Guo J, et al: Effect of fasudil hydrochloride, a protein kinase inhibitor, on cerebral vasospasm and delayed cerebral ischemic symptoms after aneurysmal subarachnoid hemorrhage, *Neurol Med Chir (Tokyo)* 46:421–428, 2006.

79. Haley EC Jr, Kassell NF, Torner JC: A randomized controlled trial of high-dose intravenous nicardipine in aneurysmal subarachnoid hemorrhage: A report of the Cooperative Aneurysm Study, *J Neurosurg* 78:537–547, 1993.

80. Schmid-Elsaesser R, Kunz M, Zausinger S, et al: Intravenous magnesium versus nimodipine in the treatment of patients with aneurysmal subarachnoid hemorrhage: A randomized study, *Neurosurgery* 58:1054–1065, 2006.

81. van den Bergh WM, Algra A, van Kooten F, et al: Magnesium sulfate in aneurysmal subarachnoid hemorrhage: A randomized controlled trial, *Stroke* 36:1011–1015, 2005.

82. Muroi C, Terzic A, Fortunati M, et al: Magnesium sulfate in the management of patients with aneurysmal subarachnoid hemorrhage: A randomized, placebo-controlled, dose-adapted trial, *Surg Neurol* 69:33–39, 2008:discussion 39.

83. Vajkoczy P, Meyer B, Weidauer S, et al: Clazosentan (AXV-034343), a selective endothelin A receptor antagonist, in the prevention of cerebral vasospasm following severe aneurysmal subarachnoid hemorrhage: Results of a randomized, double-blind, placebo-controlled, multicenter phase IIa study, *J Neurosurg* 103:9–17, 2005.

84. Barth M, Capelle HH, Munch E, et al: Effects of the selective endothelin A (ET(A)) receptor antagonist clazosentan on cerebral perfusion and cerebral oxygenation following severe subarachnoid hemorrhage: Preliminary results from a randomized clinical series, *Acta Neurochir (Wien)* 149:911–918, 2007:discussion 918.

85. Tseng MY, Czosnyka M, Richards H, et al: Effects of acute treatment with pravastatin on cerebral vasospasm, autoregulation, and delayed ischemic deficits after aneurysmal subarachnoid hemorrhage: A phase II randomized placebo-controlled trial, *Stroke* 36:1627–1632, 2005.

86. Tseng MY, Hutchinson PJ, Czosnyka M, Richards H, et al: Effects of acute pravastatin treatment on intensity of rescue therapy, length of inpatient stay, and 6-month outcome in patients after aneurysmal subarachnoid hemorrhage, *Stroke* 38:1545–1550, 2007.

87. Lynch JR, Wang H, McGirt MJ, et al: Simvastatin reduces vasospasm after aneurysmal subarachnoid hemorrhage: Results of a pilot randomized clinical trial, *Stroke* 36:2024–2026, 2005.

88. Kramer AH, Gurka MJ, Nathan B, et al: Statin use was not associated with less vasospasm or improved outcome after subarachnoid hemorrhage, *Neurosurgery* 62:422–427, 2008:discussion 427–430.

89. Haley EC Jr, Kassell NF, Alves WM, et al: Phase II trial of tirilazad in aneurysmal subarachnoid hemorrhage: A report of the Cooperative Aneurysm Study, *J Neurosurg* 82:786–790, 1995.

90. Lanzino G, Kassell NF, Dorsch NW, et al: Double-blind, randomized, vehicle-controlled study of high-dose tirilazad mesylate in women with aneurysmal subarachnoid hemorrhage. Part I: A cooperative study in Europe, Australia, New Zealand, and South Africa, *J Neurosurg* 90:1011–1017, 1999.

91. Asano T, Takakura K, Sano K, et al: Effects of a hydroxyl radical scavenger on delayed ischemic neurological deficits following aneurysmal subarachnoid hemorrhage: Results of a multicenter, placebo-controlled double-blind trial, *J Neurosurg* 84:792–803, 1996.

92. Taneda M: Effect of early operation for ruptured aneurysms on prevention of delayed ischemic symptoms, *J Neurosurg* 57:622–628, 1982.

93. Levy ML, Rabb CH, Zelman V, Giannotta SL: Cardiac performance enhancement from dobutamine in patients refractory to hypervolemic therapy for cerebral vasospasm, *J Neurosurg* 79:494–499, 1993.

94. Levy ML, Giannotta SL: Cardiac performance indices during hypervolemic therapy for cerebral vasospasm, *J Neurosurg* 75:27–31, 1991.

95. Solomon RA, Fink ME, Lennihan L: Early aneurysm surgery and prophylactic hypervolemic hypertensive therapy for the treatment of aneurysmal subarachnoid hemorrhage, *Neurosurgery* 23:699–704, 1988.

96. Sandham JD, Hull RD, Brant RF, et al: A randomized, controlled trial of the use of pulmonary-artery catheters in high-risk surgical patients, *N Engl J Med* 348:5–14, 2003.

97. Cully MD, Larson CP Jr, Silverberg GD: Hetastarch coagulopathy in a neurosurgical patient, *Anesthesiology* 66:706–707, 1987.

98. Damon L, Adams M, Stricker RB, Ries C: Intracranial bleeding during treatment with hydroxyethyl starch, *N Engl J Med* 317:964–965, 1987.

99. Trumble ER, Muizelaar JP, Myseros JS, et al: Coagulopathy with the use of hetastarch in the treatment of vasospasm, *J Neurosurg* 82:44–47, 1995.

100. Treib J, Haass A, Pindur G: Coagulation disorders caused by hydroxyethyl starch, *Thromb Haemost* 78:974–983, 1997.

101. Komotar RJ, Zacharia BE, Otten ML, et al: Controversies in the endovascular management of cerebral vasospasm after intracranial aneurysm rupture and future directions for therapeutic approaches, *Neurosurgery* 62:897–905, 2008:discussion 905–907.

102. Fandino J, Kaku Y, Schuknecht B, et al: Improvement of cerebral oxygenation patterns and metabolic validation of superselective intraarterial infusion of papaverine for the treatment of cerebral vasospasm, *J Neurosurg* 89:93–100, 1998.

103. Elliott JP, Newell DW, Lam DJ, et al: Comparison of balloon angioplasty and papaverine infusion for the treatment of vasospasm following aneurysmal subarachnoid hemorrhage, *J Neurosurg* 88:277–284, 1998.

104. Miller JA, Cross DT, Moran CJ, et al: Severe thrombocytopenia following intraarterial papaverine administration for treatment of vasospasm, *J Neurosurg* 83:435–437, 1995.

105. McAuliffe W, Townsend M, Eskridge JM et al: Intracranial pressure changes induced during papaverine infusion for treatment of vasospasm, *J Neurosurg* 83:430–434, 1995.

106. Mathis JM, DeNardo A, Jensen ME, et al: Transient neurologic events associated with intraarterial papaverine infusion for subarachnoid hemorrhage-induced vasospasm, *AJNR Am J Neuroradiol* 15:1671–1674, 1994.

107. Pritz MB: Pupillary changes after intracisternal injection of papaverine, *Surg Neurol* 41:281–282, 1994:discussion 283.

108. Fraticelli AT, Cholley BP, Losser MR, et al: Milrinone for the treatment of cerebral vasospasm after aneurysmal subarachnoid hemorrhage, *Stroke* 39:893–898, 2008.

109. Keuskamp J, Murali R, Chao KH: High-dose intraarterial verapamil in the treatment of cerebral vasospasm after aneurysmal subarachnoid hemorrhage, *J Neurosurg* 108:458–463, 2008.

110. Goodson K, Lapointe M, Monroe T, Chalela JA: Intraventricular nicardipine for refractory cerebral vasospasm after subarachnoid hemorrhage, *Neurocrit Care* 8:247–252, 2008.

111. Hanggi D, Beseoglu K, Turowski B, Steiger HJ: Feasibility and safety of intrathecal nimodipine on posthaemorrhagic cerebral vasospasm refractory to medical and endovascular therapy, *Clin Neurol Neurosurg* 110:784–790, 2008.

112. Thomas JE, Rosenwasser RH, Armonda RA, et al: Safety of intrathecal sodium nitroprusside for the treatment and prevention of refractory cerebral vasospasm and ischemia in humans, *Stroke* 30:1409–1416, 1999.

113. Jarus-Dziedzic K, Zub W, Warzecha A, et al: Early cerebral hemodynamic alternations in patients operated on the first, second and third day after aneurysmal subarachnoid hemorrhage, *Neurol Res* 30:307–312, 2008.

114. Chang HS, Hongo K, Nakagawa H: Adverse effects of limited hypotensive anesthesia on the outcome of patients with subarachnoid hemorrhage, *J Neurosurg* 92:971–975, 2000.

115. Buckland MR, Batjer HH, Giesecke AH: Anesthesia for cerebral aneurysm surgery: Use of induced hypertension in patients with symptomatic vasospasm, *Anesthesiology* 69:116–119, 1988.

116. Van Hemelrijck J, Fitch W, Mattheussen M, et al: Effect of propofol on cerebral circulation and autoregulation in the baboon, *Anesth Analg* 71:49–54, 1990.

117. Marx W, Shah N, Long C, et al: Sufentanil, alfentanil, and fentanyl: Impact on cerebrospinal fluid pressure in patients with brain tumors, *J Neurosurg Anesthesiol* 1:3–7, 1989.

118. Sperry RJ, Bailey PL, Reichman MV, et al: Fentanyl and sufentanil increase intracranial pressure in head trauma patients, *Anesthesiology* 77:416–420, 1992.

119. Trindle MR, Dodson BA, Rampil IJ: Effects of fentanyl versus sufentanil in equianesthetic doses on middle cerebral artery blood flow velocity, *Anesthesiology* 78:454–460, 1993.

120. Mayer N, Weinstabl C, Podreka I, Spiss CK: Sufentanil does not increase cerebral blood flow in healthy human volunteers, *Anesthesiology* 73:240–243, 1990.

121. Weinstabl C, Mayer N, Richling B, et al: Effect of sufentanil on intracranial pressure in neurosurgical patients, *Anaesthesia* 46:837–840, 1991.

122. Mayberg TS, Lam AM, Eng CC, et al: The effect of alfentanil on cerebral blood flow velocity and intracranial pressure during isoflurane-nitrous oxide anesthesia in humans, *Anesthesiology* 78:288–294, 1993.

123. Werner C, Kochs E, Bause H, et al: Effects of sufentanil on cerebral hemodynamics and intracranial pressure in patients with brain injury, *Anesthesiology* 83:721–726, 1995.

124. de Nadal M, Munar F, Poca MA, et al: Cerebral hemodynamic effects of morphine and fentanyl in patients with severe head injury: Absence of correlation to cerebral autoregulation, *Anesthesiology* 92:11–19, 2000.

125. Baker KZ, Ostapkovich N, Sisti MB, et al: Intact cerebral blood flow reactivity during remifentanil/nitrous oxide anesthesia, *J Neurosurg Anesthesiol* 9:134–140, 1997.

126. Warner DS, Hindman BJ, Todd MM, et al: Intracranial pressure and hemodynamic effects of remifentanil versus alfentanil in patients undergoing supratentorial craniotomy, *Anesth Analg* 83:348–353, 1996.

127. Guy J, Hindman BJ, Baker KZ, et al: Comparison of remifentanil and fentanyl in patients undergoing craniotomy for supratentorial space-occupying lesions, *Anesthesiology* 86:514–524, 1997.

128. Kapila A, Glass PS, Jacobs JR, et al: Measured context-sensitive half-times of remifentanil and alfentanil, *Anesthesiology* 83:968–975, 1995.

129. Lanier WL, Milde JH, Michenfelder JD: Cerebral stimulation following succinylcholine in dogs, *Anesthesiology* 64:551–559, 1986.

130. Kovarik WD, Mayberg TS, Lam AM, et al: Succinylcholine does not change intracranial pressure, cerebral blood flow velocity, or the electroencephalogram in patients with neurologic injury, *Anesth Analg* 78:469–473, 1994.

131. Manninen PH, Mahendran B, Gelb AW, Merchant RN: Succinylcholine does not increase serum potassium levels in patients with acutely ruptured cerebral aneurysms, *Anesth Analg* 70:172–175, 1990.

132. Lotto ML, Banoub M, Schubert A: Effects of anesthetic agents and physiologic changes on intraoperative motor evoked potentials, *J Neurosurg Anesthesiol* 16:32–42, 2004.

133. Lanier WL, Stangland KJ, Scheithauer BW, et al: The effects of dextrose infusion and head position on neurologic outcome after complete cerebral ischemia in primates: Examination of a model, *Anesthesiology* 66:39–48, 1987.

134. Lam AM, Winn HR, Cullen BF, Sundling N: Hyperglycemia and neurological outcome in patients with head injury, *J Neurosurg* 75:545–551, 1991.

135. Prakash A, Matta BF: Hyperglycaemia and neurological injury, *Curr Opin Anaesthesiol* 21:565–569, 2008.

136. Levin R, Hesselvik JF, Kourtopoulos H, Vavruch L: Local anesthesia prevents hypertension following application of the Mayfield skull-pin head holder, *Acta Anaesthesiol Scand* 33:277–279, 1989.

137. Matta BF, Lam AM, Mayberg TS, et al: A critique of the intraoperative use of jugular venous bulb catheters during neurosurgical procedures, *Anesth Analg* 79:745–750, 1994.

138. Moss E, Dearden NM, Berridge JC: Effects of changes in mean arterial pressure on SjO$_2$ during cerebral aneurysm surgery, *Br J Anaesth* 75:527–530, 1995.

139. Clavier N, Schurando P, Raggueneau JL, Payen DM: Continuous jugular bulb venous oxygen saturation validation and variations during intracranial aneurysm surgery, *J Crit Care* 12:112–119, 1997.

140. Rozet I, Newell DW, Lam AM: Intraoperative jugular bulb desaturation during acute aneurysmal rupture, *Can J Anaesth* 53:97–100, 2006.

141. Eng CC, Lam AM, Byrd S, Newell DW: The diagnosis and management of a perianesthetic cerebral aneurysmal rupture aided with transcranial Doppler ultrasonography, *Anesthesiology* 78:191–194, 1993.

142. Moore JK, Chaudhri S, Moore AP, Easton J: Macroglossia and posterior fossa disease, *Anaesthesia* 43:382–385, 1988.

143. Lam AM, Vavilala MS: Macroglossia: Compartment syndrome of the tongue? *Anesthesiology* 92:1832–1835, 2000.

144. Lam AM, Mayberg TS, Eng CC, et al: Nitrous oxide-isoflurane anesthesia causes more cerebral vasodilation than an equipotent dose of isoflurane in humans, *Anesth Analg* 78:462–468, 1994.

145. Roald OK, Forsman M, Heier MS, Steen PA: Cerebral effects of nitrous oxide when added to low and high concentrations of isoflurane in the dog, *Anesth Analg* 72:75–79, 1991.

146. Artru AA, Lam AM, Johnson JO, Sperry RJ: Intracranial pressure, middle cerebral artery flow velocity, and plasma inorganic fluoride concentrations in neurosurgical patients receiving sevoflurane or isoflurane, *Anesth Analg* 85:587–592, 1997.

147. Kuroda Y, Murakami M, Tsuruta J, et al: Blood flow velocity of middle cerebral artery during prolonged anesthesia with halothane, isoflurane, and sevoflurane in humans, *Anesthesiology* 87:527–532, 1997.

148. Cho S, Fujigaki T, Uchiyama Y, et al: Effects of sevoflurane with and without nitrous oxide on human cerebral circulation: Transcranial Doppler study, *Anesthesiology* 85:755–760, 1996.

149. Gupta S, Heath K, Matta BF: Effect of incremental doses of sevoflurane on cerebral pressure autoregulation in humans, *Br J Anaesth* 79:469–742, 1997.

150. From RP, Warner DS, Todd MM, Sokoll MD: Anesthesia for craniotomy: A double-blind comparison of alfentanil, fentanyl, and sufentanil, *Anesthesiology* 73:896–904, 1990.

151. Mutch WA, Ringaert KR, Ewert FJ, et al: Continuous opioid infusions for neurosurgical procedures: A double-blind comparison of alfentanil and fentanyl, *Can J Anaesth* 38:710–716, 1991.

152. Tankisi A, Rasmussen M, Juul N, Cold GE: The effects of 10 degrees reverse Trendelenburg position on subdural intracranial pressure and cerebral perfusion pressure in patients subjected to craniotomy for cerebral aneurysm, *J Neurosurg Anesthesiol* 18:11–17, 2006.

153. Sahar A, Tsipstein E: Effects of mannitol and furosemide on the rate of formation of cerebrospinal fluid, *Exp Neurol* 60:584–591, 1978.

154. Ravussin P, Archer DP, Tyler JL, et al: Effects of rapid mannitol infusion on cerebral blood volume: A positron emission tomographic study in dogs and man, *J Neurosurg* 64:104–113, 1986.

155. Manninen PH, Lam AM, Gelb AW, Brown SC: The effect of high-dose mannitol on serum and urine electrolytes and osmolality in neurosurgical patients, *Can J Anaesth* 34:442–446, 1987.

156. Rozet I, Tontisirin N, Muangman S, et al: Effect of equiosmolar solutions of mannitol versus hypertonic saline on intraoperative brain relaxation and electrolyte balance, *Anesthesiology* 107:697–704, 2007.

157. Barker J: An anaesthetic technique for intracranial aneurysms [letter], *Anaesthesia* 30:557–558, 1975.

158. Olivar H, Bramhall JS, Rozet I, et al: Subarachnoid lumbar drains: A case series of fractured catheters and a near miss, *Can J Anaesth* 54:829–834, 2007.

159. Hitchcock ER, Tsementzis SA, Dow AA: Short- and long-term prognosis of patients with a subarachnoid haemorrhage in relation to intraoperative period of hypotension, *Acta Neurochir (Wien)* 70:235–242, 1984.

160. Jabre A, Symon L: Temporary vascular occlusion during aneurysm surgery, *Surg Neurol* 27:47–63, 1987.

161. Momma F, Wang AD, Symon L: Effects of temporary arterial occlusion on somatosensory evoked responses in aneurysm surgery, *Surg Neurol* 27:343–352, 1987.

162. Mooij JJ, Buchthal A, Belopavlovic M: Somatosensory evoked potential monitoring of temporary middle cerebral artery occlusion during aneurysm operation, *Neurosurgery* 21:492–496, 1987.

163. Ellegala DB, Day AL: Ruptured cerebral aneurysms, *N Engl J Med* 352:121–124, 2005.

164. Suzuki J: *Temporary occlusion of trunk arteries of the brain during surgery*, In *Treatment of Cerebral Infection: Experimental and Clinical Study.* New York, 1987, Springer-Verlag.

165. Ogilvy CS, Carter BS, Kaplan S, et al: Temporary vessel occlusion for aneurysm surgery: Risk factors for stroke in patients protected by induced hypothermia and hypertension and intravenous mannitol administration, *J Neurosurg* 84:785–791, 1996.

166. Lavine SD, Masri LS, Levy ML, Giannotta SL: Temporary occlusion of the middle cerebral artery in intracranial aneurysm surgery: Time limitation and advantage of brain protection, *J Neurosurg* 87:817–824, 1997.

167. Taylor CL, Selman WR, Kiefer SP, Ratcheson RA: Temporary vessel occlusion during intracranial aneurysm repair, *Neurosurgery* 39:893–905, 1996:discussion 905–906.

168. Edelman GJ, Hoffman WE, Charbel FT: Cerebral hypoxia after etomidate administration and temporary cerebral artery occlusion, *Anesth Analg* 85:821–825, 1997.

169. Samson D, Batjer HH, Bowman G, et al: A clinical study of the parameters and effects of temporary arterial occlusion in the management of intracranial aneurysms, *Neurosurgery* 34:22–28, 1994:discussion 28–29.

170. Warner DS, Takaoka S, Wu B, et al: Electroencephalographic burst suppression is not required to elicit maximal neuroprotection from pentobarbital in a rat model of focal cerebral ischemia, *Anesthesiology* 84:1475–1484, 1996.

171. Hashimoto T, Young WL, Aagaard BD, et al: Adenosine-induced ventricular asystole to induce transient profound systemic hypotension in patients undergoing endovascular therapy: Dose-response characteristics, *Anesthesiology* 93:998–1001, 2000.

172. Groff MW, Adams DC, Kahn RA, et al: Adenosine-induced transient asystole for management of a basilar artery aneurysm: Case report, *J Neurosurg* 91:687–690, 1999.

173. Minamisawa H, Nordstrom CH, Smith ML, Siesjo BK: The influence of mild body and brain hypothermia on ischemic brain damage, *J Cereb Blood Flow Metab* 10:365–374, 1990.

174. Busto R, Dietrich WD, Globus MY, Ginsberg MD: The importance of brain temperature in cerebral ischemic injury, *Stroke* 20:1113–1114, 1989.

175. Bernard SA, Gray TW, Buist MD, et al: Treatment of comatose survivors of out-of-hospital cardiac arrest with induced hypothermia, *N Engl J Med* 346:557–563, 2002.

176. Hypothermia after Cardiac Arrest Study Group: Mild therapeutic hypothermia to improve the neurologic outcome after cardiac arrest, *N Engl J Med* 346:549–556, 2002.

177. Mack WJ, Ducruet AF, Angevine PD, et al: Deep hypothermic circulatory arrest for complex cerebral aneurysms: Lessons learned, *Neurosurgery* 60:815–827, 2007.

178. Stone JG, Goodman RR, Baker KZ, et al: Direct intraoperative measurement of human brain temperature, *Neurosurgery* 41:20–24, 1997.

179. Crowder CM, Tempelhoff R, Theard MA, et al: Jugular bulb temperature: Comparison with brain surface and core temperatures in neurosurgical patients during mild hypothermia, *J Neurosurg* 85:98–103, 1996.

180. Manninen PH, Patterson S, Lam AM, et al: Evoked potential monitoring during posterior fossa aneurysm surgery: A comparison of two modalities, *Can J Anaesth* 41:92–97, 1994.

181. Lam AM, Keane JF, Manninen PH: Monitoring of brainstem auditory evoked potentials during basilar artery occlusion in man, *Br J Anaesth* 57:924–928, 1985.

182. Neuloh G, Schramm J: Monitoring of motor evoked potentials compared with somatosensory evoked potentials and microvascular Doppler ultrasonography in cerebral aneurysm surgery, *J Neurosurg* 100:389–399, 2004.

183. Horiuchi K, Suzuki K, Sasaki T, et al: Intraoperative monitoring of blood flow insufficiency during surgery of middle cerebral artery aneurysms, *J Neurosurg* 103:275–283, 2005.

184. Quinones-Hinojosa A, Alam M, et al: Transcranial motor evoked potentials during basilar artery aneurysm surgery: Technique application for 30 consecutive patients, *Neurosurgery* 54:916–924, 2004:discussion 924.

185. Sekimoto K, Nishikawa K, Ishizeki J, et al: The effects of volatile anesthetics on intraoperative monitoring of myogenic motor-evoked potentials to transcranial electrical stimulation and on partial neuromuscular blockade during propofol/fentanyl/nitrous oxide anesthesia in humans, *J Neurosurg Anesthesiol* 18:106–111, 2006.

186. Leipzig TJ, Morgan J, Horner TG, et al: Analysis of intraoperative rupture in the surgical treatment of 1694 saccular aneurysms, *Neurosurgery* 56:455–468, 2005.

187. Batjer H, Samson D: Intraoperative aneurysmal rupture: Incidence, outcome, and suggestions for surgical management, *Neurosurgery* 18:701–707, 1986:l.

188. Elijovich L, Higashida RT, Lawton MT, et al: Predictors and outcomes of intraprocedural rupture in patients treated for ruptured intracranial aneurysms: The CARAT study, *Stroke* 39:1501–1506, 2008.

189. Raabe A, Nakaji P, Beck J, et al: Prospective evaluation of surgical microscope-integrated intraoperative near-infrared indocyanine green videoangiography during aneurysm surgery, *J Neurosurg* 103:982–989, 2005.

190. Imizu S, Kato Y, Sangli A, et al: Assessment of incomplete clipping of aneurysms intraoperatively by a near-infrared indocyanine green-video angiography (Niicg-Va) integrated microscope, *Minim Invasive Neurosurg* 51:199–203, 2008.

191. Thal GD, Szabo MD, Lopez-Bresnahan M, Crosby G: Exacerbation or unmasking of focal neurologic deficits by sedatives, *Anesthesiology* 85:21–25, 1996:discussion 29A-30A.

192. Dias MS, Sekhar LN: Intracranial hemorrhage from aneurysms and arteriovenous malformations during pregnancy and the puerperium, *Neurosurgery* 27:855–865, 1990:discussion 865–866.

193. Minielly R, Yuzpe AA, Drake CG: Subarachnoid hemorrhage secondary to ruptured cerebral aneurysm in pregnancy, *Obstet Gynecol* 53:64–70, 1979.

194. Gaist D, Pedersen L, Cnattingius S, Sorensen HT: Parity and risk of subarachnoid hemorrhage in women: A nested case-control study based on national Swedish registries, *Stroke* 35:28–32, 2004.

195. Marshman LA, Aspoas AR, Rai MS, Chawda SJ: The implications of ISAT and ISUIA for the management of cerebral aneurysms during pregnancy, *Neurosurg Rev* 30:177–180, 2007:discussion 180.

196. Kofke WA, Wuest HP, Mc Ginnis LA: Cesarean section following ruptured cerebral aneurysm and neuroresuscitation, *Anesthesiology* 60:242–245, 1984.

197. Newman B, Lam AM: Induced hypotension for clipping of a cerebral aneurysm during pregnancy: A case report and brief review, *Anesth Analg* 65:675–678, 1986.

198. Willoughby JS: Sodium nitroprusside, pregnancy and multiple intracranial aneurysms, *Anaesth Intensive Care* 12:358–360, 1984.

199. Lam AM, Gelb AW: Cardiovascular effects of isoflurane-induced hypotension for cerebral aneurysm surgery, *Anesth Analg* 62:742–748, 1983.

200. Newman B, Gelb AW, Lam AM: The effect of isoflurane-induced hypotension on cerebral blood flow and cerebral metabolic rate for oxygen in humans, *Anesthesiology* 64:307–310, 1986.

201. Palahniuk RJ, Shnider SM: Maternal and fetal cardiovascular and acid-base changes during halothane and isoflurane anesthesia in the pregnant ewe, *Anesthesiology* 41:462–472, 1974.

202. Burns PD, Linder RO, Drose VE, Battaglia F: The placental transfer of water from fetus to mother following the intravenous infusion of hypertonic mannitol to the maternal rabbit, *Am J Obstet Gynecol* 86:160–167, 1963.

203. Battaglia F, Prystowsky H, Smisson C, et al: Fetal blood studies. XIII: The effect of the administration of fluids intravenously to mothers upon the concentrations of water and electrolytes in plasma of human fetuses, *Pediatrics* 25:2–10, 1960.

204. Drake CG: Giant intracranial aneurysms: Experience with surgical treatment in 174 patients, *Clin Neurosurg* 26:12–95, 1979.

205. Solomon RA, Smith CR, Raps EC, et al: Deep hypothermic circulatory arrest for the management of complex anterior and posterior circulation aneurysms, *Neurosurgery* 29:732–737, 1991:discussion 737–738.

206. Drake CG, Barr HW, Coles JC, Gergely NF: The use of extracorporeal circulation and profound hypothermia in the treatment of ruptured intracranial aneurysm, *J Neurosurg* 21:575–581, 1964.

207. Manninen PH, Cuillerier DJ, Nantau WE, Gelb AW: Monitoring of brainstem function during vertebral basilar aneurysm surgery: The use of spontaneous ventilation, *Anesthesiology* 77:681–685, 1992.

208. Baumgartner WA, Silverberg GD, Ream AK, et al: Reappraisal of cardiopulmonary bypass with deep hypothermia and circulatory arrest for complex neurosurgical operations, *Surgery* 94:242–249, 1983.

209. Spetzler RF, Hadley MN, Rigamonti D, et al: Aneurysms of the basilar artery treated with circulatory arrest, hypothermia, and barbiturate cerebral protection, *J Neurosurg* 68:868–879, 1988.

210. Thomas AN, Anderton JM, Harper NJ: Anaesthesia for the treatment of a giant cerebral aneurysm under hypothermic circulatory arrest, *Anaesthesia* 45:383–385, 1990.

211. Levati A, Tommasino C, Moretti MP, et al: Giant intracranial aneurysms treated with deep hypothermia and circulatory arrest, *J Neurosurg Anesthesiol* 19:25–30, 2007.

212. Williams MD, Rainer WG, Fieger HG Jr, et al: Cardiopulmonary bypass, profound hypothermia, and circulatory arrest for neurosurgery, *Ann Thorac Surg* 52:1069–1074, 1991:discussion 1074–1075.

213. Silverberg GD, Reitz BA, Ream AK: Hypothermia and cardiac arrest in the treatment of giant aneurysms of the cerebral circulation and hemangioblastoma of the medulla, *J Neurosurg* 55:337–346, 1981.

214. Stone JG, Young WL, Marans ZS, et al: Consequences of electroencephalographic-suppressive doses of propofol in conjunction with deep hypothermic circulatory arrest, *Anesthesiology* 85:497–501, 1996.

215. Camboni D, Philipp A, Schebesch KM, Schmid C: Accuracy of core temperature measurement in deep hypothermic circulatory arrest, *Interact Cardiovasc Thorac Surg* 7:922–924, 2008.

216. Patterson RH Jr, Ray BS: Profound hypothermia for intracranial surgery: Laboratory and clinical experiences with extracorporeal circulation by peripheral cannulation, *Ann Surg* 156:377–393, 1962.

217. Pollick C, Cujec B, Parker S, Tator C: Left ventricular wall motion abnormalities in subarachnoid hemorrhage: an echocardiographic study, *J Am Coll Cardiol* 12:600–605, 1988.

218. Mayer SA, LiMandri G, Sherman D, et al: Electrocardiographic markers of abnormal left ventricular wall motion in acute subarachnoid hemorrhage, *J Neurosurg* 83:889–896, 1995.

219. Kuroiwa T, Morita H, Tanabe H, Ohta T: Significance of ST segment elevation in electrocardiograms in patients with ruptured cerebral aneurysms, *Acta Neurochir* 133:141–146, 1995.

220. Szelenyi A, Langer D, Kothbauer K, et al: Monitoring of muscle motor evoked potentials during cerebral aneurysm surgery: Intraoperative changes and postoperative outcome, *J Neurosurg* 105:675–681, 2006.

221. Mizoi K, Yoshimoto T: Permissible temporary occlusion time in aneurysm surgery as evaluated by evoked potential monitoring, *Neurosurgery* 33:434–440, 1993:discussion 440.

222. Schramm J, Koht A, Schmidt G, et al: Surgical and electrophysiological observations during clipping of 134 aneurysms with evoked potential monitoring, *Neurosurgery* 26:61–70, 1990.

223. Manninen PH, Lam AM, Nantau WE: Monitoring of somatosensory evoked potentials during temporary arterial occlusion in cerebral aneurysm surgery, *J Neurosurg Anesthesiol* 2:97–104, 1990.

224. Kidooka M, Nakasu Y, Watanabe K, et al: Monitoring of somatosensory-evoked potentials during aneurysm surgery, *Surg Neurol* 27:69–76, 1987.

225. Symon L, Wang AD: Costa e Silva IE, Gentili F: Perioperative use of somatosensory evoked responses in aneurysm surgery, *J Neurosurg* 60:269–275, 1984.

226. Hanel RA, Spetzler RF: Surgical treatment of complex intracranial aneurysms, *Neurosurgery* 62:SHC1289–SHC1297, 2008:discussion SHC1297–SCH1299.

227. Lawton MT, Raudzens PA, Zabramski JM, Spetzler RF: Hypothermic circulatory arrest in neurovascular surgery: Evolving indications and predictors of patient outcome, *Neurosurgery* 43:10–20, 1998:discussion 20–21.

228. Greene KA, Marciano FF, Hamilton MG, et al: Cardiopulmonary bypass, hypothermic circulatory arrest and barbiturate cerebral protection for the treatment of giant vertebrobasilar aneurysms in children, *Pediatr Neurosurg* 21:124–133, 1994.

229. Ausman JI, Malik GM, Tomecek FJ, et al: Hypothermic circulatory arrest and the management of giant and large cerebral aneurysms, *Surg Neurol* 40:289–298, 1993.

230. Gonski A, Acedillo AT, Stacey RB: Profound hypothermia in the treatment of intracranial aneurysms, *Aust N Z J Surg* 56:639–643, 1986.

231. McMurtry JG, Housepian EM, Bowman FO Jr, Matteo RS: Surgical treatment of basilar artery aneurysms: Elective circulatory arrest with thoracotomy in 12 cases, *J Neurosurg* 40:486–494, 1974.

232. Sundt TM Jr, Pluth JR, Gronert GA: Excision of giant basilar aneurysm under profound hypothermia: Report of case, *Mayo Clin Proc* 47:631–634, 1972.

233. Michenfelder JD, Kirklin JW, Uihlein A, et al: Clinical experience with a closed-chest method of producing profound hypothermia and total circulatory arrest in Neurosurgery, *Ann Surg* 159:125–131, 1964.

234. Woodhall B, Sealy WC, Hall KD, Floyd WL: Craniotomy under conditions of quinidine-protected cardioplegia and profound hypothermia, *Ann Surg* 152:37–44, 1960.

Chapter 14

INTERVENTIONAL NEURORADIOLOGY: ANESTHETIC MANAGEMENT

William L. Young • Christopher F. Dowd

Interventional neuroradiology (INR) is the most common name given to the discipline that uses endovascular procedures to treat vascular conditions of the central nervous system. Other names for the field are neurointerventional surgery, surgical neuroangiography, and endovascular neurosurgery. INR is firmly established in the management of cerebrovascular disease, a watershed event perhaps being the International Subarachnoid Aneurysm Trial, which provided level 1 evidence that aneurysm coiling has advantages over surgical clipping of intracranial aneurysms.[1]

The discussion in this chapter emphasizes perioperative and anesthetic management strategies to prevent complications and to minimize their effects if they occur. We further assume that the primary imaging technology is catheter angiography, although magnetic resonance imaging may one day augment or supplant this practice.[2] Planning of the anesthetic and perioperative management is predicated on an understanding of the goals of the therapeutic intervention and anticipation of potential problems.

The anesthetic concerns of particular importance for INR procedures are (1) maintaining the patient's immobility during the procedure to facilitate imaging; (2) either enabling rapid recovery from anesthesia at the end of the operation to facilitate neurologic examination and monitoring or providing for intermittent evaluation of neurologic function during the procedure; (3) managing anticoagulation; (4) treating and managing sudden unexpected procedure-specific complications during the procedure, such as hemorrhage or vascular occlusion, which may involve manipulating systemic or regional blood pressures; (5) guiding the medical management of critical care patients during transport to and from radiology suites; and (6) recognizing self-protection issues related to radiation safety.[3,4]

PREOPERATIVE PLANNING AND PATIENT PREPARATION

Baseline blood pressure and cardiovascular reserve should be assessed carefully. This almost axiomatic statement is particularly important for several reasons. Blood pressure manipulation is commonly required, and treatment-related perturbations should be anticipated. Therefore, a clear sense of the patient's baseline blood pressure needs to be established. One must keep in mind that "autoregulation" as presented in the textbooks is a description of a population; individual patients are likely to vary considerably, a concept based on the historical observations that underlie our modern notions of autoregulatory behavior.[5,6] To state the issue another way: When looking at the usual autoregulation curve,

one should bear in mind that each point on that curve has a 95% confidence interval (CI) associated with it—in both x and y directions.

For procedures involving the blood supply to the central nervous system, beat-to-beat blood pressure monitoring is useful, considering the rapid time constants in this setting for changes in systemic or cerebral hemodynamics. In those cases in which intra-arterial catheters are used, the concordance between blood pressure cuff and intra-arterial readings must be considered; preoperative blood pressure range is likely to be known through blood pressure cuff values.

Preoperative administration of calcium channel blockers for prophylaxis for cerebral ischemia may be used and can affect hemodynamic management. In addition, these agents or transdermal nitroglycerin is sometimes used to lower the chance of catheter-induced vasospasm.

Radiologic contrast media are well known to cause allergic reactions.[7] There seems to be no difference in the propensity to cause anaphylactoid reactions between the older and newer agents. However, newer agents provide a much lower osmolar load and therefore preserve intravascular volume in the event of an allergic crisis. The patient's previous experience with radiologic imaging that may have included administration of contrast agents should be inquired about. As intraprocedural systemic heparinization is commonly used in INR, protamine sulfate is also often used to reverse the anticoagulant effect of heparin. Protamine is also known to cause allergic reactions. In the history, items of interest include history of prior anticoagulation, coagulation disorders, protamine allergy (related items include protamine insulin use, fish allergy, and prior vasectomy), recent steroid use, and contrast agent reactions (including general atopy and iodine/shellfish allergies).

Patients who give a history of significant contrast agent reactions can be treated with steroids the day prior to the procedure, and antihistamines can be given shortly before the procedure. The treatment of severe allergic response is reviewed in general textbooks and prominently features use of adrenergic agonists, such as epinephrine.

A number of considerations regarding the *anesthetizing location* should be borne in mind. Both wall and tank oxygen should be available. All the usual anesthetizing location considerations should be provided, including adequate lighting, electrical power, and ready access to a phone line (dedicated if at all possible). The access to emergency equipment must be proximate and immediate. One configuration of a modern neuroradiology suite and associated images are shown in Figure 14-1. Magnetic resonance imaging and conventional angiography units are sometimes combined in one setting (Fig. 14-2).

A fundamental knowledge of radiation safety is essential for all staff members working in an INR suite as well as a critical

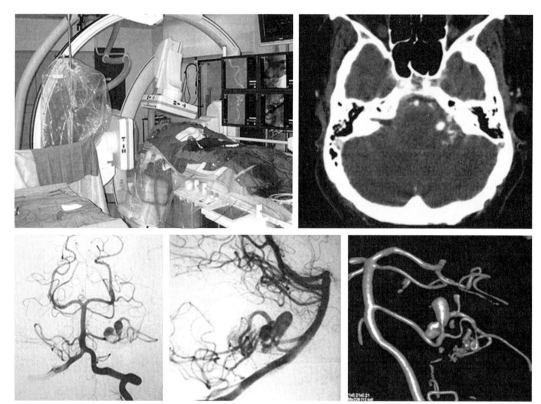

Figure 14–1 State-of-the-art neuroangiography suite (*top left*) has the capability to perform computed tomography (*top right*), biplane angiography (*bottom left and middle*), and three-dimensional reconstructed rotational angiography (*bottom right*). These views show a small cerebellar arteriovenous malformation with recently ruptured feeding artery aneurysms (see Fig, 14-6).

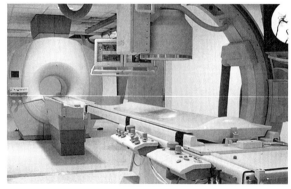

Figure 14–2 Photograph of an interventional radiology suite that combines rotational angiography with MRI capability, allowing immediate transfer of the patient from one modality to the other. The image intensifier for the angiography unit is seen in the foreground; the bore of the magnet and MR gantry is seen in the background. (*Courtesy of Alastair Martin, PhD.*)

part of preoperative planning. It is probably reasonable to assume that the x-ray machine is always on. There are three sources of radiation in the INR suite: *direct radiation* from the X-ray tube, *leakage* (through the collimators' protective shielding), and *scattered radiation* (reflected from the patients and the area surrounding the body part to be imaged). The amount of exposure decreases proportionally to the inverse of the square of the distance from the source of radiation (inverse square law). Digital subtraction angiography delivers considerably more radiation than fluoroscopy.

Optimal protection involves the use of lead aprons, thyroid shields, and radiation exposure badges. The lead aprons should be periodically evaluated for any cracks in the lead lining that may allow accidental radiation exposure. Movable lead glass screens may provide additional protection for the anesthesia team. Clear communication between the INR and anesthesia teams is also crucial for limiting radiation exposure. With proper precautions, the anesthesia team should be exposed to far less than the annual recommended limit for health care workers.

Anesthetic Technique

Choice of Anesthetic Technique

Most centers routinely involved in INR use general endotracheal anesthesia for procedures that are complex or of long duration. Choice of anesthetic technique varies among centers, with no clear superior method, and generally follows the dictates of the well-described considerations for operative neuroanesthesia.

Secure intravenous IV access should be available with adequate extension tubing to allow drug and fluid administration at maximal distance from the image intensifier during fluoroscopy. Access to intravenous or arterial catheters can be difficult when the patient is draped with the arms restrained at the sides; connections should be secure. Primary anesthetic or vasoactive agent infusions should be given through proximal ports with minimal dead space.

Monitoring

In addition to standard monitors specified by the American Society of Anesthesiologists, capnography sampling via the sampling port of the nasal cannula is useful for IV sedation.

A pulse oximetry probe can be placed on the great toe of the leg that will receive the femoral introducer sheath, to provide an early warning of femoral artery obstruction or distal thromboembolism.

For intracranial procedures and postoperative care, beat-to-beat arterial pressure monitoring and blood sampling can be facilitated by placement of an arterial line. A side port of the femoral artery introducer sheath can be used, but the sheath is usually removed immediately after the procedure. In a patient who requires continuous blood pressure monitoring or frequent blood sampling postoperatively, it is convenient to have a separate radial arterial blood pressure catheter. Electrophysiologic monitoring is not commonly used; it is more likely to be of use in procedures involving the spinal cord or its circulation.[8]

With a coaxial or triaxial catheter system, arterial pressure at the carotid artery, the vertebral artery, and the distal cerebral circulation can be measured. Pressures in these distal catheters usually underestimate systolic and overestimate diastolic pressure; however, mean pressures are reliable. Bladder catheters assist in fluid management as well as patient comfort; a significant volume of heparinized flush solution and radiographic contrast agent may be used.

General Anesthesia

Primary reasons for employing general anesthesia in INR are to minimize motion artifacts and to improve the quality of the image. Relative normocapnia or modest hypocapnia consistent with the safe conduct of positive-pressure ventilation should be maintained, unless intracranial pressure is a concern. The specific choice of anesthesia may be guided primarily by other cardiovascular and cerebrovascular considerations. There is no clear superiority of one modern anesthetic over another in terms of pharmacologic protection against neuronal injury. Total intravenous anesthetic techniques, or combinations of inhalational and intravenous methods, may optimize rapid emergence. An argument could be made for avoiding N_2O because of the possibility of introducing air emboli into the cerebral circulation and also because of reports that this agent worsens outcome after experimental brain injury.

It is important to distinguish two general settings in which hyperventilation is used in anesthetic practice. First, it is used to treat intracranial hypertension. Hyperventilation is an important mainstay of the management of an intracranial catastrophe to acutely reduce cerebral blood volume (Box 14-1). The second and far more common application is to provide brain relaxation after the skull is open, with the intent of providing better surgical access and, presumably, a lesser degree of brain retraction for a given surgical approach. The former indication may be critical in crisis management; the latter is not relevant to endovascular procedures. Therefore, $PaCO_2$ management should aim at normocapnia or mild hypocapnia to the extent consistent with the safe conduct of positive-pressure ventilation. If a patient has increased intracranial pressure, prophylactic mild hypocapnia may be indicated during induction and maintenance of anesthesia.

There are some special circumstances for which induced *hypercapnia* may be indicated, such as embolization of extracranial vascular malformations, which drain into the intracranial venous system. In these cases, induction of hypercapnia can promote high venous outflow from the cerebral venous system and help minimize the risk of inadvertent movement of embolic material into the intracranial compartment (discussed later).

Intravenous Sedation

For cases managed with an unsecured airway, routine evaluation of the potential ease of laryngoscopy in an emergency situation should take into account that direct access to the airway may be limited by table or room logistics. Recent pterional craniotomy can sometimes result in impairment of temporomandibular joint mobility.

For IV sedation cases, careful padding of pressure points and working with the patient to obtain final comfortable positioning may assist in the patient's ability to tolerate a long period of lying supine and motionless, decreasing the requirement for sedation, anxiolysis, and analgesia. The possibility of pregnancy in women and a history of adverse reactions to radiographic contrast agents should be explored.

Intravenous sedation in aneurysm management is used most often for patients coming for interim follow-up angiography to assess the necessity for re-treatment after primary coiling. If further treatment is indicated, the technique can be converted to general anesthesia. Goals of anesthetic choice for intravenous sedation are to alleviate pain, anxiety, and discomfort, provide patient immobility, and allow rapid recovery. There may be a discomfort associated with injection of contrast media into the cerebral arteries (burning) and with distention or traction on them (headache). A long period of lying motionless can cause significant discomfort.

A variety of sedation regimens is available, and specific choices are based on the experience of the practitioner and the goals of anesthetic management. Common to all intravenous sedation techniques is the potential for upper airway obstruction. Placement of a nasopharyngeal airway may cause troublesome bleeding in anticoagulated patients and is generally avoided.

Dexmedetomidine is a newer agent that may have applicability in the INR setting. A potent, selective α_2-agonist with sedative, anxiolytic, and analgesic properties, it has now received regulatory approval for sedation. Dexmedetomidine is especially noteworthy for its ability to produce a state of patient tranquility without depressing respiration. However, there are two caveats to consider. Its effects on cerebral perfusion are still unclear.[9] More importantly, there is a tendency for patients managed with dexmedetomidine to have relatively low blood pressure in the postoperative recovery period.[10] Because patients with aneurysmal subarachnoid hemorrhage (SAH) may be critically dependent on the adequacy of collateral perfusion pressure, regimens that may result in blood pressure decreases should be used with great caution.

There is a phenomenon worth mentioning that is inadequately characterized and, perhaps accordingly, lacks a good terminology. It is well known that patients, even with full recovery of a prior fixed neurologic deficit, may emerge from anesthesia with a re-emergence of a previously repaired deficit.[11] These observations are consistent with functional neuroimaging studies that suggest "rewiring" (an inadequately mechanistic metaphor) occurs to compensate for neurologic injury.[12] Why anesthetics cause a temporary reversal of the repair or compensatory process is unknown. For example, Thal and colleagues[11] showed that small doses of either midazolam or fentanyl induced transient focal motor deterioration in patients with prior motor deficits. Lazar and associates[13] demonstrated with more sophisticated methodology that not only motor, but also language and spatial, functions can be affected by this process. Indeed, they extended their observations to include patients who had suffered recent transient cerebral ischemic episodes and were neurologically intact as shown by normal diffusion-weighted imaging findings; in this study, midazolam caused reappearance of prior focal deficits that had been transient and fully resolved.[14]

The point to be made for the purpose of this discussion is that there are potentially important effects of IV sedative agents that may complicate neurologic monitoring, especially if functional testing of endovascular manipulations is desirable.

Anticoagulation

Heparin

Careful management of coagulation is required to prevent thromboembolic complications during and after the procedure. Generally, after a baseline activated clotting time is obtained, intravenous heparin (approximately 70 units/kg) is given to a target prolongation of 2 to 3 times the baseline value. Then heparin can be given continuously or as an intermittent bolus with hourly monitoring of activated clotting time. For the occasional case of refractoriness, adequate anticoagulation, switching from bovine to porcine heparin, or vice versa, should be considered. If antithrombin III deficiency is suspected, administration of fresh frozen plasma may be necessary.

Direct Thrombin Inhibitors

Heparin-induced thrombocytopenia is a rare but important adverse event in heparin anticoagulation. Development of heparin-dependent antibodies after initial exposure leads to a prothrombotic syndrome. In high-risk patients, direct thrombin inhibitors can be applied, with the realization that adverse events are inherent to their use, such as anaphylaxis. Direct thrombin inhibitors inhibit free and clot-bound thrombin, and their effect can be monitored by either an activated partial thromboplastin time or activated clotting time. Lepirudin and bivalirudin, a synthetic derivative, have half-lives of 40 to 120 minutes and about 25 minutes, respectively. Because these drugs undergo renal elimination, dose adjustments may be needed in patients with renal dysfunction. Argatroban is an alternative agent that undergoes primarily hepatic metabolism. One report has described bivalirudin as a potential alternative to heparin during INR procedures for intravenous anticoagulation and intra-arterial thrombolysis.[15]

Antiplatelet Agents

Although still controversial in the acute setting,[16] antiplatelet agents (aspirin, the glycoprotein IIb/IIIa receptor antagonists, and the thienopyridine derivatives) are increasingly being used for cerebrovascular disease management[17] and may be of use for acute treatment of thromboembolic complications.[18] Abciximab (ReoPro) has been used to treat thromboembolic complications. Activation of the platelet membrane glycoprotein IIb/IIIa leads to fibrinogen binding and is a final common pathway for platelet aggregation. Abciximab, eptifibatide, and tirofiban are glycoprotein IIb/IIIa receptor antagonists. The long duration and potent effect of abciximab also increase the likelihood of major bleeding. The smaller-molecule agents, eptifibatide and tirofiban, are competitive blockers with shorter half-lives of about 2 hours. Thienopyridine derivatives (ticlopidine and clopidogrel) bind to the platelet's adenosine diphosphate receptor, permanently altering the receptor; therefore, the duration of action is the lifespan of the platelet. Clopidogrel is commonly added to the antiplatelet regimen for procedures that require placement of devices (e.g., stents, coiling or stent-assisted coiling) primarily in patients who have not had an acute event, such as those with unruptured aneurysms.

Reversal of Anticoagulation

At the end of the procedure or at occurrence of hemorrhagic complication, heparin anticoagulation may be reversed with protamine. Because there is no specific antidote for the direct thrombin inhibitors or the antiplatelet agents, biologic half-life is one of the major considerations in drug choice, and platelet transfusion is a nonspecific therapy, should reversal be indicated. There is no currently available accurate test to measure platelet function in patients taking the newer antiplatelet drugs. Desmopressin (DDAVP) has been reported to shorten the prolonged bleeding time of individuals taking antiplatelet agents, such as aspirin and ticlopidine. There are also increasingly more reports on the use of specific clotting factors, such as recombinant factor VIIa and factor IX complex, to rescue severe life-threatening bleeding, including intracranial hemorrhage uncontrolled by standard transfusion therapy. The safety and efficacy of these coagulation factors remain to be investigated.

DELIBERATE HYPERTENSION

During acute arterial occlusion or vasospasm, the only practical way to increase collateral blood flow may be an augmentation of the collateral perfusion pressure by raising the systemic blood pressure. The circle of Willis is a primary collateral pathway in cerebral circulation. However, in as many as 21%

of otherwise normal subjects, the circle may not be complete. There are also secondary collateral channels that bridge adjacent major vascular territories, most importantly for the long circumferential arteries that supply the hemispheric convexities. These pathways are known as the pial-to-pial collateral or leptomeningeal pathways.

The extent to which the blood pressure has to be raised depends on the condition of the patient and the nature of the disease. Typically, during deliberate hypertension, the systemic blood pressure is raised by 30% to 40% above baseline in the absence of some direct outcome measure, such as resolution of ischemic symptoms or imaging evidence of improved perfusion. Phenylephrine, usually the first-line agent for deliberate hypertension, is titrated to achieve the desired level of blood pressure. The electrocardiogram and ST segment monitor should be carefully inspected for signs of myocardial ischemia.

The risk of causing hemorrhage into an ischemic area must be weighed against the benefits of improving perfusion, but augmentation of blood pressure in the presence of acute cerebral ischemia is probably protective in most settings. There is also a risk of rupturing an aneurysm or arteriovenous malformation (AVM) with induction of hypertension. There are no data that speak to this risk directly, other than older case series that report rupture during anesthetic induction in the range of about 1% that was presumably due to acute hypertension. For AVMs, cautious extrapolation of observations for head-frame application suggests the rarity of AVM rupture from acute blood pressure increases. Szabo and colleagues[19] measured blood pressure changes noninvasively in 56 conscious, unpremedicated patients undergoing local anesthetic injection and pin insertion; the maximum mean arterial pressure was 118±7 mm Hg, representing an increase of 37% from baseline. These researchers concluded that since none of their 56 patients, nor any of the more than 1000 patients treated in similar fashion, suffered a hemorrhage, moderate arterial hypertension does cause spontaneous AVM hemorrhage.[19]

DELIBERATE HYPOTENSION

The two primary indications for induced hypotension are (1) to test cerebrovascular reserve in patients undergoing carotid occlusion and (2) to slow flow in a feeding artery of a brain AVM before injecting glue (sometimes termed "flow arrest"). The most important factor in choosing a hypotensive agent is the ability to safely and expeditiously achieve the desired reduction in blood pressure while keeping the patient physiologically stable, and, if the patient is awake, not to interfere with neurologic assessment.

The choice of agent should be determined by the experience of the practitioner, the patient's medical condition, and the goals of the blood pressure reduction in a particular clinical setting. Intravenous adenosine has been used to induce transient cardiac pause and may be a viable method of partial flow arrest.[20]

MANAGEMENT OF NEUROLOGIC AND PROCEDURAL CRISES

A well thought-out plan, coupled with rapid and effective communication between the anesthesia and radiology teams, is critical for good outcomes in INR. The primary responsibility of the anesthesia team is to preserve gas exchange and, if indicated, secure the airway. Simultaneous with airway management, the first branch in the decision-making algorithm is for the anesthesiologist to communicate with the INR team and determine whether the problem is hemorrhagic or occlusive.

In the setting of vascular occlusion, the goal is to increase distal perfusion by means of blood pressure augmentation with or without direct thrombolysis. If the problem is hemorrhagic, immediate cessation of heparin and reversal of anticoagulation with protamine is indicated. As an emergency reversal dose, 1 mg protamine can be given for each 100 units of initial heparin dosage that resulted in therapeutic anticoagulation. The activated clotting time can then be used to fine-tune the final protamine dose. Complications of protamine administration include hypotension, true anaphylaxis, and pulmonary hypertension. With the advent of newer long-acting direct thrombin inhibitors such as bivalirudin, new strategies for emergency reversal of anticoagulation need to be developed.

Bleeding catastrophes are usually heralded by headache, nausea, vomiting, and vascular pain related to the area of perforation. Sudden loss of consciousness is not always due to intracranial hemorrhage. Seizures, due to contrast media reaction or transient ischemia, and the resulting postictal state, can also result in an obtunded patient. In the anesthetized or comatose patient, the sudden onset of bradycardia and hypertension (Cushing response) or the endovascular therapist's diagnosis of extravasation of contrast agent may be the only clues to a developing hemorrhage. Most cases of vascular rupture can be managed in the angiography suite. The INR team can attempt to seal the rupture site endovascularly and abort the procedure; a ventriculostomy catheter may be placed emergently in the angiography suite. Some authorities suggest that ventriculostomy catheters should be placed prior to the procedure in selected high-risk patients, for example, those with ventriculomegaly.[21] After the procedure, the patient with suspected rupture requires evaluation with computed tomography, but emergency craniotomy is usually not indicated.

SPECIFIC PROCEDURES

Table 14-1 summarizes representative procedures in INR.

Intracranial Aneurysm Ablation

The two basic approaches for INR therapy of cerebral aneurysms are occlusion of proximal parent arteries and obliteration of the aneurysmal sac. With the publication of the International Subarachnoid Aneurysm Trial,[22] coil embolization of intracranial aneurysms has become a routine first-choice therapy for many lesions (Fig. 14-3). Patients with unruptured aneurysm or for whom stent placement is contemplated may be started on antiplatelet agents preoperatively. Inflation of a temporary balloon catheter may be used to aid in placement of coils in selected cases (Fig. 14-4).

There is great interest in the development of stent-assisted coiling methods (Fig. 14-5). Placement of embolic coils within a target aneurysm may be difficult if the aneurysm has a wide neck. Stent-supported coiling is designed to provide a scaffold for the containment of the coils within the aneurysm sac and to provide continued patency of the parent artery. Aggressive antiplatelet therapy, currently using both aspirin and clopidogrel, must accompany the performance of stent-assisted

Table 14–1   Interventional Neuroradiologic Procedures and Primary Anesthetic Considerations

Procedure	Possible Anesthetic Considerations
Therapeutic embolization of vascular malformation:	
Intracranial AVM	Deliberate hypotension, postprocedure NPPB
Dural arteriovenous fistula	Existence of venous hypertension; deliberate hypercapnia
Extracranial AVM	Deliberate hypercapnia
Carotid cavernous fistula	Deliberate hypercapnia, postprocedure NPPB
Cerebral aneurysms	Aneurysmal rupture, blood pressure control*
Ethanol sclerotherapy of arteriovenous or venous malformations	Brain swelling, airway swelling, hypoxemia, hypoglycemia, intoxication from ethanol, cardiorespiratory arrest
Balloon angioplasty and stenting of occlusive cerebrovascular disease	Cerebral ischemia, deliberate hypertension, concomitant coronary artery disease, bradycardia, hypotension
Balloon angioplasty of cerebral vasospasm secondary to aneurysmal subarachnoid hemorrhage	Cerebral ischemia, blood pressure control*
Therapeutic carotid occlusion for giant aneurysms and skull base tumors	Cerebral ischemia, blood pressure control*
Thrombolysis of acute thromboembolic stroke	Postprocedure intracranial hemorrhage (NPPB), concomitant coronary artery disease, blood pressure control*
Intra-arterial chemotherapy of head and neck tumors	Airway swelling, intracranial hypertension
Embolization for epistaxis	Airway control

AVM, arteriovenous malformation; NPPB, normal perfusion pressure breakthrough.
*Blood pressure control refers to deliberate hypotension or hypertension.

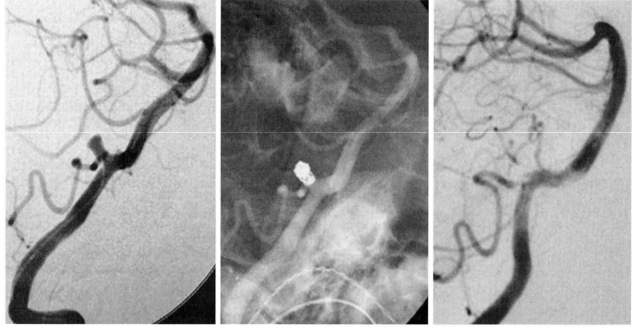

Figure 14–3   Small ruptured posterior inferior cerebellar artery (PICA) aneurysm, before (*left*) and after (*middle* and *right*) successful endovascular treatment with detachable platinum coils, with preservation of the parent PICA. The *left* and *right* views show subtracted images. The *middle* view shows an unsubtracted image to demonstrate coil mass.

coiling procedures owing to the risk of thromboembolic complications. Stent placement requires more instrumentation and manipulation, probably increasing the ever-present intraprocedural risk of parent vessel occlusion, thromboembolism, or vascular rupture.

Anesthetic management should proceed with the usual considerations employed in the care of a patient with an intracranial aneurysm.[23] Patients with aneurysmal SAH often have either increased intracranial pressure or decreased intracranial compliance, secondary to the mass of SAH, parenchymal injury from ischemia or hydrocephalus.

The anesthesiologist should be prepared for aneurysmal rupture and acute SAH at all times, from spontaneous rupture of a leaky sac to direct injury of the aneurysm wall by the vascular manipulation, perianeurysmal thrombus formation, or arterial branch occlusion. The morbidity and mortality

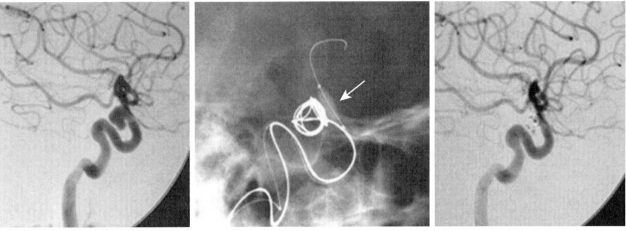

Figure 14–4 Wide-necked supraclinoid internal carotid artery aneurysm *(left)* successfully treated using temporary placement of a balloon (*arrow, middle*) to support placement of coils properly within the aneurysm sac (*right*). There are two catheters in the vascular lumen, one to deliver the coils and one to temporarily inflate the balloon.

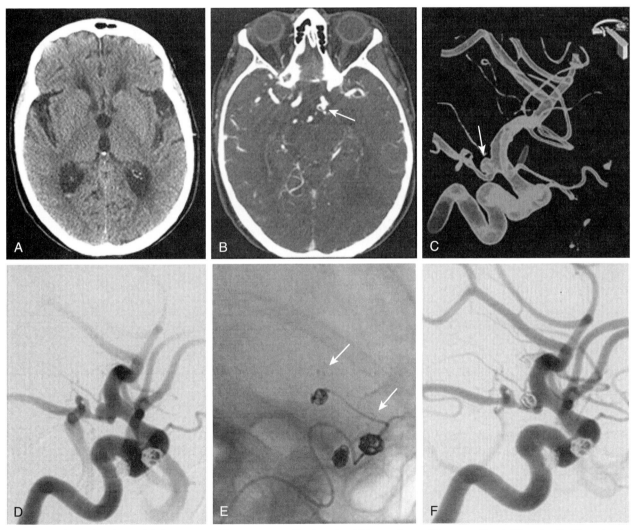

Figure 14–5 The patient is an elderly woman with a recent small subarachnoid hemorrhage. CT scans without (**A**) and with (**B**) contrast agent demonstrate blood layering in the occipital horn of the right lateral ventricle and a small, wide-necked aneurysm at the origin of the left posterior communicating (PComm) artery (*arrow*). **C,** A three-dimensional reconstruction of a rotational angiogram shows the aneurysm at the PComm origin (*arrow*). **D, E,** and **F,** Lateral views of a left internal carotid angiogram show successful treatment of the PComm aneurysm using stent-supported coiling. (Note that two contralateral internal carotid aneurysms had already been treated with endovascular coiling.) In **E,** the ends of the stent (*arrows*) are radiodense.

of intraprocedural rupture is high. One report found that, in the 5% of the studied coiling cases, 63% of patients with intraprocedural rupture had periprocedural death or disability compared with 15% of those without intraprocedural rupture.[24]

If a rupture occurs, anticoagulation must be immediately reversed. A Cushing response (hypertension and bradycardia) may develop. Cerebral perfusion pressure should be maintained at adequate levels. Emergency placement of a ventriculostomy should be considered, and an emergency computed tomography scan should be obtained to assess for sequelae of the perforation or rupture.

Angioplasty of Cerebral Vasospasm from Aneurysmal Subarachnoid Hemorrhage

Roughly one out of four patients with SAH has symptomatic vasospasm. Angioplasty, either mechanical (balloon) or pharmacologic (intra-arterial vasodilators), may be used as a treatment.[25] Angioplasty is ideally done in patients in whom the symptomatic lesion has already been surgically clipped and for patients in the early course of symptomatic ischemia in order to prevent hemorrhagic transformation of an ischemic region. The use of balloon angioplasty has been suggested as a prophylactic measure, but its efficacy has not been demonstrated.[26]

There are two options for vasospasm. First, a balloon catheter is inserted under fluoroscopic guidance into the spastic segment and inflated to mechanically distend the constricted area. It is also possible to perform a "pharmacologic" angioplasty by direct intra-arterial infusion. Historically, papaverine was the first widely used agent, but there has been growing appreciation that it has serious toxic central nervous system effects.[27,28] Calcium channel or entry blockers (CCB/CEBs), such as nicardipine and verapamil, are now being used, and a number of studies are appearing in the literature, primarily small case series.[29-33] Intravenous nimodipine has also been reported.[34,35] Intra-arterial vasodilators may have systemic effects (bradycardia and hypotension) that may be profound and may work at cross-purposes with the goals of maintaining adequate perfusion pressure. Typically, the effects of CCB/CEBs can be offset by concomitant vasopressor therapy, but this approach may not always be effective. Because the CCB/CEBs also vasodilate the pulmonary circulation, a loss of hypoxic pulmonary vasoconstriction may worsen oxygenation in susceptible patients.[36,37] Seizure activity is a potential complication of the intra-arterial injection of CCB/CEBs.[38]

Although calcium is the most direct treatment for overdose of CCB/CEBs, there are theoretical reasons to avoid increasing plasma, and potentially brain extracellular fluid, levels of calcium in the setting of ongoing cerebral ischemia. There may be promise in the use of lipid emulsion therapy for ameliorating toxicity from lipid-soluble agents.[39-41]

A number of case series have described the use of milrinone, a phosphodiesterase inhibitor.[42-44] It may be the case that superior vasodilation can be achieved with this drug, with fewer systemic side effects. Finally, there is great interest in the use of statins (hydroxymethylglutaryl coenzyme A reductase inhibitors).[45-48] There are no large well-controlled trials for angioplasty, either mechanical or chemical, which would also be an important area to study systematically. Other agents are fasudil (inhibitor of kinases, including protein kinase C) and colforsin (adenylate cyclase activator). The topic of endovascular vasospasm has been reviewed in depth,[49] and a review of

the general principles of intra-arterial drug administration has been published.[50]

Patients who come for angioplasty are often critically ill with a variety of challenging comorbidities, including neurocardiac injury, volume overload from triple-H (hypervolemia, hypertension, and hemodilution) therapy, hydrocephalus, brain injury from recent craniotomy, and residual effects of the presenting hemorrhage. Procedural complications include arterial rupture, reperfusion hemorrhage, thromboembolism, and arterial dissection.

In symptomatic patients, it is common to induce generous increases above baseline mean arterial pressure in the range of 30% to 50%. If the aneurysm is unsecured, this target may be tempered. Phenylephrine is a useful agent, but if myocardial dysfunction is present from neurogenic injury, an inotrope may be appropriate. Unless increased intracranial pressure is being targeted, hyperventilation should be avoided.

Carotid Test Occlusion and Therapeutic Carotid Occlusion

Large fusiform aneurysms of the cavernous segment of the internal carotid artery (ICA) may be treated by proximal vessel occlusion. Also, some aggressive skull base tumors may encase the ICA, and preoperative intentional, controlled ICA occlusion may help the surgeon provide optimal resection. To assess the consequences of carotid occlusion in anticipation of surgery, the surgeon may schedule the patient for a test occlusion, in which cerebrovascular reserve is evaluated in several ways. A multimodal combination of angiographic, clinical, and physiologic tests can be used to arrive at the safest course of action for a given patient's clinical circumstances. The judicious use of deliberate hypotension can improve the sensitivity of the test.[51] The most important factor in choosing a hypotensive agent is the ability to safely and expeditiously achieve the desired reduction in blood pressure while keeping the patient physiologically stable. The choice of agent should be determined by the experience of the practitioner, the patient's medical condition, and the goals of the blood pressure reduction in a particular clinical setting.

Brain Arteriovenous Malformations

Also called cerebral or pial AVMs, brain AVMs (BAVMs) are typically large, complex lesions made up of a tangle of abnormal vessels (called the *nidus*) frequently containing several discrete fistulas served by multiple feeding arteries and draining veins. The goal of therapeutic embolization is to obliterate as many of the fistulas and their respective feeding arteries as possible (Figs. 14-6 and 14-7). BAVM embolization is usually an adjunct to surgery or radiotherapy. The primary reason to treat a BAVM is to prevent future spontaneous hemorrhage. Those patients with BAVMs that have not previously ruptured may have a low risk of bleeding[52,53] and may be at a higher risk for invasive treatment.[54,55] A randomized controlled trial sponsored by the National Institute of Neurological Disorders and Stroke is currently studying the long-term benefit of treating unruptured BAVMs.[56,57]

The cyanoacrylate glues offer relatively "permanent" closure of abnormal vessels. *N*-Butyl cyanoacrylate (NBCA) is a low-viscosity liquid monomer that polymerizes to a solid form upon contact with ionic solutions, including blood and saline, but not 5% dextrose in water. Passage of glue into a draining vein can result in acute hemorrhage;

PRE-EMBO   EMBO   POST-EMBO

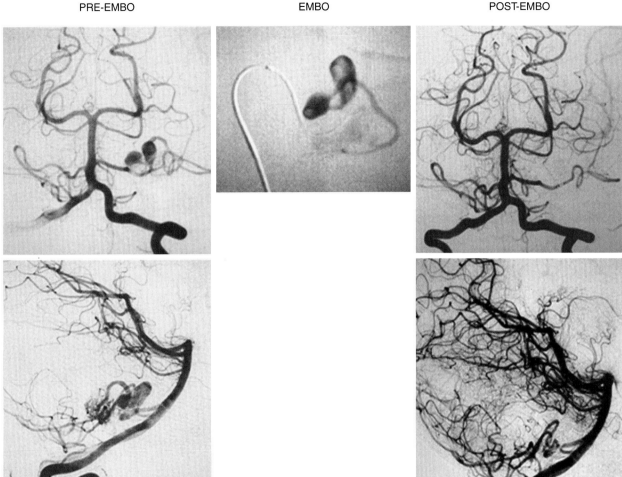

Figure 14–6 Embolization of the cerebellar arteriovenous malformation shown in Fig. 14-1. *Left,* Pre-embolization angiography shows anteroposterior (*top*) and lateral (*bottom*) projections. *Middle,* Slightly magnified view of microcatheter placement through the left anterior inferior cerebellar artery into the proximal feeding artery aneurysm sac, with subsequent elimination of the aneurysm complex after placement of detachable platinum coils. *Right,* Post-embolization views.

in smaller patients, pulmonary embolism of glue can be symptomatic. For these reasons, deliberate hypotension may increase safety of glue delivery. There is no compelling reason to choose any particular method to achieve the hypotension. The flow through the fistula is a pressure-dependent phenomenon.[58]

A major drawback to the use of *N*-butyl cyanoacrylate is that it is adhesive, with the potential to inadvertently glue the catheter to the injected polymer. Onyx Liquid Embolic System (ev3, Inc., Plymouth, MN), a new, nonadhesive liquid embolic agent consisting of ethylene-vinyl alcohol copolymer and tantalum powder in a dimethyl sulfoxide solvent, theoretically may reduce the overall complication rates for use of *N*-butyl cyanoacrylate,[59,60] although aggressive therapy may have intrinsic risks. The agent or its vehicle, dimethyl sulfoxide, may have unusual adverse effects[61]; dimethyl sulfoxide can cause a garlic-like taste and odor on the breath and skin that may last several hours and may be alarming to the patient.

Although less durable, polyvinyl alcohol microsphere embolization is also commonly used. If surgery is planned within days after polyvinyl alcohol embolization, the rate of recanalization is low. Ethanol has also been used as an agent but has many untoward effects, including induction of brain edema (see later).[62]

Even in the absence of clinically detectable deficits, subclinical injury can result from BAVM embolization. There is a high incidence of abnormal findings that are detectable on postprocedure magnetic resonance imaging examination; for example, 22% of patients showed ischemic lesions on postprocedure images in one series.[63] Intraoperative management should take this trend into consideration.

For AVM evaluation, some centers use superselective Wada testing prior to therapeutic embolization to test the eloquence of regions adjacent to the lesion. It is important to consider using a sedation regimen for such cases that will minimally affect cognitive or motor findings (see previous comments regarding reappearance phenomena). The purpose of such testing is to establish treatment risk in individual patients. Interestingly, Wada testing, functional imaging studies, and intrasurgical cortical mapping have shown redistribution of language and memory to unpredictable regions.[64,65] Further, developmental cognitive history in these patients indicates that most will have had at least some learning problems during their school-age years with varying severity,[66] reflecting a time when brain reorganization may have been occurring.

Some centers may measure feeding artery or draining vein pressures to assist in evaluating risk for future hemorrhage, if the lesion is not treated.[3,67,68] High pressure is associated with

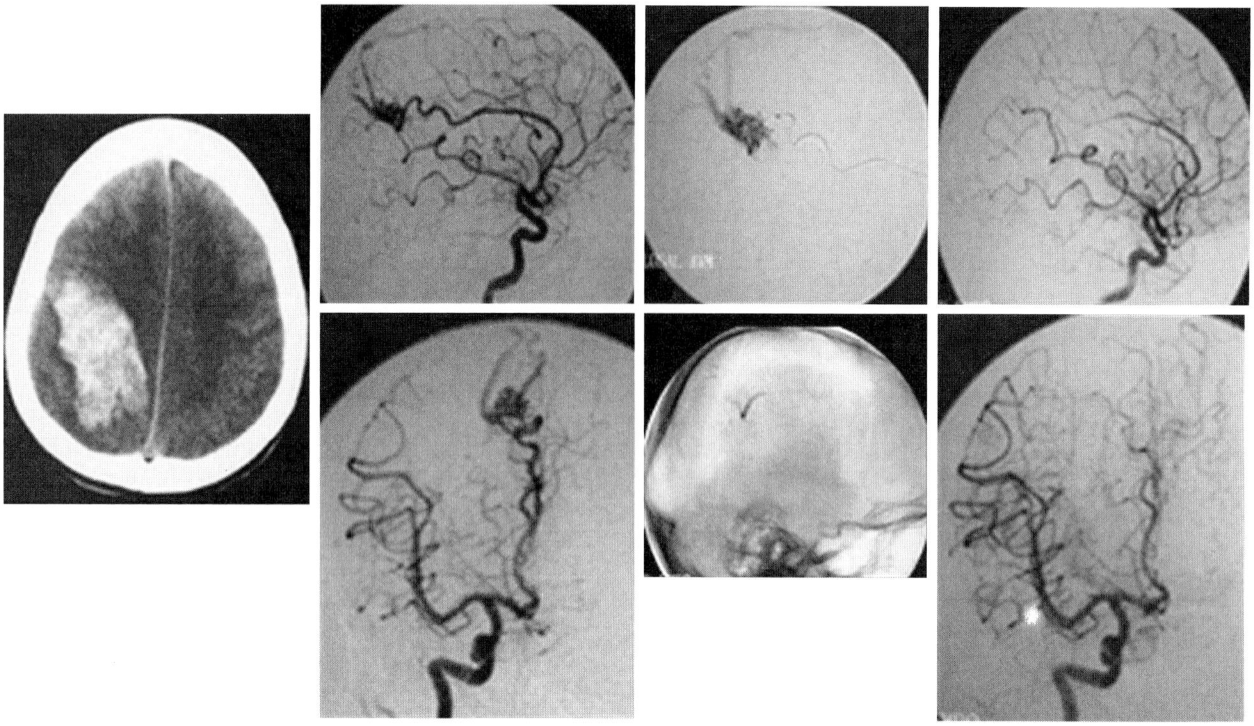

PRE EMBO POST

Figure 14–7 Endovascular treatment of a ruptured right parietal arteriovenous malformation (AVM). *Left,* CT scan shows acute parenchymal hemorrhage. Pre-embolization (PRE), mid-embolization (EMBO), and post-embolization (POST) angiographs show placement of a flow-directed microcatheter into the feeding artery and embolization using cyanoacrylate glue, with complete eradication of the AVM. Pre- and post-embolization images are lateral (*top*) and anteroposterior (*bottom*) projections. *Middle* views show the microcatheter in the AVM during progressive occlusion; both are lateral projections.

hemorrhagic presentation. Delayed transit of contrast media might be a surrogate for high intranidal pressure.[69,70]

Dural Arteriovenous Fistulas

A dural arteriovenous fistula (DAVF) is an acquired arteriovenous shunt in the wall of a dural venous sinus. The etiology of DAVFs is unclear, although some believe that many DAVFs result from venous dural sinus stenosis or occlusion, opening of potential arteriovenous shunts, and subsequent recanalization. Intracranial DAVF accounts for about 10% to 15% of all intracranial vascular malformations. Symptoms vary according to the sinus involved. Venous hypertension of pial veins is a risk factor for intracranial hemorrhage. DAVFs may be fed by multiple meningeal vessels, and therefore, multistaged embolization is often necessary. Dural arteriovenous fistulas can induce markedly raised venous pressure and diminished net cerebral perfusion pressure. Therefore, the presence of venous hypertension should be factored into management of systemic arterial and cerebral perfusion pressure. This is a critical aspect of DAVF perioperative management. It is often assumed that the venous hypertension induces the angiogenic phenotype by acting through its cause, cerebral ischemia, but newer evidence suggests that venous hypertension may be a direct stimulus for angiogenesis.[71] DAVFs are unique in that there are promising animal models of their pathogenesis,[72,73] unlike for most other hemorrhagic brain diseases.

Other rare adverse events have included trigeminocardiac reflex and asystolic arrest due to high vagal tone after glue injection. Such reflexes, if they occur, are usually amenable to anticholinergic prophylaxis or treatment.[74]

Vein of Galen Malformations

Vein of Galen malformation is a special case of an intracranial arteriovenous shunt that is beyond the scope of this review.[75,76] The malformations are relatively uncommon but complicated lesions that are present in infants and require a multidisciplinary approach. Patients may have intractable congestive heart failure, intractable seizures, hydrocephalus, and mental retardation. Several approaches have been attempted, both transarterial and transvenous. In infants with high-output failure, preexisting right-to-left shunts, and pulmonary hypertension, a relatively small pulmonary glue embolism can be fatal.

Craniofacial Venous Malformations

A craniofacial venous malformation is a congenital disorder of venous maldevelopment. In addition to causing significant cosmetic deformities, it may impinge on the upper airway and interfere with swallowing. Many of these lesions are resistant to conventional surgery, cryosurgery, or laser surgery. In the INR procedure, sclerosing agents, such as USP grade 95% ethanol opacified with contrast agent, is injected percutaneously into the lesion under fluoroscopic guidance, resulting in a chemical burn to the lesion and eventually shrinking it. Sclerotherapy alone may be adequate treatment or may be combined with surgery.[77]

This therapy has several inter-reactions with anesthetic management.[3] Because marked swelling occurs immediately after ethanol injection, the ability of the patient to maintain a patent airway postoperatively must be carefully considered.[77]

Desaturation is frequently noted on the pulse oximeter after the injection. Cardiopulmonary arrest has been reported.[62] One theory is that ethanol induces severe pulmonary precapillary vasospasm, but the relationship between this and the more common hypoxemic response is not clear. The predictable intoxication and other side effects of ethanol may be evident after emergence from anesthesia, particularly postemergence agitation in children.

Venous malformations of the face or dural fistulas have the potential to drain into intracerebral veins or sinuses. If the Pa_{CO_2} is raised to 50 to 60 mm Hg, cerebral venous outflow will greatly exceed extracranial venous outflow, and the pressure gradient will favor movement of a sclerosing agent, chemotherapeutic agent, or glue away from vital intracranial drainage pathways. Although actual pressure gradients have never been studied, increased intracranial outflow is readily demonstrable in clinical practice with angiography. Addition of CO_2 gas to the inspired gas mixture is the easiest and safest way to achieve hypercapnia. Airway collapse and atelectasis are prevented by maintaining adequate tidal volume. However, hypoventilation may be employed if CO_2 gas is not available; in this case, addition of positive end-expiratory pressure may be useful to maintain oxygenation.

Angioplasty and Stenting for Atherosclerotic Lesions

Angioplasty and stenting for treatment of atherosclerotic stenoses of the cervical, vertebral, and intracranial arteries continues to supplant open surgical management (Fig. 14-8).[78,79] Risk of distal thromboembolism is a potential complication of this procedure. Intravascular filters and balloons, collectively called "distal protection devices," have been developed to theoretically prevent distal intracranial embolization of thrombus or plaque that may become dislodged during deployment of the stent or angioplasty balloon at the carotid bifurcation. These distal protection devices have come into common use for carotid stenting, although the procedure-related complications of the use of such protection devices (carotid dissection or occlusion, device-induced arterial spasm, thrombus formation) have not been well studied. There are multiple ongoing trials to compare the utility of stenting with that of carotid endarterectomy for extracranial carotid disease. The Stenting and Angioplasty with Protection in Patients at High Risk for Endarterectomy (SAPPHIRE) trial, a hybrid randomized controlled registry trial,[80] suggested non-inferiority of stenting and angioplasty in comparison with carotid endarterectomy. The majority of lesions in this trial were asymptomatic ICA lesions treated with nickel titanium (Nitinol) stents and use of emboli protection. The rates for stroke, death, and acute myocardial infarction within the first 30 days were 9.8% for carotid endarterectomy and 4.7% for stenting and angioplasty ($P = .09$). The EVA-3S (endarterectomy versus stenting in patients with symptomatic severe carotid stenosis) Trial[81] studied patients with symptomatic ICA stenosis greater than 60%. This cohort did not have severe coronary artery disease. The trial was stopped prematurely after the inclusion of 527 patients "for reasons of both safety and futility."[81] The 30-day stroke-or-death rate was 3.9% for carotid endarterectomy versus 9.6% for stenting and angioplasty; the endpoint, incidence of any stroke-or-death at 6 months, was 6.1% versus 11.7%, respectively, with no difference in 30-day rate of acute myocardial infarction.

Preparation for anesthetic management in the patient undergoing angioplasty and stenting may include placement of transcutaneous pacing leads, in case of severe bradycardia or asystole from carotid body stimulation during angioplasty. Intravenous atropine or glycopyrrolate may also be used in an attempt to mitigate bradycardia, which almost invariably occurs to some extent with inflation of the balloon. This powerful chronotropic response may be difficult or impossible to prevent or control by conventional means. Adverse effects of increasing myocardial oxygen demand need to be considered in antibradycardia interventions.

Potential complications of the procedure include vessel occlusion, perforation, dissection, spasm, thromboemboli, occlusion of adjacent vessels, transient ischemic episodes, and stroke. As with carotid endarterectomy, there is about a 5% risk of symptomatic cerebral hemorrhage or brain swelling after carotid angioplasty.[82]

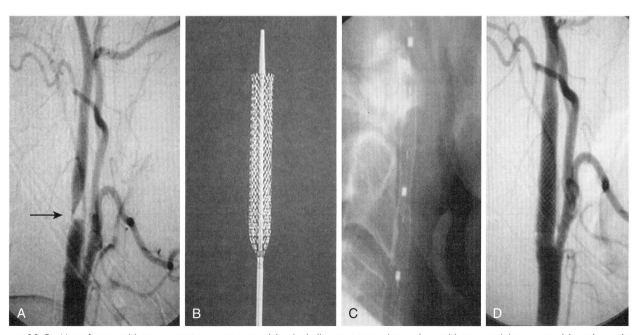

Figure 14–8 Use of a carotid artery stent restores normal luminal diameter to an internal carotid artery origin narrowed by atherosclerosis. **A,** Stenosis at arrow. **B,** Stent before deployment on catheter system. **C,** Stent expanded in situ. **D,** Catheter removed; luminal diameter is now restored.

Although the etiology of this syndrome is unknown, it has been associated with cerebral hyperperfusion, and it may be related to poor postoperative blood pressure control.

Thrombolysis and Thrombectomy of Acute Thromboembolic Stroke

In acute occlusive stroke, it is possible to recanalize the occluded vessel by superselective intra-arterial thrombolytic therapy. Thrombolytic agents can be delivered in high concentration through a microcatheter navigated close to the clot (Fig. 14-9). Neurologic deficits may be reversed without additional risk of secondary hemorrhage if treatment is completed within several hours from the onset of ischemia in the carotid territory, and somewhat longer for ischemia in the vertebrobasilar territory. Intra-arterial thrombolysis is currently an "off-label" use of these agents. Furland and coworkers[83] found that despite a higher frequency of early symptomatic hemorrhagic complications, treatment with intra-arterial pro-urokinase within 6 hours of the onset of acute ischemic stroke with middle cerebral artery occlusion significantly improved clinical outcome at 90 days.

A newer and promising approach is the use of mechanical retrieval devices to physically remove the offending thromboembolic material from the intracranial vessel, as reviewed by Smith and associates.[84,85] Such devices appear to be efficacious in recanalizing occluded vessels, and early restoration of flow appears to reduce the volume of infarcted brain (Fig. 14-10).

Both tissue plasminogen activator and mechanical retrieval have an inherent risk of promoting hemorrhagic transformation, just as in the case of IV thrombolysis. This is an important area for investigation because hemorrhagic transformation, or its threat, has great impact on clinical practice. Tissue plasminogen activator promotes expression and activity of matrix metalloproteinase-9 (MMP-9), a key protease for tissue remodeling that is also involved in various kinds of vascular injury that can damage the neurovascular unit and promote hemorrhage.[86] Tissue plasminogen activator can increase MMP-9 expression in brain endothelium, acting through the low-density lipoprotein receptor–related protein (LRP), and promotes up-regulation after focal cerebral ischemia.[87] Patient MMP-9 plasma levels are also increased after treatment.[88]

Details of anesthetic management for thrombolysis and thrombectomy are reviewed elsewhere.[89] Briefly, there are a number of challenges in hyperacute care of a patient population that is generally elderly and has common medical comorbidities, especially if little knowledge of patient history is available prior to treatment. The choice of IV or general

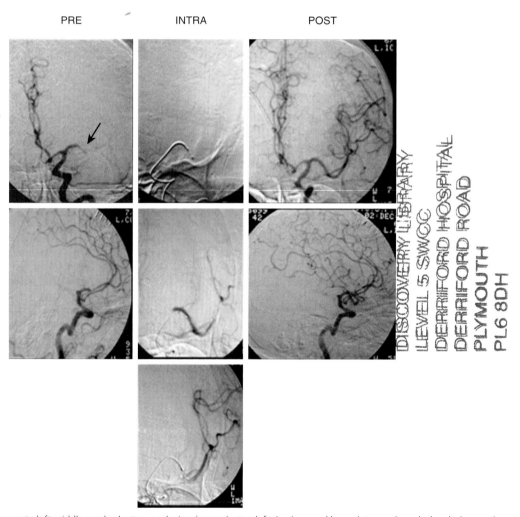

Figure 14–9 Patient with an acute left middle cerebral artery occlusion (*arrow* in *top left* view) caused by an iatrogenic embolus during angiography. *Left,* Left internal carotid angiography is shown (PRE); *top* is anteroposterior projection, and *bottom* is lateral projection. *Middle,* Immediate microcatheter placement into the clot allowed successful thrombolysis using tissue plasminogen activator (TPA) (INTRA). Top image shows microcatheter in position; middle and bottom images show contrast injection during course of thrombolysis. *Right,* Corresponding left internal carotid artery after successful TPA thrombolysis and restoration of arterial flow to the left middle cerebral territory.

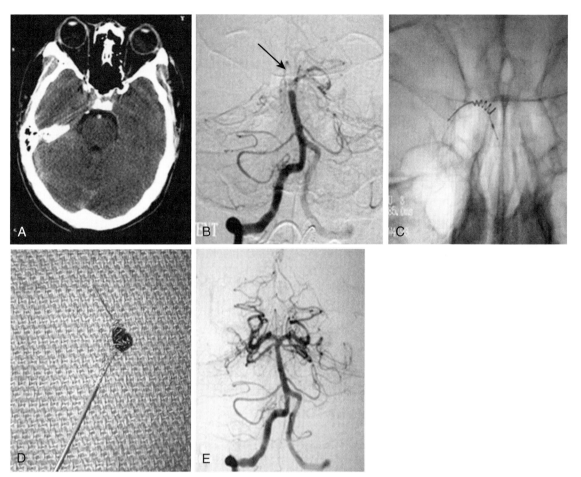

Figure 14–10 Acute basilar artery occlusion from an embolus caused by a traumatic dissection of the vertebral artery. **A,** CT scan demonstrates only a dense basilar artery, indicating its occlusion. **B,** The thrombus obstructs flow at the top of the basilar artery (*arrow*). **C,** Corkscrew-shaped clot retrieval device is seen in place on unsubtracted anteroposterior image. **D,** Clot was removed by means of this retrieval device. **E,** Flow is restored to the basilar artery, leaving the patient without neurologic deficit.

anesthesia must be carefully considered, depending on local practices, and the potential for patient agitation must be weighed against the ability to monitor neurologic status. Intravascular volume management may be challenging for several reasons. There is a very high incidence of systemic hypertension in patients with vasculopathy, who may be further volume-depleted because of an acute ictus. This fact complicates management to address the need to maintain mean arterial pressure at supranormal levels because of inadequate collateral perfusion secondary to the acute arterial obstruction. The risk of vessel rupture or clot propagation is omnipresent.

POSTOPERATIVE MANAGEMENT

Patients undergoing endovascular surgery pass the immediate postoperative period in a monitored setting so they can be watched for signs of hemodynamic instability or neurologic deterioration. Control of blood pressure (e.g., induced hypertension, if indicated) may be necessary during transport and postoperative recovery. In particular, patients who have received treatment of extracranial carotid disease are prone to postprocedural hemodynamic instability, like patients who have undergone carotid endartectomy.[90]

Abrupt restoration of normal systemic pressure to a chronically hypotensive (ischemic) vascular bed may overwhelm autoregulatory capacity and result in hemorrhage or swelling,

this is termed normal perfusion pressure breakthrough.[82,91-94] The pathogenetic mechanism is unclear, but it is probably not simply a hemodynamic effect, and the loss of neurovascular unit integrity is probably related to the pathways involved in post-reperfusion hemorrhage in the setting of acute stroke (described previously).

Nonetheless, cerebral hyperemia is probably exacerbated by uncontrolled increases in systemic arterial blood pressure. In the absence of collateral perfusion pressure inadequacy, fastidious attention to preventing hypertension is warranted. Patients with complicated situations may first be sent for computed tomography or some other kind of tomographic imaging; critical care management may have to be extended during transport and imaging. Symptomatic hyperemic complications are more uncommon than "silent" hyperemic states; with the greater use of more sensitive magnetic resonance imaging, ischemic events are probably more common than previously suspected.[63]

FUTURE DIRECTIONS

For the overall management approach to the patient with cerebrovascular disease, there is accelerating interest in and discussion of the appropriate management of asymptomatic or unruptured lesions. Anesthesiologists are not traditionally caught on the horns of these management dilemmas—at least directly. However, optimal provision of perioperative care and effective resource allocation would benefit from active involvement of all practitioners involved in the management of patients with such conditions.

The indications for invasive therapy for unruptured AVMs[56] and aneurysms[95,96] are currently undergoing critical discussion. Although it is generally agreed that ruptured lesions need treatment, the aggregate risks for treating all patients with unruptured lesions may exceed the potential benefit from protecting against future hemorrhage. For example, the previously described international multicenter randomized controlled trial sponsored by the National Institute of Neurological Disorders and Stroke known as A Randomized Trial of Unruptured Brain Arteriovenous Malformations, will test whether functional outcome and the risk of spontaneous AVM rupture at 5 years for best medical therapy is superior to procedural intervention, whether embolization, microsurgical resection, or radiosurgery.[57] Similarly, the International Study of Unruptured Intracranial Aneurysms (ISUIA) study is a longstanding effort to document the natural history and treatment outcomes for unruptured lesions.[95,97] A randomized controlled study to compare endovascular treatment with conservative management, the Trial of Endovascular Aneurysm Management (TEAM) has also begun.[98]

Future research directions for vascular disease of the brain present opportunities for neuroanesthesia, perioperative management, and neurocritical care. Basic or translational questions include the effect of the interaction of angiogenesis and vascular remodeling on pathogenesis and clinical course. Growing evidence suggests that some of these lesions undergo active angiogenesis and vascular remodeling during the patients' adult life. This new concept—active angiogenesis and vascular remodeling in intracranial vascular malformations—may generate new clinical paradigms in which pharmacologic interventions are proposed to stabilize these abnormal blood vessels and prevent further growth or hemorrhage. Research on intracranial vascular malformations has been focusing on identifying the roles of angiogenic and anti-angiogenic factors in the pathophysiology.[99]

Abnormal vascular remodeling mediated by inflammatory cells has been identified as a key pathologic component of various vascular diseases, including abdominal aortic aneurysms, brain arteriovenous malformations and atherosclerosis.[100-103] This concept may provide a new treatment strategy utilizing agents to inhibit inflammation or cytokines produced by inflammatory cells such as matrix metalloproteinases. On the basis of findings of observational studies that analyzed human intracranial aneurysms and of experimental studies that utilized animal models, an emerging concept suggests that a key component of the pathophysiology of intracranial aneurysms is sustained abnormal vascular remodeling coupled with inflammation.[104-106]

Consistent with a background contribution of a ubiquitous process such as inflammation, aneurysmal disease may be better conceived of as a process, rather than an event. For example, the long-term durability of aneurysm treatment is often assumed. There is growing appreciation that our traditional notion of "disease treatment" should not necessarily be construed as a "cure," although it may be in many cases. Although treatment clearly reduces new rupture rates, there is a measurable rebleeding rate after treatment (surgery or coiling).[1] The risk of further hemorrhage continues for up to 30 years after SAH.[107] The Dutch ASTRA group, reporting on follow-up computed tomography angiography on 610 patients 1 to 15 years after

surgical clipping of ruptured aneurysms, found a 16% incidence of new aneurysms.[108] In 24 patients, aneurysms were present at the site of the previous clipping and in 3 of these, the postoperative angiogram had shown complete aneurysm occlusion. Taken together with observations that a significant fraction of aneurysms enlarge over time,[107-109] this finding indicates that aneurysmal disease may be a process characterized by generalized vascular dysfunction rather than a sporadic focal event.

Pro-inflammatory influence on disease susceptibility[110,111] and clinical course[112-114] appears to apply to AVMs as well. Tissue interleukin-6 (IL-6) expression is associated with IL-6-174G>C genotype and linked to downstream targets involved in angiogenesis and vascular instability.[115] Further, interleukin-6 was found to induce MMP-3 and MMP-9 expression and activity in the mouse brain and to increase proliferation and migration of cerebral endothelial cells. Taken together, such observations are consistent with the hypothesis that inflammatory processes influence angiogenic and proteolytic activity, thus contributing to the pathogenesis of intracranial hemorrhage.

In the future, identification of genetic risk factors has the potential to predict to be developed to help predict new intracranial hemorrhage in the natural course after presentation,[112,113] or used in risk-stratification for postoperative complications.[116] Genetic variation can also potentially provide information related to the risk of development of post–intracranial hemorrhage complications, particularly vasospasm after SAH.[117,118] Genetic variation or plasma biomarker assays.[119-121] have the developmental potential to affect multiple aspects of perioperative management.

Acknowledgments

The authors would like to thank the members of the UCSF Brain AVM Study Project and the Center for Cerebrovascular Research (www.avm.ucsf.edu) for the opportunities to learn more about cerebrovascular disease and anesthetic management; John Pile-Spellman, Lawrence Litt, Tomoki Hashimoto, Chanhung Z. Lee, Michael T. Lawton, Randall T. Higashida, and Van Halbach for their insights and collaboration on efforts to advance knowledge in this area.

REFERENCES

1. Molyneux AJ, Kerr RS, Yu LM, et al: International Subarachnoid Aneurysm Trial (ISAT) of neurosurgical clipping versus endovascular coiling in 2143 patients with ruptured intracranial aneurysms: A randomised comparison of effects on survival, dependency, seizures, rebleeding, subgroups, and aneurysm occlusion, *Lancet* 366:809–817, 2005.
2. Omary RA, Unal O, Koscielski DS, et al: Real-time MR imaging-guided passive catheter tracking with use of gadolinium-filled catheters, *J Vasc Interv Radiol* 11:1079–1085, 2000.
3. Young WL, Pile-Spellman J: Anesthetic considerations for interventional neuroradiology, *Anesthesiology* 80:427–456, 1994.
4. Young WL, Pile-Spellman J, Hacein-Bey L, Joshi S: Invasive neuroradiologic procedures for cerebrovascular abnormalities: Anesthetic considerations, *Anesthesiol Clin N Am* 15:631–653, 1997.
5. Strandgaard S, Olesen J, Skinhoj E, Lassen NA: Autoregulation of brain circulation in severe arterial hypertension, *BMJ* 1(5852):507–510, 1973.
6. Drummond JC: The lower limit of autoregulation: Time to revise our thinking? *Anesthesiology* 86:1431–1433, 1997.
7. Goldberg M: Systemic reactions to intravascular contrast media: A guide for the anesthesiologist, *Anesthesiology* 60:46–56, 1984.
8. Sala F, Beltramello A, Gerosa M: Neuroprotective role of neurophysiological monitoring during endovascular procedures in the brain and spinal cord, *Neurophysiol Clin* 37:415–421, 2007.
9. Drummond JC, Dao AV, Roth DM, et al: Effect of dexmedetomidine on cerebral flow velocity, cerebral metabolic rate, and carbon dioxide response in normal humans, *Anesthesiology* 108:225–232, 2008.

10. Arain SR, Ebert TJ: The efficacy, side effects, and recovery characteristics of dexmedetomidine versus propofol when used for intraoperative sedation, *Anesth Analg* 95:461–466, 2002.

11. Thal GD, Szabo MD, Lopez-Bresnahan M, Crosby G: Exacerbation or unmasking of focal neurologic deficits by sedatives, *Anesthesiology* 85:21–25, 1996.

12. Chollet F, DiPiero V, Wise RJ, et al: The functional anatomy of motor recovery after stroke in humans: A study with positron emission tomography, *Ann Neurol* 29:63–71, 1991.

13. Lazar RM, Fitzsimmons BF, Marshall RS, et al: Reemergence of stroke deficits with midazolam challenge, *Stroke* 33:283–285, 2002.

14. Lazar RM, Fitzsimmons BF, Marshall RS, et al: Midazolam challenge reinduces neurological deficits after transient ischemic attack, *Stroke* 34:794–796, 2003.

15. Harrigan MR, Levy EI, Bendok BR, Hopkins LN: Bivalirudin for endovascular intervention in acute ischemic stroke: Case report, *Neurosurgery* 54:218–222, 2004.

16. Ciccone A, Abraha I, Santilli I: Glycoprotein IIb-IIIa inhibitors for acute ischaemic stroke, *Cochrane Database Syst Rev* (4)2006:CD005208.

17. Hashimoto T, Gupta DK, Young WL: Interventional neuroradiology—anesthetic considerations, *Anesthesiol Clin N Am* 20:347–359, 2002:vi.

18. Fiorella D, Albuquerque FC, Han P, McDougall CG: Strategies for the management of intraprocedural thromboembolic complications with abciximab (ReoPro), *Neurosurgery* 54:1089–1097, 2004.

19. Szabo MD, Crosby G, Sundaram P, et al: Hypertension does not cause spontaneous hemorrhage of intracranial arteriovenous malformations, *Anesthesiology* 70:761–763, 1989.

20. Hashimoto T, Young WL, Aagaard BD, et al: Adenosine-induced ventricular asystole to induce transient profound systemic hypotension in patients undergoing endovascular therapy: Dose-response characteristics, *Anesthesiology* 93:998–1001, 2000.

21. Connolly ES Jr, Lavine SD, Meyers PM, et al: Intensive care unit management of interventional neuroradiology patients, *Neurosurg Clin N Am* 16:541–545, 2005:vi.

22. Molyneux A, Kerr R, Stratton I, et al: International Subarachnoid Aneurysm Trial (ISAT) of neurosurgical clipping versus endovascular coiling in 2143 patients with ruptured intracranial aneurysms: A randomised trial, *Lancet* 360:1267–1274, 2002.

23. Drummond JC, Patel PM: Neurosurgical anesthesia. In Miller RD, editor: *Anesthesia*, vol 2, ed 5, New York, 2000, Churchill Livingstone, pp 1895–1933.

24. Elijovich L, Higashida RT, Lawton MT, et al: Predictors and outcomes of intraprocedural rupture in patients treated for ruptured intracranial aneurysms: The CARAT study, *Stroke* 39:1501–1506, 2008.

25. Newell DW, Eskridge JM, Mayberg MR, et al: Angioplasty for the treatment of symptomatic vasospasm following subarachnoid hemorrhage, *J Neurosurg* 71:654–660, 1989.

26. Zwienenberg-Lee M, Hartman J, Rudisill N, et al: Effect of prophylactic transluminal balloon angioplasty on cerebral vasospasm and outcome in patients with Fisher grade III subarachnoid hemorrhage: Results of a phase II multicenter, randomized, clinical trial, *Stroke* 39:1759–1765, 2008.

27. Smith WS, Dowd CF, Johnston SC, et al: Neurotoxicity of intra-arterial papaverine preserved with chlorobutanol used for the treatment of cerebral vasospasm after aneurysmal subarachnoid hemorrhage, *Stroke* 35:2518–2522, 2004.

28. Fogarty-Mack P, Pile-Spellman J, Hacein-Bey L, et al: Superselective intra-arterial papaverine administration: Effect on regional cerebral blood flow in patients with arteriovenous malformations, *J Neurosurg* 85:395–402, 1996.

29. Feng L, Fitzsimmons BF, Young WL: Intra-arterially administered verapamil as adjunct therapy for cerebral vasospasm: Safety and 2-year experience, *AJNR Am J Neuroradiol* 23:1284–1290, 2002.

30. Tejada JG, Taylor RA, Ugurel MS, et al: Safety and feasibility of intra-arterial nicardipine for the treatment of subarachnoid hemorrhage–associated vasospasm: Initial clinical experience with high-dose infusions, *AJNR Am J Neuroradiol* 28:844–848, 2007.

31. Avitsian R, Fiorella D, Soliman MM, Mascha E: Anesthetic considerations of selective intra-arterial nicardipine injection for intracranial vasospasm: A case series, *J Neurosurg Anesthesiol* 19:125–129, 2007.

32. Badjatia N, Topcuoglu MA, Pryor JC, et al: Preliminary experience with intra-arterial nicardipine as a treatment for cerebral vasospasm, *AJNR Am J Neuroradiol* 25:819–826, 2004.

33. Mazumdar A, Rivet DJ, Derdeyn CP, et al: Effect of intra-arterial verapamil on the diameter of vasospastic intracranial arteries in patients with cerebral vasospasm, *Neurosurg Focus* 21:E15, 2006.

34. Biondi A, Ricciardi GK, Puybasset L, et al: Intra-arterial nimodipine for the treatment of symptomatic cerebral vasospasm after aneurysmal subarachnoid hemorrhage: Preliminary results, *AJNR Am J Neuroradiol* 25:1067–1076, 2004.

35. Hui C, Lau KP: Efficacy of intra-arterial nimodipine in the treatment of cerebral vasospasm complicating subarachnoid haemorrhage, *Clin Radiol* 60:1030–1036, 2005.

36. Stiefel MF, Heuer GG, Abrahams JM, et al: The effect of nimodipine on cerebral oxygenation in patients with poor-grade subarachnoid hemorrhage, *J Neurosurg* 101:594–599, 2004.

37. Devlin JW, Coplin WM, Murry KR, et al: Nimodipine-induced acute hypoxemia: Case report, *Neurosurgery* 47:1243–1246, 2000.

38. Westhout FD, Nwagwu CI: Intra-arterial verapamil-induced seizures: Case report and review of the literature, *Surg Neurol* 67:483–486, 2007.

39. Tebbutt S, Harvey M, Nicholson T, Cave G: Intralipid prolongs survival in a rat model of verapamil toxicity, *Acad Emerg Med* 13:134–139, 2006.

40. Bania TC, Chu J, Perez E, et al: Hemodynamic effects of intravenous fat emulsion in an animal model of severe verapamil toxicity resuscitated with atropine, calcium, and saline, *Acad Emerg Med* 14:105–111, 2007.

41. Gueret G, Pennec JP, Arvieux CC: Hemodynamic effects of intralipid after verapamil intoxication may be due to a direct effect of fatty acids on myocardial calcium channels, *Acad Emerg Med* 14:761, 2007.

42. Romero CM, Morales D, Reccius A, et al: Milrinone as a rescue therapy for symptomatic refractory cerebral vasospasm in aneurysmal subarachnoid hemorrhage, *Neurocrit Care* 11:165–171,2009.

43. Fraticelli AT, Cholley BP, Losser MR, Maurice JP, Payen D: Milrinone for the treatment of cerebral vasospasm after aneurysmal subarachnoid hemorrhage, *Stroke* 39:893–898, 2008.

44. Arakawa Y, Kikuta K, Hojo M, et al: Milrinone for the treatment of cerebral vasospasm after subarachnoid hemorrhage: Report of seven cases, *Neurosurgery* 48:723–728, 2001.

45. Trimble JL, Kockler DR: Statin treatment of cerebral vasospasm after aneurysmal subarachnoid hemorrhage, *Ann Pharmacother* 41:2019–2023, 2007.

46. Tseng MY, Hutchinson PJ, Czosnyka M, et al: Effects of acute pravastatin treatment on intensity of rescue therapy, length of inpatient stay, and 6-month outcome in patients after aneurysmal subarachnoid hemorrhage, *Stroke* 38:1545–1550, 2007.

47. Tseng MY, Hutchinson PJ, Turner CL, et al: Biological effects of acute pravastatin treatment in patients after aneurysmal subarachnoid hemorrhage: A double-blind, placebo-controlled trial, *J Neurosurg* 107:1092–1100, 2007.

48. Lynch JR, Wang H, McGirt MJ, et al: Simvastatin reduces vasospasm after aneurysmal subarachnoid hemorrhage: Results of a pilot randomized clinical trial, *Stroke* 36:2024–2026, 2005.

49. Sayama CM, Liu JK, Couldwell WT: Update on endovascular therapies for cerebral vasospasm induced by aneurysmal subarachnoid hemorrhage, *Neurosurg Focus* 21:E12, 2006.

50. Joshi S, Emala CW, Pile-Spellman J: Intra-arterial drug delivery: A concise review, *J Neurosurg Anesthesiol* 19:111–119, 2007.

51. Marshall RS, Lazar RM, Pile-Spellman J, et al: Recovery of brain function during induced cerebral hypoperfusion, *Brain* 124:1208–1217, 2001.

52. Stapf C, Mast H, Sciacca RR, et al: Predictors of hemorrhage in patients with untreated brain arteriovenous malformation, *Neurology* 66:1350–1355, 2006.

53. Kim H, Sidney S, McCulloch CE, et al: Racial/ethnic differences in longitudinal risk of intracranial hemorrhage in brain arteriovenous malformation patients, *Stroke* 38:2430–2437, 2007.

54. Wedderburn CJ, van Beijnum J, Bhattacharya JJ, et al: Outcome after interventional or conservative management of unruptured brain arteriovenous malformations: A prospective, population-based cohort study, *Lancet Neurol* 7:223–230, 2008.

55. Lawton MT, Du R, Tran M, et al: Effect of presenting hemorrhage on outcome after microsurgical resection of brain arteriovenous malformations, *Neurosurgery* 56:485–493, 2005.

56. Stapf C, Mohr JP, Choi JH, et al: Invasive treatment of unruptured brain arteriovenous malformations is experimental therapy, *Curr Opin Neurol* 19:63–68, 2006.

57. National Institute of Neurological Disorders and Stroke (NINDS): A Randomized Trial of Unruptured Brain AVMs (ARUBA), 2007. Information available at http://clinicaltrials.gov/ct2/show/NCT00389181?term=brain+malformation&rank=6.

58. Gao E, Young WL, Pile-Spellman J, et al: Deliberate systemic hypotension to facilitate endovascular therapy of cerebral arteriovenous malformations: a computer modeling study, *Neurosurg Focus* 2:e3, 1997.

59. van Rooij WJ, Sluzewski M, Beute GN: Brain AVM embolization with Onyx, *AJNR Am J Neuroradiol* 28:172–177, 2007.

60. Linfante I, Wakhloo AK: Brain aneurysms and arteriovenous malformations: Advancements and emerging treatments in endovascular embolization, *Stroke* 38:1411–1417, 2007.

61. Murugesan C, Saravanan S, Rajkumar J, et al: Severe pulmonary oedema following therapeutic embolization with Onyx for cerebral arteriovenous malformation, *Neuroradiology* 50:439–442, 2008.

62. Yakes WF, Rossi P, Odink H: How I do it: Arteriovenous malformation management, *Cardiovasc Intervent Radiol* 19:65–71, 1996.

63. Cronqvist M, Wirestam R, Ramgren B, et al: Endovascular treatment of intracerebral arteriovenous malformations: Procedural safety, complications, and results evaluated by MR imaging, including diffusion and perfusion imaging, *AJNR Am J Neuroradiol* 27:162–176, 2006.

64. Lazar RM, Marshall RS, Pile-Spellman J, et al: Interhemispheric transfer of language in patients with left frontal cerebral arteriovenous malformation, *Neuropsychologia* 38:1325–1332, 2000.

65. Lazar RM, Marshall RS, Pile-Spellman J, et al: Anterior translocation of language in patients with left cerebral arteriovenous malformations, *Neurology* 49:802–808, 1997.

66. Lazar RM, Connaire K, Marshall RS, et al: Developmental deficits in adult patients with arteriovenous malformations, *Arch Neurol* 56:103–106, 1999.

67. Henkes H, Gotwald TF, Brew S, et al: Intravascular pressure measurements in feeding pedicles of brain arteriovenous malformations, *Neuroradiology* 48:182–189, 2006.

68. Duong DH, Young WL, Vang MC, et al: Feeding artery pressure and venous drainage pattern are primary determinants of hemorrhage from cerebral arteriovenous malformations, *Stroke* 29:1167–1176, 1998.

69. Todaka T, Hamada J, Kai Y, et al: Analysis of mean transit time of contrast medium in ruptured and unruptured arteriovenous malformations: A digital subtraction angiographic study, *Stroke* 34:2410–2414, 2003.

70. Norris JS, Valiante TA, Wallace MC, et al: A simple relationship between radiological arteriovenous malformation hemodynamics and clinical presentation: A prospective, blinded analysis of 31 cases, *J Neurosurg* 90:673–679, 1999.

71. Zhu Y, Lawton MT, Du R, et al: Expression of hypoxia-inducible factor-1 and vascular endothelial growth factor in response to venous hypertension, *Neurosurgery* 59:687–696, 2006.

72. Lawton MT, Jacobowitz R, Spetzler RF: Redefined role of angiogenesis in the pathogenesis of dural arteriovenous malformations, *J Neurosurg* 87:267–274, 1997.

73. Terada T, Higashida RT, Halbach VV, et al: Development of acquired arteriovenous fistulas in rats due to venous hypertension, *J Neurosurg* 80:884–889, 1994.

74. Lv X, Li Y, Lv M, et al: Trigeminocardiac reflex in embolization of intracranial dural arteriovenous fistula, *AJNR Am J Neuroradiol* 28:1769–1770, 2007.

75. Fullerton HJ, Aminoff AR, Ferriero DM, et al: Neurodevelopmental outcome after endovascular treatment of vein of Galen malformations, *Neurology* 61:1386–1390, 2003.

76. Lasjaunias PL, Chng SM, Sachet M, et al: The management of vein of Galen aneurysmal malformations, *Neurosurgery* 59:S184–S194, 2006:discussion S183–S113.

77. Lasjaunias P, Berenstein A: Endovascular treatment of the craniofacial lesions, In: Golzarian J, Sun S, and Sharafuddin MJ, editors: *Surgical Neuroangiography*, vol 2, Heidelberg, 1987, Springer-Verlag, pp 389–397.

78. Higashida RT, Meyers PM, Connors JJ 3rd, et al; American Society of Interventional and Therapeutic Neuroradiology; Society of Interventional Radiology; American Society of Neuroradiology: Intracranial angioplasty & stenting for cerebral atherosclerosis: A position statement of the American Society of Interventional and Therapeutic Neuroradiology, Society of Interventional Radiology, and the American Society of Neuroradiology, *AJNR Am J Neuroradiol* 26:2323–2327, 2005.

79. Goodney PP, Schermerhorn ML, Powell RJ: Current status of carotid artery stenting, *J Vasc Surg* 43:406–411, 2006.

80. Yadav JS, Wholey MH, Kuntz RE, et al; Stenting and Angioplasty with Protection in Patients at High Risk for Endarterectomy Investigators: Protected carotid-artery stenting versus endarterectomy in high-risk patients, *N Engl J Med* 351:1493–1501, 2004.

81. Mas JL, Chatellier G, Beyssen B, et al; EVA-3S Investigators: Endarterectomy versus stenting in patients with symptomatic severe carotid stenosis, *N Engl J Med* 355:1660–1671, 2006.

82. Meyers PM, Higashida RT, Phatouros CC, et al: Cerebral hyperperfusion syndrome after percutaneous transluminal stenting of the craniocervical arteries, *Neurosurgery* 47:335–343, 2000.

83. Furlan A, Higashida R, Wechsler L, et al: Intra-arterial prourokinase for acute ischemic stroke: The PROACT II study: A randomized controlled trial. Prolyse in Acute Cerebral Thromboembolism, *JAMA* 282:2003–2011, 1999.

84. Smith WS: Safety of mechanical thrombectomy and intravenous tissue plasminogen activator in acute ischemic stroke. Results of the multi Mechanical Embolus Removal in Cerebral Ischemia (MERCI) trial, part I, *AJNR Am J Neuroradiol* 27:1177–1182, 2006.

85. Smith WS, Sung G, Starkman S, et al: MERCI Trial Investigators: Safety and efficacy of mechanical embolectomy in acute ischemic stroke: Results of the MERCI trial, *Stroke* 36:1432–1438, 2005.

86. Wang X, Lee SR, Arai K, et al: Lipoprotein receptor-mediated induction of matrix metalloproteinase by tissue plasminogen activator, *Nat Med* 9:1313–1317, 2003.

87. Tsuji K, Aoki T, Tejima E, et al: Tissue plasminogen activator promotes matrix metalloproteinase-9 upregulation after focal cerebral ischemia, *Stroke* 36:1954–1959, 2005.

88. Horstmann S, Kalb P, Koziol J, et al: Profiles of matrix metalloproteinases, their inhibitors, and laminin in stroke patients: Influence of different therapies, *Stroke* 34:2165–2170, 2003.

89. Lee CZ, Litt L, Hashimoto T, Young WL: Physiological monitoring and anesthesia considerations of the acute ischemic stroke patient, *J Vasc Interv Radiol* 15:S13–S19, 2004.

90. Qureshi AI, Luft AR, Sharma M, et al: Frequency and determinants of postprocedural hemodynamic instability after carotid angioplasty and stenting, *Stroke* 30:2086–2093, 1999.

91. Young WL, Kader A, Ornstein E, et al: Cerebral hyperemia after arteriovenous malformation resection is related to "breakthrough" complications but not to feeding artery pressure. Columbia University AVM Study Project, *Neurosurgery* 38:1085–1093, 1996.

92. Abou-Chebl A, Yadav JS, Reginelli JP, et al: Intracranial hemorrhage and hyperperfusion syndrome following carotid artery stenting: Risk factors, prevention, and treatment, *J Am Coll Cardiol* 43:1596–1601, 2004.

93. Abou-Chebl A, Reginelli J, Bajzer CT, Yadav JS: Intensive treatment of hypertension decreases the risk of hyperperfusion and intracerebral hemorrhage following carotid artery stenting, *Catheter Cardiovasc Interv* 69:690–696, 2007.

94. Kang HS, Han MH, Kwon OK, et al: Intracranial hemorrhage after carotid angioplasty: A pooled analysis, *J Endovasc Ther* 14:77–85, 2007.

95. Wiebers DO, Whisnant JP, Huston J 3rd, et al: Unruptured intracranial aneurysms: Natural history, clinical outcome, and risks of surgical and endovascular treatment, *Lancet* 362:103–110, 2003.

96. Wiebers DO: Patients with small, asymptomatic, unruptured intracranial aneurysms and no history of subarachnoid hemorrhage should generally be treated conservatively, *Stroke* 36:408–409, 2005.

97. Unruptured intracranial aneurysms—risk of rupture and risks of surgical intervention: International Study of Unruptured Intracranial Aneurysms Investigators, *N Engl J Med* 339:1725–1733, 1998.

98. Raymond J, Meder JF, Molyneux AJ, et al: Trial on endovascular treatment of unruptured aneurysms (TEAM): Study monitoring and rationale for trial interruption or continuation, *J Neuroradiol* 34:33–41, 2007.

99. Hashimoto T, Young WL: Roles of angiogenesis and vascular remodeling in brain vascular malformations, *Semin Cerebrovasc Dis Stroke* 4:217–225, 2004.

100. Hashimoto T, Wen G, Lawton MT, et al: Abnormal expression of matrix metalloproteinases and tissue inhibitors of metalloproteinases in brain arteriovenous malformations, *Stroke* 34:925–931, 2003.

101. Knox JB, Sukhova GK, Whittemore AD, Libby P: Evidence for altered balance between matrix metalloproteinases and their inhibitors in human aortic diseases, *Circulation* 95:205–212, 1997.

102. Goodall S, Crowther M, Hemingway DM, et al: Ubiquitous elevation of matrix metalloproteinase-2 expression in the vasculature of patients with abdominal aneurysms, *Circulation* 104:304–309, 2001.

103. Loftus IM, Naylor AR, Goodall S, et al: Increased matrix metalloproteinase-9 activity in unstable carotid plaques: A potential role in acute plaque disruption, *Stroke* 31:40–47, 2000.

104. Chyatte D, Bruno G, Desai S, Todor DR: Inflammation and intracranial aneurysms, *Neurosurgery* 45:1137–1146, 1999.

105. Frosen J, Piippo A, Paetau A, et al: Remodeling of saccular cerebral artery aneurysm wall is associated with rupture: Histological analysis of 24 unruptured and 42 ruptured cases, *Stroke* 35:2287–2293, 2004.

106. Hashimoto T, Meng H, Young WL: Intracranial aneurysms: Links between inflammation, hemodynamics and vascular remodeling, *Neurol Res* 28:372–380, 2006.

107. Juvela S, Porras M, Poussa K: Natural history of unruptured intracranial aneurysms: probability of and risk factors for aneurysm rupture, *J Neurosurg* 93:379–387, 2000.

108. Wermer MJ, van der Schaaf IC, Velthuis BK, et al; ASTRA Study Group. et al: Follow-up screening after subarachnoid haemorrhage: Frequency and determinants of new aneurysms and enlargement of existing aneurysms, *Brain* 128:2421–2429, 2005.

109. Mangrum WI, Huston J 3rd, Link MJ, et al: Enlarging vertebrobasilar nonsaccular intracranial aneurysms: Frequency, predictors, and clinical outcome of growth, *J Neurosurg* 102:72–79, 2005.

110. Simon M, Franke D, Ludwig M, et al: Association of a polymorphism of the ACVRL1 gene with sporadic arteriovenous malformations of the central nervous system, *J Neurosurg* 104:945–949, 2006.

111. Pawlikowska L, Tran MN, Achrol AS, et al: Polymorphisms in transforming growth factor-ß–related genes *ALK1* and *ENG* are associated with sporadic brain arteriovenous malformations, *Stroke* 36:2278–2280, 2005.

112. Achrol AS, Pawlikowska L, McCulloch CE, et al: Tumor necrosis factor-alpha-238G>A promoter polymorphism is associated with increased risk of new hemorrhage in the natural course of patients with brain arteriovenous malformations, *Stroke* 37:231–234, 2006.

113. Pawlikowska L, Poon KY, Achrol AS, et al: Apoliprotein E epsilon2 is associated with new hemorrhage risk in brain arteriovenous malformation, *Neurosurgery* 58:838–843, 2006.

114. Kim H, Hysi PG, Pawlikowska L, et al: Common variants in interleukin-1-beta gene are associated with intracranial hemorrhage and susceptibility to brain arteriovenous malformation, *Cerebrovasc Dis* 27:176–182, 2009.

115. Chen Y, Pawlikowska L, Yao JS, et al: Interleukin-6 involvement in brain arteriovenous malformations, *Ann Neurol* 59:72–80, 2006.

116. Achrol AS, Kim H, Pawlikowska L, et al: TNF-alpha polymorphism is associated with intracranial hemorrhage (ICH) after arteriovenous malformation (AVM) treatment [abstract], *Stroke* 38:597–598, 2007.

117. Starke RM, Kim GH, Komotar RJ, et al: Endothelial nitric oxide synthase gene single-nucleotide polymorphism predicts cerebral vasospasm after aneurysmal subarachnoid hemorrhage, *J Cereb Blood Flow Metab* 28:1204–1211, 2008.

118. Ko NU, Rajendran P, Kim H, et al: Endothelial nitric oxide synthase polymorphism (-786T→C) and increased risk of angiographic vasospasm after aneurysmal subarachnoid hemorrhage, *Stroke* 39:1103–1108, 2008.

119. Sanchez-Peña P, Pereira AR, Sourour NA, et al: S100B as an additional prognostic marker in subarachnoid aneurysmal hemorrhage, *Crit Care Med* 36:2267–2273, 2008.

120. Castellanos M, Leira R, Serena J, et al: Plasma metalloproteinase-9 concentration predicts hemorrhagic transformation in acute ischemic stroke, *Stroke* 34:40–46, 2003.

121. Tung PP, Olmsted EA, Kopelnik A, et al: Plasma B-type natriuretic peptide levels are associated with early cardiac dysfunction after subarachnoid hemorrhage, *Stroke* 36:1567–1569, 2005.

Chapter 15

ANESTHETIC CONSIDERATIONS FOR SURGICAL RESECTION OF BRAIN ARTERIOVENOUS MALFORMATIONS

William L. Young • Pekka Talke • Michael T. Lawton

Surgical management of brain arteriovenous malformations (AVMs) is one of the most challenging in neurosurgery and, despite the relative rarity of the disease, the subject of a disproportionately large portion of the literature on surgical cerebrovascular disease. Perioperative and anesthetic management is optimal when the anesthetist has familiarity with the strategic goals of therapy and some familiarity with AVM pathophysiology. This chapter summarizes these topics and discusses specific neuroanesthetic issues regarding care of these patients. Although the fundamentals of providing perioperative care are similar to those for patients with other neurovascular conditions, there are some important considerations unique to AVMs.

CLINICAL BEHAVIOR

Brain AVMs are a relatively uncommon but important source of neurologic morbidity in young adults.[1] The basic morphology is of a vascular mass, called the *nidus*, that directly shunts blood between the arterial and venous circulations without a true capillary bed. Hemodynamic alterations include variable degrees of high flow through the feeding arteries, nidus, and draining veins as well as venous hypertension.[2] The nidus is a complex tangle of abnormal, dilated channels, not clearly artery or vein, with intervening gliosis.

AVMs may exert a deleterious effect on brain function through several mechanisms, including mass effects (e.g., hematoma, edema, or gradually expanding abnormal vascular structures such as venous aneurysms), metabolic depression (diaschisis), and seizure activity. The most common presentation and source of morbidity, however, is spontaneous intracranial hemorrhage (ICH), which occurs in about one half of all patients with AVMs.

The risk of spontaneous ICH without treatment is commonly estimated to be approximately 2% to 4% per year for all patients,[3] but the rate varies widely, depending on what ICH risk factors are present. The best-studied risk factors are a presentation with ICH, deep location, and venous drainage pattern.[4,5] Factors such as small size of lesion and advanced age are less robust; others, such as aneurysms, are harder to define accurately.[6] High intranidal pressure, as measured with direct puncture of feeding arteries or during superselective angiography, is associated with hemorrhage presentation.[7]

Clinical presentation with ICH appears to be the strongest risk factor for *future hemorrhage*.[5] There are a number of reports concerning other risk factors,[1,8-14] but few that have prospectively assessed future hemorrhage risk.[4,5,15-18] As mentioned, the risk of spontaneous ICH has been estimated in retrospective and prospective observational studies to range from 2% to 4% per year (see Kim and associates[5]). However, depending on a number of risk factors, the range of yearly bleeding risk varies widely, estimated to range from less than 1% to more than 30% per year.[4]

Approximately 10% of patients with AVMs also have intracranial aneurysms. One should note, however, that the converse is not true; the detection rate of AVMs in patients with aneurysms is closer to the detection rate of AVMs in the general population. Intracerebral hemorrhage from aneurysms is usually associated with subarachnoid hemorrhage, whereas AVMs more commonly bleed into the ventricle or into parenchyma. This difference probably accounts for the uncommon occurrence of vasospasm in patients with AVMs. Spontaneous hemorrhage during the perioperative period as a result of variations in systemic blood pressure is probably less likely as well, owing to a "buffering" effect of the fistula on changes in systemic pressure.[19]

The morbidity of spontaneous AVM hemorrhage is controversial,[20,21] but estimates run from very low to as high as 25% to 50%.[21-31] The latest prospective' longitudinal study data suggest that earlier estimates may be overestimates and that hemorrhage, either at initial presentation or during follow-up of untreated patients with AVM, appears to carry a lower morbidity than ICH from other causes.[32]

Consistent with the risk factors described previously, the primary reason to treat a patient with an AVM is to protect against future spontaneous ICH, although more rarely, treatment may be undertaken for control of progressive neurologic deficits or intractable seizures. Lacking any specific medical therapies for this purpose, treatment options are currently limited to some kind of surgical ablation (i.e., resection or radiotherapy). There are three modes for treatment of AVMs: endovascular embolization, radiosurgery, and microsurgical excision. Treatment strategies, especially for complex lesions, frequently involve more than one modality. In general, endovascular therapy is performed as a preparatory adjunct to surgery. Through the use of various glues or other embolic materials, the blood supply to the nidus can be reduced, most commonly in several stages. This reduction has the theoretical advantage of allowing surrounding brain regions to adapt to the circulatory changes. As a preoperative adjunct, embolization is thought to facilitate operative removal of an AVM with less bleeding and seems to be associated with better surgical

264

outcome. Embolization can also eliminate deep vascular pedicles that might be difficult to control surgically.

The risks of invasive therapy can be estimated with scales adapted for different treatment modalities, most importantly for surgery and radiotherapy.[33,34] Neurosurgeons are confident in their recommendations for microsurgical resection with most low-grade AVMs (Spetzler-Martin grades I to III), on the basis of numerous reports detailing excellent results.[35] However, all treatment modalities—endovascular therapy, surgery, and radiosurgical therapy—continue to be reported as carrying a substantial risk of disability.[21,36-40]

For example, a meta-analysis from 25 sources of 2425 patients who were undergoing invasive treatment[39] described an aggregate mortality of 3.3% and permanent morbidity of 8.6%, ranging from 1.5% to 18.7%.[39] Protection from spontaneous ICH by partial, noncurative endovascular embolization therapy has been suggested[41] but does not have rigorous support.[17,42] Presurgical embolization, thought to enhance safety of surgical resection, has its own inherent morbidity, varying from 4% to 9%.[39,43] A multicenter overview of endovascular AVM therapy (commissioned by the 2005 World Federation of Interventional and Therapeutic Neuroradiology meeting) revealed stable frequencies of self-reported treatment-related complications in numerous well-established international centers usually in the range of 9% to 12%[44-50] but as high as 22%.[51]

It is worthwhile noting that those risk factors that raise the risk associated with leaving the lesion untreated (i.e., increase the risk of spontaneous hemorrhage) do overlap with those characteristics that increase risk of surgical intervention, but they are not the same. The most widely used surgical risk score is the Spetzler-Martin scheme.[52] Any deep venous drainage increases surgical risk, but only exclusively deep venous drainage appears to influence rupture risk.[10] Larger size is an important component of greater surgical risk[53] but does not affect natural history risk or may even represent a protective effect owing to low intranidal pressure with high-flow lesions. Eloquence, an important attribute of where the AVM is located, strongly influences surgical risk, but it has no effect on natural history risk. The point here is that in a discussion of "high-risk lesions," it is important to specify whether one is talking about natural history or treatment risk.

Radiosurgical treatment offers a means to treat surgically inaccessible lesions and appears to be useful for smaller lesions. It is less efficacious for lesions more than 2 to 3 cm in largest dimension.[54-57] Further, patients who have undergone radiosurgical treatment are still exposed to the risk of new bleeding until the AVM is obliterated, usually after a course of 2 to 3 years, termed the *latency period*.[1] During the latency period, risk for ICH may decrease in patients who presented with hemorrhage, but not in those with unruptured AVMs at presentation.[58] The frequency of neurologic complications from radiotherapy of brain AVMs is generally similar to the complication rate from surgical and endovascular treatment. The investigators in the Randomized Trial of Unruptured Brain AVMs[59] performed a systematic review of the literature from 1990 or later of prospective studies with at least 30 patients, which yielded 16 studies on 3854 patients undergoing radiosurgery and a mean rate of treatment-related permanent neurologic deficits in the range of 6% to 7%; obliteration rates, completeness of removal, and type of follow-up varied greatly.

The most controversial aspect of treatment is offering potentially high-risk invasive therapy to patients whose lesions have not yet ruptured. Patients with unruptured lesions are at highest risk for postoperative deficits.[53] The presenting hemorrhage may, in effect, perform some of the dissection, in that the hemorrhage cavity is an attractive approach to the lesion. Further, patients who are recovering from a hemorrhage-induced deficit may not have reached the final level of spontaneous recovery, which may continue into the postoperative period, thus masking operative injury. One of the major developments in the field has been the start of the Randomized Trial of Unruptured Brain AVMs,[60] an international randomized controlled trial to test whether best medical therapy or procedural intervention results in superior outcomes.

ETIOLOGY AND PATHOGENESIS

The genesis of AVMs has been enigmatic. Unlike the association of antecedent head trauma or other injuries with the pathogenesis of dural arteriovenous fistulas, environmental risk factors for AVMs are lacking. There is remarkably little evidence for the common assertion that AVMs are congenital lesions that result from embryonic maldevelopment during the fourth to eighth week, if one considers the high utilization of prenatal ultrasonography (vein of Galen lesions are not true AVMs). Further, there have been multiple reports of AVMs that grow or regress, including de novo AVM formation (see Du and colleagues[61]). Inciting events might include the sequelae of even relatively modest injury from an otherwise unremarkable episode of trauma, infection, inflammation, irradiation, compression, or some underlying structural defect.[62] In susceptible individuals, one might posit some degree of localized venous hypertension[63] from microvascular thrombosis, perhaps associated with a state of relative thrombophilia.[64] All of these events may synergize and involve some underlying development defect that otherwise does not come to clinical attention. The scarce data available on longitudinal assessment of AVM growth suggest that approximately 50% of cases of AVMs display interval growth.[65] Consistent with growth is the finding of a many-fold higher endothelial proliferation rate (through immunohistochemical methods for Ki-67 antigen) in AVM surgical specimens than in control brain tissue.[65]

Available evidence points toward an active angiogenic and inflammatory lesional phenotype rather than a static congenital anomaly. A host of abnormal signals is present in the lesional tissue.[66,67] A prominent feature of the AVM phenotype is relative overexpression of vascular endothelial growth factor-A (VEGF-A) at both the messenger RNA and protein levels. Extrapolation from animals indicates that VEGF may contribute to the hemorrhagic tendency of AVMs.[68] Other upstream factors that may contribute to AVM formation are homeobox genes, such as excess proangiogenic Hox D3 and deficient antiangiogenic Hox A5.[69] The vascular phenotype of AVM tissue may be explained, in part, by inadequate recruitment of peri-endothelial support structure, which is mediated by angiopoietins and Tie-2 (tyrosine kinase with immunoglobulin and EGF homology domains 2) signaling. For example, angiopoietin-2 (Ang-2), which allows loosening of cell-to-cell contacts, is overexpressed in the perivascular region in AVM vascular channels.[70]

Vascular remodeling is facilitated by proteases and is necessary to form the enlarged vascular elements in the nidus of an AVM. A key downstream consequence of VEGF and other angiogenic activity is matrix metalloproteinase (MMP) expression. MMP-9 is of particular interest and has been found in AVMs at levels that are orders of magnitude higher than in control tissue.[71,72] Inflammatory markers that are overexpressed include myeloperoxidase and interleukin-6,[73] as well as higher immunoglobulin levels that control the brain, perhaps suggesting lymphocytic contributions.[74]

Brain AVMs are usually sporadic but sometimes familial.[75] The most promising candidate genes and pathways for brain AVM pathogenesis relate to hereditary hemorrhagic telangiectasia (HHT), an autosomal dominant disorder of mucocutaneous fragility and AVMs in various organs including the brain. There are now at least five genes associated with HHT,[76-78] but the two main subtypes of HHT (HHT1 and HHT2) are caused by loss-of-function mutations in two genes originally implicated in transforming growth factor-β (TGF–β) signaling pathways (Fig. 15-1).[79] The first is endoglin (ENG), which codes for an accessory protein of TGF-β receptor complexes. The second is activin-like kinase 1 (ALK1, or ACVLR1), which codes for a transmembrane kinase also thought to participate in TGF-β signaling. Data now suggest that ALK1 may also signal through bone morphogenetic protein-9 and that endoglin can potentiate the signal.[80,81]

As a class, the inherited AVMs in HHT have some distinguishing morphologic features, such as smaller size, multiplicity, and more superficial location, but are generally similar to the sporadic lesions and cannot be distinguished individually on the basis of their angioarchitecture.[82,83] Together, about 10% of patients with HHT1 or HHT2 display brain AVMs. This 10% figure is some 1000 times higher than the prevalence for brain AVMs in the normal population (about 10/100,000 or 0.01%).[84] Therefore, one could view frank mutations in ALK1 and ENG as "hyper-risk" factors for the brain AVM phenotype.

Such greatly elevated risk of brain AVM development in the mendelian disorders raises the possibility that germline *sequence variants* of these and other genes may likewise pose a significant risk for *sporadic* development of brain AVM. An intronic single-nucleotide polymorphism in *ALK1* has been associated with twofold higher risk of the development of sporadic brain AVM,[85] a finding replicated in an independent cohort.[86,87] This polymorphism probably causes in-frame exon skipping and may result in an ALK1 protein variant that lacks a transmembrane domain. An intriguing but unproven mechanism would be excess soluble receptor in the extracellular matrix that binds ligand and prevents it from signaling normally.

It is highly unlikely that a single polymorphic gene is responsible for AVM formation. Rather, it is mostly likely some combination of (1) an inciting event or developmental defect, (2) some genetic alteration in either ALK1 or ENG signaling or a closely related pathway, and (3) a set of modifier genes or conditions. For example, multiple genetic loci appear to control VEGF-induced angiogenesis.[88,89] Such a "conspiracy" of factors is suggested by the observations that endoglin-deficient mice spontaneously form vascular dysplasia[90] and that the response can be amplified with viral transduction to overexpress VEGF in the mouse brain.[91]

CEREBRAL CIRCULATORY CHANGES IN PATIENTS WITH ARTERIOVENOUS MALFORMATIONS

There are two primary characteristics of the cerebral circulatory changes brought about by AVMs. Rapid shunt flow results in a higher total amount of bulk through the AVMs. This increased flow results in cerebral arterial hypotension along the path of the shunt. Patients with AVMs have a progressive decrease in arterial pressure that proceeds from the circle of Willis to the AVM nidus (Fig. 15-2).[92] The corollary of this observation is that circulatory beds in parallel with the shunt system will be perfused at lower-than-normal pressures even if flow remains relatively normal.

In patients with large, high-flow AVMs, there may be normal brain regions in which cerebral arterial hypotension is below the range of normal autoregulation. Despite significant cerebral arterial hypotension, a majority of patients are free from ischemic symptoms. Hypotensive normal brain regions can be demonstrated to have normal rates of tissue perfusion, implying some adaptive change in total cerebrovascular resistance.

This phenomenon may be explained by "adaptive autoregulatory displacement."[93] In vascular territories adjacent to AVMs, the lower limit of the autoregulation curve appears to be shifted to the left, which is opposite to the effect of chronic systemic (essential) arterial hypertension on the cerebral autoregulation curve.[94] This adaptive shift to the left places the lower limit at a level considerably lower than the lower limit postulated for the normal brain (50 or 60 mm Hg).[95,96] Therefore, the presence of chronic hypotension does not necessarily result in vasoparalysis in the arteriolar resistance bed. There is generally a preserved responsiveness to CO_2 before and after surgical resection, which lends further support to the notion of intact autoregulatory capacity.[94]

Historically, it has been believed that it is not the AVM itself but rather decreased perfusion pressure in adjacent, functional tissue that is responsible for both pretreatment *ischemic* and

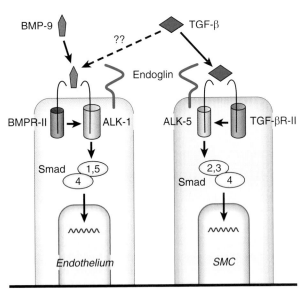

Figure 15–1 Transforming growth factor-β (TGF-β) superfamily signaling may be an important aspect of sporadic arteriovenous malformation (AVM) pathogenesis. TGF-β signals through a complex, tissue-specific set of receptors and intracellular signals. Loss-of-function mutations in at least two of these receptors proteins (endoglin and activin receptor–like kinase-1[ALK-1]) result in hereditary hemorrhagic telangiectasia, with a high prevalence of solid-organ AVMs, including those in brain. The relative roles of bone morphogenetic protein-9 (BMP-9) and TGF-β, and their cell type specificity, are currently controversial. Smad, proteins that modulate the activity of TGFs; smooth muscle cell; TGF-βR-II, TGF-β receptor 2. *(Adapted from Young WL: Clinical Neuroscience Lectures. Munster, IN, Cathenart Publishing, 2007.)*

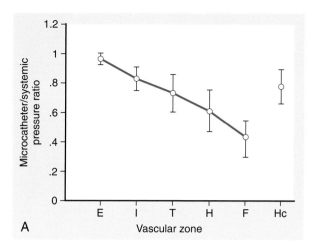

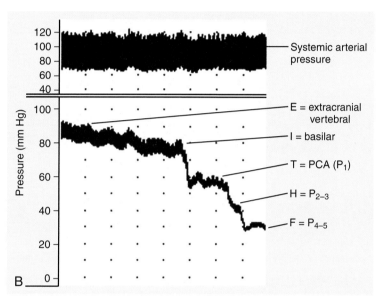

Figure 15–2 A, Pressure ratios in zones E, I, T, H, F and Hc compared with clinical observations (see Box 15-1). The predicted values of our model for the medium arteriovenous malformation are close to the mean values of the experimental observations of Fogarty-Mack and colleagues.[92] E,Extracranial: systemic pressure at level of coaxial catheter in extracranial vertebral artery or internal carotid artery; I, Intracranial: supraclinoid internal carotid artery or basilar artery; T , Transcranial Doppler insonation site: A_1, M_1, or P_1; H, halfway: arbitrarily "halfway" between T and the feeding artery; F, feeder in this model; Hc, contralateral distal arterial pressure. **B,** The continuous pressure tracing in a 40-year-old man who presented with seizures and had a left-sided, 3.5 × 2.5 × 7.0 cm temporal-occipital AVM fed by branches of the middle cerebral artery and the posterior cerebral artery (PCA). This tracing documents the pressure in the vertebral artery (E), basilar artery (I), P1 segment of the PCA (T), P2-P3 segment (H), and P4-P5 segment (F). Note the gradual decline in pressure, which is accentuated at major branch points. Further, all areas distal to the P1 (zone T), which irrigates a large area of normal, eloquent tissue, are relatively hypotensive. *(Adapted from Fogarty-Mack P, Pile-Spellman J, Hacein-Bey L, et al: The effect of arteriovenous malformations on the distribution of intracerebral arterial pressures. AJNR Am J Neuroradiol 1996;17:1443-1449.)*

post-treatment *hyperemic* symptoms, namely cerebral steal and normal perfusion pressure breakthrough (NPPB). Although these concepts are widely discussed, there is limited anecdotal evidence supporting their existence.

Cerebral steal has been suggested as an explanation for focal neurologic deficits in patients with AVMs; steal is assumed to be attributable, by inference, to local hypotension and hypoperfusion. It has been postulated that arteriolar vascular resistance in territories adjacent to AVMs is at or near a state of maximal vasodilation, and therefore steal ensues if perfusion pressure decreases. Although cerebral arterial hypotension in normal brain areas is common in patients with AVMs, clinical presentations with focal neurologic deficits are rare (10%). Moreover, there is no relation between local hypotension and focal neurologic deficits.[97] It is likely that local mass effects from the abnormal vessels of the AVMs are more important

than local hemodynamic failure in accounting for symptomatic focal neurologic deficits unrelated to intracerebral hemorrhage or seizure activity.

The intraoperative appearance of diffuse bleeding from the operative site or brain swelling and the postoperative occurrence of hemorrhage or swelling have been attributed to NPPB or "hyperemic" complications. There are difficulties in studying NPPB-type complications. First, the criteria used by different investigators appear to be very heterogeneous. Second, the incidence of this type of postoperative complication is probably lower than 5%.[98] The increase in global cerebral blood flow after AVM resection appears to be associated with NPPB-type complications, but there is no relationship with preoperative regional arterial hypotension.[98] NPPB is attributed to cerebral hyperemia due to repressurization of previously hypotensive regions. This theory assumes that chronic dilatation of vessels

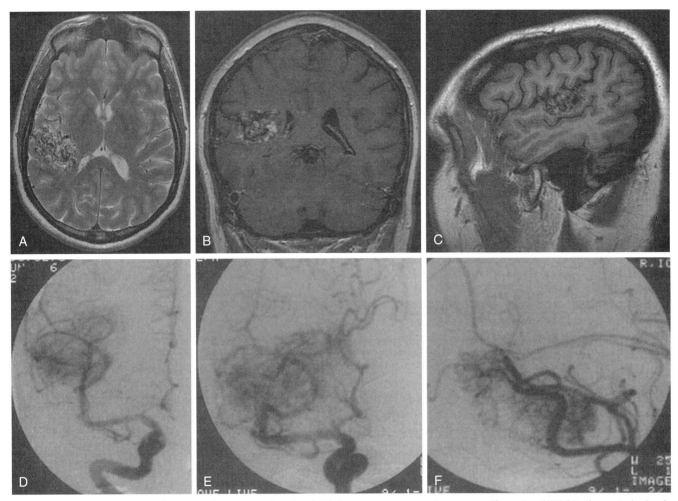

FIGURE 15–3 **A** to **C,** Preoperative magnetic resonance imaging (MRI) demonstrates an arteriovenous malformation (AVM) in the posterior insular and superior temporal cortex. **A,** T2-weighted axial image; **B,** T1-weighted coronal image with gadolinium enhancement; **C,** T1-weighted sagittal image. **D** to **F,** Preoperative angiography shows this Spetzler-Martin grade III AVM with feeding arteries originating from insular branches of the middle cerebral artery. Right internal carotid artery injection, anteroposterior view **(D)**, anterior oblique view **(E)**, and lateral view **(F)**.

in hypotensive or ischemic territory leads to a loss of autoregulation.[95] However, several observations contradict this theory. First, cerebral hyperemia after an AVM resection is global and is not limited to the ipsilateral side of the AVM.[98] Second, there is no relationship between cerebral blood flow changes after resection and the degree of arterial hypotension induced by AVM shunts.[98] Third, in hypotensive regions, autoregulatory response is not impaired but is intact and shifted to the left.[94] Finally, cerebrovascular reactivity to carbon dioxide is preserved after AVM resection,[99] suggesting that the vessels in previously hypotensive territories are not paralyzed. All of these considerations notwithstanding, postoperative brain swelling and hemorrhage will be favored by uncontrolled systemic blood pressure. Although the mechanisms are still unclear, it seems reasonable to hypothesize that barrier integrity in the circulation is compromised by excessive protease activity or growth factor elaboration, as is probably the case in the setting of post-reperfusion hemorrhage after ischemic stroke.[100]

The states of "steal" and "normal perfusion pressure breakthrough" probably do exist in some minority of cases, but they are the exception rather than the rule. As regards perioperative management, the diagnosis of NPPB should be a diagnosis of exclusion after all other correctable causes for malignant brain swelling or bleeding have been excluded. In addition to other supportive and resuscitative measures, prevention of postoperative hypertension may be useful in preventing and treating this syndrome.

PERIOPERATIVE ANESTHETIC MANAGEMENT

Patients with AVMs often undergo several diagnostic (computed tomography, magnetic resonance imaging, positron emission tomography) and therapeutic (interventional neuroradiology, radiosurgery, neurosurgery) procedures that may require anesthesia. Anesthetic management of these patients follows general goals of neuroanesthesia to maintain adequate cerebral perfusion pressure and to prevent increases in intracranial pressure, and it focuses on preventing and managing serious perioperative complications such as intracranial bleeding and NPPB. The following discussion of perioperative anesthetic management concentrates on anesthesia for neuroradiologic and intraoperative procedures. A representative case is illustrated in Figures 15-3 to 15-6.

Preoperative Management

AVM resection is rarely an emergency procedure, unless there is a need for immediate surgical evacuation of an intracranial hematoma. Thus, a careful review of the patient's preoperative

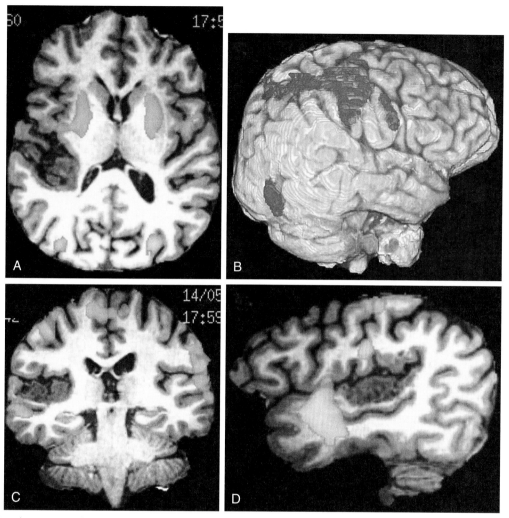

FIGURE 15–4 **A** and **B,** Functional magnetic resonance imaging (fMRI) localizes left-hand motor function by acquiring images with the patient tapping the left fingers. Axial **(A)** and three-dimensional reconstructed **(B)** images, with involved cortex shown in *orange*. **C** and **D,** Functional MRI localizes tongue motor function by acquiring images with the patient moving the tongue. Coronal **(C)** and sagittal **(D)** views, with involved cortex shown in *orange*. Even though this AVM was considered eloquent from its anatomic location, fMRI demonstrated some separation from these motor functions and facilitated the decision to resect it.

status and assessment of potential intraoperative difficulties should be possible. Most patients present with ICH, new seizures, or neurologic deficits. Preexisting medical conditions should be optimized. The impact of any neurologic dysfunction, possible use of antiseizure medications, the location (eloquent areas) and size of the AVM (possibility for significant blood loss), and intraoperative neurophysiologic monitoring should be factored into the anesthetic management plan regarding choice of monitoring, vascular access, anesthetic agents, vasoactive drugs, muscle relaxants, and perioperative airway control.

Intraoperative Management

Monitoring

In addition to routine monitors—electrocardiogram, pulse oximeter, end-tidal CO_2, and temperature—central venous catheters should be considered for use during resection of large AVMs when there is a high risk for significant intraoperative blood loss. Intra-arterial catheters are routinely used during AVM resection for continuous, direct blood pressure monitoring and arterial blood sampling. Because hypertensive

episodes are not commonly associated with AVM rupture, intra-arterial catheters are often placed after induction of anesthesia.[101] During AVM embolization, continuous intra-arterial blood pressure monitoring helps in the diagnosis and treatment of AVM rupture. Fortunately, these potentially devastating complications are rare (1%-2%).[102]

Unfortunately, our ability to routinely monitor the central nervous system lags far behind our ability to monitor other systems, and the development of suitable technologies is still in its infancy. Somatosensory evoked potential, motor evoked potential (MEP), and electroencephalographic monitoring may be used intraoperatively, and direct cerebral blood flow monitoring has been proposed by several groups (see Chapter 2). At present, this is an institution-specific endeavor and is not routinely performed. Jugular venous saturation monitoring has been proposed as an index of throttling of the shunt fraction through the fistula.[103] Continuous noninvasive hemoglobin monitoring has now been approved and may become useful in operations with significant intraoperative blood loss.

Transduction of intravascular pressures in the operative field may aid the surgeon in differentiating arterial and venous structures. In certain cases, it may assist in the decision whether a draining vein interfering with surgical access

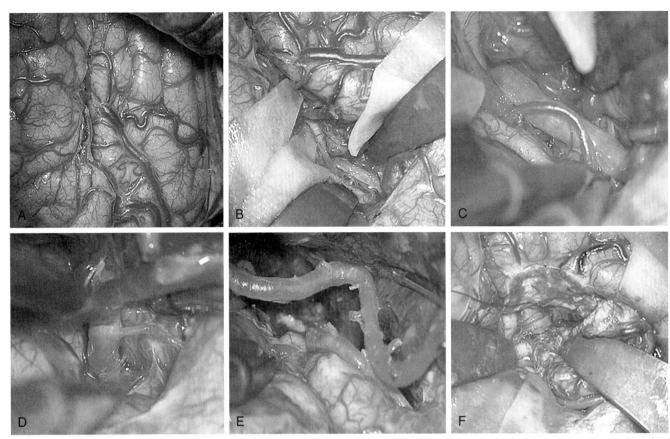

FIGURE 15–5 **A,** Intraoperative photograph shows that the arteriovenous malformation (AVM) does not reach the brain surface. Wide splitting of the distal Sylvian fissure revealed the feeding middle cerebral arteries **(B)**, with the AVM located on the temporal side of the fissure **(C,** superior). Feeding arteries were branches from the middle cerebral artery **(D)**, which was pruned or skeletonized to preserve distal blood flow to the angular cortex **(E)**. After devascularization of the AVM, its deep plane was dissected **(F)**, and the nidus was removed.

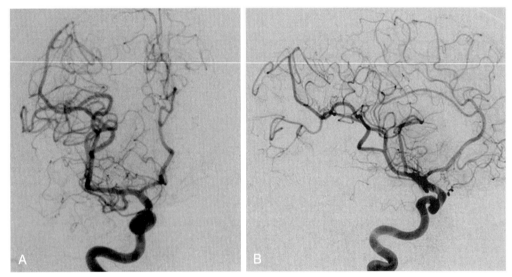

FIGURE 15–6 Postoperative angiography shows complete resection of the arteriovenous malformation, with preservation of *en passage* arteries. Right internal carotid artery injection, anteroposterior **(A)** and lateral **(B)** views.

to the nidus can be sacrificed. Proximal arterial pressure is measured during a temporary occlusion of the vein; failure of the pressure to change implies that alternate venous pathways are sufficient to prevent distention of the nidus and rupture. Technically, direct puncture of feeding arteries and draining veins in the operative field using 26-gauge needles is a simple procedure with minimal risk.

Vascular Access

The likelihood for significant intraoperative blood loss should be discussed preoperatively with the neurosurgeon. Multiple large-bore intravenous accesses for rapid blood administration and availability of appropriate blood products are mandatory. Preoperative planning should include consideration of a central venous catheter for both monitoring and provision of vasoactive drugs.

Anesthetic Technique

CHOICE OF AGENTS

Scientific literature provides minimal guidance regarding anesthetic management of patients with AVMs. Choice of anesthetic agents varies widely among institutions and is made largely to follow basic neuroanesthesia principles and account for coexisting diseases. Descriptions of the neuroanesthesia techniques most commonly used at the University of California at San Francisco, can be found on our website (neuroanesthesia.ucsf.edu).

Intracranial pressure control, which is often discussed in regard to the anesthetic care of neurosurgical patients, is usually not an issue with the patient with an AVM who is coming for elective resection, because the lesion does not displace, but rather replaces, normal brain structures. Nonetheless, such a patient may have decreased intracranial compliance, especially if significant venous hypertension is present, so the usual caveats about avoiding anesthetic techniques that result in significant cerebral vasodilation is a reasonable choice.

Patients undergoing AVM embolization at our institution routinely receive a general anesthetic. During embolization procedures, the anesthetic goals are to keep the patient immobile with adequate cerebral perfusion pressure and to plan for immediate postprocedure neurologic examination (see Chapter 14). In addition to these goals, during AVM resection, the anesthetic technique should minimize brain volume in order to reduce retractor-induced cerebral ischemia. For both procedures, there should also be a plan to treat potential complications, such as intracerebral hemorrhage during embolization and significant bleeding and/or brain swelling during and after surgery (see later).

Neurologically intact patients may be premedicated with benzodiazepines (midazolam). Propofol, thiopental, or etomidate can be used to induce anesthesia, propofol being most commonly used. Maintenance of anesthesia can be achieved with varying combinations of propofol, a narcotic, and an inhalation anesthetic. Total intravenous anesthetic techniques or combinations of inhalational and intravenous methods may optimize rapid emergence from anesthesia and allow somatosensory evoked potential and motor evoked potential monitoring. There is no evidence that the choice of an inhalation anesthetic, narcotic, or muscle relaxant has an intrinsic, independent effect on outcome.

Some centers use barbiturate loading during the resection of AVM for metabolic suppression to afford additional protection against cerebral ischemia, resulting in perhaps a greater degree of brain relaxation and protection against acute hyperemia.[104] Barbiturates can be titrated to an electroencephalographic end point of burst suppression. The main prices to be paid for barbiturate use are delayed emergence from anesthesia and forgoing of an early postoperative neurologic examination. There is no evidence that outcome is affected.

NONPHARMACOLOGIC CEREBRAL PROTECTION

The goals of modern neuroanesthesia should optimize brain-protective therapy. A number of basic considerations will maximize nonpharmacologic cerebral protection (Box 15-1). There are two general types of damage towards which protective efforts are guided, neurosurgical (anatomic) trespass and anesthetic (physiologic) trespass. Possible mechanisms of

BOX 15–1	*Nonpharmacologic Brain Protection*
Relaxed brain	Good head position
	Cerebrospinal fluid drainage
	Diuretics/osmotherapy
	Avoidance of excessive cerebral vasodilators
	Modest hypocapnia
Controlled systemic and cerebral hemodynamics	Euvolemia
	Optimal cerebral perfusion pressure
Fluid and electrolyte management	Isotonicity
	Euglycemia
Temperature management	Toleration of modest hypothermia intraoperatively
	Postoperative prevention of hyperthermia
Controlled emergence	Tailored awakening
	Autonomic control

injury from the neurosurgeon include brain retraction, direct vascular injury (ischemia, thrombosis, venous occlusion), and mechanical disruption of neuronal tissue or white matter tracts. Anesthetic injury may result from systemic hypotension or hypertension, decreased O_2 content, hypo-osmolarity, and hyperglycemia. It must be stressed that mechanisms of damage are interactive. For example, modest amounts of brain retraction coupled with modest reduction of systemic blood pressure may have synergistic effects on neurologic outcome.

Management goals should include provision for a relaxed brain (to reduce retractor-induced ischemia); control of systemic and cerebral hemodynamics; avoidance of hypotonicity, hyperglycemia, and hyperthermia; and timely emergence from anesthesia without significant hypertension, tachycardia, or coughing.

Brain Relaxation during Surgery

Interventions that reduce brain volume may help ameliorate retractor-induced ischemia. Adequate brain relaxation begins with good head position to promote intracranial venous drainage. The least amount of flexion and rotation necessary for the surgical approach should be planned with the surgeon. A rule of thumb might be given as two finger-breadths of space between the mandible and clavicle (not the sternum) after the head is positioned in rigid pin fixation. The head of the table should be elevated slightly to prevent venous engorgement.

Cerebrospinal fluid removal is an effective means of brain relaxation. It is obtained by insertion of a lumbar intrathecal catheter or ventricular drainage. Osmotic diuretic therapy with mannitol (0.5-1.0 g/kg) with or without furosemide is widely applied. The most important consideration for intraoperative anesthetic choice is the avoidance of cerebral vasodilators (moderate- to high-dose inhalation anesthetics). Modest hypocapnia should be used sparingly as an adjunct to brain relaxation, and the Pa_{CO_2} levels should be dropped below 30 mm Hg only for a specific indication.

Control of Systemic and Cerebral Hemodynamics

EUVOLEMIA AND BLOOD PRESSURE CONTROL

Euvolemia is the goal of modern neuroanesthesia fluid management. Adequate volume status to maintain stable hemodynamics, especially with the application of induced hypotension and the potential for rapid blood loss, may require liberal fluid administration. Although some anesthesiologists do use limited amounts of hetastarch, its use in neuroanesthesia is controversial owing to its potential to induce coagulopathy. Most of our patients receive mannitol at the beginning of surgery to increase serum osmolarity, so perioperatively we administer mainly lactated Ringer's solution. Many authorities recommend isotonic fluid replacement during neurosurgical procedures.

Control of cerebral hemodynamics begins with control of systemic arterial pressure, which in turn is predicated on adequate cardiac preload (euvolemia). Iatrogenic dehydration, as practiced in years past, has no place in modern neurosurgical practice. Indeed, in the setting of a potential for rapid, significant intraoperative hemorrhage, it is clearly deleterious. A large amount of shunting of blood through the AVM reduces blood pressure of the feeding and adjacent arteries. Marginally perfused areas may be critically dependent on collateral perfusion pressure. Maintenance of low blood pressure may be inadequate and results in infarction if unrecognized.

During manipulation of the intracranial contents or their vascular supply, the anesthesiologist should strive to maintain the optimal cerebral perfusion pressure, that is, the highest clinically acceptable blood pressure for the particular clinical circumstance. We achieve this goal by minimizing the use of propofol and inhalation anesthetics with a low-dose phenylephrine infusion when necessary. Brain relaxation is probably also served by maintenance of normal arterial pressure (cerebral blood volume is kept to a minimum by autoregulatory vasoconstriction).[105]

Anesthesiologists have a major role in preventing and treating retractor-related cerebral ischemia, cerebral ischemia secondary to poor cerebral perfusion, intraoperative hemorrhage, and postoperative edema. There may be marginally perfused areas adjacent to an AVM that are critically dependent on collateral perfusion pressure. Although such areas may be secondary to the hemodynamic effects of the shunt, they are more likely due to mass effect from the vascular structures of the nidus or the residua of a prior hemorrhage. The cause notwithstanding, prolonged systemic hypotension might result in infarction, if unrecognized. Thus, cerebral perfusion pressure should be maintained at close to normal values unless there is an indication for inducing hypotension to control hemorrhage.

INDUCED HYPOTENSION

In contrast to the current trend to maintain normotension during intracranial aneurysm clipping, induced hypotension may be useful during AVM resection in case of significant intraoperative bleeding. This is especially pertinent to large AVMs that have a deep arterial supply. Bleeding from these small, deep-feeding vessels may be difficult to control, and decreasing arterial pressure facilitates surgical hemostasis. The subject of induced hypotension is discussed extensively in the neuroanesthesia literature.

During uncontrolled bleeding the surgeon may be forced to place clips blindly in an attempt to stem hemorrhage. In this event, barbiturate therapy (thiopental) may be indicated and could be used as a means of, or as an adjunct to, inducing mild or moderate temporary arterial blood pressure reduction until bleeding is brought under control. Induction of systemic hypotension with a pure vasodilator has theoretical disadvantages. In the setting of emergency intracranial vascular occlusion to control hemorrhage, the distal perfusion field of the occluded artery will have little or no opportunity to recruit collateral flow from neighboring (relatively vasodilated) normal arterial supply regions. However, the clinician should use whatever means he or she is comfortable and adept with to expeditiously reduce blood pressure as demanded by the clinical situation.

Fluid Management

There is a convincing body of evidence that serum osmolarity strongly influences water movement into both normal and damaged brain tissues.[106] Even mildly hypotonic fluids such as lactated Ringer's solution (without mannitol), if given in sufficient quantity, may aggravate brain swelling more than do isotonic crystalloids or colloids. Isotonic fluid replacement with blood, saline, or hetastarch after forebrain ischemia in the rat appears to yield similar results in terms of cerebral edema formation.[107] The most important point is that fluid should never be withheld at the expense of a stable cardiovascular status. Serum osmolarity can be easily monitored if large volumes of crystalloid are administered. The influence of colloid oncotic pressure on the formation of brain edema is still a controversial topic.[108-110] Results of one experimental study indicate that a reduction of colloid oncotic pressure without decreased osmolarity may exacerbate post-traumatic brain edema.[108] Aggressive administration of isotonic crystalloids may worsen brain edema by decreasing colloid oncotic pressure.[108] Although there are no perioperative outcome data to support the use of one fluid over another, it is advisable, on the basis of available data, to avoid perioperative hypo-osmolarity.

There is considerable evidence that glucose aggravates cerebral injury not only in animals but also in humans.[111,112] Perioperative stress and the use of steroids may contribute to intraoperative and postoperative hyperglycemia. In fact, the evidence for the use of steroids for cerebrovascular surgery is lacking, although many teams use them.

In the absence of clear guidelines, the most rational approach is to avoid glucose-containing fluids unless there is a specific indication for them. One such indication would be a diabetic patient receiving insulin therapy. In this case, "tight" rather than "loose" control of serum glucose seems reasonable. Despite the compelling animal data, the lack of specific clinical outcome data would suggest that overaggressive lowering of glucose levels is not worth risking hypoglycemia in an anesthetized patient. A reasonable but arbitrary target might be to prevent renal spillage of glucose in the range of 180 mg/100 mL.

Use of Hypothermia

Mild hypothermia (with core temperature decreases as little as 1.5°-3° C) has been shown to provide dramatic cerebral protection against ischemic insult in animal models.[113] This protective effect is greater than would be expected from metabolic suppression alone and may be related to a decrease in excitatory neurotransmitter release from ischemic cells.[114] Although randomized controlled clinical trials have shown the favorable result of mild hypothermia in patients with severe traumatic brain injury and cardiac arrest, the efficacy of prophylactic mild hypothermia during craniotomy has not been validated.[115,116]

Anesthetized patients can be easily cooled to 33° to 34° C, although complete intraoperative rewarming may be difficult to achieve.[117] Even mild levels of hypothermia are not without potential risk.[118] Passive rewarming is associated with peripheral vasoconstriction, shivering, and subsequent increases in oxygen consumption and myocardial work. Drug metabolism is decreased, prolonging the effect of even short-acting anesthetic drugs. Moderate hypothermia ($<33°$ C) has other well-documented potential effects, including increased susceptibility to infection, cardiac arrhythmias, and ischemia, hypocoagulability, thrombocytopenia, impairment of platelet aggregation, and activation of fibrinolysis, all of which reverse with rewarming.[117,119] Most of these adverse effects have been observed in patients leaving the operating room while still hypothermic. It is unclear whether the potential benefits of cerebral protection gained from mild hypothermia and partial rewarming are offset by the hypothermia-induced systemic physiologic stress, particularly if shivering occurs upon emergence from anesthesia. Postoperative shivering can be significantly attenuated by intraoperative administration of meperidine or α_2 agonists (clonidine, dexmedetomidine).[120]

A conservative recommendation would be mild body temperature reduction ($34°-35°$ C) until closure is imminent, followed by active rewarming. Careful temperature monitoring should continue throughout the perioperative period; hyperthermia must be avoided as it potentiates ischemic damage.[121]

Emergence from Anesthesia and Initial Recovery

A particularly challenging aspect of the perioperative care of patients with AVMs is emergence from anesthesia and initial recovery. A moderate phenylephrine-induced blood pressure augmentation (20%-30% above normal mean arterial pressure) may be needed during drying of the operative bed to inspect for hemostasis. After hemostasis is achieved and anesthetic agents are reduced or discontinued, antihypertensive agents such as labetalol can be used to keep the patient's blood pressure within 10% below the patient's baseline values. Control of systemic hemodynamics is of critical importance during the emergence phase as the patient makes the transition from the anesthetized to the conscious state.[122] Administration of α_2 agonists (clonidine, dexmedetomidine) before the end of anesthesia can attenuate the emergence-induced stress response (hypertension, tachycardia).[123]

We would emphasize that, without firm outcome data indicating the superiority of one drug regimen or another, the choice of agent to manipulate blood pressure must be placed in the context of the clinical situation (e.g., avoiding β-adrenergic blockers in the patient with bronchospastic airway disease or the use of nitroglycerin in the patient with coronary artery disease) and the experience of the practitioner.

The most sensitive monitor of cerebral function remains the neurologic examination. A prompt emergence from anesthesia ensures that drug residua are not confused with and do not obscure focal neurologic damage. Delayed emergence may require emergency computed tomography to rule out brain swelling and bleeding. However, a long procedure with massive fluid resuscitation, a complicated intraoperative course, and surgery in a patient with a preexisting neurologic deficit may be indications for postoperative sedation and mechanical ventilation. There is no ideal regimen for maintaining postoperative sedation and blood pressure control. Use of dexmedetomidine has gained popularity owing to the combination of its sympatholytic and sedative effects with the ability to arouse the patient to allow postoperative neurologic examination.

OPERATIVE CONSIDERATIONS FOR AVOIDING COMPLICATIONS

Intraoperative complications with AVMs challenge the neurosurgeon like no other lesion in the brain. Bleeding can erupt quickly to fill the surgical field, obscure critical anatomy, and impede microdissection. Bleeding arteries can be difficult to control, particularly when they are thin, friable perforating arteries resisting coagulation with bipolar cautery. Hemorrhage into the brain can damage it and compromise patient outcome. Worst of all, uncontrollable bleeding can force dangerous or hasty maneuvers. Bleeding demands reactions from the anesthesiologist to replace volume, transfuse blood, maintain blood pressure, and sometimes correct coagulation disturbances.

Surgical complications are best avoided with judicious patient selection. The combination of AVM size, deep venous drainage, and eloquence of adjacent brain that comprises the Spetzler-Martin grading scale provides a preliminary assessment of surgical risks,[33] with low-grade AVMs (grade I-III) having acceptably low morbidity rates and high-grade AVMs (grade IV-V) having unacceptably high morbidity and mortality rates. As helpful as this simple grading scale is, it is crude at best and demands more thorough assessment of other factors: grade III subtype, patient presentation and age, deep perforating artery supply, diffuseness of the nidus margin and functional eloquence.

The dividing line between operability and nonoperability of an AVM probably runs not cleanly between grades III and IV but rather between subtypes of the third grade.[124] Our experience has demonstrated that medium-sized AVMs (3-6 cm diameter) in eloquent locations have morbidity rates resembling those of grade IV AVMs more than those of other grade III AVMs. In contrast, small AVMs (<3 cm diameter) with deep venous drainage and in eloquent locations, as well as other medium-sized AVMs away from eloquent locations, have the morbidity rates expected for grade III lesions. Therefore, the surgeon must beware of grade III AVMs that are larger and in eloquent areas, and perhaps should manage them more conservatively.

Presentation with hemorrhage is an important factor because it not only indicates AVMs with high risk of re-hemorrhage but also facilitates surgery.[53] Hematomas help separate an AVM from adjacent brain, completing some of the neurosurgeon's dissection preoperatively. Evacuation of hematoma also creates working space around the AVM that can minimize transgression of normal brain to reach the nidus or access to a deep nidus that might otherwise have been unreachable. Hemorrhage can also obliterate some of an AVM's arterial supply, reducing its flow and the risk of bleeding during resection. Hemorrhage can be damaging to brain tissue, and young age and plasticity can enhance a patient's ability to recover neurologic function. Even with unruptured AVMs, youth can enhance recovery from deficits caused by surgery.

Other anatomy predicts the likelihood of intraoperative bleeding and neurologic outcomes. For example, compact AVMs with tightly woven arteries and veins often have distinct borders that separate cleanly from the adjacent brain, whereas diffuse AVMs with ragged borders and intermixed brain force the neurosurgeon to establish a dissection plane that can extend into the normal brain. Deep perforating arteries are thin, fragile, and difficult to occlude with cautery. Bleeding during surgery can escape into deep white matter tracts and cause significant deficits. These clues to intraoperative bleeding can be found on angiography and used during the selection process.

The Spetzler-Martin grading scale defines *eloquence* as anatomic locations whose injury would result in a discrete neurologic deficit, such as the motor and somatosensory strips, visual cortex, speech areas, thalamus, and brainstem. However, structural anatomy does not always indicate functional anatomy with AVMs, because the brain often relocates functions if they lie too close to an AVM. For example, the presence of an AVM in the central sulcus may cause relocation of motor function anteriorly from the precentral gyrus into the premotor cortex. In more dramatic cases, left hemispheric functions like speech can be moved to the opposite hemisphere or rearranged in the ipsilateral hemisphere.[125,126] Therefore, we have found that preoperative imaging with functional MRI more precisely localizes neurologic function, allowing us to replace anatomic eloquence with individualized functional eloquence. These radiologic adjuncts better define the surgical risks and refine patient selection.

Even in the most carefully selected patients, intraoperative complications and catastrophes occur. Stroke from occlusion of an artery to the normal brain occurs silently unless detected on intraoperative neurophysiologic monitoring. This complication can happen when an artery feeding the nidus is occluded too early, compromising branches to the normal brain that originate between the point of occlusion and the AVM. En passage arteries transmit branches to the AVM and distal branches to the brain downstream. These en passage arteries must be skeletonized or pruned to allow occlusion of only those that supply the AVM, thereby preserving distal perfusion. Uninvolved arteries can also be mistaken for AVM feeding arteries. The neurosurgeon must rely on thorough analysis of the preoperative angiograms, thorough inspection of subtle anatomic features, and precise arterial occlusion at the point of entry into the nidus. Unexpected brain swelling during a long procedure may be an indication of an evolving stroke.

Bleeding is encountered most frequently along the deep plane of dissection, after the nidus has been dissected circumferentially. The deep penetrating arteries are typically encountered along this border and can resist coagulation with bipolar cautery. Visualization of these deep feeding arteries is often compromised by the overlying bulk of the nidus, and with stereotypical cone-shaped AVMs, this final plane is often deep below the cortical surface. The tip of the nidus can reach the ventricle, and bleeding from ventricular arteries can be difficult to identify, can rapidly fill the ventricle, and can cause the brain to herniate outward. With all these hazards along this deep plane, the neurosurgeon must approach this last stage of the dissection with the utmost concentration. Complete dissection of the nidus on all sides is accomplished before surgery moves to the deep plane, arteries resisting cautery are occluded with microclips, ventricular tips of AVMs are encircled to make sure that feeding arteries are effectively closed, and any bleeding is meticulously controlled before the dissection proceeds.

In addition to bleeding along the deep plane, frank rupture of the AVM can also occur. One of the tenets of AVM surgery is to dissect circumferentially, encircling the AVM but never violating it. AVM rupture can occur when the plane of dissection is too close. Bleeding is brisk, and the nidus cannot be cauterized like a feeding artery. The rupture site is tamponaded with hemostatic agents to control the bleeding and enable the neurosurgeon to continue working. If the dissection plane is too tight, a portion of the nidus can be separated from the AVM as a remnant. Such remnants typically have arterial input but lack venous outflow, which predisposes them to rupturing either during surgery or shortly thereafter. An area that is unusually bloody may be a sign of retained AVM, and a wider path of dissection must be established around this area. Another tenet of AVM surgery is to occlude all the feeding arteries before occluding the draining vein. Occasionally, an arterialized draining vein is mistaken for a feeding artery and occluded early, compromising venous outflow, pressuring the AVM, and precipitating rupture. The neurosurgeon must recognize this dangerous state and quickly remove the AVM. A ruptured, bleeding AVM is less tense and angry, and the neurosurgeon has a limited time window during which to continue working through the bleeding. The anesthesiologist must keep pace with this blood loss during these situations.

Significant intraoperative or postoperative brain swelling may occur after AVM resection, as previously discussed. If there is no identifiable cause—for instance, undiagnosed rupture or obstructed venous drainage from thrombosis or occlusion—treatment is symptomatic, consisting of such maneuvers as hyperventilation, administration of mannitol, and tight blood pressure control.

The threat of bleeding and catastrophe is ever-present in AVM surgery. Intraoperative excitement is rarely associated with good outcomes. The best AVM surgery is steady and meticulous for the neurosurgeon and quiet and unexciting for the anesthesiologist. The neurosurgeon and the anesthesiologist must make preparations to deal with the worst of complications while working continuously to avoid them.

REFERENCES

1. Arteriovenous Malformation Study Group: Arteriovenous malformations of the brain in adults, *N Engl J Med* 340:1812–1818, 1999.
2. Young WL: Intracranial arteriovenous malformations: Pathophysiology and hemodynamics. In Jafar JJ, Awad IA, Rosenwasser RH, editors: *Vascular Malformations of the Central Nervous System*, New York, 1999, Lippincott Williams & Wilkins, pp 95–126.
3. Choi JH, Mohr JP: Brain arteriovenous malformations in adults, *Lancet Neurol* 4:299–308, 2005.
4. Stapf C, Mast H, Sciacca RR, et al: Predictors of hemorrhage in patients with untreated brain arteriovenous malformation, *Neurology* 66:1350–1355, 2006.
5. Kim H, Sidney S, McCulloch CE, et al: Racial/ethnic differences in longitudinal risk of intracranial hemorrhage in brain arteriovenous malformation patients, *Stroke* 38:2430–2437, 2007.
6. Stapf C, Mohr JP, Pile-Spellman J, et al: The effect of concurrent arterial aneurysms on the risk of hemorrhagic presentation in brain arteriovenous malformations [abstract], *Stroke* 32:337-c, 2001.
7. Duong DH, Young WL, Vang MC, et al: Feeding artery pressure and venous drainage pattern are primary determinants of hemorrhage from cerebral arteriovenous malformations, *Stroke* 29:1167–1176, 1998.
8. Spetzler RF, Hargraves RW, McCormick PW, et al: Relationship of perfusion pressure and size to risk of hemorrhage from arteriovenous malformations, *J Neurosurg* 76:918–923, 1992.
9. Miyasaka Y, Kurata A, Tokiwa K, et al: Draining vein pressure increases and hemorrhage in patients with arteriovenous malformation, *Stroke* 25:504–507, 1994.
10. Kader A, Young WL, Pile-Spellman J, et al: The influence of hemodynamic and anatomic factors on hemorrhage from cerebral arteriovenous malformations, *Neurosurgery* 34:801–807, 1994.
11. Brown RD Jr, Wiebers DO, Forbes GS: Unruptured intracranial aneurysms and arteriovenous malformations: Frequency of intracranial hemorrhage and relationship of lesions, *J Neurosurg* 73:859–863, 1990.
12. Marks MP, Steinberg GK, Norbash AM, Lane B: Characteristics predictive of hemorrhage in AVMs [abstract], *Stroke* 24:184, 1993.
13. Marks MP, Lane B, Steinberg GK, Chang PJ: Hemorrhage in intracerebral arteriovenous malformations: Angiographic determinants, *Radiology* 176:807–813, 1990.

14. Batjer H, Suss RA, Samson D: Intracranial arteriovenous malformations associated with aneurysms, *Neurosurgery* 18:29–35, 1986.

15. Mast H, Young WL, Koennecke HC, et al: Risk of spontaneous haemorrhage after diagnosis of cerebral arteriovenous malformation, *Lancet* 350:1065–1068, 1997.

16. Halim AX, Johnston SC, Singh V, et al: Longitudinal risk of intracranial hemorrhage in patients with arteriovenous malformation of the brain within a defined population, *Stroke* 35:1697–1702, 2004.

17. Stefani MA, Porter PJ, terBrugge KG, et al: Large and deep brain arteriovenous malformations are associated with risk of future hemorrhage, *Stroke* 33:1220–1224, 2002.

18. Kim H, Sidney S, Johnston SC, et al: Racial/ethnic differences in longitudinal risk of intracranial hemorrhage in brain arteriovenous malformation patients [abstract], *Stroke* 38:468, 2007.

19. Gao E, Young WL, Pile-Spellman J, et al: Cerebral arteriovenous malformation feeding artery aneurysms: A theoretical model of intravascular pressure changes after treatment, *Neurosurgery* 41:1345–1356, 1997.

20. Fleetwood IG, Steinberg GK: Arteriovenous malformations, *Lancet* 359:863–873, 2002.

21. Hartmann A, Mast H, Mohr JP, et al: Morbidity of intracranial hemorrhage in patients with cerebral arteriovenous malformation, *Stroke* 29:931–934, 1998.

22. Forster DM, Steiner L, Hakanson S: Arteriovenous malformations of the brain: A long-term clinical study, *J Neurosurg* 37:562–570, 1972.

23. Ondra SL, Troupp H, George ED, Schwab K: The natural history of symptomatic arteriovenous malformations of the brain: A 24-year follow-up assessment, *J Neurosurg* 73:387–391, 1990.

24. Svien HJ, McRae JA: Arteriovenous anomalies of the brain: Fate of patients not having definitive surgery, *J Neurosurg* 23:23–28, 1965.

25. Waltimo O: The change in size of intracranial arteriovenous malformations, *J Neurol Sci* 19:21, 1973.

26. Fults D, Kelly DL Jr: Natural history of arteriovenous malformations of the brain: A clinical study, *Neurosurgery* 15:658–662, 1984.

27. Luessenhop AJ, Rosa L: Cerebral arteriovenous malformations: Indications for and results of surgery, and the role of intravascular techniques, *J Neurosurg* 60:14–22, 1984.

28. Brown RD Jr, Wiebers DO, Forbes G, et al: The natural history of unruptured intracranial arteriovenous malformations, *J Neurosurg* 68:352–357, 1988.

29. Perret G, Nishioka H: Report on the cooperative study of intracranial aneurysms and subarachnoid hemorrhage. Section VI: Arteriovenous malformations: An analysis of 545 cases of cranio-cerebral arteriovenous malformations and fistulae reported to the cooperative study, *J Neurosurg* 25:467–490, 1966.

30. Perret G: The epidemiology and clinical course of arteriovenous malformations. In Pia HW, Gleave JRW, Grote E, Zierski J, editors: *Cerebral Angiomas: Advances in Diagnosis and Therapy*, New York, 1975, Springer-Verlag, pp 21–26.

31. Graf CJ, Nibbelink DW: Cooperative study of intracranial aneurysms and subarachnoid hemorrhage. Report on randomized treatment study: Intracranial surgery, *Stroke* 5:559–561, 1974.

32. Choi JH, Mast H, Sciacca RR, et al: Clinical outcome after first and recurrent hemorrhage in patients with untreated brain arteriovenous malformation, *Stroke* 37:1243–1247, 2006.

33. Spetzler RF, Martin NA: A proposed grading system for arteriovenous malformations, *J Neurosurg* 65:476–483, 1986.

34. Pollock BE, Flickinger JC: A proposed radiosurgery-based grading system for arteriovenous malformations, *J Neurosurg* 96:79–85, 2002.

35. Lawton MT, Hamilton MG, Spetzler RF: Multimodality treatment of deep arteriovenous malformations: Thalamus, basal ganglia, and brain stem, *Neurosurgery* 37:29–36, 1995.

36. Hartmann A, Stapf C, Hofmeister C, et al: Determinants of neurological outcome after surgery for brain arteriovenous malformation, *Stroke* 31:2361–2364, 2000.

37. Hartmann A, Pile-Spellman J, Stapf C, et al: Risk of endovascular treatment of brain arteriovenous malformations, *Stroke* 33:1816–1820, 2002.

38. ApSimon HT, Reef H, Phadke RV, Popovic EA: A population-based study of brain arteriovenous malformation: Long-term treatment outcomes, *Stroke* 33:2794–2800, 2002.

39. Castel JP, Kantor G: Postoperative morbidity and mortality after microsurgical exclusion of cerebral arteriovenous malformations. Current data and analysis of recent literature, *Neurochirurgie* 47:369–383, 2001.

40. Morgan MK, Rochford AM, Tsahtsarlis A, et al: Surgical risks associated with the management of Grade I and II brain arteriovenous malformations, *Neurosurgery* 54:832–837, 2004.

41. Meisel HJ, Mansmann U, Alvarez H, et al: Effect of partial targeted N-butyl-cyano-acrylate embolization in brain AVM, *Acta Neurochir (Wien)* 144:879–887, 2002.

42. Wikholm G, Lundqvist C, Svendsen P: The Goteborg cohort of embolized cerebral arteriovenous malformations: A 6-year follow-up, *Neurosurgery* 49:799–806, 2001.

43. Taylor CL, Dutton K, Rappard G, et al: Complications of preoperative embolization of cerebral arteriovenous malformations, *J Neurosurg* 100:810–812, 2004.

44. Goto K: Ectatic and occlusive diseases of the venous drainage system of cerebral arteriovenous malformations (AVMs) with emphasis on spectacular shrinking neurological deficits after embolization, *Interv Neuroradiol* 11(Suppl 1):95–118, 2005.

45. Bhattacharya J, Jenkins S, Zampakis P, et al: Endovascular treatment of AVMs in Glasgow, *Interv Neuroradiol* 11(Suppl 1):73–80, 2005.

46. Campos J, Biscoito P, Sequeira P, Batista A: Intra-arterial embolization in the analysis of five years (2000–2005) in the treatment of brain arteriovenous malformations, *Interv Neuroradiol* 11(Suppl 1):81–94, 2005.

47. Vinuela F, Duckwiler G, Jahan R, Murayama Y: Therapeutic management of cerebral arteriovenous malformations: Present role of interventional neuroradiology, *Interv Neuroradiol* 11(Suppl 1):13–29, 2005.

48. Ozanne A, Alvarez H, Rodesch G, Lasjaunias P: Management of brain AVMs at Bicêtre: A comparison of two patient cohorts treated in 1985-1995 and 1996-2005, *Interv Neuroradiol* 11(Suppl 1):31–36, 2005.

49. Klurfan P, Gunnarsson T, Haw C, ter Brugge K: Endovascular treatment of brain arteriovenous malformations: The Toronto experience, *Interv Neuroradiol* 1(Suppl 1):51–56, 2005.

50. Beltramello A, Zampieri P, Ricciardi G, et al: Combined treatment of brain AVMs: Analysis of five years (2000-2004) in the Verona experience, *Interv Neuroradiol* 11(Suppl 1):63–72, 2005.

51. Raymond J, Iancu D, Weill A, et al: Embolization as one modality in a combined strategy for the management of cerebral arteriovenous malformations, *Interv Neuroradiol* 11(Suppl 1):57–62, 2005.

52. Spetzler RF, Martin NA: A proposed grading system for arteriovenous malformations. 1986, *J Neurosurg* 108:186–193, 2008.

53. Lawton MT, Du R, Tran M, et al: Effect of presenting hemorrhage on outcome after microsurgical resection of brain arteriovenous malformations, *Neurosurgery* 56:485–493, 2005.

54. Pollock BE, Flickinger JC, Lunsford LD, et al: Hemorrhage risk after stereotactic radiosurgery of cerebral arteriovenous malformations, *Neurosurgery* 38:652–659, 1996.

55. Pollock BE, Flickinger JC, Lunsford LD, et al: Factors that predict the bleeding risk of cerebral arteriovenous malformations, *Stroke* 27:1–6, 1996.

56. Pollock BE, Flickinger JC, Lunsford LD, et al: Factors associated with successful arteriovenous malformation radiosurgery, *Neurosurgery* 42:1239–1244, 1998.

57. Flickinger JC, Kondziolka D, Lunsford LD, et al: A multi-institutional analysis of complication outcomes after arteriovenous malformation radiosurgery, *Int J Radiat Oncol Biol Phys* 44:67–74, 1999.

58. Maruyama K, Kawahara N, Shin M, et al: The risk of hemorrhage after radiosurgery for cerebral arteriovenous malformations, *N Engl J Med* 352:146–153, 2005.

59 Hartmann A, Marx P, Schilling AM, et al: Neurologic complications following radiosurgical treatment of brain arteriovenous malformations [abstract], Valencia, Spain, May 2003, Presented at 12th European Stroke Conference.

60. National Institute of Neurological Disorders and Stroke (NINDS): A Randomized Trial of Unruptured Brain AVMs (ARUBA). Available at http://clinicaltrials.gov/ct/show/NCT00389181.

61. Du R, Hashimoto T, Tihan T, et al: Growth and regression of an arteriovenous malformation in a patient with hereditary hemorrhagic telangiectasia: Case report, *J Neurosurg* 106:470–477, 2007.

62. Mullan S, Mojtahedi S, Johnson DL, Macdonald RL: Embryological basis of some aspects of cerebral vascular fistulas and malformations, *J Neurosurg* 85:1–8, 1996.

63. Lawton MT, Jacobowitz R, Spetzler RF: Redefined role of angiogenesis in the pathogenesis of dural arteriovenous malformations, *J Neurosurg* 87:267–274, 1997.

64. Singh V, Smith WS, Lawton MT, et al: Thrombophilic mutation as a new high-risk feature in DAVF patients [abstract], *Ann Neurol* 60(Suppl 3):S30, 2006.

65. Hashimoto T, Mesa-Tejada R, Quick CM, et al: Evidence of increased endothelial cell turnover in brain arteriovenous malformations, *Neurosurgery* 49:124–131, 2001.

66. Hashimoto T, Young WL: Roles of angiogenesis and vascular remodeling in brain vascular malformations, *Semin Cerebrovasc Dis Stroke* 4:217–225, 2004.

67. Hashimoto T, Lawton MT, Wen G, et al: Gene microarray analysis of human brain arteriovenous malformations, *Neurosurgery* 54:410–423, 2004.

68. Lee CZ, Xue Z, Zhu Y, et al: Matrix metalloproteinase-9 inhibition attenuates vascular endothelial growth factor-induced intracranial hemorrhage, *Stroke* 38:2563–2568, 2007.

69. Chen Y, Xu B, Arderiu G, et al: Retroviral delivery of homeobox d3 gene induces cerebral angiogenesis in mice, *J Cereb Blood Flow Metab* 24:1280–1287, 2004.

70. Hashimoto T, Lam T, Boudreau NJ, et al: Abnormal balance in the angiopoietin-tie2 system in human brain arteriovenous malformations, *Circ Res* 89:111–113, 2001.

71. Hashimoto T, Wen G, Lawton MT, et al: Abnormal expression of matrix metalloproteinases and tissue inhibitors of metalloproteinases in brain arteriovenous malformations, *Stroke* 34:925–931, 2003.

72. Chen Y, Fan Y, Poon KY, Achrol AS, et al: MMP-9 expression is associated with leukocytic but not endothelial markers in brain arteriovenous malformations, *Front Biosci* 11:3121–3128, 2006.

73. Chen Y, Zhu W, Bollen AW, et al: Evidence for inflammatory cell involvement in brain arteriovenous malformations, *Neurosurgery* 62:1340–1349, 2008.

74. Shenkar R, Shi C, Check IJ, et al: Concepts and hypotheses: Inflammatory hypothesis in the pathogenesis of cerebral cavernous malformations, *Neurosurgery* 61:693–702, 2007.

75. Inoue S, Liu W, Inoue K, et al: Combination of linkage and association studies for brain arteriovenous malformation, *Stroke* 38:1368–1370, 2007.

76. Gallione CJ, Richards JA, Letteboer TG, et al: *SMAD4* mutations found in unselected HHT patients, *J Med Genet* 43:793–797, 2006.

77. Bayrak-Toydemir P, McDonald J, Akarsu N, et al: A fourth locus for hereditary hemorrhagic telangiectasia maps to chromosome 7, *Am J Med Genet A* 140:2155–2162, 2006.

78. Cole SG, Begbie ME, Wallace GM, Shovlin CL: A new locus for hereditary haemorrhagic telangiectasia (HHT3) maps to chromosome 5, *J Med Genet* 42:577–582, 2005.

79. Marchuk DA, Srinivasan S, Squire TL, Zawistowski JS: Vascular morphogenesis: Tales of two syndromes, *Hum Mol Genet* 12:R97–R112, 2003.

80. Scharpfenecker M, van Dinther M, Liu Z, et al: BMP-9 signals via ALK1 and inhibits bFGF-induced endothelial cell proliferation and VEGF-stimulated angiogenesis, *J Cell Sci* 120:964–972, 2007.

81. David L, Mallet C, Mazerbourg S, et al: Identification of BMP9 and BMP10 as functional activators of the orphan activin receptor-like kinase 1 (ALK1) in endothelial cells, *Blood* 109:1953–1961, 2007.

82. Matsubara S, Mandzia JL, ter Brugge K, et al: Angiographic and clinical characteristics of patients with cerebral arteriovenous malformations associated with hereditary hemorrhagic telangiectasia, *AJNR Am J Neuroradiol* 21:1016–1020, 2000.

83. Maher CO, Piepgras DG, Brown RD Jr, et al: Cerebrovascular manifestations in 321 cases of hereditary hemorrhagic telangiectasia, *Stroke* 32:877–882, 2001.

84. Berman MF, Sciacca RR, Pile-Spellman J, et al: The epidemiology of brain arteriovenous malformations, *Neurosurgery* 47:389–396, 2000.

85. Pawlikowska L, Tran MN, Achrol AS, et al: Polymorphisms in transforming growth factor-ß-related genes *ALK1* and *ENG* are associated with sporadic brain arteriovenous malformations, *Stroke* 36:2278–2280, 2005.

86. Simon M, Franke D, Ludwig M, et al: Association of a polymorphism of the *ACVRL1* gene with sporadic arteriovenous malformations of the central nervous system, *J Neurosurg* 104:945–949, 2006.

87. Simon M, Schramm J, Ludwig M, Ziegler A, Author reply to letter by Young WL, et al: Arteriovenous malformation, *J Neurosurg* 106:732–733, 2007.

88. Rogers MS, D'Amato RJ: The effect of genetic diversity on angiogenesis, *Exp Cell Res* 312:561–574, 2006.

89. Shaked Y, Bertolini F, Man S, et al: Genetic heterogeneity of the vasculogenic phenotype parallels angiogenesis: Implications for cellular surrogate marker analysis of antiangiogenesis, *Cancer Cell* 7:101–111, 2005.

90. Satomi J, Mount RJ, Toporsian M, et al: Cerebral vascular abnormalities in a murine model of hereditary hemorrhagic telangiectasia, *Stroke* 34:783–789, 2003.

91. Xu B, Wu YQ, Huey M, et al: Vascular endothelial growth factor induces abnormal microvasculature in the endoglin heterozygous mouse brain, *J Cereb Blood Flow Metab* 24:237–244, 2004.

92. Fogarty-Mack P, Pile-Spellman J, Hacein-Bey L, et al: The effect of arteriovenous malformations on the distribution of intracerebral arterial pressures, *AJNR Am J Neuroradiol* 17:1443–1449, 1996.

93. Kader A, Young WL: The effects of intracranial arteriovenous malformations on cerebral hemodynamics, *Neurosurg Clin N Am* 7:767–781, 1996.

94. Young WL, Pile-Spellman J, Prohovnik I, et al: Columbia University AVM Study Project: Evidence for adaptive autoregulatory displacement in hypotensive cortical territories adjacent to arteriovenous malformations, *Neurosurgery* 34:601–610, 1994.

95. Spetzler RF, Wilson CB, Weinstein P, et al: Normal perfusion pressure breakthrough theory, *Clin Neurosurg* 25:651–672, 1978.

96. Nornes H, Grip A: Hemodynamic aspects of cerebral arteriovenous malformations, *J Neurosurg* 53:456–464, 1980.

97. Mast H, Mohr JP, Osipov A, et al: "Steal" is an unestablished mechanism for the clinical presentation of cerebral arteriovenous malformations, *Stroke* 26:1215–1220, 1995.

98. Young WL, Kader A, Ornstein E, et al: Cerebral hyperemia after arteriovenous malformation resection is related to "breakthrough" complications but not to feeding artery pressure. Columbia University AVM Study Project, *Neurosurgery* 38:1085–1093, 1996.

99. Young WL, Prohovnik I, Ornstein E, et al: The effect of arteriovenous malformation resection on cerebrovascular reactivity to carbon dioxide, *Neurosurgery* 27:257–267, 1990.

100. Rosell A, Lo EH: Multiphasic roles for matrix metalloproteinases after stroke, *Curr Opin Pharmacol* 8:82–89, 2008.

101. Szabo MD, Crosby G, Sundaram P, et al: Hypertension does not cause spontaneous hemorrhage of intracranial arteriovenous malformations, *Anesthesiology* 70:761–763, 1989.

102. Jayaraman MV, Marcellus ML, Hamilton S, et al: Neurologic complications of arteriovenous malformation embolization using liquid embolic agents, *AJNR Am J Neuroradiol* 29:242–246, 2008.

103. Katayama Y, Tsubokawa T, Hirayiama T, Himi K: Continuous monitoring of jugular bulb oxygen saturation as a measure of the shunt flow of cerebral arteriovenous malformations, *J Neurosurg* 80:826–833, 1994.

104. Spetzler RF, Martin NA, Carter LP, et al: Surgical management of large AVM's by staged embolization and operative excision, *J Neurosurg* 67:17–28, 1987.

105. Rosner MJ: Cerebral perfusion pressure: Link between intracranial pressure and systemic circulation. In Wood JH, editor: *Cerebral Blood Flow: Physiologic and Clinical Aspects*, New York, 1987, McGraw-Hill, pp 425–448.

106. Zornow MH, Todd MM, Moore SS: The acute cerebral effects of changes in plasma osmolality and oncotic pressure, *Anesthesiology* 67:936–941, 1987.

107. Warner DS, Boehland LA: The effects of iso-osmolal hemodilution on post-ischemic brain water content in the rat, *Anesthesiology* 68:86–91, 1988.

108. Drummond JC, Patel PM, Cole DJ, Kelly PJ: The effect of the reduction of colloid oncotic pressure, with and without reduction of osmolality, on post-traumatic cerebral edema, *Anesthesiology* 88:993–1002, 1998.

109. Kaieda R, Todd MM, Warner DS: Prolonged reduction in colloid oncotic pressure does not increase brain edema following cryogenic injury in rabbits, *Anesthesiology* 71:554–560, 1989.

110. Kaieda R, Todd MM, Cook LN, Warner DS: Acute effects of changing plasma osmolality and colloid oncotic pressure on the formation of brain edema after cryogenic injury, *Neurosurgery* 24:671–678, 1989.

111. Lanier WL: Glucose management during cardiopulmonary bypass: Cardiovascular and neurologic implications, *Anesth Analg* 72:423–427, 1991.

112. Lam AM, Winn HR, Cullen BF, Sundling N: Hyperglycemia and neurological outcome in patients with head injury, *J Neurosurg* 75:545–551, 1991.

113. Busto R, Dietrich WD, Globus MY-T, et al: Small differences in intraischemic brain temperature critically determine the extent of ischemic neuronal injury, *J Cereb Blood Flow Metab* 7:729–738, 1987.

114. Busto R, Dietrich WD, Globus MY-T, Ginsberg MD: The importance of brain temperature in cerebral ischemic injury, *Stroke* 20:1113–1114, 1989.

115. Clifton GL, Allen S, Barrodale P, et al: A phase II study of moderate hypothermia in severe brain injury, *J Neurotrauma* 10:263–271, 1993:discussion 273.

116. Marion DW, Penrod LE, Kelsey SF, et al: Treatment of traumatic brain injury with moderate hypothermia, *N Engl J Med* 336:540–546, 1997.

117. Baker KZ, Young WL, Stone JG, et al: Deliberate mild intraoperative hypothermia for craniotomy, *Anesthesiology* 81:361–367, 1994.

118. Sessler DI: Complications and treatment of mild hypothermia, *Anesthesiology* 95:531–543, 2001.

119. Frank SM, Beattie C, Christopherson R, et al: Unintentional hypothermia is associated with postoperative myocardial ischemia. The Perioperative Ischemia Randomized Anesthesia Trial Study Group, *Anesthesiology* 78:468–476, 1993.

120. Stapelfeldt C, Lobo EP, Brown R, Talke PO: Intraoperative clonidine administration to neurosurgical patients, *Anesth Analg* 100:226–232, 2005.
121. Chen H, Chopp M: Effect of mild hyperthermia on the ischemic infarct volume after middle cerebral artery occlusion in the rat, *Neurology* 41:1133–1135, 1991.
122. Morgan MK, Sekhon LH, Finfer S, Grinnell V: Delayed neurological deterioration following resection of arteriovenous malformations of the brain, *J Neurosurg* 90:695–701, 1999.
123. Talke P, Chen R, Thomas B, et al: The hemodynamic and adrenergic effects of perioperative dexmedetomidine infusion after vascular surgery, *Anesth Analg* 90:834–839, 2000.
124. Lawton MT: UCSF Arteriovenous Malformation Study Project: Spetzler-Martin grade III arteriovenous malformations: Surgical results and a modification of the grading scale, *Neurosurgery* 52:740–748, 2003.
125. Lazar RM, Marshall RS, Pile-Spellman J, et al: Anterior translocation of language in patients with left cerebral arteriovenous malformations, *Neurology* 49:802–808, 1997.
126. Lazar RM, Marshall RS, Pile-Spellman J, et al: Interhemispheric transfer of language in patients with left frontal cerebral arteriovenous malformation, *Neuropsychologia* 38:1325–1332, 2000.

Chapter 16

OCCLUSIVE CEREBROVASCULAR DISEASE: ANESTHETIC CONSIDERATIONS

Ian A. Herrick • Randall T. Higashida • Adrian W. Gelb

The popularity of carotid endarterectomy (CEA) has shifted repeatedly since its introduction in the early 1950s. The number of procedures performed annually rose steadily until 1985, when CEA was ranked the third most common operation performed in the United States (Fig. 16-1).[1] However, by 1991, the popularity of the procedure had decreased dramatically owing to the absence of properly designed prospective studies supporting the efficacy of the procedure[2] and the wide variation in reported morbidity and mortality. Following reports from several large, well-designed, randomized trials[3-5] confirming its efficacy in selected patients, the popularity of CEA again increased, and by 1996, the number of procedures performed in the United States exceeded that reported in 1985.

Current surgical guidelines for CEA[6-8] define an important role for this operation in the prevention of stroke, and evidence suggests that the availability of well-founded clinical guidelines has influenced practice.[9] It has been estimated that approximately 103,000 to 117,000 CEA inpatient procedures continue to be performed in the United States annually.[10] Although CEA remains the gold standard and the most commonly performed surgical procedure for the prevention of stroke, considerable progress has also been made since the turn of the century in relation to the emergence of carotid angioplasty and stenting (CAS) procedures.[11-14] Although current emphasis remains focused on the inclusion of patients undergoing CAS procedures in the numerous trials and registries, carotid stenting procedures are performed in centers around the world where interventional neuroradiologic expertise is available. It has been reported that 7000 to 10,000 CAS procedures were performed in the United States in 2006.[7]

It is anticipated that both CEA and CAS will remain important treatments for the prevention of stroke. Directed at patients with advanced cerebrovascular disease, both operations represent challenging procedures from the anesthesiologist's perspective because many of the patients are elderly and have significant coexisting disease involving other organ systems. This chapter reviews the anesthetic considerations for, and management of, patients undergoing CEA and briefly explores the roles for CEA and CAS procedures for the prevention of stroke.

PHYSIOLOGIC CONSIDERATIONS

Carotid revascularization procedures involve the manipulation of the blood supply to the brain. As a consequence, the rationale and recommendations for the management of patients undergoing these procedures are founded on a clear understanding of neurovascular anatomy and physiology.

The brain is highly active metabolically but is essentially devoid of oxygen and glucose reserves, making it dependent on the continuous delivery of oxygen and glucose by the cerebral circulation. Cerebral blood flow (CBF) is provided by the internal carotid arteries (approximately 80%) and the vertebral arteries (approximately 20%). These major arteries anastomose at the base of the brain to form the circle of Willis, which provides the primary collateral vascular channel between the cerebral hemispheres. However, other collateral channels between the intracranial and extracranial circulations (e.g., through the orbit) may become well developed in patients with occlusive disease of the internal carotid artery.

CBF depends on cerebral perfusion pressure (CPP) and cerebral vascular resistance (CVR) according to the following equation:

$$CBF = CPP - CVR$$

where *CPP* represents the difference between mean arterial blood pressure and intracranial pressure or central venous pressure, whichever is greater, and *CVR* is a function of blood viscosity and the diameter of the cerebral vessels. Normally CBF is autoregulated in response to cerebral metabolic requirements, a process common to many specialized vascular beds. During CEA, however, optimization of CBF is hampered by the fact that the only factors readily amenable to intraoperative manipulation are arterial blood pressure and arterial carbon dioxide tension (Pa_{CO_2}), which affect CPP and CVR, respectively. Confounding this situation, our current understanding of the physiology of CBF is incomplete. For example, much of our understanding of cerebral hemodynamic changes during anesthesia is based on the assessment of changes that occur in larger vessels using techniques such as computed tomography (single-photon emission computed tomography [SPECT]) or transcranial Doppler ultrasonography (TCD) studies.[15-17] However, later work using orthogonal polarization spectral imaging of the sublingual microcirculation[18] suggests that the flow observed in larger vessels after the induction of anesthesia may not parallel changes in flow observed in the capillary network. These findings raise questions about our ability to predict microvascular perfusion consistently on the basis of the dynamic behavior of large vessels.

Carbon Dioxide Tension

CBF is exquisitely sensitive and directly related to Pa_{CO_2}. CBF changes 1 to 2 mL/100 g/min for every 1–mm Hg change in Pa_{CO_2} within the range from 20 to 80 mm Hg. The most appropriate level of Pa_{CO_2} during CEA has not been definitively

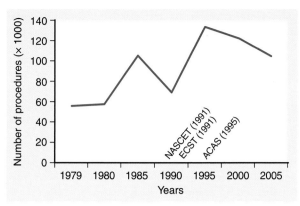

Figure 16–1 Trends in the number of carotid endarterectomy procedures performed in the United States (1979-2005). ACAS, Asymptomatic Carotid Atherosclerosis Study; ECST, European Carotid Surgery Trial; NASCET, North American Symptomatic Carotid Endarterectomy Trial. *(Adapted from American Heart Association Statistics Committee and Stroke Statistics Subcommittee. Heart Disease and Stroke Statistics 2008 Update. Circulation 2008;117;e25-e146. Available at http://circ. ahajournals.org/cgi/content/full/117/4/e25.)*

established. Hypocapnia has been advocated on the premise that vasoconstriction in areas of normal (CO_2-responsive) brain will potentially divert blood flow toward ischemic regions, the "Robin Hood" effect.[19,20] Conversely, deliberate hypercapnia has been postulated to increase global CBF and as a consequence may improve perfusion to potentially ischemic regions.[21] However, both concepts have been criticized on the grounds that studies of regional cerebral blood flow during carotid cross-clamping have demonstrated that the regional CBF response to changes in $Paco_2$ is not entirely predictable.[22] Cerebral autoregulation has been reported to be completely lost during carotid cross-clamping under hypercapnic conditions and partially lost during hypocapnia, illustrating the relatively greater importance of blood pressure control during CEA. Furthermore, increasing $Paco_2$ causes vasodilation in normal brain and has been reported to result in a potential steal of blood flow from ischemic zones in up to 23% of patients.[22] A similar steal phenomenon has also been reported during CEA in association with cerebral vasodilatation that accompanies the administration of volatile anesthetic drugs such as sevoflurane.[23]

Compounding decisions regarding the appropriate management of $Paco_2$ during CEA is the fact that other disease processes also may alter the response to changes in arterial carbon dioxide tension. For example, patients with diabetes mellitus, a common condition among patients presenting for CEA, have been reported to display impairment of cerebrovascular responsiveness to hypercapnia during anesthesia with propofol, sevoflurane, or isoflurane.[24,25] Although the level of impairment was observed to be related to the severity of the diabetes (i.e., glycosylated hemoglobin value and extent of retinopathy), the level of impairment observed among individual patients was not consistently predictable.

In the absence of a clear clinical benefit associated with either hypercapnia or hypocapnia, or a readily available means to titrate either to a cerebrovascular effect, the most prudent approach to the ventilatory management of patients undergoing CEA is maintenance of normocapnia. This is accomplished by reference to preoperative arterial blood gas measurements or, if these are not available, by ventilating to a $Paco_2$ value that produces a normal pH in a patient who does not have a coexisting metabolic acidosis. This approach attempts to achieve a balance between the optimization of CBF and the avoidance of cerebral steal.

Blood Pressure

Normally, CBF is maintained relatively constant within the range of mean arterial blood pressure, from approximately 50 to 150 mm Hg. Beyond this range the limit of vasomotor activity is exceeded and CBF becomes directly dependent on changes in CPP. In patients with preexisting chronic hypertension, both the upper and lower limits of autoregulation are shifted toward higher pressures.

A deliberate increase in intraoperative blood pressure has been advocated during CEA on the basis of the premise that autoregulation will maintain normal CBF in areas of healthy brain while flow will be increased in areas of the brain that are hypoperfused owing to vasomotor paralysis or atherosclerotic narrowing.[21] The CBF response to changes in $Paco_2$ is depressed in patients with cerebrovascular disease as well as during carotid cross-clamping (as discussed previously), suggesting that blood vessels distal to regions of atherosclerotic narrowing are operating near the limits of autoregulatory vasodilation.[26] Under these conditions, improvement in CBF is likely to depend on increases in CPP. Higher stump pressures and reversal of ischemic changes on the electroencephalogram (EEG) have been reported in response to induced hypertension during cross-clamping.[19,27]

However, deliberate hypertension is not devoid of risk. Excessive increases in CPP may cause cerebral hemorrhage or edema formation in regions of the brain that have lost autoregulation ability. In addition, patients most at risk for development of cerebral ischemia—those with inadequate collateral blood flow—have been shown to be the least responsive to induced hypertension.[28] However these patients are most in need of any safe maneuver, including judicious induced hypertension, that may increase flow to the ischemic region. In patients with ischemic heart disease, systemic vasoconstriction may lead to an adverse myocardial oxygen balance. The incidence of myocardial ischemia has been reported to be higher among patients who receive phenylephrine infusions or metaraminol to increase blood pressure during CEA.[29,30]

On the basis of the available evidence, the routine intraoperative elevation of blood pressure above the patient's normal level is not recommended. Instead, the extent and patency of the collateral circulation should be discussed prior to induction of anesthesia. In patients with good collaterals, careful maintenance of blood pressure within the normal preoperative range is recommended. Spontaneous increases in systolic blood pressure of up to 20% above normal at the time of cross-clamping are acceptable. In patients with poor collaterals, blood pressure may be cautiously increased up to about 20% to 30% above baseline, with consideration of the concerns previously described. Excessive spontaneous increases may reflect cerebral ischemia, a possibility that should be considered before the increase in blood pressure is controlled pharmacologically.

PREOPERATIVE CONSIDERATIONS

Carotid endarterectomy and carotid stenting procedures are interventions designed to reduce the risk of stroke among patients with advanced cerebrovascular disease. In view of the fact that most patients presenting for these procedures are elderly and many have coronary artery disease, arterial hypertension, peripheral vascular disease, chronic obstructive pulmonary disease, diabetes mellitus, renal insufficiency, or a combination of such conditions (Table 16-1),[31] it is not surprising that these treatments also carry substantial risk of death or serious morbidity. The benefit of these procedures resides in the fact that for the majority of patients with advanced disease, the risk of stroke or death without intervention is higher than the risk associated with the procedure. As a consequence, appropriate selection and optimization of candidates for these procedures represent important opportunities to mitigate perioperative risk.

Patient Selection

Overwhelming evidence supports the efficacy of CEA combined with best medical therapy for the prevention of stroke among appropriately selected patients. Two large multicenter randomized trials conducted in North America[3] and Europe[4] two decades ago validated the role of CEA in the treatment of patients with symptomatic high-grade carotid disease. Current American Heart Association (AHA) guidelines recommend CEA in symptomatic patients with carotid stenosis of 50% to 99% if the risk of perioperative stroke or death is less than 6%.[7,8,32] Pooled data from the major CEA trials involving symptomatic patients with stenosis greater than 50% confirm these recommendations and show that the number of patients needed to treat (NNT) to prevent 1 stroke over a 2-year period is 9 for men and 36 for women.[8] Benefit is also greater in older rather than younger patients, particularly those older than 75 years, with an NNT value of 5.

For asymptomatic patients the data are less robust. The risk of stroke is lower in asymptomatic patients than in patients with symptomatic disease, and as a consequence, the benefit of surgical intervention is realized only if the procedure can be performed with a lower 30-day risk of stroke and death. AHA guidelines[6,33] recommend CEA for asymptomatic patients with carotid stenosis of 60% to 99% if the perioperative risk of stroke or death is less than 3%.

It is noteworthy, in relation to perioperative risk, that the studies upon which many of these recommendations are based

include stringent exclusion criteria that eliminated patients with significant comorbid conditions. As a consequence, current recommendations for CEA are also influenced by clinical factors that may modify the risk and the potential for benefit (stroke prevention), such as life expectancy, age, gender, the presence of coexisting medical conditions, and the outcome performance of the surgeon and surgical team who perform the procedure. For example, several investigators have reported a positive correlation between outcome and the number of procedures performed in individual centers.[34-36] In view of the trend toward public disclosure of outcome data for a variety of procedures including CEA,[37,38] renewed interest will be focused on ensuring that all members of the care team are collaboratively committed to achieving best practices in relation to patient selection, preoperative assessment and optimization, and perioperative management and care for patients undergoing CEA.

The Role for Carotid Angioplasty and Stenting

Since the 1980s there has been an exponential increase in interest and use of endovascular approaches to treating carotid artery stenosis. This increase has paralleled the growth in the use of these techniques in other vascular specialties, especially in the coronary and peripheral vascular beds. Further impetus has come from advances in the development of catheter, balloon, stent, and endovascular emboli-trapping devices and has been encouraged by recognition of the many potential advantages of endovascular approaches, particularly in high-risk patients (Box 16-1). Perceived benefits of an endovascular approach are that it is minimally invasive, it avoids surgical wounds and their complications, and it can generally be accomplished with local anesthesia and sedation.

The technique employs standard endovascular approaches from a transfemoral arterial approach. Patients are routinely premedicated with aspirin (ASA) 325 mg and clopidogrel 75 mg 3 to 5 days prior to the procedure. A diagnostic catheter is advanced under fluoroscopic guidance, and the vascular anatomy of the aorta, neck, and head is imaged. Once the vessel to be treated is fully defined, an 8 F guiding catheter or 6 F long sheath is placed from the femoral artery and proximal to the lesion in the middle or low cervical common carotid artery. After systemic heparinization is given (70-100 units/kg) and an activated clotting time value is confirmed to be increased to about two times baseline value, a fine (e.g. 0.014-inch) steerable guidewire, often in combination with a distal filter protection device, is advanced across the stenosis

---

Table 16–1 Medical Characteristics of the 2256 Patients Eligible for Inclusion in the North American Symptomatic Carotid Endarterectomy Trial

Medical Condition (Based on History)	Symptomatic Patients (%)
Angina	24
Previous myocardial infarction	20
Hypertension	60
Claudication	15
Smoker:	
Current	37
Previous	40
Diabetes mellitus	19

Adapted from North American Symptomatic Carotid Endarterectomy Trial: Methods, patient characteristics, and progress. Stroke 1991;22:711-720.

BOX 16–1 *Potential Indications for Carotid Angioplasty-Stent*

Previous carotid endarterectomy
Contralateral carotid artery occlusion
Previous radical neck dissection or radiation therapy to neck region
Target lesion above C2 (level of jaw) or low cervical carotid lesions
Carotid dissection
Tandem lesions with ≥70% stenosis, intracranial stenosis, or occlusion
Significant cardiorespiratory comorbidity
Requires concurrent major cardiac or aortic surgery
Inability to extend neck
Contralateral laryngeal nerve palsy
At risk for wound infection (e.g., immunosuppressed, tracheostomy)

and deployed 2 to 4 cm distal to the lesion to be treated. The distal filter devices are expandable umbrella-like devices that are deployed distal to the stenosis to trap emboli released during the angioplasty and stent deployment; their benefits are still subject to ongoing trials.

The appropriate size (e.g. 2.5-4 mm × 40 mm) angioplasty balloon is then placed across the stenosis and, once positioned, is inflated to high pressure (up to 8-12 atm [this isn't an acronym, it's the abbreviation for "atmospheres"]) for 60 to 120 seconds to predilate the stenotic lesion. Aggressive balloon dilation may increase the risk of complications, and residual stenosis is mostly related to calcification, which does not resolve with repeated dilations. Thereafter, a nitinol self-expanding stent of appropriate length (2-4 cm) and diameter (4-10 mm) is deployed across the lesion to completely bridge and cover the plaque in both the cervical internal and common carotid arteries. Following stent deployment, a larger balloon that matches the normal luminal diameter of the cervical internal carotid artery or the common carotid arteries is then used to dilate the lesion to more than 80% to 90% of the normal lumen, to ensure that maximal restoration to normal vessel size is achieved. Following final balloon angioplasty across the stented lesion, the distal filter protection device is recaptured and withdrawn.

A post-stent angiogram is then obtained to ensure restoration of normal luminal diameter, full patency of the stent, and maintenance of normal filling of the more distal intracranial blood vessels. The patient is then rechecked neurologically, and in most instances, a femoral arterial closure device is placed to ensure hemostasis. Patients are usually monitored in the neurointensive care unit or other high-dependency monitoring room for 24 hours; if stable, they are discharged home with prescriptions for ASA 325 mg indefinitely and clopidogrel 75 mg for at least 6 weeks after the stenting procedure.

The safety and efficacy of endovascular approaches for carotid stenting has been a subject of much interest.[39,40] Unfortunately, comparative analysis of studies performed before 1999 is confounded by inconsistencies in the sample populations, lesion characteristics, endovascular techniques, and outcome.[41] However, the overall reported rate of technical success was greater than 95%, with acceptably low morbidity and mortality, a finding that prompted randomized well-controlled trials. A summary of the salient features and findings of these trials (some are ongoing) follows.

The *Carotid and Vertebral Transluminal Angioplasty Study (CAVATAS)*[42] was a large, prospective, randomized, multicenter trial comparing CEA with carotid angioplasty and stenting. Subjects were 504 patients with a symptomatic stenosis at 70% or greater and were randomly assigned to undergo either angioplasty and stenting or surgery. There was no significant difference between the groups in the risk of stroke or death related to either procedure or the rate of disabling stroke or death within 30 days of treatment, which was 6% in both groups. Preliminary analysis of long-term survival, up to 3 years after randomization, has found no difference in the rate of ipsilateral stroke or any disabling stroke. However, the rate of re-stenosis in the endovascular group (18%) was twice that in the surgical cohort (9%).

The *Stenting and Angioplasty with Protection in Patients at High Risk for Endarterectomy (SAPPHIRE)* trial[12,43] was a multicenter, prospective, randomized study that compared carotid artery stenting using an embolic protection device with surgical endarterectomy in 747 patients with specific comorbidities including greater than 50% symptomatic stenosis or

greater than 80% asymptomatic stenosis. Primary endpoints were a composite of death, stroke, or myocardial infarction at 30 days and ipsilateral stroke or death within 1 year. The study concluded that stenting with distal embolic protection is not inferior to endarterectomy ($P = .004$). It just narrowly missed showing statistical superiority of stenting ($P = .053$). Overall the risk of stroke, death, or myocardial infarction at 30 days was 39% lower with stenting. The risk of ipsilateral stroke or death was 7.9% lower with stenting at 1 year. The SAPPHIRE trial is the first to demonstrate the efficacy of distal embolic filtration protection in a high-risk population. Nevertheless, the study remains controversial because 55% of patients were excluded from randomization as poor surgical candidates, more than 20% in each treatment group had recurrent stenosis, and the inclusion of myocardial infarction in the composite endpoint obscures the effects of stroke and death, which were primary endpoints in other trials.

EVA-3S, the *Endarterectomy vs. Angioplasty in Severe Carotid Stenosis Study*,[44] was designed to compare carotid stenting with or without distal embolic protection and endarterectomy. Primary endpoints were recurrent stroke or death within 30 days or 4 years. The trial was prematurely halted because of safety concerns and futility, because the 30-day stroke or death rates were 3.5% after endarterectomy and 9.6% after stenting. This study was criticized because the physicians involved in the carotid stenting group were inadequately trained and physician participation in the study required experience with fewer than five cases.

SPACE, the *Stent-Protected Percutaneous Angioplasty of the Carotid vs. Endarterectomy* trial,[45] was a prospective, randomized, multicenter trial of carotid stenting and endarterectomy in patients with severe symptomatic carotid stenosis.[45] The per-protocol analysis showed equivalent periprocedural complication rates with that for carotid stenting being 6.84% and that for endarterectomy being 6.34%.

CREST, the *Carotid Revascularization: Endarterectomy vs. Stent Trial*,[46,47] is sponsored by the National Institute of Neurological Disorders and Stroke. It is a prospective, randomized, multicenter trial being conducted in symptomatic and asymptomatic patients. The primary endpoint consists of stroke, death, or myocardial infarction within 30 days, or ipsilateral stroke within 60 days of the procedure. This is an important trial that will define the role of carotid artery stenting for primary and secondary stroke prevention in the United States. The trial completed enrollment in 2008, but results will not be known for 18 to 24 months after that.

In summary, although carotid angioplasty and stenting has become quite well integrated into clinical practice, ongoing clinical trials will further define the most suitable patients, the long-term patency rates, and the benefits of embolic protection devices. However, on the basis of the preceding studies, the Clinical Expert Consensus Document on Carotid Stenting, sponsored by five cardiovascular and radiologic professional societies, states that "carotid artery stenting is a reasonable alternative to CEA, particularly in patients at high risk for CEA" but "there is insufficient evidence to support CAS in high risk patients with asymptomatic stenosis <80% or in any patient without high risk features."[47] At present CEA remains the gold standard.

Preanesthesia Assessment

In all patients presenting for CEA, preexisting medical conditions should be optimized prior to surgery. However, achieving this goal is likely to become increasingly challenging because current evidence suggests that outcome is improved by timely access to surgery. On the basis of a combined 5-year analysis of patients in the North American Symptomatic Carotid Endarterectomy Trial (NASCET) and European Carotid Surgery Trial (ECST) who had symptomatic stenosis 50% or greater, the benefit of CEA is highest (greatest risk reduction for perioperative stroke or death) when the procedure is performed within 2 weeks of the cerebral ischemic event.[48] These investigators report that the NNT is 5 if patients were randomly assigned to therapy within 2 weeks of the last transient ischemic attack (TIA) and 125 if they were randomly assigned more than 12 weeks after the last TIA. Furthermore, the benefit from surgery declines significantly more rapidly in women than in men. Although many centers will be challenged to achieve surgery within 2 weeks of the onset of symptoms, these data provide a clear incentive to ensure that preoperative assessment and optimization is conducted in an efficient and timely manner once the decision to proceed to surgery has been made.

The preoperative visit should include an assessment of the patient's state of health based on history, pertinent physical examination, and chart review. The head and neck should be examined to identify potential airway problems or evidence of positional ischemia. Catheter angiography or magnetic resonance angiography should also be reviewed to identify patients at higher risk due to high-grade contralateral carotid disease or poor collateral circulation.

Special attention should be directed toward the assessment of coexisting disease. A variety of indices have been proposed over the years to assist with the identification of patients at risk for development of perioperative complications. The risk stratification scheme for patients undergoing CEA that was proposed and validated by Sundt and colleagues[49,50] combines medical, neurologic, and radiologic risk factors to determine the perioperative risk of major complications (Tables 16-2 and 16-3). The scheme has been in widespread use for many years and continues to provide a helpful overview of factors that contribute to perioperative complications.

A 2006 comparison of the reliability of several perioperative risk indices as predictors of postoperative complications following CEA is particularly relevant to the assessment of these patients.[51] Evaluating postoperative complications including death, stroke, cardiac and noncardiac medical complications,

minor neurologic events, and wound complications, Press and associates[51] compared four indices widely used to predict risk in patients undergoing noncardiac surgery—American Society of Anesthesiologists index,[52] the index proposed by Goldman and colleagues,[53] the index proposed by Detsky and associates,[54] and the Revised Cardiac Risk (RCR) Index[55]—and two indices developed specifically in relation to risk associated with CEA—that proposed by Halm and coworkers[56] and that proposed by Tu and associates.[57] All indices performed similarly as predictors of noncardiac medical complications and, with the exception of the Tu index, as predictors of perioperative cardiac complications. The Halm index, Tu index, and RCR Index were reported to be the most reliable predictors of the combined risk of stroke or death (Tables 16-4 and 16-5). The Halm index and the RCR Index were identified as the most reliable predictors across the range of major and minor perioperative complications studied. The investigators note that the superior performance of the Halm index was expected because their study was conducted using the patient data from which the index was derived. In contrast to the RCR Index and Halm index, the index proposed by Tu and colleagues[57] was derived from a study of Canadian patients undergoing CEA and reported a lower incidence of coronary artery disease but a substantially higher burden of symptomatic carotid disease (69% vs. 31%) and a consequently higher death and stroke rate. It is not clear whether the index proposed by Tu and associates[57] represent a more reliable predictor in circumstances in which the majority of patients presenting for CEA have symptomatic disease.

Although the risk-stratification scheme developed by Sundt and colleagues[49,50] was not included in the comparison, it is noteworthy that the scheme has a number of factors in common with the indices proposed by both Tu and Halm.

Table 16–3   Risk Factors Used in Risk Stratification for Patients Undergoing Carotid Endarterectomy

Type of Risk	Risk Factors
Medical risk	Angina
	Myocardial infarction (<6 months)
	Congestive heart failure
	Severe hypertension (>180/110 mm Hg)
	Chronic obstructive lung disease
	Age >70 years
	Severe obesity
Neurologic risk	Progressing deficit
	New deficit (<24 hours)
	Frequent daily transient ischemic attacks
	Multiple cerebral infarcts
Angiographic risk	Contralateral carotid artery occlusion
	Internal carotid artery siphon stenosis
	Proximal or distal plaque extension
	High carotid bifurcation
	Presence of soft thrombus

Adapted from Sundt TM Jr, Sandok BA, Whisnant JP: Carotid endarterectomy: Complications and preoperative assessment of risk. Mayo Clinic Proc 1975;50:301-306.

Table 16–2   Preoperative Risk Stratification for Patients Undergoing Carotid Endarterectomy

Risk Group	Characteristics	Total Morbidity and Mortality (%)
1	Neurologically stable, no major medical or angiographic risk	1
2	Neurologically stable, significant angiographic risk, no major medical risk	2
3	Neurologically stable, major medical risk, major angiographic risk	7
4	Neurologically unstable, major medical or angiographic risk	10

Adapted from Sundt TM Jr, Sandok BA, Whisnant JP: Carotid endarterectomy: Complications and preoperative assessment of risk. Mayo Clinic Proc 1975;50:301-306.

The presence of significant heart disease (especially active coronary artery disease or a history of congestive heart failure) or the presence of significant contralateral carotid disease (particularly carotid occlusion) should be viewed with particular caution in patients presenting for CEA. Similarly, consistent with the risk factors identified by Sundt and colleagues,[49,50] Halm and coworkers[56] note that patients with unstable ischemic neurologic symptoms, who were excluded from the patient population upon which their index was developed (e.g., crescendo TIAs and stroke-in-evolution), face a particularly ominous prognosis in relation to CEA, with combined rates of death and stroke of 28.6% and 57.1%, respectively, on the basis of this study experience.[56]

Cardiac complications have been reported to be a primary source of mortality associated with CEA.[58-60] As noted previously, a number of factors have been reported to increase perioperative cardiac morbidity and mortality. Some investigators have advocated routine coronary angiography[59] prior to CEA; however, little evidence supports the premise that routine preoperative coronary angiography, and consequent prophylactic coronary revascularization, improves cardiac outcome in patients with stable disease.[61-63] It seems more reasonable to assume that all patients presenting for CEA have atherosclerotic heart disease and to evaluate perioperative risk in relation to each patient's functional status. Current recommendations support the consideration of additional noninvasive testing, such as exercise stress testing, dobutamine stress echocardiography, and dipyridamole myocardial perfusion imaging, in patients scheduled for CEA (intermediate-risk surgery) with one or more risk factors for perioperative cardiac complications and poor functional capacity.[62] Testing should be directed toward patients for whom the results are likely to influence perioperative management. Patients with active cardiac conditions, such as unstable coronary artery disease, congestive heart failure, significant arrhythmias, or severe valvular disease, require preoperative evaluation and treatment.[63] These high-risk patients may be considered for CEA staged or combined with a coronary artery bypass graft (CABG) procedure.

Available evidence remains inadequate to allow definitive conclusions to be drawn regarding the staging of CEA with CABG surgery. Despite many individual accounts of experience with staged or combined procedures, the most recent (2007) American College of Cardiology / American Heart Association guidelines on carotid stenting[7] provides the following recommendations:

> "In patients who require CABG, the risk of perioperative stroke is 4-fold higher in those with a past history of TIA or stroke and 10-fold higher in asymptomatic patients with carotid stenosis greater than 75%. Patients being considered for cardiac surgery should undergo a preoperative carotid duplex exam if any of the following are present: carotid bruit, age greater than 65 years, peripheral arterial disease, history of TIA or stroke, smoking, or left main coronary artery disease. Patients with a significant carotid stenosis are candidates for carotid revascularization. The timing and sequence of revascularization are influenced by the symptom status of the patient, the severity of disease, and the urgency of revascularization."

Table 16–4 Multivariate Odds Ratios (ORs) for Complications after Carotid Endarterectomy. Based on the Revised Cardiac Risk Index

Revised Cardiac Risk Index (n - 2893)	OR for Major Cardiac Complications (95% Confidence Interval)*
1. High-risk type of surgery	2.4 (1.3-4.2)
2. Ischemic heart disease	2.4 (1.3-4.2)
3. History of congestive heart failure	1.9 (1.1-3.5)
4. History of cerebrovascular disease	3.2 (1.8-6.0)
5. Insulin therapy for diabetes mellitus	3.0 (1.3-7.1)
6. Preoperative serum creatinine level (>2.0 mg/dL)	3.0 (1.4-6.8)

Data from Lee TH, Marcantonio ER, Mangione CM, et al: Derivation and prospective validation of a simple index for prediction of cardiac risk of major noncardiac surgery. Circulation 1999;100:1043-1049.

Table 16–5 Multivariate Odds Ratios for Complications after Carotid Endarterectomy. Based on the Halm and the TU Indices

Index	OR for Death and Stroke (95% CI)*	OR for Fatal + Nonfatal Stroke (95% CI)
Halm Index (n = 1972)		
Stroke as indication for surgery	3.06 (1.68-5.58)	2.96 (1.57-5.60)
Active coronary artery disease	3.59 (1.56-8.27)	4.07 (1.76-9.44)
Contralateral stenosis (>50%)	2.22 (1.28-3.83)	2.18 (1.22-3.88)
Tu Index (n = 6038)		
History of stroke or transient ischemic attack(s) (<6 months)	1.75 (1.39-2.20)	1.84 (1.42-2.39)
Contralateral carotid occlusion	1.72 (1.25-2.38)	Not applicable
History of atrial fibrillation	1.89 (1.29-2.76)	1.83 (1.18-2.83)
History of congestive heart failure	1.80 (1.15-2.81)	1.86 (1.12-3.08)
History of diabetes	1.28 (1.01-1.63)	Not applicable

CI, confidence interval; OR, odds ratio.
*"Death and stroke" indicates the 30-day rate of death and nonfatal stroke combined.
Data from Halm EA, Hannan EL, Rojas M, et al: Clinical and operative predictors of outcomes of carotid endarterectomy. J Vasc Surg 2005;42: 420-428; and Tu JV, Wang H, Bowyer B, et al: Risk factors for death or stroke after carotid endarterectomy: Observations from the Ontario Carotid Endarterectomy Registry. Stroke 2003;34:2568-2573.

CABG alone is reasonable for patients with asymptomatic carotid stenosis and critical left main disease, refractory acute coronary syndromes, or other indications for urgent CABG. In contrast, patients with recent (less than 2 weeks) TIA and carotid stenosis greater than 50% should be considered for urgent CEA, if CABG can be safely deferred for several days.

The most recent guidelines[64] suggest that CEA is recommended before or concomitant to CABG in patients with symptomatic carotid stenosis greater than 50% or asymptomatic carotid stenosis greater than 80%. The risks of simultaneous CEA and CABG are not clearly higher than the risks of separate surgery and include death in 4.7%, stroke in 3.0%, and MI in 2.2%. If the procedures are to be staged, complication rates are lower when carotid revascularization precedes CABG. For patients who can defer CABG for 4 to 5 weeks, enrollment in one of the high-risk CAS registries is a potential option. Since CAS patients are treated with clopidogrel for one month, it is best to defer CABG for 5 weeks."

Reviews of the national experiences with CEA and CEA combined with CABG from the United States[65] and Canada[66] support these recommendations. Both studies reported a higher procedural risk of stroke and death for the combined procedure (9.5%-13%, respectively). Mortality rates in both studies were similar to the risk of death following CABG surgery alone but, in contrast to the statistics reported in the ACC/AHA guidelines,[64] the risk of stroke was substantially higher for the combined procedure (5.4%-6.8%) than the risk of stroke following CABG alone (1.4%-1.8%). Hence, with the appropriate indications, combined CEA and CABG can be undertaken relatively safely with a modest increase in risk (particularly for stroke) that must be weighed against the anticipated benefits on an individual basis.

Over the past decade, considerable interest has also focused on pharmacologic interventions that may reduce the risk of perioperative cardiac events in high-risk patient groups. The aim of therapy is to mitigate perioperative conditions that lead to myocardial supply-demand imbalances or to promote stabilization of the coronary plaque and thereby reduce the incidence of ischemic events. β-Blockers, statins, and aspirin are the most prominent drugs used in this manner.

β-Blockers have attracted widespread interest since early reports were published demonstrating a marked reduction in the risk of perioperative myocardial infarction with their use.[67] However, subsequent studies have not consistently supported these results. The latest AHA guidelines for the perioperative assessment and care of patients undergoing noncardiac surgery support call for (1) the perioperative continuation of β-blockers for patients undergoing long-term β-blocker therapy for established indications, such as the treatment of angina, hypertension, and arrhythmias, and (2) the use of β-blockers for patients undergoing vascular surgery with high cardiac risk owing to documentation of ischemia by preoperative testing.[68] The guidelines also cautiously endorse the use of β-blocker therapy in patients with multiple risk factors who are scheduled for vascular surgical procedures. However, the writers of the guidelines note that little information is available to guide decisions regarding the choice of β-blocker drug, the ideal target population, duration of preoperative titration, or route of administration. In addition, practical concerns, such as how, when, how long, and by whom perioperative β-blocker therapy should ideally or practically be implemented, remain unaddressed and it remains unclear whether harm may be associated with β-blocker therapy in low-risk patients. Supporting these concerns, the study group for the Perioperative

Ischemic Evaluation (POISE) study[69] reported that perioperative administration of extended-release metoprolol (100 mg administered orally commencing 2-4 hours preoperatively) to high-risk patients undergoing noncardiac surgery (including major vascular procedures but excluding CEA) reduced the incidence of perioperative myocardial infarction but was associated with higher incidence of death, nonfatal stroke, and clinically significant hypotension and bradycardia than found in patients receiving placebo therapy.

In view of the controversy generated by the results of the POISE study and pending an opportunity for a review of the AHA recommendations concerning the perioperative administration of β-blockers, thoughtful commentary on this issue has suggested that practitioners should continue to apply the AHA guideline on the continuation of treatment for patients undergoing long-term β-blocker therapy for established indications because preoperative discontinuation of established β-blocker treatment has been shown to be associated with increased risk.[70,71] However, the results of the POISE study would suggest that initiating β-blocker therapy in the acute preoperative period may be inappropriate. Patients with ischemic heart disease or other established conditions for which β-blockers are indicated should commence therapy well in advance of the scheduled procedure.[70] Although patients undergoing CEA were not included in the POISE study, the latter advice would seem particularly prudent for patients scheduled for CEA, given the nature of the procedure and the attending risk of stroke, until further evidence is available to clarify the issue in this group of patients.

The AHA guidelines for the perioperative evaluation and care of patients undergoing noncardiac surgical procedures support the continuation of statin therapy in patients who are taking these medications prior to surgery.[68] The guidelines also suggest that statin use might be considered for patients undergoing vascular surgery with or without risk factors and for patients undergoing intermediate-risk procedures (which would include CEA) who have at least one clinical risk factor for perioperative cardiac complications. Perioperative cardiac benefits are believed to relate to plaque-stabilizing properties as well as antioxidant and anti-inflammatory effects. Similar effects have been reported in relation to carotid plaque.[72,73] Statin therapy has been reported to reduce the risk of perioperative stroke or death in patients undergoing CEA[74,75]; however, these benefits appear to be limited to symptomatic patients and do not appear to substantially reduce the incidence of adverse cardiac events.[68] Existing evidence would therefore suggest that the perioperative use of statin therapy is more likely to be beneficial in patients with CEA and a high risk of stroke rather than with cardiac complications.

Most patients who present for CEA are currently taking low-dose ASA as medical therapy for the prevention of stroke. Evidence is less clear with respect to a potential beneficial effect on cardiac outcome, although some evidence suggests that preoperative ASA withdrawal may be associated with a higher risk of adverse cardiac events.[73] In view of its beneficial effects in relation to stroke prevention, most surgeons performing CEA prefer that patients keep taking low-dose ASA throughout the perioperative period.

Several studies have reported that uncontrolled or inadequately controlled preoperative arterial hypertension (systolic blood pressure >150-170 mm Hg) increases the risk of postoperative hypertension and adverse neurologic outcome after CEA.[76,77] Aggressive perioperative control of blood pressure in patients undergoing CEA, including adequate preoperative treatment of hypertension, has been associated with improved outcome.[78] A review of the patient's blood pressure record to establish a baseline blood pressure range often provides a useful aid to intraoperative hemodynamic management.

For patients with diabetes mellitus, blood glucose levels should be carefully managed throughout the perioperative period to avoid both hypo- and hyperglycemia. Following acute stroke, current clinical and experimental evidence suggests that hyperglycemia lowers the neuronal ischemic threshold, may increase ischemic volume, and is associated with higher morbidity and mortality.[62,79,80] Similar findings have also been reported specifically in association with CEA; higher risks for stroke, myocardial infarction, and death have been associated with the presence of hyperglycemia—defined as a blood glucose level greater than 200 mg/dL (11.1 mmol/L)—at the time of surgery.[81] These findings support recommendations for tight perioperative glycemic control in diabetic patients presenting for CEA.

Hypoglycemia also represents a deleterious condition for the brain. The past several years have seen an increasing trend toward very tight glycemic control among hospitalized patients with diabetes (as well as hyperglycemic patients without a history of diabetes) following reports indicating that the aggressive management of glucose levels is associated with improved outcome among critically ill medical and surgical patients.[82-84] However, it has also been noted that the development of hypoglycemia is a significant risk when aggressive glycemic control is adopted.[85,86] In view of these concerns, perioperative management of blood glucose levels in diabetic patients presenting for CEA should probably be more conservative, in keeping with the recommendations of the AHA guidelines for the management of acute stroke suggesting that blood glucose levels should be maintained in the range of 140 to 185 mg/dL (7.8-10.3 mmol/L).[62]

ANESTHETIC MANAGEMENT

Intraoperative Monitoring

In view of the high incidence of coronary artery disease in patients undergoing CEA, the electrocardiogram (ECG) is monitored with an emphasis on the detection of ischemia. Use of a five-lead ECG with continuous monitoring of leads II and V_5 is common practice, and automated ST segment monitoring is a useful adjunct. A study of postoperative cardiac ischemic events among 185 patients who had had vascular surgery reported that lead V_3 or V_4 detects ischemic changes more consistently than V_5.[87] These investigators suggest that the use of lead V_4 may be preferable for detecting perioperative ischemia because its signal is more commonly isoelectric on baseline recordings. Furthermore, they advocate the use of multiple-lead monitoring in the perioperative period for patients at risk for cardiac ischemia, on the basis of the observation that monitoring two precordial leads (V_3 and V_4, V_3 and V_5, or V_4 and V_5) improved the sensitivity for detecting cardiac ischemia to more than 90%, compared with 66% with the use of lead V_5 alone.

An intra-arterial cannula placed with the use of local analgesia before the induction of anesthesia (regional or general) permits continuous monitoring of blood pressure throughout the perioperative period and facilitates sampling of arterial blood for blood gas analyses. Alternatively, in low-risk patients, a rapidly cycling (1-minute intervals) noninvasive blood pressure device can be used during induction, and the arterial cannula can be placed before commencement of surgery. Central venous pressure, pulmonary capillary wedge pressure, cardiac output, transesophageal echocardiography and urine output are not routinely monitored, but monitoring can be considered for high-risk patients.

Oxygenation is monitored continuously with a pulse oximeter. Placement of an esophageal stethoscope after induction of general anesthesia facilitates monitoring of core temperature as well as ventilation, because the chest is not readily accessible during surgery. End-tidal CO_2 monitoring, validated relative to an arterial blood gas sample, facilitates the continuous maintenance of Pa_{CO_2} within the patient's normal range. For patients who undergo CEA under regional anesthesia or local infiltration, the use of nasal prongs with a CO_2 sampling port allows the provision of supplemental oxygen and the measurement of expired CO_2. The CO_2 measurements obtained in this manner do not consistently correlate with end tidal CO_2 values but do provide a useful aid in monitoring respiratory rate and rhythm in situations in which the patient's face and chest may be partially obscured by surgical drapes.

Choice of Anesthetic Technique

CEA can be performed safely with use of either general anesthesia or regional anesthesia (including local anesthetic infiltration). General anesthesia represents the most popular anesthetic technique for CEA.[88-90] Advocates of general anesthesia cite patient comfort, airway security, and the more expedient management of ventilation, autonomic reflexes, and potential intraoperative complications as prominent advantages. However, general anesthesia is typically more expensive in terms of anesthetic agents used than regional anesthesia, and its use forfeits the ability to monitor neurologic status in the awake patient. Regional anesthesia is popular in some centers, and extensive experience has been reported with its use.[91] Advocates of regional anesthesia endorse the superior neurologic monitoring afforded by an awake patient as a major advantage. The technique is generally less expensive than general anesthesia, and some studies report shorter length of hospital stay and lower risk of complications in association with regional anesthesia and awake monitoring. Performing major surgery with use of regional anesthesia requires the focus of the entire operating room team being committed to the needs of the awake patient; airway and ventilation are not readily controlled, and the management of intraoperative complications, such as stroke, seizure, airway obstruction, hypoventilation, and confusion or agitation, can be more challenging, including intraoperative conversion to general anesthesia.

Despite the relative merits of the two techniques and enthusiastic advocates for each, there is little evidence, from the results of the large randomized trials, to suggest that outcome following CEA is substantially affected by the choice of regional versus general anesthesia. Subgroup analysis of patients enrolled in the NASCET[88] and the ECST[89] revealed no difference in outcome associated with the use of local or regional anesthesia, although the number of patients who underwent CEA under regional block was small in both studies (7% and 3.4%, respectively). Similarly, a later review of the literature comparing CEA performed with use of either regional or general anesthesia, which involved 48 studies and 25,622 operations, reported that analysis of the 41 methodologically less robust, nonrandomized trials showed a reduced risk of death, stroke, myocardial infarction, and pulmonary complications in favor of regional anesthesia.[91,92] However, these findings were not supported by the results of the seven prospective, randomized trials that met methodologic criteria, which did not identify a difference between the two techniques in relation to stroke, myocardial infarction, or the use of shunts. A statistically insignificant trend favoring regional anesthesia was noted for the rates of local hemorrhage at the operative site and death from all causes (Table 16-6).[92]

Given these results, it seems appropriate to conclude that outcome following CEA is likely more dependent on patient selection, preoperative optimization of comorbid conditions, and an experienced and committed surgical team than on the choice of anesthetic technique. Supporting this premise, Calligaro and colleagues[93] described their experience converting from general to regional anesthesia for CEA. Reporting on the results of 401 carotid endarterectomies (216 general anesthesia, 185 cervical plexus block) performed over a 6-year period in which a conversion from general to regional anesthesia was performed, these investigators reported a similar stroke mortality rate (<2%) with each technique. Interestingly, they also commented that a satisfactory surgical environment for performing CEA with regional anesthesia was intimately dependent on a committed group of anesthesiologists who provided a consistent and standardized approach to managing the patient.

Regional Anesthesia

Superficial and deep cervical plexus blocks are the most common regional anesthetic techniques for CEA. The superficial cervical plexus block is performed by injection of local anesthetic subcutaneously along the posterior border of the sternocleidomastoid muscle, where the cutaneous branches of the plexus fan out to innervate the skin of the lateral neck. The deep cervical plexus block is a paravertebral block of the C2-C4 nerve roots. The technique involves injecting local anesthetic at the vertebral foramina (transverse processes) of the C2, C3, and C4 vertebra to block neck muscles, fascia, and the greater occipital nerve. A 2007 review of the published experience with deep and superficial cervical plexus blocks for CEA since 1974 reported that although the absolute incidence of block-related serious (life-threatening) complications is very low, essentially all

serious complications were associated with the deep component of the block.[94] In addition, conversion to general anesthesia as a consequence of inadequate block was five times more common when a deep cervical block technique was used. The investigators in this review suggest that the use of the superficial cervical block technique is safer and technically less challenging and should be the preferred regional anesthetic option for CEA, citing evidence from two randomized comparisons that the two techniques are equally effective.[95,96] Both blocks have been described in detail (including local anesthetic infiltration)[97,98] and should be reviewed before they are performed.

Monitors of a patient under regional anesthesia should include continuous electrocardiography, pulse oximetry, capnography, and an arterial cannula placed with use of local anesthesia. Supplemental oxygen should be provided with a mask or nasal prongs positioned to avoid the site of surgery. Traditionally, carefully titrated sedation using small, repeated, intravenous doses of fentanyl (10-25 µg), midazolam (0.5-2 mg), or both represents a popular and well-established approach to ensuring that the patient is comfortable and cooperative during the operation. Propofol, a reasonable alternative to midazolam, is typically administered as a low-dose continuous infusion (0.3-1.0 mg/kg/hr). Provisions should be available to convert to general anesthesia if intraoperative conditions warrant.

The use of sedating central α_2 receptor agonists, such as clonidine and dexmedetomidine, during CEA with regional anesthesia has also been reported. Both drugs provide effective sedation and modest analgesia with minimal respiratory depression. Limited published experience with these drugs in the context of CEA has generally been favorable, with marked attenuation of sympathetic stress responses and variably beneficial effects on intraoperative hemodynamic control (e.g., reduced need for intervention for hypertension or tachycardia).[99-101] However, a higher incidence of postoperative hypotension requiring intervention has been noted,[99] and transient hypertension, hypotension, and bradycardia have been described in association with the infusion of dexmedetomidine in other settings. Although early evidence suggests that these drugs may have a role in the management of patients undergoing CEA, further study is needed before they can be advocated for routine use.[102,103]

Table 16-6 Risk of Complications after Carotid Endarterectomy Performed with Local or General Anesthesia*

| Outcome | No. Events/No. Operations | | Odds Ratio | 95% Confidence Interval |
	Local Anesthesia	General Anesthesia		
All deaths	1/280	6/274	0.23	0.05-1.02
Stroke	6/280	6/274	1.01	0.32-3.18
Stroke and death	7/280	11/274	0.63	0.25-1.62
Myocardial infarction	4/280	5/274	0.77	0.21-2.88
Local hemorrhage	4/223	14/221	0.31	0.12-0.79
Nerve injury	4/167	2/166	1.98	0.39-9.97
Artery shunted	56/223	60/221	0.68	0.40-1.14

*Based on review of data from seven randomized trials of carotid endarterectomy.
Adapted from Rerkasem K, Bond R, Rothwell PM: Local versus general anaesthetic for carotid endarterectomy. Stroke 2005;36:169-170.

General Anesthesia

Traditionally, a variety of drugs has been used satisfactorily to induce general anesthesia for CEA, including thiopental, midazolam, propofol, and etomidate. As is the case in most other areas of anesthetic practice, propofol is likely the most popular induction drug at present. A supplemental opioid such as fentanyl (2 to 5 μg/kg) or sufentanil (0.5 to 1.0 μg/kg), administered intravenously, is often included in the induction sequence. Remifentanil is also a suitable opioid to supplement anesthesia induction. Whether this agent is administered as a bolus (0.2-0.5 μg/kg) or as an infusion (0.05 to 0.2 μg/kg/min), its short half-life facilitates titration of anesthesia during the relatively unstimulating period of surgical preparation and draping that follows intubation.

Tracheal intubation is usually performed after the administration of a nondepolarizing neuromuscular blocking drug. Because many of the currently popular neuromuscular blocking drugs possess favorable hemodynamic profiles, the choice of drug is rarely a clinically important issue. Succinylcholine is a reasonable alternative in most circumstances, although it is contraindicated in patients who have experienced a recent paretic cerebral infarct. The hemodynamic response to tracheal intubation can be attenuated by the administration of intravenous lidocaine (1-1.5 mg/kg), additional opioid, or supplemental hypnotic drug, or the addition of a volatile anesthetic before intubation. An armored endotracheal tube, although not essential, may be of benefit because its flexibility facilitates its positioning without impinging on the surgical field.

Anesthesia is typically maintained with a volatile anesthetic supplemented with an opioid. Alternatively, total intravenous anesthesia (TIVA) using a propofol infusion combined with a supplemental opioid such as remifentanil or fentanyl is also popular for maintenance anesthesia. Any of the currently available vapors, isoflurane, desflurane, or sevoflurane, may be used. The agents used and doses will be influenced by the use of electrophysiologic monitoring, because evoked potentials may become depressed as the hypnotic dose increases.

The limited literature available comparing anesthetic drugs during CEA is composed largely of small clinical studies comparing combinations of these drugs in relatively small numbers of patients. At present there is no clear basis to support a strong preference among the drug options in terms of outcome. Intraoperative hemodynamic stability and cardiac status have been reported to be similar during isoflurane, desflurane, and sevoflurane anesthesia.[104] The use of remifentanil and sevoflurane or desflurane is reported to be associated with earlier emergence from anesthesia than the use of fentanyl and isoflurane, but the difference extends only into the immediate postoperative period (e.g., 15-30 minutes).[104,105] Remifentanil combined with propofol appears to be associated with fewer episodes of intraoperative hypertension than fentanyl combined with propofol,[106] but reviews of published experience with remifentanil suggest that although patients receiving remifentanil have a lower incidence of intraoperative hypertension, they are more prone to hypotension and bradycardia.[107,108] Finally, the question has been raised whether the modest benefits reported to favor remifentanil-propofol anesthesia over isoflurane-fentanyl anesthesia for CEA justify the substantially higher cost of anesthesia using the former agents.[109]

Nitrous oxide has been popular as a supplemental anesthetic for CEA for many years. The favorable hemodynamic profile associated with nitrous oxide permits a reduction in the dose of other anesthetic drugs with less favorable hemodynamic characteristics, particularly during periods with minimal surgical stimulation, and its low solubility coefficient facilitates a prompt emergence at the conclusion of surgery. However, the use of nitrous oxide during CEA remains controversial because of conflicting reports, largely from animal model studies, that it may cause an increase in CBF and cerebral metabolic rate, reduce the neuroprotective potential of other drugs, and have neurotoxic properties under some circumstances (e.g., developing brain and prolonged exposure).[110-115] However, a detrimental effect of nitrous oxide on neurologic outcome in humans, particularly following CEA, has been difficult to establish. Later evidence suggests that nitrous oxide may be neuroprotective in the rat at low inspired concentrations (50%),[116] that it does not cause a significant increase in cerebral blood volume or global cerebral metabolic rate in human volunteers,[117] and that its use during aneurysm surgery, in a population at high risk for ischemic sequelae, was not associated with a higher risk of ischemic complications.[118,119] Nitrous oxide continues to be used by some anesthesiologists during CEA, although its popularity is declining as a consequence of the availability of other short-acting anesthetic drugs such as sevoflurane, desflurane, and remifentanil as well as reports that its use during major surgical procedures is associated with a higher incidence of other postoperative complications, including postoperative fever, wound infection, pneumonia, pulmonary atelectasis, and severe nausea or vomiting.[120]

Irrespective of the specific choice of anesthetic drugs, the anesthetic goal during CEA is to provide a relatively light level of general anesthesia because the procedure is typically not highly stimulating. Some surgeons routinely infiltrate the wound with local anesthetic at the beginning of the operation, further reducing the depth of general anesthesia needed. Neuromuscular blockade is often maintained throughout the procedure and, as discussed, mechanical ventilation is adjusted to maintain end tidal CO_2 at normocapnic levels.

Hypertension most often arises in response to visceral pain associated with traction or distortion of the carotid artery or surrounding structures and typically responds to local anesthetic infiltration of the carotid sheath or deepening of the level of anesthesia. When this measure is inadequate, blood pressure should be controlled with an intravenous antihypertensive drug such as esmolol or labetalol.

Hypotension, bradycardia, or both may also accompany traction on the carotid artery during surgical dissection. These responses represent the parasympathetic output of the baroreflex, where the traction is "misinterpreted" as an increase in blood pressure. This response can usually be attenuated by local anesthetic blockade of the carotid sinus nerve. Episodes of hypotension during other phases of the operation are treated by reduction of the depth of anesthesia, infusion of intravenous fluid or, if necessary, administration of a vasopressor such as phenylephrine (0.5-1.0 μg/kg) to maintain blood pressure. Ephedrine (5-10 mg IV) is a reasonable alternative to phenylephrine, particularly for hypotension associated with bradycardia.

Before carotid cross-clamping, heparin (75-100 units/kg) is administered intravenously. Application of the carotid clamps is often associated with a rise in blood pressure, a baroreflex due to loss of stretch of the vessel wall. Mild increases in arterial pressure are acceptable (up to approximately 20% above preoperative levels), but excessive increases should be controlled. Excessive increases may also indicate inadequate cerebral perfusion.

Intravenous fluids are administered according to maintenance requirements. Blood loss during CEA is typically minimal, although the potential for hemorrhage exists. Because temporary cerebral ischemia may be aggravated by hyperglycemia or hypoglycemia, as discussed previously, intraoperative glycemic management should include the judicious use of glucose-containing solutions and intraoperative glucose monitoring for patients at risk for these complications.

Cerebral Protection

Interest in elucidating putative neuroprotective properties associated with many drugs used in anesthesia spans several decades. Most drugs used to induce anesthesia, including barbiturates, benzodiazepines, etomidate, propofol, ketamine, and the volatile agents, have been investigated in a variety of animal models and under a wide range of experimental conditions of global and regional ischemia. All of these drugs have been reported to bestow a modest degree of protection under appropriate experimental conditions (see Chapter 1).[121-124]

Patients undergoing CEA are at risk for development of cerebral ischemia; hence, it is appealing to speculate that an additional margin of safety may be achieved by administering anesthetic drugs that protect the brain from ischemic injury. Although some anesthesiologists prefer to administer additional intravenous anesthetic drugs, or to increase the depth of anesthesia, before carotid cross-clamping on the basis of the assumption that some degree of protection may be realized,[125,126] there is no evidence to suggest that this practice influences outcome in the context of CEA.

Neurologic Monitoring

A reliable means of monitoring the patient's intraoperative neurologic status has long been considered to be a key facet of intraoperative care during CEA to enable the identification of intraoperative embolic complications and, more importantly, to evaluate neurologic tolerance to carotid cross-clamping. There seems little doubt that an awake, cooperative patient provides a highly sensitive and specific means of monitoring intraoperative neurologic status. Many surgeons who prefer to perform CEA with local anesthesia cite the ability to validate management decisions at the time of cross-clamping on the basis of the patient's objective neurologic response as a key advantage associated with the technique.

In contrast, the broad popularity of general anesthesia for CEA has generated enthusiasm for evaluating other monitoring techniques that can identify patients at risk of neurologic injury during general anesthesia. Neurologic monitoring during CEA is based on the following premises: (1) the monitor is able to accurately identify patients at risk for development of intraoperative cerebral ischemia and (2) with identification, interventions can be instituted (e.g., placement of an internal shunt, increase CPP) to prevent irreversible neuronal injury and thereby improve outcome. Despite intense interest, both premises remain controversial.[127-130]

Traditionally, the EEG has been the most extensively used monitor of neurologic function during CEA (see Chapter 7).[131,132] Extensive evidence generated over several decades of clinical use during CEA supports a strong correlation between EEG changes and critical alterations in CBF.[133-135] The EEG is sensitive to adverse hemodynamic and embolic complications

associated with CEA, and most patients who experience an adverse neurologic event will be identified (low false-negative rate).[136,137] However, the few prospective studies available in which intervention was not initiated in response to EEG changes[138,139] suggest that many patients experience intraoperative EEG changes that do not correlate with neurologic outcome, which is the clinically relevant endpoint (high false-positive rate). Nevertheless, EEG remains a popular technique for monitoring neurologic function during CEA, but its routine use requires expertise for technical support and real-time interpretation.

Evoked potentials, especially somatosensory evoked potentials (SSEPs), have been used during CEA and some are now using motor evoked potentials, too (see Chapter 7). The measurement of SSEPs during CEA remains inadequately validated as a means of identifying patients at risk for adverse neurologic outcome, with many conflicting reports concerning its reliability for this application. A systematic review of 3136 patients from 15 studies conducted prior to 1998 concluded that SSEP changes were unreliable predictors of neurologic outcome and were not suitable for identifying patients who would benefit from intervention (selective shunt insertion).[140] Exemplifying the controversy, others have reported that SSEP monitoring provides superior ischemia detection during CEA.[141] However, compared with EEG monitoring, most evidence would suggest that SSEP monitoring does not improve accuracy, it is less robust during general anesthesia, and the standards for SSEP monitoring and its interpretation are less well established.

TCD is a well-established technology for assessing intraoperative cerebral blood flow in large intracranial vessels (see Chapter 8). During CEA, changes in velocity are generally considered to reflect similar changes in blood flow, provided that the arterial $PaCO_2$ remains constant.[142,143] The unique perspective on the cerebral circulation made available noninvasively with TCD makes it an appealing technique for monitoring CBF during CEA. However, TCD does not directly measure cerebral function or ischemia, the equipment tends to be cumbersome, and the results are operator dependent. TCD has also been used to detect shunt malfunction during CEA.[144]

In addition to measuring flow velocity, TCD is a sensitive method for detecting cerebral emboli that may accompany carotid manipulation, cross-clamping, and shunt insertion and can aid in the etiologic distinction between hemodynamic and embolic causes of neurologic deterioration at the time of cross-clamping. In addition, prospective studies have reported a correlation between the number of emboli detected during carotid dissection and the risk of adverse neurologic outcome and radiologic evidence of cerebral injury.[145,146] Several investigators have extended the application of TCD monitoring into the postoperative period and have reported a high incidence of microemboli originating in the ipsilateral carotid artery in the hours following CEA. Microemboli have been linked to a higher incidence of stroke among patients with symptomatic and asymptomatic carotid stenosis,[147,148] and some evidence suggests that a high incidence of microemboli after CEA (more than 50 embolic signals per hour) is associated with increased risk for subsequent stroke.[149-151] The administration of antiplatelet agents (Dextran-40[150,152,153] and, more recently, the selective platelet glycoprotein IIb/IIIa receptor antagonist tirofiban[154,155]) in the early postoperative period has been reported to substantially reduce the number of microembolic events identified with postoperative TCD among high-risk patients. These therapies remain investigational, pending randomized trials to validate their efficacy in the prevention of postoperative stroke, because they are not devoid of risk. Multiple-organ failure and intracerebral hemorrhage have been reported in association with the administration of dextran-40 following CEA.[150] However, if validation of these drugs is forthcoming, it would provide an opportunity for pharmacologic neuroprotection in the postoperative period and establish a clear indication for TCD monitoring for the identification of high-risk patients who are most likely to benefit from these antiplatelet therapies.

Carotid stump pressure (CSP) is the mean arterial pressure measured in the carotid stump (the internal carotid artery cephalad to the common carotid cross-clamp) after cross-clamping of the common and external carotid arteries. This measurement reflects pressure transmitted in a retrograde fashion through the ipsilateral carotid artery and has been postulated to provide a useful indicator of the adequacy of collateral circulation. Moore and associates[156,157] initially reported that CSP values less than 25 mm Hg correlated with cross-clamp intolerance and suggested that this level of CSP represented the threshold for adequate cerebral perfusion. However, despite the conceptual appeal and technical simplicity of the technique, CSP measurements are generally not popular as a sole index of the adequacy of cerebral perfusion, for the following reasons: (1) inadequate validation as a useful predictor of outcome, (2) controversy related to the level of stump pressure that reflects inadequate collateral circulation, and (3) evidence that the pressure measurements are influenced by the choice of anesthetic.[158-160]

Investigators continue to study CSP as a means of assessing the adequacy of cerebral perfusion after cross-clamping, but the studies continue to yield conflicting results. Moritz and colleagues,[161] for example, found a CSP of 40 mm Hg to have a sensitivity of 100% and a specificity of 75% for identifying cross-clamp intolerance among patients undergoing CEA under regional anesthesia (awake neurologic assessment). In contrast, Hans and Jareunpoon[162] reported a sensitivity of 57% and a specificity of 97% using a CSP value of 40 mm Hg under similar clinical conditions (CEA performed with regional anesthesia) and concluded that CSP monitoring lacked adequate sensitivity to reliably identify patients who require shunt placement. As a result of this continuing controversy, CSP monitoring is used in some centers but primarily as an adjuvant technique combined with another modality, such as EEG.

Cerebral near-infrared spectroscopy (NIRS) is a relatively new neurologic monitoring technique in relation to CEA that uses infrared spectrometry to estimate cerebral oxyhemoglobin saturation. Although the technology for in vivo measurement of cerebral oxygenation has been available for 30 years, its application during CEA has been sporadic.[163] Like the familiar pulse oximeter, the cerebral oximeter emits light in the near-infrared range that penetrates the scalp and cranium. Because oxyhemoglobin and deoxyhemoglobin have distinct infrared absorption spectra, their relative proportions can be measured. In contrast to pulse oximeters, which use pulse-gated changes in optical density to measure arterial oxygen saturation, cerebral oximeters emit light continuously and measure the oxygen saturation of arterial, venous, and capillary hemoglobin in the superficial cerebral cortex. Because 75% of cortical blood volume is venous, cerebral oximetry reflects predominantly venous hemoglobin saturation.[163-165]

Near-infrared spectroscopy provides a convenient, portable, noninvasive measurement of regional cerebral venous oxyhemoglobin saturation (rSo_2) based on monitoring of a small sample of cortical vessels typically over the frontal lobe(s). However, it is unclear whether such regional measurements consistently reflect physiologic changes in other areas of the brain; measurements are influenced by small changes in sensor placement, patient age, hemoglobin concentration, and some contribution from non-brain sources; also, the technique is subject to high interpatient variability.[166,167] In addition, an ischemic threshold value for rSo_2 monitoring has not been established to date in relation to CEA. To compensate for these limitations, the technique is typically used to monitor trends in rSo_2, and several investigators have reported that during CEA, a change in rSo_2 value of 20% from baseline is associated with a negative predictive value of 97% and a positive predictive value of 35% for cerebral ischemic complications.[168,169] These data suggest that the technique provides reassurance when cross-clamping is not accompanied by a significant change in regional oxygenation but does not consistently identify patients at risk of ischemic injury when measurements decline in excess of 20%.

The intraoperative measurement of CBF with intra-arterial xenon has been very useful as an investigational tool for defining the critical CBF levels associated with other monitoring techniques and anesthetic drugs.[170-175] However, because of the perception of high costs associated with the equipment (basic scintillation detector technology is actually quite cheap) and technical support, the technique has traditionally been used in only a few centers. Despite extensive experience with the technique to validate other monitors, its reliability as a predictor of outcome after CEA remains controversial.[138,139]

Although each of these monitoring techniques can identify conditions that are associated with a higher risk of ischemic complications during CEA (reductions in cerebral blood flow or oxygenation, disturbances in neuronal metabolic activity), a completely reliable method for accurately predicting neurologic outcome following CEA has yet to be identified. Interventions currently available in response to evidence of cerebral ischemia include (1) raising CPP by administering systemic vasopressor drugs such as phenylephrine (discussed previously) and (2) protecting the brain by restoring internal carotid blood flow through placement of a carotid shunt. Although the use of some form of intraoperative neurologic monitoring (or combination) remains popular during CEA, there is little adequately validated evidence that any of these techniques or the use of shunts definitively improves outcome.[176-178] As a consequence, the use of carotid artery shunting and the choice of intraoperative monitoring technique largely depends on the preference and experience of the individual surgeon and the expertise of the surgical team.

Emergence from Anesthesia

Heparin is often not reversed after closure of the arteriotomy. If hemostasis is inadequate at the time of wound closure, a small dose of protamine (0.5 mg/kg) may be given intravenously. Depth of anesthesia is adjusted so that the patient can be promptly extubated at the end of surgery to avoid prolonged coughing and straining. A small dose of opioid (e.g., fentanyl 0.5 to 1.0 μg/kg, remifentanil (0.2-0.5 μg/kg or the continuation of a remifentanil infusion at very low dose), or lidocaine (1 to 1.5 mg/kg) given before emergence from anesthesia often attenuates coughing but temporarily deepens the level of anesthesia. Hemodynamic responses associated with emergence and extubation should be anticipated and treated. Drugs such as esmolol and nitroglycerine offer short durations of action, which can be useful for controlling hemodynamic changes during emergence and in the early postoperative period. Longer-acting antihypertensives such as labetalol, hydralazine, and metoprolol can be used effectively to control hypertension that persists in the post-anesthesia care unit.

Postoperative Care

The intra-arterial cannula is maintained during the initial postoperative period to permit continuous blood pressure monitoring and blood sampling for arterial blood gas analyses. All patients receive supplemental oxygen, and the adequacy of oxygenation is monitored by pulse oximetry. Bilateral CEA, which is a high–neurologic-risk procedure not often performed, is associated with changes in the chemical control of ventilation.[179] Resting Pa_{CO_2} rises by about 5 mm Hg, and the ventilatory and cardiovascular responses to hypoxemia are abolished. Provision of supplemental oxygen and close monitoring of ventilatory status is particularly important in patients undergoing this procedure.

Postoperative hemodynamic instability is common after CEA. Determining the exact incidence is confounded by differing definitions used in the studies. Hypotension occurs in approximately 10% and hypertension in up to 50% of patients who have undergone CEA.[180] Hemodynamic fluctuations are postulated to be related to carotid baroreceptor dysfunction.[181,182] CEA performed with a technique that spares the carotid sinus nerve is associated with a higher incidence of postoperative hypotension, postulated to be due to increased exposure of the carotid sinus to the higher arterial pressure following removal of the atheromatous plaque.[183,184] This hypotension is associated with a marked decrease in systemic vascular resistance and is treated with intravenous fluid administration or, if necessary, the administration of vasopressor drugs, such as phenylephrine.[185] Intraoperative local anesthetic blockade of the carotid sinus nerve has been advocated to prevent, or attenuate, hypotension after CEA, but the effectiveness of this treatment is controversial.[183,184,186]

Hypertension after CEA is less well understood and has been reported to be more common in patients with preoperative hypertension, particularly poorly controlled or uncontrolled hypertension, and to occur more often after procedures in which the carotid sinus is denervated (surgical division or local anesthetic blockade).[77,181,186] Hypertension after sinus nerve–sparing CEA has been postulated to be caused by temporary dysfunction of the baroreceptor or nerve due to intraoperative trauma.[181] Mild rises in postoperative blood pressure are acceptable (up to approximately 20% above preoperative normotensive levels), but marked increases should be treated with antihypertensive drugs.

Other causes of hemodynamic instability after CEA are myocardial ischemia or infarction, dysrhythmias such as atrial fibrillation, hypoxia, hypercarbia, pneumothorax, pain, confusion, stroke, and distention of the urinary bladder.

Complications

Major postoperative complications after CEA are stroke, myocardial infarction, death, and the hyperperfusion syndrome.

Stroke

The majority of strokes (approximately two thirds) complicating CEA have been reported to occur in the postoperative period and appear to be related primarily to technical factors resulting in carotid occlusion (thrombosis or intimal flap) or emboli originating at the surgical site rather than to hemodynamic factors.[187-189] Approximately one third of strokes resulting from CEA occur intraoperatively. Most of these occur during carotid manipulation or cross-clamping and are embolic in nature. For example, in a review of 2024 carotid endarterectomies, Rockman and colleagues[190] found 13% of strokes manifesting within the first 24 hours to be related to clamping ischemia and 63% to be thromboembolic (in addition, intracerebral hemorrhage contributed to 13% of perioperative strokes, and 11% had no relationship to the operated artery, being due to embolic events of cardiac origin, for instance). Thus, very few intraoperative strokes are hemodynamic in origin. Intraoperative neurologic function monitoring is directed toward the identification of the relatively small group of patients in whom potentially reversible, hemodynamically induced ischemia develops.

Myocardial Infarction

Given the high incidence of concomitant coronary artery disease in patients undergoing CEA, it is not surprising that myocardial infarction represents a major cause of morbidity and mortality after CEA. It was previously believed that myocardial infarction was more common than stroke, but studies conducted over the past two decades have found the converse to be true. *The Cochrane systematic review of more than 15,000 patients found postoperative myocardial infarction to occur in 2.2% and stroke in 3.3%.*[91] Unfortunately, whether the myocardial infarct resulted in death is not clear in many reports, because stroke and death are lumped together. This fact suggests that better preoperative preparation and intraoperative management has been beneficial. However one should not be complacent because a rise in cardiac troponin level of more than 0.5 ng/mL has been found in 13% of patients undergoing CEA.[191]

Death

Stroke and myocardial infarction represent the major causes of perioperative mortality associated with CEA. As emphasized previously, operative risk is affected by patient selection, the experience of the surgeon, and the institution where the surgery is performed.[32,35,36] *The American Heart Association guidelines for CEA recommend that the combined risk for death or stroke associated with CEA should not exceed 3% for asymptomatic patients and 5% for symptomatic patients.*[5,6] These recommendations, with a durability spanning more than a decade of analysis and review, remain the gold standard against which other surgical interventions, such as CAS, are compared.[7,14] Patients with unstable neurologic or cardiac conditions who are undergoing urgent CEA or CEA combined with CABG and patients who present with complex conditions such as reoperation for recurrent stenosis have proportionally higher perioperative risk.

Hyperperfusion Syndrome

An increase in CBF has been reported to occur frequently after CEA and has been reported after CAS procedures as well.[192,193] Typically the magnitude of this increase is relatively small (less than 35%); however, in severe cases, rises in CBF can exceed 200% of preoperative levels and can be associated with greater morbidity and mortality.[172,194-196] There is no accepted definition of what absolute level of CBF increase should be considered "hyperperfusion." Knowledge of the underlying metabolic rate would be necessary to understand relative "excess" flow states. Clinically, hyperperfusion syndrome would be diagnosed in patients with all or part of the clinical triad ipsilateral headache, seizures, and focal neurologic symptoms that arise in the absence of cerebral ischemia. Features of hyperperfusion syndrome include headache (usually unilateral), face and eye pain, cerebral edema, seizures, and intracerebral hemorrhage.[194,195] The frequency of irreversible injury ranges from 0.4% to 7.7% in patients in whom the hyperperfusion syndrome develops.[197]

The syndrome is postulated to occur after perfusion is restored to an area of the brain that has lost its autoregulation ability because of chronically decreased CBF and is typically accompanied by postoperative hypertension. Patients at greatest risk include those with reduced preoperative hemispheric CBF (e.g., those with bilateral high-grade carotid stenoses, unilateral high-grade carotid stenosis with poor collateral cross-flow, or unilateral carotid occlusion with contralateral high-grade stenosis). Very low intraoperative distal (stump) pressure after cross-clamping may identify patients at increased risk for development of postoperative hyperperfusion.[197] Histologically, the hyperperfusion syndrome has features very similar to those of hypertensive encephalopathy. Patients at risk for this syndrome should be monitored closely in the perioperative period, and blood pressure should be meticulously controlled, at normal or slightly below normal levels, until autoregulation is reestablished, typically over a period of several days. Adhiyaman and Alexander[194] have suggested that blood pressure should preferably be reduced through the use of drugs such as labetalol and clonidine, which do not increase CBF, rather than angiotensin-converting enzyme inhibitors, calcium channel blockers, or vasodilators like nitroprusside and nitroglycerine, but they acknowledge that there is no evidence favoring any particular drug.

Other Complications

Other complications associated with CEA are hematoma formation and cranial nerve palsies. Postoperatively, patients should be monitored carefully for evidence of wound hematoma (i.e., neck swelling), which may progress rapidly to airway obstruction and death. From analysis of NASCET surgical outcome data, the incidence of postoperative wound hematoma has been reported to be 7% (approximately 45% of hematomas are classified as moderate to severe, involving delayed discharge and/or reoperation), and the occurrence of wound hematoma has been reported to represent a significant risk factor for perioperative stroke and death.[88] Evidence of an expanding wound hematoma should be managed as an emergency with re-intubation and surgical exploration.

The incidence of cranial nerve palsies following CEA has been reported to be 5% to 12%.[88,198,199] On the basis of NASCET and ECST results, the hypoglossal nerve, vagus nerve, and branches of the facial nerve are the most common cranial nerves injured during CEA, and their injury may manifest as dysphagia. Most events are thought to be related to traction injury, and increasing duration of the surgical procedure (>2 hours) has been reported to raise the risk of cranial nerve injury.[198] Injuries to laryngeal nerves (recurrent or superior laryngeal nerves) have also been reported. When these deficits were specifically assessed with postoperative laryngoscopic examination, vocal cord dysfunction (reduction of or absence of unilateral vocal cord movement) was reported in 4% of patients after CEA; this complication typically manifests as hoarseness.[199] Although cranial nerve injuries rarely lead to airway compromise following CEA, anesthesiologists should be cognizant that vocal cord dysfunction and swallowing difficulties are not uncommon after these procedures. Cranial nerve palsies following CEA are typically temporary, resolving within several months. Of the cranial nerve injuries reported in the ECST, 92% resolved within 4 months of surgery and 8% were permanent (persisting beyond 2 years).[198] Prolonged resolution of recurrent laryngeal nerve injuries has been reported, with recovery of full function occurring up to 36 months after surgery.[199]

SUMMARY

The past decade has witnessed a continuing effort to refine our understanding of the role of CEA for the prevention of stroke and the patients most likely to benefit from this procedure. Although CEA remains the gold standard for the surgical treatment of cerebrovascular occlusive disease, the continuing development of carotid angioplasty and stenting techniques has extend the treatment options for patients at high risk for stroke. Anesthesiologists will continue to be challenged to provide care for this elderly population of patients, who commonly present with multiple comorbid conditions. Preoperative assessment and the optimization of comorbidities are increasingly emphasized as a key component of achieving the best outcome. The role of the anesthesiologist in the care of these patients will continue to expand as opportunities to mitigate perioperative risk evolve. This chapter has reviewed the anesthetic management of patients undergoing CEA, highlighting areas of current consensus as well as controversy in relation to patient selection, risk assessment, preoperative management, the choice of anesthetic technique, monitoring, and perioperative care and complications.

REFERENCES

1. Alpert JN: Extracranial carotid artery—current concepts of diagnosis and management, *Tex Heart Inst J* 18:93–97, 1991.
2. Dyken ML: Carotid endarterectomy studies: A glimmering of science, *Stroke* 17:355–357, 1986.
3. Beneficial effect of carotid endarterectomy in symptomatic patients with high-grade carotid stenosis: North American Symptomatic Carotid Endarterectomy Trial Collaborators, *N Engl J Med* 325:445–453, 1991.
4. MRC European Carotid Surgery Trial: Interim results for symptomatic patients with severe (70-99%) or with mild (0-29%) carotid stenosis. European Carotid Surgery Trialists' Collaborative, *Lancet* 337:1235–1243, 1991.
5. Endarterectomy for asymptomatic carotid artery stenosis: Executive Committee for the Asymptomatic Carotid Atherosclerosis Study, *JAMA* 273:1421–1428, 1995.
6. Biller J, Feinberg WM, Castaldo JE, et al: Guidelines for carotid endarterectomy: A statement for healthcare professionals from a Special Writing Group of the Stroke Council, American Heart Association, *Circulation* 97:501–509, 1998.
7. 2007 Clinical Expert Consensus Document on Carotid Stenting: The American College of Cardiology Foundation Task Force on Clinical Expert Consensus Documents, *Vascular Medicine* 12:35–83, 2007.
8. Rothwell PM, Eliasziw M, Gutnikov SA, et al: Analysis of pooled data from the randomised controlled trials of endarterectomy for symptomatic carotid stenosis, *Lancet* 361:107–116, 2003.
9. Halm EA, Tuhrim S, Wang JJ, et al: Has evidence changed practice? Appropriateness of carotid endarterectomy after the clinical trials, *Neurology* 68:187–194, 2007.

10. Rosamond W, Flegal K, Furie K, et al; The American Heart Association Statistics Committee and Stroke Statistics Subcommittee. Heart disease and stroke statistics—2008 update: A report from the American Heart Association Statistics Committee and Stroke Statistics Subcommittee, *Circulation* 117:e25–e146, 2008.

11. Atkins MD, Bush RL: Embolic protection devices for carotid artery stenting: Have they made a significant difference in outcomes? *Semin Vasc Surg* 20:244–251, 2007.

12. Gurm HS, Yadav JS, Fayad P, et al: SAPPHIRE Investigators: Long-term results of carotid stenting versus endarterectomy in high-risk patients, *N Engl J Med* 358:1572–1579, 2008.

13. van der Vaart MG, Meerwaldt R, Reijnen MM, et al: Endarterectomy or carotid artery stenting: The quest continues, *Am J Surg* 95:259–269, 2008.

14. Coward LJ, Featherstone RL, Brown MM: Safety and efficacy of endovascular treatment of carotid artery stenosis compared with carotid endarterectomy: A Cochrane systematic review of the randomized evidence, *Stroke* 36:905–911, 2005.

15. Cenic A, Craen RA, Lee TY, Gelb AW: Cerebral blood volume and blood flow responses to hyperventilation in brain tumors during isoflurane or propofol anesthesia, *Anesth Analg* 94:661–666, 2002.

16. Ohmori S, Iwama H: An induction dose of propofol does not alter cerebral blood flow determined by single-photon-emission computed tomography, *J Anesth* 14:61–67, 2000.

17. Conti A, Iacopino DG, Fodale V, et al: Cerebral hemodynamic changes during propofol-remifentanil or sevoflurane anaesthesia: Transcranial Doppler study under bispectral index monitoring, *Br J Anaesth* 97:333–339, 2006.

18. Koch M, De Backer D, Vincent JL, et al: Effects of propofol on human microcirculation, *Br J Anaesth* 101:473–478, 2008.

19. Fourcade HE, Larson P, Ehrenfeld WK, et al: The effects of CO_2 and systemic hypertension on cerebral perfusion pressure during carotid endarterectomy, *Anesthesiology* 33:383–390, 1970.

20. Lassen NA, Palvolgyi R: Cerebral steal during hypercapnia and the inverse reaction during hypocapnia observed by the 133xenon technique in man, *Scand J Lab Clin Invest* 22(S102):13D, 1968.

21. Wells BA, Keats AS, Cooley DA: Increased tolerance to cerebral ischemia produced by general anesthesia during temporary carotid occlusion, *Surgery* 54:216–223, 1963.

22. Boysen G, Ladegaard-Pedersen HJ, Henriksen H, et al: The effects of $PaCO_2$ on regional cerebral blood flow and internal carotid arterial pressure during carotid clamping, *Anesthesiology* 35:286–300, 1971.

23. McCulloch TJ, Thompson CL, Turner MJ: A randomized crossover comparison of the effects of propofol and sevoflurane on cerebral hemodynamics during carotid endarterectomy, *Anesthesiology* 106:56–64, 2007.

24. Kadoi Y, Hinohara H, Kunimoto F, et al: Diabetic patients have an impaired cerebral vasodilatory response to hypercapnia under propofol anesthesia, *Stroke* 34:2399–2403, 2003.

25. Kadoi Y, Takahashi K, Saito S, Goto F: The comparative effects of sevoflurane versus isoflurane on cerebrovascular carbon dioxide reactivity in patients with diabetes mellitus, *Anesth Analg* 103:168–172, 2006.

26. Yamamoto M, Meyer JS, Sakai F, et al: Aging and cerebral vasodilator responses to hypercarbia. Responses in normal aging and in persons with risk factors for stroke, *Arch Neurol* 37:489–496, 1980.

27. Hansebout RR, Blomquist G, Gloor P, et al: Use of hypertension and electroencephalographic monitoring during carotid endarterectomy, *Can J Surg* 24:304–307, 1981.

28. Boysen G, Engell HC, Henriksen H: The effect of induced hypertension on internal carotid artery pressure and regional cerebral blood flow during temporary carotid clamping for endarterectomy, *Neurology* 22:1133–1144, 1972.

29. Smith JS, Roizen MF, Cahalan MK, et al: Does anesthetic technique make a difference? Augmentation of systolic blood pressure during carotid endarterectomy: Effects of phenylephrine versus light anesthesia and of isoflurane versus halothane on the incidence of myocardial ischemia, *Anesthesiology* 69:846–855, 1988.

30. Riles TS, Kopelman I, Imparato AM: Myocardial infarction following carotid endarterectomy: A review of 683 operations, *Surgery* 85:249–252, 1979.

31. North American Symptomatic Carotid Endarterectomy Trial: Methods, patient characteristics, and progress, *Stroke* 22:711–720, 1991.

32. Moore WS, Barnett HJM, Beebe HG, et al: Guidelines for carotid endarterectomy: A multidisciplinary consensus statement from the ad hoc committee, American Heart Association, *Stroke* 26:188–201, 1995.

33. Chambers B, Donnan G, Chambers B: Carotid endarterectomy for asymptomatic carotid stenosis, *Cochrane Database Syst Rev* (4)2005:CD001923.

34. Nazarian SM, Yenokyan G, Thompson RE, et al: Statistical modeling of the volume-outcome effect for carotid endarterectomy for 10 years of a statewide database, *J Vasc Surg* 48:343–350, 2008.

35. Holt PJ, Poloniecki JD, Loftus IM, Thompson MM: Meta-analysis and systematic review of the relationship between hospital volume and outcome following carotid endarterectomy, *Eur J Vasc Endovasc Surg* 33:645–651, 2007.

36. Killeen SD, Andrews EJ, Redmond HP, Fulton GJ: Provider volume and outcomes for abdominal aortic aneurysm repair, carotid endarterectomy, and lower extremity revascularization procedures, *J Vasc Surg* 45:615–626, 2007.

37. Shearer A, Cronin C: The State-of-the-Art of Online Hospital Public Reporting: A Review of Fifty-One Websites, 2nd ed. Easton, MD, Delmarva Foundation, 2005. Available at http://www.delmarvafoundation. org/newsAndPublications/pressReleases/2005/08_18_05.pdf.

38. Center for Medical Consumers. Surgery volume reports 2000. A special report on carotid endarterectomy. Available at http://medicalconsume rs.org/2002/01/01/2002-select-surgery-procedures-report/last accessed Sept 24/08–pdf of reoport appended.

39. Samuelson RM, Yamamoto J, Levy EI, et al: The argument to support broader application of extracranial carotid artery stent technology, *Circulation* 116:1602–1610, 2007.

40. LoGerfo FW: Carotid stents: Unleashed, unproven, *Circulation* 116:1596–1601, 2007.

41. Ederle J, Featherstone RL, Brown MM: Percutaneous transluminal angioplasty and stenting for carotid artery stenosis, *Cochrane Database Syst Rev* (4)2007:CD000515.

42. Endovascular versus surgical treatment in patients with carotid stenosis in the Carotid and Vertebral Artery Transluminal Angioplasty Study (CAVATAS): A randomized trial, *Lancet* 357:1729–1737, 2001.

43. Yadav J, Wholey M, Kuntz KM, et al: Protected carotid-artery stenting versus endarterectomy in high-risk patients, *N Engl J Med* 351:1493–1501, 2004.

44. Mas JL, Chatellier G, Beyssen B, et al: for EVA-3S Investigators: Endarterectomy versus stenting in patients with symptomatic severe carotid stenosis, *N Engl J Med* 355:1660–1671, 2006.

45. SPACE Collaborative Group, Ringleb PA, Allenberg J, Brückmann H, et al: 30 day results from the SPACE trial of stent-protected angioplasty versus carotid endarterectomy in symptomatic patients: A randomised non-inferiority trial, *Lancet* 368:1239–1247, 2006.

46. Hobson RW, Howard VJ, Roubin GS, et al; for the CREST Investigators: Carotid artery stenting is associated with increased complications in octogenarians: 30-day stroke and death rates in the CREST lead-in phase, *J Vasc Surg* 40:1106–1611, 2004.

47. Bates ER, Babb JD, Casey DE Jr, et al; American College of Cardiology Foundation Task Force; American Society of Interventional & Therapeutic Neuroradiology; Society for Cardiovascular Angiography and Interventions; Society for Vascular Medicine and Biology; Society for Interventional Radiology: ACCF/SCAI/SVMB/SIR/ASITN 2007 Clinical expert consensus document on carotid stenting, *Vasc Med* 12:35–83, 2007.

48. Rothwell PM, Eliasziw M, Gutnikov SA, et al: Endarterectomy for symptomatic carotid stenosis in relation to clinical subgroups and timing of surgery, *Lancet* 363:915–924, 2004.

49. Sundt TM Jr, Sandok BA, Whisnant JP: Carotid endarterectomy: Complications and preoperative assessment of risk, *Mayo Clin Proc* 50:301–306, 1975.

50. Sundt TM Jr, Whisnant JP, Houser OW, et al: Prospective study of the effectiveness and durability of carotid endarterectomy, *Mayo Clin Proc* 65:625–635, 1990.

51. Press MJ, Chassin MR, Wang J, et al: Predicting medical and surgical complications of carotid endarterectomy: Comparing the risk indexes, *Arch Intern Med* 166:914–920, 2006.

52. American Society of Anesthesiologists: New classification of physical status, *Anesthesiology* 24:111, 1963.

53. Goldman L, Caldera DL, Nussbaum SR, et al: Multifactorial index of cardiac risk in noncardiac surgical procedures, *N Engl J Med* 297:845–850, 1977.

54. Detsky AS, Abrams HB, Forbath N, et al: Cardiac assessment for patients undergoing noncardiac surgery: A multifactorial clinical risk index, *Arch Intern Med* 146:2131–2134, 1986.

55. Lee TH, Marcantonio ER, Mangione CM, et al: Derivation and prospective validation of a simple index for prediction of cardiac risk of major noncardiac surgery, *Circulation* 100:1043–1049, 1999.

56. Halm EA, Hannan EL, Rojas M, et al: Clinical and operative predictors of outcomes of carotid endarterectomy, *J Vasc Surg* 42:420–428, 2005.

57. Tu JV, Wang H, Bowyer B, et al: Risk factors for death or stroke after carotid endarterectomy: Observations from the Ontario Carotid Endarterectomy Registry, *Stroke* 34:2568–2573, 2003.

58. Riles TS, Kopelman I, Imparato AM: Myocardial infarction following carotid endarterectomy: A review of 683 operations, *Surgery* 85:249–252, 1979.

59. Hertzer NR, Lees CD: Fatal myocardial infarction following carotid endarterectomy, *Ann Surg* 194:212–218, 1981.

60. Towne JB, Weiss DG, Hobson RW: First phase report of cooperative Veterans Administration asymptomatic carotid stenosis study—operative morbidity and mortality, *J Vasc Surg* 11:252–259, 1990.

61. Olympio MA: The preoperative evaluation for symptomatic carotid endarterectomy: A debated issue, *J Neurosurg Anesth* 8:310–313, 1996.

62. Adams HP, del Zoppo G, Alberts MJ, et al; American Heart Association/American Stroke Association Stroke Council; American Heart Association/American Stroke Association Clinical Cardiology Council; American Heart Association/American Stroke Association Cardiovascular Radiology and Intervention Council; Atherosclerotic Peripheral Vascular Disease Working Group; Quality of Care Outcomes in Research Interdisciplinary Working Group: Guidelines for the early management of adults with ischemic stroke: A guideline from the American Heart Association/American Stroke Association Stroke Council, Clinical Cardiology Council, Cardiovascular Radiology and Intervention Council, and the Atherosclerotic Peripheral Vascular Disease and Quality of Care Outcomes in Research Interdisciplinary Working Groups: The American Academy of Neurology affirms the value of this guideline as an educational tool for neurologists. Stroke 38:1655–1711, 2007.

63. Poldermans D, Hoeks SE, Feringa HH: Pre-operative risk assessment and risk reduction before surgery, *J Am Coll Cardiol* 51:1913–1924, 2008.

64. Eagle KA, Guyton RA, Davidoff R, et al; American College of Cardiology; American Heart Association: ACC/AHA 2004 guideline update for coronary artery bypass graft surgery: Summary article:A Report of the American College of Cardiology/American Heart Association Task Force on Practice Guidelines (Committee to Update the 1999 Guidelines for Coronary Artery Bypass Graft Surgery). Circulation. 2004;110:1168–1176. Available at http://www.cardiosource.com/guidelines/guidelines/cabg/summary.pdf

65. Dubinsky RM, Lai SM: Mortality from combined carotid endarterectomy and coronary artery bypass surgery in the US, *Neurology* 68:195–197, 2007.

66. Hill MD, Shrive FM, Kennedy J, et al: Simultaneous carotid endarterectomy and coronary bypass surgery in Canada, *Neurology* 64:1435–1437, 2005.

67. Poldermans D, Boersma E, Bax JJ, et al: The effect of bisoprolol on perioperative mortality and myocardial infarction in high-risk patients undergoing vascular surgery, *N Engl J Med* 341:1789–1794, 1999.

68. Fleisher LA, Beckman JA, Brown KA, et al; American College of Cardiology/American Heart Association Task Force on Practice Guidelines (Writing Committee to Revise the 2002 Guidelines on Perioperative Cardiovascular Evaluation for Noncardiac Surgery); American Society of Echocardiography; American Society of Nuclear Cardiology; Heart Rhythm Society; Society of Cardiovascular Anesthesiologists; Society for Cardiovascular Angiography and Interventions; Society for Vascular Medicine and Biology; Society for Vascular Surgery: ACC/AHA 2007 guidelines on perioperative cardiovascular evaluation and care for noncardiac surgery: a report of the American College of Cardiology/American Heart Association Task Force on Practice Guidelines (Writing Committee to Revise the 2002 Guidelines on Perioperative Cardiovascular Evaluation for Noncardiac Surgery): Developed in collaboration with the American Society of Echocardiography, American Society of Nuclear Cardiology, Heart Rhythm Society, Society of Cardiovascular Anesthesiologists, Society for Cardiovascular Angiography and Interventions, Society for Vascular Medicine and Biology, and Society for Vascular Surgery. Circulation 2007;116;e418–e499.

69. POISE Study Group, Devereaux PJ, Yang H, Yusuf S, Guyatt G, et al: Effects of extended-release metoprolol succinate in patients undergoing non-cardiac surgery (POISE trial): A randomized controlled trial, *Lancet* 371:1839–1847, 2008.

70. Sear JW, Giles JW, Howard-Alpe G, Foex P: Perioperative beta-blockade, 2008: What does POISE tell us, and was our earlier caution justified? *Br J Anaesth* 101:135–138, 2008.

71. Fleisher LA, Poldermans D: Perioperative β blockade: Where do we go from here? *Lancet* 371:1813–1814, 2008.

72. Crisby M, Nordin-Fredriksson G, Shah PK, Yano J, et al: Pravastatin treatment increases collagen content and decreases lipid content, inflammation, metalloproteinases, and cell death in human carotid plaques: Implications for plaque stabilization, *Circulation* 103:926–933, 2001.

73. Poldermans D, Hoeks SE, Feringa HH: Pre-operative risk assessment and risk reduction before surgery, *J Am Coll Cardiol* 51:1913–1924, 2008.

74. McGirt MJ, Woodworth GF, Brooke BS, et al: Hyperglycemia independently increases the risk of perioperative stroke, myocardial infarction and death after carotid endarterectomy, *Neurosurgery* 58:1066–1073, 2006.

75. Kennedy J, Quan H, Buchan AM, et al: Statins are associated with better outcomes after carotid endarterectomy in symptomatic patients, *Stroke* 36:2072–2076, 2005.

76. Gelb AW, Herrick IA: Preoperative hypertension does predict post-carotid endarterectomy hypertension, *Can J Neurol Sci* 17:95–96, 1990.

77. Towne JB, Bernhard VM: The relationship of postoperative hypertension to complications following carotid endarterectomy, *Surgery* 88:575–580, 1980.

78. Skudlarick JL, Mooring SL: Systolic hypertension and complications of carotid endarterectomy, *South Med J* 75:1563–1565, 1982.

79. Baird TA, Parsons MW, Phanh T, Butcher KS, et al: Persistent post-stroke hyperglycemia is independently associated with infarct expansion and worse clinical outcome, *Stroke* 34:2208–2214, 2003.

80. McCormick MT, Muir KW, Gray CS, Walters MR: Management of hyperglycemia in acute stroke: How, when, and for whom? *Stroke* 39:2177–2185, 2008.

81. McGirt MJ, Woodworth GF, Brooke BS, et al: Hyperglycemia independently increases the risk of perioperative stroke, myocardial infarction and death after carotid endarterectomy, *Neurosurgery* 58:1066–1073, 2006.

82. Van den Berghe G, Wouters P, Weekers F, et al: Intensive insulin therapy in critically ill patients, *N Engl J Med* 345:1359–1367, 2001.

83. Van den Berghe G, Wilmer A, Hermans G, et al: Intensive insulin therapy in the medical ICU, *N Engl J Med* 354:449–461, 2006.

84. Inzucchi SE: Management of hyperglycemia in the hospital setting, *N Engl J Med* 355:1903–1911, 2006.

85. Varghese P, Gleason V, et al: Hypoglycemia in hospitalized patients treated with antihyperglycemic agents, *J Hosp Med* 2:234–240, 2007.

86. Wiener RS, Wiener DC, Larson RJ: Benefits and risks of tight glucose control in critically ill adults: A meta-analysis, *JAMA* 300:933–944, 2008.

87. Landesberg G, Mosseri M, Wolf Y, et al: Perioperative myocardial ischemia and infarction: Identification by continuous 12-lead electrocardiogram with online ST-segment monitoring, *Anesthesiology* 96:264–270, 2002.

88. Ferguson GG, Eliasziw M, Barr HW, et al: The North American Symptomatic Carotid Endarterectomy Trial: Surgical results in 1415 patients, *Stroke* 30:1751–1758, 1999.

89. Bond R, Warlow CP, Naylor AR, et al: Variation in surgical and anaesthetic technique and associations with operative risk in the European carotid surgery trial: Implications for trials of ancillary techniques, *Eur J Vasc Endovasc Surg* 23:117–126, 2002.

90. Cheng MA, Theard MA, Tempelhoff R: Anesthesia for carotid endarterectomy: A survey, *J Neurosurg Anesth* 9:211–216, 1997.

91. Rerkasem K, Bond R, Rothwell PM: Local versus general anaesthesia for carotid endarterectomy, *Cochrane Database Syst Rev* (2)2004:CD000126.

92. Rerkasem K, Bond R, Rothwell PM: Local versus general anaesthetic for carotid endarterectomy, *Stroke* 36:169–170, 2005.

93. Calligaro KD, Dougherty MJ, Lombardi J, et al: Converting from general anesthesia to cervical block anesthesia for carotid endarterectomy, *Vasc Surg* 35:103–106, 2001.

94. Pandit JJ, Satya-Krishna R, Gration P: Superficial or deep cervical plexus block for carotid endarterectomy: A systematic review of complications, *Br J Anaesth* 99:159–169, 2007.

95. Pandit JJ, Bree S, Dillon P, et al: A comparison of superficial versus combined (superficial and deep) cervical plexus block for carotid endarterectomy: A prospective, randomized study, *Anesth Analg* 91:781–786, 2000.

96. Stoneham MD, Doyle AR, Knighton JD, et al: Prospective, randomized comparison of deep or superficial cervical plexus block for carotid endarterectomy surgery, *Anesthesiology* 89:907–912, 1998.

97. Chaikof EL, Dodson TF, Thomas BL, et al: Four steps to local anesthesia for endarterectomy of the carotid artery, *Surg Gynecol Obstet* 177:308–310, 1993.

98. Murphy TM: Somatic blockade of the head and neck. In Cousins MJ, Bridenbaugh PO, editors: *Neural Blockade in Clinical Anesthesia and Management of Pain*, 3rd ed, Philadelphia, 1998, Lippincott-Raven, pp 489–514.

99. McCutcheon CA, Orme RM, Scott DA, et al: A comparison of dexmedetomidine versus conventional therapy for sedation and hemodynamic control during carotid endarterectomy performed under regional anesthesia, *Anesth Analg* 102:668–675, 2006.

100. Schneemilch CE, Bachmann H, Ulrich A, et al: Clonidine decreases stress response in patients undergoing carotid endarterectomy under regional anesthesia: A prospective, randomized, double-blinded, placebo-controlled study, *Anesth Analg* 103:297–302, 2006.

101. Bekker AY, Basile J, Gold M, et al: Dexmedetomidine for awake carotid endarterectomy: Efficacy, hemodynamic profile, and side effects, *J Neurosurg Anesthesiol* 16:126–135, 2004.

102. Carollo DS, Nossaman BD, Ramadhyani U: Dexmedetomidine: A review of clinical applications, *Curr Opin Anaesthesiol* 21:457–461, 2008.

103. Gerlach AT, Dasta JF: Dexmedetomidine: An updated review, *Ann Pharmacother* 41:245–252, 2007.

104. Umbrain V, Keeris J, D'Haese J, et al: Isoflurane, desflurane and sevoflurane for carotid endarterectomy, *Anaesthesia* 55(11):1052–1057, 2000.

105. Wilhelm W, Schlaich N, Harrer J, et al: Recovery and neurological examination after remifentanil-desflurane or fentanyl-desflurane anaesthesia for carotid artery surgery, *Br J Anaesth* 86(1):44–49, 2001.

106. Kostopanagiotou G, Markantonis SL, Polydorou M, et al: Recovery and cognitive function after fentanyl or remifentanil administration for carotid endarterectomy, *J Clin Anesth* 17:16–20, 2005.

107. Komatsu R, Turan AM, Orhan-Sungur M, et al: Remifentanil for general anaesthesia: A systematic review, *Anaesthesia* 62:1266–1280, 2007.

108. Fodale V, Schifilliti D, Pratico C, Santamaria LB: Remifentanil and the brain, *Acta Anaesthesiol Scand* 52:319–326, 2008.

109. Jellish WS, Sheikh T, Baker WH, et al: Hemodynamic stability, myocardial ischemia, and perioperative outcome after carotid surgery with remifentanil/propofol or isoflurane/fentanyl anesthesia, *J Neurosurg Anesth* 15:176–184, 2003.

110. Algotsson L, Messeter K, Rosen I, et al: Effects of nitrous oxide on cerebral haemodynamics and metabolism during isoflurane anaesthesia in man, *Acta Anaesthesiol Scand* 36:46–52, 1992.

111. Hansen TD, Warner DS, Todd MM, et al: Effects of nitrous oxide and volatile anesthetics on cerebral blood flow, *Br J Anaesth* 63:290–295, 1989.

112. Hartung J, Cottrell JE: Nitrous oxide reduces thiopental-induced prolongation of survival in hypoxic and anoxic mice, *Anesth Analg* 66:47–52, 1987.

113. Pelligrino DA, Miletich DJ, Hoffman WE, Albrecht RF: Nitrous oxide markedly increases cerebral cortical metabolic rate and blood flow in the goat, *Anesthesiology* 60:405–412, 1984.

114. Ikonomidou C, Bosch F, Miksa M, et al: Blockade of NMDA receptors and apoptotic neurodegeneration in the developing brain, *Science* 283:70–74, 1999.

115. Jevtovic-Todorovic V, Hartman RE, Izumi Y, et al: Early exposure to common anesthetic agents causes widespread neurodegeneration in the developing rat brain and persistent learning deficits, *J Neurosci* 23:876–882, 2003.

116. Haelewyn B, David HN, Rouillon C, et al: Neuroprotection by nitrous oxide: facts and evidence, *Crit Care Med* 36:2651–2659, 2008.

117. Reinstrup P, Ryding E, Ohlsson T, et al: Regional cerebral metabolic rate (positron emission tomography) during inhalation of nitrous oxide 50% in humans, *Br J Anaesth* 100:66–71, 2008.

118. McGregor DG, Lanier WL, Pasternak JJ, et al: Effect of nitrous oxide on neurologic and neuropsychological function after intracranial aneurysm surgery, *Anesthesiology* 108:568–579, 2008.

119. Culley DJ, Crosby G: Nitrous oxide in neuroanesthesia, *Anesthesiology* 108:553–554, 2008.

120. Myles PS, Leslie K, Chan MTV, et al: Avoidance of nitrous oxide for patients undergoing major surgery: A randomized controlled trial, *Anesthesiology* 107:221–231, 2007.

121. Head BP, Patel P: Anesthetics and brain protection, *Curr Opin Anaesthesiol* 20:395–399, 2007.

122. Koerner IP, Brambrink AM: Brain protection by anesthetic agents, *Curr Opin Anaesthesiol* 19:481–486, 2006.

123. Kawaguchi M, Furuya H, Patel PM: Neuroprotective effects of anesthetic agents, *J Anesth* 19:150–156, 2005.

124. Sanders RD, Ma D, Maze M: Anaesthesia induced neuroprotection, *Best Pract Res Clin Anaesthesiol* 19:461–474, 2005.

125. Melgar MA, Mariwalla N, Madhusudan H, Weinand M: Carotid endarterectomy without shunt: The role of cerebral metabolic protection, *Neurol Res* 27:850–856, 2005.

126. Durward QJ, Ragnarsson TS, Reeder RF, et al: Carotid endarterectomy in nonagenarians, *Arch Surg* 140:625–628, 2005.

127. Drader KS, Herrick IA: Carotid endarterectomy: Monitoring and its effect on outcome, *Anesthesiol Clin N Am* 15:613–629, 1997.

128. Craen RA, Gelb AW, Eliasziw M, et al: Anesthesia monitoring and neurologic outcome in carotid endarterectomy: NASCET results, *J Neurosurg Anesth* 5:303, 1993.

129. Bond R, Rerkasem K, Rothwell PM: Routine or selective carotid artery shunting for carotid endarterectomy (and different methods of monitoring in selective shunting). Cochrane Database Syst Rev2002;(2):CD000190.

130. Guarracino F: Cerebral monitoring during cardiovascular surgery, *Curr Opin Anaesthesiol* 21:50–54, 2008.

131. Cheng MA, Theard MA, Tempelhoff R: Anesthesia for carotid endarterectomy: A survey, *J Neurosurg Anesth* 9:211–216, 1997.

132. Craen RA, Gelb AW, Eliasziw M, et al: Anesthesia for carotid endarterectomy: The North American practice at 50 centres. NASCET Study Results, *Anesth Analg* 76:S61, 1993.

133. Sundt TM Jr, Sharbrough FW, Anderson RE, et al: Cerebral blood flow measurements and electroencephalograms during carotid endarterectomy, *J Neurosurg* 41:310–320, 1974.

134. Sundt TM Jr, Sharbrough FW, Piepgras DG, et al: Correlation of cerebral blood flow and electroencephalographic changes during carotid endarterectomy: With results of surgery and hemodynamics of cerebral ischemia, *Mayo Clin Proc* 56:533–543, 1981.

135. Sundt TM: Jr: The ischemic tolerance of neural tissue and need for monitoring and selective shunting during carotid endarterectomy, *Stroke* 14:93–98, 1983.

136. Redekop G, Ferguson GG: Correlation of contralateral stenosis and intraoperative electroencephalogram change with risk of stroke during carotid endarterectomy, *Neurosurgery* 30:191–194, 1992.

137. Plestis KA, Loubser P, Mizrahi EM, et al: Continuous electroencephalographic monitoring and selective shunting reduces neurologic morbidity rates in carotid endarterectomy, *J Vasc Surg* 25:620–628, 1997.

138. Morawetz RB, Zeiger HE, McDowell HA Jr, et al: Correlation of cerebral blood flow and EEG during carotid occlusion for endarterectomy (without shunting) and neurologic outcome, *Surgery* 96:184–189, 1984.

139. Zampella E, Morawetz RB, McDowell HA, et al: The importance of cerebral ischemia during carotid endarterectomy, *Neurosurg* 29:727–731, 1991.

140. Wober C, Zeitlhofer J, Asenbaum S, et al: Monitoring of median nerve somatosensory evoked potentials in carotid surgery, *J Clin Neurophysiol* 15:429–438, 1998.

141. Rowed DW, Houlden DA, Burkholder LM, Taylor AB: Comparison of monitoring techniques for intraoperative cerebral ischemia, *Can J Neurol Sci* 31:347–356, 2004.

142. Murkin JM, Lee DH: Noninvasive measurement of cerebral blood flow: Techniques and limitations, *Can J Anaesth* 38:805–808, 1991.

143. Markwalder TM, Grolimund P, Seiler RW, et al: Dependency of blood flow velocity in the middle cerebral artery on end-tidal carbon dioxide partial pressure—a transcranial ultrasound Doppler study, *J Cereb Blood Flow Metab* 4:368–372, 1984.

144. Naylor AR, Wildsmith JA, McClure J, et al: Transcranial Doppler monitoring during carotid endarterectomy, *Br J Surg* 1001;78:1264–1268.

145. Jansen C, Ramos LM, van Heesewijk JP, et al: Impact of microembolism and hemodynamic changes in the brain during carotid endarterectomy, *Stroke* 25:992–997, 1994.

146. Ackerstaff RG, Jansen C, Moll FL, et al: The significance of microemboli detection by means of transcranial Doppler ultrasonography monitoring in carotid endarterectomy, *J Vasc Surg* 21:963–969, 1995.

147. Molloy J, Markus HS: Asymptomatic embolization predicts stroke and TIA risk in patients with carotid artery stenosis, *Stroke* 30:1440–1443, 1999.

148. Siebler M, Kleinschmidt A, Sitzer M, et al: Cerebral microembolism in symptomatic and asymptomatic high-grade internal carotid artery stenosis, *Neurology* 44:615–618, 1994.

149. Levi CR, O'Malley HM, Fell G, et al: Transcranial Doppler detected cerebral microembolism following carotid endarterectomy: High microembolic signal loads predict postoperative cerebral ischaemia, *Brain* 120:621–629, 1997.

150. Lennard N, Smith J, Dumville J, et al: Prevention of postoperative thrombotic stroke after carotid endarterectomy: The role of transcranial Doppler ultrasound, *J Vasc Surg* 26:579–584, 1997.

151. van der Schaaf IC, Horn J, Moll FL, Ackerstaff RG: Transcranial Doppler monitoring after carotid endarterectomy, *Ann Vasc Surg* 19:19–24, 2005.

152. Levi CR, Stork JL, Chambers BR, et al: Dextran reduces embolic signals after carotid endarterectomy, *Ann Neurol* 50:544–547, 2001.

153. Robless PA, Tegos TJ, Okonko D, et al: Platelet activation during carotid endarterectomy and the antiplatelet effect of Dextran 40, *Platelets* 13:231–239, 2002.

154. Junghans U, Siebler M: Cerebral microembolism is blocked by tirofiban, a selective nonpeptide platelet glycoprotein IIb/IIIa receptor antagonist, *Circulation* 107:2717–2721, 2003.

155. van Dellen D, Tiivas CA, Jarvi K, et al: Transcranial Doppler ultrasonography-directed intravenous glycoprotein IIb/IIIa receptor antagonist therapy to control transient cerebral microemboli before and after carotid endarterectomy, *Br J Surg* 95:709–713, 2008.

156. Moore WS, Hall AD: Carotid artery back pressure: A test of cerebral tolerance to temporary carotid occlusion, *Arch Surg* 99:702–710, 1969.

157. Moore WS, Yee JM, Hall AD: Collateral cerebral blood pressure: An index of tolerance to temporary carotid occlusion, *Arch Surg* 106:521–523, 1973.

158. McKay RD, Sundt TM, Michenfelder JD, et al: Internal carotid artery stump pressure and cerebral blood flow during carotid endarterectomy: Modification by halothane, enflurane and Innovar, *Anesthesiology* 45:390–399, 1976.

159. Modica PA, Tempelhoff R: A comparison of computerized EEG with internal carotid artery stump pressure for detection of ischemia during carotid endarterectomy, *J Neurosurg Anesth* 1:211–218, 1989.

160. Whitley D, Cherry KJ: Predictive value of carotid artery stump pressures during carotid endarterectomy, *Neurosurg Clin N Am* 7:723–732, 1996.

161. Moritz S, Kasprzak P, Arlt M, et al: Accuracy of cerebral monitoring in detecting cerebral ischemia during carotid endarterectomy: A comparison of transcranial Doppler sonography, near-infrared spectroscopy, stump pressure, and somatosensory evoked potentials, *Anesthesiology* 107:563–569, 2007.

162. Hans SS, Jareunpoon O: Prospective evaluation of electroencephalography, carotid artery stump pressure, and neurologic changes during 314 consecutive carotid endarterectomies performed in awake patients, *J Vasc Surg* 45:511–515, 2007.

163. Wolf M, Ferrari M, Quaresima V: Progress of near-infrared spectroscopy and topography for brain and muscle clinical applications, *J Biomed Opt* 12:062104, 2007.

164. McCormick PW, Stewart M, Goetting MG, et al: Regional cerebrovascular oxygen saturation measured by optical spectroscopy in humans, *Stroke* 22:596–602, 1991.

165. Ferrari M, Mottola L, Quaresima V: Principles, techniques, and limitations of near infrared spectroscopy, *Can J Appl Physiol* 29:463–487, 2004.

166. Lam JM, Smielewski P, al-Rawi P, et al: Internal and external carotid contributions to near-infrared spectroscopy during carotid endarterectomy, *Stroke* 28:906–911, 1997.

167. Kishi K, Kawaguchi M, Yoshitani K, et al: Influence of patient variables and sensor location on regional cerebral oxygen saturation measured by INVOS 4100 near-infrared spectrophotometers, *J Neurosurg Anesthesiol* 15:302–306, 2003.

168. Samra SK, Dy EA, Welch K, et al: Evaluation of a cerebral oximeter as a monitor of cerebral ischemia during carotid endarterectomy, *Anesthesiology* 93:964–970, 2000.

169. Mille T, Tachimiri ME, Klersy C, et al: Near infrared spectroscopy monitoring during carotid endarterectomy: Which threshold value is critical? *Eur J Vasc Endovasc Surg* 27:646–650, 2004.

170. Sharbrough FW, Messick JM, Sundt TM: Correlation of continuous electroencephalograms with cerebral blood flow measurements during carotid endarterectomy, *Stroke* 4:674–683, 1973.

171. Sundt TM Jr, Sharbrough FW, Anderson RE, et al: Cerebral blood flow measurements and electroencephalograms during carotid endarterectomy, *J Neurosurg* 41:310–320, 1974.

172. Sundt TM Jr, Sharbrough FW, Piepgras DG, et al: Correlation of cerebral blood flow and electroencephalographic changes during carotid endarterectomy: With results of surgery and hemodynamics of cerebral ischemia, *Mayo Clin Proc* 56:533–543, 1981.

173. Messick JM Jr, Casement B, Sharbrough FW, et al: Correlation of regional cerebral blood flow (rCBF) with EEG changes during isoflurane anesthesia for carotid endarterectomy: Critical rCBF, *Anesthesiology* 66:344–349, 1987.

174. Michenfelder JD, Sundt TM, Fode N, et al: Isoflurane when compared to enflurane and halothane decreases the frequency of cerebral ischemia during carotid endarterectomy, *Anesthesiology* 67:336–340, 1987.

175. Grady RE, Weglinski MR, Sharbrough FW, Perkins WJ: Correlation of regional cerebral blood flow with ischemic electroencephalographic changes during sevoflurane-nitrous oxide anesthesia for carotid endarterectomy, *Anesthesiology* 88:892–897, 1998.

176. Bond R, Rerkasem K, Rothwell PM: Routine or selective carotid artery shunting for carotid endarterectomy (and different methods of monitoring in selective shunting), *Cochrane Database Syst Rev* (2)2002:CD000190.

177. Sloan MA: Prevention of ischemic neurologic injury with intraoperative monitoring of selected cardiovascular and cerebrovascular procedures: Roles of electroencephalography, somatosensory evoked potentials, transcranial Doppler, and near-infrared spectroscopy, *Neurol Clin* 24:631–645, 2006.

178. Whiten C, Gunning P: Carotid endarterectomy: Intraoperative monitoring of cerebral perfusion, (In press, corrected proof) Current Anaesthesia & Critical Care 20:42–45, 2009.

179. Wade JG, Larson CP, Hickey RF, et al: Effect of carotid endarterectomy on carotid chemoreceptor and baroreceptor function in man, *N Engl J Med* 15:823–829, 1970.

180. O'Connor CJ, Tuman KJ: Anesthetic considerations for carotid artery surgery. In Kaplan JA, Lake CL, Murray MJ, editors: *Vascular Anesthesia*, 2nd ed, St. Louis, 2004, Churchill Livingstone.

181. Bove EL, Fry WJ, Gross WS, et al: Hypotension and hypertension as consequences of baroreceptor dysfunction following carotid endarterectomy, *Surgery* 85:633–637, 1979.

182. Nouraei SA, Al-Rawi PG, Sigaudo-Roussel D, et al: Carotid endarterectomy impairs blood pressure homeostasis by reducing the physiologic baroreflex reserve, *J Vasc Surg* 41:631–637, 2005.

183. Cafferata HT, Merchant RF, DePalma RG: Avoidance of postcarotid endarterectomy hypertension, *Ann Surg* 196:465–472, 1982.

184. Pine R, Avellone JC, Hoffman M, et al: Control of postcarotid endarterectomy hypotension with baroreceptor blockade, *Am J Surg* 147:763–765, 1984.

185. Prough DS, Scuderi PE, McWhorter JM, et al: Hemodynamic status following regional and general anesthesia for carotid endarterectomy, *J Neurosurg Anesth* 1:35–40, 1989.

186. Gottlieb A, Satariano-Hayden P, Schoenwald P, et al: The effect of carotid sinus nerve blockade on hemodynamic stability after carotid endarterectomy, *J Cardiothorac Vasc Anesth* 11:67–71, 1997.

187. Krul JMJ, van Gijn J, Ackerstaff RGA, et al: Site and pathogenesis of infarcts associated with carotid endarterectomy, *Stroke* 20:324–328, 1989.

188. Steed DL, Peitzman AB, Grundy BL, et al: Causes of stroke in carotid endarterectomy, *Surgery* 92:634–641, 1982.

189. Sieber FE, Toung TJ, Diringer MM, et al: Factors influencing stroke outcome following carotid endarterectomy [abstract], *Anesth Analg* 70:S370, 1990.

190. Rockman CB, Jacobowitz GR, Lamparello PJ, et al: Immediate reexploration for the perioperative neurologic event after carotid endarterectomy: Is it worthwhile? *J Vasc Surg* 32:1062–1070, 2000.

191. Motamed C, Motamed-Kazerounian G, Merle JC, et al: Cardiac troponin I assessment and late cardiac complications after carotid stenting or endarterectomy, *J Vasc Surg* 41:769–774, 2005.

192. Rijbroek A, Boellaard R, Vermeulen EG, et al: Hemodynamic changes in ipsi- and contralateral cerebral arterial territories after carotid endarterectomy using positron emission tomography, *Surg Neurol* 71:668–676, 2009:discussion 676.

193. Abou-Chebl A, Yadav JS, Reginelli JP, et al: Intracranial haemorrhage and hyperperfusion syndrome following carotid artery stenting, *J Am Coll Cardiol* 43:1596–1601, 2004.

194. Adhiyaman V, Alexander S: Cerebral hyperperfusion syndrome following carotid endarterectomy, *Q J Med* 100:239–244, 2007.

195. Schroeder T, Sillesen H, Sorensen O, et al: Cerebral hyperperfusion following carotid endarterectomy, *J Neurosurg* 66:824–829, 1987.

196. Schroeder T: Hemodynamic significance of internal carotid artery disease, *Acta Neurol Scand* 77:353–372, 1998.

197. Yoshimoto T, Shirasaka T, Yoshizumi T, et al: Evaluation of carotid distal pressure for prevention of hyperperfusion after carotid endarterectomy, *Surg Neurol* 63:554–557, 2005.

198. Cunningham EJ, Bond R, Mayberg MR, et al: Risk of persistent cranial nerve injury after carotid endarterectomy, *J Neurosurg* 101:445–448, 2004.

199. Ballotta E, Da Giau G, Renon L, et al: Cranial and cervical nerve injuries after carotid endarterectomy: A prospective study, *Surgery* 125:85–91, 1999.

Chapter 17

AWAKE CRANIOTOMY, EPILEPSY, MINIMALLY INVASIVE, AND ROBOTIC SURGERY

Armin Schubert • Michelle Lotto

AWAKE CRANIOTOMY

Awake craniotomy is performed when tissue resection requires mapping of eloquent cortical tissue located in close proximity to the area to be resected. This may be necessary for either brain tumor removal or resection of ictal foci during epilepsy surgery, in which this technique may also be helpful to avoid anesthetic-related interference with intraoperative brain mapping. Awake craniotomy also potentially causes fewer complications. Patients with good preoperative functional status undergoing uncomplicated tumor resection with this technique have hospital stays of only 1 day.[1,2] The technique is associated with acceptable patient satisfaction, 8% to 37% of patients having amnesia about having been awake during surgery. The most frequent complaints are about pain from the head holder, inadequate local anesthesia, and position on the operating table.[3]

Anesthetic Technique

The anesthetic technique for "awake" craniotomy is more aptly described as variable-depth general anesthesia with periods of wakefulness. Various institutions and anesthetists have reported on favored techniques for "awake" craniotomies, including periods of general anesthesia with use of a laryngeal mask airway[4] or endotracheal intubation; alternatively, deep sedation with discontinuation of anesthesia for the period of speech or memory testing has been described[5,6] and found safe.[7] Despite the development of multiple approaches to the problem, the awake craniotomy remains one of the more challenging techniques of anesthesia, and no method is without its pitfalls and limitations.

Critical Success Factors

Components of successful technique include appropriate patient selection, thorough preoperative psychological preparation, solid rapport between patient and anesthesiologist, comfort in patient positioning, appropriate scalp block, proper anesthetic selection, and continuous team communication. In our clinical experience, patients who do best are well motivated, mature, and free of alcohol and drug abuse. Little guidance exists in the literature about patient factors, although lack of maturity, hypertension, and alcohol abuse are mentioned anecdotally as risk factors for sedation failure.[8]

Psychological Preparation

Preoperative consultation and discussion of expectations with the patient should have a significant impact on the anxiety of the patient undergoing neurologic surgery. Planned awake craniotomy should always be preceded by a realistic description of what the patient will experience, including expected discomforts, level of cooperation desired, and tasks that will be performed for speech and memory testing, and the possibility of events that may require rapid interventions, such as conversion to general anesthesia. It is important that the anesthesiologist develop good rapport with the patient during the preoperative period. The interview should include an assessment of the patient's ability to cooperate during a planned awake procedure. Patients who are too young, are mentally impaired, have personality disorders (particularly those involving anxiety), behavioral problems, or difficult airways should not be considered for "awake" craniotomy. The age cutoff utilized at our institution varies according to the individual adolescent's maturity. We recommend that children younger than 14 years not be considered, although the developmental status of the individual should be assessed.[9]

Positioning

Patients are best placed in the full lateral position to allow adequate access to the airway and avoid back or pressure point pain after prolonged positioning. The patient should be allowed to assist in finding the most comfortable head and body position for the procedure, so that risk of positioning injury is minimized. Excellent access to the patient's face and extremities is required. The drapes must be appropriately tented to allow access to the patient's face for both patient safety and adequate sensorimotor, speech, and memory testing. Pillows are placed between the patient's legs, between the back and the back support, and in front of the patient, who is allowed "hug" the pillow in front. Potential pressure points are padded with foam or soft blankets. Figure 17-1 demonstrates a configuration for operating room setup that we have found useful. Patient position is stabilized with the use of a deflatable beanbag or a backrest fixed to the operating table, augmented by taping of the patient to the table. Although some surgeons choose to use a pin-type head holder to minimize head movement, the holder is not attached to the bed but is placed on a foam doughnut for comfort.

Anesthetic Options

There are no prospective data showing that one anesthetic approach is preferable to another for awake craniotomy. Some patients can tolerate the entire procedure with only light sedation; others may require what has also been referred to as "asleep-awake-asleep" anesthetic protocols. Neuroleptanalgesia with droperidol (0.15 mg/kg) and fentanyl

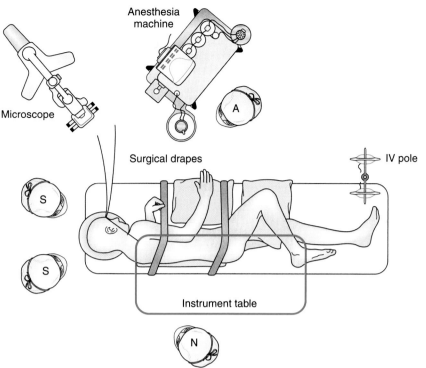

Figure 17–1 Operating room setup for right-sided craniotomy performed for the awake patient. Note the arrangement of the surgical drapes, which ensures access to the patient's face. The pin holder is not shown. A, anesthesiologist; N, nurse; S, surgeon. *(From Schubert A: Epilepsy Surgery. Clinical Neuroanesthesia, 2nd ed. Cleveland, OH, Cleveland Clinic Press, 2006, p 66.)*

(0.5-0.75 μg/kg) was popular in the 1980s.[10] In the United States and Europe this regimen has been all but abandoned because of the association of prolonged sedation, seizures, and the risk of prolonged QT interval–related cardiac rhythm disturbances, as identified in a "black box warning" issued by the U.S. Federal Drug Administration. Propofol infusion with various opioids and, more recently, the central nervous system–specific α_2 agonist dexmedetomidine has been successfully used for awake craniotomy.

Regardless of anesthetic technique, excellent scalp local anesthesia is required for patient comfort. Escalating the patient's sedation to supplement an inadequate scalp block should be avoided because doing so would needlessly increase the risk of airway obstruction and oversedation during cognitive testing. Two reports have described the technique utilized for local scalp anesthesia during craniotomy.[11,12] Individually blocking the auriculotemporal, zygomaticotemporal, supraorbital, supratrochlear, lesser occipital, and greater occipital nerves is necessary to provide complete analgesia of the scalp. This technique uses less local anesthetic and may therefore prevent toxicity. Ropivacaine and levobupivacaine can be safely used up to doses of 4.5 mg/kg[13] and 2.5 mg/kg, respectively.[14] These blocks achieve peak plasma concentrations approximately 15 minutes after injection.

After monitors are applied, we begin light sedation in the supine position for placement of urinary and arterial catheters. Infusion rates of sedatives are increased, and bolus doses of a short-acting sedative, such as propofol 10 to 20 mg, are administered during the placement of the scalp block and Mayfield head-pin holder. Anesthetics are then adjusted to induce general anesthesia with spontaneous ventilation. Frequently, a nasal airway is necessary to ensure airway patency.

The development of short-acting rapidly titratable intravenous agents has made total intravenous anesthetic (TIVA) a viable choice for the awake craniotomy.[15] Propofol-only anesthesia with spontaneously breathing patients has been described as safe. Propofol is begun with a bolus of 0.5 mg/kg and continued at a rate of 75-250 μg/kg/min.[7] We have used a combination of propofol (75-150 μg/kg/min) and either alfentanil (0.25-0.75 μg/kg/min) or fentanyl (0.5-1 μg/kg/hr). These agents are discontinued 15 to 20 minutes prior to the testing period. During testing, the opioid infusion may be restarted at a low dose to maintain an analgesic background. Alfentanil is known to induce epileptiform discharges in the hippocampal area and so should be used with caution in patients with complex partial epilepsy.[16] At conventional doses, remifentanil may cause severe hypopnea in the spontaneously ventilating patient; dosing should be in the range of 0.01-0.05 μg/kg/min.[17] In a comparison with continuous remifentanil infusion, propofol infusion combined with intermittent fentanyl yielded similar patient satisfaction, recall, and intraoperative complications, although a few more patients experienced reversible respiratory depression with propofol.[18] Time of emergence from sedation for intraoperative testing with the use of remifentanil-propofol is on the order of 9 minutes.[19] It should be remembered that remifentanil's intraoperative analgesic effect must be replaced with longer-acting analgesics before emergence in order to minimize emergence excitement and hyperalgesia.

Dexmedetomidine has now gained favor owing to its unique property of inducing sedation with minimal respiratory effects.[20] It offers both anxiolytic and analgesic qualities. Whether it possesses anticonvulsant and brain-protective properties in humans remains to be demonstrated. This agent is given as a loading dose of 1 μg/kg over 10 to 15 minutes and then infused at 0.2 to 0.6 μg/kg/hr for the remainder of the procedure. Doses are higher in children. Dexmedetomidine can be used as a sole sedative agent and in combination with other agents such as fentanyl.[21] We prefer to use a low-dose propofol infusion (25 to 75 μg/kg/min) that can be titrated to the desired sedation depth. Others have reported good experience with remifentanil combined with dexmedetomidine.[22] Propofol and dexmedetomidine are discontinued 15 to 20 minutes before intraoperative stimulation of motor and speech areas, to allow adequate time for the patient's emergence from sedation. Experience with dexmedetomidine has demonstrated that some patients require more intense effort to be roused from dexmedetomidine sedation (a physical stimulus such as sternal rub and calling of the patient's name). However, once roused and engaged, the patient remains able to cooperate with cognitive testing. At least one institution has reported difficulty with cognitive testing in patients receiving dexmedetomidine during Wada testing. It is possible the excessive sedation was due to the use of additional sedative agents, such as benzodiazepines, in combination with dexmedetomidine. Some practitioners continue dexmedetomidine during testing, albeit at a lower dose. Dexmedetomidine is known to have a significant synergistic effect, and the sedative effect will be greater when this agent is used in combination with other sedative agents.[23]

Brain Mapping and Cognitive Testing

Patients may be temporarily confused while emerging for the testing portion of the procedure. During this time it is prudent to engage the patient continually in a calming voice and to have personnel available to restrain the patient's movement. Once the patient is sufficiently awake to cooperate reliably (usually 15 to 20 minutes after stopping of the anesthetic), brain mapping is accomplished. Brain mapping procedures may include direct cortical stimulation to identify functional brain areas, cortical evoked potentials (EPs) to distinguish motor from sensory cortex, and electrocorticography (ECoG) to identify seizure foci. During cortical stimulation, the patient may be distressed by strange sensations and involuntary movements. Reassurance and comforting words go a long way, but mild sedation is occasionally also provided. More seriously, a seizure may be precipitated, which it requires prompt termination as well as assurance of a patent airway and adequate ventilation. Surgical resection then proceeds while the patient either completes verbal tasks (speech area assessment) or performs motor tasks (motor area assessment).

Surgical resection is stopped or modified at the first sign of speech difficulty or motor weakness. After completion of the brain functional testing, sedation is again deepened to the point of unresponsiveness as necessary. This lower depth is frequently necessary because of increased surgical stimulation during scalp closure and because many patients have exceeded their limits of tolerance toward the end of a lengthy surgical procedure during which their cooperation was intermittently needed.

Adverse Events and Management

During sedation for "awake" craniotomy, complications such as seizures, respiratory depression, nausea, vomiting, and agitation can be managed safely by the experienced anesthesiologist. Airway obstruction, hypercarbia, and hypoxemia may occur during deep sedation or general anesthesia without mechanical ventilation. The rate of conversion to general anesthesia has been reported to be 2%.[5] Skucas and Artru[7] reported that hypoxemic events occurred at a rate of 18.4% for asleep-awake-asleep techniques at their institution, compared with less than 1% for general anesthesia with tracheal intubation and mechanical ventilation. Similarly, hypertensive and hypotensive episodes were more prevalent. Transient respiratory depression is much more prevalent with propofol than with dexmedetomidine-based techniques, in which it is virtually absent.[5] Reducing anesthetic dose and inserting an oral cuffed, oropharyngeal,[24] nasal, or laryngeal mask airway

may become necessary. Titrating sedative dose to a respiratory rate of 12 breaths/min is a useful rule of thumb to avoid excessive respiratory depression. Dexmedetomidine was used successfully to rescue a patient unable to tolerate awake brain mapping after a propofol-remifentanil sedation regimen.[25]

The risk of vomiting is present in a heavily sedated patient with an unprotected airway. The incidence of nausea and vomiting is 4% for mixed sedation techniques[26] and even less for use of propofol.[7] To guard against nausea and vomiting, prophylactic administration of antiemetics is advisable. Once symptoms occur, they can be controlled with a 5' hydroxytryptamine (5-HT-3) receptor antagonist, such as metoclopramide 10 mg. Nausea can also result from inadequate analgesia of dural attachments and meningeal vessels; an additional local anesthetic should be administered by the surgeon and supplemented by intravenous analgesia.

Brain swelling can be an issue, especially in patients with intracranial mass effect. Spontaneous ventilation, through maintenance of negative intrathoracic pressure and promotion of cerebral venous outflow, assists in keeping the brain slack. The administration of mannitol or furosemide may become necessary in some cases. Sudden movement is certainly undesirable during craniotomy; it may be associated with straining and resultant brain swelling as well as with injury to scalp and soft tissues from the head pins. Sudden movement is most likely a result of seizures, startling responses during emergence, or delirium; it must be anticipated during awake craniotomy, and appropriate management strategies employed. In our experience, small predrawn boluses of propofol administered into a patent intravenous line and flushed immediately are effective to stop patient movement.

Compared with neuroleptanalgesia, propofol sedation techniques have a much lower intraoperative seizure risk. Still, a 4.9% incidence of seizures was reported with cortical mapping in an unselected series of 610 awake craniotomies.[1] Seizures may occur from electrical stimulation during brain mapping or from a patient's underlying condition. Immobilization of the head may be dangerous in these situations. Seizure activity (especially with direct cortical stimulation) can be treated with propofol (0.75-1.25 mg/kg), or thiopental (1.0-1.5 mg/kg), depending on the need for subsequent electroencephalograph (EEG) recording. At the end of the procedure, benzodiazepines and phenytoin may also be used.

EPILEPSY SURGERY

Epilepsy is a disease that pervasively and negatively affects patients' lifestyle, intellectual and social development, employment, economic status, and general health. It is prevalent in 0.5% to 2.2% of the general population.[27] Because 30% to 40% of cases of epilepsy do not respond adequately to pharmacologic intervention,[28] more than 400,000 people still have medically uncontrolled epilepsy in the United States. Medically uncontrolled epilepsy should lead to an assessment of surgical treatment options. However, only 10% to 30% of the patients with seizures refractory to medical management are appropriate candidates for seizure surgery, and only 1% eventually undergo the procedure.

Epilepsy is classified as partial epilepsy, generalized epilepsy, and pseudoseizures. *Partial epilepsy* denotes a focal onset in the brain. Partial seizures are *complex* when they spread into other brain regions and are associated with loss of consciousness; they are *simple* when they stay localized and are nearly asymptomatic. *Generalized seizures* have no focal onset and are either inhibitory (which include "absence" or "petit mal" and atonic seizures) or excitatory (tonic, clonic, or myoclonic). Tonic-clonic seizures are also referred to as convulsive or "grand mal" seizures. *Pseudoseizures* are conversion reactions with motor activity that mimic a seizure but with no EEG evidence of epileptic activity.

Surgical management of epilepsy has become widely accepted for patients in whom medical management fails. Despite the potential emergence of alternative surgical interventions such as vagal nerve stimulation and thalamic deep brain stimulation, resection of the seizure focus, for example, temporal lobectomy via open craniotomy, is still the mainstay of surgical treatment. With surgical intervention, lifestyle improves, although most patients continue anticonvulsant therapy. Chin and colleagues[29] reported that the rate of employment improved only modestly in their group of 375 patients, from 39.5% fully employed status preoperatively to 42.8% postoperatively; the rate of part-time employment nearly doubled, however, from 6.9% to 12.4%.[29]

Anesthetic selection is key to successful intraoperative mapping of the epileptic foci or identification of eloquent tissue during resection of epileptogenic tissue. Anesthetic agents vary widely and in a confusing manner with respect to their proconvulsant and anticonvulsant effects, yet the latter must be taken into consideration in the design of an anesthetic regimen for epilepsy surgery. Pharmacologic interactions between anticonvulsant medications and anesthetic drugs must also be taken into account. Optimal anesthetic care plan development considers intraoperative goals of the surgeon and neurophysiologist as well as the pharmacology of the patient's antiepileptic medications and the anesthetic agents. Good communication among the anesthesiologist, surgeon, and neurophysiologist is critical in achieving patient safety and a successful procedure. An overview of the anesthetic care for epilepsy surgery is presented here, with a focus on the pharmacology of common anesthetic agents and their potential effects on patient experience as well as the success of the surgical procedure.

Pharmacology of Anesthetic Agents

Given the modification of neuronal transmission generated by anesthetic agents, it is not surprising that these drugs can have significant effects on central nervous system excitation events. However, the literature describing the proconvulsant versus anticonvulsant effects of many anesthetic agents can be confusing and seemingly contradictory. The mechanisms behind the conflicting convulsant effects of these agents are not completely understood. It may be that the ratio of affected inhibitory or excitatory neurons in both the cortical and subcortical brain structures changes with depth of sedation. EEG recordings support altering the activation and inhibition of the cerebral cortex with administration of anesthetic agents. For example, during light sedation, cortical activation with higher-frequency beta activity predominates, which then progresses to slow-wave activity as sedative or anesthetic depth increases.[30]

To make matters even more complex, several induction agents, such as propofol and thiopental, can induce myoclonic movements not associated with EEG excitatory activity, whereas others, such as etomidate and methohexital, have been shown to generate both myoclonus and EEG-documented epileptiform activity in patients.[31,32]

Sedative-Hypnotic Agents

As a group, sedative-hypnotic agents have the greatest variation and most confusing profile as far as effects on epileptogenic activity. Most of the agents can generate neuroexcitatory effects when used at low doses and neurodepressive effects when used at higher doses. Motor stimulatory phenomena, such as myoclonus, opisthotonus, and tonic-clonic activity, may occur with varying frequency in both epileptic and nonepileptic patients during induction with these agents, but only a few agents actually produce cortical electrical activity suggestive of seizures.

Methohexital, etomidate, and ketamine are known to activate EEG seizure activity when administered to patients with a history of epilepsy.[33,34] Motor activity may not occur with the induction of abnormal spike wave activity. Etomidate, methohexital, and ketamine have been used to assist with activation of ictal foci during intraoperative ECoG.[35-38] These agents may also generate nonepileptic myoclonic activity during induction[39,40] that can be mistaken for epileptic convulsions.

Etomidate has a dichotomous effect on seizure thresholds, producing EEG-confirmed epileptic activity when used as an induction agent in epileptic patients as well as producing burst suppression and breaking status epilepticus when administered in higher doses.[41,42] Ketamine appears to have a dose-dependent threshold for seizure generation, with most reported cases of clinical seizure activity occurring when doses larger than 4 mg/kg are administered.[43,44] In patients undergoing anterior temporal lobe resection for intractable epilepsy, dexmedetomidine was found to reduce ECoG median frequency but did not affect seizure spike activity during sevoflurane anesthesia.[45]

Despite an early report of seizure induction with propofol injection, propofol has had a good safety record and low epileptogenic potential when used in patients undergoing epilepsy surgery. The anticonvulsant properties of propofol are fairly well established, although the antiepileptic effect may be shorter acting after discontinuation of propofol in comparison with thiopental.[46] The short-acting antiepileptic nature of propofol can be useful for sedation during epileptic procedures. Propofol decreases the frequency of epileptogenic spikes and quiets existing seizure foci, particularly in the lateral and mesial temporal areas.[47] However, propofol may generate beta EEG activity, obscuring spike wave activity for up to 20 minutes after discontinuation of the infusion (Fig. 17-2).[11,48] Therefore, propofol infusions should be discontinued 20 to 30 minutes prior to ECoG monitoring to facilitate interpretation of ECoG readings and successful location of the ictal foci.[49] Propofol also causes myoclonic movements during anesthesia induction.

Barbiturates and benzodiazepines have substantiated anticonvulsive properties and are recommended for treatment of refractory status epilepticus.[50]

Volatile Inhalational Agents and Nitrous Oxide

The epileptogenic potential of isoflurane, desflurane, and halothane appears low, and there have been no reported seizures when used in isolation.[51] However, there are rare reports of myoclonic activity with a normal EEG. Convulsions with spike and wave activity on EEG have been reported with combinations of isoflurane and nitrous oxide (N_2O).[52,53] Although N_2O has been associated with seizure generation when used to supplement other agents, it appears to be fairly inert in both the development and the treatment of seizure activity in

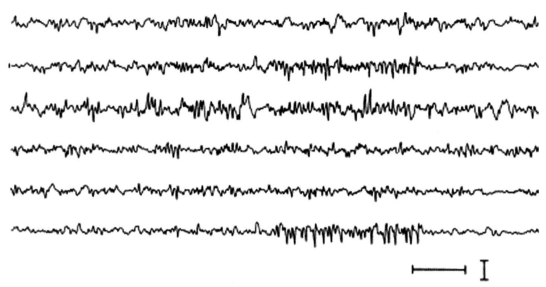

Figure 17–2 β-electroencelographic activation 10 minutes after propofol injection (right temporal and central convexity). *(From Ebrahim ZY, Schubert A, Van Ness P, et al: The effect of propofol on the electroencephalogram of patients with epilepsy. Anesth Analg 1994;78:275-279.)*

humans.[54] Both N_2O and isoflurane have been used for many years at multiple institutions with a good safety record in epileptic patients.

Enflurane, used either with or without nitrous oxide, has been the most common offender, with reports of intraoperative and postoperative myoclonus and EEG-demonstrated epileptiform activity in both epileptic and nonepileptic patient populations.[12,34,35,54,55] The incidence of EEG spike wave production with enflurane appears to be dose dependent. The end-tidal concentration that triggers maximum epileptiform activity is reduced during hypocapnia. Enflurane has fallen out of favor as new inhalational agents have become available, and it is now rarely used clinically in the United States. Enflurane should be avoided in patients with epilepsy unless the desired effect is to trigger seizures during ECoG.

Sevoflurane, but not desflurane,[51] has been reported to generate convulsions as well as electrical spike waves in both epileptic and nonepileptic patients.[56,57] The frequency of spike wave activity with sevoflurane increases with dose escalation and hyperventilation (Fig. 17-3).[51,58] Hisada and colleagues[59] reported that widespread neuroexcitatory activity associated with sevoflurane did not facilitate seizure focus localization in patients with temporal lobe epilepsy.[59] Hyperventilation decreases the prediction specificity of leads with ictal spikes and should be employed cautiously during ECoG.[60]

Analgesics

The effects of opioids on seizure threshold vary with opioid drug class. Synthetic opioids such as alfentanil, fentanyl, sufentanil, and the newer remifentanil are commonly used in neurosurgical anesthesia owing to their short duration of action and their ability to minimize cortical effects through continuous infusion. High doses of synthetic opioids have proepileptic properties. Bolus doses of synthetic opioids, such as alfentanil and remifentanil, increase spike wave activity in the interictal foci of patients undergoing intraoperative ECoG.[61,62] In fact, bolus doses of these agents are used to facilitate location of the ictal cortex through stimulation of spike wave phenomenon with concomitant depression of background EEG. Alfentanil 30 μg/kg has been found to be more effective for this purpose than remifentanil 1 μg/kg.[63] Fentanyl has been associated with epileptiform electrical activity in subcortical nonictal cortical tissue; therefore we avoid the dosing range in which epileptogenic properties have been observed (17-25 μg/kg).[64] The clinical history of the use of synthetic opioids in large numbers of epileptic patients undergoing ablative procedures suggests that synthetic opioids can be used safely in this patient population without a significant increase in the risk of perioperative seizures. Morphine and hydromorphone used at clinically relevant doses do not appear to have significant proconvulsant activity.[54]

Muscle Relaxants

Long-term anticonvulsant therapy with phenytoin, carbamazepine, or both is associated with resistance to the effect of nondepolarizing neuromuscular blockers, including pancuronium, vecuronium,[65-67] metocurine, cisatracurium, and rocuronium, but less so with atracurium.[68,69] The etiology of this phenomenon is likely both pharmacodynamic and pharmacokinetic.[70,71]

Anesthetic Management

Goals

In providing perioperative care for the patient undergoing epilepsy surgery, the anesthesiologist aims to give a continuum of critical care throughout the perioperative period. Preoperatively, the status of both the patient's neurologic and medical comorbidities needs to be assessed. Intraoperatively, the common goals of neurosurgical anesthesia apply, including control of brain bulk, cerebral blood flow, systemic blood pressure, and emergence from anesthesia to allow for early postoperative neurologic examination. For procedures that require seizure induction for localization of epileptic foci, the anesthesiologist is concerned with selecting the most effective agent and avoiding induction of a prolonged epileptogenic event and potential patient injury. In the postoperative period, seizures may have to be treated, neurologic status monitored, and depressed consciousness evaluated.

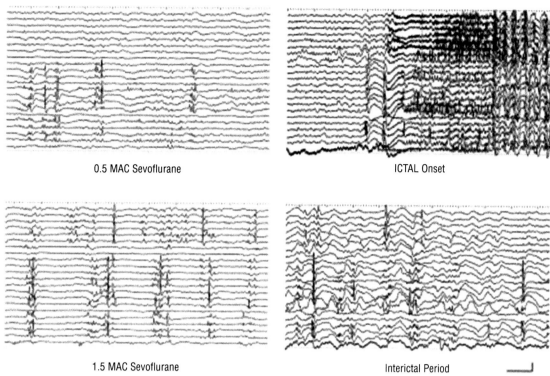

0.5 MAC Sevoflurane

ICTAL Onset

1.5 MAC Sevoflurane

Interictal Period

Figure 17–3 Effect of sevoflurane on electroencephalogram (EEG).). At 0.5 minimum alveolar concentration (MAC) sevoflurane, EEG is comparable to pre-ictal awake EEG. At 1.5 MAC sevoflurane, EEG is similar to interictal periods before anesthesia. NV, normoventilation. *(From Kurita N, Kawaguchi M, Hoshida T, et al: The effects of sevoflurane and hyperventilation on electrocorticogram spike activity in patients with refractory epilepsy. Anesth Analg 2005;101:517-523.)*

Preoperative Evaluation

NEUROLOGIC HISTORY

The nature and manifestations of the patient's seizures should be inquired about preoperatively. Epileptic activity can occasionally be difficult to discriminate from psychomotor behavior sometimes displayed during emergence delirium. Familiarity with the patient's seizure pattern promotes recognition and awareness of perioperative seizures. In all cases, the anesthesiologist should maintain a high level of suspicion for an epileptic etiology in a patient who has prolonged emergence from anesthesia, poor responsiveness, or repetitive motor movements in the postoperative period. Small case series suggest that significant pneumocephalus may be seen for up to 1 month after craniotomy.[72] Avoidance of nitrous oxide in patients in whom intracranial electrodes have recently been placed would thus be prudent.

CONCOMITANT MEDICAL AND SURGICAL CONDITIONS

Many patients presenting for epilepsy surgery are relatively young and fit from a cardiovascular and respiratory standpoint. Any patient with a significant end-organ dysfunction or complex past medical history should undergo a comprehensive preoperative anesthetic evaluation prior to surgery. Open craniotomy is considered a moderate-risk procedure (indicating a less than 5% risk of cardiac events) with regard to its taxing effects on the cardiovascular system of the patient.[73]

Several rare medical conditions associated with epilepsy may present significant challenges to the anesthesiologist. Von Recklinghausen's disease (neurofibromatosis) is inherited through an autosomal dominant gene and affects 1 in 300 births. Patients with neurofibromatosis may have intracranial

tumors as well as airway compromise from tumors involving the respiratory tract or from cranial nerve involvement. Pulmonary status may be compromised from chronic aspiration syndrome, pulmonary fibrosing alveolitis, pulmonary hypertension, and cor pulmonale. Tuberous sclerosis is rarer in such patients but is associated with such serious problems as cardiac dysrhythmias, intracardiac tumors, cerebral embolization, renal dysfunction, and arterial aneurysms. Intracardiac tumors occur in 18% of adults and 58% of children with tuberous sclerosis, so patients with this disease should undergo a thorough preoperative cardiac evaluation, including echocardiography.

MEDICATION HISTORY

Medication history is important for preoperative laboratory test selection and prediction of intraoperative drug interactions. Certain anticonvulsants significantly elevate dose requirements for both nondepolarizing muscle blockers[70] and opioids.[75] Both phenytoin and carbamazepine are associated with resistance to nondepolarizing neuromuscular blockade and elevated liver function parameters. The direct relationship between the number of anticonvulsants a patient receives and the dose of fentanyl required for intraoperative anesthetic maintenance[75] further suggests that anticonvulsant therapy predisposes to resistance to opioids. Elevations in hepatic enzyme concentrations are prevalent (γ-glutamyl transpeptidase is elevated in 75% and alanine aminotransferase in 25% of patients receiving anticonvulsant therapy).[76] Asymptomatic laboratory abnormalities should not cause cancellation of the surgery because elevated liver function parameters are almost always a predictable result of anticonvulsant therapy. Sedation and lethargy are common side effects of many antiepileptic agents, including newer agents such as lamotrigine and oxcarbazepine, and may potentiate the central nervous system–depressant effects of anesthetics. Chronic topiramate intake has been associated with intraoperative metabolic acidosis.[77] Carbamazepine may cause a severe depression of the hemopoietic system and cardiac toxicity in rare cases. This drug's metabolism is materially slowed by erythromycin and cimetidine, drugs that may be administered perioperatively. Topiramate is associated with an asymptomatic non–anion gap acidosis.[78] Likewise, a ketogenic diet, sometimes used as an adjunct anticonvulsant therapy, predisposes patients to metabolic acidosis. Valproic acid therapy results in dose-related thrombocytopenia and platelet dysfunction.[79] On the basis of a review of over 300 craniotomy cases, however, additional bleeding risk during surgery is likely to be low in a patient taking valproic acid.[80]

PSYCHOLOGICAL PREPARATION

Because intraoperative ECoG commonly requires a significant reduction in the dose of sedative-hypnotic agents for adequate EEG monitoring, patients should be prepared for the possibility of intraoperative awareness even when this procedure is performed with use of a general endotracheal anesthetic technique. The patient should be reassured that this experience is usually described as a painless awareness of voices or other sensations. Patients and their families need to understand that this awareness is expected and that there are other risks, such as perioperative seizure, nausea, vomiting, and airway compromise. Empathy and consideration for the psychological frailties of patients with epilepsy are in order. Epilepsy has a pervasive effect on patients and is associated with higher incidence of cognitive dysfunction, affective disorders, suicide, neuroses, and personality disorders.

Diagnostic Surgical Procedures for Intractable Epilepsy

Placement of epidural ("peg") electrodes requires multiple bur-holes and can be a lengthy procedure, depending on the number of electrodes to be placed. "Depth" electrodes for exploring subcortical regions of the brain require stereotactic placement. The procedure usually is uneventful and not associated with significant bleeding. A general anesthetic is most frequently used. Unless further monitoring is indicated for a medical comorbidity, only routine noninvasive monitoring is employed.

Implantation of subdural grid electrodes requires a full craniotomy. Because EEG recording or stimulation is done postoperatively in an epilepsy monitoring unit, a standard anesthetic technique is appropriate without special consideration for suppression of EEG components. As with any full craniotomy procedure, significant bleeding may occur from dural sinuses. This requires large-gauge intravenous catheters and direct arterial access. The anesthetic regimen should be constructed to allow rapid emergence of the patient from anesthesia for timely neurologic assessment. The electrode plates to be implanted are quite bulky and require brain shrinkage. Because hyperventilation may precipitate seizure activity, this intervention should be employed only briefly as necessary to facilitate surgical exposure, with preferential reliance on ancillary measures such as diuretics. Furthermore, hyperventilation may be less effective in patients with complex partial seizures, who may have lower CO_2 reactivity of cerebral blood flow than normal patients.[81]

Resection of Epileptogenic Brain Regions under General Anesthesia

Anesthetic planning for epileptogenic brain resection procedures depends greatly upon the need for intraoperative brain mapping for seizure foci localization. Resection of epileptic foci with use of general anesthesia without brain mapping has goals similar to those of most open craniotomy procedures. These goals are to ensure lack of patient awareness, immobility, and hemodynamic stability, to facilitate brain relaxation, to ensure rapid emergence so that neurologic status can be assessed, and to suppress perioperative seizures. Benzodiazepine premedication can be given if an EEG recording is not planned. Antihistamines can activate seizure foci in patients with epilepsy and should be avoided as premedicants. Multiple studies have investigated the potential benefits of one anesthetic technique over another for providing hemodynamic stability, good brain relaxation, and rapid emergence for evaluation of the patient's neurologic examination. Many anesthetic combinations have been used with success. TIVA with propofol may have the benefit of providing lower intracranial pressures and better brain relaxation than isoflurane or sevoflurane administered at more 0.5 minimum alveolar concentration (MAC) in patients undergoing craniotomy with intracranial mass lesions.[82] However, these benefits may be less clinically significant when lower MAC doses of such volatile agents are used.[83] The ultra–short-acting opioid remifentanil more consistently allows for rapid emergence and early neurologic examination than other opioids.[84-87] Remifentanil has also been associated with better brain relaxation than fentanyl; however, this feature has not been a consistent finding in comparison studies.[88,89] Use of remifentanil also requires replacement of its intraoperative analgesic effect with longer-acting opioids prior to emergence. No prospective studies have been sufficiently powered to allow determination of the impact of anesthetic technique on neurologic outcome after craniotomy.

Additional goals for anticipated use of intraoperative brain mapping include avoidance of drugs that will interfere with monitoring of seizure spikes and prevention of unwanted generalization of interictal spike wave activity. Barbiturate and benzodiazepine premedication should be avoided because it may elevate the seizure threshold, making ECoG recording of epileptogenic activity more difficult. In children, rectal thiopental may be used.[71] An intubation dose of short-acting barbiturate during anesthesia induction is not contraindicated, but barbiturates should be avoided later in the procedure, as should intravenous lidocaine. Despite an isolated report of N_2O-related diminution of epileptic foci during intraoperative ECoG,[81] N_2O can be used for these procedures. Ebrahim and colleagues[49] recommended that propofol administration must be stopped 15 to 20 minutes prior to ECoG because it elicits high-frequency beta EEG activity for as long as 30 minutes after discontinuation, although other investigators have reported that this type of EEG activity did not prevent ECoG interpretation.[90] The use of low concentrations of isoflurane or desflurane is permissible, provided that these agents can be eliminated well before the start of corticography. Isoflurane may decrease the frequency and spatial distribution of epileptogenic spikes, although whether this effect persists at low concentrations is unclear.[91] Low-dose sevoflurane would be preferred, given its mild proconvulsant properties and short duration of action. When no potent inhaled anesthetics are in use, scopolamine, droperidol, and increased opioid dosing can be substituted to prevent intraoperative recall with virtually no effect on the EEG. Mild to moderate hypocapnia (PaCO2 30-35 mm Hg), however, is often necessary to assist in brain volume control and brain relaxation. If hyperventilation must be initiated during sevoflurane anesthesia, the anesthesiologist should be aware that the specificity of ictal lead prediction may diminish.[60]

If cortical motor area stimulation is necessary for the surgeon to accomplish safe resection, particular attention must be paid to the management and dosage of neuromuscular blocking agents. As a general rule, neuromuscular blockade should be minimal to allow motor stimulation. If moderate residual neuromuscular block persists, a small dose of anticholinesterase can be administered to achieve its complete reversal.

Cortical stimulation for localization as well as light anesthesia and brain manipulation may lead to intraoperative seizures. Treatment of seizure activity during ongoing intraoperative ECoG therefore requires the use of short-acting anticonvulsants (such as methohexital) as one weighs the therapeutic goals of gross seizure control against the potential for interference with critical electrocortical monitoring.

When intraoperative EEG recordings fail to reveal seizure spikes, and in consultation with the surgeon and the electroencephalographer, the anesthesiologist administers anesthetics known to promote epileptiform discharges. These include methohexital (25-50 mg),[35,55] alfentanil (20 µg/kg),[16,92] and etomidate (0.2 mg/kg),[34] all of which may be administered to help activate dormant foci. Alfentanil is the most effective of these agents, provoking abnormal EEG spike activity in 83% of patients, compared with 50% for methohexital.[16] However, controversy exists over the correlation of pharmacologically elicited seizure spikes with the patients' native epileptogenic foci.[93]

Severe bradycardia has been reported during amygdalahippocampectomy that is not seen during routine anterior temporal lobe resection. This problem is thought to be the result of surgical limbic system stimulation resulting in enhanced neural vagal activity.[94,95]

Cerebral Hemispherectomy

On occasion, the seizure foci are so diffuse as to require resection of substantial portions of an entire cerebral hemisphere. Frequently, this procedure is performed in children and can be associated with significant morbidity and mortality related to massive blood loss, electrolyte and metabolic disturbances, coagulopathy, cerebral hemorrhage, and seizures. Hemispherectomy requires a very large craniectomy, which increases the chance of bleeding and tearing of dural sinuses. Air embolism also has been reported and may lead to serious morbidity. Kofke and associates[96] compared three different surgical techniques (anatomical, functional, and lateral) for hemispherectomy. Lateral hemispherectomy was associated with the lowest intraoperative blood loss, the shortest intensive care stay, and the lowest complication rate. Functional hemispherectomy had the highest rate of reoperation, whereas patients undergoing anatomical hemispherectomy had the longest hospital stays, greatest requirement for cerebrospinal fluid (CSF) diversion, and highest postoperative fever. Patients with cortical dysplasia had the largest intraoperative blood loss.[96]

Continuous monitoring of blood pressure by arterial catheter is required, as is central venous access and monitoring of cardiac filling pressure. In addition, pressor and inotropic infusions should be readily available to combat low cardiac

output states.[78] Brian and coworkers[97] report a series of 10 patients, aged 3 months to 12 years, whose intraoperative blood replacement amounted to 1.5 blood volumes on average. In 7 of the patients, a coagulopathy developed intraoperatively, requiring administration of platelets, fresh frozen plasma, or both. Progressive hypokalemia requiring replacement occurred in 4 of the patients. Hypothermia and metabolic acidosis was observed in 5 patients. Urine output was a poor indicator of volume status because of frequent massive glycosuria. Zuckerberg and colleagues[98] report several children younger than 5 years in whom severe decreases in cardiac index, bradycardia, increased systemic vascular resistance (SVR), and an alveolar-to-arterial gradient suggestive of neurogenic pulmonary edema developed after hemispherectomy with extensive subcortical resection. Removal of the endotracheal tube at the conclusion of procedures with large-volume resuscitation and with a high potential for postoperative complications would therefore seem unwise. Postoperative hemodynamic instability is common, and the airway may be compromised by seizure activity. Early postoperative recovery is best accomplished in an intensive care environment. As has been reported in adults,[99] children undergoing major brain resection become hypercoagulable as early as during dural closure.[100] Although the clinical significance of this finding is debated, thrombotic complications should be anticipated.

Vagal Nerve Stimulator Placement

Patients with refractory seizures who are not candidates for seizure focus resection may be considered for vagus nerve stimulator placement. Vagus nerve stimulation has been shown to reduce seizure frequency; the mechanism of action is still not entirely understood but likely involves central projections of the vagus nerve to the locus ceruleus and amygdala.[101] More than 32,000 such devices have been implanted worldwide. The stimulator device is placed in the mid-cervical neck area to avoid cardiac vagal branches, which arise more proximally; it is placed on the left side to reduce the risk of severe sinus bradycardia—the left vagus nerve innervates the atrioventricular node, whereas the right vagus nerve innervates the sinus node. The procedure is frequently performed on an outpatient basis. Rare and short-lived intraoperative bradycardia, presumably from retrograde stimulation, has been reported with test stimulation.[102] In addition, patients frequently experience hoarseness and coughing from stimulation of the recurrent laryngeal nerve and the sensation of a constricted throat from superior laryngeal nerve activation. Unilateral vocal cord paralysis has been reported as well, as has a predisposition to chronic pulmonary aspiration.[103] Anesthetic management involves many of the considerations relevant for cranial epilepsy surgery without the need for brain mapping. Preoperative seizure control should be optimized, anticonvulsant medications and their potential interaction with anesthetic agents reviewed, proconvulsant anesthetics avoided, and airway symptoms anticipated.

Emergence from Anesthesia and Postoperative Management

The incidence of complications after intracranial neurosurgery remains substantial.[104] Nausea and vomiting occur in 30% to 50% of cases; neurologic deterioration occurs in 8% to 10% of patients, for approximately one-half of whom the deterioration is permanent. Respiratory morbidity occurs in

3% to 8%, whereas cardiovascular complications are found in 5% to 19% of patients. Patients with epilepsy are generally healthy from a cardiovascular perspective, seizures, but impaired mental function and the effect of large craniotomy procedures with substantive brain resection can combine to put them at significant postoperative risk.

Because of preoperative tapering of anticonvulsants and perioperative drug interactions, patients may be at higher risk for development of postoperative seizures. Anticonvulsant blood levels must be checked frequently, and doses adjusted accordingly, to continue appropriate maintenance of anticonvulsant therapy postoperatively. When a seizure occurs, adequacy of oxygenation and ventilation must be ensured with appropriate measures to secure airway patency. The first step should be ventilation with 100% oxygen via bag and mask. If necessary, the airway is secured by a laryngeal mask airway or tracheal intubation. In adults, the seizure may be stopped with thiopental 1 to 1.5 mg/kg, lorazepam 2 to 5 mg, diazepam 5 to 10 mg administered over 2 to 3 minutes, or midazolam 2 to 4 mg. If seizure activity recurs, phenytoin is begun at 50 mg/min to a total dose of 20 mg/kg, assuming the patient has not previously been treated with phenytoin. Intractable status epilepticus is treated with general anesthesia using isoflurane, barbiturates, or propofol.

Anticonvulsant medications are associated with drowsiness and lethargy. It is our clinical experience that patients with epilepsy emerge from anesthesia more slowly than neurologically normal individuals. Intraoperative loading of phenytoin for treatment of seizures may increase the risk of delayed emergence from general anesthesia. This tendency can be exacerbated in patients with epilepsy and mental handicaps who are also undergoing therapy with the anticonvulsants mentioned. During the course of aggressive medical therapy and in the postoperative period, blood levels of phenytoin and carbamazepine may rise into the toxic range.[96]

Intracranial bleeding occurs in a small percentage of patients, so that neurologic status must be closely and continuously monitored during recovery. Coughing and systemic hypertension should be avoided and promptly treated so as not to precipitate or aggravate intracranial bleeding. Prophylactic administration of antinauseants is effective[105] and advisable. Other postoperative neurologic complications of temporal lobe surgery include memory and visual field deficits. Patients with temporary subdural grid electrode implants may suffer cerebral edema[106] occasionally necessitating emergency reexploration.

MINIMALLY INVASIVE CRANIAL NEUROSURGERY

Background and Anesthetic Goals

In step with technologic advances in imaging, computing, and optics, the field of minimally invasive neurosurgery has evolved rapidly with regard to indications and applications. The potential benefit of minimally invasive neurosurgery results from enhanced patient safety, shorter hospital stay, reduced invasiveness, and lower postoperative morbidity in compared with open surgical procedures. Table 17-1 describes the most common indications for cranial disease. General goals for anesthetic management are to (1) keep the patient immobile, (2) ensure safe, rapid emergence from anesthesia for prompt neurologic assessment, (3) minimize

postoperative complications, (4) facilitate intraoperative neurophysiologic monitoring techniques, and (5) collaborate in the management of intracranial pressure (ICP).

Whether the procedure requires general anesthesia or monitored anesthesia care preoperative evaluation should be as thorough and comprehensive as for other surgical procedures. Immobility is crucial to the success of minimally invasive procedures. The choice of neuromuscular blocking drugs and the methods for monitoring their effects are critically important, because immobilization must be complete yet also rapidly reversible. Head fixation is required for some procedures, and movement during use of head pins must be scrupulously avoided. Procedures are of variable duration, depending on the neuropathology being treated. It is generally more difficult for the anesthesiologist to keep track of surgical progress in minimally invasive neurosurgical procedures than during conventional craniotomy. The anesthesia team must maintain a dialogue with surgical team members about the progress of the procedure while also closely observing the surgical video screens, the surgical field, and neurologic and anesthetic monitoring systems.

Table 17–1	Indications for Minimally Invasive Surgery on the Central Nervous System*
Diagnosis	**Intervention**
Hydrocephalus	Third ventriculostomy for aqueductal stenosis,[196] fourth-ventricular outlet obstruction,[197] or pineal neoplasm[198] Septostomy[199] Endoscopic ventriculoperitoneal shunts[200,201]
Colloid cysts	Endoscopic removal[202]
Arachnoid cysts	Fenestration[203]
Hematoma	Endoscopic drainage for subdural,[204] intracerebral[205]
Brain abscess	Endoscopic drainage[206] Image-guided stereotactic drainage[207]
Pituitary tumor	Endoscopic transnasal hypophysectomy[208]
Periventricular tumor	Biopsy[209]
Cranial synostosis	Endoscopic strip craniectomy[210]
Cerebral aneurysm	Endoscopy-assisted microsurgery[211]
Acoustic neuroma	Endoscopy-assisted microsurgery[212]
Arteriovenous malformation	Endoscope-assisted surgery[213,214]
Parkinson's disease,[215] behavioral disorders,[216,217] essential tremor[218]	Deep brain stimulation (uses stereotaxis)
Spinal disease (syringomyelia, palmar hyperhidrosis, disk herniation, spine deformities, instability, tumors)	Syringostomy[219] Transthoracic endoscopic sympathectomy[220] Arthroscopic microdiskectomy[221] Lumbar diskectomy[191] Video-assisted thoracoscopic surgery[167,222] Kyphoplasty[223] Spinal fusion[165] Tumor resection[182,224,225] Spine trauma[226]

*Superscript numbers refer to chapter references.

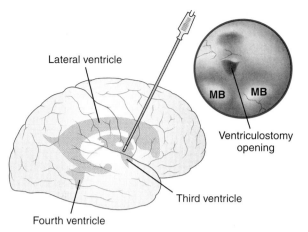

Figure 17–4 Endoscopic third ventriculostomy and endoscopic view of the floor of the third ventricle. MB, Mammillary body.

Labels on figure: Lateral ventricle; MB; MB; Ventriculostomy opening; Third ventricle; Fourth ventricle.

Neuroendoscopy

Neuroendoscopy is increasingly applied in the treatment of noncommunicating hydrocephalus and intraventricular pathology. A low rate of operative mortality (0%-1%) has been reported. However, the incidence of intraoperative and postoperative complications ranges widely, from 5% to 30%.[107-109] The technique employs burr-hole access to the cranium with placement of a rigid or flexible scope through the frontal cortex into the ventricle (Fig. 17-4). Adequate visualization requires continuous irrigation of the ventricles with warmed normal saline or lactated Ringer's solution accompanied by drainage of CSF and irrigating fluid through the scope or the bur-hole. The procedure has been successfully used for third ventriculostomy, tumor biopsy, cyst removal and fenestration, and fulguration of the choroids plexus. It has had its most prominent application in the treatment of noncommunicating hydrocephalus via third ventriculostomy. The surgeon establishes a connection between the third ventricle and the subtentorial subarachnoid space by endoscopically fenestrating the floor of the third ventricle (Fig 17-4). The surgical risk of third ventriculostomy is approximately 5% for significant morbidity,[110] with an overall success rate of 60% to 90%.[111,112]

PREOPERATIVE ISSUES

Patients presenting for ventriculostomy may have prior shunt placements with existing shunt tubing routed from the cranium to peritoneal, pleural, or central vascular locations. Patients with hydrocephalus or a primary lesion resulting in obstruction of CSF pathways may present with symptoms of elevated ICP, such as vomiting, headache, confusion, and obtundation. Patients presenting with prolonged nausea and vomiting may have significant dehydration or electrolyte abnormalities requiring correction prior to surgery. The patient's neurologic status and examination should be documented prior to induction. Patients may present with varying levels of consciousness, depending on the intracranial pathology and severity of hydrocephalus. Preoperative sedatives should be used with caution and are best avoided in patients with depressed consciousness.

INTRAOPERATIVE CONCERNS

Although the bur-hole approach to neuroendoscopy makes it amenable to local anesthesia and sedation,[113] general anesthesia is preferable to ensure patient immobility. After induction, the patient is positioned in neurosurgical head pins and the anesthesia team is at the patient's side (Fig. 17-5). Direct arterial pressure monitoring is advisable owing to the high incidence of hemodynamic perturbations during these procedures.[114] Delayed emergence has been reported to occur in up to 15% of patients undergoing neuroendoscopy.[108] Therefore, benzodiazepines or other agents that may contribute to prolonged postoperative sedation are avoided. The anesthetic goals should center on intraoperative immobilization, cardiovascular stability, and rapid emergence for early neurologic examination. Shunt location should be determined when central line placement is required; otherwise, unintended puncture of the peripheral shunt tubing may occur. Nitrous oxide poses the risk of diffusion into and expansion of ventricular air bubbles and should not be used. The burr-hole incision creates minimal postoperative pain, so small doses of short-acting narcotics are appropriate.

Despite the minimal brain penetration required with use of the endoscope, the pressure generated by the continuous irrigation system can create significant intraoperative events owing to intracranial circulatory insufficiency.[115] Measuring the pressure inside the neuroendoscope is technically easy and may be helpful because it has been shown to correlate with ICP and cerebral perfusion pressure.[108,115] Cardiovascular instability, bradyarrhythmias, and ventricular irritability are most commonly reported, occurring in 28% to 32% of patients,[108,109] with bradydysrhythmias occurring in as many as 41%.[116] These events are thought to be generated by heightened autonomic output in response to brain shifts generated by ICP changes related to irrigation and CSF drainage, to irrigation jets directed at hypothalamic nuclei, or both. The majority of these events are self-limiting and rapidly improve with release of ICP upon removal of the endoscope and drainage of irrigant from the burr-hole. However, severe bradycardia leading to cardiac arrest requiring cardiopulmonary resuscitation has also been reported.[117,118] Intraoperative bradycardia, possibly due to distortion of the posterior hypothalamus, can occur.[119]

It is important to understand that the selection and volume of irrigating fluid can affect the CSF composition and might cause an increase in postoperative morbidity neuroendoscopic procedures.[120] The use of body-temperature normal saline as irrigating fluid has been advocated.[121] However, normal saline irrigation in volumes larger than 500 mL may cause CSF acidosis,[120] and use of lactated Ringer's irrigation has been found to result in postoperative hyperkalemia.[119] Significant intraoperative bleeding can occur from vessel injury and may require abandonment of the procedure secondary to poor visualization. Injury to the basilar artery or perforating artery, the most feared surgical complication during third ventriculostomy, has resulted in intraoperative death.[107,122] Pneumocephalus and transient herniation syndromes due to CSF drainage and irrigation have also been reported.[110] A preexisting patent ventriculoatrial shunt could theoretically predispose to venous air embolism if pneumocephalus were to develop after endoscopy. If bleeding cannot be controlled, emergency conversion to open craniotomy should be anticipated, and appropriate preparations made.

POSTOPERATIVE CONCERNS

Mounting experience demonstrates that close postoperative monitoring is imperative in patients who have undergone neuroendoscopy. Transient neurologic deficits are the most common postoperative complication, occurring in 8% to 38%

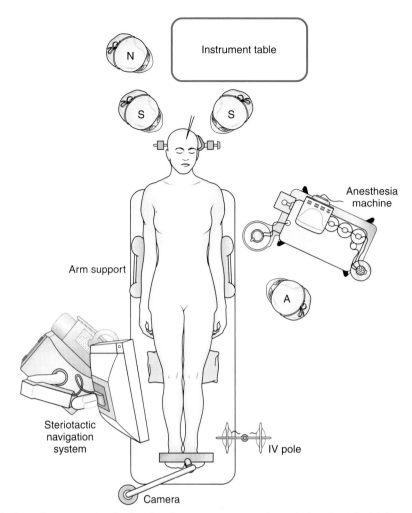

Figure 17–5 Operating room setup for functional neurosurgery procedures. A, Anesthesiologist; N, nurse; S, surgeon.

of patients.[107,108] Common problems in the immediate post-operative period include delayed emergence, hyperkalemia,[119] confusion, transient pupillary dysfunction, transient hemiplegia, and memory loss.[107,108,123] High pressure levels inside the endoscope are reportedly associated with delayed arousal and a higher rate of postoperative complications.[108] Careful control of irrigating pressure therefore may reduce postoperative risk and avoid delayed emergence. Respiratory arrest has been reported in infants during the first hours after neuroendoscopy, necessitating the use of apnea monitors.[124] Postoperative monitoring of serum electrolyte levels is warranted because diabetes insipidus and hypothalamic dysfunction have been reported in multiple series of patients undergoing endoscopic surgery.[107,123,125] Late infectious complications, such as meningitis and ventriculitis, have significantly contributed to morbidity, so patients should be monitored for signs of central nervous system infection.[107,109]

Endoscopic Transsphenoidal Hypophysectomy

The surgical technique for minimally invasive pituitary surgery gains access to the pituitary gland without brain retraction (Fig. 17-6). This technique is associated with lower morbidity (injury to optic chiasm and frontal lobes, diabetes insipidus) and mortality than open craniotomy via the subfrontal approach and is cosmetically more acceptable because it creates no scars.[126] Traditionally, incisions were made

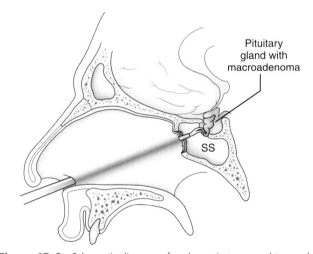

Figure 17–6 Schematic diagram of endoscopic transnasal transsphenoidal hypophysectomy. SS, sphenoid sinus.

sublabially via the sublabial transeptal (SLTS) approach. These days, the dissection is carried out entirely intranasally (endoscopic endonasal or MIPS approach). A wide and clearer surgical view, shorter hospital stay, reduced need for nasal packing, and a relatively short operating time, especially for recurrent cases, have been reported for the minimally invasive technique.[127,128] Further improvements in accuracy and tissue invasiveness have been gained through the use of navigation technology.[129]

PREOPERATIVE CONCERNS

The patient with pituitary disease requires careful preoperative evaluation to exclude the presence of panhypopituitarism, acromegaly, Cushing's disease, hypothyroidism, and hyperthyroidism. The endocrinologic evaluation should be studied in detail. Preoperative preparation may require administration of glycopyrrolate to decrease airway secretions if fiberoptic airway instrumentation is deemed necessary for acromegalic patients, administration of replacement hormones in patients with panhypopituitarism, and careful attention to the potential for preoperative electrolyte and metabolic (hyperglycemia) abnormalities.

INTRAOPERATIVE CONCERNS

In the transsphenoidal approach for hypophysectomy, blood pressure should be monitored closely. Severe hypertension may occur as a result of nasal injection or topical application of epinephrine.[130,131] The injection should be stopped immediately, and esmolol, nitroglycerin, of both should be administered. If reflex bradycardia occurs from epinephrine-induced hypertension, the urge to administer anticholinergic drugs should be resisted. There is also a need for repeated blood studies, including arterial blood gas, glucose, sodium and osmolarity measurements, to monitor endocrine disturbances. Sevoflurane and desflurane are similar to isoflurane in the potential to sensitize the human myocardium to the arrhythmogenic effect of exogenously administered epinephrine. Both may be used safely.[132,133] The airway may be in jeopardy upon emergence from anesthesia because of nasal packing or acromegalic features, especially large tongue, so excessive intraoperative narcotization is undesirable. Hemorrhagic complications during endoscopic transsphenoidal surgery are similar to those for a microsurgical transsphenoidal approach.[134] Major intraoperative bleeding leading to formation of pseudoaneurysm of the internal carotid artery has been reported.[135]

POSTOPERATIVE CONCERNS

Emergence from anesthesia should be rapid to allow assessment of visual function and accomplished with minimal coughing to avoid bleeding. Nevertheless, premature extubation must be avoided. Patients are at risk for aspiration of blood pooled in the pharynx and stomach during surgery. The airway may be obstructed from laryngospasm or obligate nasal breathing, requiring the use of artificial airway devices. Several cases of negative pressure pulmonary edema have been reported with these procedures. The presenting signs of acute hematoma (sudden blindness and ophthalmoplegia along with loss of consciousness and hypotension) should be carefully monitored in immediate postoperative period. Diabetes insipidus is uncommon with this approach and is generally a transient phenomenon.

Endoscopic Strip Craniectomy

The development of endoscopic surgery has advanced markedly, especially for the treatment of craniosynostosis in infants. The concept of using minimally invasive surgery to remold the skull is not new, dating back to the early part of the twentieth century, when neurosurgeons performed strip craniectomies to remove the abnormal, premature suture fusions. Today

the endoscopic cranial vault remodeling technique involves more than a simple strip craniectomy through a small endoscopic port. It is a wide sutural excision combined with lateral osteotomies and osteoectomies that allow for normalization of the cranial skeleton. The endoscopic surgery is combined postoperatively with helmet molding therapy to normalize the calvarial form completely.

Endoscopic cranial vault remodeling has several distinct advantages over conventional reconstruction techniques. The endoscopic approach reduces scarring and alopecia risks, reducing operative time, blood loss, and hospital stay. Mean operative time is less than 1 hour, compared with approximately 3 hours for the conventional open approach. Instead of a typical 5-day postoperative course with an intensive care admission, patients undergoing endoscopic surgery are being discharged on the first postoperative day.[136] More than 90% of patients undergoing open calvarial surgery require transfusion,[137] compared with 10% of those receiving endoscopic surgery.[136] Shorter operative time, reduced hospital stay, use of fewer blood products, and the elimination of internal plating systems all add up to a decrease in overall cost of the procedure.

One disadvantage of endoscopic procedures is that the surgery needs to be performed at a young age, preferably before 4 months. The reason is that the cranial bones in child this young are thin enough to allow osteotomies with endoscopic shears. In addition, there is less bleeding with bone cutting owing to the underdevelopment of the cancellous space between the two cortices of the skull. Lastly, endoscopic cranial vault remodeling involves the added expense of the cranial orthotic molding helmet as well as the prolonged and frequent postoperative follow-up (8 to 15 months) to ensure that cranial form is normalizing.

PREOPERATIVE CONCERNS

Patients presenting for endoscopic strip craniectomy are usually younger than 6 months. Ideally, the surgery should be scheduled past the physiologic nadir of the infant's hematocrit value, which occurs between the second and third month of life. Some centers give recombinant erythropoietin at a dose of 600 IU/kg/wk for three weeks prior to surgery to build up the preoperative hematocrit.[138] Preoperative laboratory analysis should include a baseline complete blood count. Although blood loss and blood transfusions are significantly decreased with endoscopic surgery, there is always the risk of significant blood loss due to injury of the sagittal sinus. A blood specimen for type and screen can be sent on the day of surgery after the placement of an intravenous cannula. If the patient has received previous blood transfusions and has potential antibody formation, a blood crossmatch should be obtained before the start of surgery.

Craniofacial anomalies may be associated with cardiac and other congenital anomalies.[139] Patients may also have a difficult airway, cervical spine abnormalities, cardiovascular problems, altered respiratory mechanics, gastroesophageal reflux, and other organ involvement. Undiagnosed obstructive sleep apnea syndrome might coexist and add to the perioperative morbidity in these children.[140] Butler and associates[141] provide an excellent review of complications with recommended pre-sedation evaluations and a checklist of potential problems for common and uncommon genetic disorders. Associated cervical spine abnormalities are of particular importance, given the patient positioning required for endoscopic strip craniectomies. Patients are placed in a modified prone position (Fig. 17-7) with the neck extended and supported by an

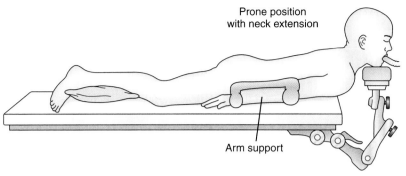

Figure 17–7 Positioning for endoscopic strip craniectomy.

inflatable bag ("sea lion" or "sphinx" position). This position may be contraindicated in patients with cervical spine anomalies. If a difficult airway is anticipated, fiberoptic intubation equipment and the laryngeal mask airway should be available. Pretreatment with glycopyrrolate (6-10 μg/kg) as an antisialagogue and to reduce the risk of gastroesophageal reflux may be indicated. Patients receiving anticonvulsants or other therapeutic agents should continue to take them during the perioperative period. Anticonvulsant levels should be checked for optimal dosing.

INTRAOPERATIVE CONCERNS

Airway control, positioning of the patient, and the potential for rapid blood loss and venous air embolization are the major issues. Most infants undergo an inhalational induction followed by placement of an intravenous cannula. Significant endotracheal tube displacement may occur with simple flexion or extension of the head. A few centimeters of movement may result in endobronchial intubation or accidental extubation of the patient when the patient is placed in the prone position.[142] One can advance the endotracheal tube into the right mainstem bronchus and then pull back until bilateral breath sounds are appreciated. The length of the tube in centimeters at the lip should be noted when taped and rechecked when the patient is in the final position. Correct endotracheal tube placement can also be confirmed by chest radiograph or fiberoptically. The anesthesiologist's access to the patient is limited, throughout the procedure, mandating the securing of appropriate venous access and monitoring devices before the patient is draped. An arterial line may not be needed owing to the short duration and minimal hemodynamic changes. Pressure points must be padded, and pressure must not be placed on bony prominences or vital structures such as the eyes.[108] Owing to the small size of the infant, minimal shifting of the position can cause significant changes in pressure points. Venous air embolism has been reported to occur in up to 82.6% of patients during surgical procedures for craniosynostosis.[143] In contrast, Tobias and colleagues[144] reported an incidence of 8% for venous air embolism with use of precordial Doppler ultrasonography monitoring during endoscopic strip craniectomy. None of the episodes of venous air embolism in the minimally invasive surgery cases resulted in hemodynamic compromise. Patients should be monitored with a precordial Doppler ultrasonography probe throughout the case.

POSTOPERATIVE CONCERNS

No infections, dural sinus tears, CSF leaks, or neurologic injuries136 were reported in a representative series of patients undergoing endoscopic strip craniectomy. Although careful monitoring is needed in the immediate postoperative period, many patients are discharged within 24 hours.

Functional Neurosurgery and Deep Brain Stimulation

Functional neurosurgery denotes surgical intervention for diseases not characterized by gross anatomic abnormalities. The functional activity of the central nervous system is tested, stimulated, or suppressed with the use of implanted electrodes delivering stimulatory or ablative current. Movement disorders, chronic pain, psychiatric disorders,[145] and, even minimally conscious states[146] have been treated with this modality. Most interventions involve sophisticated targeting of small and deep brain structures. Targeting methods include stereotactic and electrophysiologic neuronavigation.

Imaging-guided placement of neurostimulators in the thalamus, globus pallidus, and subthalamic nucleus has received considerable attention as an effective modality for treatment of refractory movement disorders such as Parkinson's disease, dystonia, and essential tremor.[147] A review of 250 patients undergoing deep brain stimulation (DBS) at one center showed Parkinson's disease to be the indication for 68% of procedures, with the remainder (32%) performed for other motor disorders.[148] Bilateral placement of DBS electrodes occurred in 68.8%. Neurostimulation provides an alternative as efficacious as basal ganglia lesioning without the same risk of permanent complications. Target localization is performed with computed tomography or magnetic resonance imaging. The precise location of stimulator lead placement is then achieved through identification of neuronal activity characteristic of the globus pallidus or subthalamic nucleus through the use of intraoperative microelectrode recordings. The external leads are later connected to an implanted programmable pulse generator.

PREOPERATIVE CONCERNS

A careful assessment of the extent of the disease and coexisting medical conditions should be made, and a history of alcohol or drug abuse, claustrophobia and previous failure of sedation should be noted. The most common comorbidities patients undergoing functional neurosurgery are cigarette smoking (88%), obesity (86%), and systemic hypertension (21%).[148] Assessment of the patient's ability to cooperate in whom MAC is contemplated and discussion with the patient about each step of the procedure are absolutely necessary. If magnetic resonance imaging will be used for the procedure, careful questions about implanted ferrous metals, pacemakers, and aneurysm clips should be asked. The planned intraoperative position should be ascertained, and the need for invasive monitoring determined on the basis of the severity of coexisting diseases and patient positioning (e.g. monitoring for air embolism).

INTRAOPERATIVE CONCERNS

During DBS surgery, assessment of changes in motor symptoms in response to brain stimulation is often used to guide appropriate placement of stimulator leads. Worse outcome has been reported in a retrospective report of patients undergoing this procedure with general anesthesia.[149] For this reason, most DBS procedures are performed while patients are awake, in the supine "beach chair" position.[148] Patients receive local anesthesia before scalp incision and a neurosurgical head-frame is used routinely. Monitoring should be performed in accordance with American Society of Anesthesiologists (ASA) guidelines.[150] Supraorbital and greater occipital nerve blocks can be used for the placement of an external head frame.[151] Medications used for treatment of motor symptoms should be withheld from these patients overnight and on the morning of surgery. Preoperative benzodiazepines, opioids, and other sedatives can affect patient cooperation and eliminate movement disorders; use of these medications interferes with the interpretation of tremor and the electrophysiologic recordings of cellular firing used to position stimulator leads. These agents should be avoided; selective and nonselective β antagonists can reduce tremor intensity in patients presenting for treatment of essential tremor and should also be avoided if possible.[152] Back pain can be a considerable problem for patients undergoing lengthy DBS procedures while awake. Spinal opioids have been reported to provide relief without interfering with electrophysiologic recordings.[153] Patients with dystonic movements may require anesthesia for reduction of uncontrolled movement during placement of stereotactic frames and performance of magnetic resonance imaging. Propofol infusion, even at sedative doses, significantly reduces uncontrolled tremor and movement in both patients with Parkinson's disease and those with dystonia.

Monitoring of sedative depth with the bispectral index does not improve time to arousal, propofol consumption, or hemodynamic stability.[154] Hypertension is a frequent intraoperative complication that may lead to intracranial bleeding.[155,156] Care should be taken to keep systolic blood pressure within 20% of baseline values during the procedure and in the immediate postoperative period. The team at our institution uses propofol sedation intraoperatively only for bur-hole placement. Alternatively, a low-dose infusion of propofol combined with remifentanil may be employed. All anesthetics are discontinued during neuronal microrecording. In our experience of 258 procedures, the overall intraoperative complication rate was 11.6%, with 5.6% being major.[148] The most common neurologic complications (3.6%) were intracranial hemorrhage and seizure. Confusion and anxiety occurred with similar frequency. Intraoperative venous air embolism,[157,158] pneumocephalus, and seizures have also been reported.[159] Patients who cannot tolerate the procedure may benefit from dexmedetomidine; it has been reported to reduce the need for antihypertensives and to provide patient comfort without interfering with electrophysiologic recordings.[160] Dexmedetomidine has also been reported to be useful for control of propofol-induced dyskinesias.[161]

POSTOPERATIVE CONCERNS

Postoperative monitoring may be warranted and should be considered even in patients receiving limited intraoperative anesthesia for stereotactic procedures. Retrospective series have reported the perioperative complication rate of surgical stereotactic treatment of movement disorders to be 3% to 5%, with intraparenchymal hematoma the most common complication.[162] Confusional symptoms have been reported in the postoperative period in 15% of patients with Parkinson's disease after DBS surgery in one series.[163] Akinetic rigid states can occur in the immediate postoperative period. The preferred method of treatment is activation of the DBS stimulator.[164] Patients with Parkinson's disease should receive their medications as soon as possible postoperatively to avoid motor fluctuations that could confound postprocedural neurologic deterioration or impair respiratory muscle strength needed to clear secretions.

MINIMALLY INVASIVE SPINE SURGERY

An alternative to open reconstructive surgery, minimally invasive techniques have been developed for a variety of spine surgery needs, such as decompression, stabilization, and sympathectomy. Common indications are listed in Table 17-1. Endoscopic approaches with thorascopic and laparoscopic assistance facilitate the approach to the anterior thoracic and lumbar spine without the risk and discomfort of open thoracotomy or laparotomy. Keyhole access surgery and percutaneous spine stabilization are used for posterior and cervical spine disease. Smaller incisions are possible through extensive use of the operating microscope, fluoroscopic guidance, stereotactic neuronavigation, and special instruments such as tubular retractors disk space dilators and special cage devices for structural support.[165] The endoscopic approach reduces the amount of muscle dissection required for access to the spine and thereby decreases postoperative pain, recovery time, and hospital stay.[166]

Video-Assisted Thoracoscopic Surgery

Video-assisted thoracoscopic surgery (VATS) has been primarily used for diagnostic and ablative surgery on the lungs and pleura. However, anterior thoracic spine release and fusion for scoliosis/kyphosis or spine trauma are now being accomplished through VATS as an alternative to open thoracotomy, as is thoracic sympathetic ganglionectomy for hyperhidrosis. After anterior release, conventional posterior spinal fusion may be added in a combined anterior and posterior approach. The advantages of the minimally invasive approach to the spine are less surgical time,[167] less acute postoperative pain, improved respiratory function, and a faster functional recovery in compared with conventional procedures.[168] Table 17-2 compares VATS with open thoracotomy.

PREOPERATIVE CONCERNS

Physicians should be cautioned against equating minimally invasive procedures with low perioperative risk. Blood loss, perioperative physiologic stress, and postoperative complications vary significantly with the type of minimally invasive spinal surgery performed. Thoracoscopically and laparoscopically assisted scoliosis correction, multilevel spinal fusions, and thoracic corpectomies should still be considered intermediate- to high-risk procedures. Preoperative evaluation must take into consideration how well patients requiring thoracoscopy will tolerate the significant cardiopulmonary effects of one-lung ventilation. Patients with long-standing idiopathic or neuromuscular kyphoscoliosis should be evaluated for restrictive lung disease and associated congenital anomalies. Some neuromuscular diseases predispose to a higher risk of malignant hyperthermia. Patients with spinal pathology associated with connective tissue disorders should be screened for systemic manifestations of the disease, such as coagulation abnormalities, fibrotic lung disease, pulmonary hypertension, and cervical spine pathology.

INTRAOPERATIVE CONCERNS

Anterior thoracic spine release through VATS is usually performed with the patient in the lateral position. The operating room arrangement for VATS is shown in Figure 17-8. The standard technique requires one-lung ventilation to facilitate the surgeons' view through the endoscope, which would otherwise be obliterated by the nondeflated lung. The possibility of prolonged one-lung ventilation should be anticipated during anterior release and multiple level fusions. Nitrous oxide should be avoided. A double-lumen endotracheal tube or bronchial blocker is used to isolate the lung. Double-lumen tubes may be difficult to place in patients with significant thoracic kyphosis because of tracheobronchial distortion.

Combined anterior-posterior fusions may require changing the double-lumen tube to a single-lumen tube in anticipation of placing the patient in the prone position. This position change creates an inherent risk of loss of the secured airway. The alternative is to withdraw the bronchial portion of the double lumen tube into the trachea but has the disadvantage of potential tube malposition during prone ventilation. We therefore prefer to change to a single-lumen tube using a tube exchanger or to use a bronchial blocker for the lateral position portion of the operation. Anesthetic and muscle relaxant restrictions required for somatosensory and motor evoked potential monitoring[169,170] can make it difficult to avoid patient coughing from carinal stimulation due to the double-lumen tube. Remifentanil is useful in this situation to improve depth of anesthesia and tolerance of the endotracheal tube[171] and to prevent patient movement.[172] Unintentional surgical entry into large blood vessels and viscera may occur. Both the anesthesia and surgical teams must be prepared for rapid conversion to open thoracotomy in case of difficulty with surgical hemostasis. The prophylactic placement of arterial and venous access lines is advocated, and blood should be available. Risk of blood loss with various VATS procedures is described in Table 17-3.

An alternative procedure involves a combined posterior and lateral chest approach in the prone position.[173] This technique entails surgical preparation of the right chest as well as the back for optimal surgical access. Lung isolation is not necessary because the lung falls away from the surgical endoscope, aided either by an atmospheric pneumothorax or by mild tension pneumothorax induced by low-pressure insufflation with carbon dioxide. Advantages include shorter procedure times because placement of double-lumen tracheal tube and confirmatory bronchoscopy are avoided as is the repositioning from the lateral to the prone position. Furthermore, a lower rate of pulmonary complications has been observed.[174]

POSTOPERATIVE CONCERNS

Intercostal neuralgia, pneumothorax, and Horner's syndrome have been reported after thoracoscopic procedures.[175] Pulmonary complications such as atelectasis may be sufficiently

Table 17–2 Comparison of Video-Assisted Thoracoscopic Surgery (VATS) with Open Thoracotomy

	VATS	Thoracotomy
Operating Time (min)	205 (80-542)	268 (210-690)
Blood Loss (ml)	327 (125-1500)	683 (250-1200)
Chest Tube (days)	1.5 (0-6)	3.5 (2.8-9.1)
Narcotics (mg/day)	3.7 (1.5-15)	20.4 (5-60)
Hospital Stay (days)	6.5 (2-24)	16.2 (5-34)
Pulmonary Dysfunction	7%	33%
Neurologica	16%	50%

From Rosenthal D, Dickman CA: Thoracoscopic microsurgical excision of herniated thoracic discs. J Neurosurg 1998;89:224-235.

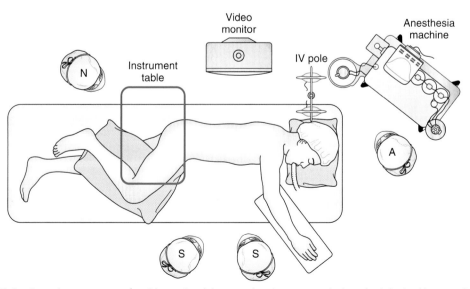

Figure 17–8 Operating room setup for video-assisted thoracoscopic spine surgery. A, Anesthesiologist; N, nurse; S, surgeon.

Table 17–3	Risk of Blood Loss in Video-Assisted Thoracoscopic Surgery	
Procedure	Blood Loss Risk	Estimated Blood Loss
Thoracic sympathectomy	Low	Minimal
Thoracic diskectomy, anterior fusion	Intermediate	< 500 mL
Spinal metastasis (12%), corpectomy, multilevel reconstruction after resection	High	>2000 mL

Data from references 227 through 229.

severe to prolong hospitalization.[176] Proper attention should be directed to appropriate chest tube management and assurance of good pulmonary toilet.

Kyphoplasty and Vertebroplasty

Kyphoplasty and vertebroplasty are similar minimally invasive percutaneous procedures developed to treat osteoporotic and osteolytic fractures of the thoracic and lumbar vertebrae. The procedures reduce pain through cementing of the fractured vertebrae with polymethylmethacrylate to reduce movement of bony fragments. Kyphoplasty is slightly more invasive than vertebroplasty in that it uses balloon tamps to reexpand the vertebrae to their original height and to create a potential space prior to cement application. Both procedures have shown short-term benefits in pain relief.[177]

PREOPERATIVE CONCERNS

Although, minimal incision and lack of significant fluid shifts make kyphoplasty and vertebroplasty low surgical risks, the patient population presents substantive anesthetic risk because of multiple comorbidities, including end-stage cardiopulmonary disease, which requires careful preoperative medical assessment and optimization. Many patients have osteoporosis secondary to long-standing steroid-dependent pulmonary or systemic inflammatory disease. Preoperative pulmonary function should be optimized, and patients should be evaluated for the need to give stress-dose steroids. Long-term opioid use is prevalent in chronic severe back pain and is associated with substantial opioid tolerance. A perioperative plan for pain control should be established.

INTRAOPERATIVE CONCERNS

Both procedures can be performed under monitored anesthesia care if the patient is a good candidate for monitored sedation. Disadvantages of MAC are the discomfort of prolonged prone positioning and limited airway access. Patients with rheumatoid arthritis may have joint contractures, which do not allow the arms to be placed over the head in the prone position. We have successfully used a padded sling under the Jackson table to support the arms of patients with severe shoulder contractures. Padding and gentle positioning are crucial in patients with severe osteoporosis. Skin lacerations and rib fractures have been reported in these patients during prone positioning.[177] The procedures require only a minimal incision and are generally well tolerated despite the acute illness level of this patient population. Arterial oxygenation decreases during vertebroplasty under sedation; the decrement in partial pressure of oxygen is related to the number of spinal segments treated.[178] It is not clear whether this relationship is the result of higher sedative doses or a greater amount of cement used. Rare occurrences of symptomatic pulmonary embolism and intraoperative death have been reported during vertebroplasty,[179,180] but no significant embolic events have yet been reported with kyphoplasty. A light anesthesia regimen using short-acting anesthetic agents is appropriate, aiming at rapid recovery to facilitate same-day discharge.

POSTOPERATIVE CONCERNS

Patients are commonly discharged on the day of surgery; however, those with end-stage pulmonary disease or severe perioperative pain may warrant closer monitoring and a hospital stay of up to 24 hours.

Endoscopic Cervical Diskectomy and Foraminotomy

Anterior microforaminotomy has long been in use for radiculopathic conditions, and has now been advocated to replace anterior vertebrectomy for removal of tumors located anterior to the spinal cord. Minimally invasive endoscopic cervical foraminotomy (MEF) is being increasingly used for cervical root decompression and results in less blood loss, shorter hospitalizations, and a much lower postoperative pain medication requirement than open cervical laminoforaminotomy.[181] Postoperative pain is minimal. Neither bony fusion nor a cervical brace are needed, and patients undergoing MEF are kept in the hospital only overnight.[182]

The prone or sitting position may be used for posterior cervical MEF. The sitting position decreases epidural venous engorgement and has been shown to entail less blood loss than MEF performed in the prone position.[183] Although venous air embolism has not been reported, it remains a potential risk. Other potential complications of MEF include the risk of dural puncture or nerve root injury with guidewires.[184] Injury to the sympathetic chain causing postoperative Horner's syndrome can occur during anterior cervical foraminotomy. However, the intraoperative complication of most concern with this approach is injury to the vertebral artery during drilling of the uncovertebral joint.[182] The risk of arterial injury is highest at the level of C6-C7. Vertebral artery injury requires intraoperative control of bleeding and postoperative angiographic assessment to assess for dissection or pseudoaneurysm formation.[184]

Microdiskectomy and Percutaneous Disk Space Treatment

Patients undergoing open lumbar microdiskectomy may be considered for spinal anesthesia.[185] The surgeon needs to feel comfortable with the notion that motor function will not be assessable immediately after the operation. Spinal anesthesia for spine surgery is virtually free of the risk of post–dural puncture headache and reduces postprocedure pain, nausea, and bleeding.[186] Isobaric bupivacaine (0.5%) with epinephrine and fentanyl has been used successfully with minimal cardiovascular effect. Postoperative pain requirements after microdiskectomy depend significantly on preoperative pain severity.[187] Combination anesthetic techniques, utilizing spinal anesthesia with supplemental epidural clonidine in combination with incision site subcutaneous bupivacaine,[188] may be of further benefit through improving postoperative pain control in these patients. Epidural anesthesia has been suggested to be an important alternative to general anesthesia[189] in terms of reducing surgical times and blood loss, providing stable intraoperative hemodynamics, and resulting in better recovery characteristics without delaying hospital discharge. Contraindications include coagulopathy, patient refusal, and lesion at the site.

Percutaneous hemonucleolysis with the use of papain as well as blind nucleotomy and laser disk decompression have largely fallen out of favor because of allergic complications, neurovascular injury, and transverse myelitis.[190] Instead, arthroscopic technology, using instruments that can be visualized, and endoscopic fiberoptic techniques are being developed and show considerably greater promise.

Minimally Invasive Spinal Fusion

Minimally invasive techniques for spinal fusion have been developed for transforaminal interbody fusion (TLIF), anterior interbody fusion (ALIF), extreme lateral interbody fusion (XLIF), and axial lumbar interbody fusion (AxiaLIF).

TLIF procedures are usually performed in the prone position. The incision is small, facilitated by microscopic technique, computer or precise fluoroscopic localization, and tubular retractors. The surgeon begins by performing a total facetectomy, after which annulotomy and diskectomy are accomplished. After the disk space is freed up, it is filled with morselized cancellous bone or a metal cage for structural support. Autologous bone from the iliac crest may be harvested. Stabilization may be augmented through the use of limited open or percutaneous pedicle screw fixation.[165]

Transperitoneal or retroperitoneal laparoscopic approaches may be used to access the lumbar spine.[191] They have been used successfully for both lumbar diskectomy and ALIF. The laparoscopic approach to the lumbar spine requires steep head-down positioning and the use of shoulder braces, which can cause brachial neurapraxia if they are placed too medially. The patient's arms may need to be crossed and placed on the anterior chest. The usual precautions for laparoscopic procedures must be followed, and potential problems, such as pulmonary barotrauma, CO_2 embolism, hypercapnia, and right main-stem intubation, anticipated. The bifurcation of the iliac vessels occurs around the level of the L4-L5 interspace; thus, an anterior laparoscopic approach to the lower lumbar disk spaces requires the mobilization of these vessels, raising the risk of laceration. Iatrogenic injury to bowel and superior hypogastric plexus has also been reported. Surgeons have reported prolonged surgical times, which has led some to prefer a mini-open procedure to laparoscopic assistance.[192]

Extreme lateral interbody fusion (XLIF) is performed in the lateral position with the operating table flexed at the interspace of interest. The surgical approach entails risk of injury to the peritoneal cavity, pleural cavity, great vessels, and lumbosacral plexus. To deal with the latter, intraoperative electromyographic monitoring may be used, which limits the use of neuromuscular blockade. If the interspace to be treated is thoracic, the potential for development of intraoperative pneumothorax should be considered.

Newer developments have made an axial approach to the lower lumbar spine possible. Axial approaches to spinal fusion are thought to have substantial biomechanical advantages.[165] This approach affords the surgeon access to the spine via the presacral space through a keyhole incision, avoiding the risks of body cavity, ligamentous, muscle, and neural plexus injury

inherent in ALIF, TLIF and XLIF. The patient is positioned prone, and extensive use of fluoroscopy and special instrumentation are required.

Robotically Assisted Spine Surgery

Robotic technology is being tested for application during spine surgery. In particular, the promises of robotic surgery are improved accuracy, reduced radiation exposure, enhanced user-friendliness, and shorter operative time. A new miniature robot system (SpineAssist; Mazor Surgical Technologies, Caesare, Israel) has been developed and tested for accurate placement of pedicle and transforaminal facet screws. It utilizes preoperatively obtained computed tomography scans of the spine and limited intraoperative fluoroscopy to guide automated pedicle screw placement. The components of the robotic system are a spinous process clamp, a minimally invasive frame, a miniature robot with arms and drill guide, and a computer console. The system's performance is not affected by the surgeon's hand motion.[193] Cadaver studies confirming the system's accuracy support its use in minimally invasive spine surgery for selected patients.[194]

CONCLUSION

Minimally invasive techniques will continue to change the practice of traditional cranial and spine surgery as they evolve further. Ongoing advances promise to be even less invasive, while facilitating surgical accuracy and outcome.[195] Although some procedures might be performed without anesthesia, anesthesiologists may be faced with entirely new risks for others. Anesthesiologists can positively contribute to overall neurologic outcome through attention to the medical condition of the patient, the idiosyncrasies of the surgical procedure, and heightened awareness of specific risks, both intraoperative and immediately postoperative.

REFERENCES

1. Serletis D, Bernstein M: Prospective study of awake craniotomy used routinely and nonselectively for supratentorial tumors, *J Neurosurg* 107:1–6, 2007.
2. Blanshard HJ, Chung F, Manninen PH, et al: Awake craniotomy for removal of intracranial tumor: Considerations for early discharge, *Anesth Analg* 92:89–94, 2001.
3. Whittle IR, Midgley S, Georges H, et al: Patient perceptions of "awake" brain tumour surgery, *Acta Neurochir (Wien)* 147:275–277, 2005.
4. Hagberg CA, Gollas A, Berry JM: The laryngeal mask airway for awake craniotomy in the pediatric patient: Report of three cases, *J Clin Anesth* 16:43–47, 2004.
5. Archer DP, McKenna JM, Morin L, Ravussin P: Conscious-sedation analgesia during craniotomy for intractable epilepsy: A review of 354 consecutive cases, *Can J Anaesth* 35:338–344, 1988.
6. Sarang A, Dinsmore J: Anaesthesia for awake craniotomy—evolution of a technique that facilitates awake neurological testing, *Br J Anaesth* 90:161–165, 2003.
7. Skucas AP, Artru AA: Anesthetic complications of awake craniotomies for epilepsy surgery, *Anesth Analg* 102:882–887, 2006.
8. Senel FC, Buchanan JM Jr, Senel AC, Obeid G: Evaluation of sedation failure in the outpatient oral and maxillofacial surgery clinic, *J Oral Maxillofac Surg* 65:645–650, 2007.
9. Klimek M, Verbrugge SJ, Roubos S, et al: Awake craniotomy for glioblastoma in a 9-year-old child, *Anaesthesia* 59:607–609, 2004.
10. Trop D: Conscious-sedation analgesia during the neurosurgical treatment of epilepsies—practice at the Montreal Neurological Institute, *Int Anesthesiol Clin* 24:175–184, 1986.

Masking of epileptiform activity by propofol during seizure surgery, *Anesthesiology* 76:652–654, 1992.
12. Girvin JP: Neurosurgical considerations and general methods for craniotomy under local anesthesia, *Int Anesthesiol Clin* 24:80–114, 1986.
13. Costello TG, Cormack JR, Hoy C, et al: Plasma ropivacaine levels following scalp block for awake craniotomy, *J Neurosurg Anesthesiol* 16:147–150, 2004.
14. Costello TG, Cormack JR, Mather LE, et al: Plasma levobupivacaine concentrations following scalp block in patients undergoing awake craniotomy, *Br J Anaesth* 94:848–851, 2005.
15. Silbergeld DL, Mueller WM, Colley PS, et al: Use of propofol (Diprivan) for awake craniotomies: Technical note, *Surg Neurol* 38:271–272, 1992.
16. Keene DL, Roberts D, Splinter WM, et al: Alfentanil mediated activation of epileptiform activity in the electrocorticogram during resection of epileptogenic foci, *Can J Neurol Sci* 24:37–39, 1997.
17. Berkenstadt H, Perel A, Hadani M, et al: Monitored anesthesia care using remifentanil and propofol for awake craniotomy, *J Neurosurg Anesthesiol* 13:246–249, 2001.
18. Manninen PH, Balki M, Lukitto K, Bernstein M: Patient satisfaction with awake craniotomy for tumor surgery: A comparison of remifentanil and fentanyl in conjunction with propofol, *Anesth Analg* 102:237–242, 2006.
19. Keifer JC, Dentchev D, Little K, et al: A retrospective analysis of a remifentanil/propofol general anesthetic for craniotomy before awake functional brain mapping, *Anesth Analg* 101:502–508, 2005.
20. Coursin DB, Coursin DB, Maccioli GA: *Dexmedetomidine. Curr Opin Crit Care* 7:221–226, 2001.
21. Souter MJ, Rozet I, Ojemann JG, et al: Dexmedetomidine sedation during awake craniotomy for seizure resection: Effects on electrocorticography, *J Neurosurg Anesthesiol* 19:38–44, 2007.
22. Bekker AY, Kaufman B, Samir H, et al: The use of dexmedetomidine infusion for awake craniotomy, *Anesth Analg* 92:1251–1253, 2001.
23. Bustillo MA, Lazar RM, Finck AD, et al: Dexmedetomidine may impair cognitive testing during endovascular embolization of cerebral arteriovenous malformations: A retrospective case report series, *J Neurosurg Anesthesiol* 14:209–212, 2002.
24. Audu PB, Loomba N: Use of cuffed oropharyngeal airway (COPA) for awake intracranial surgery, *J Neurosurg Anesthesiol* 16:144–146, 2004.
25. Moore TA, Markert JM, Knowlton RC: Dexmedetomidine as rescue drug during awake craniotomy for cortical motor mapping and tumor resection, *Anesth Analg* 102:1556–1558, 2006.
26. Manninen PH, Tan TK: Postoperative nausea and vomiting after craniotomy for tumor surgery: A comparison between awake craniotomy and general anesthesia, *J Clin Anesth* 14:279–283, 2002.
27. Kelvin EA, Hesdorffer DC, Bagiella E, et al: Prevalence of self-reported epilepsy in a multiracial and multiethnic community in New York City, *Epilepsy Res* 77:141–150, 2007.
28. Bazil CW: Comprehensive care of the epilepsy patient-controlled, comorbidity, and cost, *Epilepsia* 45:3–12, 2004.
29. Chin PS, Berg AT, Spencer SS, et al: Employment outcomes following resective epilepsy surgery, *Epilepsia* 48:2253–2257, 2007.
30. Kiersey DK, Bickford RG, Faulconer A Jr: Electro-encephalographic patterns produced by thiopental sodium during surgical operations: Description and classification, *Br J Anaesth* 23:141–152, 1951.
31. Modica PA, Tempelhoff R, White PF: Pro- and anticonvulsant effects of anesthetics (part II), *Anesth Analg* 70:433–444, 1990.
32. Reddy RV, Moorthy SS, Dierdorf SF, et al: Excitatory effects and electroencephalographic correlation of etomidate, thiopental, methohexital, and propofol, *Anesth Analg* 77:1008–1011, 1993.
33. Rockoff MA, Goudsouzian NG: Seizures induced by methohexital, *Anesthesiology* 54:333–335, 1981.
34. Ebrahim ZY, DeBoer GE, Luders H, et al: Effect of etomidate on the electroencephalogram of patients with epilepsy, *Anesth Analg* 65:1004–1006, 1986.
35. Hufnagel A, Burr W, Elger CE, et al: Localization of the epileptic focus during methohexital-induced anesthesia, *Epilepsia* 33:271–284, 1992.
36. Rysz A, Bachanski M, Bidzinski J, Bacia T: The comparison of ketamine with methohexital and thiopental in the intraoperative EEG in drug-resistant epilepsy, *Neurol Neurochir Pol* 32:237–245, 1998.
37. Hansen HC, Drenck NE: Generalised seizures after etomidate anaesthesia, *Anaesthesia* 43:805–806, 1988.
38. Nicoll K, Callender J: Etomidate-induced convulsion prior to electroconvulsive therapy, *Br J Psychiatry* 177:373, 2000.
39. Huter L, Schreiber T, Gugel M, Schwarzkopf K: Low-dose intravenous midazolam reduces etomidate-induced myoclonus: A prospective, randomized study in patients undergoing elective cardioversion, *Anesth Analg* 105:1298–1302, 2007.
40. Freyer DR, Schwanda AE, Sanfilippo DJ, et al: Intravenous methohexital for brief sedation of pediatric oncology outpatients: Physiologic and behavioral responses, *Pediatrics* 99:E8, 1997.
41. Opitz A, Marschall M, Degan R, et al: General anesthesia in patients with epilepsy and status epilepticus. In Delgado-Escueta AV, Wasterlain CG, Treiman DM, editors: *Advances in Neurology: Status Epilepticus, Mechanisms of Brain Damage and Treatment*, New York, 1983, Raven Press, pp 531–535.
42. Yeoman P, Hutchinson A, Byrne A, et al: Etomidate infusions for the control of refractory status epilepticus, *Intensive Care Med* 15:255–259, 1989.
43. Bennett DR, Madsen JA, Jordan WS, et al: Ketamine anesthesia in brain-damaged epileptics: Electroencephalographic and clinical observations, *Neurology* 23:449–460, 1973.
44. Kugler J, Doenicke A: Ketamine—anticonvulsive and proconvulsive actions, *Anaesthetist* 43:S2–S7, 1994.
45. Oda Y, Toriyama S, Tanaka K, et al: The effect of dexmedetomidine on electrocorticography in patients with temporal lobe epilepsy under sevoflurane anesthesia, *Anesth Analg* 105:1272–1277, 2007.
46. Wood PR, Browne GP, Pugh S: Propofol infusion for the treatment of status epilepticus, *Lancet* 1(8583):480–481, 1988.
47. Rampil IJ, Lopez CE, Laxer KD, Barbaro NM: Propofol sedation may disrupt interictal epileptiform activity from a seizure focus, *Anesth Analg* 77:1071–1073, 1993.
48. Awad IA, Nayel MH: Epilepsy surgery: Introduction and overview, *Clin Neurosurg* 38:493–513, 1992.
49. Ebrahim ZY, Schubert A, Van Ness P, et al: The effect of propofol on the electroencephalogram of patients with epilepsy, *Anesth Analg* 78:275–279, 1994.
50. Walker M: Status epilepticus: An evidence based guide, *BMJ* 331:673–677, 2005.
51. Vakkuri AP, Seitsonen ER, Jantti VH, et al: A rapid increase in the inspired concentration of desflurane is not associated with epileptiform encephalogram, *Anesth Analg* 101:396–400, 2005.
52. Hymes JA: Seizure activity during isoflurane anesthesia, *Anesth Analg* 101:396–400, 1985.
53. Harrison JL: Postoperative seizures after isoflurane anesthesia, *Anesth Analg* 64:367–368, 1986.
54. Modica PA, Tempelhoff R, White PF: Pro- and anticonvulsant effects of anesthetics (part I), *Anesth Analg* 70:303–315, 1990.
55. Wyler AR, Ritchey ET, Atkinson RA, Hermann BP: Methohexital activation of epileptogenic foci during acute electrocorticography, *Epilepsia* 28:490–494, 1987.
56. Schultz B, Schultz A, Grouven U, Korsch G: Epileptiform EEG activity: Occurrence under sevoflurane and not during propofol application, *Anaesthetist* 50:43–45, 2001.
57. Woodforth IJ, Hicks RG, Crawford MR, et al: Electroencephalographic evidence of seizure activity under deep sevoflurane anesthesia in a non-epileptic patient, *Anesthesiology* 87:1579–1582, 1997.
58. Watts AD, Herrick IA, McLachlan RS, et al: The effect of sevoflurane and isoflurane anesthesia on interictal spike activity among patients with refractory epilepsy, *Anesth Analg* 89:1275–1281, 1999.
59. Hisada K, Morioka T, Fukui K, et al: Effects of sevoflurane and isoflurane on electrocorticographic activities in patients with temporal lobe epilepsy, *J Neurosurg Anesthesiol* 13:333–337, 2001.
60. Kurita N, Kawaguchi M, Hoshida T, et al: The effects of sevoflurane and hyperventilation on electrocorticogram spike activity in patients with refractory epilepsy, *Anesth Analg* 101:517–523, 2005.
61. Wass CT, Grady RE, Fessler AJ: The effects of remifentanil on epileptiform discharges during intraoperative electrocorticography in patients undergoing epilepsy surgery, *Epilepsia* 42:1340–1344, 2001.
62. Cascino GD, So EL, Sharbrough FW, et al: Alfentanil-induced epileptiform activity in patients with partial epilepsy, *J Clin Neurophysiol* 10:520–525, 1993.
63. McGuire G, El-Beheiry H, Manninen P, et al: Activation of electrocorticographic activity with remifentanil and alfentanil during neurosurgical excision of epileptogenic focus, *Br J Anaesth* 91:651–655, 2003.
64. Tempelhoff R, Modica PA, Bernardo KL, Edwards I: Fentanyl-induced electrocorticographic seizures in patients with complex partial epilepsy, *J Neurosurg* 77:201–208, 1992.
65. Koenig HM, Hoffman WE: The effect of anticonvulsant therapy on two doses of rocuronium-induced neuromuscular blockade, *J Neurosurg Anesthesiol* 11:86–89, 1999.
66. Richard A, Girard F, Girard DC, et al: Cisatracurium-induced neuromuscular blockade is affected by chronic phenytoin or carbamazepine treatment in neurosurgical patients, *Anesthesiology* 100:538–544, 2005.

17 • AWAKE CRANIOTOMY, EPILEPSY, MINIMALLY INVASIVE, AND ROBOTIC SURGERY

313

67. Ornstein E, Matteo RS, Young WL, Diaz J: Resistance to metocurine-induced neuromuscular blockade in patients receiving phenytoin, *Anesthesiology* 63:294–298, 1985.

68. Spacek A, Neiger FX, Spiss CK, Kress HG: Atracurium-induced neuromuscular block is not affected by chronic anticonvulsant therapy with carbamazepine, *Acta Anaesthesiol Scand* 41:1308–1311, 1997.

69. Tempelhoff R, Modica PA, Jellish WS, Spitznagel EL Jr: Resistance to atracurium-induced neuromuscular blockade in patients with intractable seizure disorders treated with anticonvulsants, *Anesth Analg* 71:665–669, 1990.

70. Ornstein E, Matteo RS, Schwartz AE, et al: The effect of phenytoin on the magnitude and duration of neuromuscular block following atracurium or vecuronium, *Anesthesiology* 67:191–196, 1987.

71. Alloul K, Whalley DG, Shutway F, et al: Pharmacokinetic origin of carbamazepine-induced resistance to vecuronium neuromuscular blockade in anesthetized patients, *Anesthesiology* 84:330–339, 1996.

72. Reasoner DK, Todd MM, Scamman FL, et al: The incidence of pneumocephalus after supratentorial craniotomy: Observations on the disappearance of intracranial air, *Anesthesiology* 80:1008–1012, 1994.

73. Eagle KA, Berger PB, Calkins H, et al: ACC/AHA guideline update for perioperative cardiovascular evaluation for noncardiac surgery—executive summary a report of the American College of Cardiology/American Heart Association Task Force on Practice Guidelines (Committee to Update the 1996 Guidelines on Perioperative Cardiovascular Evaluation for Noncardiac Surgery), *Circulation* 105:1257–1267, 2002.

74. Watson GH: Cardiac rhabdomyomas in tuberous sclerosis, *Ann N Y Acad Sci* 615:50–57, 1991.

75. Tempelhoff R, Modica PA, Spitznagel EL Jr: Anticonvulsant therapy increases fentanyl requirements during anaesthesia for craniotomy, *Can J Anaesth* 37:327–332, 1990.

76. Wall M, Baird-Lambert J, Buchanan N, et al: Liver function tests in persons receiving anticonvulsant medications, *Seizure* 1:187–190, 1992.

77. Rodriguez L, Valero R, Fabregas N: Intraoperative metabolic acidosis induced by chronic topiramate intake in neurosurgical patients, *J Neurosurg Anesthesiol* 20:67–68, 2008.

78. Soriano SG, Bozza P: Anesthesia for epilepsy surgery in children, *Childs Nerv Syst* 22:834–843, 2006.

79. Gidal B, Spencer N, Maly M, et al: Valproate-mediated disturbance of hemostasis: Relationship to dose and plasma concentration, *Neurology* 44:1418–1422, 1994.

80. Anderson GD, Lin YX, Berge C, Ojemann GA: Absence of bleeding complications in patients undergoing cortical surgery while receiving valproate treatment, *J Neurosurg* 87:252–256, 1997.

81. Artru AA, Lettich E, Colley PS, et al: Nitrous oxide: Suppression of focal epileptiform activity during inhalation and spreading of seizure activity following withdrawal, *J Neurosurg Anesthesiol* 2:189–193, 1990.

82. Peterson KD, Landsfeldt U, Cold GE, et al: Intracranial pressure and cerebral hemodynamic in patients with cerebral tumors: A randomized prospective study of patients subjected to craniotomy in propofol-fentanyl, isoflurane-fentanyl, or sevoflurane-fentanyl anesthesia, *Anesthesiology* 98:329–336, 2003.

83. Todd MM, Warner DS, Sokoll MD, et al: A prospective, comparative trial of three anesthetics for elective supratentorial craniotomy, *Anesthesiology* 78:1005–1020, 1993.

84. Coles JP, Leary TS, Monteiro JN, et al: Propofol anesthesia for craniotomy: A double-blind comparison of remifentanil, alfentanil, and fentanyl, *J Neurosurg Anesthesiol* 12:15–20, 2000.

85. Balakrishnan G, Raudzens P, Samra SK, et al: A comparison of remifentanil and fentanyl in patients undergoing surgery for intracranial mass lesions, *Anesth Analg* 91:163–169, 2000.

86. Gerlach K, Uhlig T, Huppe M, et al: Remifentanil-propofol versus sufentanil-propofol anaesthesia for supratentorial craniotomy: A randomized trial, *Eur J Anaesthesiol* 20:813–820, 2003.

87. Sneyd JR, Whaley A, Dimpel HL, et al: An open, randomized comparison of alfentanil, remifentanil and alfentanil followed by remifentanil in anaesthesia for craniotomy, *Br J Anaesth* 81:361–364, 1998.

88. Gelb AW, Salevsky F, Chung F, et al: Remifentanil with morphine transitional analgesia shortens neurological recovery compared to fentanyl for supratentorial craniotomy, *Can J Anaesth* 50:946–952, 2003.

89. Guy J, Hindman BJ, Baker KZ, et al: Comparison of remifentanil and fentanyl in patients undergoing craniotomy for supratentorial space-occupying lesions, *Anesthesiology* 86:514–524, 1997.

90. Herrick IA, Craen RA, Gelb AW, et al: Propofol sedation during awake craniotomy for seizures: Patient-controlled administration versus neurolept analgesia, *Anesth Analg* 84:1285–1291, 1997.

91. Ito BM, Sato S, Kufta CV, et al: Effect of isoflurane and enflurane on the electrocorticogram of epileptic patients, *Neurology* 38:924–928, 1988.

92. Cascino GD, Sharbrough FW, So EL, et al: Intraoperative alfentanil hydrochloride in temporal lobe epilepsy: Correlation with MRI-based volume studies, *Epilepsia* 33:85, 1992.

93. Fiol ME, Torres F, Gates JR, Maxwell R: Methohexital (Brevital) effect on electrocorticogram may be misleading, *Epilepsia* 31:524–528, 1990.

94. Sato K, Shamoto H, Yoshimoto T: Severe bradycardia during epilepsy surgery, *J Neurosurg Anesthesiol* 13:329–332, 2001.

95. Sinha PK, Neema PK, Manikandan S, et al: Bradycardia and sinus arrest following saline irrigation of the brain during epilepsy surgery, *J Neurosurg Anesthesiol* 16:160–163, 2004.

96. Kofke WA, Tempelhoff R, Dasheiff RM: Anesthesia for epileptic patients and for epilepsy surgery. In Cottrell JE, Smith DS, editors: *Anesthesia and Neurosurgery*, St. Louis, 1994, Mosby, pp 495–524.

97. Brian JE Jr, Deshpande JK, McPerson RW: Management of cerebral hemispherectomy in children, *J Clin Anesth* 2:91–95, 1990.

98. Zuckerberg AL, Tobin JR, Fleisher L, et al: The physiopathological consequences of cerebral hemispherectomy in children, *Anesthesiology* 79:A1187, 1993.

99. Abrahams JM, Torchia MB, McGarvey M, et al: Perioperative assessment of coagulability in neurosurgical patients using thromboelastography, *Surg Neurol* 58:5-11, 2002.

100. Goobie SM, Soriano SG, Zurakowski D, et al: Hemostatic changes in pediatric neurosurgical patients as evaluated by thrombelastograph, *Anesth Analg* 93:887–892, 2001.

101. Ramani R: Vagus nerve stimulation therapy for seizures, *J Neurosurg Anesthesiol* 20:29–35, 2008.

102. Ardesch JJ, Buschman HP, van der Burgh PH, et al: Cardiac responses of vagus nerve stimulation: Intraoperative bradycardia and subsequent chronic stimulation, *Clin Neurol Neurosurg* 109:849–852, 2007.

103. Zalvan C, Sulica L, Wolf S, et al: Laryngopharyngeal dysfunction from the implant vagal nerve stimulator, *Laryngoscope* 113:221–225, 2003.

104. Manninen PH, Raman SK, Boyle K, et al: Early postoperative complications following neurosurgical procedures, *Can J Anaesth* 46:7–14, 1999.

105. Madenoglu H, Yildiz K, Dogru K, et al: Randomized, double-blinded comparison of tropisetron and placebo for prevention of postoperative nausea and vomiting after supratentorial craniotomy, *J Neurosurg Anesthesiol* 15:82–86, 2003.

106. Onal C, Otsubo H, Araki T, et al: Complications of invasive subdural grid monitoring in children with epilepsy, *J Neurosurg* 98:1017–1026, 2003.

107. Schroeder HW, Niendorf WR, Gaab MR: Complications of endoscopic third ventriculostomy, *J Neurosurg* 96:1032–1040, 2002.

108. Fabregas N, Lopez A, Valero R, et al: Anesthetic management of surgical neuroendoscopies: Usefulness of monitoring the pressure inside the neuroendoscope, *J Neurosurg Anesthesiol* 12:21–28, 2000.

109. Ambesh SP, Kumar R: Neuroendoscopic procedures: anesthetic considerations for a growing trend: A review, *J Neurosurg Anesthesiol* 12:262–270, 2000.

110. Brockmeyer D, Abtin K, Carey L, Walker ML: Endoscopic third ventriculostomy: An outcome analysis, *Pediatr Neurosurg* 28:236–240, 1998.

111. Cinalli G, Salazar C, Mallucci C, et al: The role of endoscopic third ventriculostomy in the management of shunt malfunction, *Neurosurgery* 43:1323–1327, 1998.

112. Hopf NJ, Grunert P, Fries G, et al: Endoscopic third ventriculostomy: Outcome analysis of 100 consecutive procedures, *Neurosurgery* 44:795–804, 1999.

113. Longatti PL, Barzoi G, Paccagnella F, et al: A simplified endoscopic third ventriculostomy under local anesthesia, *Minim Invasive Neurosurg* 47:90–92, 2004.

114. van Aken J, Struys M, Verplancke T, et al: Cardiovascular changes during endoscopic third ventriculostomy, *Minim Invasive Neurosurg* 46:198–201, 2003.

115. Fabregas N, Valero R, Carrero E, et al: Episodic high irrigation pressure during surgical neuroendoscopy may cause intermittent intracranial circulatory insufficiency, *J Neurosurg Anesthesiol* 13:152–157, 2001.

116. El Dawlatly AA, Murshid WR, Elshimy A, et al: The incidence of bradycardia during endoscopic third ventriculostomy, *Anesth Analg* 91:1142–1144, 2000.

117. Fukuhara T, Vorster S, Luciano M: Risk factors for failure of endoscopic third ventriculostomy for obstructive hydrocephalus, *Neurosurgery* 46:1100–1109, 2000.

118. Handler M, Abbott R III, Lee M: A near-fatal complication of endoscopic third ventriculostomy: Case report, *Neurosurgery* 33:525–527, 1994.

119. Anandh B, Madhusudan Reddy KR, Mohanty A, et al: Intraoperative bradycardia and postoperative hyperkalemia in patients undergoing endoscopic third ventriculostomy, *Minim Invasive Neurosurg* 45:154–157, 2002.

120. Salvador L, Valero R, Carrero E, et al: Cerebrospinal fluid composition modification after neuroendoscopic procedures, *Minim Invasive Neurosurg* 50:51–55, 2007.

121. El Dawlatly AA: Blood biochemistry following endoscopic third ventriculostomy, *Minim Invasive Neurosurg* 47:47–48, 2004.

122. McLaughlin MR, Wahlig JB, Kaufmann AM, Albright AL: Traumatic basilar aneurysm after endoscopic third ventriculostomy: Case report, *Neurosurgery* 41:1400–1403, 1997.

123. Choi J, Kim D, Kim S: Endoscopic surgery for obstructive hydrocephalus, *Yonsei Med J* 40:600–607, 1999.

124. Enya S, Masuda Y, Terui K: Respiratory arrest after a ventriculoscopic surgery in infants: Two case reports, *Masui* 46:416–420, 1997.

125. Teo C, Jones R: Management of hydrocephalus by endoscopic third ventriculostomy in patients with myelomeningocele, *Pediatr Neurosurg* 25:57–63, 1996.

126. Schubert A: Pituitary surgery. In Schubert A, editor: *Clinical Neuroanesthesia*, Newton, MA, 1997, Butterworth-Heinemann, pp 69–80.

127. Nasseri SS, Kasperbauer JL, Strome SE, et al: Endoscopic transnasal pituitary surgery: Teport on 180 cases, *Am J Rhinol* 15:281–287, 2001.

128. Tada Y, Koike S, Ohta N, et al: Endoscopic transnasal transsphenoidal surgery for pituitary tumors—intranasal procedures, *Nippon Jibiinkoka Gakkai Kaiho* 103:212–218, 2000.

129. Citardi MJ, Batra PS: Intraoperative surgical navigation for endoscopic sinus surgery: Rationale and indications, *Curr Opin Otolaryngol Head Neck Surg* 15:23–27, 2007.

130. Chelliah YR, Manninen PH: Hazards of epinephrine in transsphenoidal pituitary surgery, *J Neurosurg Anesthesiol* 14:43–46, 2002.

131. Pasternak JJ, Atkinson JL, Kasperbauer JL, Lanier WL: Hemodynamic responses to epinephrine-containing local anesthetic injection and to emergence from general anesthesia in transsphenoidal hypophysectomy patients, *J Neurosurg Anesthesiol* 16:189–195, 2004.

132. Navarro R, Weiskopf RB, Moore MA, et al: Humans anesthetized with sevoflurane or isoflurane have similar arrhythmic response to epinephrine, *Anesthesiology* 80:545–549, 1994.

133. Moore MA, Weiskopf RB, Eger EI, et al: Arrhythmogenic doses of epinephrine are similar during desflurane or isoflurane anesthesia in humans, *Anesthesiology* 79:943–947, 1993.

134. Cavallo LM, Briganti F, Cappabianca P, et al: Hemorrhagic vascular complications of endoscopic transsphenoidal surgery, *Minim Invasive Neurosurg* 47:145–150, 2004.

135. Cappabianca P, Briganti F, Cavallo LM, de Divitiis E: Pseudoaneurysm of the intracavernous carotid artery following endoscopic endonasal transsphenoidal surgery, treated by endovascular approach, *Acta Neurochir (Wien)* 143:95–96, 2001.

136. Jimenez DF, Barone CM, Cartwright CC, Baker L: Early management of craniosynostosis using endoscopic-assisted strip craniectomies and cranial orthotic molding therapy, *Pediatrics* 110:97–104, 2002.

137. Faberowski LW, Black S, Mickle JP: Blood loss and transfusion practice in the perioperative management of craniosynostosis repair, *J Neurosurg Anesthesiol* 11:167–172, 1999.

138. Helfaer MA, Carson BS, James CS, et al: Increased hematocrit and decreased transfusion requirements in children given erythropoietin before undergoing craniofacial surgery, *J Neurosurg* 88:704–708, 1998.

139. Bermejo E, Felix V, Lapunzina P, Galan E, et al: Craniofacial dyssynostosis: Description of the first four Spanish cases and review, *Am J Med Genet A* 132:41–48, 2005.

140. Pijpers M, Poels PJ, Vaandrager JM, et al: Undiagnosed obstructive sleep apnea syndrome in children with syndromal craniofacial synostosis, *J Craniofac Surg* 15:670–674, 2004.

141. Butler MG, Hayes BG, Hathaway MM, Begleiter ML: Specific genetic diseases at risk for sedation/anesthesia complications, *Anesth Analg* 91:837–855, 2000.

142. Sugiyama K, Yokoyama K: Displacement of the endotracheal tube caused by change of head position in pediatric anesthesia: Evaluation by fiberoptic bronchoscopy, *Anesth Analg* 82:251–253, 1996.

143. Faberowski LW, Black S, Mickle JP: Incidence of venous air embolism during craniectomy for craniosynostosis repair, *Anesthesiology* 92:20–23, 2000.

144. Tobias JD, Johnson JO, Jimenez DF, et al: Venous air embolism during endoscopic strip craniectomy for repair of craniosynostosis in infants, *Anesthesiology* 95:340–342, 2001.

145. Rasche D, Rinaldi PC, Young RF, Tronnier VM: Deep brain stimulation for the treatment of various chronic pain syndromes, *Neurosurg Focus* 21:E8, 2006.

146. Schiff ND, Giacino JT, Kalmar K, et al: Behavioural improvements with thalamic stimulation after severe traumatic brain injury, *Nature* 448:600–603, 2007.

147. Venkatraghavan L, Manninen P, Mak P, et al: Anesthesia for functional neurosurgery: Review of complications, *J Neurosurg Anesthesiol* 18:64–67, 2006.

148. Khatib R, Ebrahim Z, Rezai A, et al: Perioperative events during deep brain stimulation: The experience at Cleveland Clinic, *J Neurosurg Anesthesiol* 20:36–40, 2008.

149. Maltete D, Navarro S, Welter ML, et al: Subthalamic stimulation in Parkinson disease: With or without anesthesia? *Arch Neurol* 61:390–392, 2004.

150. American Society of Anesthesiologists Task Force on Sedation and Analgesia by Non-Anesthesiologists: Practice guidelines for sedation and analgesia by non-anesthesiologists, *Anesthesiology* 96:1004–1017, 2002.

151. Watson R, Leslie K: Nerve blocks versus subcutaneous infiltration for stereotactic frame placement, *Anesth Analg* 92:424–427, 2001.

152. Zesiewicz TA, Elble R, Louis ED, et al: Practice parameter: Therapies for essential tremor: report of the Quality Standards Subcommittee of the American Academy of Neurology, *Neurology* 64:2008–2020, 2005.

153. Feltracco P, Ori C: A new look at the paravertebral block: A percutaneous video-assisted technique, *Reg Anesth Pain Med* 32:538–539, 2007.

154. Schulz U, Keh D, Barner C, et al: Bispectral index monitoring does not improve anesthesia performance in patients with movement disorders undergoing deep brain stimulating electrode implantation, *Anesth Analg* 104:1481–1487, 2007.

155. Binder DK, Rau G, Starr PA: Hemorrhagic complications of microelectrode-guided deep brain stimulation, *Stereotact Funct Neurosurg* 80:28–31, 2003.

156. Binder DK, Rau GM, Starr PA: Risk factors for hemorrhage during microelectrode-guided deep brain stimulator implantation for movement disorders, *Neurosurgery* 56:722–732, 2005.

157. Deogaonkar A, Avitsian R, Henderson JM, Schubert A: Venous air embolism during deep brain stimulation surgery in an awake supine patient, *Stereotact Funct Neurosurg* 83:32–35, 2005.

158. Moitra V, Permut TA, Penn RM, Roth S: Venous air embolism in an awake patient undergoing placement of deep brain stimulators, *J Neurosurg Anesthesiol* 16:321–322, 2004.

159. Santos P, Valero R, Arguis MJ, et al: Preoperative adverse events during stereotactic microelectrode-guided deep brain surgery in Parkinson's disease, *Rev Esp Anestesiol Reanim* 51:523–530, 2004.

160. Rozet I, Muangman S, Vavilala MS, et al: Clinical experience with dexmedetomidine for implantation of deep brain stimulators in Parkinson's disease, *Anesth Analg* 103:1224–1228, 2006.

161. Deogaonkar A, Deogaonkar M, Lee JY, et al: Propofol-induced dyskinesias controlled with dexmedetomidine during deep brain stimulation surgery, *Anesthesiology* 104:1337–1339, 2006.

162. Beric A, Kelly PJ, Rezai A, et al: Complications of deep brain stimulation surgery, *Stereotact Funct Neurosurg* 77:73–78, 2001.

163. Herzog J, Volkmann J, Krack P, et al: Two-year follow-up of subthalamic deep brain stimulation in Parkinson's disease, *Mov Disord* 18:1332–1337, 2003.

164. Dagtekin O, Berlet T, Gerbershagen HJ, et al: Anesthesia and deep brain stimulation: Postoperative akinetic state after replacement of impulse generators, *Anesth Analg* 103:784, 2006.

165. Shen FH, Samartzis D, Khanna AJ, Anderson DG: Minimally invasive techniques for lumbar interbody fusions, *Orthop Clin North Am* 38:373–386, 2007.

166. Regan JJ, Yuan H, McAfee PC: Laparoscopic fusion of the lumbar spine: Minimally invasive spine surgery: A prospective multicenter study evaluating open and laparoscopic lumbar fusion, *Spine* 24:402–411, 1999.

167. Huang EY, Acosta JM, Gardocki RJ, et al: Thoracoscopic anterior spinal release and fusion: Evolution of a faster, improved approach, *J Pediatr Surg* 37:1732–1735, 2002.

168. Kokoska ER, Gabriel KR, Silen ML: Minimally invasive anterior spinal exposure and release in children with scoliosis, *JSLS* 2:255–258, 1998.

169. Banoub M, Tetzlaff JE, Schubert A: Pharmacologic and physiologic influences affecting sensory evoked potentials, *Anesthesiology* 99:716–737, 2003.

170. Lotto ML, Banoub M, Schubert A: Effects of anesthetic agents and physiologic changes on intraoperative motor evoked potentials, *J Neurosurg Anesthesiol* 16:32–42, 2004.

171. Boulesteix G, Simon L, Lamit X, et al: Intratracheal intubation without muscle relaxant with the use of remifentanil-propofol, *Ann Fr Anesth Reanim* 18:393–397, 1999.

172. Maurtua M, Deogaonkar A, Katz E, et al: Does remifentanil prevent movement during neurosurgical stimulation in the absence of neuromuscular blockade? Preliminary results from a randomized trial, *J Neurosurg Anesthesiol* 16:363, 2004.

173. Engum SA: Minimal access thoracic surgery in the pediatric population, *Semin Pediatr Surg* 16:14–26, 2007.

174. Sucato DJ, Elerson E: A comparison between the prone and lateral position for performing a thoracoscopic anterior release and fusion for pediatric spinal deformity, *Spine* 28:2176–2180, 2003.

175. Lai YT, Yang LH, Chio CC, Chen HH: Complications in patients with palmar hyperhidrosis treated with transthoracic endoscopic sympathectomy, *Neurosurgery* 41:110–113, 1997.

176. McAfee PC, Regan JR, Zdeblick T, et al: The incidence of complications in endoscopic anterior thoracolumbar spinal reconstructive surgery: A prospective multicenter study comprising the first 100 consecutive cases, *Spine* 20:1624–1632, 1995.

177. Coumans JV, Reinhardt MK, Lieberman IH: Kyphoplasty for vertebral compression fractures: 1-year clinical outcomes from a prospective study, *J Neurosurg Spine* 99:44–50, 2003.

178. Uemura A, Numaguchi Y, Matsusako M, et al: Effect on partial pressure of oxygen in arterial blood in percutaneous vertebroplasty, *Am J Neuroradiol* 28:567–569, 2007.

179. Childers JC Jr: Cardiovascular collapse and death during vertebroplasty, *Radiology* 228:902–903, 2003.

180. Yoo KY, Jeong SW, Yoon W, Lee J: Acute respiratory distress syndrome associated with pulmonary cement embolism following percutaneous vertebroplasty with polymethylmethacrylate, *Spine* 29:E294–E297, 2004.

181. Fessler RG, Khoo LT: Minimally invasive cervical microendoscopic foraminotomy: An initial clinical experience, *Neurosurgery* 51:37–45, 2002.

182. Jho HD, Ha HG: Anterolateral approach for cervical spinal cord tumors via an anterior microforaminotomy: Technical note, *Minim Invasive Neurosurg* 42:1–5, 1999.

183. King AG, Mills TE, Loe WA Jr, et al: Video-assisted thoracoscopic surgery in the prone position, *Spine* 25:2403–2406, 2000.

184. Perez-Cruet MJ, Fessler RG, Perin NI: Review: Complications of minimally invasive spinal surgery, *Neurosurgery* 51:26–36, 2002.

185. Dagher C, Narchi P, Naccache N, et al: Regional anesthesia for lumbar disc surgery, *Anesthesiology* 89 (3A) Sept. 1998: A44.

186. Tetzlaff JE, Dilger JA, Kodsy M, et al: Spinal anesthesia for elective lumbar spine surgery, *J Clin Anesth* 10:666–669, 1998.

187. Fogarty P, Abalos A, Haas D, et al: Postoperative narcotic requirement following lumbar microdiscectomy is related to pre-operative pain, not to intraoperative ketorolac or bupivacaine, *Anesth Analg* 86 (2s) 1988: s6.

188. Jellish WS, Thalji Z, Stevenson K, Shea J: A prospective randomized study comparing short- and intermediate-term perioperative outcome variables after spinal or general anesthesia for lumbar disk and laminectomy surgery, *Anesth Analg* 83:559–564, 1996.

189. Demirel CB, Kalayci M, Ozkocak I, et al: A prospective randomized study comparing perioperative outcome variables after epidural or general anesthesia for lumbar disc surgery, *J Neurosurg Anesthesiol* 15:185–192, 2003.

190. Mathews HH, Long BH: Minimally invasive techniques for the treatment of intervertebral disk herniation, *J Am Acad Orthop Surg* 10:80–85, 2002.

191. Henry LG, Cattey RP, Stoll JE, Robbins S: Laparoscopically assisted spinal surgery, *JSLS* 1:341–344, 1997.

192. Liu JC, Ondra SL, Angelos P, et al: Is laparoscopic anterior lumbar interbody fusion a useful minimally invasive procedure? *Neurosurgery* 51:155–158, 2002.

193. Lieberman IH, Togawa D, Kayanja MM, et al: Bone-mounted miniature robotic guidance for pedicle screw and translaminar facet screw placement: Part I: Technical development and a test case result, *Neurosurgery* 59:641–650, 2006.

194. Togawa D, Kayanja MM, Reinhardt MK, et al: Bone-mounted miniature robotic guidance for pedicle screw and translaminar facet screw placement: Part 2: Evaluation of system accuracy, *Neurosurgery* 60:ONS 129–139, 2007.

195. Jain R, Kato Y, Sano H, et al: Micromanipulator: Effectiveness in minimally invasive neurosurgery, *Minim Invasive Neurosurg* 46:235–239, 2003.

196. Feng H, Huang G, Liao X, et al: Endoscopic third ventriculostomy in the management of obstructive hydrocephalus: An outcome analysis, *J Neurosurg* 100:626–633, 2004.

197. Mohanty A, Anandh B, Kolluri V, Praharaj SS: Neuroendoscopic third ventriculostomy in the management of fourth ventricular outlet obstruction, *Minim Invasive Neurosurg* 42:18–21, 1999.

198. Robinson S, Cohen AR: The role of neuroendoscopy in the treatment of pineal region tumors, *Surg Neurol* 48:360–365, 1997.

199. Hamada H, Hayashi N, Kurimoto M, et al: Neuroendoscopic septostomy for isolated lateral ventricle, *Neurol Med Chir* 43:582–587, 2003.

200. Kestle JR, Drake JM, Cochrane DD, et al: Lack of benefit of endoscopic ventriculoperitoneal shunt insertion: A multicenter randomized trial, *J Neurosurg* 98:284–290, 2003.

201. Villavicencio AT, Leveque JC, McGirt MJ, et al: Comparison of revision rates following endoscopically versus nonendoscopically placed ventricular shunt catheters, *Surg Neurol* 59:375–379, 2003.

202. Lewis AI: Endoscopic management of colloid cysts, *Neurosurgery* 44:232, 1999.

203. Levy ML, Wang M, Aryan HE, et al: Microsurgical keyhole approach for middle fossa arachnoid cyst fenestration, *Neurosurgery* 53:1138–1144, 2003.

204. Rodziewicz GS, Chuang WC: Endoscopic removal of organized chronic subdural hematoma, *Surg Neurol* 43:569–572, 1995.

205. Karakhan VB, Khodnevich AA: Endoscopic surgery of traumatic intracranial haemorrhages, *Acta Neurochir Suppl (Wien)* 61:84–91, 1994.

206. Fritsch M, Manwaring KH: Endoscopic treatment of brain abscess in children, *Minim Invasive Neurosurg* 40:103–106, 1997.

207. Boviatsis EJ, Kouyialis AT, Stranjalis G, et al: CT-guided stereotactic biopsies of brain stem lesions: Personal experience and literature review, *Neurol Sci* 24:97–102, 2003.

208. An H, Wang L, Liu Y: Endoscopic transnasal sphenoidal approach in hypophysectomy, *Zhonghua Er Bi Yan Hou Ke Za Zhi* 35:367–368, 2000.

209. Yurtseven T, Ersahin Y, Demirtas E, Mutluer S: Neuroendoscopic biopsy for intraventricular tumors, *Minim Invasive Neurosurg* 46:293–299, 2003.

210. Cartwright CC, Jimenez DF, Barone CM, Baker L: Endoscopic strip craniectomy: A minimally invasive treatment for early correction of craniosynostosis, *J Neurosci Nurs* 35:130–138, 2003.

211. Kalavakonda C, Sekhar LN, Ramachandran P, Hechl P: Endoscope-assisted microsurgery for intracranial aneurysms, *Neurosurgery* 51:1119–1126, 2002.

212. Tan C, Brookes GB: The endoscopic technique utilized in removal process of acoustic neuroma by retrosigmoid approach, *Lin Chuang Er Bi Yan Hou Ke Za Zhi* 17:25–26, 2003.

213. Yamada S, Iacono RP, Mandybur GT, et al: Endoscopic procedures for resection of arteriovenous malformations, *Surg Neurol* 51:641–649, 1999.

214. Otsuki T, Jokura H, Nakasato N, Yoshimoto T: Stereotactic endoscopic resection of angiographically occult vascular malformations, *Acta Neurochir Suppl (Wien)* 61:98–101, 1994.

215. Benabid AL: Deep brain stimulation for Parkinson's disease, *Curr Opin Neurobiol* 13:696–706, 2003.

216. Cosyns P, Gabriels L, Nuttin B: Deep brain stimulation in treatment refractory obsessive compulsive disorder, *Verh K Acad Geneeskd Belg* 65:385–399, 2003.

217. Temel Y, Visser-Vandewalle V: Surgery in Tourette syndrome, *Mov Disord* 19:3–14, 2004.

218. Rehncrona S, Johnels B, Widner H, et al: Long-term efficacy of thalamic deep brain stimulation for tremor: Double-blind assessments, *Mov Disord* 18:163–170, 2003.

219. Huewel N, Perneczky A, Urban V, Fries G: Neuroendoscopic technique for the operative treatment of septated syringomyelia, *Acta Neurochir Suppl (Wien)* 54:59–62, 1992.

220. Fredman B, Olsfanger D, Jedeikin R: Thorascopic sympathectomy in the treatment of palmar hyperhidrosis: Anaesthetic implications, *Br J Anaesth* 79:113–119, 1997.

221. Heikkinen ER: Whole body" stereotaxy: Application of stereotactic endoscopy to operations of herniated lumbar discs, *Acta Neurochir Suppl (Wien)* 54:89–92, 1992.

222. Anand N, Regan JJ: Video-assisted thoracoscopic surgery for thoracic disc disease: Classification and outcome study of 100 consecutive cases with a 2-year minimum follow-up period, *Spine* 27:871–879, 2002.

223. Krasna MJ, Jiao X, Eslami A, et al: Thoracoscopic approach for spine deformities, *J Am Coll Surg* 197:777–779, 2003.

224. McLain RF: Spinal cord decompression: An endoscopically assisted approach for metastatic tumors, *Spinal Cord* 39:482–487, 2001.

225. Rosenthal D, Marquardt G, Lorenz R, Nichtweiss M: Anterior decompression and stabilization using a microsurgical endoscopic technique for metastatic tumors of the thoracic spine, *J Neurosurg* 84:565–572, 1996.

226. Khoo LT, Beisse R, Potulski M: Thoracoscopic-assisted treatment of thoracic and lumbar fractures: A series of 371 consecutive cases, *Neurosurgery* 51:104–117, 2002.

227. Rosenthal D, Dickman CA: Thoracoscopic microsurgical excision of herniated thoracic discs, *J Neurosurg* 89:224–235, 1998.

228. Huang TJ, Hsu RW, Sum CW, Liu HP: Complications in thoracoscopic spinal surgery: A study of 90 consecutive patients, *Surg Endosc* 13:346–350, 1999.

229. Huang TJ, Hsu RW, Liu HP, et al: Video-assisted thoracoscopic surgery to the upper thoracic spine, *Surg Endosc* 13:123–126, 1999.

Chapter 18

PERIOPERATIVE MANAGEMENT OF ADULT PATIENTS WITH SEVERE HEAD INJURY

Audrée A. Bendo

EPIDEMIOLOGY OF HEAD INJURY

A *traumatic brain injury* (TBI) is defined as a blow or jolt to the head or a penetrating head injury that disrupts the function of the brain. TBI is one of the most serious, life-threatening conditions in trauma victims. It is a leading cause of disability and death in children and adults. An estimated 1.5 million people sustain TBIs every year in the United States.[1] Of these, more than 50,000 people die annually as a result of TBI, and another 80,000 people become impaired or disabled for life. TBI is a leading cause of disability in the United States, affecting approximately 5.3 million people. TBI-related disability has a devastating effect on the lives of the injured individuals and their families and results in a tremendous cost to hospital systems and society for rehabilitation and chronic care of these individuals.

Head injury occurs most often in adolescents, young adults, and people older than 75 years. In all age groups, males are affected two times more often than females and are more likely to sustain severe head injury. The leading causes of TBI are falls, motor vehicle crashes, and assaults.[1] Blasts are a leading cause of TBI among active duty military personnel in war zones.[1] On April 28, 2008, the 110th United States Congress passed a bill to provide for the expansion and improvement of TBI programs (Public Law 110-206), such as research funding for therapeutic interventions and development of practice guidelines for rehabilitation.

HEAD INJURY GUIDELINES

In 1995, recognizing the need to standardize care to improve outcome in head-injured patients, the Brain Trauma Foundation approved guidelines for the initial resuscitation of the patient with severe head injury and the treatment of intracranial hypertension.[2] A task force was formed in 1998 to review and update the scientific evidence for the guidelines. These evidence-based guidelines for the management of severe TBI were published in 2000[3,4] and then updated in 2007 (Box 18-1).[5] This extensive review of the literature recommends three standards based on Class I evidence and several guidelines based on Class II evidence.

Results of the Corticosteroid Randomization After Significant Head Injury (CRASH) trial, which studied the effect of early administration of methylprednisolone on outcome after head injury in 10,008 adults, were published in 2005.[6] This was an international randomized, placebo-controlled trial on the effect of early administration of 48-hour infusion of methylprednisolone on the risk of death and disability after head injury. The CRASH trial revealed a higher risk of death within 2 weeks of injury in the group receiving corticosteroids than in the group receiving placebo, as well as a higher risk of death or severe disability.[6] The trial investigators concluded that "corticosteroids should not be used routinely in the treatment of head injury."[6]

Evidence-based guidelines for prehospital management of TBI[7,8] and for pediatric brain injury[9] have also been published, and in March 2006, surgical management guidelines were published.[10] However, unlike the writers of the severe TBI management guidelines,[3,5] the writers of the surgical management guidelines report no controlled clinical trials in the literature to support different forms of surgical management or surgical versus conservative therapy. As with the other published guidelines for the management of severe TBI, they state that "this is a document in evolution," and revisions will be made as new knowledge is gained.[10]

CLASSIFICATION OF HEAD INJURY

Classification of severe head injury is based on the Glasgow Coma Scale (GCS) (Table 18-1), which defines neurologic impairment in terms of eye opening, speech, and motor function.[11,12] The total score that can be obtained is 15, and severe head injury is determined by a score of 8 or less persisting for 6 hours or more. The GCS and Glasgow Outcome Scale permit comparison between series of traumatically head-injured patients on the basis of initial clinical presentation and eventual outcome.[13] The prognosis after head injury depends on the type of lesion sustained, the age of the patient, and the severity of the injury as defined by the GCS. In general, mortality is closely related to the initial score on the GCS. For any given lesion and score, however, the elderly have a poorer outcome than do younger patients.[14,15]

Following head trauma, the primary injury results from the biomechanical effect of forces applied to the skull and brain at the time of the insult and are manifested within milliseconds. Currently, there is no treatment for the primary injury. Secondary injury occurs in the minutes, hours, or days after the impact and represents complicating processes initiated by the primary injury, such as ischemia, brain swelling and edema, intracranial hemorrhage, intracranial hypertension, and herniation. The common denominator of secondary injury is cerebral hypoxia with ischemia (Box 18-2). Factors that aggravate the initial injury include hypoxia, hypercarbia, hypotension, anemia, and hyperglycemia. These contributing factors to secondary injury are preventable. Seizures, infection, and sepsis that may occur hours to days after injury would further aggravate brain damage and must also be prevented or treated promptly.

BOX 18–1 *Recommendations from Guidelines for the Management of Severe Traumatic Brain Injury (TBI)*

Standards Based on Class I Evidence

- If intracranial pressure (ICP) is normal, avoid prolonged hyperventilation therapy ($Paco_2 < 25$ mm Hg).
- The use of steroids is not recommended for improving outcome or reducing ICP.
- Prophylactic use of anticonvulsants does not prevent late post-traumatic seizures.

Guidelines Based on Class II Evidence

- All regions should have an organized trauma care system.
- Avoid or immediately correct hypotension (systolic blood pressure <90 mm Hg) and hypoxia (Sao_2 <90% or Pao_2 <60 mm Hg).
- Indications for ICP monitoring include Glasgow Coma Scale score of 3 to 8 with abnormal computed tomography findings or two or more of the following adverse features: age >40 yrs, motor posturing, and systolic blood pressure <90 mm Hg.
- Initiate treatment for ICP at an upper threshold above 20 mm Hg.
- The cerebral perfusion pressure (CPP) value to target lies within the range of 50 to 70 mm Hg. Aggressive attempts to maintain CPP above 70 mm Hg should be avoided because of the risk of acute respiratory distress syndrome.
- Avoid using prophylactic hyperventilation ($Paco_2 \leq 25$ mm Hg) therapy during the first 24 hours after severe TBI.
- Mannitol is effective for controlling raised ICP after severe TBI, in doses ranging from 0.25 to 1 g/kg.
- High-dose barbiturate therapy may be considered in hemodynamically stable, salvageable patients who have severe TBI and whose intracranial hypertension is refractory to maximal medical and surgical ICP-lowering therapy.
- Provide nutritional support (140% of resting energy expenditure in patients without respiratory paralysis and 100% of resting energy expenditure in patients with it), using enteral or parenteral formulas containing at least 15% of calories as protein by day 7 after injury.

Adapted from Bullock RM, Chesnut RM, Clifton GL, et al: Guidelines for the management of severe traumatic brain injury. J Neurotrauma 2000;17: 449-554; Robertson CS: Management of cerebral perfusion pressure after traumatic brain injury. Anesthesiology 2001;95:1513-1517; and Guidelines for the management of severe traumatic brain injury, 3rd ed. The Brain Trauma Foundation, American Association of Neurological Surgeons; Congress of Neurological Surgeons. J Neurotrauma 2007;24:S1-106.

Table 18–1 Modified Glasgow Coma Scale*

Feature	Point(s)
Eye Opening	
Spontaneously	4
To verbal command	3
To pain	2
None	1
Best Verbal Response	
Oriented, conversing	5
Disoriented, conversing	4
Inappropriate words	3
Incomprehensible sounds	2
No verbal response	1
Best Motor Response	
Obeys verbal commands	6
Localizes to pain	5
Flexion or withdrawal	4
Abnormal flexion (decorticate)	3
Extension (decerebrate)	2
No response (flaccid)	1

*Total scores: mild head injury = 13-15 points; moderate = 9-12 points; severe ≤8 points.
Adapted from Teasdale G, Jennett B: Assessment of coma and impaired consciousness: A practical scale. Lancet 1974;2:81; and Jennett B: Assessment of the severity of head injury. J Neurol Neurosurg Psychiatry 1976;39:647.

Secondary insults complicate the course of more than 50% of head-injured patients.[5] An outcome study using data from the Traumatic Coma Data Bank revealed that hypotension occurring after head injury is profoundly detrimental, with more than 70% of patients with hypotension experiencing

---

BOX 18–2 *Secondary Insults that Can Contribute to Hypoxic and/or Ischemic Brain Damage*

Systemic

Hypoxemia
Hypotension
Anemia
Hypocarbia
Hypercarbia
Pyrexia
Hyponatremia
Hypoglycemia
Hyperglycemia

Intracranial

Hematoma
Raised intracranial pressure
Seizures
Infection
Vasospasm

---

significant morbidity and mortality (Table 18-2).[14] Furthermore, the combination of hypoxia and hypotension is significantly more detrimental than that of hypotension alone; more than 90% of patients who had both of these experienced a severe outcome or died. These findings confirm the importance of avoiding hypovolemic shock in head-injured patients. The management goal in head-injured patients is to initiate timely and appropriate therapy to prevent secondary brain injury. When the initial injury is not fatal, subsequent neurologic damage and systemic complications should be preventable in most patients.

Primary injury or biomechanical trauma to brain parenchyma consists of concussion, contusion, laceration, and hematoma. Not all severely head-injured patients require surgery. Generalized brain injury with edema or contusion is a common finding, whether or not a surgically correctable mass

Table 18–2 Impact of Hypoxia and Hypotension* on Outcome after Severe Head Injury (Defined as Glasgow Coma Scale Score ≤ 8)

Secondary Insults	Number of Patients	Outcome (% of Patients)		
		Good or Moderate	Severe or Vegetative	Dead
Total number of cases	699	43	21	37
Neither insult	456	51	22	27
Hypoxia (Pao_2 <60 mm Hg)	78	45	22	33
Hypotension (systemic blood pressure <90 mm Hg)	113	26	14	60
Both	52	6	19	75

*At time of hospital arrival.
Data adapted from Moppett IK: Traumatic brain injury: Assessment, resuscitation and early management. Br J Anaesth 2007;99:18-31.

lesion is present. *Diffuse cerebral swelling* occurs because of sudden intracerebral congestion and hyperemia. Twenty-four hours or more after the initial insult, cerebral edema develops in the extracellular spaces of the white matter. Nonoperative treatment of diffuse cerebral swelling involves hyperventilation, diuresis with mannitol and furosemide, and barbiturates in conjunction with intracranial pressure (ICP) monitoring.

Depressed skull fractures and acute epidural, subdural, and intracerebral hematomas usually require craniotomy. Chronic subdural hematomas are often evacuated through burr holes. *Depressed skull fractures* under lacerations should be elevated and debrided within 24 hours to minimize the risk of infection. Bony fragments and penetrating objects should not be manipulated in the emergency department (ED), because they may be tamponading a lacerated vessel or dural sinus.

Traumatic epidural hematoma is an infrequent complication of head injury, usually the result of a motor vehicle accident. The initial injury tears middle meningeal vessels or dural sinuses and causes unconsciousness. When a spasm and clot occur in the vessel(s), the bleeding stops and the patient recovers, experiencing a lucid interval. Over the next several hours, the vessel bleeds and the patient rapidly deteriorates (especially with arterial bleeding). In rapidly deteriorating conditions, treatment should not be delayed to await radiologic evaluation; emergency evacuation is necessary. Venous epidural hematomas develop more slowly, and there may be time for diagnostic testing.

The clinical presentation of *acute subdural hematomas* ranges from minimal deficits to unconsciousness and signs of a mass lesion (hemiparesis, unilateral decerebration, and pupillary enlargement). A lucid interval may occur. The most common cause of subdural hematoma is trauma, but it may occur spontaneously and is associated with coagulopathies, aneurysms, and neoplasms. It is considered acute if the patient becomes symptomatic within 72 hours, subacute if symptoms appear between 3 and 15 days, and chronic with symptoms after 2 weeks. *Subacute* or *chronic subdural hematoma* is usually observed in patients older than 50 years. There may be no history of head trauma. The clinical presentation in these patients may vary from focal signs of brain dysfunction to a depressed level of consciousness or development of an organic brain syndrome. Intracranial hypertension is usually associated with acute subdural hematoma. Intensive medical therapy to correct elevated ICP and control brain edema and swelling may be required before, during, and after hematoma evacuation.

In patients with *intracerebral hematomas*, the clinical picture may vary from minimal neurologic deficits to deep coma.

Large, solitary intracerebral hematomas should be evacuated. Lesions causing delayed neurologic deterioration from fresh hemorrhage are also evacuated but carry a poor prognosis. Depending on the extent of cerebral injury, patients with intracerebral hematomas may require intensive medical therapy to control intracranial hypertension and cerebral edema. *Coup and contrecoup injuries* usually cause cerebral contusion and intracerebral hemorrhage. In general, contused brain tissue is not removed; occasionally, however, contused tissue over the frontal or temporal poles may be removed to control edema formation and prevent herniation.

EMERGENCY THERAPY

Perioperative management of the head-injured patient focuses on aggressive stabilization of the patient and avoidance of systemic and intracranial insults that cause secondary neuronal injury (see Box 18-2). Secondary brain injury complicates the course of the majority of head-injured patients, adversely influencing outcome. The need to improve care of these patients in the field and ED has been recognized with the development of guidelines, improvement of emergency response services, and better training of providers.[7] The goals of emergency therapy in the field and ED are to prevent and treat all secondary insults and, ultimately, to improve outcome in patients with TBI.

Prehospital Management

Emergency therapy should begin at the site of the accident and in the ambulance. According to the Brain Trauma Foundation's Guidelines for Prehospital Management of Traumatic Brain Injury,[7] emergency medical service (EMS) providers should be trained to follow an established algorithm for assessment and treatment of TBI. The first priority is initiation of a basic resuscitation protocol that prioritizes the ABCs (airway, breathing, and circulation), assessment, and treatment. The patient's airway is maintained, and blood pressure is supported. The EMS provider performs an assessment for appropriate triage of the patient and all necessary therapy to stabilize the patient prior to transport. It is recommended that the severely injured patient (GCS score <9) be taken directly to a level I trauma center "with 24 hour scanning capability, operating room, prompt neurosurgical care and the ability to monitor intracranial pressure and treat intracranial hypertension as delineated in the Guidelines for the Management of Severe Head Injury."[7] Optimal results for patients with intracranial hematomas require surgical evacuation within 2 to 4 hours of the injury.[16] Therefore, direct transport to a neurosurgical center is crucial for such patients.

The prehospital management guidelines published in 2002[7] and 2008[8] are accepted as the standard for management by prehospital and ED clinicians. Currently, there is insufficient data to support any standard recommendations for prehospital assessment, treatment, transport, and destination. Subsequent to the initial publication of these guidelines, the results of several studies have questioned whether outcome is improved by following them.[17-19] These studies support the direct transfer of patients with severe TBI to a level I or level II trauma center, but controversy remains regarding whether patient outcome is improved by paramedic intubations in the field or mode of transport.[19] Randomized, controlled trials are currently under way in Australia and other countries to determine whether or not physician involvement in advanced interventions at the accident scene will decrease the rate of death and severe disability in patients with severe head injury.

Emergency Department Management

All patients with head injury require full diagnostic evaluation with complete history and neurologic examination. Not all patients require radiologic examination. Two comprehensive studies have resulted in the development of two slightly different sets of rules for determining whether or not a patient with minor head injury must undergo computed tomography (CT) scanning.[20,21] These are the Canadian and New Orleans CT scanning rules for minor head injury (Box 18-3). An unenhanced CT scan is the radiologic procedure of choice in acute

TBI. A spiral CT of the head and craniocervical junction is useful in the patients with more severe TBI and potential high cervical spine injuries.

The majority of head-injured patients seen in the ED are classified as having *mild head injuries* (GCS score 13-15). Most of these patients recover without incident or may have neuropsychological sequelae. These patients are sent home with a care giver and instructions only if they have had no history of loss of consciousness, no vomiting or amnesia, normal neurologic findings, and minimal, if any, subgaleal swelling. A small percentage of patients with a GCS score of 13 to 15 on arrival deteriorate and require neurosurgical intervention (for additional references, see Gopinath and colleagues[16]).

Implementation of ED protocols and the use of the Canadian or New Orleans CT scanning rules for minor head injury should help identify the subgroup of patients at risk of deterioration.[20,21] Patients with *moderate head injury* (GCS score 9-12) are able to follow simple commands in the ED, but they can deteriorate rapidly. These patients require emergency CT scanning and admission for observation with serial neurologic examinations, even if the initial CT scan is normal. Patients with *severe head injury* (GCS score ≤ 8) require full Advanced Trauma Life Support (ATLS) resuscitation and stabilization in the ED, CT scanning of the head and cervical spine, and, often, surgical management.

Emergency Therapy for Severe Traumatic Brain Injury

The neurologic status and concomitant injuries of patients with severe TBI should be assessed prior to tracheal intubation. These patients are intubated to protect the airway from aspiration and to ensure adequate ventilation and avoidance of hypoxia, hypocapnia, and hypercarbia. The incidence of cervical spine injuries in surviving victims of head injury is 1% to 3% in adults and 0.5% in children.[22,23] Victims of head-first falls or high-speed motor vehicle accidents have a 10% or greater chance of cervical spine fractures. Radiographic evaluation with a cross-table lateral view can miss 20% of cervical spine fractures.[23] To improve the reliability of radiographic evaluation, anteroposterior and odontoid views, in addition to a lateral view, have been recommended. Reportedly, this combination misses only 7% of fractures.[22] When a cervical spine fracture has not been excluded by radiographic evaluation, cervical alignment with in-line stabilization is recommended during emergency intubation.[23-25]

When facial fractures and soft tissue edema prevent direct visualization of the larynx, a fiberoptic intubation or intubation with an illuminated stylet or intubating laryngeal mask airway may be attempted. In the patient with severe facial and/or laryngeal injuries, a cricothyrotomy may be required. Nasal intubations are avoided in the patient with suspected basal skull fracture, severe facial fractures, or bleeding diathesis. Basal skull fractures are strongly suspected when the patient has tympanic cavity hemorrhage, otorrhea, petechiae on the mastoid process (Battle's sign), and petechiae around the eyes (panda sign). Nasal intubation of a patient with basal skull fractures can introduce contaminated material directly into the brain and so is best avoided.

For patients with facial injuries, the simplest and most expeditious approach to intubation is preoxygenation, followed by rapid-sequence anesthesia induction with cricoid pressure and maintenance of in-line stabilization. All head-injured patients are assumed to have a full stomach. Awake,

---

BOX 18–3 *Computed Tomography Scanning Rules for Minor Head Injury*

Canadian Rules*

High risk (for neurological intervention)
- GCS score <15 at 2h after injury
- Suspected open or depressed skull fracture
- Any sign of basal skull fracture
- Vomiting ≥ two episodes
- Age ≥ 65 years

Medium risk (for brain injury on CT)
- Amnesia before impact > 30 min
- High risk mechanism of injury

New Orleans Rules†

Short-term memory deficits (persistent anterograde amnesia with GCS score 15)
Intoxication (drug alcohol)
Physical evidence of trauma above the clavicles
Age > 60 years
Seizure (suspected or witnessed)
Headache
Vomiting
Coagulopathy

---

*Stiell IG, Wells GA, Vandemheen K, et al: The Canadian CT head rule for patients with minor head injury, Lancet 357:1391–1396, 2001.
†Haydel MJ, Preton CA, Mills TJ, et al: Indications for computed tomography in patients with minor head injury, N Engl L Med 343: 100–105, 2000.

oral intubation without anesthetic agents may be possible in the severely injured patient, but it is difficult in the awake or uncooperative, combative patient. Depending on the patient's cardiovascular status, virtually any of the intravenous anesthesia induction agents can be used. The choice of muscle relaxants for emergency intubation in a neurosurgical patient has been the subject of controversial discussion for many years. Succinylcholine can increase ICP. However, in the setting of acute airway compromise, full stomach, and the need to perform subsequent neurologic examinations, the benefits of rapid onset and elimination of succinylcholine may outweigh the risk of transiently increasing ICP.[26]

After control of the airway has been achieved in the head-injured patient, attention should focus on resuscitation of the cardiovascular system. Transient hypotension after head injury is not uncommon, but sustained hypotension usually results from hemorrhage secondary to other systemic injuries. These injuries must be sought and aggressively treated with fluids, blood, and inotropic and vasopressor drugs, when necessary.

When multiple trauma complicates head injury, there is no ideal crystalloid resuscitation fluid. A major concern during resuscitation is the development of cerebral edema. Animal investigations reveal that total serum osmolality is a key factor in brain edema formation.[27,28] When serum osmolality is reduced, cerebral edema develops in normal and abnormal brain. This occurs because the blood-brain barrier is relatively impermeable to sodium. Solutions containing sodium in concentrations lower than that in serum cause water movement into the brain, increasing brain water. Thus, hypo-osmolar solutions (0.45% NaCl and lactated Ringer's solution) are more likely than iso-osmolar fluids (0.9% saline) to increase brain water content. Large-volume fluid resuscitation with iso-osmolar crystalloids reduces colloid oncotic pressure and increases peripheral tissue edema. However, in animal investigations, the brain behaves differently from other tissues, and profound lowering of colloid oncotic pressure with maintenance of serum osmolality does not result in edema in normal brain[27] or in some head-injury models.[28,29] These results can be explained by the unique structure of the blood-brain barrier and the fact that colloid oncotic pressure gradients generate weak forces in comparison with osmolar gradients.[27]

Some doubt has been cast on the applicability of these laboratory findings to clinical practice. The cryogenic injury model used in these experiments may not be equivalent to head injury in patients. In head-injured patients, the capillary permeability of the brain may be rendered similar to that of peripheral tissues when the blood-brain barrier is damaged. In addition, the time course of these experiments did not allow observation of edema developing 24 to 48 hours after initial resuscitation, which occurs in head-injured patients. An investigation using the percussive head injury model in rats has shown that reduction in colloid oncotic pressure can aggravate cerebral edema under certain conditions.[30] Therefore, it seems reasonable in clinical practice to avoid a profound reduction in colloid oncotic pressure. Iso-osmolar colloid solutions, such as 5% albumin and 6% hetastarch, have been recommended to maintain oncotic pressure and intravascular volume. However, fresh whole blood, when available, is the ideal colloid resuscitation fluid for hypovolemic patients with TBI and ongoing blood loss.

There is continuing controversy about the selection of resuscitation fluids in patients with TBI after the report of the post hoc follow-up study on the Saline versus Albumin Fluid Evaluation (SAFE) Study.[31] This randomized, controlled trial compared 4% albumin with 0.9% saline for fluid management in critically ill trauma patients. The subset of patients with TBI who received albumin resuscitation had substantially worse outcomes than patients with TBI who received saline resuscitation. The findings in this study suggest that saline may be preferable to albumin during the acute resuscitation of patients with severe TBI.

Hypertonic saline solutions (3%, 7.5%) can be very useful for low-volume resuscitation in the head-injured patient because they lower ICP, raise blood pressure, and may improve regional cerebral blood flow (CBF).[32,33] Hypertonic saline produces an osmotic diuretic effect on the brain that is similar to that of other hyperosmolar solutions (e.g., mannitol). However, a randomized controlled trial did not show a significant improvement in neurologic outcome when prehospital resuscitation with hypertonic saline was compared with conventional fluid resuscitation.[34] Hypertonic saline therapy may be more effective than other diuretics in certain clinical conditions, for example, in patients with refractory intracranial hypertension or those who require brain debulking and maintenance of intravascular volume.[35,36] With long-term use of hypertonic sodium, there is concern about the physiologic implications of elevated serum sodium values, such as a depressed level of consciousness and seizures. More studies are required to determine dose-response curves and the safety and efficacy of these solutions.

During fluid resuscitation of the head-injured patient, the goals are to maintain serum osmolality, avoid profound reduction in colloid oncotic pressure, and restore circulating blood volume. Immediate therapy is directed at preventing hypotension and maintaining cerebral perfusion pressure (CPP) above 60 mm Hg.[5] When indicated, an ICP monitor is inserted to guide fluid resuscitation and prevent severe elevations in ICP. The current recommendation is to restore circulating blood volume to normovolemia with glucose-free isotonic crystalloids. Glucose-containing solutions are avoided to enhance perioperative glycemic control. In both animal and human studies, evidence suggests that hyperglycemia at the time of cerebral ischemia worsens outcome.[37,38] Substantial blood loss requires transfusion with crossmatched or fresh whole blood. A minimum hematocrit value between 30% and 33% is recommended to maximize oxygen transport.

Hypertension, tachycardia, and increased cardiac output often develop in patients with isolated head trauma, especially young adults. Electrocardiographic abnormalities and fatal arrhythmias have been reported. The hyperdynamic circulatory responses and electrocardiographic changes may result from a surge in epinephrine that accompanies head injury. Either labetalol or esmolol can be used to control hypertension and tachycardia in this situation.

In some patients, severe intracranial hypertension precipitates reflex arterial hypertension and bradycardia (Cushing's triad). A reduction in systemic blood pressure in these patients can further aggravate cerebral ischemia by reducing CPP. Systemic blood pressure must be lowered cautiously when intracranial hypertension is severe. In such cases, a reduction of ICP may interrupt this reflex response.

During stabilization of head-injured patients, including control of airway and systemic blood pressure, therapeutic interventions to control intracranial hypertension are instituted (Box 18-4). Management of intracranial hypertension

---

BOX 18–4 *Treatment of Intracranial Hypertension in Severe Traumatic Brain Injury (Glasgow Coma Scale Score ≤8)*

1. Insert intracranial pressure monitor
2. Maintain cerebral perfusion pressure between 50 and 70 mm Hg

First-Tier Therapy

- Ventricular drainage (if available)
- Mannitol 0.25-1 g/kg IV (may repeat if serum osmolarity < 320 mOsm/L and patient is euvolemic)
- Hyperventilation to achieve $Paco_2$ value of 30-35 mm Hg

Second Tier-Therapy

- Hyperventilation to $Paco_2$ < 30 mm Hg (Sjo_2, $AVDo_2$ and/or CBF monitoring is recommended)
- High-dose barbiturate therapy
- Consider hypothermia
- Consider hypertensive therapy
- Consider decompressive craniectomy

Adapted from Bullock R, Chesnut R, Clifton G, et al: Guidelines for the management of severe head injury. The Brain Trauma Foundation, American Association of Neurological Surgeons, Joint Section on Neurotrauma and Critical Care. J Neurotrauma 1996;13:641-734; Bullock RM, Chesnut RM, Clifton GL, et al: Guidelines for the management of severe traumatic brain injury. J Neurotrauma 2000;17:449-554; and Guidelines for the management of severe traumatic brain injury, 3rd ed. The Brain Trauma Foundation, American Association of Neurological Surgeons; Congress of Neurological Surgeons. J Neurotrauma 2007;24:S1-S106.

BOX 18–5 *Preanesthesia Assessment of the Head-Injured Patient*

Airway (cervical spine)
Breathing: ventilation and oxygenation
Circulatory status
Associated injuries
Neurologic status (Glasgow Coma Scale)
Preexisting chronic illness
Circumstances of the injury:

- Time of injury
- Duration of unconsciousness
- Associated alcohol or drug use

Data from Bendo AA, Kass IS, Hartung J, Cottrell JE: Anesthesia for neurosurgery. In Barash PG, Cullen BF, Stoelting RK (eds): Clinical Anesthesia, 5th ed. Philadelphia, Lippincott Williams & Wilkins, 2006, pp. 746-789.

---

is crucial because CPP is directly related to both mean arterial pressure and ICP. The following measures are instituted to acutely reduce intracranial hypertension:

1. The head is elevated 15 degrees and kept in a neutral position to facilitate cerebral venous and cerebrospinal fluid drainage.
2. Mannitol, 0.25-1 g/kg, is administered to lower ICP acutely. Alternatively, hypertonic saline may be administered.[39-41]
3. After tracheal intubation, the patient is given a muscle relaxant and mechanically ventilated to a $Paco_2$ value of 35 mm Hg. When there is evidence of transtentorial herniation, hyperventilation to a $Paco_2$ value of 30 mm Hg should be instituted because hyperventilation can rapidly and effectively reduce ICP. Hyperventilation to a $Paco_2$ lower than 30 mm Hg, barbiturate therapy, and cerebrospinal fluid drainage may be considered when other measures have failed.[2,3,5]
4. Appropriate monitoring must be instituted, and hypotension must be avoided.

Mechanical hyperventilation to a $Paco_2$ value of 25 to 30 mm Hg was routinely employed in head-injured patients on the basis of an assumption that hyperventilation, by reducing CBF, would reduce ICP, thereby preserving CPP and CBF. Clinical investigations suggest that head-injured patients are ischemic within the first 24 hours of injury.[42-44] In these patients, hyperventilation may further diminish CBF and aggravate cerebral ischemia.[45] Published guidelines for the management of severe traumatic brain injury no longer recommend hyperventilation to a $Paco_2$ of 25 to 30 mm Hg as a first-tier therapy.[3,5] In fact, current guidelines recommend avoiding the use of prophylactic hyperventilation ($Paco_2$ ≤35 mm Hg) therapy during the first 24 hours after severe TBI.[3,5] When hyperventilation is initiated for control of intracranial hypertension, the $Paco_2$ value should be maintained in the range of 30 to 35 mm Hg in order to accomplish ICP control while minimizing the associated risk of ischemia. Hyperventilation to $Paco_2$ values less than 30 mm Hg should be considered only when second-tier therapy of refractory intracranial hypertension is required. Continuous measurement of jugular bulb oxygen saturation or CBF monitoring is recommended during hyperventilation to guide therapy.[3,5] In emergency situations, hyperventilation should continue in patients in whom the clinical control of intracranial hypertension is the primary concern. However, when the clinical situation no longer requires it or there is evidence of cerebral ischemia, normocapnic ventilation should be instituted.

Mannitol is considered the standard for hyperosmolar therapy and is recommended as a first-tier therapy for treating increased ICP. However, a 2007 Cochrane systematic review found "insufficient reliable evidence to make recommendations on the use of mannitol in the management of patients with traumatic brain injury."[46] After publication of this review, a meta-analysis of 18 studies was conducted to analyze the dose-response relationship between mannitol and ICP.[47] This meta-analysis revealed a significant difference in ICP reduction between patients in whom the initial ICP was higher than 30 mm Hg and those in whom it was lower, but it did not provide specific information regarding the mannitol dose-response curve. There was only a weak linear relationship between the change in ICP and mannitol dose. The investigators attributed this weakness to variation in protocols and patients within and among studies and highlighted the need for definitive well-designed studies to answer this important question.[47]

Anesthetic Management

A management priority for all head-injured patients is the rapid diagnosis with CT of an expanding mass lesion that requires immediate surgical evacuation. Intracranial mass lesions such as acute extradural hematoma, subdural hematoma, intracerebral hematoma, and hemorrhagic contusion are surgically evacuated by craniotomy as soon as possible, but preferably no more than 4 hours after injury. When these patients are brought to the operating room, there is usually minimal time available for preanesthetic assessment. Information that should be obtained preoperatively is described in Box 18-5. Anesthetic management is a continuation of the initial resuscitation, including airway management, fluid and electrolyte balance, and ICP control. The routine monitors used for major neurosurgical procedures are applied.

Major goals of anesthetic management are to improve cerebral perfusion and oxygenation, to avoid secondary damage, and to provide adequate surgical conditions. CPP (which is equal to mean arterial pressure [MAP] minus ICP) should be maintained between 60 and 110 mm Hg, especially prior to surgical opening of the dura. If ICP rises to a greater extent than mean arterial pressure, CPP is reduced, and the brain becomes ischemic. Uncontrolled increases in ICP can result in herniation and death. Therefore, drugs and techniques that raise ICP are avoided in these patients.

The choice of anesthetic agents depends on the condition of the patient. In the hemodynamically stable patient with severe intracranial hypertension, narcotics in conjunction with a thiopental infusion (2 to 3 mg/kg/hr) and a nondepolarizing muscle relaxant can be administered with oxygen and air. In patients with less severe intracranial hypertension, anesthesia can be maintained with various combinations of benzodiazepines, narcotics, and a sub–minimum alveolar concentration (sub-MAC) concentration of a potent inhalation agent. Anesthetic management is directed at avoidance of secondary brain injury. Intraoperative hypotension secondary to blood loss or precipitated by anesthetic drugs must be avoided with appropriate volume expansion. Because the brain's response to injury in the first 24 hours is more often hypoperfusion, aggressive hyperventilation and drugs that can exacerbate cerebral ischemia also should be avoided. Propofol may reduce cerebral blood flow more than cerebral metabolism and thereby can produce ischemia under certain conditions, especially during hyperventilation.[48,49] Throughout intraoperative management, the anesthesiologist enhances cerebral homeostasis by maintaining oxygen delivery (hematocrit 30%-35% and normal cardiac output), serum glucose level (80-150 mg/dL[3] is recommended), and normal electrolyte balance and by implementing temperature management.

Intraoperative brain swelling or herniation from the operative site may complicate hematoma decompression. Such causes as improper patient positioning, contralateral intracerebral hematoma, venous drainage obstruction from packing, and acute hydrocephalus from intraventricular hemorrhage must be eliminated. In this setting, the adequacy of hyperventilation must also be verified. A large alveolar-arterial CO_2 gradient may exist, so that end-tidal CO_2 may not reflect arterial CO_2. The respiratory system and equipment should be reviewed to ensure normal peak inspiratory and expiratory pressures. Hemopneumothorax, high intra-abdominal pressures, a kinked endotracheal or expiratory tube, or a stuck expiratory valve can produce marked peak inspiratory or expiratory pressures as well as hypoxemia and hypercarbia. Fluid and electrolyte balance must be reevaluated in patients with cerebral swelling. Mannitol loses its effect after 1 to 3 hours, so a second mannitol bolus to increase osmolarity may be necessary. Volume overload and hyponatremia may also cause cerebral swelling and must be corrected. If cerebral swelling persists, the anesthetic should be converted to opioid and thiopental infusions with oxygen and air. Thiopental may be given in a series of boluses over 5 to 10 minutes to a total dose of 5-25 mg/kg, followed by an infusion of 4 to 10 mg/kg/hr. To avoid barbiturate-induced myocardial depression and hypotension, it may be necessary to increase preload and add a vasopressor or inotrope such as phenylephrine or dopamine. Malignant brain swelling may require removal of brain tissue and temporary scalp closure with a loose dural patch to minimize ICP after closure.

Emergence of a patient with TBI from anesthesia usually involves transporting an intubated, ventilated, and anesthetized patient to the critical care unit. Even in an uncomplicated craniotomy for evacuation of hematoma, a period of postoperative ventilation is recommended because brain swelling is maximal 12 to 72 hours after injury. Hypertension and coughing or bucking of the patient on the endotracheal tube should be avoided because either can lead to significant intracranial bleeding. Labetalol or esmolol can be used to treat hypertension, and supplemental barbiturates are given to sedate the patient.

Cerebral Protection

Reducing the cerebral metabolic rate for oxygen (CMR_{O_2}) is the mainstay of pharmacologic brain protection, and barbiturate administration is the only such intervention that has proved useful in humans. However, level II evidence does not support the use of prophylactic barbiturate administration to achieve electroencephalographic burst suppression. High-dose barbiturate administration is recommended to control elevated ICP refractory to maximum medical and surgical treatment but should be administered only in hemodynamically stable patients.

When ischemia reduces supply, hypothermia remains the *sine qua non* for reducing oxygen demand. A reduction of body temperature to 33° to 35° C may confer cerebral protection. Although results of clinical trials of moderate hypothermia after head injury have been encouraging, none has shown statistically significant improvement in outcome.[50] The multi-institutional study of postoperative mild hypothermia in patients with head injury was terminated by its safety monitoring board after 392 patients were enrolled.[51] The results showed no difference in mortality between hypothermic and normothermic treatments, and hypothermic patients experienced more medical complications. Subgroup analysis revealed that younger patients (≤45 years) who were hypothermic on admission and assigned to the hypothermic group tended to have better outcomes than those assigned to the normothermic group. A new study looking at this group with an earlier induction of hypothermia and more consistent critical care was initiated; however, patient enrollment was recently stopped.[52]

It remains unclear whether there is a therapeutic window of opportunity for inducing protective post injury hypothermia. When induction of hypothermia is elected, meticulous care is necessary to avoid adverse side effects such as hypotension, cardiac arrhythmias, coagulopathies, and infections. Rewarming should be carried out slowly.[53] In this population, there is no doubt that hyperthermia is strongly associated with poor outcome.[53]

Decompressive Craniectomy

Decompressive craniectomy is an advanced treatment option for ICP control in patients with diffuse brain swelling refractory to maximal medical management. It decreases ICP by reducing volume constraints on the cranial contents. A wide bilateral frontotemporal craniectomy, duratomy, and duraplasty may be performed. Although decompressive craniectomy decreases ICP, it may not improve neurologic outcome. Therefore, its use is controversial. There are two ongoing randomized, controlled clinical trials—the Randomised Evaluation of Surgery with Craniectomy for Uncontrollable Elevation of Intra-Cranial Pressure (RESCUEicp study) in Europe and The DECRA Trial: Early Decompressive Craniectomy in Patients With Severe Traumatic Brain Injury in Australia—to determine whether decompressive craniectomy is more effective in improving outcome than maximal medical therapy in adults.[54]

Systemic Sequelae

The systemic effects of head injury are diverse and can complicate management. They include cardiopulmonary problems (airway obstruction, hypoxemia, shock, acute respiratory distress syndrome, neurogenic pulmonary edema, electrocardiographic changes), hematologic problems (disseminated intravascular coagulation), endocrine problems (pituitary dysfunction, e.g., diabetes insipidus, syndrome of inappropriate antidiuretic hormone secretion), metabolic problems (nonketotic hyperosmolar hyperglycemic coma), and gastrointestinal problems (stress ulcers, hemorrhage).

Aspiration pneumonia, fluid overload, and trauma-related acute respiratory distress syndrome are common causes of pulmonary dysfunction in head-injured patients. A fulminant pulmonary edema may also occur. Neurogenic pulmonary edema is characterized by marked pulmonary vascular congestion, intra-alveolar hemorrhage, and a protein-rich edema fluid. Specific features of this syndrome are its rapid onset, its relationship to hypothalamic lesions, and the ability to prevent or attenuate it by α-blockers and central nervous system depressants. Neurogenic pulmonary edema is thought to result from massive sympathetic discharge from injured brain secondary to intracranial hypertension. Traditional therapy for pulmonary edema of cardiac origin is ineffective, and the outcome is often fatal. Therapy consists of immediate pharmacologic or surgical relief of intracranial hypertension, supportive respiratory care, and careful fluid management.

In head-injured patients, several clotting abnormalities may be present. Disseminated intravascular coagulation has been reported after mild and severe brain trauma and anoxic brain damage, and it presumably develops after release of brain tissue thromboplastin into the systemic circulation. Treatment of the underlying disease process usually results in spontaneous recovery of the coagulation defects. Occasionally, administration of cryoprecipitate, fresh frozen plasma, platelet concentrates, and blood may be required.

Anterior pituitary insufficiency after head injury is a rare occurrence. However, patients exhibiting post-traumatic diabetes insipidus may have a delayed impairment of anterior pituitary hormones, requiring replacement therapy. Posterior pituitary dysfunction occurs more frequently after head trauma. Diabetes insipidus may occur after craniofacial trauma and basal skull fracture. Its clinical presentation involves polyuria, polydipsia, hypernatremia, high serum osmolality, and dilute urine. Commonly, post-traumatic diabetes insipidus is transient, and treatment is based on water replacement. If the patient cannot maintain fluid balance, exogenous vasopressin may be administered. The syndrome of inappropriate antidiuretic hormone secretion is associated with hyponatremia, serum and extracellular fluid hypo-osmolality, renal excretion of sodium, urine osmolality greater than serum osmolality, and normal renal and adrenal function. The patient has symptoms and signs of water intoxication (anorexia, nausea, vomiting, irritability, personality changes, and neurologic abnormalities). This syndrome usually begins 3 to 15 days after trauma, lasting no more than 10 to 15 days with appropriate therapy. Treatment includes water restriction with or without hypertonic saline.

Many factors in neurosurgical patients predispose to nonketotic hyperosmolar hyperglycemic coma, such as steroids, prolonged mannitol therapy, hyperosmolar tube feedings, phenytoin, and limited water replacement. Diagnostic criteria for nonketotic hyperosmolar hyperglycemic coma are hyperglycemia, glucosuria, absence of ketosis, plasma osmolality greater than 330 mOsm/kg, dehydration, and central nervous system dysfunction. Hypovolemia and hypertonicity are the immediate threats to life. Serum sodium levels may be high, normal, or low, depending on the state of hydration. The serum potassium level is low. Serial laboratory tests are essential. Once sodium deficits are replaced and blood pressure and urine output are stable, water deficits are replaced with 0.45% saline. Hyperglycemia usually responds to relatively small doses of insulin. Intermittent furosemide therapy may be given for prophylaxis of cerebral edema in a patient who is elderly, has type 2 diabetes, or has compromised renal function.

CRITICAL CARE

In the critical care unit, the main objectives are to improve recovery from primary brain injury by preventing secondary injury and maintaining cerebral homeostasis. This requires provision of optimal systemic support for cerebral energy metabolism and adequate CPP, and normalizing of ICP for the injured brain. Prompt recognition and treatment of systemic complications that contribute to secondary injury are essential to management of the head-injured patient.[55] To achieve them, multimodality systemic and cerebral monitoring should be instituted. Monitoring of ICP, CPP, and CBF (or transcranial Doppler ultrasonography or laser Doppler flowmetry) should be standard practice. Monitors of cerebral oxygenation, such as jugular bulb oximetry and brain tissue Po_2, and brain metabolism can provide more specific information for managing cerebral hypoxia and ischemia.[56] There is controversy concerning the best management protocol for improving outcome in patients with TBI.[5,56] A management protocol that uses individualized assessment and a multi-targeted approach to provide therapy and reduce the risk of iatrogenic injuries is gaining acceptance.

SUMMARY

Guidelines for the management of patients with severe traumatic brain injury were published by the Brain Trauma Foundation in 1996.[2] Revisions to the guidelines were published in 2000 in a document that discusses various management protocols and treatments in light of supporting evidence.[3] Management updates are being published on the Worldwide Web as new information is made available and the guidelines are revised.[5] Publication of these recommendations, guidelines, and standards by the Brain Trauma Foundation reflects an ongoing effort to improve outcome in this high-risk population through evidence-based management and standardized care.

However, several management recommendations are based only on level II or III evidence, and not all recommendations, when implemented, have improved outcome. Therefore, to address these unresolved clinical concerns, large multicenter randomized trials are under way or being planned. There is no doubt that the growing awareness of perioperative risk and prevention of secondary injury in this population from the time of injury through critical care has the potential to improve outcome. The challenge is to reduce both mortality and disability in this vulnerable patient population.

REFERENCES

1. The Brain Trauma Foundation. Facts about TBI in the USA. 2007. Available at http://www.braintrauma.org/site/TBI_Facts.
2. Bullock R, Chesnut R, Clifton G, et al: Guidelines for the management of severe traumatic brain injury. The Brain Trauma Foundation, American Association of Neurological Surgeons, Joint Section on Neurotrauma and Critical Care, *J Neurotrauma* 13:641–734, 1996.
3. Bullock RM, Chesnut RM, Clifton GL, et al: Guidelines for the management of severe traumatic brain injury, *J Neurotrauma* 17:449–554, 2000.
4. Robertson CS: Management of cerebral perfusion pressure after traumatic brain injury, *Anesthesiology* 95:1513–1517, 2001.
5. Guidelines for the management of severe traumatic brain injury, 3rd ed. The Brain Trauma Foundation, American Association of Neurological Surgeons; Congress of Neurological Surgeons, *J Neurotrauma* 24: S1–S106, 2007.
6. Edwards P, Arango M, Balica L, et al: Crash Trial Collaborators: Final results of MRC CRASH, a randomized placebo controlled trial of intravenous corticosteroid in adults with head injury—outcomes at 6 months, *Lancet* 365:1957–1959, 2005.
7. Gabriel EJ, Ghajar J, Jagoda A, et al: Brain Trauma Foundation: Guidelines for prehospital management of traumatic brain injury, *J Neurotrauma* 19:111–174, 2002.
8. Badjatia N, Carney N, Crocco TJ, et al: Brain Trauma Foundation; BTF Center for Guidelines Management: Guidelines for prehospital management of traumatic brain injury, ed 2, Prehospital Emerg Care 12: S1–S52, 2008.
9. Adelson PD, Bratton SL, Carney NA, et al; American Association for Surgery of Trauma; Child Neurology Society; International Society for Pediatric Neurosurgery; International Trauma Anesthesia and Critical Care Society; Society of Critical Care Medicine; World Federation of Pediatric Intensive and Critical Care Societies: Guidelines for the acute medical management of severe traumatic brain injury in infants, children, and adolescents. *Pediatr Crit Care Med* 4(Supp):S1–S75, 2003.
10. Bullock MR, Chesnut R, Ghajar J, et al: The Brain Trauma Foundation and the Congress of Neurological Surgeons: Guidelines for the surgical management of traumatic brain injury, *Neurosurgery Supplement* 58:S2-1,S2-62, 2006.
11. Teasdale G, Jennett B: Assessment of coma and impaired consciousness: A practical scale, *Lancet* 2(7872):81, 1974.
12. Jennett B: Assessment of the severity of head injury, *J Neurol Neurosurg Psychiatry* 39:647, 1976.
13. Jennett B, Bond MR: Assessment of outcome after severe brain damage, *Lancet* 1(7905):480, 1975.
14. Chesnut RM, Marshall LF, Klauber MR, et al: The role of secondary brain injury in determining outcome from severe head injury, *J Trauma* 34:216–222, 1993.
15. Moppett IK: Traumatic brain injury: Assessment, resuscitation and early management, *Br J Anaesth* 99:18–31, 2007.
16. Gopinath SP, Robertson CS: Management of Severe Head Injury. In Cottrell JE, Smith DS, editors: *Anesthesia and Neurosurgery*, ed 4, St. Louis, MO, 2001, Mosby, pp 663–691.
17. Härtl R, Gerber LM, Iacono L, et al: Direct transport within an organized state trauma system reduces mortality in patients with severe traumatic brain injury, *J Trauma* 60:1250–1256, 2006.
18. Bernard SA: Paramedic intubation of patients with severe head injury: A review of current Australian practice and recommendations for change, *Emerg Med Australas* 18:221–228, 2006.
19. Davis DP, Fakhry SM, Wang HE, et al: Paramedic rapid sequence intubation for severe traumatic brain injury: Perspectives from an expert panel, *Prehosp Emerg Care* 11:1–8, 2007.
20. Stiell IG, Wells GA, Vandemheen K, et al: The Canadian CT head rule for patients with minor head injury, *Lancet* 357:1391–1396, 2001.
21. Haydel MJ, Preton CA, Mills TJ, et al: Indications for computed tomography in patients with minor head injury, *N Engl J Med* 343:100–105, 2000.
22. Hastings RH: Marks JD:. Airway management for trauma patients with potential cervical spine injuries, *Anesth Analg* 73:471–482, 1991.
23. Crosby ET: Airway management in adults after cervical spine trauma, *Anesthesiology* 104:1293–1318, 2006.
24. Hoffman JR, Mower WR, Wolfson AB, et al: Validity of a set of clinical criteria to rule out injury to the cervical spine in patients with blunt trauma, *N Engl J Med* 343:94, 2000.
25. Lennarson PJ, Smith D, Todd MM, et al: Segmental cervical spinal motion during orotracheal intubation of the intact and injured spine with and without external stabilization, *J Neurosurg* 92(Spine 2):201–206, 2000.
26. Bendo AA, Kass IS, Hartung J, Cottrell JE: Anesthesia for neurosurgery. In Barash PG, Cullen BF, Stoelting RK, editors: *Clinical Anesthesia*, ed 5, Philadelphia, 2006, Lippincott Williams & Wilkins, pp 746–789.
27. Zornow MH, Todd MM, Moore SS: The acute cerebral effects of changes in plasma osmolality and oncotic pressure, *Anesthesiology* 67:936, 1987.
28. Kaieda R, Todd MM, Cook LN, et al: Acute effects of changing plasma osmolality and colloid oncotic pressure on the formation of brain edema after cryogenic injury, *Neurosurgery* 24:671, 1989.
29. Kaieda R, Todd MM, Warner DS: Prolonged reduction in colloid oncotic pressure does not increase brain edema following cryogenic injury in rabbits, *Anesthesiology* 72:554, 1989.
30. Drummond JC, Patel PM, Cole DJ, et al: The effect of the reduction of colloid oncotic pressure, with and without reduction of osmolality, on post-traumatic cerebral edema, *Anesthesiology* 88:993, 1998.
31. SAFE Study Investigators; Australian and New Zealand Intensive Care Society Clinical Trials Group; Australian Red Cross Blood Service; George Institute for International Health; Myburgh J, Cooper DJ, Finfer S, et al: Saline or albumin for fluid resuscitation in patients with hypotension and severe traumatic brain injury, *N Engl J Med*; 357: 874–884, 2007.
32. Vassar MJ, Fischer RP, O'Brien RE, et al: A multicenter trial for resuscitation of injured patients with 7.5% sodium chloride, *Arch Surg* 128:1003, 1993.
33. Prough DS, Whitley JM, Taylor CL, et al: Regional cerebral blood flow following resuscitation from hemorrhagic shock with hypertonic saline, *Anesthesiology* 75:319, 1991.
34. Cooper DJ, Myles PS, McDermott FT, et al: Prehospital hypertonic saline resuscitation of patients with hypotension and severe traumatic brain injury, *JAMA* 291:1350–1357, 2004.
35. Qureshi AI, Suarez JI: Use of hypertonic saline solutions in treatment of cerebral edema and intracranial hypertension, *Crit Care Med* 28:3301, 2000.
36. Vialet R, Albanese J, Thomachot L, et al: Isovolume hypertonic solutes (sodium chloride or mannitol) in the treatment of refractory posttraumatic intracranial hypertension: 2 ml/kg 7% saline is more effective than 2 ml/kg 20% mannitol, *Crit Care Med* 31:1683, 2003.
37. Wass CT, Lanier WL: Glucose modulation of ischemic brain injury: Review and clinical recommendations, *Mayo Clin Proc* 71:801–812, 1996.
38. Bilotta F, Giovannini F, Caramia R, Rosa G: Glycemia management in neurocritical care patients: A review, *J Neurosurg Anesthesiol* 20:2–9, 2009.
39. White H, Cook D, Venkatesh B: The use of hypertonic saline for treating intracranial hypertension after traumatic brain injury, *Anesth Analg* 102:1836, 2006.
40. Rozet I, Tontisirin N, Muangman S, et al: Effect of equiosmolar solutions of mannitol versus hypertonic saline on intraoperative brain relaxation and electrolyte balance, *Anesthesiology* 107:697, 2007.
41. McDonough DL, Warner DS: Hypertonic saline for craniotomy? *Anesthesiology* 107:689, 2007.
42. Orbits WD, Linguist TW, Jaggy JL, et al: Cerebral blood flow and metabolism in comatose patients with acute head injury: Relationship to intracranial hypertension, *J Neurosurg* 61:241, 1984.
43. Mislead JP, Marabou A, Ward JD, et al: Adverse effects of prolonged hyperventilation in patients with severe head injury: A randomized clinical trial, *J Neurosurg* 75:731, 1991.
44. Martin NA, Patwardhan RV, Alexander MJ, et al: Characterization of cerebral hemodynamic phases following severe head trauma: Hypoperfusion, hyperemia, and vasospasm, *J Neurosurg* 87:9, 1997.
45. Stringer WA, Hasso AN, Thompson JR, et al: Hyperventilation-induced cerebral ischemia in patients with acute brain lesions: Demonstration by xenon-enhanced CT, *AJNR Am J Neuroradiol* 14:475, 1993.
46. Wakai A, Roberts I, Schierhout G: Mannitol for acute traumatic brain injury, *Cochrane Database Syst Rev* (1):CD001049, 2007.
47. Sorani MD, Manley GT: Dose-response relationship of mannitol and intracranial pressure: A meta-analysis, *J Neurosurg* 108:80–87, 2008.

48. Cenic A, Craen RA, Lee TY, Gelb AW: Cerebral blood volume and blood flow responses to hyperventilation in brain tumors during isoflurane or propofol anesthesia, *Anesth Analg* 94:661–666, 2002.

49. Adembri C, Venturi L, Pellegrini-Giampietro DE: Neuroprotective effects of propofol in acute cerebral injury, *CNS Drug Rev* 13:333–351, 2007.

50. Peterson K, Carson S, Carney N: Hypothermia treatment for traumatic brain injury: A systematic review and meta-analysis, *J Neurotrauma* 25:62, 2008.

51. Clifton GL, Miller ER, Choi SC, et al: Lack of effect of induction of hypothermia after acute brain injury, *N Engl J Med* 344:556, 2001.

52. Clifton GL, Drever P, Valadka A, et al: Multicenter trial of early hypothermia in severe brain injury, *J Neurotrauma* 26(3):393-397, 2009.

53. Polderman KH: Induced hypothermia and fever control for prevention and treatment of neurologic injuries, *Lancet* 371:1955, 2008.

54. Toussaint CP, Origitano TC: Decompressive craniectomy review of indication, outcome, and implication, *Neurosurg Quart* 18:45, 2008.

55. Mazzeo AT, Kunene NK, Choi S, et al: Quantification of ischemic events after severe traumatic brain injury in humans: A simple scoring system, *J Neurosurg Anesthesiol* 18:170, 2006.

56. Huang S-J, Hong W-C, Han Y-Y, et al: Clinical outcome of severe head injury in different protocol-driven therapies, *J Clin Neurosci* 14:449, 2007.

Chapter 19

PEDIATRIC NEUROANESTHESIA AND CRITICAL CARE

Sulpicio G. Soriano • Michael L. McManus

Technical advances in neurosurgery have dramatically improved the outcome in pediatric patients with surgical lesions of the central nervous system. Most of these developments are modifications of techniques used in adults. The perioperative management should be based on developmental stage of the neurosurgical patient throughout the preoperative, intraoperative, and postoperative periods. The aim of this chapter is to highlight these age-dependent differences and their effects on the management of the pediatric neurosurgical patient.

DEVELOPMENTAL CONSIDERATIONS

Age-dependent differences in cerebrovascular physiology and cranial bone development distinguish the infants and children from adults. Cerebral blood flow is coupled tightly to metabolic demand, and both increase proportionally immediately after birth. Wintermark and colleagues[1] determined the effect of age on cerebral blood flow (CBF).[1] Using computed tomography perfusion techniques, they reported that CBF peaked between 2 and 4 years and settled at 7 to 8 years (Fig. 19-1). These changes mirror changes in neuroanatomical development. The autoregulatory range of blood pressure in a normal newborn is between 20 and 60 mm Hg,[2] which reflects the relatively low cerebral metabolic requirements and blood pressure during the perinatal period. More importantly, the slope of the autoregulatory curve drops and rises significantly at the lower and upper limits of the curve, respectively (Fig. 19-2). Neonates are especially vulnerable to cerebral ischemia and intraventricular hemorrhage owing to this narrow autoregulatory range.

Full-term healthy neonates have the ability to autoregulate their cerebral circulation, but premature neonates do not.[3] Tsuji and associates[3] demonstrated that in sick premature neonates, there is a linear correlation between CBF and systemic blood pressure. This pattern of cerebral blood flow pressure-passivity occurs in premature neonates with low gestational age and birth weight and systemic hypotension. Therefore, tight blood pressure control is essential in the management of neonates to minimize both cerebral ischemia and intraventricular hemorrhage. Vavilala and coworkers[4] demonstrated that the lower limit of cerebral autoregulation was equivalent among older and younger children. They also observed that children younger than 2 years have lower autoregulatory reserve because of their relatively low baseline mean arterial pressures and may be at greater risk of cerebral ischemia.

Adults and infants differ in the percentage of cardiac output directed to the brain. CBF is 10% to 20% of the cardiac output during the first 6 months and peaks at 55% between the second and fourth years.[1] Cerebral blood flow settles to the adult levels of 15% by 7 to 8 years. The head of the infant and child also accounts for a large percentage of the body surface area and blood volume (Fig. 19-3). This feature places the young child at risk for significant hemodynamic instability during neurosurgical procedures.

The infant cranial vault is also in a state of flux. Open fontanelles and cranial sutures lead to a compliant intracranial space (Fig. 19-4). The mass effect of a slow-growing tumor or insidious hemorrhage is often masked in an infant by a compensatory increase in intracranial volume due to widening of the fontanelles and cranial sutures. However, as in adults, acute increases in cranial volume due to massive hemorrhage or an obstructed ventricular system cannot be attenuated by expansion of the immature cranial vault and often result in life-threatening intracranial hypertension.[5]

Neonates and infants have functionally immature organ systems. The neonatal renal system is characterized by a decreased glomerular filtration rate and concentrating ability. These changes result in diminished excretion of saline and water and limit the neonate's ability to compensate for fluctuations in fluid and solute loads. Drugs that are renally excreted may have a prolonged half-life. Hepatic function is also diminished in neonates, and metabolism of drugs may be delayed owing to decreased activity of hepatic enzymes. Total body water drops from 85% in premature infants to 65% in adults, whereas body fat content increases from less than 1% in premature infants to 15% in term infants and 35% in adults. The total protein level follows a similar trend. Therefore, hydrophilic drugs have more binding sites, and hydrophobic drugs fewer, in infants. The constellation of these factors should prompt the clinician generally to decrease the weight-adjusted dose and frequency of administration of drugs given to the newborn.

PREOPERATIVE EVALUATION AND PREPARATION

Given the systemic effects of general anesthesia and the physiologic stress of surgery, an organ system review is essential for identifying coexisting disease, and anticipating potential physiologic derangements increase the risk of perioperative complications.[6] General perioperative concerns in infants and children are listed in Table 19-1. Preoperative laboratory tests should be tailored to the proposed neurosurgical procedure. Given the risk of significant blood loss associated with surgery, the hematocrit, prothrombin time, and partial thromboplastin time should be measured to uncover any insidious hematologic disorder. Patients with suprasellar pathology should

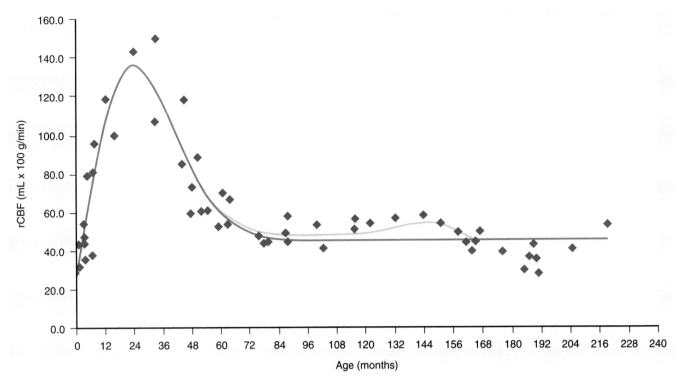

Figure 19–1 Age-related evolution of global average regional cerebral blood flow (rCBF) values. *(From Wintermark M, Lepori D, Cotting J, et al: Brain perfusion in children: evolution with age assessed by quantitative perfusion computed tomography. Pediatrics 2004;113:1642-1652.)*

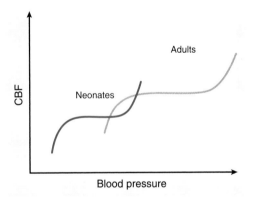

Figure 19–2 Autoregulation of cerebral blood flow (CBF) in children. The slope of the autoregulatory curve drops and rises significantly at the lower and upper limits of the curve, respectively, and is shifted to the left in the neonate and small child.

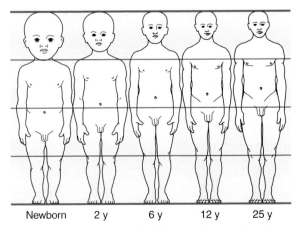

Figure 19–3 The head size and surface area is proportionately greater in infants than in adults. y, years.

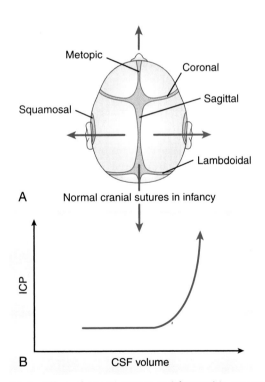

Figure 19–4 Effect of cranial sutures and fontanel in neonates and infants. A. The open fontanelles and cranial sutures permit slow expansion of the intracranial volume. B. Initially the compliant skull of the neonate minimizes insidious increases in intracranial volume. B, However, acute increases in intracranial volume (hemorrhage and obstructed ventriculoperitoneal shunt) lead to rapid rises in intracranial pressure (ICP). CSF, cerebrospinal fluid.

undergo an endocrinologic evaluation.[7] Typed and cross-matched blood should be ordered prior to all craniotomies. Table 19-2 matches special concerns in pediatric patients with neurologic problems. Endocrinologists may be needed to help optimize the patient's condition before surgery and to assist in postoperative management.

Closed-claim analysis studies have revealed that, for all forms of operative management, neonates and infants are at higher risk for morbidity and mortality than other age groups.[8,9] Respiratory and cardiac-related events account for a majority of these complications. Given the urgent nature of many pediatric neurosurgical procedures, a thorough preoperative evaluation may be difficult. A complete airway examination is essential, because some craniofacial anomalies may require specialized techniques to secure the airway.[10] Congenital heart disease may not be apparent immediately after birth and may complicate the perioperative course of the neonate undergoing an emergency neurosurgical procedure. Therefore, echocardiography can be helpful in the assessment of the heart, especially in the neonate, and a pediatric cardiologist should evaluate a patient with suspected cardiac problems in order to optimize cardiac function prior to surgery.

Perioperative anxiety plays a significant role in the care of the pediatric neurosurgical patient. These issues are related to the cognitive development and age of the child (Table 19-3). Preoperative sedatives given prior to the induction of anesthesia can ease the transition from the preoperative holding area to the operating room.[11] Midazolam administered orally is particularly effective in relieving anxiety and producing amnesia. If an indwelling intravenous catheter is in place, midazolam can be slowly titrated to achieve sedation.

Preoperative fasting regimens have dramatically evolved over the years and vary according to local preferences.[12] The purpose of limiting oral intake is to minimize the risk of pulmonary aspiration of gastric contents. However, prolonged fasting periods can potentially result in both hypovolemia and hypoglycemia, which in turn can lead to hemodynamic and metabolic instability during anesthesia. Although the scientific validity of many recommendations has not been investigated, a common guideline is given in Table 19-4.

INTRAOPERATIVE MANAGEMENT

Induction of Anesthesia

The patient's preoperative status dictates the appropriate technique and drugs for induction of anesthesia. General anesthesia can be induced with sevoflurane and nitrous oxide with oxygen. A nondepolarizing muscle relaxant is then administered after intravenous (IV) access has been established to facilitate intubation of the trachea. Pancuronium is an ideal muscle relaxant for neonates and infants because it produces tachycardia, which counters the parasympathetic effect of laryngoscopy. If the patient already has an IV catheter, anesthesia can be induced with a sedative-hypnotic drug such as thiopental (5-8 mg/kg) or propofol (3-4 mg/kg). Patients who are vomiting or have recently ingested food or fluids are at risk for aspiration pneumonitis and so should undergo

Table 19–1 General Perioperative Concerns in Infants and Children

Condition	Anesthetic Implications
Congenital heart disease	Hypoxia, arrhythmias, and cardiovascular instability; paradoxical air emboli
Prematurity	Postoperative apnea
Gastrointestinal reflux	Aspiration pneumonia
Upper respiratory tract infection	Laryngospasm, bronchospasm, hypoxia, pneumonia
Craniofacial abnormality	Difficulty with airway management

Table 19–2 Common Perioperative Concerns for Infants and Children with Neurologic Problems

Condition	Anesthetic Implications
Denervation injuries	Hyperkalemia after succinylcholine, Resistance to nondepolarizing muscle relaxants, abnormal response to nerve stimulation
Long-term anticonvulsant therapy	Hepatic and hematologic abnormalities Increased metabolism of anesthetic agents
Arteriovenous malformation	Potential congestive heart failure
Neuromuscular disease	Malignant hyperthermia Respiratory failure Sudden cardiac death
Chiari malformation	Apnea Aspiration pneumonia
Hypothalamic or pituitary lesions	Diabetes insipidus Hypothyroidism Adrenal insufficiency

Table 19–3 Developmental Factors Affecting the Pediatric Patient in the Perioperative Period

Age Group	Concerns
Infants (0-9 months)	None; will separate easily from parents
Preschoolers (9 months–5 years)	Stranger anxiety; difficulty with separation from parents
Grade schoolers (6-12 years)	Fear of needles/pain
Adolescence (>12 years)	Anxiety about surgery and self-image

Table 19–4 Common Fasting Guidelines For Pediatric Patients

Fasting Time (Hours)	Substance to be Withheld
2	Clear liquids
4	Breast milk
6	Formula
8	Solid food

rapid-sequence induction of anesthesia with thiopental or propofol, followed immediately with a rapid-acting muscle relaxant and cricoid pressure. Rocuronium can be used when succinylcholine is contraindicated, such as for patients with spinal cord injuries or paretic extremities; in these instances, succinylcholine can result in sudden, catastrophic hyperkalemia. Etomidate and ketamine are often used to induce anesthesia in hemodynamically compromised patients, because these drugs are less likely to cause hypotension than thiopental or propofol. However, central nervous system excitation and increased intracranial pressure (ICP), respectively, have been associated with these drugs, which may not be appropriate for many neurosurgical patients.

Airway Management

Developmental changes in airway anatomy have a significant effect on management of the pediatric airway. The infant's larynx is funnel-shaped, being narrowest at the level of the cricoid ring. This feature puts the infant at risk for subglottic obstruction secondary to mucosal swelling after prolonged endotracheal intubation with a tight-fitting endotracheal tube. Cuffed endotracheal tubes can be used, but the cuff pressure should be checked frequently and adjusted to minimize tracheal injury. Because the trachea is relatively short, an endotracheal tube can easily migrate into a mainstem bronchus if the infant's head is flexed, as it will be for a suboccipital approach to the posterior fossa or the cervical spine (Fig. 19-5). Therefore, great care should be devoted to ensuring proper position of the endotracheal tube during tracheal intubation, and the anesthesiologist should auscultate both lung fields to rule out inadvertent intubation of a mainstem bronchus after final positioning of the patient. Nasotracheal tubes are best suited for situations when the patient will be prone, because they are easier to secure in these situations, and when postoperative mechanical ventilation is anticipated.[13] Furthermore, orotracheal tubes can kink at the base of the tongue when the head is flexed, resulting in airway obstruction and direct pressure injury to the tongue.

Timing of tracheal extubation sometimes presents a challenge after neurosurgical procedures. Infants, particularly those with the Chiari malformation,[14] and older children after procedures in the posterior fossa[15] may exhibit intermittent apnea, vocal cord paralysis, or other irregularities before resuming a stable respiratory pattern. Significant airway edema and postoperative obstruction can complicate prone procedures or operations involving significant blood loss and large volume replacement. Finally, preexisting pulmonary dysfunction, as in infants with bronchopulmonary dysplasia or older children with neuromuscular disease, may force delays in extubation because of respiratory insufficiency. In these cases, standard tracheal extubation criteria and the presence of an endotracheal tube air leak of less than 20 cm H_2O can assist the clinician in appropriate decision-making.[16,17] When lingual or supraglottic swelling suggests obstruction, direct laryngoscopy can be reassuring. When swelling is significant, head-up positioning and gentle forced diuresis usually requires postoperative ventilation in the intensive care unit and improves conditions within 24 hours.

Positioning

The diminutive size of the neonate or infant requires careful preoperative planning to allow adequate access to the patient for both the neurosurgeon and anesthesiologist (Table 19-5). The prone position is commonly used for posterior fossa and spinal cord surgery. Although the sitting position has been used less often in pediatric patients, it may be appropriate for obese patients, who may be difficult to ventilate in the prone position. In addition to the physiologic sequelae of the prone position, a whole spectrum of compression and stretch injuries has been reported. Padding under the chest and pelvis can support the torso. It is important to ensure free abdominal wall motion because greater intra-abdominal pressure can impair ventilation, cause compression of the vena cava, and increase epidural venous pressure and bleeding. Soft rolls are generally used to elevate and support the lateral chest wall and hips to minimize the increases in abdominal and thoracic pressure. In addition, this elevation permits a Doppler probe to be on the chest without pressure.

Many neurosurgical procedures are performed with the head slightly elevated to facilitate venous and cerebrospinal fluid drainage from the surgical site. However, superior sagittal sinus pressure decreases with increasing head elevation and increases the likelihood of venous air embolism (VAE).[18]

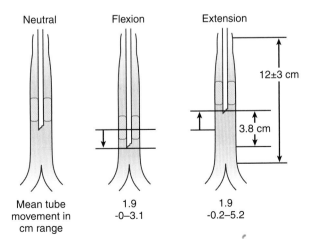

Figure 19-5 Effect of head flexion and extension on endotracheal tube position. Note that flexion of the neck causes the endotracheal to migate towards a mainstem bronchus. While neck extension can lead to dislodgement of the endotracheal from the trachea.

Neutral	Flexion	Extension
		12±3 cm
		3.8 cm
Mean tube movement in cm range	1.9 -0–3.1	1.9 -0.2–5.2

Table 19–5	**Physiologic Effects of Positioning in All Patients**
Position	**Physiologic Effect**
Head elevated	Enhanced cerebral venous drainage
	Decreased cerebral perfusion pressure (potential cerebral blood flow decrease)
	Increased venous pooling in lower extremities
	Postural hypotension
Head down	Increased cerebral venous and intracranial pressure
	Decreased functional residual capacity (lung function)
	Decreased lung compliance
Prone	Venous congestion of face, tongue, and neck
	Decreased lung compliance
	Increased abdominal pressure can lead to compression of the vena cava
Lateral decubitus	Decreased compliance of down-side lung

Extreme head flexion can cause brainstem compression in patients with posterior fossa pathology, such as a mass lesion or Arnold-Chiari malformation. However, significant rotation of the head can impede venous return through the jugular veins, leading to impairment of cerebral perfusion and increases in ICP and venous bleeding.

Vascular Access

Owing to limited access to the patient during neurosurgical procedures, optimal intravenous access is mandatory prior to the start of surgery. Typically two large-bore venous cannulas are sufficient for most craniotomies. Should initial attempts fail, central venous cannulation may be necessary. Use of the femoral vein avoids the risk of pneumothorax associated with subclavian catheters and does not interfere with cerebral venous return, as use of jugular vein catheters might. Furthermore, femoral catheters are more easily accessible to the anesthesiologist during operations on the head. Because significant blood loss and hemodynamic instability can occur during craniotomies, cannulation of the radial artery would provide direct blood pressure monitoring and sampling for blood gas analysis. Other useful arterial sites in infants and children are the dorsalis pedis artery and posterior tibial artery.

Maintenance of Anesthesia

Potent, volatile anesthetic agents are administered by inhalation. Sevoflurane has virtually replaced halothane as the principal anesthetic for induction of anesthesia in infants and children.[19] Changing the inspired concentration of the drug can rapidly alter anesthetic depth. Intravenous anesthetics are categorized as sedative-hypnotic or opioid. These drugs are also potent cerebral metabolic depressants but do not cause cerebrovasodilation. Therefore, they are closer to "ideal" anesthetics. Fentanyl is the opioid most commonly used in this setting. The half-lives of fentanyl and other related synthetic opioids, including sufentanil, increase with repeated dosing or prolonged infusions and require hepatic metabolism, which is immature in neonates. As a result, the narcotic effects, such as respiratory depression and sedation, of these drugs may be prolonged. Remifentanil is a unique opioid that is rapidly cleared by plasma esterases. This makes it, when administered at a rate of 0.2 to 1.0 µg/kg/min, an ideal opioid for rapid emergence from anesthesia.[20,21] However, this rapid recovery is often accompanied by delirium and inadequate analgesia.[22,23]

Nevertheless, the choice of anesthetic agents for maintenance of anesthesia has been shown not to affect the outcome of neurosurgical procedures when properly administered.[24] The most commonly used technique during neurosurgery consists of an opioid (fentanyl or remifentanil) along with inhaled nitrous oxide (70%) and low-dose (0.2%-0.5%) isoflurane. However, the routine use of nitrous oxide in neurosurgical patients is not universally accepted. The incidence of awareness under anesthesia has been reported to be 0.8% in children, a value higher than in adults.[25] Routine administration of a benzodiazepine like midazolam (0.5 mg/kg PO [by mouth] or 0.1 mg/kg IV) should provide some amnesia of perioperative events and minimize patient anxiety. Deep neuromuscular blockade with a nondepolarizing muscle relaxant is maintained to avoid patient movement and minimize the amounts of anesthetic agents needed. Patients who have undergone long-term anticonvulsant therapy will require larger doses of muscle relaxants and narcotics because of induced enzymatic metabolism of these agents (Fig. 19-6).[26] Muscle relaxants should be withheld or their effects permitted to wear off when assessment of motor function during neurosurgery is planned.

Intraoperative Fluid and Electrolyte Management

Hemodynamic stability during intracranial surgery requires careful maintenance of intravascular volume and electrolytes. Because CBF constitutes 55% of total cardiac output in 2- to 4-year old patients,[1] sudden blood loss or venous air embolus can rapidly deteriorate to cardiovascular collapse. Therefore, normovolemia should be maintained throughout the procedure. Estimation of the patient's blood volume is essential in determining the amount of allowable blood loss and the time to transfuse blood. Blood volume depends on the age and size of the patient, as delineated in Table 19-6. Normal saline is commonly used as the maintenance fluid during neurosurgery because it is mildly hyperosmolar (308 mOsm/kg) and should minimize cerebral edema. However, rapid infusion of large quantities of normal saline (>60 mL/kg) can be associated with hyperchloremic acidosis.[27] Given the relatively large blood volume of the neonate or infant, the maintenance rate of fluid administration depends on the weight of the patient (Table 19-7). Significant blood loss is likely in most craniotomies in infants and children, so the maximum allowable blood loss should be determined in advance so the anesthesiologist will know when blood should be transfused to the patient. However, there are no guidelines on threshold for transfusing blood and the decision to transfuse should be dictated by the type of surgery, underlying medical condition of the patient,

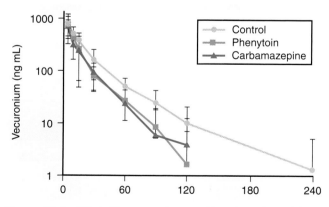

Figure 19–6 Effect of long-term therapy with anticonvulsants (phenytoin, carbamazepine) on the half-life of the muscle relaxant vecuronium. Vecuronium plasma concentrations are plotted against time after a single bolus dose of vecuronium (0.15 mg/kg). Mean ± SD values are plotted for groups taking both anticonvulsants and the control group.

Table 19–6	**Estimated Blood Volume in Children**
Age	**Estimated Blood Volume (mL/kg)**
Preterm neonate	100
Full-term neonate	90
≤1 year	80
1-12 years	75
Adolescents and adults	70

Table 19–7	**Rate of Maintenance Fluid Administration**
Weight (kg)	Rate
≤10	4 mL/kg/hr
10-20	40 mL + 2 mL/kg/hr for every kg over 10 kg
≥20	60 mL + 1 mL/kg/hr for every kg over 20 kg

and potential for additional blood loss, both intraoperative and postoperative. Hematocrit values of 21% to 25% should provide some impetus for blood transfusion. Packed red blood cells (10 mL/kg) will raise the hematocrit by 10%. Initially, blood losses should be replaced with 3 mL of normal saline for each 1 mL of lost blood or a colloid solution such as 5% albumin equal to the amount of blood loss. Depending on the extent and length of the surgical procedure and exposure of vascular beds, additional fluid administration at 3 to 10 mL/kg/hr may be necessary.

Pediatric patients, particularly infants, are at particular risk for hypoglycemia. Small premature infants, who have limited reserves of glycogen and limited gluconeogenesis, require continuous infusions of glucose at 5 to 6 mg/kg/min to maintain serum levels. Surgery elicits a stress response, and children are generally able to maintain normal serum glucose levels without exogenous glucose administration.[28] The stress of surgery and critical illness and resulting insulin resistance can produce hyperglycemia which in turn may be associated with neurologic injury.[29] Because inadvertent hypoglycemia is clinically less important in adults than in children, tight glycemic control has been widely recommended.[30] In pediatrics, hyperglycemia has been linked to poor outcome, but it remains unclear that tight control offers significant benefits.[31,32] Limited evidence now suggests that tight glycemic control may carry undue risk of hypoglycemia, and newer data are less supportive of this practice in all populations.[33] It is prudent, therefore, to remain mindful of the particular vulnerabilities of children and, until pediatric trials can provide better guidance, follow a conservative approach that keeps randomly measured serum glucose levels below 180 mg/dL. In any case hyperglycemia is always best avoided, because it may exacerbate neurologic injury if ischemia occurs.

Brain swelling can be managed initially with hyperventilation and elevation of the head above the heart. Should these maneuvers fail, mannitol can be given at a dose of 0.25 to 1.0 g/kg IV. This agent will transiently alter cerebral hemodynamics and raise serum osmolality by 10 to 20 mOsm/kg.[34] However, repeated dosing of mannitol can lead to extreme hyperosmolality, renal failure, and further brain edema.[35] Furosemide is a useful adjunct to mannitol for decreasing acute cerebral edema and has been shown in vitro to prevent the rebound swelling due to mannitol.[35,36] All diuretics interfere with the ability to use urine output as a guide to intravascular volume status.

Monitoring

Hemodynamic Monitoring

Patients undergoing major craniotomy and spine surgery are at risk of sudden hemodynamic instability due to hemorrhage, VAE, herniation syndromes, or manipulation of cranial

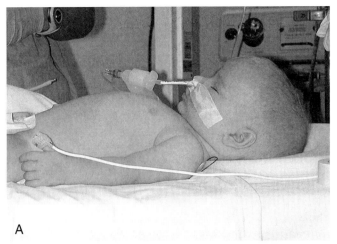

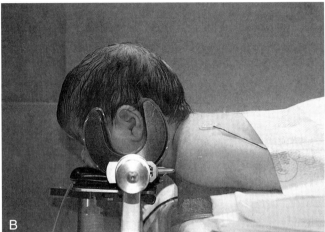

Figure 19–7 Supine (**A**) and prone (**B**) positioning for an infant. Note that the infant's head lies at a higher plane than the rest of the body. This feature increases the likelihood of venous air embolism during craniotomy.

nerves. The potential for cerebral hypoperfusion generally warrants placement of an arterial cannula for continuous blood pressure monitoring. This canula also provides access for sampling for serial measurements of blood gases, electrolytes, glucose, and hematocrit. Though it may initially appear counterintuitive, small patient size decreases the threshold for insertion of an arterial catheter, because small children cannot tolerate blood loss as adults can.

The utility of central venous catheterization remains controversial. Cannulation of the jugular or subclavian vein with multiple-orifice catheters in adults is often preferred, particularly when VAE is anticipated. However, these multiple-orifice catheters are too large for infants and most small children and are not used in pediatric settings. Furthermore, monitoring of the central venous pressure may not accurately reflect intravascular volume in small children, particularly in the prone position.[37] Therefore the risks of a central venous catheter may outweigh its benefits. One study reported that in infants, even when VAE occurred, a single-orifice central venous catheter was not often successful for aspirating air, presumably because of the high resistance of the small-gauge catheters used in these patients.[38]

Venous air emboli have been detected during many craniotomies in infants and children, primarily because the head of a small child is large in relation to the rest of body and rests above the heart in either the prone or supine position

(Fig. 19-7).[39,40] Standard neurosurgical positioning often includes elevation of the patient's head to optimize cerebral venous drainage. However, this maneuver can increase the risk for air entrainment into the venous system through open venous channels in bone and sinuses.[18] Patients with cardiac defects and the potential for right-to-left shunting, such as patent foramen ovale and patent ductus arteriosus, are at risk for paradoxical air emboli, leading to cerebral and myocardial infarction. A precordial Doppler ultrasound device can detect minute VAE and should be routinely used in conjunction with an end-tidal carbon dioxide analyzer and arterial catheter in all craniotomies in order to detect VAE early, before significant hemodynamic instability develops. The Doppler probe is best positioned on the anterior chest, usually just over or to the right of the sternum at the fourth intercostal space (i.e., the nipple line). An alternative site on the posterior thorax can be used in infants in the prone position who weigh approximately 6 kg or less.[41] In addition to the characteristic changes in Doppler sounds, sudden decreases in end-tidal CO_2, dysrhythmias, ischemic changes in the electrocardiogram, or a combination, can occur with VAE.

Neurophysiologic Monitoring

Advances in neurophysiologic monitoring have enhanced the ability to safely perform more definitive neurosurgical resections in functional areas of the brain and spinal cord. However, the depressant effects of many anesthetic agents limit the utility of these monitors. A major part of preoperative planning should include a thorough discussion of the modality and type of neurophysiologic monitoring to be used during any surgical procedure. In general, electrocorticography (ECoG) and electroencephalography (EEG) can be used when anesthesia is achieved with low levels of volatile anesthetics. Spinal cord and peripheral nerve surgery may require electromyography (EMG) and detection of muscle movement as an endpoint. Therefore, muscle relaxants should be avoided or their effects permitted to dissipate during the monitoring period.

Monitors of Cerebral Oxygenation

The primary cause of cerebral ischemia in infants and children is cerebral hypoperfusion secondary to systemic arterial hypotension, especially when accompanied by intracranial hypertension. The three potential clinical intraoperative modalities for monitoring cerebral ischemia are (1) EEG, (2) transcranial Doppler ultrasonography (TCD) and (3) cerebral oximetry. However, routine use of these monitoring modalities often presents technical difficulties with positioning and recording owing to the proximity of the surgical field.

Detection of Seizure Foci

ECoG is typically recorded continuously on a polygraph via grid and strip electrodes placed on the surface of the brain after the dura is opened. Some epileptogenic foci are in close proximity to cortical areas controlling speech, memory, motor, or sensory function, so monitoring of the patient with electrophysiologic responses is frequently utilized to minimize iatrogenic injury to these areas.[42-44] Cortical stimulation of the motor strip in a child under general anesthesia requires either EMG or direct visualization of muscle movement. Neuromuscular blockade should be used cautiously, less than two twitches in the train-of-four monitoring, in this situation. Cortical stimulation using a dual-channel

stimulator is possible. Epileptogenic activity may be evident from either clearly documented electrographic seizures or EEG spike activity, which consists of either interictal spikes of 50 to 80 msec or sharp waves of 80 to 200 msec. During anesthesia, the use of low concentrations of volatile anesthetics and opioids alone should not depress ECoG and EEG signals.

Awake Craniotomy

Surgical resection of epileptogenic foci in functional areas of the brain can lead to significant neurologic deficits in patients under general anesthesia. Neural function is best assessed in an awake and cooperative patient.[45] Positioning of the patient is critical for the success of this technique. The patient should be in a semilateral position to allow patient comfort as well as surgical and airway access (Fig. 19-8). Motor and sensory cortices are localized by induction of motor movements or sensory changes by cortical stimulation. Language function is tested by eliciting speech arrest with cortical stimulation. Verbal memory is tested by stimulating the hippocampus or lateral temporal cortex. In children undergoing craniotomy with local anesthesia and propofol and fentanyl for sedation and analgesia during resections in eloquent areas of the brain, Soriano and colleagues[46] found that propofol, when discontinued 20 minutes before monitoring, did not interfere with the ECoG and that cooperative children older than 10 years were able to withstand the procedure without incident. Other anesthetic regimens such as remifentanil-propofol and dexmedetomidine have been reported.[47,48] However, it is imperative that candidates for an awake craniotomy be mature and psychologically prepared to participate in this procedure. Therefore, patients who are developmentally delayed or have a history of severe anxiety or psychiatric disorders should not be considered for an awake craniotomy. Very young patients cannot be expected to cooperate for these procedures and usually require general anesthesia with extensive neurophysiologic monitoring to minimize inadvertent resection of the eloquent cortex.

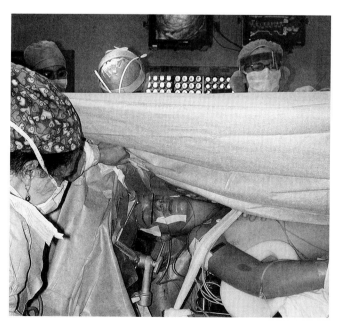

Figure 19–8 Positioning the patient for an awake craniotomy. Note that there is clear access to the patient to facilitate neuropsychological testing.

Monitoring Spinal Cord and Nerve Root Integrity

Surgery on the spinal cord and nerve roots exposes the patient to ischemic and traumatic injury. The risk for the development of a neural injury during the resection of a spinal cord or nerve root tumor can be difficult to assess but can be exacerbated by compression of the vascular supply of the cord and resection of the tumor itself. Similarly, brainstem surgery places vital nuclei and spinal pathways at risk of ischemia and direct damage. These factors justify the need for intraoperative neurologic monitoring.

Somatosensory Evoked Potentials

Somatosensory evoked potentials (SSEPs) primarily assess the integrity of the dorsal (sensory) pathways of the spinal cord.[49] SSEP monitoring provides real-time examination of spinal tracts at risk during surgical manipulation of the spinal cord. Helmers and Hall[50] reported their experience with SSEP monitoring in children undergoing orthopaedic and neurosurgical procedures. These investigators noted that the SSEP monitoring data derived from pediatric patients appear to be more sensitive to the depressant effects of general anesthesia. Cortical responses were less reliable in children younger than 10 years and in those with myelodysplasia or cerebral palsy. Although the SSEPs obtained from these patients demonstrated attenuated cortical responses, relatively robust signals were recorded from the cervical spine. Helmers and Hall[50] recommended that isoflurane and nitrous oxide levels should be maintained below 0.6% and 50%, respectively.

Motor Evoked Potentials

The major drawback of SSEP monitoring is that it cannot reliably monitor the integrity of the ventral (motor) pathways. Assessment of motor function is limited by the depressant effect of general anesthetics. One such modality is the motor evoked potential, which uses magnetic stimulation of the motor cortex and detection of the action potential in the corresponding muscle groups. All volatile anesthetic agents, including nitrous oxide, have a dose-dependent depressant effect on motor evoked potentials. Ketamine, propofol, or etomidate infusions appear to preserve the motor evoked potential and have been used routinely.[51]

Nerve Root Monitoring

Neurosurgical procedures for tethered spinal cord syndrome and spasticity often employ EMG monitoring during identification and dissection of the nerve roots. The tethered spinal cord syndrome due to spinal dysraphism is associated with conditions such as myelomeningocele, lipoma of the filum terminalis, spina bifida occulta, and adhesions from prior spinal surgery. Visualization and identification of functional nerve roots may be difficult and may result in an inadvertent injury during the surgical dissection. EMG monitoring can be helpful for identifying functional nerve roots. Placement of the EMG electrodes in the external anal and urethral (in girls) sphincter allows continuous monitoring of the nerve roots supplying the pudendal nerves (S2-S4). Inserting a balloon manometer into the bladder and recording changes in pressure during stimulation can assess detrusor muscle function. Movement and evoked action potentials of the anterior tibialis and sural muscles can also be detected visually and by EMG. Muscle contractions can be readily observed with the use of clear sterile plastic drapes. Muscle relaxation must be discontinued to enable detection of motor activity. Volatile anesthetics and opioids do not appear to interfere with muscle action potentials, and the patient should be deeply anesthetized for this monitoring because direct nerve root stimulation often elicits a significant sympathetic response from pain.

SPECIAL ISSUES

Neonatal Emergencies

Most neonatal surgery is performed on an emergency basis, increasing risks in the perioperative period due to undiagnosed congenital anomalies and, in premature neonates, persistence of the transitional circulation. In addition, there is a more than 10-fold increase in perioperative morbidity and mortality in neonates than in other pediatric patients.[8] Congestive heart failure can occur in neonates with large cerebral arteriovenous malformations, and this condition requires aggressive hemodynamic support. More commonly, intracranial right to left shunting occurs through a patent ductus arteriosus or foramen ovale that has not yet closed. Management of the neonatal respiratory system may be difficult because of the diminutive size of the airway, craniofacial anomalies, laryngotracheal lesions, and acute (hyaline membrane disease, retained amniotic fluid) or chronic (bronchopulmonary dysplasia) disease. Because these conditions are in a state of flux, they should be addressed preoperatively so as to minimize perioperative morbidity.

The neonatal central nervous system is capable of sensing pain and mounting a stress response after a surgical stimulus, and premature infants require anesthesia for painful procedures.[52] However, immature neonatal organ systems are highly sensitive to anesthetic agents. Neonatal myocardial function is particularly sensitive to both inhaled and intravenous anesthetics, and these agents must be administered judiciously to block surgical stress response without causing myocardial depression. An opioid-based anesthetic is generally the most stable hemodynamic technique for neonates. However, neonatal hepatic and renal systems are not fully developed, so neonates anesthetized with a narcotic technique often have delayed emergence from anesthesia and may require postoperative mechanical ventilation.

Closure of a myelomeningocele or encephalocele presents special problems. Positioning the patient for tracheal intubation may rupture the membranes covering the spinal cord or brain. Careful padding of the lesion by elevation of the neonate on top of soft supports with a hollow center minimizes the chance of rupture of the fragile membranes. In some cases intubation of the neonate's trachea in the left lateral decubitus position may be necessary. General anesthesia should be provided to optimize surgical condition and minimize pain.[52] The use of spinal anesthesia for closure of small myelomeningoceles has been advocated by a highly specialized group who have integrated regional anesthesia in neonatal surgery,[53] but this practice has not been universally accepted. Most surgical closures of simple myelomeningoceles have relatively minimal blood loss. Large lesions may require significant dissection of cutaneous tissue to cover the defect, however, posing larger risks for blood loss and hemodynamic instability. Advances in the management of myelomeningoceles have led to early intervention in the intrauterine period.[54] The management of the fetus and mother during fetal surgery has been reviewed extensively elsewhere.[55,56]

Craniosynostosis

Remodeling of craniosynostosis is likely to have the best result if done early in life.[57] However, the procedure can be associated with loss of a significant percentage of an infant's blood volume, with greater losses occurring when more sutures are involved.[40] VAE often occurs and should be minimized by maintenance of adequate intravascular blood volume. Early detection with continuous precordial Doppler ultrasonography can enable treatment to be instituted before large amounts of air are entrained. When hemodynamic instability does occur, the operating table can be placed in the Trendelenburg position. This maneuver will augment the patient's blood pressure and prevent further entrainment of intravascular air. Special risks exist in neonates and young infants, in whom potential right-to-left cardiac mixing lesions can result in arterial emboli. Because neuroendoscopic techniques are designed to minimize surgical incision, dissection, and blood loss, less aggressive fluid replacement and invasive hemodynamic monitoring is becoming the norm. The application of endoscopic techniques for craniosynostosis repair has resulted in significantly less morbidity. Endoscopic strip craniectomy involves insertion of an endoscope through a small scalp incision and resection of the fused cranial sutures. This minimally invasive approach is associated with decreased blood loss, less surgical time, and improved postoperative recovery in neonates and infants.[58-60] Tobias and colleagues[61] reported a significantly lower incidence of VAE during endoscopic strip craniectomy in comparison with the open procedure. However, this approach is indicated only for patients younger than 2 months and for straightforward strip craniectomies.

Hydrocephalus

Hydrocephalus is the most common condition confronting the pediatric neurosurgical team. Hemorrhage (intraventricular or subarachnoid hemorrhage in the neonate), congenital problems (aqueductal stenosis) trauma, infection, or tumors (especially in the posterior fossa) lead to hydrocephalus. Unless the etiology of the hydrocephalus can be definitively treated, management entails surgical placement of a ventricular drain or ventriculoperitoneal shunt. Occasionally the distal end of the shunt must be placed in the right atrium or pleural cavity, usually because of inability of the peritoneal cavity to absorb cerebrospinal fluid. Acute obstruction of these shunts should be treated urgently to avoid a lethal rise in ICP in the relatively small cranial vault of the infant and child. Intracranial hypertension manifests as vomiting and places the patient at risk for pulmonary aspiration, in which case rapid-sequence induction should be performed.

Hydrocephalus often produces large, dilated scalp veins in infants, and these can be used for induction of anesthesia if necessary. Anesthesia should be established with a rapid-sequence induction technique and tracheal intubation with cricoid pressure. If intravenous access cannot be established, an inhalation induction with sevoflurane and gentle cricoid pressure may be an alternative, though less desirable, method of induction. Once an intravenous catheter is inserted, hyperventilation is instituted, the patient's respiratory muscles are paralyzed, the trachea is intubated, and anesthesia is maintained with a balanced nitrous oxide–narcotic technique or low concentrations of isoflurane. The possibility of VAE during placement of the distal end of a ventriculo-atrial shunt should always be kept in mind. Postoperatively, patients should be observed carefully because altered mental status and recent peritoneal incision put them at high risk for pulmonary aspiration once feedings are begun.

Tumors

Because the majority of intracranial tumors in children occur in the posterior fossa, cerebrospinal fluid flow is often obstructed, and intracranial hypertension and hydrocephalus are often present. Most neurosurgeons approach this region with the child in the prone position. The patient's head is generally secured with a Mayfield head frame, although pins used in small children can cause severe skin lacerations, skull fractures, dural tears, and intracranial hematomas.[62] Elevation of the bone flap can result in sinus tears, massive blood loss, or VAE. Surgical resection of tumors in the posterior fossa can also lead to brainstem or cranial nerve damage. Table 19-8 lists some of the signs of encroachment on these structures. Damage to the respiratory centers and cranial nerves can lead to apnea and airway obstruction after extubation of the patient's trachea. Small children requiring stereotactically guided radiosurgery need general anesthesia to tolerate the procedures. Special head frames devised to allow airway manipulations should be used in these patients.[63]

Craniopharyngiomas, the most common perisellar tumors in children and adolescents, may be associated with hypothalamic and pituitary dysfunction. Steroid replacement therapy (with dexamethasone or hydrocortisone) is generally administered because the integrity of the hypothalamic-pituitary-adrenal axis may be uncertain. In addition, diabetes insipidus occurs preoperatively in some patients and is a common postoperative problem. Nocturnal enuresis may result in preoperative hypovolemia. If diabetes insipidus does not exist preoperatively, it usually does not develop until the postoperative period. This is because there appears to be an adequate reserve of antidiuretic hormone in the posterior pituitary gland capable of functioning for many hours even when the hypothalamic-pituitary stalk is damaged intraoperatively. Surgical exposure to the sella is performed between the frontal lobes in infants and young children and transnasally in adolescent. Although diabetes insipidus occurs primarily after surgery, serum electrolytes should be frequently measured to detect its development.

Table 19–8	**Effect of Surgical Brainstem Manipulation**	
Brainstem Area	Signs	Changes Seen on Monitoring
Cranial nerve (CN) V	Hypertension, bradycardia	Arterial pressure, electrocardiography (ECG)
CN VII	Facial muscle movement	Electromyography
CN X	Hypotension, bradycardia	Arterial pressure, ECG
Pons, medulla	Arrhythmias, hypotension/ hypertension, tachycardia/ bradycardia, irregular breathing pattern	ECG, arterial pressure, end-tidal carbon dioxide monitor

Epilepsy

Surgical treatment has become a viable option for many patients with medically intractable epilepsy. Two major considerations should be kept in mind. Long-term administration of anticonvulsant drugs, such as phenytoin and carbamazepine, induces rapid metabolism and clearance of several classes of anesthetic agents, including neuromuscular blockers and opioids.[64] Therefore, the anesthetic requirements for these drugs are increased, so close monitoring of their effect and frequent redosing are needed. General anesthetics can compromise the sensitivity of intraoperative neurophysiologic monitors used to guide the actual resection of the epileptogenic focus.[65] Furthermore, if cortical stimulation is used to mimic the seizure pattern or identify areas on the motor strip, neuromuscular blockade should be antagonized. Implantable ECoG leads—grids and strips—are laid on the cortical surface in order to detect and localize the seizure focus.

After emergence from anesthesia, patients undergoing epilepsy surgery are typically monitored in a specialized EEG unit, and the seizure focus is mapped out. A second craniotomy is necessary for removal of ECoG grids and strips used for invasive EEG monitoring and subsequent resection of the seizure focus. It is important to avoid administration of nitrous oxide until the dura is opened, because intracranial air can persist up to 3 weeks after a craniotomy, and nitrous oxide can cause rapid expansion of air cavities and result in tension pneumocephalus.[66]

Vascular

Vascular anomalies are rare in infants and children. Most of these conditions are congenital lesions that manifest early in life. Large cerebral arteriovenous shunts in neonates may be associated with high-output congestive heart failure and require vasoactive support. They are usually vein of Galen malformations but sometimes true pial arteriovenous malformations. Initial treatment of a high-flow fistula often consists of intravascular embolization in the radiologic suite.[67] In extraordinary circumstances, microsurgical resection might be considered and would be associated with massive blood loss, requiring several IV access sites as well as invasive hemodynamic monitoring. Acute interruption of any sort of intracranial fistula or shunt may lead to dramatic hemodynamic changes, including sudden hypertension with hyperemic cerebral edema.[68] Vasodilators such as labetalol and nitroprusside may be necessary to control a hypertensive crisis.

Moyamoya syndrome is a rare chronic vaso-occlusive disorder of the internal carotid arteries that manifests as transient ischemic attacks, recurrent strokes, or both in childhood. The etiology is unknown, but the syndrome can be associated with prior intracranial irradiation, neurofibromatosis, Down syndrome, and a variety of hematologic disorders. The anesthetic management of patients with this syndrome is directed at optimizing cerebral perfusion.[69] It includes ensuring generous preoperative hydration and maintaining the blood pressure within the patient's preoperative levels. Maintenance of normocapnia is essential as well, because both hypercapnia and hypocapnia can lead to steal phenomenon from the ischemic region and further aggravate cerebral ischemia,[70] although the pathophysiology of "steal" is largely speculative. A nitrous oxide and narcotic–based anesthetic technique provides a stable level of anesthesia for the patient with moyamoya syndrome and is compatible with intraoperative

EEG monitoring. Once the patient emerges from anesthesia, the same maneuvers that optimize cerebral perfusion should be extended into the postoperative period. The patient should receive IV fluids to maintain adequate cerebral perfusion and should be given adequate narcotics to avoid hyperventilation induced by pain and crying.

Trauma

Pediatric head trauma requires a multiple-organ approach to minimizing morbidity and mortality.[71] A small child's head is often the point of impact in injuries, but other organs can also be damaged. Basic life support algorithms should be immediately applied to ensure a patent airway and adequate respiration and circulation. Because the head-to-torso ratio is great in infants and younger children, acceleration-deceleration injuries are more common in the pediatric population and lead to more diffuse brain and upper cervical spine injuries. Immobilization of the cervical spine is important to avoid secondary spinal cord injury with manipulation of the patient's airway until radiographs confirm absence of cervical spine injury. Therefore, an unstable cervical spine should be immobilized with cervical traction during laryngoscopy for tracheal intubation. Blunt abdominal trauma and long bone fractures often occur with head injury and can be major sources of blood loss. To ensure tissue perfusion during the operative period, the patient's blood volume should be restored with crystalloid solutions or blood products. Ongoing blood loss can lead to coagulopathies and should be treated with specific blood components.

Infants with shaken baby syndrome are often presented with a myriad of chronic and acute subdural hematomas.[72] As with all traumatic events, the presence of other coexisting injuries, fractures, and abdominal trauma should be identified. Small children undergoing craniotomy for the evacuation of either epidural or subdural hematoma are at risk for significant blood loss and VAE. Postoperative treatment includes the management of intracranial hypertension and, in severe cases, determination of brain death.

Pediatric head injury management is currently based on few randomized trials and draws heavily from data derived from adult series; evidence-based management is still evolving in this area. Therefore fundamental knowledge of age-related differences in cerebrovascular physiology and anatomy is essential in the application of adult-based head trauma protocols in pediatric patients. In 2003, a multispecialty group of pediatric neurosurgeons and intensivists published "Guidelines for the acute medical management of severe traumatic brain injury in infants, children, and adolescents."[73] This document is a comprehensive evidence-based review of controversial management issues in the care of the head-injured pediatric patient.

Spine Surgery

Spinal dysraphism is the primary indication for laminectomies in pediatric patients. Many of these patients have a history of a meningomyelocele closure followed by several corrective operations. The patients have been exposed to latex products and often demonstrate hypersensitivity to latex. Latex allergy can manifest as a severe anaphylactic reaction, heralded by hypotension and wheezing with or without a rash, and should be rapidly treated by removal of the source of latex and administration of fluid and vasopressors.[74] Patients at risk for latex allergy should be managed in a latex-free environment.

Tethered cord release entails EMG monitoring to help identify functional nerve roots. EMG of the anal sphincter and muscles of the lower extremities is performed intraoperatively to minimize inadvertent injury to nerves innervating these muscle groups.[75] Neuromuscular blockade should be discontinued or antagonized to allow accurate EMG monitoring. Insertion of an epidural catheter by the surgeon under direct vision can provide a conduit for the administration of local anesthetics and opioids for the management of postoperative pain. Severe spasticity associated with cerebral palsy can be surgically alleviated by a selective dorsal rhizotomy, which reduces spasticity by surgically dividing dorsal rootlets to diminish the afferent input to motor neurons in the spinal cord, thus decreasing the hyperactive reflexes associated with spastic diplegia. Pathologic rootlets are identified by directly stimulating them and noting the corresponding muscle action potential with EMG. Exaggerated action potentials can be elicited in innervated as well as other distal muscle groups. These abnormal rootlets are partially sectioned to decrease afferent nerve conduction. However, these rootlets can potentially contain sensory and proprioceptive fibers.

The Hoffman reflex, a measure of motor neuron excitability, is significantly increased in children with spastic diplegia. This response can be evoked by direct stimulation of the nerve root followed by recording of the direct efferent muscle response and the Hoffman reflex. The reflex represents the reflex potential emanating from the motor neurons of the spinal cord.[76] The use of the Hoffman reflex as a guide for measuring the relative degree of spinal reflex hyperactivity during partial sectioning of the pathologic rootlets is more precise. Anesthetic agents limit the utility of the Hoffman reflex as an intraoperative monitor of spinal reflex activity; inhalational agents, nitrous oxide, barbiturates, and benzodiazepines all depress it.[77] An opioid-based anesthetic technique with intermittent doses of ketamine or propofol does not appear to suppress the reflex. Because the EMG is the observed endpoint, muscle relaxation should be avoided.

Neuroendoscopy

Technologic advances in minimally invasive endoscopic surgery have entered the neurosurgical arena. The anesthetic considerations for these evolving techniques are the same as for any other neurosurgical procedures, as discussed in this chapter.[78] Endoscopic third ventriculoscopy has became an accepted procedure for the treatment of obstructive hydrocephalus in infants and children.[79] Despite the relative safety of this procedure, bradycardia and other arrhythmias have been reported to occur during it in conjunction with use of irrigation fluids and manipulation of the floor of the third ventricle.[80,81]

Neuroradiology

Advances in imaging technology have provided less invasive procedures to diagnose and treat lesions in the central nervous system. Most neuroradiologic studies, such as computed tomography and magnetic resonance imaging, can be accomplished with use of light sedation. Recommendations published by consensus groups of anesthesiologists and pediatricians can serve as guidelines for managing patients undergoing neuroradiologic procedures.[82,83] General anesthesia is typically used in patients who are uncooperative or have coexisting medical problems and for potentially painful procedures, such as intravascular embolization of vascular lesions.[67]

POSTOPERATIVE CARE

General Considerations

Although a few selected patients may be safely managed in alternative settings, neurosurgical patients generally require postoperative treatment in an intensive care unit until cardiorespiratory stability and neurologic recovery are ensured. In high-volume centers, specialized neurocritical care teams can improve patient outcomes for children.[84] Once the patient is in the intensive care unit, optimal care begins with a clear delineation of responsibilities and thorough "handoff" from the neurosurgical and anesthesia teams to the responsible intensive care professionals. Clear communication of patient history, medications, operative events, and anticipated course is essential.

All new arrivals require physiologic and neurologic assessment, the latter sometimes necessitating repeated examinations to ensure normal awakening from anesthesia. Although tracheal extubation and initial neurologic assessment are ideally accomplished in the operating room, this approach may not be possible in unstable patients, those who are slow to awaken, those in whom large fluid shifts are anticipated, or if comorbidities mandate otherwise. In these settings, intermittent lightening of sedation and frequent examinations are necessary to reassure the intensivist that all is well.

Respiratory Support

Postoperative mechanical ventilation aims to support alveolar gas exchange while permitting ongoing neurologic assessment. In most cases, a triggered mode, which allows continuous assessment of respiratory drive, is preferable over controlled ventilation. Pressure support ventilation, even in neonates, offers a convenient means of providing needed support without losing respiratory control as a marker of neurologic function. In patients with severe lung disease, extrapolations from the Acute Respiratory Distress Syndrome Network trial suggest a low–tidal volume, pressure-limited approach.[85] However, neurointensivists are left to balance the potential advantages of this strategy against ICP considerations and the risks attendant to CO_2 retention. In patients for whom positive end-expiratory pressure is necessary to reverse hypoxemia, small animal models have suggested that a setting as low as 10 cm H_2O may impair venous return and decrease cerebral compliance.[86] Nonetheless, when mean arterial pressure is maintained, adult series clearly demonstrate that modest levels of positive end-expiratory pressure (10-12 cm H_2O)[87,88] and even high-frequency oscillatory ventilation[89] can safely reverse hypoxemia without significant impact on the cerebral circulation. In young infants, in whom fontanels and sutures are open, there is no association between mean airway and ICP values.[90] Finally, although heavy sedation, controlled ventilation, and neuromuscular blockade are employed more often in the care of critically ill children than of adults, the efficacy of this in the setting of high ICP is unknown. Thus, although the practice can be beneficial, there are insufficient data to recommend its routine use.[91]

Hemodynamic Support

Hemodynamic support aims to avoid hypotension, maintain adequate cerebral perfusion pressure, and minimize injury from transient changes in pressure. In neonates and premature infants, the lower limit of pressure autoregulation is approximately 30 mm Hg, or around the fifth percentile for gestational age.[92,93] In sick neonates, intermittent pressure passivity is present and can predispose to hemorrhage.[94,95] In the smallest patients, therefore, a fine balance is required. Even in very-low-birth-weight infants, both dopamine and epinephrine are effective in supporting systemic pressure and restoring cerebral blood flow.[92]

When increased ICP is present, critical cerebral perfusion pressure for preschool children (2-6 years) is approximately 50 mm Hg, rising to 55 to 60 mm Hg in older children. Although lower levels are powerful predictors of poor outcome,[96,97] intentional increases beyond these levels are controversial because complications of therapy (fluid overload, acute respiratory distress syndrome) may begin to negate any benefits.[98] When cerebral perfusion pressure is low and ICP remains high despite all medical management, decompressive craniectomy may have a more favorable outcome in children than adults.[99]

Fluid Management

Meticulous fluid management is critical in the care of neurosurgical patients. Small size, immature renal function, and variable intake make fluid and electrolyte imbalances common in pediatrics. These vulnerabilities are further magnified in neurosurgical patients by the disruption of normal homeostatic controls. For example, nonosmotic secretion of antidiuretic hormone makes hyponatremia common after neurosurgery, despite the intraoperative use of fluids that are high in sodium and isotonic—or slightly hypertonic—to plasma (lactated Ringer's solution, 272 mOsm/L; normal saline, 310 mOsm/L). Overall, more than 10% of all children experience postoperative hyponatremia,[100] and this fraction is likely much higher after neurosurgery. Elevations of antidiuretic hormone can result from a variety of stimuli ranging from pain and nausea to fluid shifts and hypovolemia. Because sudden, unrecognized drops in serum sodium levels can provoke seizures, it is prudent to monitor electrolyte values closely throughout the perioperative period. When significant hyponatremia occurs, seizures may be treated with hypertonic saline and free water excesses addressed through fluid restriction and administration of diuretics.[101] Because of these risks, many clinicians avoid hypotonic solutions altogether in the perioperative period.[102]

The syndrome of cerebral salt wasting is also common in children and can be seen after head trauma and all manner of neurosurgical procedures. As it has become more commonly appreciated, the syndrome has been diagnosed with increasing frequency and reported in association with meningitis,[103] calvarial remodeling,[104,105] tumor resection,[106] and even hydrocephalus. The syndrome can be easily confused with other entities,[107] but a retrospective review put its incidence at 11.3 per 1000 procedures.[106] In affected patients, the mean duration of symptoms was 6 days, with a range of 1 to 5 days. Cerebral salt wasting, the result of excessively high levels of atrial or brain natriuretic peptide,[108] is marked by hyponatremia, hypovolemia, and excessive urinary excretion of sodium. Because these peptides also block steroidogenesis, cerebral

salt wasting is typically accompanied by mineralocorticoid deficiency.[109,110] The classic treatment involves saline administration, but more rapid resolution has been achieved with fludocortisone.[110,111]

Diabetes insipidus is a well-known complication of surgical procedures involving or adjacent to the pituitary and hypothalamus. It is most commonly seen in association with craniopharyngioma, for which it is a presenting symptom in 40% of cases.[112] Diabetes insipidus is recognized from a rising serum sodium value (>150 mg/dL) accompanied by copious (>4 mL/kg/hr) output of dilute urine. Urine output is unchecked, so severe dehydration and hypovolemia may result. Because there are a variety of successful approaches to DI management, a standardized protocol is helpful when postoperative care is multidisciplinary. Patients who are unconscious, who are unable to take oral fluids, or whose normal thirst mechanisms are impaired are best managed with a continuous infusion of arginine vasopressin. One effective protocol employs maximal antidiuresis and strict limitation of intravenous fluids (Fig. 19-9).[113] This strategy avoids the pitfalls of titrating drug dosage to urine output and recognizes that renal blood flow remains adequate in the normovolemic child receiving maximal antidiuresis. Because urine output is minimal (0.5 mL/kg/min), other clinical markers of volume status must be followed closely. After recovery from surgery and anesthesia, the awake and thirsty patient may be easily transitioned to oral fluids and desmopressin.

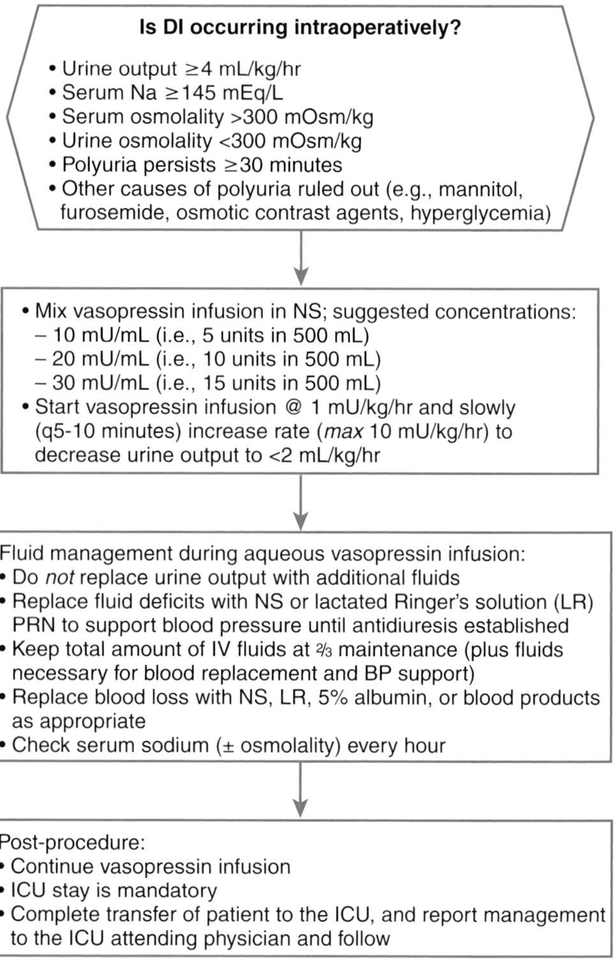

Is DI occurring intraoperatively?

- Urine output ≥4 mL/kg/hr
- Serum Na ≥145 mEq/L
- Serum osmolality >300 mOsm/kg
- Urine osmolality <300 mOsm/kg
- Polyuria persists ≥30 minutes
- Other causes of polyuria ruled out (e.g., mannitol, furosemide, osmotic contrast agents, hyperglycemia)

↓

- Mix vasopressin infusion in NS; suggested concentrations:
  - 10 mU/mL (i.e., 5 units in 500 mL)
  - 20 mU/mL (i.e., 10 units in 500 mL)
  - 30 mU/mL (i.e., 15 units in 500 mL)
- Start vasopressin infusion @ 1 mU/kg/hr and slowly (q5-10 minutes) increase rate (*max* 10 mU/kg/hr) to decrease urine output to <2 mL/kg/hr

↓

Fluid management during aqueous vasopressin infusion:
- Do *not* replace urine output with additional fluids
- Replace fluid deficits with NS or lactated Ringer's solution (LR) PRN to support blood pressure until antidiuresis established
- Keep total amount of IV fluids at ⅔ maintenance (plus fluids necessary for blood replacement and BP support)
- Replace blood loss with NS, LR, 5% albumin, or blood products as appropriate
- Check serum sodium (± osmolality) every hour

↓

Post-procedure:
- Continue vasopressin infusion
- ICU stay is mandatory
- Complete transfer of patient to the ICU, and report management to the ICU attending physician and follow

Figure 19–9 Algorithm for perioperative management of diabetes insipidus (DI). BP, blood pressure; ICU, intensive care unit; NS, normal saline.

Sedation

Pain control and sedation present unique challenges in the pediatric intensive care unit. Ideally, postoperative neurosurgical patients are comfortable, awake, and cooperative with their care. In pediatric patients, however, these goals can be mutually exclusive, and some level of sedation is often necessary to ensure a safe recovery. The ideal sedation regimen would include short-acting or reversible agents that can be withdrawn intermittently to permit neurologic assessment, but a single agent suitable for children has yet to be developed. Some agents suitable for adults are unsuitable in children, and some agents used widely in pediatrics are less useful in adults.

For example, propofol is a potent, ultra–short-acting sedative-hypnotic that is extremely useful in adult neurocritical care.[114] It has only limited utility in pediatrics, however, because of its association with a fatal syndrome of bradycardia, rhabdomyolysis, metabolic acidosis, and multiple-organ failure when it is used over extended periods in small children.[115] Although the mechanism of this syndrome remains unclear, it appears related to both the duration of therapy and the cumulative dose. These difficulties are much less common in adults,[116] probably owing to the use of lower doses per kilogram of body weight. Some centers have advocated the use of propofol in pediatric patients under strict controls, but the agent is generally limited to operative anesthesia,[117] procedural sedation,[118,119] and continuous infusions of limited duration.

A newer agent, dexmedetomidine, offers many of the advantages of propofol as an ultra–short-acting, single-agent sedative to be used in the postoperative period. Unlike with propofol, apnea is not a problem and spontaneous breathing is easily maintained with use of dexmedetomidine. At this writing, studies involving children are preliminary, but the drug appears to be safe and effective when used for periods of 24 hours or less.[120] The pharmacokinetics of dexmedetomidine in infants and children are similar to the published values for adults. Opioid cross-tolerance makes it a useful agent for treatment of fentanyl or morphine withdrawal.[121] Transient increases in blood pressure can be seen with boluses, followed by hypotension and bradycardia as sedation deepens. In our experience, both hypotension and hypertension can occasionally be observed with long-term dexmedetomidine infusions, and a withdrawal syndrome results when extended infusions are discontinued. Further experience and vetting will be necessary to determine the proper place for this agent in the routine perioperative care of neurosurgical patients.

By far the mainstay of sedation in the pediatric intensive care unit remains a combination of narcotic and benzodiazepine administered via continuous infusion.[122] Titration to a validated sedation score is advised, and regular drug holidays help ensure that excessive sedation is avoided.[123,124] If chemical paralysis must be used to control ICP or facilitate mechanical ventilation, use of a neuromuscular blockade monitor helps avoid prolonged blockade and weakness.[125] Infants and children receiving sedative infusions for more than 3 to 5 days are subject to tolerance and experience symptoms of withdrawal when infusions are discontinued.[126]

Seizures

Seizures are a common manifestation of neurologic illness in pediatric patients. In the child with unexplained altered mental status, nonconvulsive status epilepticus should also be considered in the differential diagnosis.[127] Prophylaxis in the perioperative period and aggressive treatment of new convulsions are well-recognized principles of care. Although phenytoin is the agent used most commonly for prophylaxis, maintaining therapeutic serum levels of this agent can be challenging.[128] Alternative agents commonly used in pediatrics include phenobarbital, carbamazepine, and valproic acid. For status epilepticus, lorazepam 0.1 mg/kg IV push over 2 minutes or diazepam 0.5 mg phenytoin sodium equivalents per kg per rectum is an effective agent. Lorazepam may be repeated after 10 minutes and accompanied by fosphenytoin 20 mg phenytoin sodium equivalents per kg IV or intramuscularly if initial doses are ineffective. Though potentially compounding respiratory depression, phenobarbital 20 mg/kg is also an effective first-line antiepileptic drug.

Refractory status epilepticus continues to present a significant challenge, and no prospective study is available to inform management.[129] Chemically induced coma remains the mainstay of care, with antiepileptics titrated to EEG burst suppression. In our institution, we typically employ pentobarbital, midazolam, or phenobarbital in bolus-infusion regimens with adjustments directed by continuous ECG. Mechanical ventilation is provided as outlined previously, and invasive monitoring is necessary because therapy usually results in hypotension and myocardial depression. Propofol is also effective in quenching seizures and inducing coma, but the propofol infusion syndrome limits its use in pediatrics.[130]

The utility of seizure prophylaxis after pediatric head trauma continues to be controversial. Although some data suggest that children may benefit more than adults from routine prophylaxis,[131] the overall risk of seizures is low after blunt injury. Thus, the added benefit of prophylaxis is small,[132] and it remains a treatment option.[133]

Intracranial Pressure

ICP monitoring is desirable in trauma and in neurosurgical patients at risk for brain swelling or sudden expansion of a mass lesion. Symptoms of increased ICP are nonspecific in children, and intermittent apnea may be the first sign in infancy. Occasionally, increased ICP may be present even when computed tomography findings are normal.[134] In babies, split sutures and bulging fontanels provide clinical evidence of rising ICP, but noninvasive quantitative measures are problematic. In our institution, intraventricular catheters are preferred for ICP monitoring because simultaneous cerebrospinal fluid drainage can provide significant therapeutic benefits.

Unfortunately, the treatment of increased ICP in infants and children is still largely driven by adult data. A notable exception, as discussed previously, is that target thresholds for mean arterial pressure and cerebral perfusion pressure vary with age. Although osmotherapy with 3% (hypertonic) saline is widely used in boluses or infusion to control ICP, it may lead to severe hypernatremia more rapidly in small children than in adults. Other elements of management extrapolated from adult data are avoidance of steroids,[135] the preference of crystalloid over colloid resuscitation fluids,[136] and the reluctance to employ hyperventilation.[137] Regarding the last, it is particularly important to recognize that small children are subject to inadvertent overventilation and that hyperventilation-associated cerebral ischemia can occur.[138,139] Careful monitoring of blood gas, minute ventilation, and end-tidal carbon dioxide tension values are therefore recommended.

Brain Death

Determination of brain death in older children is similar to that in adults, but the diagnosis is difficult in infancy. The Uniform Determination of Death Act defines death as "irreversible cessation of circulatory and respiratory function or irreversible cessation of all functions of the entire brain, including the brainstem." Diagnosis requires normothermia, normotension, normal systemic oxygenation, and the absence of confounding toxins or medications. The examination seeks to establish the complete absence of cortical and brainstem function. An apnea test (documenting the absence of respiratory effort despite P_{CO_2} >60 torr) is conducted last, because elevated P_{CO_2} may exacerbate neurologic injury. To establish irreversibility, age-related observation periods are necessary. For premature neonates and infants younger than 7 days, no such period has been established. For infants 1 to 8 weeks of age, our institution uses two examinations and two isoelectric electroencephalograms performed 48 hours apart. In infants 2 to 12 months of age, two clinical examinations separated by 24 hours are required. Patients older than 1 year undergo examinations 6 to 12 hours apart, or 24 hours if the proximate cause of death is hypoxia-ischemia. Cerebral single photon emission computed tomography with technetium Tc 99m ECD (ethyl cysteinate dimer) is used to document the absence of cerebral perfusion when confounding factors complicate the clinical diagnosis.

SUMMARY

The perioperative management of pediatric neurosurgical patients presents many challenges to neurosurgeons, anesthesiologists, and intensivists. Many conditions are unique to small children. A basic understanding of age-dependent variables and of the interaction of anesthetic and surgical procedures is essential in minimizing perioperative morbidity and mortality at all stages of care.

REFERENCES

1. Wintermark M, Lepori D, Cotting J, et al: Brain perfusion in children: Evolution with age assessed by quantitative perfusion computed tomography, *Pediatrics* 113:1642–1652, 2004.
2. Pryds O: Control of cerebral circulation in the high-risk neonate, *Ann Neurol* 30:321–329, 1991.
3. Tsuji M, Saul JP, du PA, et al: Cerebral intravascular oxygenation correlates with mean arterial pressure in critically ill premature infants, *Pediatrics* 106:625–632, 2000.
4. Vavilala MS, Lee LA, Lam AM: The lower limit of cerebral autoregulation in children during sevoflurane anesthesia, *J Neurosurg Anesthesiol* 15:307–312, 2003.
5. Shapiro K, Marmarou A, Shulman K: Characterization of clinical CSF dynamics and neural axis compliance using the pressure-volume index: I: The normal pressure-volume index, *Ann Neurol* 7:508–514, 1980.
6. *Anesthesia and Pain Management for the Pediatrician*, Baltimore, 1999, The Johns Hopkins University Press.
7. Hopper N, Albanese A, Ghirardello S, Maghnie M: The pre-operative endocrine assessment of craniopharyngiomas, *J Pediatr Endocrinol Metab* 19(Suppl 1):325–327, 2006.
8. Cohen MM, Cameron CB, Duncan PG: Pediatric anesthesia morbidity and mortality in the perioperative period, *Anesth Analg* 70:160–167, 1990.
9. Morray JP, Geiduschek JM, Ramamoorthy C, et al: Anesthesia-related cardiac arrest in children: Initial findings of the Pediatric Perioperative Cardiac Arrest (POCA) Registry, *Anesthesiology* 93:6–14, 2000.
10. Nargozian CD: The difficult airway in the pediatric patient with craniofacial anomaly, *Anesthesiol Clin North Am* 16:839–852, 1999.
11. McCann ME, Kain ZN: Management of perioperative anxiety in children, *Anesth Analg* 93:98–105, 2001.
12. Ferrari LR, Rooney FM, Rockoff MA: Preoperative fasting practices in pediatrics, *Anesthesiology* 90:978–980, 1999.
13. Spiekermann BF, Stone DJ, Bogdonoff DL, Yemen TA: Airway management in neuroanaesthesia, *Can J Anaesth* 43:820–834, 1996.
14. Cochrane DD, Adderley R, White CP, et al: Apnea in patients with myelomeningocele, *Pediatr Neurosurg* 116:232–239, 1990.
15. Cochrane DD, Gustavsson B, Poskitt KP, et al: The surgical and natural morbidity of aggressive resection for posterior fossa tumors in childhood, *Pediatr Neurosurg* 20:19–29, 1994.
16. Foland JA, Super DM, Dahdah NS, Mhanna MJ: The use of the air leak test and corticosteroids in intubated children: A survey of pediatric critical care fellowship directors, *Respir Care* 47:662–666, 2002.
17. Mhanna MJ, Zamel YB, Tichy CM, Super DM: The "air leak" test around the endotracheal tube, as a predictor of postextubation stridor, is age dependent in children, *Crit Care Med* 30:2639–2643, 2002.
18. Grady MS, Bedford RF, Park TS: Changes in superior sagittal sinus pressure in children with head elevation, jugular venous compression, and PEEP, *J Neurosurg* 65:199–202, 1986.
19. Lerman J: Inhalational anesthetics, *Paediatr Anaesth* 14:380–383, 2004.
20. German JW, Aneja R, Heard C, Dias M: Continuous remifentanil for pediatric neurosurgery patients, *Pediatr Neurosurg* 33:227–229, 2000.
21. Chiaretti A, Pietrini D, Piastra M, et al: Safety and efficacy of remifentanil in craniosynostosis repair in children less than 1 year old, *Pediatr Neurosurg* 33:83–88, 2000.
22. Guy J, Hindman BJ, Baker KZ, et al: Comparison of remifentanil and fentanyl in patients undergoing craniotomy for supratentorial space-occupying lesions, *Anesthesiology* 86:514–524, 1997.
23. Gelb AW, Salevsky F, Chung F, et al: Remifentanil with morphine transitional analgesia shortens neurological recovery compared to fentanyl for supratentorial craniotomy, *Can J Anaesth* 50:946–952, 2003.
24. Todd MM, Warner DS, Sokoll MD, et al: A prospective, comparative trial of three anesthetics for elective supratentorial craniotomy, *Anesthesiology* 78:1005–1020, 1993.
25. Davidson AJ, Huang GH, Czarnecki C, et al: R: Awareness during anesthesia in children: A prospective cohort study, *Anesth Analg* 100:653–661, 2005.
26. Soriano SG, Sullivan LJ, Venkatakrishnan K, et al: Pharmacokinetics and pharmacodynamics of vecuronium in children receiving phenytoin or carbamazepine for chronic anticonvulsant therapy, *Br J Anaesth* 86:223–229, 2001.
27. Scheingraber S, Rehm M, Sehmisch C, Finsterer U: Rapid saline infusion produces hyperchloremic acidosis in patients undergoing gynecologic surgery [see comments], *Anesthesiology* 90:1265–1270, 1999.
28. Sandstrom K, Nilsson K, Andreasson S, et al: Metabolic consequences of different perioperative fluid therapies in the neonatal period, *Acta Anaesthesiol Scand* 37:170–175, 1993.
29. Van den BG, Schoonheydt K, Becx P, et al: Insulin therapy protects the central and peripheral nervous system of intensive care patients, *Neurology* 64:1348–1353, 2005.
30. Van den BG, Wilmer A, Milants I, Wouters PJ, et al: Intensive insulin therapy in mixed medical/surgical intensive care units: Benefit versus harm, *Diabetes* 55:3151–3159, 2006.
31. Branco RG, Tasker RC: Glycemic level in mechanically ventilated children with bronchiolitis, *Pediatr Crit Care Med* 8:546–550, 2007.
32. Klein GW, Hojsak JM, Rapaport R: Hyperglycemia in the pediatric intensive care unit, *Curr Opin Clin Nutr Metab Care* 10:187–192, 2007.
33. Kitabchi AE, Umpierrez G, Fisher JN, et al: Thirty years of personal experience in hyperglycemic crises: Diabetic ketoacidosis, and hyperglycemic hyperosmolar state, *J Clin Endocrinol Metab* 93:1541–1552, 2008.
34. Soriano SG, McManus ML, Sullivan LJ, et al: Cerebral blood flow velocity after mannitol infusion in children, *Can J Anaesth* 43:461–466, 1996.
35. McManus ML, Soriano SG: Rebound swelling of astroglial cells exposed to hypertonic mannitol, *Anesthesiology* 88:1586–1591, 1998.
36. Thenuwara K, Todd MM, Brian JE Jr: Effect of mannitol and furosemide on plasma osmolality and brain water, *Anesthesiology* 96:416–421, 2002.
37. Soliman DE, Maslow AD, Bokesch PM, et al: Transoesophageal echocardiography during scoliosis repair: Comparison with CVP monitoring, *Can J Anaesth* 45:925–932, 1998.
38. Cucchiara RF, Bowers B: Air embolism in children undergoing suboccipital craniotomy, *Anesthesiology* 57:338–339, 1982.
39. Harris MM, Yemen TA, Davidson A, et al: Venous embolism during craniectomy in supine infants, *Anesthesiology* 67:816–819, 1987.

40. Faberowski LW, Black S, Mickle JP: Incidence of venous air embolism during craniectomy for craniosynostosis repair, *Anesthesiology* 92: 20–23, 2000.

41. Soriano SG, McManus ML, Sullivan LJ, et al: Doppler sensor placement during neurosurgical procedures for children in the prone position, *J Neurosurg Anesthesiol* 6:153–155, 1994.

42. Haglund MM, Berger MS, Shamseldin M, et al: Cortical localization of temporal lobe language sites in patients with gliomas, *Neurosurgery* 34:567–576, 1994, discussion 576.

43. Adelson PD, Black PM, Madsen JR, et al: Use of subdural grids and strip electrodes to identify a seizure focus in children, *Pediatr Neurosurg* 22:174–180, 1995.

44. Ojemann SG, Berger MS, Lettich E, Ojemann GA: Localization of language function in children: Results of electrical stimulation mapping, *J Neurosurg* 98:465–470, 2003.

45. Penfield W: Combined regional and general anesthesia for craniotomy and cortical exploration: Part I: Neurosurgical considerations, *Anesth Analg* 33:145–155, 1954.

46. Soriano SG, Eldredge EA, Wang FK, et al: The effect of propofol on intraoperative electrocorticography and cortical stimulation during awake craniotomies in children, *Paediatr Anaesth* 10:29–34, 2000.

47. Keifer JC, Dentchev D, Little K, et al: A retrospective analysis of a remifentanil/propofol general anesthetic for craniotomy before awake functional brain mapping, *Anesth Analg* 101:502–508, 2005.

48. Ard J, Doyle W, Bekker A: Awake craniotomy with dexmedetomidine in pediatric patients, *J Neurosurg Anesthesiol* 15:263–266, 2003.

49. Banoub M, Tetzlaff JE, Schubert A: Pharmacologic and physiologic influences affecting sensory evoked potentials: Implications for perioperative monitoring, *Anesthesiology* 99:716–737, 2003.

50. Helmers SL, Hall JE: Intraoperative somatosensory evoked potential monitoring in pediatrics, *J Pediatr Orthop* 14:592–598, 1994.

51. Lotto ML, Banoub M, Schubert A: Effects of anesthetic agents and physiologic changes on intraoperative motor evoked potentials, *J Neurosurg Anesthesiol* 16:32–42, 2004.

52. Anand KJ, Hickey PR: Pain and its effects in the human neonate and fetus, *N Engl J Med* 317:1321–1329, 1987.

53. Viscomi CM, Abajian JC, Wald SL, et al: Spinal anesthesia for repair of meningomyelocele in neonates, *Anesth Analg* 81:492–495, 1995.

54. Sutton LN, Sun P, Adzick NS: Fetal neurosurgery, *Neurosurgery* 48:124–142, 2001.

55. Gaiser RR, Kurth CD: Anesthetic considerations for fetal surgery, *Semin Perinatol* 23:507–514, 1999.

56. O'Hara IB, Kurth CD: Anesthesia for fetal surgery. In Greeley WJ, editor: *Pediatric Anesthesia*, Philadelphia, 1999, Churchill Livingstone, pp 15.1–15.11.

57. Shillito J Jr: A plea for early operation for craniosynostosis, *Surg Neurol* 37:182–188, 1992.

58. Jimenez DF, Barone CM: Endoscopic craniectomy for early surgical correction of sagittal craniosynostosis, *J Neurosurg* 88:77–81, 1998.

59. Johnson JO, Jimenez DF, Barone CM: Blood loss after endoscopic strip craniectomy for craniosynostosis, *J Neurosurg Anesthesiol* 12:60, 2000.

60. Jimenez DF, Barone CM, Cartwright CC, Baker L: Early management of craniosynostosis using endoscopic-assisted strip craniectomies and cranial orthotic molding therapy, *Pediatrics* 110:97–104, 2002.

61. Tobias JD, Johnson JO, Jimenez DF, et al: Venous air embolism during endoscopic strip craniectomy for repair of craniosynostosis in infants, *Anesthesiology* 95:340–342, 2001.

62. McClain CD, Soriano SG, Goumnerova LC, et al: Detection of unanticipated intracranial hemorrhage during intraoperative magnetic resonance image–guided neurosurgery: Report of two cases, *J Neurosurg* 106:398–400, 2007.

63. Stokes MA, Soriano SG, Tarbell NJ, et al: Anesthesia for stereotactic radiosurgery in children, *J Neurosurg Anesthesiol* 7:100–108, 1995.

64. Soriano SG, Martyn JA: Antiepileptic-induced resistance to neuromuscular blockers: Mechanisms and clinical significance, *Clin Pharmacokinet* 43:71–81, 2004.

65. Eldredge EA, Soriano SG, Rockoff MA: Neuroanesthesia. *Neurosurg Clin N Am* 6:505–520, 1995.

66. Reasoner DK, Todd MM, Scamman FL, Warner DS: The incidence of pneumocephalus after supratentorial craniotomy: Observations on the disappearance of intracranial air, *Anesthesiology* 80:1008–1012, 1994.

67. Burrows PE, Robertson RL: Neonatal central nervous system vascular disorders, *Neurosurg Clin N Am* 9:155–180, 1998.

68. Morgan MK, Sekhon LH, Finfer S, Grinnell V: Delayed neurological deterioration following resection of arteriovenous malformations of the brain, *J Neurosurg* 90:695–701, 1999.

69. Soriano SG, Sethna NF, Scott RM: Anesthetic management of children with moyamoya syndrome, *Anesth Analg* 77:1066–1070, 1993.

70. Kuwabara Y, Ichiya Y, Sasaki M, et al: Response to hypercapnia in moyamoya disease: Cerebrovascular response to hypercapnia in pediatric and adult patients with moyamoya disease, *Stroke* 28:701–707, 1997.

71. Lam WH, MacKersie A: Paediatric head injury: Incidence, aetiology and management, *Paediatr Anaesth* 9:377–385, 1999.

72. Duhaime AC, Christian CW, Rorke LB, Zimmerman RA: Nonaccidental head injury in infants—the "shaken-baby syndrome" [see comments], *N Engl J Med* 338:1822–1829, 1998.

73. Adelson PD, Bratton SL, Carney NA, et al: American Association for Surgery of Trauma; Child Neurology Society; International Society for Pediatric Neurosurgery; International Trauma Anesthesia and Critical Care Society; Society of Critical Care Medicine; World Federation of Pediatric Intensive and Critical Care Societies Guidelines for the acute medical management of severe traumatic brain injury in infants, children, and adolescents, *Pediatr Crit Care Med* 4:1–75, 2003.

74. Holzman RS: Clinical management of latex-allergic children, *Anesth Analg* 85:529–533, 1997.

75. Legatt AD, Schroeder CE, Gill B, Goodrich JT: Electrical stimulation and multichannel EMG recording for identification of functional neural tissue during cauda equina surgery, *Childs Nerv Syst* 8:185–189, 1992.

76. Logigian EL, Wolinsky JS, Soriano SG, et al: H reflex studies in cerebral palsy patients undergoing partial dorsal rhizotomy [see comments], *Muscle Nerve* 17:539–549, 1994.

77. Soriano SG, Logigian EL, Scott RM, et al: Nitrous oxide depresses the H-reflex in children with cerebral palsy, *Anesth Analg* 80:239–241, 1995.

78. Johnson JO, Jimenez DF, Tobias JD: Anaesthetic care during minimally invasive neurosurgical procedures in infants and children, *Paediatr Anaesth* 12:478–488, 2002.

79. Rekate HL: Selecting patients for endoscopic third ventriculostomy, *Neurosurg Clin N Am* 15:39–49, 2004.

80. El-Dawlatly AA, Murshid WR, Elshimy A, et al: The incidence of bradycardia during endoscopic third ventriculostomy, *Anesth Analg* 91:1142–1144, 2000.

81. El-Dawlatly AA, Murshid W, Alshimy A, et al: Arrhythmias during neuroendoscopic procedures, *J Neurosurg Anesthesiol* 13:57–58, 2001.

82. American Academy of Pediatrics Committee on Drugs: Guidelines for monitoring and management of pediatric patients during and after sedation for diagnostic and therapeutic procedures, *Pediatrics* 89:1110–1115, 1992.

83. Practice guidelines for sedation and analgesia by non-anesthesiologists: A report by the American Society of Anesthesiologists Task Force on Sedation and Analgesia by Non-Anesthesiologists, *Anesthesiology* 84:459–471, 1996.

84. Bell MJ, Carpenter J, Au AK, et al: Development of a pediatric neurocritical care service, *Neurocrit Care* 10:4–10, 2009.

85. Ventilation with lower tidal volumes as compared with traditional tidal volumes for acute lung injury and the acute respiratory distress syndrome. The Acute Respiratory Distress Syndrome Network, *N Engl J Med* 342:1301–1308, 2000.

86. Feldman Z, Robertson CS, Contant CF, et al: Positive end expiratory pressure reduces intracranial compliance in the rabbit, *J Neurosurg Anesthesiol* 9:175–179, 1997.

87. Caricato A, Conti G, Della CF, et al: Effects of PEEP on the intracranial system of patients with head injury and subarachnoid hemorrhage: The role of respiratory system compliance, *J Trauma* 58:571–576, 2005.

88. Huynh T, Messer M, Sing RF, et al: Positive end-expiratory pressure alters intracranial and cerebral perfusion pressure in severe traumatic brain injury, *J Trauma* 53:488–492, 2002.

89. Bennett SS, Graffagnino C, Borel CO, James ML: Use of high frequency oscillatory ventilation (HFOV) in neurocritical care patients, *Neurocrit Care* 7:221–226, 2007.

90. Stewart AR, Finer NN, Peters KL: Effects of alterations of inspiratory and expiratory pressures and inspiratory/expiratory ratios on mean airway pressure, blood gases, and intracranial pressure, *Pediatrics* 67:474–481, 1981.

91. Adelson PD, Bratton SL, Carney NA, et al: Use of sedation and neuromuscular blockade in the treatment of severe pediatric traumatic brain injury, *Pediatr Crit Care Med* 4:S34–S37, 2003.

92. Munro MJ, Walker AM, Barfield CP: Hypotensive extremely low birth weight infants have reduced cerebral blood flow, *Pediatrics* 114:1591–1596, 2004.

93. Seri I: Management of hypotension and low systemic blood flow in the very low birth weight neonate during the first postnatal week, *J Perinatol* 26(Suppl 1):S8–S13, 2006.

94. Soul JS, Hammer PE, Tsuji M, et al: Fluctuating pressure-passivity is common in the cerebral circulation of sick premature infants, *Pediatr Res* 61:467–473, 2007.

95. Wong FY, Leung TS, Austin T, et al: Impaired autoregulation in preterm infants identified by using spatially resolved spectroscopy, *Pediatrics* 121:e604–e611, 2008.

96. Chambers IR, Jones PA, Lo TY, et al: Critical thresholds of intracranial pressure and cerebral perfusion pressure related to age in paediatric head injury, *J Neurol Neurosurg Psychiatry* 77:234–240, 2006.

97. Carter BG, Butt W, Taylor A: ICP and CPP: Excellent predictors of long term outcome in severely brain injured children, *Childs Nerv Syst* 24:245–251, 2008.

98. Huang SJ, Hong WC, Han YY, et al: Clinical outcome of severe head injury using three different ICP and CPP protocol-driven therapies, *J Clin Neurosci* 13:818–822, 2006.

99. Sahuquillo J, Arikan F: Decompressive craniectomy for the treatment of refractory high intracranial pressure in traumatic brain injury, *Cochrane Database Syst Rev* (1)2006:CD003983.

100. Au AK, Ray PE, McBryde KD, et al: Incidence of postoperative hyponatremia and complications in critically-ill children treated with hypotonic and normotonic solutions, *J Pediatr* 152:33–38, 2008.

101. Porzio P, Halberthal M, Bohn D, Halperin ML: Treatment of acute hyponatremia: Ensuring the excretion of a predictable amount of electrolyte-free water, *Crit Care Med* 28:1905–1910, 2000.

102. Choong K, Kho ME, Menon K, Bohn D: Hypotonic versus isotonic saline in hospitalised children: A systematic review, *Arch Dis Child* 91:828–835, 2006.

103. Celik US, Alabaz D, Yildizdas D, et al: Cerebral salt wasting in tuberculous meningitis: Treatment with fludrocortisone, *Ann Trop Paediatr* 25:297–302, 2005.

104. Levine JP, Stelnicki E, Weiner HL, et al: Hyponatremia in the postoperative craniofacial pediatric patient population: A connection to cerebral salt wasting syndrome and management of the disorder, *Plast Reconstr Surg* 108:1501–1508, 2001.

105. Byeon JH, Yoo G: Cerebral salt wasting syndrome after calvarial remodeling in craniosynostosis, *J Korean Med Sci* 20:866–869, 2005.

106. Jimenez R, Casado-Flores J, Nieto M, Garcia-Teresa MA: Cerebral salt wasting syndrome in children with acute central nervous system injury, *Pediatr Neurol* 35:261–263, 2006.

107. Singh S, Bohn D, Carlotti AP, et al: Cerebral salt wasting: Truths, fallacies, theories, and challenges, *Crit Care Med* 30:2575–2579, 2002.

108. Berger TM, Kistler W, Berendes E, et al: Hyponatremia in a pediatric stroke patient: Syndrome of inappropriate antidiuretic hormone secretion or cerebral salt wasting? *Crit Care Med* 30:792–795, 2002.

109. Sakarcan A, Bocchini J Jr: The role of fludrocortisone in a child with cerebral salt wasting, *Pediatr Nephrol* 12:769–771, 1998.

110. Papadimitriou DT, Spiteri A, Pagnier A, et al: Mineralocorticoid deficiency in post-operative cerebral salt wasting, *J Pediatr Endocrinol Metab* 20:1145–1150, 2007.

111. Taplin CE, Cowell CT, Silink M, Ambler GR: Fludrocortisone therapy in cerebral salt wasting, *Pediatrics* 118:e1904–e1908, 2006.

112. Di RC, Caldarelli M, Tamburrini G, Massimi L: Surgical management of craniopharyngiomas—experience with a pediatric series, *J Pediatr Endocrinol Metab* 19(Suppl 1):355–366, 2006.

113. Wise-Faberowski L, Soriano SG, Ferrari L, et al: Perioperative management of diabetes insipidus in children, *J Neurosurg Anesthesiol* 16:200–205, 2004.

114. Hutchens MP, Memtsoudis S, Sadovnikoff N: Propofol for sedation in neuro-intensive care, *Neurocrit Care* 4:54–62, 2006.

115. Cray SH, Robinson BH, Cox PN: Lactic acidemia and bradyarrhythmia in a child sedated with propofol [see comments], *Crit Care Med* 26:2087–2092, 1998.

116. Kumar MA, Urrutia VC, Thomas CE, et al: The syndrome of irreversible acidosis after prolonged propofol infusion, *Neurocrit Care* 3:257–259, 2005.

117. Hertzog JH, Dalton HJ, Anderson BD, et al: Prospective evaluation of propofol anesthesia in the pediatric intensive care unit for elective oncology procedures in ambulatory and hospitalized children, *Pediatrics* 106:742–747, 2000.

118. Vardi A, Salem Y, Padeh S, et al: Is propofol safe for procedural sedation in children? A prospective evaluation of propofol versus ketamine in pediatric critical care, *Crit Care Med* 30:1231–1236, 2002.

119. Wheeler DS, Vaux KK, Ponaman ML, Poss BW: The safe and effective use of propofol sedation in children undergoing diagnostic and therapeutic procedures: Experience in a pediatric ICU and a review of the literature, *Pediatr Emerg Care* 19:385–392, 2003.

120. Diaz SM, Rodarte A, Foley J, Capparelli EV: Pharmacokinetics of dexmedetomidine in postsurgical pediatric intensive care unit patients: Preliminary study, *Pediatr Crit Care Med* 8:419–424, 2007.

121. Tobias JD: Dexmedetomidine to treat opioid withdrawal in infants following prolonged sedation in the pediatric ICU, *J Opioid Manag* 2:201–205, 2006.

122. Rhoney DH, Murry KR: National survey on the use of sedatives and neuromuscular blocking agents in the pediatric intensive care unit, *Pediatr Crit Care Med* 3:129–133, 2002.

123. Marx CM, Smith PG, Lowrie LH, et al: Optimal sedation of mechanically ventilated pediatric critical care patients, *Crit Care Med* 22:163–170, 1994.

124. Ista E, van DM, Tibboel D, de HM: Assessment of sedation levels in pediatric intensive care patients can be improved by using the COMFORT "behavior" scale, *Pediatr Crit Care Med* 6:58–63, 2005.

125. Dulin PG, Williams CJ: Monitoring and preventive care of the paralyzed patient in respiratory failure, *Crit Care Clin* 10:815–829, 1994.

126. Tobias JD: Tolerance, withdrawal, and physical dependency after long-term sedation and analgesia of children in the pediatric intensive care unit, *Crit Care Med* 28:2122–2232, 2000.

127. Abend NS, Dlugos DJ: Nonconvulsive status epilepticus in a pediatric intensive care unit, *Pediatr Neurol* 37:165–170, 2007.

128. Wolf GK, McClain CD, Zurakowski D, et al: Total phenytoin concentrations do not accurately predict free phenytoin concentrations in critically ill children, *Pediatr Crit Care Med* 7:434–439, 2006.

129. Riviello JJ Jr, Holmes GL: The treatment of status epilepticus, *Semin Pediatr Neurol* 11:129–138, 2004.

130. Schor NF, Riviello JJ Jr: Treatment with propofol: The new status quo for status epilepticus? *Neurology* 65:506–507, 2005.

131. Tilford JM, Simpson PM, Yeh TS, et al: Variation in therapy and outcome for pediatric head trauma patients, *Crit Care Med* 29:1056–1061, 2001.

132. Young KD, Okada PJ, Sokolove PE, et al: A randomized, double-blinded, placebo-controlled trial of phenytoin for the prevention of early posttraumatic seizures in children with moderate to severe blunt head injury, *Ann Emerg Med* 43:435–446, 2004.

133. Adelson PD, Bratton SL, Carney NA, et al: The role of anti-seizure prophylaxis following severe pediatric traumatic brain injury, *Pediatr Crit Care Med* 4:S72–S75, 2003.

134. Adelson PD, Bratton SL, Carney NA, et al: Indications for intracranial pressure monitoring in pediatric patients with severe traumatic brain injury, *Pediatr Crit Care Med* 4:S19–S24, 2003.

135. Edwards P, Arango M, Balica L, et al: CRASH trial collaborators: Final results of MRC CRASH, a randomised placebo-controlled trial of intravenous corticosteroid in adults with head injury-outcomes at 6 months *Lancet*, 365:1957–1959, 2005.

136. Myburgh J, Cooper DJ, Finfer S, et al: Saline or albumin for fluid resuscitation in patients with traumatic brain injury, *N Engl J Med* 357:874–884, 2007.

137. Adelson PD, Bratton SL, Carney NA, et al: Use of hyperventilation in the acute management of severe pediatric traumatic brain injury, *Pediatr Crit Care Med* 4:S45–S48, 2003.

138. Skippen P, Seear M, Poskitt K, et al: Effect of hyperventilation on regional cerebral blood flow in head-injured children, *Crit Care Med* 25:1402–1409, 1997.

139. Stringer WA, Hasso AN, Thompson JR, et al: Hyperventilation-induced cerebral ischemia in patients with acute brain lesions: demonstration by xenon-enhanced CT, *AJNR Am J Neuroradiol* 14:475–484, 1993.

Chapter 20

NEUROSURGICAL DISEASES AND TRAUMA OF THE SPINE AND SPINAL CORD: ANESTHETIC CONSIDERATIONS

Gary R. Stier • Cassie L. Gabriel • Daniel J. Cole

The first descriptions of spine disorders were recorded nearly 4000 years ago in Egypt, when patients with such afflictions were left bedridden and death was considered unavoidable. One of the first extensive series on surgery of the spine was reported by Elsberg in 1925, in which the surgical treatment of spinal cord tumors was described.[1] Since those early reports, spine surgery has made remarkable advancements, particularly since the 1980s. As surgical techniques have matured, complex operations are being performed on spine diseases once thought incurable. Moreover, increasingly older patients with multiple comorbidities are presenting for spine procedures. Consequently, the anesthetic approach to patients scheduled for spine surgery must consider the following issues: preoperative risk assessment, the specific spine pathology being treated, basic knowledge of spine anatomy and imaging modalities, the surgical procedure planned, an awareness of the specific spine disorder being treated, potential airway difficulties, patient positioning, anesthetic choices, intraoperative medical management decision-making (blood replacement, blood salvage, hemodynamic goals, pulmonary function), and postoperative airway concerns and pain management. This chapter discusses these issues.

ANATOMY

The anatomy of the spine can be divided into that pertaining to the vertebral bony column and the contents of the vertebral canal.[2]

Vertebral Column

The vertebral column is composed of 33 vertebrae. In adult life this number is functionally reduced to 24 presacral vertebrae, the sacrum, and the coccyx. The presacral vertebrae consist of 7 cervical, 12 thoracic, and 5 lumbar bones. The 5 sacral and 4 coccygeal vertebrae fuse early in development. The vertebral column normally exhibits four curves in the anteroposterior (AP) plane. The two forward curves, or lordoses, are in the cervical and lumbar areas, and the two posterior curves, or kyphoses, are in the thoracic and sacral areas. The combination of these curves gives the normal bony spine the characteristic S shape when viewed from the side (Fig. 20-1).

Each of the individual "standard" vertebrae that make up the vertebral column is a single bony structure consisting of a large body, bilateral pedicles, bilateral lamina, bilateral transverse processes, a spinous process, and four articular processes (Fig. 20-2). The two pedicles laterally, the two lamina posteriorly, and the body anteriorly together form the vertebral canal in which lies the spinal cord. The segmental nerves exit between the vertebrae through the intervertebral foramina. The four articular processes mate with corresponding processes on the vertebrae above and below to form the facet joints. The facet joint articulations provide posterior stability, and the body articulations provide anterior and vertical stability. In addition, the facet joints provide flexion, extension, and lateral rotation of the spine.

The first two cervical vertebrae, C1 and C2, differ in structure from the standard vertebrae (Fig. 20-3). C1, the atlas, is ring-shaped and wider than the other vertebrae. The superior articular surfaces are configured to articulate with the two occipital condyles located at the base of the skull on either side of the foramen magnum. The atlas is composed of anterior and posterior arches, each possessing a tubercle while sharing lateral masses. The atlas has no spinous processes or body. C2, the axis, possesses a body that projects superiorly as the dens (odontoid process) (see Fig. 20-3), and a short bifid spinous process. The axis has two large flat superior articular facets. The transverse ligament of the atlas holds the dens in place, preventing horizontal movement of the atlas.

The anterior longitudinal ligament and the posterior longitudinal ligament (see Fig. 20-2) extend from the base of the skull and atlas to the sacrum. The anterior ligament is attached to the anterior surface of the vertebrae and intervertebral disks. The posterior ligament is attached to the posterior surface of the vertebrae and the intervertebral disks and lies within the vertebral canal. These two ligaments provide extension and flexion stability to the vertebral column. The supraspinal and interspinal ligaments join the spinous processes at each level, providing additional flexion stability. The ligamentum flavum unites the vertebral laminae at each level and forms part of the posterior border of the intervertebral foramen.

The intervertebral disks are fibrocartilaginous joints composed of an interior nucleus pulposus surrounded and enclosed by a tough anulus fibrosus (Fig. 20-4). Together, these two components provide a strong attachment between adjacent vertebrae but allow some movement. In addition, the disks act as very efficient shock absorbers.

The facet joints are synovial joints, which are paired and compose part of the posterior elements of the vertebral column. With the intervertebral disks they form the remaining articulations of the vertebrae with each other. As posterior elements, the facet joints allow flexion of the spine. The facet joints of the cervical region are less rigid, thus allowing greater flexion of the neck.

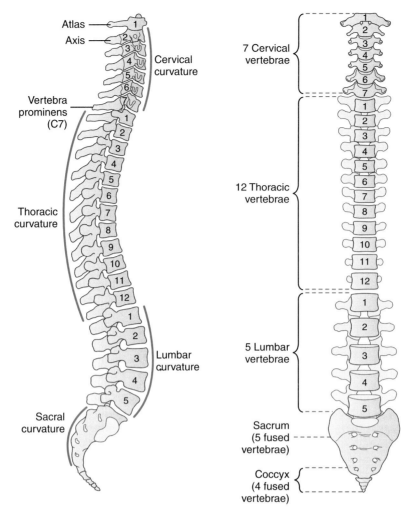

Figure 20–1 Vertebral column showing 24 presacral vertebrae, sacrum, coccyx, and curvatures of the adult vertebral column. Note that the first coccygeal vertebra has fused with the sacrum. Most vertebral columns are 72 to 75 cm long; about one fourth of this length is contributed by the fibrocartilaginous intervertebral disks. The vertebral column supports the skull and transmits the weight of the body through the pelvis to the lower limbs. *(From Moore KL: Clinically Oriented Anatomy, 2nd ed, Baltimore, Williams & Wilkins, 1985, p 566.).*

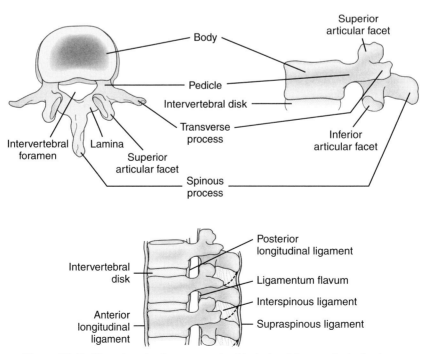

Figure 20–2 Normal anatomic components of typical vertebrae and spinal column.

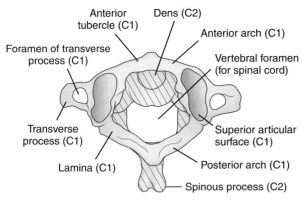

View from above

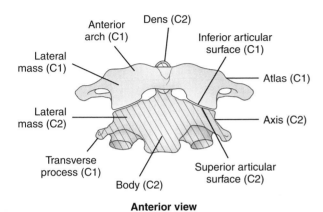

Anterior view

Figure 20–3 C1 and C2 cervical vertebrae, viewed from above and in anterior view.

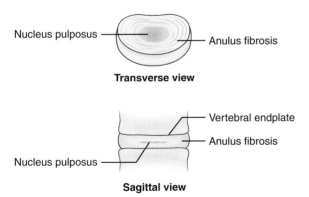

Transverse view

Sagittal view

Figure 20–4 Transverse and sagittal images of an intervertebral disk.

Spinal Cord

The spinal cord is contained within the confines of the vertebral canal. The anteroposterior (AP) diameter of the cervical cord constitutes about 40% of the diameter of the cervical canal, decreasing in diameter with neck extension. The spinal cord is contiguous with the brainstem at the foramen magnum, and in the adult it extends to the conus medullaris at about the level of the first or second lumbar vertebra. The filum terminale attaches the end of the conus to the first coccygeal segment of the bony spine. The cord exhibits two

prominent bulges in the cervical and lumbar areas, which correspond to the origins of the nerves to the upper and lower extremities, respectively. A cross section of the cord reveals a mixture of white matter and gray matter (Fig. 20-5). The gray matter, in the shape of an H, surrounds the central canal and contains the cell bodies of the spinal neurons.

The dorsal horns are associated with sensory functions, including pain, position sense, touch, and temperature. The ventral horns contain neurons associated with motor functions and spinal reflexes. The surrounding white matter contains the myelinated and unmyelinated fibers that communicate with higher and lower centers, including the brainstem and cerebral cortex. The descending motor pathways travel in the white matter located in the lateral and ventral areas of the cord. The corticospinal tract conducts all primary motor impulses. The vestibulospinal and rubrospinal tracts also participate in motor function and are located in the ventral and lateral areas of white matter, respectively. The dorsal areas of white matter contain the dorsal column tracts, the spinothalamic tracts, and the spinoreticular tracts, among others. These pathways transmit sensory information to higher cord segments and the brain.

The sympathetic nervous system is also segmental and traverses the length of the vertebral column in two chains anterior to the bony spine (Fig. 20-6).[3] Segmental communication is accomplished at each spinal segment via the communicating ramus of each segmental spinal nerve. The segmental spinal nerves are made up of the confluence of a dorsal root and a ventral root at each level (see Fig. 20-6).

A nerve emerges from each side of the spinal cord; thus they are paired. The dorsal roots conduct sensory information, including pain. All nerve cell bodies of afferent axons are located in the dorsal root ganglion. The ventral roots conduct primarily motor and efferent information from the cord to the periphery. The two roots combine in the spinal nerve as they traverse the vertebral foramen. The nerve then divides into three rami: dorsal, ventral, and communicating. The ventral ramus continues as the primary spinal nerve, the dorsal ramus innervates the paraspinous muscles of the back and the facet joints at each level, and the communicating ramus provides segmental neuronal connections to the sympathetic chains.

The spinal nerves have a particular relationship to the respective spinal vertebrae (Fig. 20-7). The spinal nerves exit the vertebral canal via the intervertebral foramina. These foramina are formed by the juxtaposition of adjoining vertebrae in the spinal column.

Spinal Cord Blood Supply

The spinal cord is supplied with blood from the aorta via the vertebral and segmental or radicular arteries; the three main arteries of the spinal cord are the single anterior spinal artery in the anterior or ventral median sulcus and two posterior spinal arteries located in the area of the dorsal nerve rootlets (Fig. 20-8). These three arteries usually arise as branches of the vertebral arteries at the base of the brainstem and traverse the entire length of the cord (Fig. 20-9). The blood flow is augmented by multiple segmental radicular and medullary arteries that enter at the intervertebral foramen (see Figs. 20-8 and 20-9).

The anterior spinal artery supplies the anterior two thirds of the cord, and the posterior spinal arteries supply the posterior one third. Below the level of the cervical cord segments,

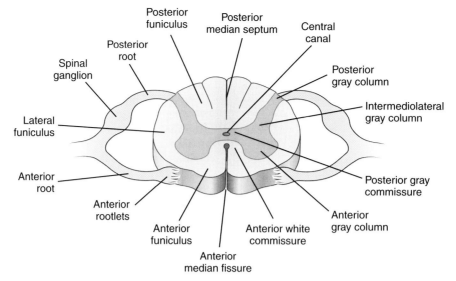

Figure 20–5 Anatomy of the spinal cord.

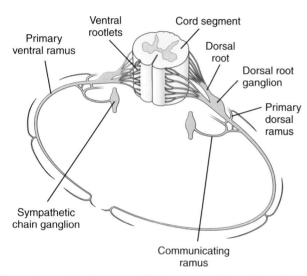

Figure 20–6 Cord segment with its roots, ganglia, and branches.

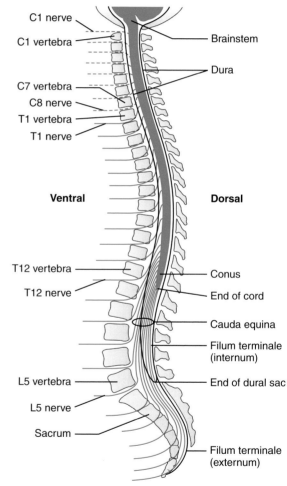

Figure 20–7 Lateral view of the relationships among spinal cord, spinal nerves, and vertebral column. Termination of the dura (dura mater spinalis) and its continuation as the filum terminale externum are shown.

additional blood supply is provided by segmental or radicular arteries that arise as branches of the aorta and enter the cord arterial system. The most consistent of these arteries is the artery of Adamkiewicz, which is the largest segmental feeder in the thoracolumbar region of the cord. It usually enters as a single vessel between the ninth and the eleventh thoracic levels and arises on the left side of the aorta.[2] This major arterial feeder vessel is thought to be the principal contributor to the arterial supply of the entire thoracic and lumbar cord distal to its entry. Loss of this artery after surgery or trauma to the aorta may produce paraplegia in the thoracic region.[4]

The arterial network of the three main blood vessels supplies blood to the interior of the cord through an extensive network of arterioles and capillaries. The density of the capillary bed reflects the metabolic demands of the different areas of the cord. Blood flow through these capillaries is very sensitive to compression of the cord, and ischemia may result.

Venous drainage of the spinal cord is through radial veins serving the parenchyma.[2] The veins feed into the coronal venous plexus or longitudinal veins on the surface of the cord, which are, in turn, drained by medullary veins that penetrate the dura adjacent to the dural penetration of the nerve roots to join the epidural venous plexus. The epidural or internal vertebral venous system drains into the external vertebral venous system, which communicates with the caval veins.

The veins in the epidural system are valveless and therefore subject to engorgement in certain normal and disease states, such as pregnancy and obesity, in which there is an increase in the intra-abdominal pressure or obstruction to venous flow through the inferior vena cava.

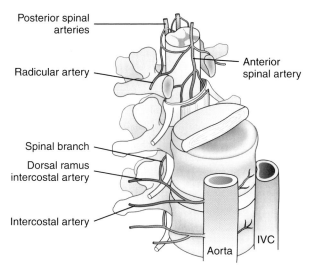

Figure 20–8 Blood supply of the spinal cord illustrating the single anterior spinal artery, paired posterior arteries, and feeding radicular branches from the aorta. IVC, inferior vena cava.

PHYSIOLOGY

Blood Flow

Spinal cord blood flow (SCBF) has been studied extensively in animal models. The values and data obtained from these studies are consistent with values obtained for the brain; average SCBF is about 60 mL/100 g/min,[5,6] including a threefold to fourfold gray matter–white matter differential in blood flow.[7] Autoregulation in the cord mimics that in the brain, with flow well maintained with a mean arterial blood pressure (MAP) of 60 to 120 mm Hg.[7] Likewise, the effects of arterial blood gas tensions are similar to those in the brain; hypoxemia and hypercapnia cause vasodilation, and hypocapnia causes vasoconstriction (Fig. 20-10).[8]

Injury to the spinal cord disturbs autoregulation of blood flow. Trauma to the cord results in a decrease in SCBF and loss of autoregulatory function.[9,10] The nature of the operative procedure itself may also have an effect on SCBF. This effect is well recognized with spinal distraction and instrumentation but may also occur during other operations, such as simple laminectomy.[11]

RADIOLOGIC CONSIDERATIONS

Imaging of the spine and spinal cord is an essential part of the diagnosis and treatment of spinal diseases. A variety of imaging modalities are available for the assessment of spinal pathology,

347

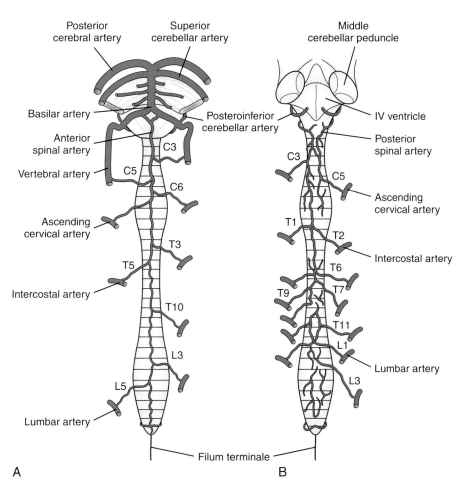

A   B

Figure 20–9 Arteries of spinal cord. **A,** Ventral aspect. **B,** Dorsal aspect. Regions most vulnerable to vascular deprivation when the contributing arteries are injured are T3-T5 and T12-L2 for anterior spinal artery and C8-T4 for dorsal circulation. Levels of entry of common radicular branches are shown (e.g., C5 and T5). Note that the spinal cord is enlarged in two regions for innervation of the limbs. Cervical enlargement extends from C4 to T1, and lumbosacral enlargement extends from L2 to S3. *(From Moore KL: Clinically Oriented Anatomy, 2nd ed. Baltimore, Williams & Wilkins, 1985, p 613.)*

the most common of which are plain radiography, computed tomography (CT), CT angiography, magnetic resonance imaging (MRI), MR angiography, bone scanning, single-photon emission computed tomography (SPECT), and positron emission tomography (PET). The choice of imaging modalities best suited for the patient depends on the history, physical findings, and differential diagnosis. A general review of the common imaging techniques used in spine disease can be found in the later section on traumatic spinal cord injury (SCI).

SURGICAL DISORDERS OF THE SPINE

Disorders of the Cervical Spine

Cervical Spondylosis

Degenerative disease of the cervical spine affects more than 90% of individuals older than 65 years. The term *cervical spondylosis* refers to the nonspecific degenerative process of the spine that results in spinal stenosis as well as neural foraminal encroachment (Fig. 20-11).[12]

In those individuals who eventually experience symptoms of cervical degenerative disease, radiculopathy is the most common. *Cervical radiculopathy* is defined as a neurologic condition characterized by dysfunction of a cervical spinal nerve, the nerve roots, or both.[13] It is most commonly caused by lateral disk herniation, osteophyte overgrowth with narrowing of the lateral foramen (termed the *lateral recess syndrome*), or cervical spinal instability caused by subluxation of a cervical vertebra (Fig. 20-12).

MRI is the imaging modality of choice in the diagnosis of cervical radiculopathy; however, MRI is not indicated in the initial stages of management because the findings will not alter treatment. In general, medical management is attempted for 4 to 6 weeks, and if the patient remains symptomatic, an MRI study is appropriate. CT is of value primarily for defining the bony anatomy in the area of the spinal canal. Surgical treatment for cervical radiculopathy is indicated for severe clinical symptoms that medical therapy has failed to control combined with a compatible MRI study demonstrating nerve compression, for the persistence of pain despite medical management for at least 6 weeks, and for the presence of an evolving neurologic deficit.[13]

Cervical Spondylotic Myelopathy

Cervical spondylotic myelopathy (CSM) is the most common type of spinal cord dysfunction in patients older than 55 years. Originally described more than 50 years ago, CSM is the result of narrowing of the cervical spinal canal due to a degenerative process or a congenital disorder. The primary pathophysiologic abnormality in CSM is a reduction in the sagittal diameter of spinal canal, with cervical myelopathy developing in nearly all patients in whom there is a greater than 30% reduction in the cross-sectional area of the cervical vertebral canal.[14,15] Typical signs and symptoms of CSM are pain in the neck, shoulder, and subscapular areas; numbness or tingling in the upper extremities; motor weakness in the upper or lower extremities; sensory changes in the lower extremities; gait disturbances; bowel and bladder dysfunction; and spasticity, hyperreflexia, and clonus typical of an upper motor neuron lesion. The most common presentation of CSM is a spastic gait. Physical findings include atrophy of the muscles of the hand, hyperreflexia, electric shock–like sensations down the arm or back after flexion of the neck (Lhermitte's sign), and sensory loss. Plain films often show evidence of osteophyte formation, kyphosis, and subluxation. MRI remains the imaging modality of choice, providing information about the

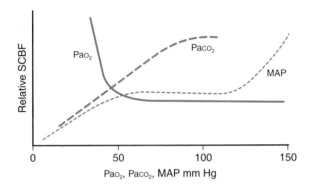

Figure 20–10 Illustration of effect of changes in $Paco_2$, Pao_2, and mean arterial pressure (MAP) on spinal cord blood flow (SCBF).

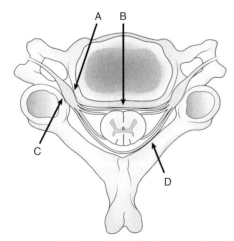

Figure 20–11 Cervical spondylosis.[12] Common sites of pathology that may result in compression of the spinal cord or nerve root: A, Lateral disk herniation or osteophyte hypertrophy; B, Central disk herniation or osteophyte formation; C, Facet joint osteophyte; D, Hypertrophy of the ligamentum flavum.

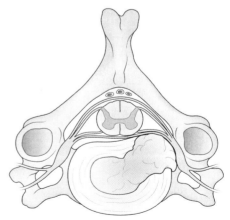

Figure 20–12 Cervical radiculopathy caused by foraminal stenosis from a posterolateral herniation of the nucleus pulposus with compression of the exiting nerve root. *(From Won DS, Herkowitz HN: Cervical radiculopathy: Posterior surgical approach. In Herkowitz HN, Garfin SR, Eismont FJ, et al [eds], Rothman-Simeone: The Spine, 5th ed. Philadelphia, Saunders-Elsevier, 2006, p 842.)*

spinal canal (demyelination, spinal cord atrophy, and edema), intervertebral disks, vertebral osteophytes, and ligaments. Treatment of CSM initially involves nonoperative therapy; however, early surgery is associated with significant improvement in the neurologic prognosis.

For patients with symptomatic spinal stenosis, anesthetic management should consider the benefits of an awake fiberoptic intubation or at least induction of general anesthesia with the head stabilized and intubation performed under fiberoptic guidance with the use of spinal cord monitoring. During these operations, spinal cord monitoring may provide useful feedback on potential SCI during the procedure and allow the operation to be modified to minimize adverse effects on spinal cord function.

Cervical Disk Herniation

Intervertebral disks are composed of a well-hydrated central nucleus pulposus surrounded by an outer anulus fibrosis. With age, the disks deteriorate, ultimately resulting in herniation when the anulus fibrosus breaks open or cracks, allowing the nucleus pulposus to extrude (see Fig. 20-12).

In the cervical spine, the most common location of the herniation is at C5-C6, followed by C6-C7, and herniation is most common in individuals older than 40 years. The symptoms of a cervical disk herniation are neck pain and radicular symptoms, which consist of shoulder, arm, or hand paresthesias or pain, and muscle weakness in a dermatomal nerve root distribution. Patients may also present with symptoms of a cervical myelopathy if the herniation is centrally located. In patients in whom a disk herniation is suspected, plain films may demonstrate a narrowed disk space, osteophytes, or subluxation of the vertebra. An MRI study is the radiologic imaging modality of choice for evaluation of a suspected herniated cervical disk (Fig. 20-13).

The primary treatment of a cervical disk herniation is medical management, at least initially. Cervical soft collars, anti-inflammatory agents, oral steroids, and physical therapy are all appropriate in the short term because more than 90% of patients with radiculopathic symptoms experience improvement with

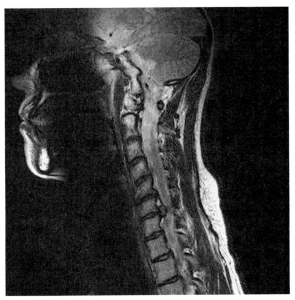

Figure 20–13 Cervical disk herniation and anterior cervical diskectomy and fusion (ACD & F). A 41-year-old woman presented with pain in the neck that radiated to the left hand and fingers. This sagittal T2-weighted magnetic resonance image shows a 6-mm disk protrusion at C6-C7.

these measures. If nonsurgical therapy fails or the patient demonstrates progressive neurologic symptoms, surgical therapy is selected, typically an anterior cervical diskectomy and fusion (ACD&F) with or without anterior cervical plating.

Complications of surgery include thoracic duct injury, cerebrospinal fluid (CSF) leak, spinal cord or nerve root injury, vertebral artery injury, perforation of the esophagus or trachea, recurrent laryngeal nerve injury (vocal cord paralysis), postoperative hematoma, and wound infection. In instances in which there is a significant postoperative hematoma, the airway should be left secured until the patient is fully awake, the hematoma is not enlarging, and there is a tracheal cuff leak.

Syringomyelia

Syringomyelia refers to the cystic cavitation of the spinal cord. Two main forms of syringomyelia have been described: communicating syringomyelia and noncommunicating syringomyelia. In communicating syringomyelia, there is primary dilatation of the central canal that is often associated with abnormalities at the foramen magnum such as tonsillar herniation (Chiari malformation) and basal arachnoiditis. In noncommunicating syringomyelia, a cyst arises within the cord substance itself and does not communicate with the central canal or subarachnoid space. Common causes of noncommunicating syringomyelia include trauma (most common), neoplasm, and arachnoiditis. In the typical presentation, an adult between the ages of 20 and 50 years complains of sensory loss (similar to central cord syndrome) in a "cape" distribution, cervical or occipital pain, wasting in the hands, and painless arthropathies. MRI is the investigation of choice and should include images of the cervical and thoracic spinal cord as well as the brain. Treatment focuses upon reestablishing normal CSF flow across the site of the injury. Therapeutic choices include a posterior decompression procedure, placement of a shunt with direct drainage of the cyst into the subarachnoid space or pleural cavity, and a percutaneous aspiration of the cyst.

Disorders of the Thoracic and Lumbar Spine

Herniated Disk

Symptomatic thoracic disk herniations are rare, with an annual incidence of 1 per 1 million patients.[16] Thoracic disk herniations occur most commonly at T8-T12, with a peak incidence between the ages of 40 and 60 years (mean, 46 years).[17] The majority of disk herniations are located centrolaterally (94%) or laterally (6%) and manifest a variety of symptoms and signs, including pain (localized, axial, or radicular), myelopathy, sensory disturbances, and bladder dysfunction.[17] The radiographic diagnosis is made through a combination of plain films and MRI. The majority of symptomatic thoracic disk herniations are effectively managed with nonoperative therapy alone. Indications for surgery include failure of a 4-to 6-week trial of medical treatment; severe, persistent radicular pain; and significant neurologic deficits, particularly if there is any progression of symptoms. Major surgical complications are uncommon; they include death from cardiopulmonary compromise, spinal instability requiring further surgery, and an increase in the severity of a preoperative paraparesis.[17]

Unlike a thoracic disk herniation, a lumbar disk herniation is very common, occurring in 2% of the general population at some time in their lives.[18] Sciatica, resulting from a herniated lumbar disk, is the most common cause of radicular leg pain in the adult working population.[19] Fortunately, the symptoms of sciatica typically resolve within 2 months from the onset in patients who are treated medically, and surgery is rarely necessary. The majority of lumbar herniations occur at the L4-L5 or L5-S1 spinal levels, most often posterolaterally, where the posterior longitudinal ligament is thinnest. The symptoms of a lumbar disk herniation range from lower back pain to radiculopathy with leg pain, weakness, and paresthesias. With a large centrally located disk herniation, the cauda equina syndrome may occur, resulting in lower back pain, bilateral lower extremity sensorimotor deficits, bladder dysfunction, sexual dysfunction, and perirectal sensory loss. The presence of the cauda equinae syndrome warrants urgent medical attention. MRI is the imaging modality of choice for suspected herniation of an intervertebral disk, as it clearly defines the local anatomy (Fig. 20-14).

The majority of patients with disk herniations are treated medically. With such treatments, more than 75% of patients recover within 6 to 8 weeks. Accepted indications for surgical therapy include the cauda equina syndrome; significant motor deficits; severe pain unresponsive to medical therapy; failure of conservative therapy after 2 to 3 months; and large extruded disk fragments.

Lumbar Spondylosis

Lumbar spondylosis is a general term referring to changes in the vertebral joint characterized by progressive degeneration of the intervertebral disk, with subsequent changes in the bones and soft tissues. Disk degeneration, spinal stenosis, and spondylolisthesis are the characteristic pathologic changes that result. The clinical spectrum of spondylosis includes spinal instability, spinal stenosis, and degenerative spondylolisthesis. Spinal stenosis, the most common of the spondylitic disorders, is a common indication for spinal surgery in adults older than 65 years.[20]

Lumbar Spinal Stenosis

The etiology of lumbar spinal stenosis may be congenital, acquired, or a combination of both. The patient with congenitally short pedicles typically has a shallow spinal canal that predisposes to spinal stenosis later in life as the typical degenerative changes in the spine occur, such as disk protrusion, facet joint degeneration and hypertrophy, and spondylolisthesis (Fig. 20-15).

Lumbar stenosis most commonly occurs at the L4-L5 spinal level, followed by the L3-L4 level. Clinical symptoms of lumbar spinal stenosis include the gradual onset of leg and buttock pain combined with lower extremity sensorineural deficits. These symptoms progress over a period of months. The initial diagnostic investigation should include AP, lateral, flexion, and extension plain films. Suggestive findings on plain films include disk space narrowing and erosion and sclerosis of the vertebral end plates. MRI, the imaging modality of choice in lumbar stenosis, typically shows degenerative changes such as facet joint and ligamentous hypertrophy, disk herniation, and nerve root impingement. The initial approach for patients with the symptoms of spinal stenosis is medical management. Surgical therapy is indicated in patients for whom conservative treatment has failed or who have severe and debilitating pain, significant motor deficits, or symptoms of myelopathy.

Degenerative Spondylolisthesis

Spondylolisthesis is a term referring to the anterior displacement of one vertebra on another in the presence of an intact neural arch (Fig. 20-16). Spondylolisthesis may be congenital or acquired. Degenerative spondylolisthesis is a common condition, particularly in individuals older than 50 years, with a reported incidence as high as 8.7%.[21] Women are affected four to six times more commonly than men.[22] The development of spondylolisthesis is associated with the presence of degenerative intervertebral disks, laxity of ligaments, and facet joint pathology.[23]

Spondylolisthesis is typically asymptomatic; however, clinical symptoms may develop and are related to the presence of spinal stenosis causing lower back pain, radiculopathy, and neurogenic claudication (lower extremity pain, paresthesias, and weakness associated with walking or standing). The evaluation of patients with spondylolisthesis incorporates clinical symptoms in combination with anatomic abnormalities detected on radiologic imaging studies, because stenosis is commonly present without symptoms.[24] The severity of spondylolisthesis is determined by evaluation of the extent of slip and the slip angle using plain films. The extent of slip is subsequently expressed as a percentage of anterior displacement

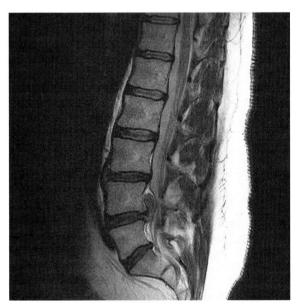

Figure 20–14 Lumbar disk herniation. A 42-year-old man complained of low back pain with radiation to the left lower extremity. This sagittal T2-weighted magnetic resonance image shows a large disk herniation at L4-L5 with the nucleus pulposis extruding 2 cm cephalad into the ventral epidural space.

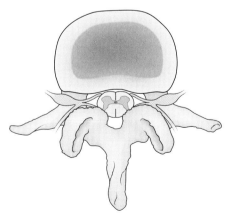

Figure 20–15 Axial view of a lumbar vertebra. Characteristic hypertrophic degenerative changes can be seen in the central canal, facet joints, and lateral recesses.

of the inferior end plate of the vertebral body above with the superior end plate of the vertebral body below.[25,26] The slip angle is generally less than 30 degrees in patients with degenerative spondylolisthesis, but it may progress in about a third of patients.

The initiating pathophysiologic event in the development of degenerative spondylolisthesis is deterioration of the intervertebral disk leading to a narrowing of the disk space, which in turn results in buckling of the ligamentum flavum with consequent microinstability of the motion segment.[27,28] Owing to the loss of normal ligamentous restriction, the vertebra develops an anterior listhesis (Fig. 20-17) or, occasionally, a posterior listhesis. Degeneration of the intervertebral disk may also result in segmental instability in the coronal plane, with a lateral listhesis (lateral slippage of the vertebra) leading to a progressive degenerative scoliosis, which is often associated with spondylolisthesis.[28]

The diagnosis of degenerative spondylolisthesis is based on plain films, including AP, lateral, flexion and extension, and oblique views. The definitive diagnosis of spondylolisthesis relies upon the lateral lumbar radiograph taken in the standing position showing the vertebral slippage (listhesis), which reduces with the supine film. In the presence of neurologic signs and symptoms, MRI of the lumbosacral spine is indicated. This modality detects the presence of ligamentous hypertrophy, spinal cord compression, nerve root impingement, pathologic disk anatomy, and synovial cysts, all of which may be the source of back pain, neurologic deficits, or both.[29]

Definitive therapy in patients with degenerative spondylolisthesis is based on the clinical signs and symptoms combined with the findings from imaging studies. In nearly all cases, nonoperative therapy is preferred for the treatment of lower back pain, with or without neurologic deficits, for at least the first 4 to 6 weeks. If conservative therapy fails, a trial of epidural steroids is appropriate. The indications for surgery include persistent or recurrent back or leg pain or neurogenic claudication, which interferes with the daily activities of life and is unresponsive to 12 weeks of nonsurgical therapy; a progressive neurologic deficit; and symptoms of spinal stenosis.[28]

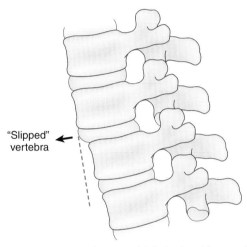

"Slipped" vertebra

Figure 20–16 Degenerative spondylolisthesis with anterior "slippage" of the cephalad vertebra over the vertebra below it.

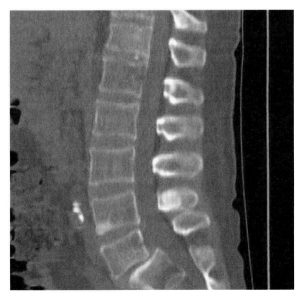

Figure 20–17 Spondylolisthesis. A 48-year-old man presented with bilateral lower extremity numbness. This midsagittal computed tomography scan of the lumbar spine shows a 1-cm anterolisthesis of L5 on S1.

Infections of the Spine

Osteomyelitis

Spinal infections may involve the vertebral body, the intervertebral disk, the neural arch, or the posterior elements. Vertebral osteomyelitis is the most common of the spinal infections, whereas epidural abscesses are relatively rare. Vertebral osteomyelitis preferentially involves the anterior and middle spinal columns. Although the treatment of vertebral osteomyelitis is usually nonsurgical, surgical intervention may at times be warranted.

Clinically, the symptoms and laboratory findings in patients with vertebral osteomyelitis are nonspecific, with little evidence of a systemic process. The diagnosis, therefore, relies upon a high index of suspicion combined with the use of radiologic imaging.[30] Bacteremic spread is the most likely route of vertebral osteomyelitis and is related to the rich arterial blood supply to the vertebral body, particularly near the longitudinal ligament.[31] Vertebral osteomyelitis most commonly affects the lumbar spine, followed by the thoracic spine, cervical spine, and sacral spine. Patients often complain of localized back pain and paravertebral muscle spasms.[32,33] Mild neurologic deficits are reported in about a third of patients,[34,35] whereas others demonstrate a severe neurologic deficit or an incomplete spinal cord syndrome. Laboratory tests demonstrate a leukocytosis in more than half of the patients, an elevation in the erythrocyte sedimentation rate, and an increase in C-reactive protein (CRP) levels.[34-36]

The initial radiologic signs of osteomyelitis are usually absent, becoming evident only after several weeks, when the early findings reveal a reduction in disk height and vertebral end plate erosions, followed by the appearance of osteolytic areas, paravertebral soft tissue shadows, and eventual vertebral body collapse. The most sensitive early radiologic imaging technique is a nuclear bone scan using technetium Tc 99m MDP (methylene diphosphonate) with single-photon emission computed tomography. This technique has a sensitivity greater than 90% in the early stages of vertebral osteomyelitis.[30] MRI, the preferred imaging modality for the diagnosis of osteomyelitis, discloses accurate detail regarding the intervertebral disk, vertebral marrow, neurologic structures, and paraspinal soft tissue pathology.[37] The typical MRI findings in vertebral osteomyelitis and diskitis include loss of end plate definition and decreased signal in the disk and adjacent vertebral bodies (Fig. 20-18).

Effective medical therapy consists of making an accurate and rapid diagnosis, followed by 4 to 6 weeks of intravenous antibiotics and an equal period of oral antibiotics. Surgical therapy is indicated for definitive identification of the causative organism, progressive neurologic deficits, spinal instability, progressive spinal deformity, or failure of medical therapy.

Epidural Abscess

Epidural abscesses are relatively rare infections, occurring in about 1 in 10,000 hospital admissions.[38] Local spread of bacteria into the epidural space is responsible for about one third of cases, and bacteremic seeding of the epidural space occurs in about 50% of cases.[38] The clinical manifestations of an epidural abscess include back pain, fever, and neurologic deficits.[38] Neurologic deficits are late manifestations of the infection, and they require rapid treatment. As in vertebral osteomyelitis, laboratory findings are nonspecific, with a leukocytosis present in two thirds of patients; however, blood culture results may be positive and patients may appear to be systemically septic.[39] Epidural abscesses are more commonly located in the posterior regions of the spine (unlike osteomyelitis, which affects the vertebral body), typically manifest in the thoracolumbar region, and often involve multiple spinal segments.

Spinal epidural abscesses are diagnosed from clinical and radiologic findings in combination with results of the culture of drainage material. Plain radiographs provide diagnostic assistance in less than 20% of the cases, although there may be evidence of coexisting osteomyelitis.[40] The radiologic imaging test of choice is MRI. This modality is able to identify the exact location and extension of the epidural infection and to detect spinal cord compression and surrounding edema. Because of its noninvasive nature with less morbidity, MRI has replaced CT myelography in most instances. Plain films, CT scans, and

radionuclide imaging may be helpful in the diagnosis but do not take the place of MRI because the findings of these other evaluations are nonspecific. Once the diagnosis is confirmed, systemic antibiotic therapy is usually combined with surgical drainage.[38,39,41] The most common surgical procedure performed for the treatment of a spinal epidural abscess is a posterior decompressive laminectomy with debridement.[38,41,42] Neurologic outcome depends on the patient's preoperative neurologic condition.

Spinal Tumors

Although an in-depth review of spinal tumors is not the intent of this discussion, a number of issues pertinent to the care of patients with spinal tumors are addressed. In the approach to spinal tumors, a simple anatomic classification divides the tumors into extradural, intradural extramedullary, and intramedullary categories (Box 20-1). Clinically, the presentation

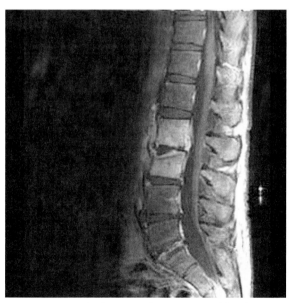

Figure 20–18 Vertebral osteomyelitis. A 50-year-old male intravenous drug abuser presented with low back pain that had lasted for 1 month. This sagittal T1-weighted magnetic resonance image of the lumbar spine obtained after contrast administration shows edema and enhancement of the L2 and L3 vertebral body marrow and loss of height and signal in the L2-L3 disk space.

BOX 20–1 *Anatomic Classification of Spinal Tumors*

Extradural

Metastasis
Chordoma
Osteochondroma
Osteoid osteoma
Osteoblastoma
Osteosarcoma
Aneurysmal bone cyst
Chondrosarcoma
Neurofibroma
Vertebral hemangioma
Giant cell tumor
Osteogenic sarcoma
Plasmacytoma
Multiple myeloma
Ewing's sarcoma
Angiolipoma

Intradural Extramedullary

Spinal meningioma
Schwannoma
Neurofibroma
Epidermoid/dermoid
Lipoma
Metastasis
Arachnoid cyst

Intramedullary

Astrocytoma
Ependymoma
Dermoid/epidermoid
Malignant glioblastoma
Teratoma
Lipoma
Neuroma
Hemangioblastoma
Ganglioglioma
Oligodendroglioma
Paraganglioma
Cholesteatoma
Metastases: melanoma, sarcoma, breast

Data from Patel N: Surgical disorders of the thoracic and lumbar spine: A guide for neurologists. J Neurol Neurosurg Psychiatry 2002;73:42-48.

of patients harboring spinal tumors includes pain, progressive spinal deformity, neurologic deficits, or a combination of all three. Radiologic imaging is invaluable in facilitating a diagnosis. The specific surgical approach to spinal tumors is guided by the particular location and size of the tumor, the effect of the tumor on the biomechanical stability of the spine, and the involvement of surrounding tissues.[43]

Extradural spinal tumors most commonly originate in the vertebral body or the epidural space. Primary tumors of this area are Ewing's sarcoma (Fig. 20-19), chordomas, chondrosarcomas, osteoid osteomas, multiple myelomas, and osteosarcomas.

The majority of extradural tumors are malignant, representing metastatic disease from the lung, breast, prostate, or hematopoietic/lymphoid tissue. Indeed, the skeletal system is a common site of metastatic disease, ranking only behind the lungs and liver in the frequency of occurrence of metastases. As many as 30% of all patients with cancer have metastasis to the spine at autopsy.[44] In the vast majority of patients, spinal metastasis involves the vertebral body and occurs through hematogenous seeding or direct extension of a paravertebral tumor. The thoracic spine is the most common location for spinal metastasis,[45,46] with pain the presenting symptom in more than 85% of cases. The pain is due to vertebral body involvement and may manifest as local constant pain arising from the mass effect on surrounding tissues, radicular pain from nerve root compression by epidural extension of the tumor, and axial pain that is mechanical in nature, being worse with motion and relieved with rest. Neurologic deficits may vary from mild radicular symptoms to spinal cord dysfunction. The neurologic deficits may occur in response to pathologic vertebral body fractures or dislocations or to progressive neural compression from tumor growth.

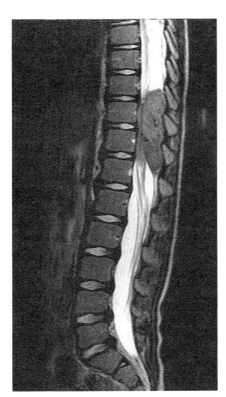

Figure 20–19 Ewing's sarcoma. A sagittal pre-contrast T2-weighted magnetic resonance image shows a 5.4 cm long by 1.6 cm heterogeneously enhancing mass located in the dorsal epidural space from T9 to T12 that is severely compressing the spinal cord.

Radiologic imaging is invaluable for assisting in the diagnosis of suspected extradural spinal metastasis. For highly vascular tumors (melanoma, hypernephroma), preoperative angiography with tumor embolization may be used to minimize intraoperative blood loss during resection of a particularly large tumor.[47-49] The treatment of metastatic disease to the spine involves primarily nonsurgical treatment, particularly in patients without neurologic compromise or spinal instability. These patients are best treated with palliative irradiation, chemotherapy, or both, depending on the tumor cell type. The indications for surgical therapy for extradural spinal disease include an unknown primary for which biopsy therefore is not possible, progressive neurologic deficits, severe pain unresponsive to medical treatment, progressive spinal deformity or instability, radioresistant tumors, and solitary tumors not responding to nonsurgical treatments.

Intradural extramedullary tumors are located within the dura but outside the substance of the spinal cord and may involve the arachnoid tissue, circulating CSF, nerve sheaths, dentate ligaments, filum terminale, and vascular structures. Tumors that arise within this space are typically benign, and more than 90% are either nerve sheath tumors or meningiomas. The nerve sheath tumors can be located at any level of the spine and are usually schwannomas or neurofibromas, which tend to localize in the dorsal or sensory nerve roots. Malignant tumors in this region of the spine are much less common and usually originate from a primary brain tumor (e.g., ependymoma or medulloblastoma) or from meningeal spread secondary to metastatic disease. The thoracic spine is the most common location for a meningioma (80%), followed by the cervical (10%-20%) and lumbar (1%-5%) regions.

The clinical presentation of a patient with an intradural extramedullary tumor is usually a myelopathy or a radiculopathy. As with extradural metastatic spinal tumors, radiologic diagnosis relies on plain films, CT, CT myelography, and MRI. Although plain films are rarely of significant value in making a diagnosis, CT provides useful detail of the spinal anatomy, with meningiomas appearing as high-density well-circumscribed intradural lesions. CT myelography is highly sensitive in delineating the location of a displaced spinal cord; however, MRI has essentially replaced CT myelography in most institutions and is now considered the imaging modality of choice. Surgery is warranted for the treatment of benign intradural extramedullary tumors such as schwannomas, meningiomas, and neurofibromas.[50]

Intramedullary tumors are located within the substance of the spinal cord. In adults, more than 80% of these tumors consist of astrocytomas and ependymomas. The typical clinical manifestations of intramedullary tumor consist of a myelopathy and sensory disturbance below the level of the spinal tumor. When the tumor is located at the level of the conus medullaris, a cauda equina syndrome is characteristic. The primary treatment for an intramedullary tumor is surgical laminectomy, followed by tumor resection or biopsy.[50]

Scoliosis

Adult scoliosis is defined as any curvature of the spine greater than 10 degrees in a skeletally mature individual. Adult scoliosis is divided into two groups. In the first group, a curve develops during adolescence (idiopathic scoliosis) but is treated only in adulthood. In the second group, the curve first manifests after skeletal maturity (termed "de novo" scoliosis).[51] Degenerative spine disease is the most common cause of de novo scoliosis, although scoliosis may occur after previous spinal surgery or in patients with osteoporosis.[52] Degenerative lumbar scoliosis occurs as part of the normal aging process that adversely affects the vertebrae, intervertebral disks, spinal ligaments, facet joints, and muscles. This degenerative process leads to wedging of vertebral bodies and disks with progressive spinal rotation and translation, most commonly involving the upper lumbar and lower thoracolumbar spine.[53] Degenerative scoliosis is common, with a prevalence reported to range from 6% to 68%[51,54] and increasing with age.[55-57] The clinical symptom that first requires medical care is back pain. Although the incidence of back pain in adults with scoliosis is similar to that found in the general population, the most common indication for eventual surgery is back pain, with 1% of patients with scoliosis requiring surgery.[53]

Thoracic scoliotic curves have a much greater adverse effect on pulmonary function than curves located in other regions of the spine. There is a direct relationship between the magnitude of the curve and the reduction in lung volumes. With thoracic curves greater than 60 degrees, and particularly those greater than 100 degrees, the patient complains of shortness of breath and dyspnea, and spirometric testing shows progressive restrictive pulmonary disease with reductions in vital capacity, forced expiratory volume in one second (FEV_1), and Pao_2 with all abnormalities being in proportion to the severity of the scoliotic curve.

Most patients with back pain related to scoliosis are effectively treated with nonsurgical therapy. At present, the indications for surgery in the setting of scoliosis include persistent back pain that medical therapy has failed to control; progressive neurologic deficits; progressive spinal deformity, particularly in the setting of worsening pulmonary function; and postural imbalance related to muscle fatigue. The surgical goals are to correct deformity without creating spinal instability and to allow early patient mobilization. Postoperative complications are not uncommon. In one report, patients older than 60 years undergoing an anterior fusion for scoliosis correction had a 64% incidence of postoperative complications, and 24% of the complications were considered major.[58] Pulmonary dysfunction was the most common major complication.[58]

Inflammatory Arthritides of the Spine

Rheumatoid Arthritis

Rheumatoid arthritis (RA) is the most common of the inflammatory diseases, affecting approximately 1% of the world's population. It is characterized by a chronic, systemic, autoimmune inflammatory state resulting in symmetrical pain, heat, swelling, and destruction in synovial joints of the hands and feet, wrists, elbows, hips, knees, ankles, and the cervical spine.[59] The T cell–mediated inflammatory state of RA affects synovial tissues throughout the body, resulting in hypertrophy of joint tissue and erosion of articular cartilage and subchondral bone.[60] The cervical spine is affected, with involvement of the synovial joints of the cervical spine, particularly those surrounding the C1-C2 articulation.[61,62] The synovitis weakens the surrounding supportive structures, resulting in axial instability that may lead to subluxation of the C1-C2 articulation and spinal cord compression. Atlantoaxial subluxation affects as many as one fourth of patients with RA and is the most common cervical spine manifestation of RA.

Clinically, patients with RA involving the cervical spine may complain of neck pain, headaches, and limitation of neck movement. In severe disease, subaxial subluxation may cause progressive cervical myelopathy with spasticity of the legs, motor weakness, and incontinence, or symptoms of nerve root compression. The diagnosis of cervical spine involvement in the setting of RA relies upon typical radiologic findings, including atlantoaxial subluxation, narrowed disk spaces, erosion of vertebral end plates, apophyseal joint erosion with blurred facets, and spinal osteoporosis.[59] A CT scan is of value for detecting the extent of cervical spine bony destruction, whereas MRI is useful for identification of spinal cord pathology and soft tissue abnormalities.

Surgery is indicated in the presence of myelopathy; severe neck pain with a neurologic deficit and excessive subluxation of C1-C2 with spinal canal stenosis, vertebral artery compromise, and spinal cord compression. Patients demonstrating symptoms of myelopathy, particularly in the presence of C1-C2 subluxation, require emergency posterior spinal decompression and fusion, with placement of screws across the C1-C2 facet joint and bone grafting. The presence of subaxial subluxation (C3-C7) warrants realignment and stabilization from a posterior approach, particularly when multiple levels are involved. An anterior approach may be appropriate as an alternative technique; it involves a decompressive corpectomy with spinal fusion with or without instrumentation.[59]

The anesthetic approach for a patient undergoing surgery for RA should take into account the airway concerns unique to these patients, including limitation of neck and temporomandibular joint movement (limiting visualization of the larynx), arthritic involvement of the cricoarytenoid joints (preoperative hoarseness and stridor) with a narrowed tracheal inlet, atlantoaxial subluxation with potential vertebral artery compromise, basilar impression (from rostral advancement of the odontoid process with compression of the spinal cord or medulla), and instability of the lower cervical spine. That said, an awake fiberoptic intubation with spinal cord monitoring may be appropriate to minimize further neurologic injury during the induction of anesthesia and positioning of the patient.

Ankylosing Spondylitis

Ankylosing spondylitis (AS) is considered the prototypical seronegative spondyloarthropathy; it is characterized by a progressive inflammatory involvement of the sacroiliac and axial skeletal joints, which may result in severe spinal deformity (Fig. 20-20). In addition to axial skeletal disease, AS involves enthesopathy (inflammation at the sites of tendon and ligamentous insertions), the presence of human leukocyte antigen (HLA-B27), and the absence of rheumatoid nodules and rheumatoid factor in serum (seronegative).[59] The disease is three times more common in men than in women.

Patients with AS may experience radicular pain that is very similar to the pain of a herniated lumbar disk. Thoracic spine involvement causes reduced movement in the costovertebral articulations and adversely affects pulmonary function. Laboratory findings are nonspecific in AS and of little diagnostic value; however, the erythrocyte sedimentation rate is increased in 80% of patients with active disease. The diagnosis is typically made on the basis of clinical criteria, including significant and persistent lower back discomfort and stiffness, particularly in the morning hours, along with limited spinal mobility and chest expansion in combination with radiographic findings

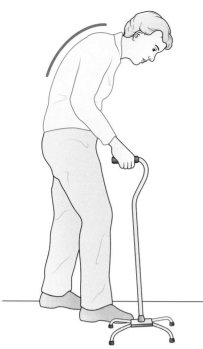

Figure 20–20 In a patient with ankylosing spondylitis, a progressive spinal curvature may eventually develop, resulting in a stooped posture from vertebral fusion.

of sacroiliitis, spinal inflammation, and ligamentous calcification. The regions of the spine most often involved in AS are the sacroiliac, costovertebral, zygapophyseal, and discovertebral joints.[59] In AS, fractures are most commonly seen in the lower cervical spine (C6-C7), although they may also occur in the lumbar and thoracic segments.[63]

Surgery is indicated for individuals with severe spinal deformities that adversely affect normal activities and in patients who have spinal instability due to spondylodiskitis or spinal fracture.[64] In patients with AS who are scheduled for corrective spine surgery or other, unrelated surgical procedures, preoperative considerations should include an assessment of pulmonary function and potential difficulties with intubation due to the severe cervical deformities seen in some patients.

Osteoporosis

Osteoporosis is a metabolic bone disease characterized by a decrease in bone mineral density and disrupted microarchitecture that leads to a higher risk of fractures, particularly of the hip, spine, and wrists. Osteoporosis affects nearly 30 million individuals in the United States, making it the most prevalent bone disease.[65,66] It is found most commonly in women after menopause but may occur in men and premenopausal women in the presence of hormonal disorders or other chronic disease states, in which case it is secondary osteoporosis. Disease states associated with secondary osteoporosis include hyperthyroidism, gastrointestinal disorders, disorders of calcium balance, and chronic steroid use.

Vertebral compression fractures, the most common complication of osteoporosis, occur most often in the thoracic and lumbar spine.[67] Development of an acute fracture manifests as acute pain localized over the affected area or referred across the chest. After the fracture heals, the patient may complain of chronic back pain. In the thoracic spine, osteoporotic fractures are located primarily in the anterior aspect of the

vertebral body, causing a compression fracture that appears as a wedge shape on plain films. The wedge-shaped vertebral body results in a dorsal kyphosis, particularly if fractures affect multiple spinal levels. In the lumbar spine, the vertebral fractures are located more evenly throughout the vertebral body, resulting in a compression fracture without the wedge shape.

The diagnosis of osteoporosis relies on a combination of clinical history, plain radiographs, bone mineral density (BMD) testing, and biochemical markers suggesting rapid bone turnover (bone-specific alkaline phosphatase). Osteoporosis is treated nonsurgically in the majority of cases. Surgical intervention is indicated in the setting of acute vertebral compression fractures associated with severe pain unresponsive to medical therapy, neurologic deficits, and in the presence of progressive spinal deformity and instability.

TRAUMA OF THE SPINE AND SPINAL CORD

Among individuals suffering general traumatic injuries, the cervical spine is involved in 4.3% of cases, the thoracolumbar spine in 6.3% of cases, and the spinal cord in 1.3%.[68,69] The most common causes of spine trauma are motor vehicle accidents, falls, violence, and sports-related injuries. Spinal injuries have a predilection for the more mobile areas of the spine, which include the cervical spine (75% of cervical spine injuries are at C3-C7) and the thoracolumbar junction (16% of thoracolumbar injuries are at the L1 junction),[69] with as many as one fifth of injuries to the spine occurring at multiple levels. In general, the goals of management of spinal trauma are: prevention of further neurologic injury; enhancement of neurologic recovery if deficits exist; neurologic decompression; and the surgical correction of spinal malalignment or deformity.

After initial evaluation and resuscitation, a more detailed neurologic examination is performed to detect the presence of neurologic deficits. Initial radiologic imaging consists of a cross-table lateral radiograph of the cervical spine, which is able to detect nearly 80% of all injuries. The lateral view must satisfactorily visualize the entire cervical spine, including the cervicothoracic junction. The addition of an AP view and an open-mouth view facilitates an accuracy of diagnosis of cervical spine injury approaching 95%.[69]

Biomechanical Considerations in Spinal Injury

An understanding of the biomechanics of spinal impact and resulting spinal injury is helpful in estimating the probability and severity of both the spinal column and SCI as well as the planning of effective therapy. Traumatic spinal injuries most commonly occur after impact forces that result in the following seven basic types of spinal trauma: hyperflexion, hyperextension, compression, rotation, shear, avulsion injuries, and a combination of these types.[69] A variant mechanistic classification of cervical spinal injuries is also illustrated (Fig. 20-21): Traumatic spinal injuries, associated neurologic sequelae, and the usual treatments are outlined in Table 20-1.

Hyperflexion

Hyperflexion injuries may be divided into flexion-compression and flexion-distraction injuries. The direction of the applied load determines the particular injury pattern. Simple flexion-compression fractures results in wedge fractures of the vertebral body that cause a loss of anterior vertebral body

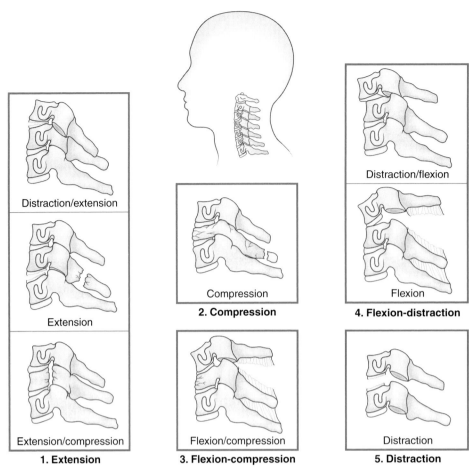

Figure 20–21 Mechanistic classification of cervical spinal injuries. This illustration of the spectrum of cervical spine injuries is based on the mechanistic classification proposed by Allen and colleagues.[250] *(From Lindsey RW, Gugala Z, Pneumaticos SG: Injury to the vertebra and spinal cord. In Moore EE, Feliciano DV, Mattox KL [eds]: Trauma, 5th ed. New York, McGraw-Hill, 2004, pp 459-492.)*

height, creating a wedge shape. These injuries are typically stable, unless significant loss of vertebral body height results. Severe flexion-distraction injuries occur from a combination of flexion and distraction loads, with the center of rotation located anteriorly. This injury results in characteristic subluxations or dislocations (Fig. 20-22) of the vertebral bodies with disruption of the posterior longitudinal ligament, causing significant spinal instability. Herniation of the intervertebral disks is commonly seen after severe flexion injuries, as is dislocation of the facet joints, particularly if enough of a rotational component is involved.

Hyperextension

Hyperextension injuries are most common in the cervical region and are a common cause of lower cervical neck injuries (see Fig. 20-22). Hyperextension injuries may result from facial or frontal trauma, whereby the forces separate the vertebral body and the adjacent lower end of the intervertebral disk. Hyperextension injuries result in disruption of the anterior and middle spinal columns in tension, reducing the AP diameter of the spinal canal and compressing the spinal cord between the posterior aspect of the vertebral body and the ligamentum flavum and lamina. Elderly individuals with cervical spondylosis are particularly susceptible to hyperextension injuries, and even moderate hyperextension may produce cord injury. The vertebral arteries may be damaged in cervical extension injuries, particularly in people with severe spondylosis. Hyperextension injuries are typically unstable owing to the disruption of the stabilizing ligamentous elements and injury to the intervertebral disks.

Compression

Compression injuries occur after impact forces containing a significant axial load (e.g., falls on the occiput) and result in wedge compression fractures, burst fractures (Fig. 20-23), and ligamentous rupture. Wedge compression fractures, most common in the thoracolumbar region, result from pure flexion injury, whereby the posterior ligamentous complex remains intact. Compression injuries with burst fractures often cause serious neurologic damage from retropulsion of bone fragments, ligaments, and disk material into the spinal canal. Compression injuries associated with flexion may produce the so-called teardrop fracture, in which the vertebra is dislocated anteriorly, with an associated avulsion of the superior aspect of the vertebra and posterior longitudinal ligament damage, usually with significant neurologic damage.

Rotation

Flexion and extension injuries that include significant rotational forces may result in severe spinal injuries, including subluxation, dislocation, and fracture-dislocations. Serious injuries to the vertebral bodies and intervertebral disks are often involved in the process (Fig. 20-24).

Rotational spinal injuries often result in severe injuries to the spinal cord and cauda equina. In particular, hyperflexion-rotation forces associated with dislocation may produce either unilateral or bilateral locked facets. Bilateral facet dislocations (locked facets) are associated with major neurologic injury and often require surgical reduction and stabilization.

Table 20–1   Selected Spinal Injuries, Associated Clinical Findings, and Treatment

Spinal Injury	Typical Clinical Findings	Treatment
Upper Cervical (C1-C2) Spine Injuries		
Atlanto-occipital dislocation	Unstable; commonly fatal; if patient survives there are neurologic deficits	Reduction, immobilization; surgical stabilization-fusion
Atlas fracture (Jefferson fracture) with intact transverse ligament	Usually stable, neurologically intact	Cervical orthosis if nondisplaced; C1-C2 fusion if displaced
Atlantoaxial dislocation/subluxation	Usually neurologically intact	Reduction and immobilization, posterior fusion if reduction fails
Isolated odontoid fracture at neck or base (type II)	Usually neurologically intact; typically unstable	Immobilization ± surgical stabilization-fusion
Axis fracture—bilateral pars interarticularis or pedicle fracture (hangman's fracture)	Usually neurologically intact	Immobilization; if severe, surgical fusion
Subaxial Cervical (C3-C7) Spine Injuries		
Axial compression Wedge compression fracture	Neurologically variable	Immobilization ± surgical stabilization-fusion
Burst fracture	Unstable; neurologically variable	Halo vest vs. surgical stabilization
Flexion compression Teardrop fracture	Unstable; neurologically variable	Usually surgical stabilization
Flexion-distraction	Unstable (disrupted posterior longitudinal ligament); neurologically variable	Surgical stabilization
Extension-distraction Hyperextension, ± fracture ± dislocation:	May or may not be stable; elderly patients with spinal stenosis; neurodeficits (central cord syndrome)	Immobilization vs. surgical decompression and stabilization
With retrolisthesis	Unstable, neurologically variable	Surgical stabilization (anterior ± posterior)
Rotation-flexion or extension Unilateral facet dislocation Bilateral facet dislocation	Unstable; disrupted posterior stabilizing elements; usually severe neurologic deficits	Reduction; surgical decompression, stabilization
Thoracolumbar Injuries		
Transverse process, spinous process, and articular process fractures	Stable; neurologically intact	Symptomatic ± orthoses
Compression fractures Wedge fracture	Unstable if severe compression (>50% loss of vertebral body height); neurologically variable	Thoracolumbosacral orthosis (TLSO) if stable; surgical stabilization if unstable
Burst fracture	Neurologically variable	TLSO ± surgical decompression and stabilization
Chance fracture (horizontal fracture through anterior-posterior bony elements)	Unstable; neurologically variable	Surgical stabilization
Flexion-distraction	Unstable if ligamentous disruption; neurologically variable	Surgical stabilization
Fracture-dislocation	Unstable; neurologically variable	Reduction; surgical stabilization
Extension-distraction	Rare (patients with metabolic bone disease); unstable; neurologic deficits common	Reduction; surgical stabilization
Penetrating missile injury	Neurologically variable; recovery poor	Symptomatic treatment

These are most often seen in the lower cervical spine (C5-C7). Fractures of the vertebral peduncles may be associated with bilateral facet dislocations. Unilateral facet dislocations may be associated with no neurologic injury; however, they may be associated with nerve root compression or an incomplete SCI.

Shear

Some degree of spinal translation is involved in most spinal injuries, including spinal fractures and ligamentous tears. The shear mechanism typically involves all three columns of the spine and is associated with a higher incidence of facet dislocation.[69]

Avulsion

Avulsion injuries are typically stable injuries. An example of such an injury is the odontoid type 1 fracture, in which the tip of the odontoid process is fractured or chipped. These fractures are stable injuries. Another example is the extension teardrop fracture.[69]

Combined

Combined injuries, resulting from various vectors of force such as axial loading, rotation, and flexion or extension, chiefly affect the cervical region and commonly produce

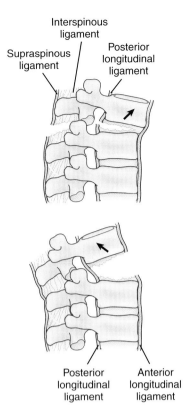

Interspinous ligament

Supraspinous ligament

Posterior longitudinal ligament

Posterior longitudinal ligament

Anterior longitudinal ligament

Figure 20–22 *Top,* Distracted vertebral body with disrupted posterior longitudinal ligament occurring after hyperflexion injury. *Bottom,* Distracted vertebral body with disrupted anterior longitudinal ligament occurring after hyperextension injury (arrows shows direction of forces).

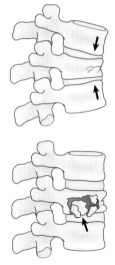

Figure 20–23 *Top,* Vertebral compression fracture (arrow). *Bottom,* Vertebral burst fracture (arrow) with retropulsion of bone fragments posteriorly into the vertebral canal.

ligamentous tears and distraction (an increase in distance between individual components of adjacent vertebrae. For example, a combined injury, or whiplash, involves rapid acceleration-deceleration forces resulting in extreme extension followed by flexion and is often associated with rotation, compression, and tearing forces. This kind of acceleration lesion distorts the spinal components, damaging the soft tissues of the neck, muscles, and anteroposterior ligaments, and sometimes involves nerve roots and disks.

Traumatic spondylolisthesis of the axis occurs with motor vehicle accidents when the driver's face or chin hits the steering

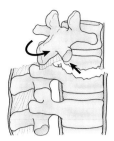

Figure 20–24 Rotation injury showing dislocated articular facts (small arrow).

wheel. The extreme hyperextension of the neck produces shear stresses on the C2-C3 vertebral units, resulting in fracture of the neural arches with dislocation between C2 and C3. However, the avulsed arches decompress the cervicomedullary junction, so patients seldom experience neurologic deficits and usually have a good prognosis.

Mid-thoracic to upper thoracic spinal injuries are much less common than injuries of the cervical or thoracolumbar regions because of the protection and fixation of the thoracic area by the rib cage and sternum. When thoracic spine injuries do occur, the SCI is typically neurologically complete. The greater mobility of the vertebral column at the thoracolumbar junction contributes significantly to the frequency of spinal injuries in this region. Injury to the thoracolumbar spinal column can result in wedge fractures of the vertebrae, with destruction of the laminae, pedicles, and facets. Protrusion of the vertebral body or disk material into the spinal cord may occur. The addition of torque results in fracture-dislocations of the vertebral column. Lumbar fractures have been reported to occur much less often and are the result of flexion and compression forces. Neurologic injuries that involve only the cauda equina have a high potential for significant neurologic recovery.

Penetrating wounds of the spine may cause significant damage, including direct and indirect spinal cord injury through transmitted energy. Many of these injuries produce damage to both the spinal cord and nerve roots as a result of associated shear stress; compression and contusion of cord tissue by bony impingement, herniated disks, or intraparenchymal bone fragments; or ischemia caused by interruption of the vascular supply. However, no consistent relationship exists between actual trauma to supporting structures and injury to the spinal cord. Thus, a patient may present with a stable spine without bony or ligamentous injury and still sustain SCI or may have serious fractures and an unstable spine without neurologic deficits. In adults, the areas most susceptible to injury are the lower cervical spine (C5 to C7) and the thoracolumbar junction (T12- L1), regions of the spine coinciding with the areas of greatest spinal column mobility.[70]

Neurologic Assessment

In patients with spinal trauma, a neurologic examination is essential in establishing a baseline of neurologic function and in facilitating the decision matrix for specific radiologic testing. Following the primary trauma survey, the neurologic evaluation process includes an assessment of mental status, an examination of the spinal column, and an evaluation of the sensorimotor function of the extremities. Initially, the clinician palpates the spine in its entirety, specifically noting tenderness, evidence of hematoma, or spinal malalignment. During examination of the patient, it is important to maintain spinal precautions at all times (i.e., log rolling, maintaining neutral

Dermatome Chart

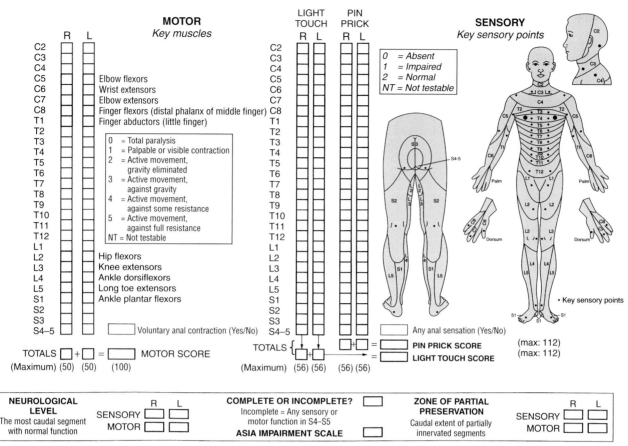

Figure 20–25 American Spinal Injury Association (ASIA) Dermatome Chart demonstrating the comprehensive neurologic evaluation system for determining the extent of neurologic injury. *(Reproduced from the American Spinal Injury Association, Atlanta, GA, with permission.)*

neck position). The neurologic examination should be accurately detailed in the medical record using the American Spinal Injury Association (ASIA) dermatome chart (Fig. 20-25).

The ASIA chart standardizes the neurologic evaluation process and facilitates the accuracy of the neurologic examination (see Fig. 20-25). In the ASIA system, neurologic assessment is performed by testing of key muscles and sensory points. For muscle testing, 10 groups are tested. The function of these muscles is graded on a 6-point scale, with 0 assigned for total paralysis and 5 points assigned for normal strength. In total, there are 100 points when the right and left sides are assessed.

The second part of the ASIA neurologic examination is the sensory score, which is based on the evaluation of 28 sensory dermatomes on the right and left sides of the body. At each of these key points, both sensitivity to pinprick and to light touch are tested and scored on a scale of 0 to 2 (0, absence of sensation; 1, impaired sensation; and 2, normal sensation). In addition to testing of the key muscles and sensory points, voluntary motor contraction of the external anal sphincter is tested by digital examination. Perirectal sensation is also tested; this sensation, along with the presence of the bulbocavernosus reflex or the anal-cutaneous reflex, is an important signal of the preservation of distal function (sacral sparing), indicating incomplete SCI and predicting a more favorable prognosis. Proprioception (position sensation) testing is considered optional but is highly recommended.

Table 20–2 American Spinal Injury Association (ASIA) Impairment Scale

ASIA Grade	Type of Injury	Definition of Type of Injury
A	Complete	No motor or sensory function
B	Incomplete	Sensory but not motor function is preserved below the level of the injury
C	Incomplete	Motor function is preserved, but majority of key muscles below the neurologic level have a muscle grade <3
D	Incomplete	Motor function is preserved, and majority of key muscles below the neurologic level have a muscle grade ≥ 3
E	Normal	Motor function and sensory function are normal

Finally, an assessment should be made of the completeness of the neurologic injury as defined by the ASIA impairment scale (Table 20-2). In this scale (formerly called the Frankel scale), the neurologic injury is divided into one of five possible grades. The term *sensory level* or *motor level* is used to define the most caudal segment of the cord with normal sensory or motor function, respectively, on both sides of the body.

The diagnosis of SCI should be considered when the following signs or symptoms are present: motor signs, such as weakness or paralysis of the extremities or trunk muscles; sensory signs, such as the absence or alteration of sensation of the trunk or extremities; bowel or bladder incontinence; abrasions, lacerations, or deformities of the spine, neck, or head region; and tenderness or pain on palpation of the spine or neck. The patient's neck or back should not be moved to determine whether it is painful but should only be palpated. An unconscious patient must be considered to have an SCI until proved otherwise. An injury to other systems (e.g., head injury) may mask an SCI; conversely, an SCI may mask other system injuries (e.g., visceral rupture or fracture of long bones).

Radiologic Considerations

The goal of imaging after spinal trauma is to recognize and quantify spinal injury as well as to aid in determining prognosis (Table 20-3). The results of radiologic tests and identification of neurologic deficits are combined with knowledge of the mechanism of injury to define the final pathologic state.

Plain Radiographs

Initial determination of spinal pathologic conditions such as fractures, dislocations, and combination injuries begins with plain radiographs. For patients with signs or symptoms of thoracic or lumbosacral injury, AP and lateral films should be taken. For the cervical spine, the most important radiographic tests include a lateral view, an AP view, and an open-mouth view of the odontoid; these three views are often called a "three-view series" (Fig. 20-26).

Supine oblique views are added when findings of the three-view series are equivocal or negative or if facet-joint dislocation is suspected. The initial images must visualize the occipitocervical junction, all seven cervical vertebrae, and the C7-T1 junction.

If all seven cervical vertebrae are not visualized, a swimmer's view should be ordered to view the lowermost cervical spine (all images collectively termed a "five-view" series). Fractures of vertebral bodies, spinous processes, and the odontoid process are usually seen on lateral plain radiographs, whereas injuries to the pedicles and facets are seen best on AP and oblique views. The AP view is the most sensitive view on which to identify lateral mass fractures of the vertebral bodies. Flexion and extension films of the cervical spine are indicated in alert patients in whom plain films demonstrated normal spinal anatomy but who either complain of persistent neck tenderness or are tender on examination and who have no neurologic symptoms. These patients may still be at risk of having suffered significant ligamentous injury.

Although a lateral cervical spine film is sensitive in detecting cervical spine trauma, it is often inaccurate in completely eliminating cervical spine injury; therefore the three-view series is considered superior to the lateral film for diagnosis of cervical spine injury.[71-73]

Computed Tomography

The spatial resolution of CT is superior to that of plain radiographs, and the axial format provides better evaluation of the spinal canal. CT provides an excellent means of imaging bone and may be the only way to properly evaluate the lower cervical area, which must be studied to the C7-T1 junction. Moreover, CT is useful for measuring spinal canal and neuroforaminal diameter, provides detail of the facet joints, and can display hematoma formation. It is usually the procedure of choice for determining compression of the spinal canal and spinal stability. CT may also be necessary to detect a unilateral jumped facet or bone fragments in the canal or root foramen.

In general, CT is performed for any injury resulting in a neurologic deficit, for fractures of the posterior arch of the cervical canal, and for fractures that may involve bony fragments in the spinal canal. CT is also indicated for the evaluation of uncertain radiographic findings, to provide details of bony injury as an aid to surgical planning, for assessment of focal cervical pain when no radiologic abnormalities are evident, to clear the lower cervical spine in symptomatic patients for whom plain films are inadequate, to assess postoperative complications of internal fixation, and to localize foreign bodies and bone fragments in relation to the spinal cord.

Magnetic Resonance Imaging

MRI has inherent advantages in the setting of spinal trauma, including the ability to image the spinal cord in any orientation and to visualize soft tissues. MRI is able to show the epidural and subarachnoid spaces, thereby providing exceptional ability to detect intraspinal ligament tears and disruptions (Fig. 20-27).

MRI is superior in the ability to directly image injury to spinal cord parenchyma, including edema, hemorrhage, myelomalacia, and lacerations. MRI also has a better capacity to evaluate the extent of spinal canal compromise from bone fragments, osteophytes, herniated disk material, or epidural hematomas. MRI is an excellent choice for directly imaging nerve root impingement in addition to detecting the presence of syrinx formation, scarring, or late compression of the cord. Although MRI can detect most vertebral fractures, it is not as sensitive as CT for this purpose. MRI is indicated in patients with incomplete neurologic deficits after traction, realignment, and immobilization of the spine and in patients who have cervical cord deficits after trauma but no demonstrated

Table 20–3	Specificity of Spine Radiologic Evaluations		
Category	Plain Radiograph	Computed Tomography	Magnetic Resonance Imaging
Bony anatomy	++	+++	++
Ligament injury	+	+	+++
Spinal canal size	0	+++	+++
Spinal cord compression	0	++	+++
Nerve root compression	0	++	+++
Hemorrhage and edema	0	+	+++
Syrinx formation	0	++	+++
Prediction of deficit	++	++	+++
Prediction of outcome	+	++	+++

0, no benefit; +, poor; ++, good; +++, very good.

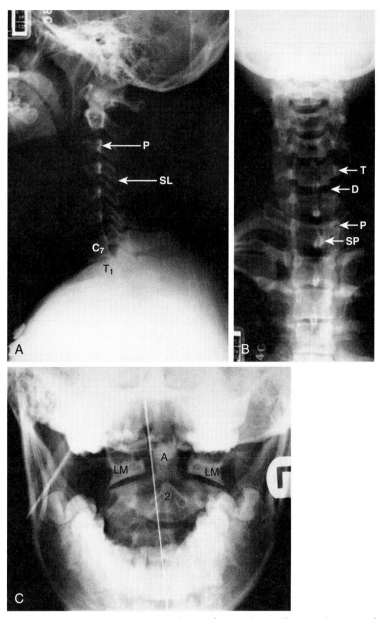

Figure 20–26 Three-view cervical spinal radiographic series. **A,** Lateral view of cervical spine showing alignment of posterior aspects of the vertebral bodies (P) and spinolaminar junction (SL). All seven cervical vertebrae (including C7) and the upper border of T1 should be visualized. **B,** Anteroposterior view showing alignment of spinous processes (SP) and vertebral bodies. Note the uniformity of disk spaces (D). Also visualized are transverse processes (T) and pedicles (P). **C,** Open-mouth (odontoid) view showing the odontoid (A). The odontoid is normally centered between the lateral masses (LM) of C1. The body of C2 (2) should be clearly visualized.

abnormalities on plain films or CT scans. MRI is indicated in a patient manifesting neurologic progression of a previously stable neurologic deficit as well as in a patient whose level of neurologic deficit appears to be above the level of apparent cervical spine injury.

Summary

Patients at risk for SCI should undergo a neurologic evaluation followed by radiologic imaging to identify and quantify abnormalities suggested by history or examination (Table 20-4). At a minimum, clearance of the cervical spine requires a three-view cervical spine series. If visualization of the cervical anatomy is inadequate, then additional evaluation is indicated. Patients with SCI may require MRI to detect intramedullary lesions, extrinsic spinal cord processes, and possible ligamentous injury.

Spinal Cord Injury

Epidemiology

The reported incidence of SCI in the United States varies from 12 to 55 patients per million population per year,[74] with a prevalence of 253,000 (range 225,000-296,000 persons).[75] Etiologic factors responsible for SCI are motor vehicle accidents (46.9%-50.4%), falls (23.7%), violence (11.2%-13.7%), sports and recreational accidents (8.7%-9.0%), and other causes (7%).[75,76] Most victims of SCI are young males between 15 and 34 years of age. The incidence of SCI declines after this period and modestly peaks again in the elderly population.[77] Spinal cord injury occurring after spinal trauma is most common in the cervical spine (55%), followed by the thoracic spine (30%), and the lumbar spine (15%). Of those individuals sustaining an SCI, incomplete tetraplegia (34.5%) is the

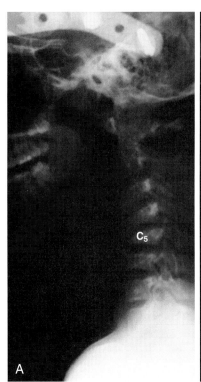
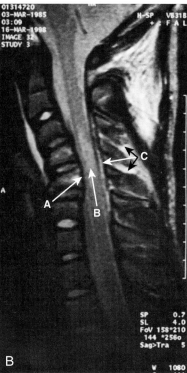

Figure 20–27 **A,** Lateral cervical spine radiograph of a patient with a flexion injury involving C5 shows malaligned posterior vertebral body lines. **B,** T2-weighted sagittal magnetic resonance image of the same patient showing probable injury to the posterior longitudinal ligament *(A),* an increased signal within the spinal cord *(B)* consistent with spinal cord injury, and a hyperintense signal involving the posterior ligamentous complex *(C).*

Table 20–4	**Summary of Appropriate Radiographic Evaluation of Cervical Spine Trauma**
Clinical Status or Findings	**Recommended Procedure**
Asymptomatic; alert, with normal physical findings	Radiographs not needed
Symptomatic; signs and symptoms of cervical injury	Three-view radiographic series
Ligamentous injury; normal plain film findings but with neck pain	Flexion and extension views (patient awake; physician in attendance) or magnetic resonance imaging
Neurologic deficit in spite of normal plain film findings	Magnetic resonance imaging
Plain films indicate craniovertebral injury involving occiput, C1, or C2	Computed tomography
Impaired sensorium; neurologic evaluation compromised	Three-view radiographic series

most common, followed in descending order by complete paraplegia (23.1%), complete tetraplegia (18.4%), and incomplete paraplegia (17.5%).[76] The probability of death following SCI is 6.3% during the first year, decreases to 1.8% during the second year, and is 0.7% to 1.3% per year thereafter, with a 12-year survival rate of 85.1%.[78] Predictors of survival include level of consciousness; presence of multiple injuries; need for respiratory assistance; lesion level; severity of neurologic injury; age; and psychological, social, and vocational variables. Leading causes of death in patients with SCI include respiratory and cardiac complications, septicemia, pulmonary embolism, and suicide.[78-80]

Terminology

In describing the severity of acute SCI, the use of correct terminology is essential. The term *pentaplegia* is used to describe high cervical spine injuries (C1) with paralysis of the lower cranial nerves and diaphragm and loss of motor and sensory function involving both upper and lower extremities. For SCI

involving C3 to C5, the term *tetraplegia* or *quadriplegia* is used; although facial and neck sensation and accessory muscle function remain intact at this level, the patient loses diaphragmatic function as well as motor and sensory function of the upper and lower extremities. For SCI involving C5 to C6, the term *tetraplegia* is still used. In this lesion, patients retain diaphragmatic function and some proximal movement of the upper extremities but nothing else. For SCI involving the T1 level and below, the term *paraplegia* is used and is most commonly associated with loss of lower extremity function. Perineal paraplegia involves loss of sacral roots (S2 to S5) only, with resulting dysfunction of the bowel, bladder, and sexual function.

Complete versus Incomplete Spinal Cord Injury

Determining whether a patient has complete or incomplete SCI is vitally important in the prediction of outcome and in surgical planning. The diagnosis of a *complete SCI* (ASIA grade A) can be made only when there is absence of all motor and sensory function distal to the level of injury for more than 48 hours. An *incomplete neurologic injury* is defined by the ASIA as the presence of any sensory or motor function in the lowest sacral segment. Determining touch and pinprick sensations in the lowest sacral dermatomes (S4, S5), such as perianal sensation, and demonstrating voluntary rectal tone (rather than reflex rectal tone) is important, as there is a favorable prognosis for recovery in patients with incomplete injuries.[81,82]

Incomplete SCI manifests as a distinct constellation of neurologic abnormalities correlating with an involvement of a distinct lesion in the spinal cord (Fig. 20-28; Table 20-5).[83]

The type of neurologic syndrome depends on the level of injury as well as the force and vector in spinal impact. The common spinal cord syndromes are the cervicomedullary syndrome, central cord syndrome, anterior cord syndrome, posterior spinal cord syndrome, the Brown-Séquard syndrome, conus medullaris syndrome, and cauda equina syndrome (see Table 20-5). The *cervicomedullary syndrome* (cervical cord to medulla syndrome) involves the upper cervical cord and brainstem; it typically occurs from excessive traction or compression due to severe dislocation with AP spinal cord compression. The distinguishing feature is sensory loss over the face, so it is important to include an examination of facial sensation in all cervical spinal injuries. A perioral distribution of sensory loss signifies a lesion in the medulla and upper cervical cord, whereas a more peripheral facial distribution of sensory loss, involving the forehead, ear, and chin, denotes a lesion in the cord at C3-C4. In addition to the facial sensory loss, there may be evidence of motor deficits with a greater loss of upper extremity function than lower extremity function (similar to the anterior cord syndrome).

The *central cord syndrome* is an acute central cervical spinal cord injury syndrome in which upper extremity weakness is greater than lower extremity weakness and there are alterations in pain and temperature sensations (as the fibers cross the midline). This syndrome is seen more often in elderly patients with cervical spinal stenosis who have extension-type injuries from falls, trauma, syringomyelia, or intrinsic cord tumor.

The *anterior cord syndrome* results from an injury to the spinal cord that spares the posterior columns. Motor and sensory functions and pain and temperature sensations are lost, but vibration and position sensation are preserved. The syndrome occurs more commonly in the cervical region and is characterized by lower motor neuron paralysis of the arms and upper motor neuron paralysis of the legs. The *posterior cord syndrome* is a rare type of incomplete syndrome that involves the posterior column primarily, resulting in loss of fine sensation and vibratory and position sensations, with preservation of pain sensation, temperature sensation, and motor function. The *Brown-Séquard syndrome* is relatively uncommon, appearing most often in the context of cervical spine injuries; it involves impairment of the lateral half of the spinal cord, sparing the other half. Clinically, there is motor paralysis and a loss of position sense ipsilateral to the lesion, with loss of sensory and temperature sensation opposite to the lesion. This syndrome is seen more often with hyperextension injuries but can be associated with flexion injuries, locked facets, compression fractures, herniated disks, and extrinsic tumors.

The *conus medullaris syndrome* involves a lesion at the level of the conus (T12-L1), where the spinal cord narrows and involves the sacral (and perhaps lumbar) cord segments. This syndrome is characterized by areflexia of the bowel and bladder, variable motor and sensory losses in the lower extremities, and sacral sensory sparing. The *cauda equina syndrome* occurs from SCI at or below the L1-L2 disk space and involves the lumbar and sacral nerve roots (L1-L5). Typical findings include variable lower motor neuron sensory and motor loss to the lower extremities and an areflexic bowel and/or bladder. The cauda equina syndrome is seen after acute central disk herniation, spinal trauma, and extrinsic neoplastic or infectious processes.

Anatomic and Physiologic Considerations

Following traumatic SCI, autoregulation of SCBF is impaired, so the adverse effects of hypotension or hypoxia are compounded (particularly when both are present), resulting in further injury. Subsequent to SCI, there is an initial catecholamine release resulting in a pressor response that contributes

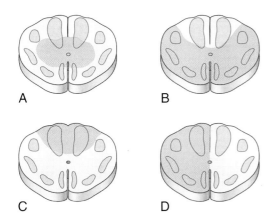

Figure 20–28 Types of spinal cord injury (*shaded areas*) that produce the four main incomplete injury patterns seen clinically. **A,** Central cord syndrome; **B,** anterior cord syndrome; **C,** posterior cord syndrome; **D,** Brown-Séquard syndrome.

Table 20–5	Incomplete Spinal Cord Injury Syndromes
Syndrome	**Clinical Findings**
Conus medullans syndrome	Areflexia of bowel and bladder; variable motor and sensory loss in lower extremities; sacral sparing
Cauda equina syndrome	Areflexia of bowel and bladder; variable motor and sensory loss in lower extremities
Cervicomedullary syndrome tetraplegia	Respiratory arrest, hypotension, anesthesia below C1 Distinguishing feature is facial sensory loss Deficits may be greater in upper than in lower extremity
Anterior cord syndrome	Loss of motor, sensory, temperature, and pain sensations Vibration and position sensations intact
Central cord syndrome	Motor impairment of upper extremities more than lower extremities Alterations in pain and temperature sensations
Posterior cord syndrome	Loss of fine, vibratory, and position sensations Motor function preserved
Brown-Séquard syndrome	Ipsilateral paralysis, loss of proprioception, touch, and vibration sensations Contralateral loss of pain and temperature sensations

to vasogenic edema.[84] After the hypertensive response, there is a phase of hypotension and reduced cardiac output. These hemodynamic changes are in part responsible for a reduction in SCBF that is observed as early as 30 to 60 minutes after injury, which preferentially affects gray matter and central white matter.[85,86] Blood flow may not return to preinjury levels for up to 24 hours. Finally, after SCI, there is a progressive decrease in oxygen tension and a loss of CO_2 responsiveness, which is correlated with neurologic outcome.[87]

Pathophysiology of Spinal Cord Injury

PRIMARY AND SECONDARY INJURY (Fig. 20-29)

Primary injury results from direct tissue destruction from blunt or penetrating forces. Such trauma is observed following vertebral fracture or dislocation, burst fractures with retropulsion of bone fragments or disk material into the spinal cord, ligamentous injury with distraction and spinal cord compression, and gunshot and knife wounds. The term *secondary injury* is simply defined as a worsening of the original injury as a result of factors other than the mechanism of the original insult. Many mechanisms for secondary injury have been proposed (Box 20-2); they are set in motion within minutes of the primary injury and may continue for days. These processes contribute to the ischemic zones observed in the gray matter and surrounding central white matter soon after SCI and explain the increases in tissue lactic acid and decreases in adenosine triphosphate (ATP) production observed.[88] Progressive ischemia is an etiologic factor in secondary degeneration; it may be worsened by edema, which reaches a maximum at 3 to 6 days and may persist for 2 weeks.

One of the first changes observed immediately after spinal injury is a loss of neurologic function (spinal cord concussion), which may occur in the absence of initial histologic changes. This effect is due in part to an efflux of K^+ into the extracellular space, which causes membrane depolarization as well as disturbances in metabolic and synaptic function.[89,90] Depolarization of the membrane stimulates the release of excitatory amino acids, which in turn facilitates further depolarization. In addition, the failure of transmembrane ionic pumps results in increases in intracellular Na^+, which stimulates the Na^+/Ca^{2+} pump to operate contrary to its normal function, that is, pumping Na^+ out of the cell and Ca^{2+} into the cell. Intracellular Ca^{2+} activates calcium-dependent proteases, phospholipases, and endonucleases, further facilitating cell damage.

Free radical–induced lipid peroxidation of neuronal and vascular cell membranes and myelin is also involved in secondary injury.[91] Finally, the release of endogenous opioids after

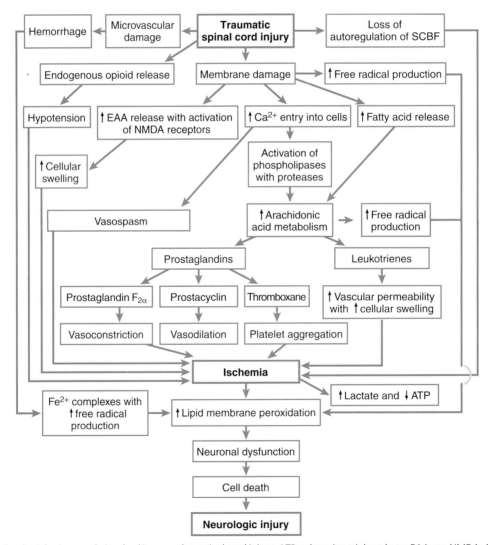

Figure 20–29 Pathophysiologic cascade involved in secondary spinal cord injury. ATP, adenosine triphosphate; EAA, xx; NMDA, *N*-methyl-D-aspartate; SCBF, spinal cord blood flow; ↑, increase; ↓, decrease.

BOX 20–2 *Secondary Mechanisms of Acute Spinal Cord Injury*

Vascular	Cellular Dysfunction	Biochemical Aberrations
Hemorrhage	↑Extracellular K⁺	↑Catecholamine release
Loss of auto regulation	↑Intracellular Ca²⁺	↑Arachidonic acid metabolism
Arteriolar occlusion	↑Intracellular Na⁺	Prostaglandins
Vasospasm	Inhibition of Na⁺/K⁺-ATPase	Thromboxanes
Edema	Lipid peroxidation	Leukotrienes
↑Vascular permeability	Increased intracellular edema	Free radicals
Hypotension	Mitochondrial failure	↑Endogenous opioid release
		↑Excitatory amino acid release
		↑Free radical formation
		Arachidonic acid metabolism
		Decompartmentalization of iron
		Hemoglobin extravasation
		Mitochondrial "leak"
		Activated neutrophils

traumatic SCI has been implicated in the pathophysiology of secondary injury.[92] However, in the definitive human study, naloxone did not improve SCI.[93] Subsequent reanalysis of the data did indicate some benefit from the use of naloxone.[94]

Spinal Cord–Protective Strategies

Minimizing secondary SCI is the most important aspect of medical therapy following any injury to the spinal cord. Early institution of pharmacologic therapies combined with surgical decompression and stabilization of the spine may result in the best outcome potential. The current use of both modalities is briefly reviewed.

PHARMACOLOGIC THERAPIES

Corticosteroids. Corticosteroids are believed to stabilize membranes, alter ionic-clearing mechanisms, improve blood flow, inhibit lipid peroxidation formation, and enhance Na⁺/K⁺-ATPase activity.[95] The membrane-stabilizing effects may prevent the release of lysosomes and excessive Ca²⁺ ionic fluxes into cells. Improvement in blood flow may be due to a reduction in tissue edema, the direct vasodilative effects of steroids, and antioxidant properties. One of the first clinical studies of corticosteroid use in SCI was the first National Acute Spinal Cord Injury Study (NASCIS I).[96] This study failed to show any benefit in neurologic recovery following steroid therapy; however, the dose regimen was thought to be inadequate.

The second National Acute Spinal Cord Injury Study (NASCIS II) was a multi-institutional, randomized, placebo-controlled, double-blind study that involved 487 patients entered into the study within 12 hours of their injuries.[93] The patients were randomly allocated to one of three treatment groups: (1) methylprednisolone, 30 mg/kg, followed by 5.4 mg/kg/hr for 23 hours; (2) naloxone, 5.4 mg/kg followed by 4 mg/kg/hr for 23 hours; or (3) placebo. No meaningful improvement in neurologic function was seen between the groups, but when the methylprednisolone results were stratified according to the timing of administration, patients treated within 8 hours of injury showed significant improvement in motor and sensory function in comparison with those given the placebo. The naloxone-treated group, however, did not show any difference in neurologic outcome. The NASCIS II results led to the common practice of administering methylprednisolone to patients within 8 hours of SCI.

NASCIS III compared the efficacy of methylprednisolone administered for 24 hours with methylprednisolone given for 48 hours or tirilazad mesylate administered for 48 hours.[95] A total of 499 patients received methylprednisolone (30 mg/kg) within 8 hours of SCI. Patients in the 24-hour group received methylprednisolone (5.4 mg/kg/hr) for 24 hours, those in the 48-hour group received methylprednisolone (5.4 mg/kg/hr) for 48 hours, and those in the tirilazad group received tirilazad mesylate 2.5 mg/kg every 6 hours for 48 hours. Patients treated with methylprednisolone for 48 hours showed greater motor recovery at 6 weeks and 6 months after injury than patients treated with the same agent for 24 hours. The effect of the 48-hour methylprednisolone regimen was most significant at 6 weeks and 6 months among patients whose therapy was initiated 3 to 8 hours after injury. Patients treated with tirilazad for 48 hours showed motor recovery rates equivalent to those of patients treated with methylprednisolone for 24 hours. The investigators concluded that patients with acute SCI who received methylprednisolone within 3 hours of injury were to remain on the treatment regimen for 24 hours. When methylprednisolone was initiated 3 to 8 hours after injury, patients were to stay on steroid therapy for 48 hours. No functional benefit was demonstrated for the use of steroid therapy in the treatment of penetrating SCI.[97]

The use of methylprednisolone after acute SCI has now been questioned. Since the original publication of both NASCIS II and III, reexamination of these trials has led to significant criticism about their conclusions. Specifically, NASCIS II has been disparaged for flaws in study design and statistical analysis, and NASCIS III results have been questioned because of concerns regarding the timing of surgery, the process of neurologic assessment, and the fact that differences in motor scores and functional outcome were clinically negligible.[98] In a reevaluation of the results and conclusions of these trials regarding primary outcomes and post-hoc comparisons, it was concluded that both NASCIS II and III failed to demonstrate meaningful differences in neurologic recovery among the placebo, 24-hour methylprednisolone, and 48-hour methylprednisolone treatment groups.[99] Moreover, in patients in NASCIS III who received a 48-hour infusion, there was a higher incidence of infections than in patients receiving a 24-hour infusion. Thus, any marginal benefit of steroid use in SCI may be nullified by the increase in infectious complications. In response to the paucity of medical evidence conclusively supporting significant clinical benefits from steroid use in either a 24-hour or 48-hour dosing regimen, most guidelines now consider the use of high-dose steroids to be a "treatment option" rather than a standard.[100,101]

Hypothermia. Extensive animal evidence supports the efficacy of hypothermia for the treatment of traumatic SCI. A review of the literature on the efficacy of hypothermia in the setting of experimental SCI determined that although the efficacy of hypothermia in improving functional outcome of mild to moderate traumatic SCI has been demonstrated, hypothermia may not be protective against severe traumatic SCI.[102] To date, little clinical evidence conclusively proves that hypothermic techniques can benefit patients with traumatic SCI. Moreover, because of significant circulatory, pulmonary, metabolic, and immunologic side effects, the routine use of hypothermia as a spinal cord protectant in the setting of traumatic SCI remains an option but cannot be considered standard therapy.

Hypertension. Hypertension is advocated by some to improve perfusion in the post-traumatic patient with hypoperfusion of the spinal cord. Although definitive data are lacking, early and aggressive intervention to maintain a mean arterial blood pressure above 85 mm Hg for the first 7 days after injury is recommended to preserve neurologic function because autoregulation is impaired.[100,103] Even though more aggressive hypertensive therapy may have advantages, it may convey a risk of further hemorrhage and edema.

Conclusion. Unfortunately, no clear benefit from any pharmacologic therapy has yet emerged to significantly reduce spinal cord damage following traumatic injury. Nonetheless, research into newer therapies focusing on neurologic regeneration and protection is receiving much attention and may ultimately prove beneficial (Box 20-3).

SURGICAL THERAPIES

Early surgical therapy following SCI may reduce neurologic injury. The decision for surgical intervention following SCI involves many considerations including (1) neurologic and radiologic evaluation; (2) the initial success of closed reduction and decompression; (3) determination of the degree of spinal column stability; (4) determination of the benefit of early open surgical decompression and stabilization; and (5) choosing the particular surgical approach (Box 20-4).

Neurologic and Radiologic Evaluation. Surgical intervention following SCI is based on the detection of neurologic deterioration obtained from frequent neurologic assessments (every 12 hours) and the extent of spinal column abnormalities detected on initial radiographic studies.

Initial Closed Reduction and Decompression. Initial therapy after SCI is directed toward prevention of further neurologic injury, because up to 25% of SCIs occur after the initial insult, either during the transport process or early in the course of treatment.[13] Spinal immobilization is initially carried out at the scene of the accident and is achieved by placing the patient on a spinal board, with immobilization of the head and neck using sandbags as well as adhesive tape on the forehead attached to each side of the board.

If radiographic films taken at the hospital reveal a spinal dislocation, closed reduction is attempted with the use of a traction device to align and immobilize the spine, decompress neural structures, and prevent further neurologic injury. Diminished pressure on the spinal cord results in improved microvascular circulation, which may reduce spinal cord edema and prevent a progressive neurologic deficit. Closed reduction is successful 70% to 80% of the time, with few reports of neurologic worsening.[104] On occasion, facets may be locked during injury, preventing reduction even with extreme traction.

Determination of Spinal Stability. The determination of spinal stability following trauma is important in planning potential surgical treatment. *Spinal stability* has been defined as the means by which the vertebral structures maintain their cohesion in all physiologic positions.[105] Instability or loss of stability is a pathologic process that, if left untreated, can lead to progressive spinal deformity, neurologic loss, and chronic pain.[106] In the setting of acute spine trauma, the clinical history, neurologic examination, and initial radiographic

---

BOX 20–3 *Current Status of Treatment After Traumatic SCI in Humans*

Accepted Benefit

None

Potential Benefit

Methylprednisolone
21-Aminosteroids
GM-1 gangliosides
Minocycline
Prostacyclin analogs
NMDA-receptor antagonists
Hypertonic saline
Platelet-activating factor antagonists
Neurite growth inhibitor antibodies
Antioxidants and free radical scavengers
Stem cell transplantation
Gene therapy
Activated macrophage implantation

Little or No Proven Benefit

Opioid antagonists
Thyrotropin-releasing hormone analogs
Arachidonic acid metabolite inhibitors
Localized hypothermia
Dimethyl sulfoxide
Hyperbaric oxygen
ε-aminocaproic acid
Calcium antagonists

BOX 20–4 *Indications for Surgical Intervention Following Traumatic Spinal Injury*

Accepted Indications for Surgery

- Progressive neurologic deterioration in an unstable spine, especially with spinal canal compromise
- Failure of closed reduction and stabilization of dislocation with residual canal narrowing of ≥ 50%
- Unstable spine with dislocated bilateral "locked" facets
- Unstable spine where nonunion is likely (e.g., ligamentous injury with vertebral body separation)
- Uncooperative patient with unstable spine risking further neurologic injury
- Compression of conus medullaris or cauda equina

Controversial Indications for Surgery

- Vertebral fractures with bony encroachment of spinal canal without neurologic findings
- Complete SCI with dislocation successfully treated with closed reduction and immobilization
- Incomplete SCI with dislocation successfully treated with closed reduction and immobilization
- Unstable spine with complete SCI (to facilitate "zonal root" recovery)
- Unstable spine with incomplete SCI (to prevent further deterioration)
- Unstable spine without neurologic deficits
- Thoracolumbar burst fractures successfully treated by closed reduction and immobilization

SCI, Spinal cord injury.

imaging should allow a reasonable determination of spinal stability.

For the upper cervical spine (C1-C2), the primary determinant of stability is the transverse atlantal ligament (TAL), which is assessed by plain radiographs and by CT. Any bony displacement beyond acceptable limits renders the spine unstable. In general, if the sagittal plane distance between the back of the anterior ring of C1 and the anterior portion of the dens is greater than 3 or 4 mm, and the sagittal plane distance between the posterior dens and the anterior portion of the posterior ring of C1 is less than 13 mm, the spine is unstable at that level.[107]

For the lower cervical spine (C3-C7), a variety of methods have been used to determine spinal stability; they include anatomic considerations that divide the spine into columns[105,108-110]; clinical considerations that correlate the magnitude of the neurologic injury with the likelihood of spinal instability[111]; and radiographic criteria that assess various measurements of spinal bony alignment, spinal canal dimensions, disk space size, and identification of the presence of major ligamentous injury.[105,108,109,112,113] Determination of major ligamentous injury is also important because adequate healing is unlikely in this setting, resulting in a chronically unstable spine with progressive kyphosis, neurologic deficits, or both.[112]

Anatomic considerations used in the assessment of spinal stability after lower cervical spine injury may be viewed in the context of either a three-column[105,110] or a two-column approach.[108,113] The Denis three-column model is a well-described method of predicting spinal instability.[110] Originally described and most commonly used for assessing thoracolumbar trauma, it has been employed in cervical injuries as well. In this model, the spinal column is divided into three longitudinal columns (Fig. 20-30). The anterior column comprises the anterior longitudinal ligament, the anterior anulus fibrosis, and the anterior half of the vertebral body. The middle column comprises the posterior half of the vertebral body, the posterior longitudinal ligament, and the posterior anulus fibrosis. The posterior column comprises the posterior bony arch with the posterior ligamentous complex. The biomechanics of the injury combined with plain films and CT scans of the spine demonstrating failure of two or all columns renders the spinal unstable.

Clinical considerations may be used to predict cervical spine stability. This approach considers the presence of a neurologic deficit to imply that the cervical spinal trauma subjected the spinal cord or nerve roots to either a vascular, mechanical, or chemical insult and that given such severe injury, the integrity of the supporting structures has been altered enough to permit further injury, thus representing an unstable spine.[107]

Use of radiographic criteria is a popular method for predicting lower cervical spine instability. In particular, radiographic abnormalities demonstrating more than 11 degrees of sagittal plane translation and more than 3.5 mm of sagittal plane translation, more than 50% compression of the vertebral body, interspinous widening, loss of facet parallelism, and loss of normal cervical lordosis indicate spinal instability. Finally, both the clinical and radiologic findings may be combined and used as part of an instability checklist, as suggested by White and Panjabi.[107] The instability checklist assigns individual points to specific radiologic and clinical findings, and then the points are summated for a total score that is used to estimate the likelihood of spinal instability. This checklist approach is very useful and can be applied to a variety of clinical scenarios.

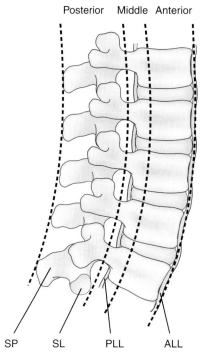

Posterior Middle Anterior

SP   SL   PLL   ALL

Figure 20–30 Spinal column stability after traumatic injury is often based on a system that divides the spine into three columns. The anterior column comprises the anterior longitudinal ligament (ALL), the anterior anulus fibrosis, and the anterior half of the vertebral body. The middle column comprises the posterior half of the vertebral body, the posterior longitudinal ligament (PLL), and the posterior anulus fibrosis. The posterior column comprises the posterior bony arch, which includes the spinolaminar junction (SL), the spinous process (SP), and the posterior ligamentous complex. Disruption of two or more of these columns indicates spinal instability.

For assessment of thoracic and lumbar spinal injury, the evaluation is very similar to the techniques described for assessing the cervical spine, and it often relies on the Denis three-column model, or an instability checklist similar to that described by White and Panjabi for cervical spinal injury.[107] In the lumbar region, the Denis three-column model is most frequently used. Ultimately, correlating neurologic findings with radiologic evidence of structural damage will best guide treatment.

Early Surgical Therapy Following Spinal Injuries. The indications and timing of surgical therapy following spinal injuries are debated. Most authorities agree that surgery is clearly indicated in any unstable spinal injury associated with evolving neurologic deficits, especially when they are associated with radiologic evidence of acute spinal canal compromise. Most would also agree that surgery is indicated for an unstable spine with dislocated bilateral "locked" facets, an unstable spine with significant ligamentous injury and vertebral body separation, and an unstable spine in an uncooperative patient who risks further neurologic injury. However, for other types of spinal injuries, the benefits and timing of surgical decompression and stabilization after SCI remain controversial. Experimental evidence strongly suggests that early decompression after SCI reduces secondary SCI and improves neurologic outcome.[115-120] Clinical studies, however, have failed to clearly demonstrate the beneficial effects of early decompression so evident in the experimental models. Later studies and literature reviews increasingly suggest that early decompression (<24 hours) may indeed facilitate a more favorable neurologic outcome, particularly in patients with incomplete injuries.[121-125] For spinal decompression therapy to be most effective, evidence suggests that decompression must occur within 24 hours, particularly in incomplete neurologic injuries. Late surgical decompression (>48 hours) offers no particular neurologic benefits other than stabilization of the spinal column, which facilitates rehabilitation therapy.

Surgical Approaches in Spinal Injury. If surgical therapy is chosen, three basic approaches may be taken: anterior, posterior, or a combination of the two. In general, anterior approaches for spinal decompression and stabilization are indicated for removal of disk material, bone, or ligamentous tissue compressing the spinal cord anteriorly. Anterior cervical instrumentation is typically used to treat unstable compression-flexion and distractive-flexion injuries, often in conjunction with a decompressive corpectomy (removal of vertebral body) if the cord is compressed (Fig. 20-31).

Posterior stabilization is indicated for significant disruption of the posterior bony or ligamentous structures of the cervical spine, particularly with minimal or no involvement of the vertebral body. Posterior fixation techniques are used to treat occipitocervical and atlantoaxial instability and for most cases of spinal instability caused by flexion injuries, including posterior ligamentous injury, anterior dislocation, bilateral facet dislocation, and simple wedge compression fractures. Flexion-rotation injuries causing unilateral facet dislocation may require posterior cervical stabilization as well, particularly if closed reduction is unsuccessful.

A combined approach is indicated for significant injuries involving both the anterior and posterior bony or ligamentous structures. Such injuries include extensive cervical injuries, such as flexion teardrop fractures, vertical compression burst fractures with significant posterior ligamentous injury, and bilateral facet dislocation with disk compression of the spinal cord.

Medical Management

PULMONARY SYSTEM

Although acute SCI can have differing effects on the pulmonary system, the level of injury often determines the magnitude of effect and the clinical course (Table 20-6; Box 20-5). Most abnormalities are the result of the adverse effects of SCI on pulmonary lung volumes and pulmonary mechanics.

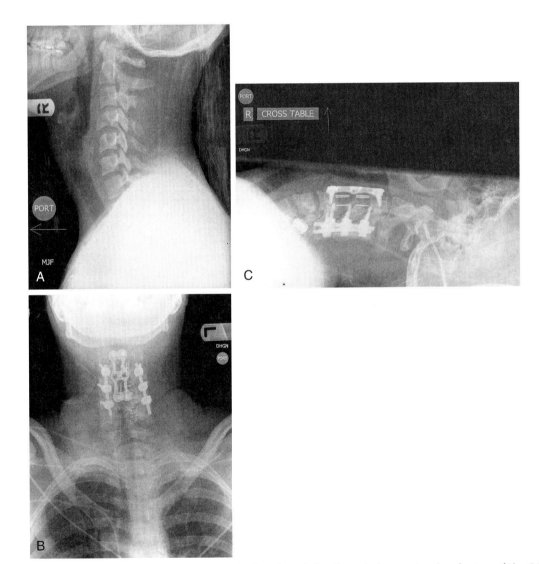

Figure 20–31 Cervical spine teardrop fracture. **A,** A preoperative lateral cervical radiograph shows a teardrop fracture of the C4 vertebral body inferiorly. **B,** An anteroposterior radiograph shows anterior plate and screw fusion from C3 to C5 with prosthetic strut grafts and posterior fusion of the same levels with bilateral pedicle screws and rods. **C,** On this postoperative lateral radiograph, the anterior plate and screws are clearly visible.

Table 20–6 Level of Spinal Cord Injury and Corresponding Respiratory Function*

Injury Level	Ventilatory Function	Cough	Relevant Comment(s)
Above C3	0	0	Paralysis of diaphragm and accessory muscles, resulting in apnea; lifelong ventilator dependence
C3-C5	0 to +	0	Partial to complete diaphragmatic paralysis; paralysis of accessory muscles; marked reduction in lung volumes with hypoxemia; recurrent atelectasis and pneumonia; prolonged mechanical ventilator dependence; probable tracheostomy; most patients will be weaned from mechanical ventilation
C5-C7	+ to ++	+ to ++	Paralysis of accessory muscles; marked reduction in volumes with hypoxemia; recurrent atelectasis and pneumonia; many patients need mechanical ventilation; possible tracheostomy
High thoracic	++	++	Partial paralysis of accessory muscles; reduction in lung volumes with atelectasis; increased incidence of pneumonia; possible need for mechanical ventilation

*Scale: 0 (no function) to +++ (normal).

BOX 20–5 *Protocol For Reduction of Pulmonary Complications in Patients with SCI*

Aggressive pulmonary hygiene
 Frequent nasotracheal suctioning
 Positional changes every 2 hours, best achieved with kinetic devices (e.g., rotational or circle beds)
 Chest percussion every 4 hours
 Assisted coughing exercises every 4 hours
 Deep breathing exercises every 4 hours
 Incentive spirometry every 4 hours
Bronchodilator therapy for assisting secretion clearance and bronchodilator effects
Early use of fiberoptic bronchoscopy in cases of lobar atelectasis secondary to retained secretions
Early institution of mechanical ventilation in those with progressive labored breathing, increasing respiratory failure (hypoxia or hypercapnia) and vital capacities <1000 ml
Close monitoring of respiratory mechanics in patients receiving mechanical ventilation with optimal use PEEP therapy and limitation of plateau pressure to <30 cm Hg

---

The normal muscles of respiration are composed of the intercostal muscles (supplied by the intercostal nerves originating from the thoracic spinal cord) and the diaphragm (supplied by cervical innervation originating from C3 to C5). The diaphragm normally contributes about 65% of the vital capacity. Injuries to the cervical cord above C3 produce nearly complete respiratory muscle paralysis. Patients with injuries to this level of the spinal cord are not able to produce a tidal breath or to cough. Consequently, these patients require emergency assistance for breathing to prevent profound hypercapnia and hypoxemia. Tetraplegic patients use the accessory muscles of breathing during tidal breathing. With inspiration, the sternum is pulled cephalad and the upper rib cage expands, increasing the upper anterior–posterior diameter, and the lower rib cage is pulled inward, resulting in a reduction in the lower rib cage transverse diameter. With cervical SCI involving levels below C3, increasing function of the diaphragm is noted. However, the persistent absence of intercostal muscle function limits expiratory muscle use, and the ability to cough remains extremely limited. Spirometric pulmonary function tests performed acutely on patients with cervical SCI show significant reductions in all lung volumes except for residual volume (which is nearly twice normal levels).[126,127] However, over the course of the first 4 to 5 months, improvement in most lung volumes can be expected to occur.

Contrary to the normal increase in vital capacity seen when healthy patients assume an upright position, patients with cervical SCI demonstrate an improvement in vital capacity when assuming the supine position. This improvement in vital capacity is secondary to a reduction in the residual volume, which occurs in the supine position and is considered to be related to the effect of gravity on the abdominal contents in the presence of paralyzed abdominal musculature.

Pulmonary mechanics are altered in cervical SCI, with decreases in lung compliance[128] and resultant increases in the work of breathing. The adverse effects on lung compliance are considered to be related to actual changes in the mechanical properties of the lung in addition to the reduction in lung volumes.[128] Gastric distention secondary to gastric atony may also be a contributory factor to the adverse effects of SCI on pulmonary mechanics. As the spinal shock state resolves (2 to 5 weeks), progressive spasticity of chest wall and abdominal muscles will assist in improving pulmonary function.

Pulmonary complications are the leading causes of morbidity and early mortality after cervical and upper thoracic SCI and are seen in as many as 75% of patients.[129] Pulmonary complications occur as a result of the alterations in respiratory mechanics and lung volumes. The reduction of lung volumes and the inability of the patient to generate an effective cough result in progressive retention of pulmonary secretions with gradual microatelectasis and lobar atelectasis, leading to incremental hypoxemia and CO_2 retention.

Other pulmonary problems are pulmonary edema (noncardiogenic, cardiogenic), aspiration pneumonitis, and coexisting blunt chest trauma (pulmonary contusions, hemothorax). The onset of pulmonary complications depends on the level of SCI. Jackson and Groomes[129] prospectively investigated the occurrence of pulmonary complications relative to the level of SCI. Overall, 84% of patients with C1 to C4 injuries, 60% of those with C5 to C8 injuries, and 65% of those with T1 to T12 injuries had respiratory complications. Ventilatory failure and aspiration were the earliest to occur (at 4.5 days) for all patients with SCI.

Kinetic therapy (i.e., rotational bed), in particular, is effective in reducing the incidence of pulmonary complications, decreasing time on the ventilator, and shortening length of stay in the intensive care unit.[130-136] For best results, kinetic therapy should be started early in the treatment of patients with acute cervical spinal cord injuries. Aggressive prevention strategies, as mentioned, reduce hospital resource utilization as well as overall morbidity and mortality.[126]

Because significant impairment in pulmonary function is seen early in patients with tetraplegia, frequent reassessments and close monitoring of diagnostic tests are imperative. During the first 1 to 3 days, significant declines in pulmonary reserve may occur before overt clinical signs are seen. In addition, although tetraplegic patients may be initially hospitalized with a functioning diaphragm, progressive cord edema may occur over the first 2 days, resulting in an ascending neurologic injury. This condition may cause a loss of diaphragmatic function with progressive respiratory failure and the need for tracheal cannulation. When the vital capacity decreases to less than 50% of predicted (2000 mL in an average adult), more frequent determinations of vital capacity must be made (e.g., every 6 hours); when the vital capacity decreases to less than 1 L, and especially if the patient is clinically dyspneic and hypoxemic, endotracheal intubation should be performed.

When mechanical ventilation is indicated, a volume-control mode of mechanical ventilation, such as assist-control or synchronized intermittent mechanical ventilation (SIMV) is initially chosen, although other choices, including pressure-limited modes, may be selected. Ventilator settings should be selected that limit the occurrence of ventilator-associated lung injury (VALI).[137-140] Typical settings are an initial tidal volume of 6 to 8 mL/kg, positive end-expiratory pressure (PEEP) of 5, an initial rate of 8 to 15 breaths/min, and a plateau pressure of ≤30 mm Hg. The positive end-expiratory pressure is added to recruit collapsed alveoli and prevent further atelectasis. In patients with cervical SCI below C4, eventual weaning from mechanical ventilation is to be expected and is facilitated when spinal shock resolves and the respiratory and abdominal muscles develop spasticity (2-3 weeks), leading to improvement in lung volumes and overall ventilatory ability. Nearly all patients with complete cervical SCI above C6 will require a tracheostomy because of the length of time on the ventilator and the difficulty with clearing secretions. In this setting, a tracheostomy should be placed early.

Pulmonary edema may be observed in patients with acute SCI, with etiologic factors including neurogenic or cardiac pulmonary edema and pulmonary contusion. Neurogenic increases in extravascular water resulting in pulmonary edema have been observed both in head injury and in SCI[141] and may be related, in part, to the initial sympathetic discharge that occurs at the time of SCI. Cardiogenic pulmonary edema may also be due to the combination of reduced myocardial inotropy, seen with high SCI, and overzealous fluid administration. Because of the hemodynamic alterations observed in SCI (hypotension, bradycardia), the usual indicators of fluid adequacy are unreliable. Chest trauma is associated with SCI and may include pulmonary contusions, rib fractures, pneumothorax, hemothorax, and acute respiratory distress syndrome. These injuries may result in prolonged mechanical ventilation with difficult weaning and delayed operative spinal intervention.

Cardiovascular System

SCI also has a profound effect on the cardiovascular system, the magnitude again depending on the level of injury. In general, complete cervical SCI has the most pronounced physiologic effects, consisting of cardiovascular instability, cardiac dysrhythmias, and ventricular dysfunction, whereas SCI below T5 results in varying degrees of hypotension caused by the functional sympathectomy below the level of injury.

Hemodynamic changes noted after SCI have been observed consistently in experimental models of SCI and include a transient severe increase in blood pressure caused by an extensive sympathetic discharge at the time of injury. The systolic blood pressure may be as high as 300 mm Hg, lasting 2 to 5 minutes,[142] with a gradual decline to values less than baseline.[85] Although the hypertensive response to SCI has been documented only in experimental models, it is generally believed to occur in humans at the time of injury and to resolve by the time medical treatment is undertaken. This sympathetic discharge may be responsible for the noncardiogenic pulmonary edema reported to occur after SCI.

After the initial period of transient hypertension has resolved, hypotension becomes the predominant hemodynamic abnormality and is present in nearly all patients with complete cervical SCI. The hypotension is related to vasodilation of the vasculature, which arises secondary to the withdrawal of sympathetic neural outflow. When an SCI occurs in the cervical region, the sympathetic receptors lose their normal input and regulation, resulting in a functional sympathetic blockade. In contrast, the parasympathetic nervous system remains intact as the vagus nerve exits from the brainstem. Consequently, after an acute injury occurs in the cervical or high thoracic spinal cord, the resulting autonomic imbalance between sympathetic and parasympathetic outflows leads to inadequate cardiac contraction and a loss of tonic vasoconstriction, with resulting hypotension, bradycardia, and hypothermia (termed *neurogenic shock*).

Spinal shock describes the phenomenon seen with physiologic or anatomic transection, or near transection, of the spinal cord; it consists of the loss of somatic motor and sensory function below the level of injury, loss of voluntary rectal contraction, and loss of sympathetic autonomic function. The more severe the functional spinal cord transection and the higher the level of injury, the greater the severity and duration of spinal shock. If the loss of motor and sensory functions resulting from spinal shock lasts longer than 1 hour, pathologic injuries to the spinal cord, as opposed to a transient concussive injury, are assumed to exist.

Sixty percent to 70% of patients demonstrate neurogenic shock after complete cervical injury.[143] The more cephalad the level of spinal injury, the more severe the physiologic derangements encountered. The most common cardiovascular abnormalities observed after an acute cervical SCI are marked bradycardia (in 71% of patients) and hypotension (in 68%). Bradycardia is present in virtually all patients with complete cervical SCI; however, it is less likely with SCI involving the thoracic and lumbar regions. Bradycardia results from the interruption of the sympathetic cardiac accelerator nerves (T1 to T4), leaving an unopposed parasympathetic influence. Bradycardia usually resolves over a 3- to 5-week period after injury. More profound degrees of bradycardia, even cardiac arrest, may occur during stimulation of the patient, such as turning or tracheal suctioning. The cardiovascular derangements remain most problematic during the first 2 weeks after an acute cervical SCI.[144] Preventive measures to avoid severe bradycardic episodes are encouraged; they include sedation, 100% oxygen before suctioning, and limiting the time allowed for suctioning. Although most episodes are effectively treated with atropine, temporary pacemaker therapy may be required.

Hypotension, defined as a systolic blood pressure below 90 mm Hg or systolic blood pressure 30% below baseline, is seen in 60% to 80% of patients with an acute cervical SCI. The optimal treatment of hypotension after SCI has yet to be defined, but it is recommended that the mean arterial pressure be maintained at ≥85 mm Hg for the first 7 days following acute SCI.[103,145] Because autoregulation is lost after SCI, aggressive use of fluids or vasoactive medications for the correction of hypotension is crucial for optimal preservation of neurologic function and reduction of secondary injury. The hypotension is in part related to the relative hypovolemia secondary to vasodilation in patients with neurogenic shock. Appropriate blood replacement should be administered as indicated to maintain a hemoglobin level of 10 g/dL in the early period of resuscitation. Caution should be exercised to limit the overall volume of fluid, because patients are prone to develop cardiogenic and noncardiogenic pulmonary edema. If hypotension persists despite adequate fluid administration, vasopressor or inotropic therapy should be promptly instituted.

Care should be taken in the administration of potent α-agonist agents because substantial increases in cardiac afterload may impair cardiac output and precipitate left ventricular failure. Accordingly, an inotropic agent is often the drug of choice for maintaining spinal cord perfusion. Invasive hemodynamic monitoring is recommended for optimal guidance in the treatment of persistent hypotension in the context of neurogenic shock. Finally, there is evidence to support improvement in neurologic outcome separate from surgical intervention in SCI patients in whom hemodynamics are managed aggressively.[103] Because spinal cord edema is maximal at 3 to 6 days after injury, blood pressure support should continue during this period.

Although isotonic crystalloid is the initial fluid of choice in the treatment of neurogenic shock, the use of hypertonic saline may be of additional benefit in the initial resuscitation phase after SCI. Experimental data have indicated that the administration of hypertonic saline after experimental SCI improves SCBF and preserves spinal cord function,[146,147] but definitive clinical studies are lacking.

Cardiac dysrhythmias are commonly observed following SCI in both experimental and clinical reports. In an experimental model of extradural SCI,[148] sinus tachycardia was noted, followed by striking electrocardiographic changes consisting of sinus pauses, a shifting sinus pacemaker, nodal escape beats, brief runs of atrial fibrillation, multifocal ventricular premature contractions, ventricular premature contractions, ventricular tachycardia, and ST-T wave changes. Atropine or bilateral vagal nerve section abolished all ectopic atrial and ventricular rhythm abnormalities but did not alter the sinus tachycardia. Propranolol abolished the tachycardia and ST-T wave changes. The investigators of the study concluded that the initial response to spinal cord compression, characterized by the marked sympathetic discharge, elicited a secondary, compensatory, parasympathetic discharge. The resulting autonomic imbalance was responsible for the cardiac dysrhythmias observed.

In a clinical report investigating the incidence of cardiovascular abnormalities in 71 consecutive patients with acute SCI who were classified as having severe cervical SCI, mild cervical SCI, or thoracolumbar SCI,[143] persistent bradycardia was observed in all 31 patients with severe acute cervical SCI, in 6 of 17 (35.3%) patients with mild cervical SCI, and in 3 of 23 (13%) patients with thoracolumbar injury. Primary cardiac arrest requiring cardiopulmonary resuscitation occurred in 16% of the 31 patients with severe cervical SCI. The frequency of bradydysrhythmias was maximal on day 4 after injury, with all abnormalities resolving over a 14-day to 6-week period. The researchers proposed that the cardiac abnormalities were caused by an acute autonomic imbalance resulting from a disruption of sympathetic pathways while the parasympathetic influences via the vagus nerve remain undisturbed. In patients with chronic SCI, the risk of cardiac dysrhythmias decreases with time from injury and eventually disappears.

GASTROINTESTINAL SYSTEM

Gastrointestinal complications are seen in up to 11% of patients after SCI; they consist of ileus, gastric distention, peptic ulcer disease, and pancreatitis.[149] Excessive gastric dilation may occur after acute SCI, resulting in gastric distention that put the patient at risk for regurgitation and aspiration. In addition, gastric distention may cause upward pressure on the diaphragm, adversely affecting ventilation. Insertion of a nasogastric tube may help in limiting distention, reducing the risk of regurgitation and minimizing adverse effects on the diaphragm and pulmonary system. Gastric emptying rates may also be decreased in patients with SCI, and patients should always be considered to be at an increased risk of gastric regurgitation.

The incidences of gastritis, ulceration, and hemorrhage are increased after SCI, particularly in patients requiring mechanical ventilation and those in whom high-dose corticosteroids have been administered. Preventive techniques that have been demonstrated to be effective include antacids, H$_2$ blockers, sucralfate, proton pump inhibitors, and enteral feedings. In general, therapy with either H$_2$ blockers or proton pump inhibitors should be instituted as prophylactic treatment upon admission and continued for 4 weeks.[150] Minimal benefits are to be expected in continuing treatment beyond this period unless specific indications exist.

Other diseases that may be seen in SCI are pancreatitis, acalculous cholecystitis, and occult acute abdomen. A high index of suspicion for acute abdomen is necessary because patients with SCI may not demonstrate the usual signs and symptoms (fever, tachycardia, pain). Patients with SCI characteristically have elevated metabolic rates and are catabolic early; therefore early nutritional supplementation is advised.

GENITOURINARY SYSTEM

During the acute stages of SCI, the bladder is flaccid. Insertion of an indwelling urinary catheter (Foley catheter) facilitates bladder emptying and allows accurate recording of urinary output. Bladder flaccidity is followed by bladder spasticity. The abnormalities with bladder emptying predispose the patient to persistent urinary problems, which include recurrent urinary tract infections, bladder stones, nephrocalcinosis, and recurrent bouts of urosepsis.

TEMPERATURE CONTROL

The body temperatures of patients with complete SCI tend to approach that of the environment because of the inability to conserve heat in cold environments by vasoconstriction or to sweat in hot ambient conditions. Consequently, such patients are prone to hypothermia in situations in which the ambient temperatures are lower than normal body temperature.

COAGULATION

Deep vein thrombosis (DVT) has been reported to occur in 40% to 100% of patients with acute SCI.[151-154] Other risk factors for DVT include advanced age, a concomitant lower extremity fracture, and lack of or delay in thromboprophylaxis.[154] Pulmonary embolism occurs in 0.5% to 4.6% of patients with SCI[151,156,157] and is the third leading cause of death in such patients.[154] Pulmonary embolism occurs more often with complete SCI and thoracic injury. The diagnosis of DVT or pulmonary embolism is made from clinical suspicion combined with support from a variety of diagnostic methods, including D-dimer levels, venography, color flow duplex imaging (CFDI), CT angiography, and pulmonary angiography. The high incidence of DVT in patients with SCI necessitates the institution of prophylactic treatment as soon after injury as is possible (i.e., 72 hours), which should be continued for a minimum of 3 months. With an effective treatment plan, the occurrence of DVT can be decreased to 5%. Consensus guidelines on the prevention of DVT in patients with SCI have been published and serve to guide therapy.[155]

HYPERREFLEXIC SYNDROMES

Hyperreflexic syndromes are muscle spasms caused by hyperactive spinal reflexes without the tempering effect of modulating cortical, brainstem, and cerebellar influences. This "mass reflex" may make the management of the unanesthetized patient difficult.

Autonomic Hyperreflexia. Autonomic hyperreflexia, which occurs in 85% of patients with spinal cord transections above T5 in whom the splanchnic outflow remains intact, is secondary to autonomic vascular reflexes, which usually begin to appear about 2 to 3 weeks after injury. Afferent impulses originating from bladder or bowel distention, childbirth, manipulations of the urinary tract, or surgical stimulation are transmitted along the pelvic, pudendal, or hypogastric nerves to the isolated spinal cord and elicit a massive sympathetic response from the adrenal medulla and sympathetic nervous system, which is no longer modulated by the normal inhibitory impulses arising from the brainstem and hypothalamus. Vasoconstriction occurs below the lesion; reflex activity of carotid and aortic baroreceptors produces vasodilation above the lesion, which is often accompanied by bradycardia, ventricular dysrhythmias, and even heart block. The hypertension may be treated with direct-acting vasodilators (e.g., sodium nitroprusside), β-blocking agents (e.g., esmolol), combination β-blockers (e.g., labetalol), calcium channel blocking agents (nicardipine), or ganglionic blocking agents (e.g.,

trimethaphan). Sedation or topical anesthesia does not appear to attenuate the hypertensive response, but deep general, epidural, or spinal anesthesia is effective.

INFECTIONS

Infections, the leading cause of death in patients with SCI, include pneumonia and urosepsis. A high index of suspicion must be maintained at all times, and appropriate clinical examinations and testing must be performed routinely.

PRESSURE ULCERS

Decubitus pressure ulcers readily develop in paralyzed patients as a result of direct pressure effects, reduced tissue perfusion, and limited mobility. The use of rotational beds, frequent patient turning, good skin care, foam padding of bony prominences, or air floatation beds can help prevent pressure ulcers. If a pressure ulcer is identified, early care is essential in healing.

LONG-TERM IMMOBILIZATION

Prolonged immobilization predisposes patients to altered calcium metabolism, resulting in painful heterotopic ossification and calcification of muscles as well as joint immobility. Early institution of active physical therapy is essential to limit joint immobility. Inactivity may lead to osteoporosis with hypercalcemia, resulting in nephrocalcinosis and secondary renal failure. Late mobilization of the patient may result in pathologic fractures.

NEUROLOGIC SYSTEM

Ten percent of patients with traumatic quadriplegia have combined head injury.[158] Following care and treatment of the patient with acute SCI, chronic medical issues arise, presenting further challenges for the medical care team, including particular relevance for perioperative management.

Summary

A synopsis of medical problems in the patient with chronic SCI can be found in Table 20-7. The perioperative care of the patient with acute SCI represents a complex challenge for

---

Table 20–7 **Summary of Medical Problems in Patients with Chronic Spinal Cord Injury (SCI)**

System	Abnormality	Relevant Comment
Cardiovascular	Autonomic hyperreflexia, decreased blood volume, orthostatic hypotension	Patient is susceptible to hypertensive crisis if SCI level is above T5; positional changes and intrathoracic pressure may cause hypotension
Respiratory	Muscle weakness, decreased respiratory drive, decreased cough	Patient is susceptible to postoperative pneumonia and may be difficult to wean from mechanical ventilation
Muscular	Proliferation of acetylcholine receptors, spasticity	Hyperkalemia from succinylcholine
Genitourinary	Recurrent urinary tract infections, altered bladder emptying	May lead to renal insufficiency, pyelonephritis, sepsis, or amyloidosis
Gastrointestinal	Gastroparesis, ileus	Patient is susceptible to aspiration
Immunologic	Urinary tract infection, pneumonia, decubitus ulcers	Watch for subtle signs of infection and sepsis; questionable risk of seeding of an infection from invasive monitoring
Skin	Decubitus ulcers	Prevention
Hematologic	Anemia, risk of deep vein thrombosis (DVT) or pulmonary embolism	DVT prophylaxis
Bone	Bone density	Osteoporosis, hypercalcemia, heterotopic ossification, and muscle calcification
Central nervous system	Chronic pain	Perioperative pain can be difficult to manage

anesthesiologists. A fundamental knowledge of the initial neurologic assessment and acute medical management strategies will facilitate the limitation of further neurologic deterioration (Box 20-6).

ANESTHETIC CONSIDERATIONS IN SPINAL SURGERY

Preoperative Evaluation and Preparation

General

Preoperative considerations derive from the overall medical condition of the patient and the specific procedure that is planned. Patients presenting for surgery of the spine may manifest peripheral neuropathy, paraplegia, or spine instability, each with its attendant complications and anesthetic considerations. A comprehensive and coordinated anesthetic plan involving the surgeon and anesthesiologist that addresses the need for neurophysiologic or invasive monitoring (or both), the optimal approach to securing the airway, patient positioning, fluid requirements, special maneuvers such as an intraoperative "wake-up" test, and timing of extubation must be formulated in advance.

Airway Evaluation

The airway of the patient presenting for elective spinal surgery under general anesthesia requires meticulous evaluation, perhaps more so than for any other operation. Particular attention should be paid to the range of motion of the neck and to the presence of any neurologic symptoms or pain during such movement.

The initial airway assessment is made by means of a general survey of the patient's head and neck. Obvious problems such as morbid obesity, short neck, cervical collars, and any breathing difficulties (e.g., stridor) should be noted. The presence of any craniofacial abnormalities may suggest a potentially difficult airway. The presence of a full beard may make mask ventilation more difficult. Mouth opening, a function of

---

BOX 20–6 *Summary of Medical Management Guidelines for Acute SCI*

Important General Points

- Any patient sustaining traumatic injuries resulting in significant head or facial injuries, severe penetrating injuries in proximity to the spine, multiple blunt trauma, crush injuries, or significant acceleration or deceleration injuries should be suspected of having an unstable spinal injury (SCI).
- Spinal injuries may occur at multiple levels. Immobilization of the head and neck should be performed until a spinal injury is excluded.

Initial Management Points

- Initial management involves limiting any further injury to the spine and spinal cord through careful immobilization of the spine. This is best accomplished initially by placing the patient on a spinal board with the neck in a neutral or slightly extended position, immobilizing the neck by placing sandbags on either side of the head, and securing the head to the spinal board by placing 3-inch adhesive tape over the forehead and attaching it to either side of the spinal board. A cervical collar also may be used but provides no further spinal protection.
- Respiratory failure should be identified rapidly, and any patient with obvious signs of respiratory distress, such as cyanosis, apnea, severe paradoxic breathing pattern, or airway obstruction, should have an oral airway placed with assisted or positive-pressure ventilation. This should be followed with endotracheal intubation via either an orotracheal or nasotracheal route stressing in-line manual immobilization (not traction). If endotracheal intubation is difficult and the patient is deteriorating, a laryngeal mask airway should be temporarily inserted until an emergency cricothyrotomy or tracheostomy can be performed.
- Hemodynamic instability is common in SCI because of the sympathectomy with resulting venous pooling. Hypotension should be identified and treated first with vasopressors, if needed, until further hemodynamic monitoring can guide therapy. As autoregulatory ability is lost after spinal cord injury, aggressive blood pressure control is essential with the goal of maintaining the blood pressure in the normal to slightly increased range (i.e., mean arterial pressure of ≥85 mm Hg). Patients with SCI are susceptible to fluid overload and pulmonary edema; thus indiscriminate administration of fluids for blood pressure support should be avoided. It is always important to consider hemorrhagic shock as the cause of hypotension and rule it out by appropriate examination and testing.
- Bradycardia is nearly universal in high spinal cord injuries and should be treated with atropine if associated with hypotension. Occasionally, a temporary pacemaker is needed.
- Gastric atony resulting in significant gastric distention is common in patients with SCI; thus a nasogastric tube for decompression is indicated early on to decrease the chances of regurgitation and to facilitate oxygenation.
- A physical examination, including a pointed neurologic examination, should focus on the patient's mental status, motor and sensory function (pinprick and light touch), and rectal tone. Frequent repeat neurologic examinations should be performed to detect deterioration in neurologic status. Following the new international standard for neurologic examination of the spinal cord–injured patient (American Spinal Injury Association grades and motor sensory scores) is important.
- Radiologic examination of the patient with potential spine injury should be carried out expeditiously. A three-view radiographic series of films including a cross-table lateral (with visualization of C7-T1) anteroposterior (AP) and odontoid (open mouth) views of the cervical spine are mandatory. Additional lateral and AP films of the thoracic and lumbar spines are indicated for multiple trauma patients with a history and physical examination suggestive of thoracolumbar injury. Computed tomography scans may be ordered early on to further identify bony spinal injuries, including spinal canal encroachment, facet joint dislocations, and occipital-C1 and C7-T1 vertebral injuries. Magnetic resonance imaging is often carried out after the initial stabilization of the patient and is superior for visualizing spinal cord parenchyma, longitudinal ligaments, nerve roots, and intervertebral disks.
- Steroid therapy is a treatment option in patients with neurologic abnormalities after acute spinal injury. The protocol involves an intravenous bolus of methylprednisolone of 30 mg/kg over 15 minutes followed 45 minutes later by either a 23-hour intravenous infusion of 5.4 mg/kg/hr if therapy is started within 3 hours of SCI, or a 47-hour infusion if therapy is started between 3 and 8 hours after SCI. Recent recommendations consider the use of steroid therapy following acute SCI to be a treatment option, rather than a standard of therapy.
- Closed reduction of spinal dislocations using various traction devices is attempted as soon as the initial examination and radiologic testing are completed.

the temporomandibular joint, should be assessed. The extent of mouth opening is often related to the ease of laryngoscopy. Limited mouth opening can make visualization of any laryngeal structures challenging. The presence of loose teeth should be noted and documented on the record. Next, the oral pharynx is examined, with special notation made of the size of the tongue in relation to the mouth opening. During mouth opening, the ability to visualize the faucial pillars, soft palate, and base of the uvula with the tongue protruded maximally (Mallampati classification) has been shown to be an accurate predictor of difficulty with direct laryngoscopy and should be documented.

Patients with rheumatoid arthritis, cervical myelopathy, or spinal cord injury are at an increased risk for further neurologic injury if a controlled approach by an experienced anesthesiologist is not performed. Moreover, the patient with moderate to severe limitation caused by mechanical or neurologic restrictions should be considered for an awake intubation under local anesthesia to minimize movement of the head and neck. If an awake intubation is considered optimal, a detailed discussion should take place with the patient, if possible, regarding the steps that will be required and in assuring the patient that care will be taken for comfort. Patients with only mild limitation of movement, in which a difficult intubation is not anticipated, may undergo anesthesia induction prior to laryngoscopy, depending on the comfort level of the anesthesiologist. However, it should always be brought to the patient's attention that the potential for further neurologic injury exists, and the option of performing an awake intubation should be offered.

For patients with spinal trauma who are presenting for elective surgery, clearance of the cervical spine to confirm stability should be performed prior to anesthesia induction. In the patient with cervical spine instability, the spine should be immobilized prior to surgery and anesthetic induction, if time allows. Several alternative means of intubating the trachea should be planned for and available in the event that airway management becomes difficult.

Pulmonary Evaluation

Patients presenting for spine surgery may have significant pulmonary disease related to the specific spine abnormality or to other risk factors, including smoking, obesity, asthma, chronic obstructive lung disease (COPD), and pulmonary tumor. In the evaluation of the pulmonary system, a focused history and physical examination are of value in eliciting evidence of pulmonary disease. A chest radiograph is indicated for any patient undergoing thoracotomy for spine surgery or for any patient with the signs and symptoms of pulmonary disease. Arterial blood gas analysis is reasonable in any patient with evidence of significant pulmonary dysfunction, with spinal deformity, or with morbid obesity.

Scoliosis may cause a significant restrictive lung defect. Pulmonary function should be optimized prior to surgical correction of scoliosis (or any major spine surgery), including deep breathing and coughing exercises, discontinuation of tobacco use, antibiotics for any evidence of purulent sputum, and optimization of breathing medications. Preoperative baseline spirometric tests (pre- and post-bronchodilator) and arterial blood gas analysis are reasonable for any patient with serious pulmonary disease and in individuals with advanced scoliosis. Upper thoracic spine surgery has a greater impact on postoperative pulmonary function than lower thoracic or lumbar spine surgery; thus, optimization of pulmonary function is particularly vital for patients undergoing a planned upper thoracic procedure.

Cardiac Evaluation

Evaluation of the cardiac system should focus on identification of heart disease and the stability of the disease. Many patients with spine abnormalities are older than 70 years and thus have an increased incidence of ischemic heart disease or the risk factors for it. A history and physical examination will identify most significant abnormalities. Cardiac risk assessment depends on the type of surgery (low, intermediate, or high risk), the level of activity, and, most importantly, the presence of key risk factors.[159]

The Revised Cardiac Risk Index (RCRI)[159] is now recommended as part of the latest American College of Cardiology/American Heart Association (ACC/AHA) 2007 guidelines on perioperative cardiovascular evaluation and care for noncardiac surgery.[160] The RCRI factors considered most predictive of perioperative cardiac morbidity and mortality are major surgery; ischemic heart disease (myocardial infarction from history or electrocardiographic evidence, angina); heart failure; use of insulin therapy; cerebrovascular disease (stroke or transient ischemic attacks); and renal insufficiency (serum creatinine >2.0 mg/dL).[159] In clinically stable patients with three or more RCRI factors and with exercise capacity that is less then 4 METS or is unknown, noninvasive preoperative stress testing may be indicated. Otherwise, perioperative heart rate control with use of β-adrenergic blocking agents is sufficient.

Patients with a history of heart failure or in whom heart failure is suspected on the basis of the presence of cardiomegaly present on chest radiograph have very high perioperative morbidity and mortality.[161] As such, these patients should undergo echocardiography (if such a study has not been done within the past year) to better define the type of cardiac pathology and overall function. For patients presenting with uncontrolled hypertension (i.e., systolic blood pressure >180 mm Hg and/or diastolic blood pressure >110 mm Hg) and known or suspected heart disease, the surgery should be postponed until adequate blood pressure control is obtained.

Neurologic Evaluation

Patients presenting for spinal surgery should be carefully evaluated for a preexisting neurologic deficit. This assessment should be documented for comparison with the postoperative condition. The neurologic deficit, its duration, and its extent may influence other organ systems, as noted previously. If possible, the patient should demonstrate positions or describe conditions that exacerbate his or her neurologic symptoms, so that precautions may be taken to avoid these movements and reduce any further insult. The presence of neurologic deficits may also alter the choice of anesthetic drugs and adjuncts, such as the use of muscle relaxants. Autonomic dysreflexia is likely in patients with SCI above T6 after 3 weeks of injury (sometimes sooner).

Laboratory Studies

The laboratory studies obtained for surgery are individualized to each patient. However, certain basic evaluations are applicable to all patients preparing to undergo spinal operation. In addition, specific studies may be indicated (Box 20-7).

Pharmacology

Patients with chronic SCI may have altered pharmacokinetics with various medications[162]; such patients generally demonstrate an increased ratio in the size of extravascular to

---

BOX 20–7 *Preoperative Laboratory Values of Interest*

Basic Laboratory Values

Hematocrit
Hemoglobin level
White blood cell count
Urinalysis

Specific Laboratory Values

Blood urea nitrogen
Serum creatinine level
Serum electrolytes
Prothrombin time
Partial thromboplastin time
Fibrinogen
Platelet count
Electrocardiogram
Chest x-ray film
Arterial blood gases
Pulmonary function tests (spirometry)

Intraoperative Monitoring Techniques for Spinal Surgery

Routine Monitoring

Electrocardiography
Blood pressure measurement (non-invasive)
Pulse oximetry
End-tidal carbon dioxide
Temperature

Invasive Monitoring

Arterial blood pressure
Central venous pressure
Pulmonary artery pressure
Urine output
Cardiac output
Mixed venous oxygen saturation
Neurophysiologic monitoring

---

intravascular albumin pools. Total body water is decreased, and body fat content is increased. However, the percentage of body weight that is represented by water can increase with extensive erosion of muscle mass.[162] Endogenous creatinine clearance does not correlate with inulin clearance in paraplegics and therefore should not be used as a measure of glomerular filtration.[162]

An important anesthetic consideration in patients with a preexisting neurologic deficit is the effect of succinylcholine on denervated muscle. Succinylcholine normally causes a muscular depolarization with resultant relaxation. In denervated muscle, motor end plate receptors proliferate, and succinylcholine then produces an exaggerated response with a very large release of potassium into the circulation.[163] This acute increase in serum potassium may cause cardiac dysrhythmias, cardiac arrest, or death. Succinylcholine should therefore be avoided in these patients.[163]

In patients with spinal cord injury, gastrointestinal motility may be impaired, and thus the bioavailability of orally administered drugs that require intact postprandial gastric emptying to be absorbed may be reduced. Drugs that undergo biotransformation and have relatively small volumes of distribution in the body when given as a single dose, such as lorazepam, are not likely to have disturbed pharmacokinetics. Intramuscular injections may have delayed absorption secondary to decreased blood flow in paralyzed muscles.

Patients with chronic neurologic dysfunction may be receiving low-dose heparin subcutaneously for prophylaxis against DVT. The decision to use regional anesthetic techniques in this instance must be tempered by the slight risk of hematoma formation and spinal cord or nerve compression and injury. Finally, opioid tolerance is often present in patients with chronic back pain and other neurologic conditions, and this possibility should be considered in the administration of perioperative opioids (i.e., larger overall doses may be required).

Premedication

The necessity for premedication and the drugs chosen depend largely on the perceived or stated level of anxiety of the patient, the medical condition of the patient, and aspects of the operation and anesthetic that may be affected. In general, premedication is optional and should be prescribed at the discretion of the anesthesiologist and the patient. A small dose of a potent intravenous benzodiazepine may be considered desirable if the patient is particularly anxious, and narcotic analgesics may be valuable if the patient is in pain.

Airway Management for Cervical Spine Surgery

Patients with disease of the cervical spine have an increased incidence of difficulty with laryngoscopy, approaching 20% in one report.[164] In particular, patients with occipito-atlanto-axial complex disease have a higher prevalence of difficulty than those with disease in the subaxial (C3-C7) cervical spine. The best single radiographic predictor of difficulty is reduced separation of the posterior elements of C1 and C2 on lateral views,[164] whereas the Mallampati classification is the best single clinical predictor of a difficult airway.[164] For patients with symptomatic spinal stenosis (cervical myelopathy), initial airway management should consider the benefits of an awake fiberoptic intubation or induction of general anesthesia with the head stabilized and intubation performed under fiberoptic guidance with the use of spinal cord monitoring. For most other patients scheduled for cervical spine surgery who have a reasonable range of motion, difficulty with intubation is no higher than with other types of surgery. For all patients with cervical spine disease, documentation of a pre-induction mental status and neurologic examination is essential to ensure that further injury has not occured during the intubation and positioning process.

One of the most challenging airways that anesthesiologists face is that of a patient with acute cervical spine injury. After a traumatic injury, patients who are awake, alert, and without neck pain or tenderness to palpation have minimal potential of cervical spine injury.[165] However, a comatose or intoxicated patient is assumed to have a cervical spine injury until a full diagnostic evaluation can be completed and expertly reviewed.[165,166] Although secondary SCI resulting from airway management techniques is a valid concern, there are few case reports of neurologic injury following tracheal intubation in patients with unstable spine injuries.[167] Indeed, it is important to first remember the ABCs of primary resuscitation. A patient with new-onset traumatic quadriplegia is likely to suffer from respiratory compromise secondary to diminished breathing mechanics, aspiration, or a concurrent head injury resulting in altered level of consciousness.

Although the indications for endotracheal intubation are well defined and usually apparent, little agreement can be found within the current literature regarding a superior approach to rapidly securing the airway while avoiding further injury in patients with acute SCI. Of more importance, a basic knowledge of airway maneuvers and the effects that such maneuvers have on craniofacial structures and cervical spine motion is vital to avoiding airway mishaps that may worsen neurologic injury.[168-170] Currently, the emphasis in airway management has shifted from a recommendation of a specific airway technique to operator expertise and managing each patient on a case-specific basis, because the current published clinical data do not show any particular technique to be superior for tracheal intubation of patients with cervical spine injuries.[171-173] Factors to consider in initial airway management of the potentially cervical spine–injured patient include urgency of airway intervention and whether there is time for adequate radiographic cervical spine evaluation; the presence of associated facial injuries or soft tissue injuries of the neck that may distort the normal airway anatomy and necessitate awake or surgical airway management; the presence of a basilar skull fracture or midface fracture that would contraindicate nasal tracheal intubation; whether the patient is awake and cooperative or possibly uncooperative as a result of alcohol or drug use; head injury; and the expertise of the operator in the different airway management techniques, including direct laryngoscopy, nasal intubation, fiberoptically assisted intubation, and surgical airway.

Maintaining a patent airway and adequate oxygenation in a patient with possible cervical spine injury may require bag-mask ventilation, an oral or nasal airway, chin lift or jaw thrust, and oral or nasotracheal intubation (which is often accomplished in a rapid-sequence manner with cricoid pressure). All of these modalities of airway support have the potential for moving the cervical spine even when a cervical collar is in place (Table 20-8).[174-177] The classic sniffing position requires flexion of the lower neck on the chest and extension of the head on the upper neck. The majority of cervical motion in anesthetized normal patients undergoing direct laryngoscopy with a Macintosh blade is extension produced at the occipitoatlantal and atlantoaxial (C1-C2) articulations. The subaxial cervical segments (C2-C5) are displaced only minimally,[174,177,179] so the risk of direct laryngoscopy may vary with the level of cervical spine injury. By inference, the upper cervical spine is at greater risk for secondary injury with laryngoscopy than the lower cervical spine, where the majority of injuries occur. Thus, patients with unstable C1 or C2 injuries might be the most vulnerable to neurologic damage from atlanto-occipital extension. However, the manner in which motion is distributed over segments adjacent to and remote from the level of cervical spine injury has not been fully studied.

Table 20–8 Airway Management Techniques and Their Effects on the Cervical Spine

Maneuver	Condition	Result
Laryngoscopy	Normal, anesthetized	• Extension at occipitoatlantal and C1-C2 articulations • C2-C5 displaced only minimally • Sniffing position-flexing lower neck on the chest and extending the head on the upper neck
	Cadaver, C5-C6 instability	• 3-4 mm widening disk space at level of injury
Straight vs. curved blade	Normal, anesthetized	• No difference in cervical spine movement
Glidescope®	Normal, anesthetized	• Overall spine movement reduced 50% at C2-C5 as compared to curved blade
Bullard laryngoscope	Normal, anesthetized, in-line stabilization	• Overall cervical spine movement reduced at C2-C5 • Less extension at occipitoatlantoaxial complex but similar occiput-C-5 extension compared with direct laryngscopy with Macintosh blade if no in-line stabilization
Augustine guide	Normal, healthy	• Less spine extension than with direct laryngoscopy
Rigid indirect laryngoscopy		• Cervical spine movements less than with direct laryngoscopy • Better visualization of the glottis than direct laryngoscopy
Intubating laryngeal mask airway		• Exerts high pressures against upper cervical vertebrae with insertion and manipulation • May produce posterior displacement of upper cervical spine • For insertion, C5 and superior spinal segments flexed <2°; during intubation, C4 and superior segments flexed <3°; little movement of the spine above C3
Cricoid pressure	Normal, anesthetized, in-line stabilization	• Single-handed cricoid pressure causes vertical displacement of neck ≈5 mm, but no spine movement
Blind nasotracheal	Cadaver, C5-C6 instability	• Up to 2 mm subluxation but no increase in disk space; intubation >5 mm subluxation when neck is stabilized anteriorly by hand pressure
Airway support		
Chin lift/jaw thrust	Cadaver, C5-C6 instability	• >5 mm widening disk space at level of injury
Oral/nasopharyngeal	Cadaver, C5-C6 instability	• ≈2 mm widening disk space at level of injury
Mask ventilation	Cadaver	• Significant anteroposterior translation displacement with maximal flexion and extension of the head

Table 20–9 Cervical Spine Immobilization Techniques

Technique	Effect on Spine Immobilization
Cervical collar, sandbags, backboard, head tape	• Very effect method of limiting flexion, extension, rotation, and lateral bending; recommended by the American College of Surgeons for effective C-spine immobilization; makes orotracheal intubation much more difficult if left in place at time of intubation
Hard and soft collar	• Little effect on spine immobilization; allows moderate amount of head and neck extension; does not effectively eliminate movement of the neck during tracheal intubation; anterior portion of collar interferes with mouth opening; increases incidence of grade III or IV laryngoscopic view; alerts medical personnel to possibility of C-spine injury
Manual in-line immobilization (MILI)	• Reduces neck movement during intubation; recommended method of reducing neck mobility during tracheal intubation; head held in neutral position without axial traction; better view of larynx when anterior aspect of collar, if present, is removed before laryngoscopy
Axial traction	• Excessive axial traction may cause distraction and subluxation
Halo brace	• Most rigid immobilization technique of all the spinal orthoses; highly effective for skeletal fixation and in limiting motion of the upper cervical spine; limits both flexion-extension and lateral bending movements of the cervical spine by 96% and axial rotation by 99%; utilized in the setting of an unstable cervical spine; does not allow any neck movement making direct laryngoscopy very difficult; fiberoptic intubation is recommended (awake or after induction)

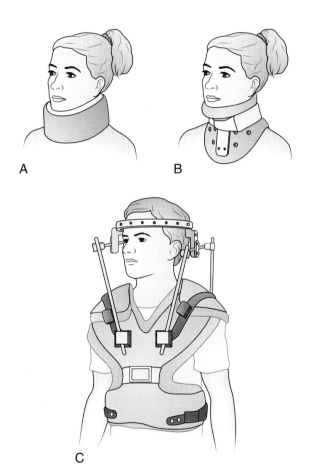

Figure 20–32 Cervical orthoses. **A,** Soft cervical collar; **B,** Philadelphia-type reinforced cervical collar; **C,** halo brace.

A significant incidence of cord injury may occur because of improper immobilization of the spine after trauma.[181] However, immobilization techniques (Table 20-9) can easily become the primary focus in resuscitation of patients at risk for cervical spine injury, delaying airway assessment, making orotracheal intubation more difficult, and endangering patients subjected to the risks of inadequate ventilation.[182] Neck-stabilizing cervical orthotic devices, such as the soft and hard collars (Fig. 20-32), do not eliminate spinal movement; however, these collars are commonly placed on patients until the cervical spine is confirmed not to be injured. While providing some degree of spine immobilization and patient comfort, such collars allow both neck flexion and extension and thus do little to eliminate cervical motion, particularly during laryngoscopy.[176,183] Moreover, the anterior portion of the collar interferes with mouth opening during orotracheal intubation and increases the incidence of difficult laryngoscopic views.[184,185] That said, the removal of these devices is recommended in combination with manual in-line immobilization (MILI), to facilitate tracheal intubation.[184,185]

Immobilization techniques can make laryngoscopy difficult. Cervical Collars, tape, and sandbags result in a poor view of the larynx (grade III or IV) on laryngoscopy in more than half (64%) of patients immobilized in this manner.[182] MILI is a technique applied to patients with known or suspected cervical spine injury to limit movement of the head and neck during direct laryngoscopy or other similar procedures. It is carried out by having an assistant positioned at the head of the bed or just to the side of the patient's head who provides immobilization of the head by using the fingers placed on the mastoid processes and the hands holding the occiput steady.[169] Unfortunately, MILI makes direct laryngoscopy more difficult. In the absence of stabilization maneuvers, the glottis is best visualized with 10 to 15 degrees of head extension; MILI reduces the typical head extension with laryngoscopy by about 4 to 5 degrees compared with no stabilization, although it is more effective than axial traction immobilization in limiting neck extension.[186] When MILI is substituted for the collar, tape, and sandbags method, however, the laryngoscopic view is improved, mainly because of increased mouth opening.[183,186] Indeed, MILI is associated with a grade 3 or 4 view in only 22% of patients, as compared with 64% in patients in whom collar, tape, and sandbags are in place.[182] MILI reduces but does not totally eliminate spine movement during laryngoscopy.[176,181-189] Fortunately, the amount of airway movement with MILI is small, though not uniformly reduced in comparison with other methods.[190-192]

As mentioned, all airway maneuvers cause some neck and cervical spine movement (see Table 20-8). Basic maneuvers, including the jaw thrust and chin lift, resulted in up to 5 mm of movement of the spine at the site of the cervical injury in a cadaver model with an unstable spine.[174] In the same model, advanced maneuvers, including placement of an orotracheal tube using a straight or curved laryngoscope blade, an esophageal obturator airway, and a nasotracheal tube, produced 3 to 4 mm of disk space enlargement.[174] Another study examining the effect of basic airway maneuvers on cervical spine movement in traumatic arrest victims noted that maximal cervical spine displacement was 2.93 mm for mask ventilation, 1.51 mm for oral intubation, and 1.20 mm for nasal intubation.[193] Mask ventilation resulted in more cervical spine movement than the other methods.

In a different study looking at spine motion occurring during intubation in a cadaver model with an intact spine and then with intubation following creation of an unstable C1-C2 segment,[194] the use of maximum neck flexion and extension maneuvers (as occurs with mask ventilation) narrowed the space available for the spinal cord (SAC) by 1.49 mm in the intact spine and by 6.06 mm in the unstable spine. Chin lift and jaw thrust reduced the SAC by 1.09 mm and 2.47 mm, respectively, and had the greatest effect in narrowing the SAC. Oral intubation and nasal intubation narrowed the SAC by 1.60 mm and 1.61 mm, respectively.[194] The researchers concluded that in an unstable C1-C2 spine injury, oral intubation had the same effect on diminution of SAC as nasotracheal intubation and that the chin lift/jaw thrust maneuvers caused the most motion and hence the greatest effect on narrowing the SAC in the C1-C2 unstable spine.[194] Rigid indirect laryngoscopy is associated with less cervical spine movement and better glottic visualization than direct laryngoscopy, with the exception of the GlideScope device.

In general, cervical spine movement during laryngoscopy is associated with the greatest degree of movement in the upper cervical spine with superior rotation of the occiput and C1 and mild inferior rotation of C3-C5. The greatest motion is at the atlanto-occipital and atlantoaxial joints.[175] The position of the cervical spine below C4 remains reasonably static during laryngoscopy.[180] Maximal movement of the spine during laryngoscopy is typically less than 5 mm with 2 to 3 mm of displacement. Such movements are very small and typically within physiologic ranges.[169] Specific blades available for direct laryngoscopy have minimal differences with respect to the effects on spine movement.[175,178,180,194-198] A newer laryngoscopic device, the GlideScope (Verathon, Inc., Bothell, WA) is a video laryngoscope incorporating a digital camera in the tip of the blade that transmits images to a display monitor via a video cable. Compared with the curved Macintosh blade, the GlideScope improves the laryngeal view by one grade in normal patients wearing cervical collars.[199] Furthermore, compared with the MacIntosh blade, the GlideScope reduces spinal movement by 50%, although the time to intubation is longer.[200]

Emergency Airway Management in the Cervical Spine–Injured Patient

For emergency situations, a variety of airway management plans are reasonable for patients with potential cervical spine injuries because no evidence shows the superiority of any individual tracheal incubation technique.[166] The urgency of intervention is a primary factor in planning airway management for patients with potential cervical spine injuries, as demonstrated in a suggested management algorithm from the American Society of Anesthesiologists (Fig. 20-33).

Patients who need immediate airway control should initially receive oxygen by bag and mask with assisted ventilation. Although all of the techniques used to relieve airway obstruction have the potential of displacing the cervical spine (see Table 20-8), oxygenation and ventilation are a higher

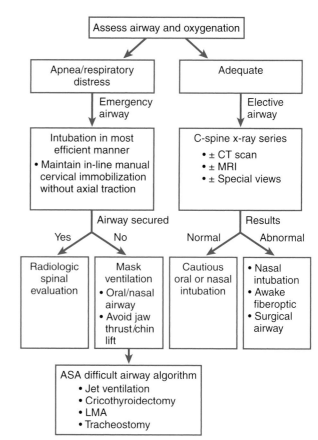

Figure 20–33 Suggested airway management algorithm for a patient with a suspected C-spine (cervical spine) injury. ASA, American Society of Anesthesiologists; CT, computed tomography; LMA, laryngeal mask airway; MRI, magnetic resonance imaging

priority than the risk of neurologic injury. Direct laryngoscopy is advocated by many writers as the method of choice for immediate airway control in patients with actual or potential cervical spine injuries, whereas others recommend that anesthesiologists choose the technique with which they have the most expertise.

If necessary, midazolam, propofol, thiopental, or etomidate may be used for sedation, and succinylcholine may be used for muscular relaxation without apparent danger of hyperkalemia if the injury is less than 24 hours old.[163] The application of single- or double-handed cricoid pressure may be used to reduce the risk of pulmonary aspiration of gastric contents.[201,202] Depending on the force applied and whether the posterior aspect of the neck is stabilized, as in bimanual application of cricoid pressure, there is a risk of vertical displacement of the neck.[201] If direct laryngoscopy fails, the patient should be ventilated by mask, and a backup method for tracheal intubation should be attempted.

As mentioned, head and neck stabilization techniques increase the difficulty of direct laryngoscopy and reduce visualization of the glottic structures. Moreover, facial edema and fractures, pharyngeal edema, and soft tissue injuries are common with cervical spine injuries, and fractures can cause hematoma and edema formation around the larynx, further increasing the difficulty of airway management. If laryngoscopy or other techniques fail and mask ventilation becomes inadequate, the practitioner should institute the American Society of Anesthesiologists difficult airway algorithm (see Fig. 20-33). Transtracheal ventilation or cricothyroidotomy may be required. The role of the laryngeal mask airway (LMA) in the cervical spine–injured patient has not been definitively determined. Although the presence of a cervical collar[201] or use of MILI of the neck[196] does not appear to interfere with placement of the LMA, it may be more difficult to position properly when MILI in combination with cricoid pressure is used. In one study,[203] not only was the LMA more difficult to place under these conditions, but also vocal cord identification through the LMA was not possible in many of the cases. This finding suggests that attempted tracheal intubation through the LMA, using a bougie or small endotracheal tube, may be extremely difficult.

If oxygenation and ventilation are initially assessed to be adequate, there is time to further evaluate the cervical spine or plan an elective method of airway management. In stable trauma patients with possible cervical spine injury who are scheduled for nonemergency surgery, the operation should be delayed until the cervical spine can be adequately assessed. If a cervical spine injury is excluded, orotracheal intubation should be initiated. If an unstable cervical spine injury is confirmed or suspected and tracheal intubation is necessary in a cooperative patient, an awake fiberoptic oral intubation, nasal intubation, or blind nasal intubation with topical anesthesia may be appropriate.

Awake intubation techniques are often unsuitable in traumatized, uncooperative patients who may be intoxicated or hemodynamically unstable. Controlled oral intubation by an experienced laryngoscopist is often used in this setting. If the patient is brought to the operating room in tongs and traction, any technique of tracheal intubation may be chosen. However, an awake fiberoptic intubation with topical anesthesia is a popular choice because the traction device prevents optimal positioning for direct laryngoscopy.

In summary, there is no evidence that any particular airway management technique is either safe or dangerous in a patient with an unstable cervical spine. Some authorities have advocated that the patient with an unstable spine injury with intact neurologic function undergo an awake tracheal intubation, if that has not already been accomplished, followed by awake positioning to allow neurologic evaluation in the planned surgical position before induction of general anesthesia. However, several retrospective studies have failed to demonstrate a higher incidence of neurologic injury in patients with cervical instability after trauma associated with intubation. The method for definitive airway control should be based primarily on the operator's skill and experience rather than on the fear of inflicting cervical cord damage. In the event that the patient is apneic, orotracheal intubation should be attempted immediately with MILI. If this approach fails or extensive maxillofacial injury is present, a surgical airway should be achieved.

Anesthesia Induction and Maintenance

Induction

Once the airway is secured, delivery of anesthesia can begin. Induction of anesthesia for spinal surgery carries the same considerations as those for any other general anesthesia. Concerns related to patient comorbidities should be addressed as appropriate. As previously noted, a major issue is often whether to induce anesthesia before or after positioning. Muscle relaxants should be used with consideration of the potential for a hyperkalemic response in the instance of succinylcholine use

in the patient sustaining a spinal cord injury. If muscle relaxants are used for induction, short-acting agents are recommended, allowing subsequent evoked response monitoring. Following intubation and securing of the endotracheal tube, the patient can be prepared for positioning.

Concerns arise regarding protection of neurologic integrity after prone positioning when an area of the bony spine is unstable and susceptible to movement during positioning.[204] If spinal instability is located in the cervical region, the patient may present for surgery with a cervical collar or in a halo immobilization or traction device. Other clinical conditions that may be present include spinal stenosis, severe root impingement by a disk fragment, and preexisting neurologic deficit. It is important that every effort be expended to keep the head and spine in a neutral position during the positioning of a patient with any of these conditions. Once the prone position has been attained, access to the head and endotracheal tube is restricted; thus, the use of a flexible armored endotracheal tube is advocated to avoid the risk of the tube kinking, which may result in difficulty with ventilation and oxygenation.

Maintenance

The anesthetic technique chosen for the majority of surgical procedures on the spine should be based primarily on the patient's underlying medical condition, the anticipated intraoperative conditions, and the preference of the anesthetist. If neurophysiologic monitoring is planned, an awareness of the effects of the various anesthetic agents on neurophysiologic testing is essential, and the anesthetic choices should be altered accordingly. Most importantly, a stable intraoperative anesthetic depth is essential so that any changes in evoked responses can be explained appropriately. An in-depth discussion of neurophysiologic monitoring techniques in the context of spine surgery is discussed in detail elsewhere in this book and is not covered in this discussion.

In addition to planning for neurophysiologic monitoring, the possibility of an intraoperative wake-up test should be determined before induction. If an intraoperative wake-up test is desired, either a total intravenous anesthesia technique or a balanced technique consisting of low doses of a volatile agent together with opioids is effective.[205] With use of such regimens, there is an associated 25% incidence of patient intraoperative awareness and recall of the awakening event; however, the recall is not regarded as unpleasant in most instances.[206]

Anesthetic Management of Patients with Acute Spinal Cord Injury

The level of SCI, severity of associated injuries, and preexisting medical conditions are factors to consider in selecting appropriate anesthetic agents and monitors for patients with acute SCI. An acute SCI that disrupts sympathetic outflow may result in neurogenic shock with myocardial depression. Disruption of the cardioaccelerator fibers and unopposed vagal stimulation may result in bradycardia, bradydysrhythmias, and atrioventricular block. The loss of the peripheral vasoconstrictive response to cold predisposes the patient to hypothermia; and positive-pressure ventilation, positioning, and anesthetic-induced myocardial depression or vasodilation in the operating room may increase circulatory instability, reduce systemic pressure, and cause deterioration in spinal cord perfusion.

The standard monitors recommended by the American Society of Anesthesiologists plus a urinary catheter, arterial catheter, and central venous or pulmonary artery catheter are characteristically used. A pulmonary artery catheter may be useful in guiding adequacy of fluid resuscitation in the patient with a high SCI and an unstable form of neurogenic shock. Cervical spine stabilization devices, inability to position the neck with lateral rotation, and possibly altered neck anatomy from a hematoma or neck edema may make obtaining venous access via the internal jugular vessels difficult and necessitate the use of the subclavian or femoral veins. Nasal temperature probes should not be placed in the patient with a basilar skull fracture or midface fracture.

Transesophageal echocardiography may be used to evaluate intraoperative myocardial function and anatomy. However, when making the decision to use this modality, one must consider several factors: the potential difficulty in placing the probe with the cervical spine immobilized; the theoretical possibility of cervical spine movement when the relatively large transesophageal echocardiography probe is placed and moved in the esophagus to obtain views; and the potential for an associated esophageal injury in trauma patients with a high SCI. These factors raise the question of whether the cervical spine should always be "cleared" before such a probe is placed.

Selecting the particular anesthetic technique for operations on the traumatized spine with acute SCI is of less importance than optimizing medical management during the procedure. To date, no evidence has been presented that conclusively favors one anesthetic agent or technique over another in the patient with acute SCI. However, maintenance of mean arterial blood pressure at or above 85 mm Hg and an adequate cardiac output have been shown to prevent secondary injury to the spinal cord.[207]

Optimization of cardiovascular function in patients with acute SCI is essential in avoiding further neurologic injury. Systemic arterial hypoxemia and hypotension (e.g., neurogenic shock) are common clinical sequelae of SCI. Loss of autoregulation coupled with hypotension and arterial hypoxemia may severely diminish spinal cord perfusion and oxygen delivery, leading to ischemia and secondary injury after the primary traumatic event. Because the inotropic and chronotropic effects of the sympathetic nervous system are attenuated or lost, such patients may be unusually sensitive to the myocardial depressant effects of anesthetics. Although α-adrenergic agents such as phenylephrine may increase systemic vascular resistance and restore blood pressure, they may do so at the expense of increased afterload and a reduction in cardiac output. Some patients are unable to increase left ventricular stoke work in response to a fluid challenge, and peripheral vasoconstriction may be detrimental.

Because the diaphragm is innervated by C3 to C5, an SCI at this level or above produces life-threatening respiratory failure. SCI at T7 to T8 or above produces respiratory impairment because abdominal and intercostal muscle strength is lost. With high spinal cord transection, there is a predisposition to hypoxemia because of a decreased functional residual capacity, greater risk of pulmonary aspiration of gastric contents secondary to impaired airway reflexes, and an inability to effectively cough, leading to decreased ability to handle secretions and increased risk of pneumonia.

The incidence of pulmonary edema in the patient with acute SCI is increased[208] and is exacerbated by fluid overload during resuscitation. Often, diuretic therapy or ventilation with positive end-expiratory pressure is required. Respiratory alkalosis produced by hyperventilation may depress the myocardium and should be avoided unless required for the management of intracranial hypertension. A gradual deterioration in respiratory function often occurs during the first few days after SCI. As a result, most patients with cervical SCI should remain intubated after spine surgery and should be transferred directly to the intensive care unit.

Spinal cord vascular responsiveness to carbon dioxide is abolished with severe SCI; therefore, normocapnia should be maintained intraoperatively. Meticulous control of intraoperative blood glucose levels is important, because hyperglycemia in the setting of critical illness has been associated with a greater morbidity and mortality. The blood glucose level above which neurologic risk is increased is unknown and likely varies among individuals. Until clinical studies provide data with clear recommendations for intraoperative glucose management of a patient with acute SCI, the prudent approach is to keep intraoperative blood glucose levels below 150 mg/dL by the avoidance of glucose-containing intravenous solutions and frequent determination of blood glucose levels. Should the patient's blood glucose value remain elevated, an insulin infusion is appropriate.

Positioning

Spine surgery typically requires that the patient be placed in one of three basic positions: supine, prone, or lateral decubitus. Each of these positions requires special considerations to prevent injury. One of the most common injuries encountered with any particular position is peripheral nerve injuries. In general, avoidance of excessive arm abduction in the supine position to less than 90 degrees, positioning of the arms and lower extremities to avoid unnecessary pressure on nerves, appropriate padding of all pressure points including chest rolls for patients in the lateral decubitus position, neutral positions of the head and hips, properly functioning automated blood pressure equipment, and postoperative assessment for nerve injuries are recommended. Care should be directed to the avoidance of extreme head extension or rotation for operations on the cervical spine. Endotracheal tube position should be confirmed after positioning of the head in extension for anterior cervical spine surgery, because the tube may move proximally in this instance.

The lateral decubitus position is used for lateral approaches to the cervical spine, anterior approaches to the upper thoracic spine, and retroperitoneal approaches to the thoracolumbar junction and lumbar spine. In the lateral position, particular care must be directed to the positioning of the dependent arm to prevent brachial plexus injury and vascular compression; the use of an axillary roll is thus recommended for most procedures in the lateral position. In addition, the nondependent arm is usually outstretched in front of the patient and should be supported on a pillow or padded armrest. The head should be positioned in a neutral position to avoid cerebral venous outflow and endotracheal tube obstruction, and it should be supported with a pillow or padded headrest.

The prone position is indicated for posterior spine surgery and is accomplished in a variety of ways (Fig. 20-34). In general, the goals of prone positioning are to:

- Provide adequate surgical exposure of the spine; this usually involves decreasing the lumbar lordotic curvature to increase the site of the interspinous spaces.
- Avoid abdominal compression, allow free movement of the abdomen, and reduce vena caval pressure, thus preventing vertebral venous engorgement and difficulties with bleeding during surgery.

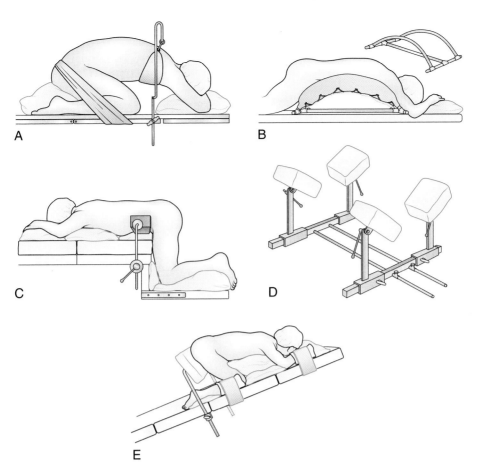

Figure 20–34 Examples of achieving the prone position for spine surgery. **A,** Kneeling prone; **B,** Wilson Frame Pad; **C,** Georgia prone; **D,** Relton-Hall frame; **E,** Seated prone.

- Avoid thoracic compression to allow easier ventilation. Increased airway pressure should be avoided because it may worsen vena caval engorgement and decrease venous return, which in turn may decrease cardiac output.
- Maintain normal positioning of the extremities. Compression or stretching of peripheral nerves or vasculature or entrapment of digits should be avoided.
- Support the head. Ocular pressure or pinching of the ears should be avoided.
- Provide liberal padding, thus avoiding pressure sores that otherwise may occur with long procedures.

Particular care must be taken when positioning the patient prone, particularly when there is spinal cord compromise or the potential for compromise. Moreover, positioning of patients who have a spinal deformity may be challenging because of the curvature of the spine. An adjustable four-posted frame operating table can be selected for such patients. For patients who have an unstable cervical spine and who are scheduled for a cervical spine operation, a halo brace or other immobilization technique may be necessary for spinal cord protection before positioning. Patients who have undergone previous coronary artery bypass surgery using vein grafts may demonstrate electrocardiographic evidence of ischemia with prone positioning and anterior chest wall pressure.[209] Attentiveness to maintaining a neutral head position is always essential during prone positioning of a patient. The arms are typically placed on arm boards attached to the side of the table and at the level of the head; care should be directed to ensure that the shoulders are free and relaxed to avoid brachial plexus injuries and that the elbows and wrists

are padded to prevent nerve compression (ulnar and median nerves).

Complications inherent to the prone position include pressure necrosis and muscle breakdown (with myoglobinuria) from prolonged compression of tissues during lengthy operations, peripheral nerve injuries due to overstretch or pressure, and blindness. Finally, postoperative visual loss is a feared complication of any surgical procedure performed with the patient in the prone position, particularly when the procedure is prolonged; this complication is discussed in more detail later.

Head Position

Basic principles of head positioning include avoidance of hyperextension, hyperflexion, and extreme rotation of the cervical spine. When surgery is being performed for a cervical spinal pathologic condition, these considerations are obvious. However, careful positioning of the head and cervical spine during operations on the thoracic and lumbar spine is also important. As mentioned, particular attention should be directed to maintaining a neutral head position when placing a patient prone. For posterior approaches to the middle to lower thoracic, lumbar, or sacral spine, the head is typically placed on soft foam or a gel pad with preconfigured cutouts or a horseshoe headrest that allows midline orientation of the face and head despite the prone position. Prior to prone positioning, the eyes should be carefully protected, and plans should be made to avoid undue ocular pressure during surgery. After turning, it is critical that the eyes be rechecked and documented to be free of any pressure. The nose should also be free from the surface of the table; otherwise pressure sores may develop. If the head is turned to one side, care must be exercised to avoid turning it too far and to avoid pressure on the ear. Hyperextension of the cervical spine is another complication of the prone position that can be avoided by placing sufficient padding under the chest.

During operations on the anterior cervical spine, it is common for the surgeon to require traction on the head to distract the cervical vertebrae for placement of the bone graft for fusion. This maneuver should be performed under the direct supervision of the surgeon, because excessive traction may result in stretching and ischemic damage to the cervical cord. Hyperflexion during cervical laminectomy using the posterior approach is a common occurrence, primarily because of the conflict between the needs of the surgeon and the physical limitations on the cervical spine. To expose the posterior cervical vertebrae high in the neck, the surgeon must often flex the head forward on the chest. This movement may put undue strain on the spine, but it also results in very restricted venous outflow from the head and face. In addition, the airway may be compromised by sharp bending of the tracheal tube in the posterior pharynx. Restriction of venous outflow from the face and head produces macroglossia and intracranial hypertension, respectively. To prevent this complication, sufficient space must be retained between the anterior angle of the mandible and the sternal notch. This space may be ascertained by the comfortable placement of at least two finger-breadths in this space at peak inspiration after positioning.

Monitoring

Physiologic Monitoring

Surgical procedures on the spine are commonly associated with significant blood loss and extended operating times. Therefore, in addition to routine monitoring, anticipated hemodynamic conditions during an extensive surgery may require more intensive monitoring (Box 20-7).

Generally, invasive monitoring of arterial blood pressure is advisable for patients with deliberately induced hypotension, prolonged surgical procedures (>4 hours) in which moderate to heavy blood loss is anticipated, significant cardiovascular and renal disease, and serious pulmonary dysfunction or intended use of intraoperative lung isolation techniques in which systemic oxygenation may be problematic. Central venous or pulmonary artery pressure monitoring is appropriate for complex surgical procedures associated with large amounts of blood loss or fluid shifts and in any patient with a history of ischemic heart disease, heart failure, valvular disease, or dysrhythmias. The inability to place invasive monitors intraoperatively, should the need arise, may also influence the decision whether to place them preoperatively.

Some debate still exists over the need to monitor patients for venous air embolism when surgery takes place in a position other than the seated position.[210] Air embolism may occur whenever the incision is elevated 5 cm or more above the level of the heart, and posterior spine approaches using the prone position result in a wound often located above that level. Indeed, venous air embolism has been reported during spine surgery, particularly in association with spine operations performed in the prone position.[211-215] The incidence of this complication is increased further during extensive surgical spine procedures associated with significant blood loss and bony dissections. That said, an increased awareness and monitoring for venous air embolism is advocated in all

instances in which the surgical site is elevated above the level of the heart. In such procedures, particularly when associated with the potential for substantial blood loss, a central venous catheter and direct arterial pressure monitoring, in addition to close monitoring of oxygenation and end-tidal carbon dioxide concentrations, are suggested.[213,214] Neurologic monitoring is covered in detail elsewhere and will not be discussed here.

Fluid Management and Blood Transfusion

Fluid management in the context of spinal surgery reflects a balance between maintaining intravascular volume to ensure adequate tissue perfusion and oxygenation of vital organs, including the spinal cord, and avoiding the venous congestion that may occur with fluid overload. Certainly, the type of surgery to be performed influences the approach to fluid replacement. Surgery involving extensive exposure of the spine with denuding of bone, such as scoliosis repair or extensive spinal fusion and instrumentation procedures, may be associated with significant blood loss.[216] Patients undergoing such procedures typically receive large amounts of asanguineous fluid in addition to multiple blood products, with resulting longer stays in the intensive care unit.[217] In patients undergoing revision posterior lumbar spine decompression, fusion, and segmental instrumentation, the number of levels fused and patient age appear to be the most significant factors predicting hospital stay, operative time, intraoperative blood loss, and transfusion therapy.[218] As expected, patients who have received large amounts of fluid or blood products have significant tissue edema, and the safety of postoperative extubation should be carefully considered before the endotracheal tube is removed.

Acute Normovolemic Hemodilution

Acute normovolemic hemodilution (ANH) involves the removal of blood from a patient immediately prior to surgery. The blood is removed into a collection bag containing an anticoagulant and is stored in the operating room at ambient temperature until it is re-infused into the patient at the conclusion of the operation once the majority of blood loss has occurred. The blood that has been removed from the patient is replaced with an appropriate volume of acellular fluid (crystalloid or colloid) to maintain a euvolemic state. Surgery is thus performed with a reduced red blood cell mass but a normal vascular volume. The goal of ANH is to reduce the patient's hematocrit to 30% prior to surgery. ANH is well tolerated in most patients because the reduced oxygen-carrying capacity of blood is compensated for by greater cardiac output and enhanced venous return owing to a reduction in viscosity. Moreover, oxygen delivery to the tissues is unaffected by hematocrit levels as low as 20%,[219-221] and cardiovascular stability does not deteriorate until hematocrit levels reach 15%.[222]

The decision to use ANH should consider the patient's underlying medical condition before the technique is implemented. Recommendations for the use of ANH have been previously published; they emphasize the use of ANH in the appropriately selected patient.[223] Patients who are considered good candidates for ANH have the following features: preoperative hemoglobin greater than 12 gm/dL; absence of clinically significant coronary, pulmonary, renal, or liver disease; absence of severe hypertension; and the absence of infection and the risk of bacteremia. Although the efficacy of ANH in reducing the use of allogeneic red blood cell transfusion is debated,[224] a number of studies have demonstrated the usefulness of ANH in decreasing the use of allogeneic blood in cases associated with significant blood loss.[224-227]

Intraoperative Cell Salvage

Intraoperative cell salvage is a technique in which blood lost during surgery is collected via suction instruments, in which it is mixed with an anticoagulant (heparin or citrate) and then sent into a collection reservoir. The salvaged blood is subsequently pumped from the collection reservoir into a centrifuge bowl. After centrifugation, the red cell pack is washed with normal saline and then is pumped back into the patient, with a final hematocrit approaching 60%. In comparison with other methods of reducing allogeneic red cell transfusion, cell salvage offers the greatest flexibility and is the most cost effective method when blood loss is substantial (i.e., >2000 mL), as occurs in major reconstructive spine operations.[228] The disadvantages are that the re-infused red cells may cause a coagulopathy from residual anticoagulant and lack of coagulation factors or platelets. Clotting factors may need to be replaced if microvascular bleeding is noted in the surgical field.

Postoperative Care

Extubation

The question whether or not to extubate the patient following spinal surgery depends largely on the particular surgical procedure performed and the clinical condition of the patient. In the majority of cases involving spinal surgery, extubation may be performed immediately upon awakening of the patient after demonstration of the usual criteria for extubation. Intubation may have to be maintained in certain cases of impaired ventilation caused by high cervical or thoracic lesions, preoperative pulmonary impairment, metabolic derangement, or persistent muscle weakness. Extubation is not necessarily imperative for the resumption of consciousness or ability to follow commands. In cases in which the operation was long (>6 hours) or the patient has significant facial edema, it is much safer to leave the patient intubated and to raise the head of the bed as least 45 degrees, and to extubate the patient in the recovery room or intensive care unit after the facial swelling has diminished. Another important factor to consider in the assessment of readiness for extubation is to check for a tracheal air leak following endotracheal cuff deflation.

Postoperative Pain Control

Major surgical operations on the spine result in significant postoperative pain.[229-236] Effective pain management is essential in order to facilitate early mobility, reduce postoperative pulmonary complications, shorten hospital length of stay, and enhance patient satisfaction. A variety of techniques are available to treat postoperative pain issues after spine surgery, with the particular surgical approach dictating the pain management method. In general, cervical spine surgery is associated with the least amount of postoperative pain, whereas spinal fusion and instrumentation procedures involving the thoracic and lumbar spine are associated with the most significant postoperative pain. Techniques of pain management that have been used include intermittent intramuscular and intravenous opioid use; continuous peripheral intravenous infusions of opioids; patient-controlled anesthesia (PCA) using intravenous opioids,[229] intrathecal opioids,[237-239] epidural analgesia (including patient-controlled epidural analgesia-PCEA)

using only opioids, opioid-local anesthetic combinations, and local anesthetic infusions alone;[232-235,240-241] intercostal blocks; paravertebral blocks; continuous wound instillation of local anesthetics via locally placed catheters[231]; non-opioid analgesics[242]; and a multimodal analgesic regimen incorporating a variety of these pain techniques.[242] With the exception of the intermittent administration of opioids (intravenous, intramuscular), all the techniques listed have been demonstrated to be efficacious in reducing postoperative pain.

Complications

Complications of spinal surgery may occur intraoperatively or postoperatively. Intraoperative complications include cardiac arrest from hypoxia while in the prone position and acute SCI from either direct trauma to the cord or distraction pressure during instrumentation, pneumothorax, and hemothorax. Postoperative complications include neurologic injury or deficit, visual loss, epidural hematoma, arachnoiditis, intravascular volume deficits, anemia, coagulopathy, CSF leak from an intraoperative dural tear, hypoxemia from atelectasis or pulmonary edema, urinary retention, ileus, atelectasis or pneumonia, and venous thrombosis. Complications specific to anterior cervical procedures include dysphagia, hoarseness, and airway obstruction from edema or neck hematoma.

Neurologic Deficit

Neurologic deficits following spinal surgery are uncommon events. In particular, the incidence of complications is highest with scoliosis repair in which spinal fusion and instrumentation is used.[243] In addition to spinal instrumentation, traction on the spinal cord during correction of the spinal deformity is a risk factor. The estimated frequency of new neurologic deficits after corrective scoliosis repair is less than 1%. When complete paralysis complicates instrumentation during scoliosis surgery, removal of the instrumentation, alteration of the corrective angle within 3 hours of discovery of the neurologic deficit, or both is important. With the advent of neurophysiologic monitoring, neurologic deficits are now being detected intraoperatively, reducing the incidence of permanent injury.

Anterior Spinal Artery Syndrome

Anterior spinal artery syndrome results from anterior central cord ischemia in the distribution of the anterior spinal artery. This condition typically manifests as motor weakness that is greater than any sensory change[244] and is due to the more central and ventral location of the motor tracts in the spinal cord, as opposed to the more dorsal and peripheral location of the sensory tracts. This syndrome results from obstruction of the feeder vessels to the anterior spinal artery, as occurs with aortic cross-clamping for repair of thoracolumbar aortic aneurysm or coarctation of the aorta. However, anterior spinal artery syndrome may also result from sustained hypoperfusion, correction of scoliosis, cervical spondylosis, disk herniation, and vertebral trauma. Treatment is aimed at relieving any existing contributory pathologic condition and providing general support.

Postoperative Visual Loss

Postoperative visual loss (POVL) is uncommon. The disorder has been reported most often following spine, cardiac, and head and neck operations. The reported estimates for blindness after spine surgery and cardiac surgery are 0.3% and 4.5%, respectively.[245,246] Most cases of POVL involve ischemic optic neuropathy, central retinal artery occlusion, or ischemic lesions in the cerebral cortex.[247] Suggested risk factors for POVL in the context of cardiac surgery include advanced age, arteriosclerosis, prolonged bypass time, plaque-related microemboli or macroemboli, postoperative anemia, and intraoperative hypotension.[248]

The etiology of POVL has not been clearly identified. Although POVL has been associated with spine surgery in the prone position, the commonly proposed etiologies, including increased intraocular pressure from the prone position, hypotension, and anemia, have not been clearly demonstrated as causative. A report by the American Society Task Force on Perioperative Blindness acknowledged that preoperative anemia, hypertension, glaucoma, carotid artery disease, obesity, diabetes, prolonged procedures, and significant blood loss may be associated with perioperative visual loss.[249] The important point is that although these disorders *may* be associated with POVL, no direct evidence of any involvement of these conditions has ever been demonstrated to be clearly causative. The Task Force members published a practice advisory for POVL associated with spine surgery that should serve to guide perioperative management (see unnumbered box in Summary).

A retrospective analysis of 93 spine procedures in which POVL occurred concluded that ischemic optic neuropathy was the most common cause of visual loss after spine surgery, that most patients were previously healthy, and that blood loss of more than 1000 mL, anesthetic duration of greater than 6 hours, or both was present in 96% of cases.[250]

In summary, POVL is uncommon after spine surgery but clearly may occur. That said, vision should be assessed after surgery once the patient is awake and alert. Any indication of deficit should be immediately followed by an ophthalmologic consultation to evaluate for possible causes. MRI should also be considered to evaluate for nonophthalmologic, intracranial causes of blindness.

Epidural Hematoma

Epidural hematomas may arise spontaneously as a result of a hypocoagulable state or trauma or from iatrogenic causes. The hematoma may exert a mass effect, with corresponding neuropathy, or it may be asymptomatic, as is often the case after the intentional epidural hematoma created as a result of epidural blood patching for post–dural puncture headache.

Deep Venous Thrombosis

DVT occurs with varying rates in orthopedic patients. Patients undergoing spine surgery appear to have a smaller risk of venous thromboembolism than those who have lower extremity surgery.[155] Nonetheless, deliberate hypotension, hypothermia, decreased cardiac output, and hypovolemia all may predispose to thrombophlebitis, increasing the patient's risk for this complication. A review of patient outcomes following lumbar spinal fusion noted a 3.7% rate of symptomatic DVT, with a 2.2% incidence of pulmonary embolism.[19] In patients with spine surgery who do not have DVT prophylaxis, the rate of DVT has been demonstrated to be as high as 18%.[227] Greater age and lumbar surgery appear to raise the postoperative risk for DVT.[230] Other proposed risk factors are anterior or combined anterior-posterior surgical approaches, surgery for tumors, prolonged operations, and decreased postoperative ambulation or activity. Some form of venous thromboembolism prophylaxis is recommended after spine surgery, whether mechanical prophylaxis or pharmacologic therapy.

Dural Tear

Interruption of the dura mater during spinal surgery is not uncommon and is often a necessary part of the operation, particularly in procedures on the cord itself. It also may occur unintentionally, especially when the surgeon is working in an area of a previous operation. The tear is usually repaired with no further sequelae. However, a CSF leak occasionally develops, which may result in a postoperative headache, fluid collections, or leaks. If drainage of CSF persists, reoperation and repair may be necessary.

Summary

Patients undergoing surgery on the spine or spinal cord present a complex challenge to anesthesiologists. A fundamental knowledge of spine anatomy facilitates an appreciation of the scheduled surgical procedure and the particular approach used by the surgeon to complete the operation. A basic understanding of radiologic imaging in the context of spinal diseases, and the indications for such tests, enhances awareness of the importance of imaging in formulating a medical and surgical treatment strategy. General familiarity with the various surgical approaches to the spine greatly augments decisions about patient positions, hemodynamic monitoring, anesthetic choices, and the potential for perioperative complications. An awareness of the medical concerns related to the common surgical diseases of the spine assists the anesthesiologist in initiating medical discussions with the surgical team and also provides a degree of comfort with the appropriateness of the planned surgery. Spine diseases may present unique management challenges, such as the unstable cervical spine in a patient with severe rheumatoid arthritis or spinal cord

---

ANESTHESIA-RELATED ISSUES IN THE MANAGEMENT OF THE ACUTE SCI PATIENT UNDERGOING SURGICAL THERAPY

- Early surgical therapy of spine injuries focuses on the limitation of secondary spinal cord injury in patients with progressive neurologic deficits due to spinal instability or in patients with the failure of closed reduction.
- Anesthetic concerns should consider a technique of securing the airway that limits spine movement.
  - Manual in-line stabilization may be indicated with direct laryngoscopy
  - An awake intubation may be the safest technique to limit neurologic injury.
- Anesthetic induction and maintenance techniques should select anesthetic agents and doses that support blood pressure and minimize cardiac depression.
- Hemodynamic monitoring is recommended for frequent determination of blood pressure, central venous pressure, arterial blood gas analysis, hemoglobin levels, and blood glucose.
- Meticulous attention to fluid management is essential to avoid fluid overload.
- Bradycardia is treated with appropriate chronotropic agents (i.e. dopamine) and hypotension is treated with fluids, to a state of euvolemia, and then the use of vasoactive medications with alpha agonist properties.
- Following surgery, extubation should be carefully considered in the context of the level of spinal injury. Patients with a spine injury resulting in an acute cervical SCI should be left intubated and transferred to the intensive care unit for further treatment.

impingement in a patient with spinal stenosis, and a more complete understanding of the pathology associated with such diseases directly affects the delivery of anesthetic care.

An in-depth comprehension of airway management in the context of spine diseases is a fundamental requirement for every anesthesiologist. Knowledge of airway manipulations and their effect on subsequent spine movement is important to facilitate better decision-making and reduce further neurologic injury, particularly in the setting of acute SCI. Following tracheal intubation, intraoperative anesthetic management of the spinal cord–injured patient should focus on maintaining adequate perfusion pressure and oxygenation. Vasoactive agents are appropriate only after ensuring adequate volume status and cardiac function. In the majority of spine operations, anesthesia induction and maintenance are achieved using a variety of accepted techniques. In the setting of major spine surgery in which the potential for injury to the spinal cord is present (i.e., correction of spinal deformities, spinal stenosis, spine stabilization procedures), the use of neurophysiologic monitoring dictates the use of a limited number of acceptable anesthetic techniques. In this context, intravenous or balanced techniques are preferred.

Decisions regarding fluid management choices during spine surgery should focus more upon the maintenance of a euvolemic state and less upon the particular fluid type. Fluid overload is associated with an increase in morbidity, and thus invasive monitoring may be appropriate in prolonged major spine operations to avoid excessive fluid administration. A sensible blood conservation strategy is facilitated by autologous blood predonation, lowering the transfusion triggers, preoperative acute normovolemic hemodilution, deliberate hypotension, and blood salvage techniques, whenever possible.

Postoperative pain control is important to increase patient satisfaction and reduce both the overall hospital length of stay and health care cost. A variety of techniques is appropriate in the postoperative setting, and they provide excellent pain control if started early and continued for 2 to 4 days postoperatively. Epidural techniques appear particularly efficacious, although other strategies are effective as well. Finally, the avoidance and early detection of perioperative complications is imperative in improving surgical outcome. In particular, reducing the risk of postoperative visual loss through meticulous attention to intraoperative detail and postoperative surveillance may avoid this devastating complication.

REFERENCES

1. Parsa AT, Miller JI: Neurosurgical diseases of the spine and spinal cord: Surgical considerations. In Cottrell JE, Smith DS, editors: *Anesthesia and Neurosurgery*, ed 4, St. Louis, 2001, Mosby, pp 531–555.
2. Moore KL, Dalley AF II: *Clinically Oriented Anatomy*, Philadelphia, 2006, Lippincott Williams & Wilkins, 477–531.
3. DeGroot J, Chusid J: *Correlative Neuroanatomy*, ed 20, East Norwalk, CT, 1988, Appleton & Lange.
4. Wolf HK, Anthony DC, Fuller GN: Arterial border zone necrosis of the spinal cord, *Clin Neuropathol* 9:60–65, 1990.
5. Goodnough LT, Rudnick S, Price TH, et al: Increased preoperative collection of autologous blood with recombinant human erythropoietin therapy, *N Engl J Med* 321:1163–1168, 1989.
6. Sandler AN, Tator CH: Effect of acute spinal cord compression injury on regional spinal cord blood flow in primates, *J Neurosurg* 45:660–676, 1976.
7. Hickey R, Albin MS, Bunegin L, et al: Autoregulation of spinal cord blood flow: Is the cord a microcosm of the brain? *Stroke* 17:1183–1189, 1986.
8. Griffiths IR: Spinal cord blood flow in dogs: II: The effect of the blood gases, *J Neurol Neurosurg Psychiatry* 36:42–49, 1973.
9. Griffiths IR: Spinal cord blood flow after acute impact injury. In Harper AM (ed): Blood Flow and Metabolism in the Brain: Proceedings of the 7th International Symposium on Cerebral Blood Flow and Metabolism, Aviemore, Scotland, June 17th-20th, 1975. New York, Churchill-Livingstone, pp 427–429.
10. Guha A, Tator CH, Rochon J: Spinal cord blood flow and systemic blood pressure after experimental spinal cord injury in rats, *Stroke* 20:372–377, 1989.
11. Anderson DK, Nicolosi GR, Means ED, et al: Effects of laminectomy on spinal cord blood flow, *J Neurosurg* 48:232–238, 1978.
12. Malcolm GP: Surgical disorders of the cervical spine: Presentation and management of common disorders, *J Neurol Neurosurg Psychiatry* 73:i34–i41, 2002.
13. Carette S, Fehlings MG: Cervical radiculopathy, *N Engl J Med* 353:392–393, 2005.
14. Greenberg MS: *Spine, Handbook of Neurosurgery*. New York, 2006, Thieme International, 289-364.
15. Yu YL, du Boulay GH, Stevens JM, et al: Computed tomography in cervical spondylotic myelopathy and radiculopathy: Visualization of structures, myelographic comparison, cord measurements, and clinical utility, *Neuroradiology* 28:221–236, 1986.
16. Rosen M, Beiner J, Kwon B, et al: Herniation of the nucleus pulposus in the cervical, thoracic, and lumbar spine. In Vaccaro AR, editor: *Spine: Core Knowledge in Orthopaedics*, Philadelphia, 2005, Elsevier-Mosby, pp 66–82.
17. Stillerman CB, Chen TC, Couldwell WT, et al: Experience in the surgical management of 82 symptomatic herniated thoracic discs and review of the literature, *J Neurosurg* 88:623–633, 1998.
18. Patel N: Surgical disorders of the thoracic and lumbar spine: A guide for neurologists, *J Neurol Neurosurg Psychiatry* 73:42–48, 2002.
19. Turner JA, Ersek M, Herron L, et al: Patient outcomes after lumbar spinal fusions, *JAMA* 268:907–911, 1992.
20. Frymoyer JW: Back pain and sciatica, *N Engl J Med* 318:291–300, 1988.
21. Iguchi T, Wakami T, Kurihara A, et al: Lumbar multilevel degenerative spondylolisthesis: Radiological evaluation and factors related to anterolisthesis and retrolisthesis, *J Spinal Disord Tech* 15:93–99, 2002.
22. Jacobsen S, Sonne-Holm S, Rovsing H, et al: Degenerative lumbar spondylolisthesis: An epidemiological perspective: The Copenhagen Osteoarthritis Study, *Spine* 32:120–125, 2007.
23. Bell GR: Degenerative spondylolisthesis. In Herkowitz HN, Garfin SR, et al: *Rothman-Simeone: The Spine*, 5th ed, Philadelphia, 2006, Saunders-Elsevier, 1027–1036.
24. Boden SD, Davis DO, Dina TS, et al: Abnormal magnetic-resonance scans of the lumbar spine in asymptomatic subjects: A prospective investigation, *J Bone Joint Surg Am* 72:403–408, 1990.
25. Shafi B, Beiner JM, Grauer JN, et al: Lumbar spondylolisthesis. In Vaccaro AR, editor: *Spine: Core Knowledge in Orthopaedics*, Philadelphia, 2005, Elsevier-Mosby, pp 157–171.
26. Wiltse LL, Winter RB: Terminology and measurement of spondylolisthesis, *J Bone Joint Surg* 65A:768–772, 1983.
27. Sengupta DK, Herkowitz HN: Degenerative spondylolisthesis: Review of current trends and controversies, *Spine* 30(Suppl):S71–S81, 2005.
28. Herkowitz HN: Spine update: Degenerative lumbar spondylolisthesis, *Spine* 20:1084–1090, 1995.
29. Vibert BT, Sliva CD, Herkowitz HN: Treatment of instability and spondylolisthesis: Surgical versus nonsurgical treatment, *Clin Orthop Rel Res* 443:222–227, 2006.
30. Basbarrini A, Bertoldi E, Mazzetti M, et al: Clinical features, diagnostic and therapeutic approaches to haematogenous vertebral osteomyelitis, *Eur Rev Med Pharmacol Sci* 9:53–66, 2005.
31. Tyrrell PN, Cassar-Pullucino VN, McCall IW: Spinal infection, *Eur Radiol* 9:1066–1077, 1999.
32. Carragee E: Pyogenic vertebral osteomyelitis, *J Bone Joint Surg* 79A:874–880, 1997.
33. Patzakis MJ, Rao S, Wilkins J, et al: Analysis of 61 cases of vertebral osteomyelitis, *Clin Orthop* 264:178–183, 1991.
34. Chelsom J, Solberg CO: Vertebral osteomyelitis at a Norwegian University Hospital 1997: Clinical features, laboratory findings and outcome, *Scand J Infect Dis* 30:147–151, 1998.
35. Nolla JM, Ariza J, Gomez-Vaquero C, et al: Spontaneous pyogenic vertebral osteomyelitis in nondrug users, *Semin Arthritis Rheum* 31:271–278, 2002.
36. Hadjipavlou AG, Mader JT, Necessari JT, et al: Hematogenous pyogenic spinal infections and their surgical management, *Spine* 13:1668–1679, 2000.
37. Love C, Patel M, Lonner BS, et al: Diagnosing spinal osteomyelitis, *Clin Nucl Med* 25:963–977, 2000.

38. Darouiche RO: Spinal epidural abscess, *N Engl J Med* 355:2012–2020, 2006.

39. Curry WT Jr, Hoh BL, Amin-Hanjani S, et al: Spinal epidural abscess: Clinical presentation, management, and outcome, *Surg Neurol* 63:364–371, 2005.

40. Grewal S, Hocking G, Wildsmith JA: Epidural abscesses, *Br J Anaesth* 96:292–302, 2006.

41. Davis DP, Wold RM, Patel RJ, et al: The clinical presentation and impact of diagnostic delays on emergency department patients with spinal epidural abscess, *J Emerg Med* 26:285–291, 2004.

42. Lu C-H, Chang W-N, Lui C-C, et al: Adult spinal epidural abscess: Clinical features and prognostic factors, *Clin Neurol Neurosurg* 104:306–310, 2002.

43. Patel N: Surgical disorders of the thoracic and lumbar spine: A guide for neurologists, *J Neurol Neurosurg Psychiatry* 73:42–48, 2002.

44. Khan SN, Donthineni R: Surgical management of metastatic spine tumors, *Orthop Clin North Am* 37:99–104, 2006.

45. Gokaslan ZL, York JE, Walsh GL, et al: Transthoracic vertebrectomy for metastatic spinal tumors, *J Neurosurg* 89:599–609, 1998.

46. Perrin R, McBroom RJ: Anterior versus posterior decompression for symptomatic spinal metastasis, *Can J Neurol Sci* 14:75–80, 1987.

47. Rafliff JK, Cooper PR: Metastatic spine tumors, *South Med J* 97:246–253, 2004.

48. Jackson RJ, Loh SC, Gokaslan ZL: Metastatic renal cell carcinoma of the spine: Surgical treatment and results, *J Neurosurg* 94(Suppl):18–24, 2001.

49. Fourney DR, Abi-Said D, Rhines LD, et al: Simultaneous anterior-posterior approach to the thoracic and lumbar spine for the radical resection of tumors followed by reconstruction and stabilization, *J Neurosurg* 94(Suppl):232–244, 2001.

50. Patterson JT, Hanbali F, Robbi L, et al: Intraspinal Tumors. In Townsend CM, Beauchamp RD, Evers BM, editors: *Townsend: Sabiston Textbook of Surgery*, ed 18, Philadelphia, 2008, Saunders-Elsevier, pp 2111–2112.

51. Vanderpool DW, James JI, Wynne-Davies R: Scoliosis in the elderly, *J Bone Joint Surg* 51:446–455, 1969.

52. Hu SS: Adult scoliosis. In Herkowitz HN, Garfin SR, et al: *Rothman-Simeone: The Spine*, ed 5, Philadelphia, 2006, Saunders-Elsevier, pp 1046–1057.

53. Ploumis A, Transfledt EE, Denis F: Degenerative lumbar scoliosis associated with spinal stenosis, *Spine J* 7:428–436, 2007.

54. Kobayashi T, Atsuta Y, Takemitsu M, et al: A prospective study of de novo scoliosis in a community based cohort, *Spine* 31:178–182, 2006.

55. Pritchett JW, Bortel DT: Degenerative symptomatic lumbar scoliosis, *Spine* 18:700–703, 1993.

56. Weinstein SL, Zavala DC, Ponseti IV: Idiopathic scoliosis: Long-term follow-up and prognosis in untreated patients, *J Bone Joint Surg Am* 63:702–712, 1981.

57. Ascani E, Bartolozzi P, Logroscino CA, et al: Natural history of untreated idiopathic scoliosis after skeletal maturity, *Spine* 11:784–789, 1986.

58. McDonnell MF, Glassman SD, Dimar JR II, et al: Perioperative complications of anterior procedures on the spine, *J Bone Joint Surg Am* 78:839–847, 1996.

59. Borenstein D: Inflammatory arthritides of the spine: Surgical versus nonsurgical treatment, *Clin Orthop Rel Res* 443:208–221, 2006.

60. Panayi GS: The immunopathogenesis of rheumatoid arthritis, *Br J Rheumatol* 32(Suppl 1):4–14, 1993.

61. Boden SD, Dodge LD, Bohlman HH, et al: Rheumatoid arthritis of the cervical spine: A long term analysis with predictors of paralysis and recovery, *J Bone Joint Surg* 75A:1282–1289, 1993.

62. Miceli-Richard C, Dougados M: NSAIDs in ankylosing spondylitis, *Clin Exp Rheumatol* 20(Suppl 28):S65–S66, 2002.

63. Broom MJ, Raycroft JF: Complications of fractures of the cervical spine in ankylosing spondylitis, *Spine* 13:763–766, 1988.

64. Szpalski M, Gunzburg R: What are the advances for surgical therapy of inflammatory disease of the spine? *Best Pract Clin Rheumatol* 16:141–154, 2002.

65. Melton LJ 3rd, Kan SH, Frye MA, et al: Epidemiology of vertebral fractures in women, *Am J Epidemiol* 129:1000–1011, 1989.

66. Cooper C, Atkinson EJ, O'Fallon WM, et al: Incidence of clinically diagnosed vertebral fractures: A population-based study in Rochester, Minnesota, 1985-1989, *J Bone Miner Res* 7:221–227, 1992.

67. Lopez LM, Grimes DA, Schulz KF, et al: Steroidal contraceptives: Effect on bone fractures in women, *Cochrane Database Syst Rev* (4):CD006033, 2006.

68. Holmes J, Miller P, Panacek E, et al: Epidemiology of thoracolumbar spine injury in blunt trauma, *Acad Emerg Med* 8:866–872, 2001.

69. Lindsey RW, Gugala Z, Pneumaticos SG: Injury to the vertebra and spinal cord. In Moore EE, Feliciano DV, Mattox KL, editors: *Trauma*, ed 5, New York, 2004, McGraw-Hill, pp 459–492.

70. Vaccaro AR: Fractures of the Cervical, Thoracic, and Lumbar Spine, New York, 2002, Marcel Dekker, Patterson RH, Arbit E: A surgical approach through the pedicle to protruded thoracic discs, *J Neurosurg* 48:768–772, 1978.

71. Ross SE, Schwab W, David ET, et al: Clearing the cervical spine: Initial radiologic evaluation, *J Trauma* 27:1055–1066, 1987.

72. MacDonald RL, Schwartz ML, Mirich D, et al: Diagnosis of cervical spine injury in motor vehicle crash victims: How many x-rays are enough? *J Trauma* 30:392–397, 1990.

73. Freemyer B, Knopp R, Piche J, et al: Comparison of five-view and three-view cervical spine series in the evaluation of patients with cervical trauma, *Ann Emerg Med* 18:818–821, 1989.

74. McDonald JW: Spinal-cord injury, *Lancet* 359:417–425, 2002.

75. The National SCI Statistical Center (NSCISC): *Facts and Figures at a Glance*, Birmingham, 2006, University of Alabama.

76. Ho CH, Wuermser L-A, Priebe MM, et al: Spinal cord injury medicine. 1: Epidemiology and classification, *Arch Phys Med Rehabil* 88(Suppl 1):S49–S54, 2007.

77. DeVivo MJ, Rutt RD, Black KJ, et al: Trends in spinal cord injury demographics and treatment outcomes between 1973 and 1986, *Arch Phys Med Rehabil* 73:424–430, 1992.

78. DeVivo MJ, Stover SL, Black KJ: Prognostic factors for 12-year survival after spinal cord injury, *Arch Phys Med Rehabil* 73:156–162, 1992.

79. Daverat P, Gagnon M, Dartigues JF, et al: Initial factors predicting survival in patients with a spinal cord injury, *J Neurol Neurosurg Psychiatry* 52:403–406, 1989.

80. Krause JS, Kjorsvig JM: Mortality after spinal cord injury: A four-year prospective study, *Arch Phys Med Rehabil* 73:558–563, 1992.

81. Waters RL, Adkins RH, Yakura JS, et al: Motor and sensory recovery following incomplete tetraplegia, *Arch Phys Med Rehabil* 75:306–311, 1994.

82. Waters RL, Adkins RH, Yakura JS, et al: Motor and sensory recovery following incomplete paraplegia, *Arch Phys Med Rehabil* 75:67–72, 1994.

83. Tator CH: Classification of spinal cord injury based on neurological presentation. In Narayan RK, Wilberger JE Jr, Povlishock JT, editors: *Neurotrauma*, New York, 1996, McGraw-Hill, pp 1059–1073.

84. Osterholm JL, Mathews GJ: Altered norepinephrine metabolism following experimental spinal cord injury. Part I: Relationship to hemorrhagic necrosis and post-wounding neurological deficits, *J Neurosurg* 36:386–394, 1972.

85. Senter HJ, Venes JL: Loss of autoregulation and posttraumatic ischemia following experimental spinal cord trauma, *J Neurosurg* 50:198–206, 1979.

86. Griffiths IR: Spinal cord blood flow after acute experimental cord injury in dogs, *J Neurol Sci* 27:247–259, 1976.

87. Ducker TB, Saleman M, Perot PL, et al: Experimental spinal cord trauma. I: Correlation of blood flow, tissue oxygen and neurologic status in the dog, *Surg Neurol* 10:60–63, 1978.

88. Nemecek S: Morphological evidence of microcirculatory disturbances in experimental spinal cord trauma, *Adv Neurol* 20:395–405, 1978.

89. Zwimpfer TJ, Berstein M: Spinal cord concussion, *J Neurosurg* 72:894–900, 1990.

90. Chesler M, Young M, Hassan AZ, et al: Elevation and clearance of extracellular K$^+$ following graded contusion of the rat spinal cord, *Exp Neurol* 125:93–98, 1994.

91. Stys PK: Anoxic and ischemic injury of myelinated axons in CNS white matter: From mechanistic concepts to therapeutics, *J Cereb Blood Flow Metab* 18:2–25, 1998.

92. Faden AI, Molineaux CJ, Rosenberger JG, et al: Endogenous opioid immunoreactivity in rat spinal cord following traumatic injury, *Ann Neurol* 17:386–390, 1985.

93. Bracken MB, Shephard MJ, Collins WF, et al: A randomized, controlled trial of methylprednisolone and naloxone in the treatment of acute spinal cord injury, *N Engl J Med* 322:1405–1411, 1990.

94. Bracken MB, Holford TR: Effects of timing of methylprednisolone or naloxone administration on recovery of segmental and long-tract neurological function in NASCIS 2, *J Neurosurg* 79:500–507, 1993.

95. Bracken MB, Shepard MJ, Holford TR, et al: Administration of methylprednisolone for 24 or 48 hours or tirilazad mesylate for 48 hours in the treatment of acute spinal cord injury: Results of the Third National Acute Spinal Cord Injury Randomized Controlled Trial. National Acute Spinal Cord Injury Study, *JAMA* 277:1597–1604, 1997.

96. Bracken MB, Collins WF, Freeman DF, et al: Efficacy of methylprednisolone in acute spinal cord injury, *JAMA* 251:45–52, 1984.

97. Levy ML, Gans W, Wijesinghe HS, et al: Use of methylprednisolone as an adjunct in the management of patients with spinal cord injury: Outcome analysis, *Neurosurgery* 39:1141–1148, 1996.

98. Sayer FT, Kronvall E, Nilsson OG: Methylprednisolone treatment in acute spinal cord injury: The myth challenged through a structured analysis of published literatures, *Spine J* 6:335–343, 2006.

99. Hurlbert RJ: Methyprednisolone for acute spinal cord injury: An inappropriate standard of care, *J Neurosurg* 93(Suppl):1, 2000.

100. Hadley MN: Management of acute central cervical spinal cord injuries, *Neurosurgery* 50(Suppl):S166–S172, 2002.

101. Consortium for Spinal Cord Medicine: *Early Acute Management in Adults with Spinal Cord Injury: A Clinical Practice Guideline for Health-Care Providers*, Washington, DC, 2007, Paralyzed Veterans of America.

102. Inamasu J, Nakamura Y, Ichikizaki K: Induced hypothermia in experimental traumatic spinal cord injury: An update, *J Neurol Sci* 209:55–60, 2003.

103. Vale FL, Burns J, Jackson AB, et al: Combined medical and surgical treatment after acute spinal cord injury: Results of a prospective pilot study to assess the merits of aggressive medical resuscitation and blood pressure measurement, *J Neurosurg* 87:239–246, 1997.

104. Podolsky S, Baraff LJ, Simon RR: Efficacy of cervical spine immobilization methods, *J Trauma* 23:461–465, 1983.

105. Louis R: Stability and instability of the cervical spine. In Kehr P, Weidner A, editors: *Cervical Spine I*, New York, 1987, Springer-Verlag, pp 21–27.

106. Glasser RS, Fessler RG: Biomechanics of cervical spine trauma. In Narayan RK, Wilberger JE Jr, Povlishock JT, editors: *Neurotrauma*, New York, 1996, McGraw-Hill, pp 1095–1112.

107. White AA III, Panjabi MM: The problem of clinical instability in the human spine: A systematic approach. In White AA III, Panjabi MM: *Clinical Biomechanics of the Spine*. ed 2, Philadelphia, 1990, Lippincott-Raven, pp 277-378.

108. Holdsworth FW: Fractures, dislocations, and fracture-dislocations of the spine, *J Bone Joint Surg Br* 45:6–20, 1963.

109. Panjabi MM, White AA III, Johnson RM: Cervical spine biomechanics as a function of transection of components, *J Biomech* 8:327–336, 1975.

110. Denis F: Spinal instability as defined by the three-column spine concept in acute spinal trauma, *Clin Orthop Rel Res* 189:65–76, 1984.

111. Bernhardt M, White AA, Panjabi MM: Biomechanical considerations of spinal stability. In Herkowitz HN, Garfin SR, Eismont FJ, et al, editors: *Rothman-Simeone: The Spine*, 5th ed, Philadelphia, 2006, Saunders-Elsevier, pp 132–156.

112. Terk MR, Hume-Neal M, Fraipont M, et al: Injury of the posterior ligament complex in patients with acute spinal trauma: evaluation by MR imaging, *AJR Am J Roentgenol* 168:1481–1486, 1997.

113. Eismont FJ, Clifford S, Goldberg M, et al: Cervical sagittal spinal canal size in spine injury, *Spine* 9:663–666, 1984.

114. Barolat G, Myklebust JB, Wenninger W: Effects of spinal cord stimulation on spasticity and spasms secondary to myelopathy, *Appl Neurophysiol* 51:29–44, 1988.

115. Dolan EJ, Tator CH, Endrenyi L: The value of decompression for acute experimental spinal cord compression injury, *J Neurosurg* 53:749–755, 1980.

116. Guha A, Tator CH, Endrenyl L, et al: Decompression of the spinal cord improves recovery after acute experimental spinal cord compression injury, *Paraplegia* 25:324–339, 1987.

117. Carlson GD, Minato Y, Okada A, et al: Early time-dependent decompression for spinal cord injury: Vascular mechanisms of recovery, *J Neurotrauma* 14:951–962, 1997.

118. Delamarter RB, Sherman J, Carr JB: Pathophysiology of spinal cord injury: Recovery after immediate delayed decompression, *J Bone Joint Surg Am* 77:1042–1049, 1995.

119. Dimar JR II, Glassman SD, Raque GH, et al: The influence of spinal canal narrowing and timing of decompression on neurologic recovery after spinal cord contusion in a rat model, *Spine* 24:1623–1633, 1999.

120. Carlson GD, Gorden CD, Oliff HS, et al: Sustained spinal cord compression. Part I: Time-dependent effect on long-term pathophysiology, *J Bone Joint Surg Am* 85:86–94, 2003.

121. Geisler F, Coleman W: Timing of surgical decompression for acute severe spinal injury: Retrospective results from a large multi-center clinical trial, *Spine J* 3:108S, 2003.

122. Papadopoulos S, Selden N, Quint D, et al: Immediate spinal cord decompression for cervical spinal injury: Feasibility and outcome, *J Trauma* 52:323–332, 2002.

123. Fehlings MG, Perrin RG: The timing of surgical intervention in the treatment of spinal cord injury: A systematic review of recent clinical evidence, *Spine* 31:S28–S35, 2006.

124. La Rosa G, Conti A, Cardali S, et al: Does early decompression improve neurological outcome of spinal cord injured patients? Appraisal of the literature using a meta-analytical approach, *Spinal Cord* 42:503–512, 2004.

125. Ball JR, Sekhon HS: Timing of decompression and fixation after spinal cord injury: When is surgery optimal? *Crit Care Res* 8:56–63, 2006.

126. McMichan JC, Michel L, Westbrook PR: Pulmonary dysfunction following traumatic quadriplegia, *JAMA* 243:528–531, 1980.

127. Ledsome JR, Sharp JM: Pulmonary function in acute cervical cord injury, *Am Rev Respir Dis* 124:41–44, 1981.

128. Scanlon PD, Loring SH, Pichurko BM, et al: Respiratory mechanics in acute quadriplegia, *Am Rev Respir Dis* 139:615–620, 1989.

129. Jackson AB Groomes TE: Incidence of respiratory complications following spinal cord injury, *Arch Phys Med Rehabil* 75:270–275, 1994.

130. Rechtine GR: II: Nonoperative management and treatment of spinal injuries, *Spine* 31:S22–S27, 2006.

131. Hildebrand F, et al: Management of polytraumatized patients with associated blunt chest trauma: A comparison of two European countries, *Injury* 36:293–302, 2005.

132. Pape HC, et al: Is early kinetic positioning beneficial for pulmonary function in multiple trauma patients? *Injury* 29:219–225, 1998.

133. Bein T, et al: Acute effects of continuous rotational therapy on ventilation-perfusion inequality in lung injury, *Intensive Care Med* 24:132–137, 1998.

134. Ahrens T, et al: Effect of kinetic therapy on pulmonary complications, *Am J Crit Care* 13:376–383, 2004.

135. Dodek P, et al: Evidence-based clinical practice guideline for the prevention of ventilator-associated pneumonia, *Ann Intern Med* 141:305–313, 2004.

136. Heyland DK, Cook DJ, Dodek M: Prevention of ventilator-associated pneumonia: Current practice in Canadian intensive care units, *J Crit Care* 17:161–167, 2002.

137. Tobin MJ: Advances in mechanical ventilation, *N Engl J Med* 344:1986–1996, 2001.

138. Gajic O, Dara SI, Mendez JL, et al: Ventilator associated lung injury in patients without acute lung injury at the onset of mechanical ventilation, *Crit Care Med* 32:1817–1824, 2004.

139. Yilmaz M, Keegan MT, Isciment R, et al: Toward the prevention of acute lung injury: Protocol-guided limitation of large tidal volume ventilation and inappropriate transfusion, *Crit Care Med* 35:1660–1666, 2007.

140. The Acute Respiratory Distress Syndrome Network: Ventilation with lower tidal volumes as compared with traditional tidal volumes for acute lung injury and the acute respiratory distress network, *N Engl J Med* 342:1301–1308, 2000.

141. Poe RH, Reisman JL, Rodenhouse TG: Pulmonary edema in cervical spinal cord injury, *J Trauma* 18:71–73, 1978.

142. Eidelberg EE: Cardiovascular response to experimental spinal cord compression, *J Neurosurg* 38:326–331, 1973.

143. Lehmann KG, Lane JG, Piepmeier JM, et al: Cardiovascular abnormalities accompanying acute spinal cord injury in humans: incidence, time course, and severity, *J Am Coll Cardiol* 10:46–52, 1987.

144. Piepmeier JM, Lehmann KB, Lane JG: Cardiovascular instability following acute cervical spinal cord trauma, *Cent Nerv Syst Trauma* 2:153–160, 1985.

145. Chang U, Lee MC, Kim DH: Posterior approach to the mid-cervical spine. In Kim DH, Henn JS, et al, editors: *Surgical Anatomy & Techniques to the Spine*, Philadelphia, 2006, Saunders-Elsevier, pp 57–64.

146. Young WF, Rosenwasser RH, Vasthare US, et al: Preservation of post-compression spinal cord function by infusion of hypertonic saline, *J Neurosurg Anesthesiol* 6:122–127, 1994.

147. Tuma RF, Vasthare US, Arfors K-E, et al: Hypertonic saline administration attenuates spinal cord injury, *J Trauma* 42:S54–S60, 1997.

148. Greenhoot JH, Mauck HP: The effect of cervical cord injury or cardiac rhythm and conduction. *Am Heart J* 83:659–662, 1972.

149. Segal JL, Milne N, Brunnemann SR: Gastric emptying is impaired in patients with spinal cord injury, *Am J Gastroenterol* 90:466–470, 1995.

150. Wuermser L-A, Chester HH, Chiodo AE, et al: Spinal cord injury medicine: 2: Acute care management of traumatic and nontraumatic injury, *Arch Phys Med Rehabil* 88(Suppl 1):S55–S61, 2007.

151. Waring WP, Karunas RS: Acute spinal cord injuries and the incidence of clinically occurring thromboembolic disease, *Paraplegia* 29:8–16, 1991.

152. Rogers FB, Cipolle MD, Velmahos G, et al: Practice management guidelines for the prevention of venous thromboembolism in trauma patients: The EAST Practice Management Guidelines Work Group, *J Trauma* 53:142–164, 2002.

153. Attia J, Ray JG, Cook DJ, et al: Deep vein thrombosis and its prevention in critically ill adults, *Arch Intern Med* 161:1268–1279, 2001.

154. Spinal Cord Injury Thromboprophylaxis Investigators: Prevention of venous thromboembolism in the acute treatment phase after spinal cord injury: A randomized, multicenter trial comparing low-dose heparin plus intermittent pneumatic compression with enoxaparin, *J Trauma* 54:1116–1126, 2003.

155. Geerts WH, Pineo GF, Heit JA, et al: Prevention of venous thromboembolism: The Seventh ACCP Conference on Antithrombotic and Thrombolytic Therapy, *Chest* 126:338S–400S, 2004.

156. Maxwell RA, Chavarria-Aguilar M, Cockerham WT, et al: Routine prophylactic vena cava filtration is not indicated after acute spinal cord injury, *J Trauma* 52:902–906, 2002.

157. Stawicki SP, Grossman MD, Cipolla J, et al: Deep venous thrombosis and pulmonary embolism in trauma patients: an overstatement of the problem? *Am Surg* 71:387–391, 2005.

158. Cassady JF Jr, Lederhaas G, Cancel DD, et al: A randomized comparison of the effects of continuous thoracic epidural analgesia and intravenous patient-controlled analgesia after posterior spinal fusion in adolescents, *Reg Anesth Pain Med* 25:246–253, 2000.

159. Lee TH, Marcantonio ER, Mangione CM, et al: Derivation and prospective validation of a simple index for prediction of cardiac risk of major noncardiac surgery, *Circulation* 100:1043–1049, 1999.

160. Fleisher LA, et al: ACC/AHA 2007 Guidelines on Perioperative Cardiovascular Evaluation and Care for Noncardiac Surgery: Executive Summary, *Circulation* 116:1971–1996, 2007.

161. Hernandez AF, Whellan DJ, Stroud S, et al: Outcomes in heart failure patients after major noncardiac surgery, *J Am Coll Cardiol* 44:1446–1453, 2004.

162. Segal JL, Brunnemann SR: Clinical pharmacokinetics in patients with spinal cord injuries, *Clin Pharmacokinet* 17:109–129, 1989.

163. Gronert GA, Theye RA: Pathophysiology of hyperkalemia induced by succinylcholine, *Anesthesiology* 43:4389–4399, 1975.

164. Calder I, Calder J, Crockard HA: Difficult direct laryngoscopy with cervical spine disease, *Anaesthesia* 50:756–763, 1995.

165. Lee LA, Roth S, Posner KL, et al: The American Society of Anesthesiologists Postoperative Visual Loss Registry: Analysis of 93 spine surgery cases with postoperative visual loss, *Anesthesiology* 105:652–659, 2006.

166. Muckart DJJ, Bhagwanjee S, van der Merwe R: Spinal cord injury as a result of endotracheal intubation in patients with undiagnosed cervical spine fractures, *Anesthesiology* 87:418–420, 1997.

167. Hastings RH, Kelley SD: Neurologic deterioration associated with airway management in a cervical spine–injured patient, *Anesthesiology* 78:580–583, 1993.

168. Crosby ET: Considerations for airway management for cervical spine surgery in adults, *Anesthesiology Clin* 25:511–533, 2007.

169. Crosby ET: Airway management in adults after cervical spine trauma, *Anesthesiology* 104:1293–1318, 2006.

170. Kitamura Y, Isono S, Suzuki N, et al: Dynamic interaction of craniofacial structures during head positioning and direct laryngoscopy in anesthetized patients with and without difficult laryngoscopy, *Anesthesiology* 107:875–883, 2007.

171. Crosby ET, Lui A: The adult cervical spine: Implications for airway management, *Can J Anaesth* 37:77–93, 1990.

172. Wood PR, Lawler PGP: Managing the airway in cervical spine injury: A review of the advanced trauma life support protocol, *Anaesthesia* 47:792–797, 1992.

173. Hastings RH: Airway management of patients with cervical spine injury, *Probl Anesth* 9:25, 1997.

174. Aprahamian C, Thompson BM, Finger WA, et al: Experimental cervical spine injury model: Examination of airway management and splinting techniques, *Ann Emerg Med* 13:584–587, 1984.

175. Sawin PD, Todd MM, Traynelis VC, et al: Cervical spine motion with direct laryngoscopy and orotracheal intubation, *Anesthesiology* 85:26–36, 1996.

176. Majernick T, Bieniek R, Houston J, et al: Cervical spine movement during orotracheal intubation, *Ann Emerg Med* 15:417–420, 1986.

177. Bivins H, Ford S, Bezmalinovic Z, et al: The effect of axial traction during orotracheal intubation of the trauma victim with an unstable cervical spine, *Ann Emerg Med* 17:25, 1988.

178. Hastings RH, Vigil AC, Hanna R, et al: Cervical spine movement during laryngoscopy with the Bullard, Macintosh, and Miller laryngoscopes, *Anesthesiology* 82:859–869, 1995.

179. Fitzgerald RD, Krafft P, Skrbensky G, et al: Excursions of the cervical spine during tracheal intubation: Blind oral intubation compared with direct laryngoscopy, *Anaesthesia* 49:111–115, 1994.

180. Horton WA, Fahy L, Charters P: Disposition of the cervical vertebrae, atlanto-axial joint, hyoid and mandible during x-ray laryngoscopy, *Br J Anaesth* 63:435–438, 1989.

181. Podolsky S, Baraff LJ, Simon RR, et al: Efficacy of cervical spine immobilization methods, *J Trauma* 23:461–465, 1983.

182. Heath KJ: The effect of laryngoscopy of different cervical spine immobilization techniques, *Anaesthesia* 49:843–845, 1994.

183. Althoff B, Goldie IF: Cervical collars in rheumatoid atlanto-axial subluxation: A radiographic comparison, *Ann Rheum Dis* 39:485–489, 1980.

184. Pennant JH, Pace NA, Gajraj NM: Role of the laryngeal mask airway in the immobile cervical spine, *J Clin Anesth* 5:226–230, 1993.

185. Goutcher CM, Lochhead V: Reduction in mouth opening with semirigid cervical collars, *Br J Anaesth* 95:344–348, 2005.

186. Hastings RH, Wood PR: Head extension and laryngeal view during laryngoscopy with cervical spine stabilization maneuvers, *Anesthesiology* 80:825–831, 1994.

187. Watts AD, Gelb AW, Bach DB, et al: Comparison of Bullard and Macintosh laryngoscopes for endotracheal intubation of patients with a potential cervical spine injury, *Anesthesiology* 87:1335–1342, 1997.

188. Walls RM: Airway management in the blunt trauma patient: How important is the cervical spine? *Can J Surg* 35:27–30, 1992.

189. Lennarson PJ, Smith DW, Sawin PD, et al: Cervical spinal motion during intubation: Efficacy of stabilization maneuvers in the setting of complete segmental instability, *J Neurosurg (Spine 2)* 94:265–270, 2001.

190. Davies G, Dealin C, Wilson A: The effect of a rigid collar on intracranial pressure, *Injury* 27:647–649, 1996.

191. Kolb JC, Summers RL, et al: Cervical collar-induced changes in intracranial pressure, *Am J Emerg Med* 17:135–137, 1999.

192. DeLorenzo RA, Olson JE, Boska M, et al: Optimal positioning for cervical immobilization, *Ann Emerg Med* 28:301–308, 1996.

193. Hauswald M, Sklar DP, Tandberg D, et al: Cervical spine movement during airway management: Cinefluoroscopic appraisal in human cadavers, *Am J Emerg Med* 9:535–538, 1991.

194. Donaldson WF III, Heil BV, Donaldson VP, Silvaggio VJ: The effect of airway maneuvers on the unstable C1-C2 segment: A cadaver study, *Spine* 22:1215–1218, 1997.

195. Lennarson PJ, Smith D, Todd MM, et al: Segmental cervical spine motion during orotracheal intubation of the intact and injured spine with and without external stabilization, *J Neurosurg (Spine 2)* 92:201–206, 2000.

196. Brimacombe J, Keller C, Kunzel KH, et al: Cervical spine motion during airway management: A cinefluoroscopic study of the posteriorly destabilized third cervical vertebrae in human cadavers, *Anesth Analg* 91:1274–1278, 2000.

197. MacIntyre PR, McLeod AD, Hurley R, et al: Cervical spine movements during laryngoscopy: Comparison of the Macintosh and McCoy laryngoscope blades, *Anaesthesia* 54:413–418, 1999.

198. Gerling MC, Davis DP, Hamilton RS, et al: Effects of cervical spine immobilization technique and laryngoscope blade selection on an unstable cervical spine in a cadaver model of intubation, *Ann Emerg Med* 36:293–300, 2000.

199. Agro F, Barzoi G, Montechia F: Tracheal intubation using a Macintosh laryngoscope or a Glidescope® in 15 patients with cervical spine immobilization, *Br J Anaesth* 90:705–706, 2003.

200. Turkstra TP, Craen RA, Pelz DM, et al: Cervical spine motion: A fluoroscopic comparison during intubation with lighted stylet, Glidescope®, and Macintosh laryngoscope. *Anesth Analg* 101:910-915, 2005.

201. Gabbott DA: The effect of single-handed cricoid pressure on neck movement after applying manual inline stabilization, *Anaesthesia* 52:586–588, 1997.

202. Hartley M: Cricoid pressure and potential spine injuries, *Anaesthesia* 48:1113, 1993.

203. Gabbott DA, Sasada MP: Laryngeal mask airway insertion using cricoid pressure and manual in-line neck stabilization, *Anaesthesia* 50:674–676, 1995.

204. Albin MS: Resuscitation of the spinal cord, *Crit Care Med* 6:270–276, 1978.

205. Raw DA, Beattie JK, Hunter JM: Anaesthesia for spinal surgery in adults, *Br J Anaesth* 91:886–904, 2003.

206. Abbott TR, Bentley G: Intraoperative awakening during scoliosis surgery, *Anaesthesia* 35:298–302, 1980.

207. Levi L, Wolf A, Belzberg H: Hemodynamic parameters in patients with acute cervical cord trauma: Description, intervention and prediction of outcome, *Neurosurgery* 33:1007–1016, 1993.

208. Poe RH, Reisman JL, Rodenhouse TG: Pulmonary edema in cervical cord injury, *J Trauma* 18:71–73, 1978.

209. Weinlander CM, Coombs DW, Plume SK: Myocardial ischemia due to obstruction of an aortocoronary bypass graft by intraoperative positioning, *Anesth Analg* 64:933–936, 1985.

210. Albin MS, Newfield P, Pautler S, et al: Atrial catheter and lumbar disc surgery, *JAMA* 239:496, 1978.

211. Ablin MS, Ritter RR, Pruett CE, et al: Venous air embolism during lumbar laminectomy in the prone position: Report of three cases, *Anesth Analg* 73:346–349, 1991.

212. Frankel AH, Holzman RS: Air embolism during posterior spinal fusion, *Can J Anaesth* 35:511–514, 1988.

213. McDouall SF, Shlugman D: Fatal venous air embolism during lumbar surgery: The tip of the iceberg? *Eur J Anaesth* 24:803–816, 2007.

214. Horlocker TT, Wedel DJ, Cucchiara RF: Venous air embolism during spinal instrumentation and fusion in the prone position, *Anesth Analg* 75:152–153, 1992.

215. McCarthy RE, Lonstein JE, Mertz JD, et al: Air embolism in spinal surgery, *J Spinal Disord* 3:1–5, 1990.

216. Lennon RL, Hosking MP, Gray JR, et al: The effects of intraoperative blood salvage and induced hypotension on transfusion requirements during spinal surgical procedures, *Mayo Clin Proc* 62:1090–1094, 1987.

217. Nahtomi-Shick O, Kostuik JP, Winters BD, et al: Does intraoperative fluid management in spine surgery predict intensive care unit length of stay? *J Clin Anesth* 13:208–212, 2001.

218. Zheng F, Cammisa FP Jr, Sandhu HS, et al: Factors predicting hospital stay, operative time, blood loss, and transfusion in patients undergoing revision posterior lumbar spine decompression, fusion, and segmental instrumentation, *Spine* 15:818–824, 2002.

219. Krämer AH, Hertzer NR, Beven EG: Intraoperative hemodilution during elective vascular reconstruction, *Surg Gynecol Obstet* 149:831–836, 1979.

220. Laks H, Pilon RN, Kloverkorn P, et al: Acute hemodilution: Its effect on hemodynamics and oxygen transport in anesthetized man, *Ann Surg* 180:103–109, 1974.

221. Rose D, Coutsoftides T: Intraoperative normovolemic hemodilution, *J Surg Res* 31:375–381, 1981.

222. Martin E, Ott E: Extreme hemodilution in the Harrington procedure, *Bibl Haemat* 47:322–337, 1981.

223. Goodnough LT, Monk TG: Autologous transfusion. In Miller RD, editor: *Miller's Anesthesia*, 6th ed, Philadelphia, 2005, Elsevier/Churchill Livingstone, pp 1831–1844.

224. Bryson GL, Laupacis A, Wells GA: for the International Study of Perioperative Transfusion: Does acute normovolemic hemodilution reduce perioperative allogeneic transfusion? A meta-analysis, *Anesth Analg* 86:9–15, 1998.

225. Brecher ME, Rosenfeld M: Mathematical and computer modeling of acute normovolemic hemodilution, *Transfusion* 34:176–179, 1994.

226. Olsfanger D, Fredman B, GoldsteinB, et al: Acute normovolaemic haemodilution decreases postoperative allogeneic blood transfusion after total knee replacement, *Br J Anaesth* 79:317–321, 1997.

227. Matot I, Scheinin O, Jurim O, et al: Effectiveness of acute normovolemic hemodilution to minimize allogeneic blood transfusion in major liver resections, *Anesthesiology* 97:794–800, 2002.

228. Waters JH: Red blood cell recovery and reinfusion, *Anesthesiol Clin N Am* 23:283–294, 2005.

229. Schenk MR, Putzier M, Kugler B, et al: Postoperative analgesia after major spine surgery: Patient-controlled epidural anesthesia versus patient-controlled intravenous analgesia, *Anesth Analg* 103:1311–1317, 2006.

230. Oda T, Fuji T, Kato Y, et al: Deep venous thrombosis after posterior spinal surgery, *Spine* 25:2962–2967, 2000.

231. Bianconi M, Ferraro L, Ricci R, et al: The pharmacokinetics and efficacy of ropivacaine continuous wound installation after spine fusion surgery, *Anesth Analg* 98:166–172, 2004.

232. Fisher CG, Belanger L, Gofton EG, et al: Prospective randomized clinical trial comparing patient-controlled intravenous analgesia with patient-controlled epidural analgesia after lumbar spinal fusion, *Spine* 28:739–743, 2003.

233. Cohen BE, Hartman MB, Wade JT, et al: Postoperative pain control after lumbar spine fusion: Patient-controlled analgesia versus continuous epidural analgesia, *Spine* 22:1892–1897, 1997.

234. Gottschalk A, Freitag M, Tank S, et al: Quality of postoperative pain using an intraoperatively placed epidural catheter after major lumbar surgery, *Anesthesiology* 101:175–180, 2004.

235. Blumenthal S, Min K, Nadig M, Borgeat A: Double epidural catheter with ropivacaine versus intravenous morphine: A comparison for postoperative analgesia after scoliosis correction surgery, *Anesthesiology* 102:175–180, 2005.

236. Lowry KJ, Tobias J, Kittle D, et al: Postoperative pain control using epidural catheters after anterior spinal fusion for adolescent scoliosis, *Spine* 26:1290–1293, 2001.

237. O'Neill P, Knickenberg C, Bogahalanda S, et al: Use of intrathecal morphine for postoperative pain relief following lumbar spine surgery, *J Neurosurg* 63:413–416, 1985.

238. Blackman RG, Reynolds J, Shively J: Intrathecal morphine: Dosage and efficacy in younger patients for control of postoperative pain following spinal fusion, *Orthopedics* 14:555–558, 1991.

239. Ross DA, Drasner K, Weinstein PR, et al: Use of intrathecally administered morphine in the treatment of postoperative pain after lumbar spine surgery: A prospective, double-blind, placebo-controlled study, *Neurosurgery* 28:700–704, 1991.

240. Joshi GP, McCarroll SM, O'Rourke K: Postoperative analgesia after lumbar laminectomy: Epidural fentanyl infusion versus patient-controlled intravenous morphine, *Anesth Analg* 80:511–514, 1995.

241. Shaw BA, Watson TC, Merzel DI, et al: The safety of continuous epidural infusion for postoperative analgesia in pediatric spine surgery, *J Pediatr Orthop* 16:374–377, 1996.

242. White PF: The changing role of non-opioid analgesic techniques in the management of postoperative pain, *Anesth Analg* 101:S5–S22, 2005.

243. MacEwan GD, Bunnel WP, Krishnaswami S: Acute neurological complications in the treatment of scoicosisi a report of the sediosis research society. *J Bone Joint Surg* 57A:404–408, 1975.

244. Sandson TA, Friedman JH: Spinal cord infarction: Report of 8 cases and review of the literature, *Medicine* 68:282–292, 1989.

245. Stevens WR, Glazer PA, Kelley SD, et al: Opthalmic complications after spinal surgery, *Spine* 22:1319–1324, 1997.

246. Shaw PJ, Bates D, Cartlidge NE, et al: Neuro-ophthalmological complications of coronary artery bypass graft surgery, *Acta Neurol Scand* 76:1–7, 1987.

247. Warner MA: Perioperative neuropathies, blindness, and positioning problems, *ASA Refresher Courses in Anesthesiology* 34:195–205, 2006.

248. Nuttall GA, Garrity JA, Dearani JA, et al: Risk factors for ischemic optic neuropathy after cardiopulmonary bypass: A matched case/control study, *Anesth Analg* 93:1410–1416, 2001.

249. Practice Advisory for Perioperative Visual Loss Associated with Spine Surgery: A report by the American Society of Anesthesiologists Task Force on Perioperative Blindness, *Anesthesiology* 104:1319–1328, 2006.

250. Allen BL, Ferquson RL, Lehmann TR, et al. A mechanistic classification of closed indirect fractures and dislocations of the lower cervical spine. *Spine* 7:1–27, 1982.

Chapter 21

NEUROLOGIC DISEASE AND ANESTHESIA

Deborah J. Culley • Meredith R. Brooks • Gregory Crosby

The primary neurodegenerative or demyelinating diseases that are the subjects of this chapter share common features. With one exception, they tend to manifest as variable degrees of neurologic impairment, they affect neuromuscular and pulmonary function, and they are relentlessly progressive and incurable. Another shared feature is that although the diseases themselves are well described, clinical anesthetic experience with them is limited and largely reported in the form of small clinical series and anecdotes. Consequently, a discussion of the anesthetic management of these diseases has inherent limitations that the prudent reader should recognize.

NEURODEGENERATIVE DISEASES

Huntington's Disease

Huntington's disease is a universally fatal neurodegenerative disorder that affects the central nervous system and results from an autosomal dominant mutation in the Huntingtin gene.[1] It is characterized by movement and psychiatric disorders as well as dementia and occurs in 5 to 7 persons per 100,000 population.[1] The genetic defect is due to a mutation in the Huntington gene IT15 on the short arm of chromosome 4, resulting in production of an abnormal form of the huntingtin protein. Huntingtin is present ubiquitously in somatic tissues, but curiously, the pathologic changes associated with Huntington's disease are limited to the brain. The mechanism by which the genetically altered protein induces the associated central nervous system changes is unknown, but prevailing theories suggest that huntingtin deposition enhances neuronal susceptibility to oxidative stress or glutamate-mediated excitotoxicity.[1] The brain of a patient with Huntington's disease undergoes progressive atrophy and gliosis that are most prominent in the basal ganglia.[1] Interestingly, striatal atrophy becomes apparent with some magnetic resonance imaging (MRI) techniques more than a decade before onset of clinical symptoms.[1] These cerebral alterations, combined with loss of gamma-aminobutyric acid–ergic neurons in the striatum, help explain the motor symptoms of Huntington's disease, but the pathophysiology of the cognitive and psychiatric alterations remains unknown.

A patient with Huntington's disease can experience symptoms at any time after infancy but usually becomes symptomatic in the late 30s or early 40s. Therefore, the diagnosis is often not established until after reproduction, although genetic testing now allows earlier diagnosis and the option of genetic counseling.[1] The motor symptoms of Huntington's disease typically begin with a lack of coordination and involuntary jerks. These uncontrollable, involuntary choreic movements (i.e., random jerking movements of the extremities, torso, face, and truncal muscles) and athetosis (i.e., slower

sinusoid writhing movements) peak after steady progression for 10 years and ultimately develop a rigid dystonic character. Dysphagia is common in advanced cases, and most patients suffer from nutritional depletion at some stage.

All patients with Huntington's disease eventually experience dementia that spares long-term memory but impairs executive functions. Other psychiatric and cognitive changes occur before, after, or at the same time as motor abnormalities and may include irritability, apathy, emotional instability, impulsiveness, and aggression. Depression is common, as is suicide, which occurs at a rate up to 10 times that of the general population. Death usually occurs within 20 years of diagnosis as a result of a fall, pneumonia, aspiration, malnutrition, or suicide.[1]

There are no specific treatments that prevent, cure, or slow the progression of Huntington's disease. Symptomatic therapy aims to control the motor and psychiatric aspects of the disorder. The only drugs proven in clinical trials to be efficacious for the treatment of chorea are amantadine, remacemide, levetiracetam, and tetrabenazine. However, they can cause bradykinesia, rigidity, depression, and sedation.[1] The affective disorders associated with Huntington's disease are often amenable to psychiatric treatment, such that polypharmacy is common. The prudent anesthesiologist will therefore be vigilant for the possibility of adverse drug interactions.

Anesthetic management for a patient with Huntington's disease is driven mostly by theory because the literature is limited to anecdotal experiences and case reports. Because patients with Huntington's disease are at increased risk of pulmonary aspiration due to pharyngeal muscle abnormalities and dysphagia, aspiration prophylaxis and precautions seem warranted, but whether administration of anesthesia to these patients further raises the risk of aspiration pneumonitis is unknown. Patients with Huntington's disease are also alleged to be at risk for prolonged respiratory depression and delayed return to consciousness after general anesthesia and have reduced requirements for midazolam.[2] Whether this risk is related to altered pharmacokinetics, due to nutritional depletion and altered protein binding, or caused by increased central nervous system sensitivity and altered pharmacodynamics is unknown. In any event, some patients with Huntington's disease experience a normal anesthetic and post-anesthetic course.[3,4]

Data concerning the response to muscle relaxants are similarly confusing. There is a higher incidence of abnormal plasma cholinesterase variants among patients with Huntington's disease, and a case report of prolonged muscle relaxation following administration of succinylcholine, but succinylcholine has been used uneventfully in other patients.[5-8] There are, however, no case reports of succinylcholine-induced hyperkalemia. With respect to nondepolarizing muscle relaxants, both abnormal and normal responses have been reported.

There are also reports of clinically significant generalized tonic muscle spasms related to shivering during emergence from anesthesia in patients with Huntington's disease,[8] suggesting that maintenance of perioperative normothermia is especially important in these patients. Some writers even recommend avoiding inhalational anesthetics to decrease the risk of postoperative shivering, although the benefit of doing so is only theoretical.[3,9] Lastly, other than being technically difficult because of the continuous uncontrollable movements, there appears to be no contraindication to regional anesthesia in the patient with Huntington's disease.[4,10]

Amyotrophic Lateral Sclerosis

Amyotrophic lateral sclerosis (ALS) is a progressive, untreatable degenerative disease of the central nervous system that involves both upper and lower motor neurons. The disease affects 1 to 2.5 persons per 100,000 population and usually manifests between 50 and 70 years of age.[11] ALS is marked by loss of motor neurons in the anterior horn of the spinal cord and of brainstem nuclei of cranial nerves V, VII, IX, X, and XII as well as degeneration of the corticospinal tracts secondary to loss of cortical motor neurons. This degeneration produces symptoms that include asymmetric muscle atrophy and weakness and bulbar abnormalities such as dysarthria, dysphagia, drooling, and an ineffective cough. The clinical course ultimately ends in paralysis, but the type depends upon whether upper or lower motor neuron lesions are more prominent. If upper motor neuron lesions predominate, the paralysis is spastic, whereas lower motor neuron lesions result in flaccidity. Both evolve over months to years and affect all striated muscle except that of cardiac and ocular origin.

The disease leads to a restrictive pulmonary defect, with progressive decreases in FVC (forced vital capacity) and FEV_1 (forced expiratory volume in the first second of expiration) as a result of muscle weakness and skeletal deformities. These changes can occur rapidly but typically are slowly progressive and lead to hypercarbia, atelectasis, and a predisposition to pneumonia.[12] Studies now suggest that survival and quality of life may be enhanced by the administration of riluzole, a glutamate release antagonist, and both respiratory and nutritional support in the form of noninvasive ventilation and placement of a gastrostomy tube.[11,12] Death usually occurs within 3 to 10 years of diagnosis owing to respiratory complications such as pneumonia, atelectasis, and aspiration.

There are no laboratory tests to confirm the diagnosis of ALS, which is usually made on the basis of both upper and lower motor neuron abnormalities in association with progressive motor dysfunction.[12] Supporting laboratory evidence includes spontaneous fibrillations, positive sharp waves, fasciculations, and decreased recruitment of motor units on electromyography (EMG). Results of nerve conduction studies are normal or reflect denervation of motor neurons without sensory involvement.

The etiology of ALS remains unknown, but glutamate-mediated excitotoxicity, genetic defects leading to free radical formation, autoimmune disease, and abnormalities in neurotrophic growth factors have all been hypothesized.[13] Ultrastructural changes in the motor neurons of patients with ALS include the presence of inclusion bodies and swelling in the proximal axon and cell body. Ultimately, these abnormal neurons are thought to undergo necrosis or apoptosis, leading to degeneration and neuronal cell loss.

Given the pathophysiology and clinical manifestations of ALS, anesthetic considerations include altered responses to muscle relaxants, ventilation impairment, bulbar dysfunction, and concerns about neurologic sequelae of regional anesthesia. Patients with ALS are predisposed to succinylcholine-induced hyperkalemia because of denervation and atrophy of skeletal muscles, so succinylcholine is best avoided in these patients.[14,15] Such patients may also have increased sensitivity to nondepolarizing muscle relaxants, suggesting either that relaxants be avoided altogether or that shorter-acting relaxants be used.[15] Progressive impairment of ventilation is another serious problem, and preoperative ventilatory impairment has been used to predict anesthetic risk. Although it would be easy to think that regional anesthesia is preferable to general anesthesia in such high-risk patients, such a practice is not established.[16] Operations have been successfully conducted with use of epidural anesthesia, but most of the patients involved did not have severe preoperative pulmonary involvement; in one reported case in which there was significant respiratory involvement, the patient required noninvasive respiratory support consisting of biphasic positive airway pressure postoperatively.[17-19] Accordingly, it may be necessary to support ventilation in the patient with ALS both during surgery and in the immediate postoperative period regardless of anesthetic technique.[20,21]

The primary concern about bulbar dysfunction is dysphagia and the risk of recurrent pulmonary aspiration.[12] For this reason, aspiration prophylaxis should be considered, but there is no evidence that this measure reduces the perioperative risk of aspiration pneumonitis in the patient with ALS. Moreover, because of the inability to swallow properly, many patients with ALS require placement of a feeding tube. This can typically be accomplished with use of regional anesthesia but may require the use of noninvasive ventilation both during and after the procedure.[21]

Lastly, there has been concern about the possibility that regional anesthesia may facilitate progression of neurodegenerative diseases such as ALS. Evidence for this concept is entirely anecdotal, however, and there are several case reports of uneventful neurologic recovery after epidural anesthesia in patients with ALS.[17-19,22] Perhaps the most one can say is that regardless of the type of anesthesia, the proximate cause of neurologic deterioration is difficult to establish in a relentlessly progressive neurologic disorder.

Parkinson's Disease

Parkinson's disease (PD) is the second most common neurodegenerative disease, second only to Alzheimer's disease. Classically considered a movement disorder secondary to degeneration of dopaminergic neurons in the basal ganglia and nigrostriatal system, PD is now recognized as a multisystem neurodegenerative process. It afflicts about 1 million Americans, or approximately 1% of patients older than 60 years, and its prevalence is projected to double in the next 15 to 20 years.[23] Fifteen years after diagnosis, 40% of patients with this disorder are living in long-term care facilities, and mortality is almost twice that of unaffected age-matched persons. Most cases are idiopathic, but environmental factors, including general anesthesia,[24] and genetic predisposition are implicated; as many as 10% to 15% of patients with PD have a first- or second-degree relative with the disorder.

The common feature of the disease is neuronal loss and gliosis of the pars compacta substantiae nigrae. By the time motor symptoms develop, 70% of the dopamine-producing cells in the striatum have degenerated, leading to a relative imbalance between the inhibitory properties of dopamine and the excitatory properties of acetylcholine within the striatum.[25] However, pathology extends beyond the striatum and dopamine. The pathologic hallmark of PD is the Lewy body, an intracellular aggregate of abnormal proteins including α-synuclein, which is present in nearly all forms.[26] This α-synuclein pathology and concomitant neurodegeneration are seen in numerous areas of the central and peripheral nervous systems, including noradrenergic, serotonergic, and cholinergic neurons of the brainstem and in the amygdala, cingulate gyrus, and neocortex. Moreover, changes in these regions may actually precede the striatal degeneration. Therefore, it is overly simplistic to regard PD only as a movement disorder.

Cardinal clinical features of the disorder are a resting rhythmic tremor, muscular rigidity, and bradykinesia.[26] These are often associated with a lack of spontaneous movement, masked facies, cogwheel rigidity, a monotonous voice, stooped posture, and a shuffling gait leading to postural instability and impaired locomotion. Not surprisingly given the widespread neurodegeneration, nonmotor features of the disease represent important sources of disability and, in long-standing PD, are often the predominant problem.[27] Autonomic dysfunction (postural hypotension), daytime sleepiness, depression, anxiety, hallucinations, and psychosis are common; dementia is almost universal in patients with long-standing disease.[28,29] In fact, after 8 years of disease, the prevalence of dementia is as high as 78%.[30]

There is no cure for PD. Therapy has focused almost exclusively on the motor aspects of the disorder, leaving cognitive and other nonmotor features unaddressed. Given that the main deficit is inadequate dopamine in the basal ganglia, pharmacologic therapy aims to increase the activity of dopamine relative to acetylcholine in this region.[26] This is typically accomplished with dopamine receptor agonists such as bromocriptine and pergolide or with levodopa (L-dopa), a prodrug that undergoes decarboxylation in both the periphery and central nervous system to produce dopamine. Peripheral conversion of levodopa to dopamine produces side effects such as nausea, vomiting, and hemodynamic instability, so combined treatment with levodopa and carbidopa, a decarboxylase inhibitor that does not cross the blood-brain barrier, is common. Levodopa is the most potent, best-tolerated agent for symptomatic therapy and it may even slow disease progression. Nevertheless, dopamine agonists are often first-line therapy because use of levodopa is associated with a higher incidence of dyskinesias, particularly in patients younger than 40 years.[23,26] Dopamine agonists have their own problems, however, including leg edema, hallucinations, somnolence, and development of impulse control disorders such as binge eating and compulsive gambling.

A variety of other drugs used to treat PD also act by altering the dopamine-acetylcholine balance in the brain.[31] Usually used for initial therapy of mild PD or as adjuncts to levodopa therapy in patients with dose-related fluctuations, benztropine and other anticholinergic agents block cholinergic transmission, and the antiviral agent amantadine alters the uptake and release of dopamine at presynaptic sites. Because monoamine oxidase is the major enzyme involved in oxidative metabolism of dopamine in the striatum, type-B monoamine oxidase inhibitors such as selegiline are sometimes employed, but this therapy remains controversial because the combination of levodopa and selegiline has been linked to increased mortality.[32] When motor complications become disabling and medical therapy fails, neurosurgical treatments such as pallidotomy and deep brain stimulation, which has the advantage of being adjustable and reversible, are considered.[33] Transplantation of fetal midbrain or stem cells into human patients with PD is another exciting alternative. The cells function and survive but begin to develop Lewy bodies and fail after about 10 years.[34,35] Indeed, some argue that pharmacologic and surgical treatments are inherently limited because they address only a late, specific event—loss of striatal dopamine neurons—in what is likely to be a widespread disease.

Perioperative management of the patient with PD is challenging. Attention should be directed toward maintenance of perioperative drug therapy, potential adverse drug interactions, and the physiologic perturbations associated with the disease. It is also important to recognize that emotional stress, which is unavoidable and difficult to address in the perioperative period, can also exacerbate PD. One major problem is that the half-life of levodopa is short (about 90 minutes).[36] Therefore, even brief interruptions in drug therapy are undesirable and can result in an acute exacerbation of the symptoms of PD or the development of neuroleptic malignant syndrome, a potentially fatal disorder that manifests as hyperthermia, akinesia, altered consciousness, muscle rigidity, and autonomic dysfunction.[37,38] Consequently, interruption of antiparkinsonian drug therapy should be as brief as possible. However, maintenance of therapy is difficult when the patient is unable to take medications by mouth for lengthy periods. Intravenous levodopa has been used successfully in the perioperative period but, without co-administration of a decarboxylase inhibitor (not yet available in intravenous form), cardiovascular side effects such as hypertension, hypotension, and arrhythmias can be anticipated. Levodopa and carbidopa are absorbed in the small intestine and thus must first traverse the stomach, making administration of tablets through a gastric tube suboptimal or ineffective because patients with PD often have delayed gastric emptying.[39,40]

In addition, the disease takes a toll on body systems that are vitally important during and after surgery. Respiratory dysfunction is especially prominent.[41,42] PD can produce restrictive lung disease secondary to chest wall rigidity, but pulmonary function tests often reveal a obstructive pattern with a characteristic sawtooth pattern on flow-volume loops that are improved but not normalized with levodopa.[42,43] Upper airway abnormalities also occur. Involuntary movements of the glottis and supraglottic structures cause intermittent airway obstruction, a condition that can be exacerbated by levodopa withdrawal.[42,44] Upper airway obstruction, laryngospasm, and respiratory arrest are documented complications of PD and may occur outside the setting of anesthesia and surgery.[42,45-47] Perhaps not surprisingly, therefore, laryngospasm has been reported postoperatively in awake patients hours after surgery.[48] Direct visualization of the larynx during such episodes reveals complete apposition of the vocal cords, requiring succinylcholine for relief.[47] Although some of these cases occurred despite maintenance of antiparkinsonian drug therapy, most followed withdrawal or pharmacologic antagonism of antiparkinsonian medication.[46,48] Indeed, not only should interruption of drug therapy be avoided, the dosage may need to be increased if airway problems persist despite otherwise adequate therapy.

Patients with PD are predisposed to aspiration because they often have severe, but asymptomatic, dysphagia and dysmotility that, in combination with upper airway abnormalities, present an especially troublesome situation.[49,50] In fact, pulmonary aspiration is a common cause of death among patients with PD. Thus, administration of antacids and prokinetic agents should be considered, but whether anesthesia actually increases the risk of aspiration in these patients is unknown. Metoclopramide must be avoided, however, because it is a dopamine receptor antagonist and could acutely exacerbate the disease. In contrast, prokinetic agents such as cisapride and domperidone, which have no effect on central dopaminergic balance, are reasonable alternatives.[51]

Other forms of nervous system dysfunction are also common. Autonomic insufficiency affects the ability of patients with PD to respond to the hypovolemia and vasodilation sometimes associated with anesthesia and surgery.[52,53] Orthostatic hypotension and thermoregulatory or genitourinary dysfunction suggest preexisting autonomic insufficiency and should heighten awareness of the potential for perioperative hemodynamic instability and altered responses to vasopressors such as noradrenaline.[54] At the level of the central nervous system, psychiatric complications such as anxiety, confusion, and even frank psychosis occur more often in patients with PD than in the general population and can be especially problematic in the perioperative period.[28,55] Because these complications are often related to or exacerbated by fluctuations in antiparkinsonian drugs, the first line of treatment is to look for and remedy reversible causes as one would in any patient with delirium.[56] Pharmacologic treatment is difficult, however, because the usual remedies (e.g., benzodiazepines for anxiety and antipsychotics for psychosis) can have severe side effects, such as oversedation and acute exacerbation of motor symptoms in elderly patients with PD.[28,55,57] In the event such treatment becomes necessary, consultation with a specialist is recommended.

Anesthetics and a number of other agents used perioperatively may affect the disease process. Volatile anesthetics can alter dopaminergic balance in the brain, but whether they exacerbate PD is unknown.[58,59] In fact, provided that the intraoperative electrophysiologic approach is based on multiple-unit recording, deep brain stimulation surgery has been performed successfully during general anesthesia using a volatile agent, suggesting that activity in dopaminergic circuits are reasonably well maintained.[60] Propofol produces both dyskinesias and ablation of resting tremor, suggesting that it has both excitatory and inhibitory effects in this patient population, but it also has been used successfully to sedate patients with PD during deep brain stimulation surgery.[61,62] Dexmedetomidine also appears to be safe and, when used for deep brain lead implantation and stimulation, has the advantage of not interfering with motor symptoms.[63] Ketamine should be used cautiously, if at all, because of potential interactions between levodopa and ketamine's sympathomimetic properties. However, in a single case report, ketamine temporarily stopped the motor symptoms of the disease.[64] Butyrophenones (e.g., droperidol) and phenothiazines, which block dopamine receptors, exacerbate PD and should be avoided.[65] In at least one case, droperidol may have induced parkinsonism in a normal patient.[66] Ondansetron, a 5-HT$_3$ serotonin receptor antagonist, appears to be safe for treatment or preventing emesis in patients with Parkinson's disease and has been used successfully to treat the psychosis of long-term levodopa therapy.[67] Although opioids are more likely to produce muscular rigidity in a patient with PD, acute dystonia has been observed only rarely, and enhancement of opioid neurotransmission during disease progression may be a compensatory mechanism that prevents motor complications.[68,69] Meperidine should be avoided in a patient taking monoamine oxidase inhibitor, however, because of the potential for development of stupor, rigidity, agitation, and hyperthermia.[70] Responses to depolarizing and nondepolarizing muscle relaxants are thought to be normal in PD, despite a single case report of succinylcholine-induced hyperkalemia.[71-73]

Finally, with the advent and increasing popularity of deep brain stimulation, issues arise about the safety of MRI or intraoperative electrocautery in patients who have PD and who have stimulator leads in place.[74,75] In the brain stimulation procedure, a thin coiled wire is implanted stereotactically in the subthalamic nucleus or globus pallidus and tunneled subcutaneously to a stimulator implanted in the chest wall. In theory, extraneous current can heat the electrode tip, causing brain tissue damage, but there is limited clinical experience with this circumstance. To reduce the risk of injury, the bipolar mode should be used if electrocautery is needed and the leads and generator should not be located between the surgical site and the ground plate. If the patient is to undergo MRI, the neurostimulator should be switched off.

Alzheimer's Disease-type Dementia

Dementia is a chronic and progressive decline in intellectual function. As such, it is distinct from normal age-related memory impairment and the acute confusion of delirium. The differential diagnosis of dementia is extensive, but Alzheimer's disease (AD) is the most common type.[76] This section therefore focuses on AD because it is the most prevalent type of dementia and because there is little evidence that the form of dementia alters perioperative considerations.

Alzheimer's disease–type dementia is a chronic neurodegenerative disease that afflicts about 4.5 million Americans, making it the seventh leading cause of death in the United States and a major public health problem.[77] AD rarely manifests before age 65 years but increases in incidence two-fold every 5 years thereafter until, by age 90 years, up to 50% of persons are affected.[77,78] The clinical diagnosis of AD is difficult because, at least early on, symptoms are often subtle and nonspecific and so not easily distinguished from those of other dementias.[77] Therefore, the definitive diagnosis is made postmortem with demonstration of gross atrophy of the cerebral cortex in conjunction with the neuropathologic hallmarks of the disease—namely, neurofibrillary tangles consisting of phosphorylated τ protein and neuritic plaques composed of β amyloid (Aβ).[77,79]

Advances in neuroimaging for amyloid plaques and biomarker discovery, particularly for Aβ and τ protein in plasma and cerebrospinal fluid, promise to enhance the ability to diagnose AD early, but there is enough overlap in the distribution and levels of these markers between demented and nondemented persons that at present none is a foolproof surrogate for a clinical or histopathologic diagnosis.[80-82]

AD is insidious, relentless, and devastating. There is a transitional phase, mild cognitive impairment, between normal aging and AD that is defined by memory complaints and objective evidence of amnesia but otherwise intact cognitive function.[83] Up to 30% of community-dwelling elders have mild cognitive impairment, which in a large percentage will ultimately convert to AD, suggesting that mild cognitive impairment is an early phase of AD.[83] Full-blown AD affects much more than memory; language, visuospatial skills, judgment, reasoning, decision-making, and ability to manage complex tasks deteriorate. In addition, behavioral and psychiatric abnormalities, such as depression, hallucinations, delusions, anxiety, aggression, and agitation, are common in the patient with AD. Ultimately, the patient becomes incapacitated to the point of being unable to perform basic activities of daily living.[77] There is currently no cure, and death usually occurs within 2 to 16 years of onset.

AD is probably the end result of a number of biologic and environmental factors.[78] There is a genetic component to the disease, as demonstrated by linkage studies revealing rare mutations in the amyloid precursor protein and presenilin genes as well as increased susceptibility to AD among carriers of the apolipoprotein gene E4 allele.[84] Most of these genetic alterations are neither necessary nor sufficient to cause AD, however, indicating that genetic susceptibility works in combination with other factors.[78] Low education level, prior history of head trauma, thyroid disease, and exposure to general anesthesia have been investigated as possible risk factors, with mixed results.[78,85,86] Because patients with dementia have a higher incidence of depression, there is also a debate as to whether depression is a risk factor for dementia or, conversely, whether subclinical dementia leads to depression.

As mentioned previously, the pathologic hallmarks of AD are extracellular plaques and intracellular neurofibrillary tangles composed of Aβ and τ protein, respectively. How Aβ and τ protein produce neurodegeneration and functional impairment is not definitively known, but free radical–mediated oxidative damage, stimulation of inflammation, energy depletion, calcium-mediated neurotoxicity, and alterations in metal homeostasis are a few of the main theories.[77,78,81,87] If the exact mechanism of injury is uncertain, the result is clear. Patients with AD have profound and accelerated cortical atrophy, synaptic loss, and reactive gliosis.[77,78,81,87] Neurotransmitter systems are damaged. These patients have fewer nicotinic cholinergic receptors and reduced acetylcholine synthesis, particularly in areas associated with memory and cognition, such as the hippocampus, basal forebrain, and cerebral cortex, and norepinephrine and serotonin are also modified.[81,87] Cerebral pro-inflammatory cascades are also activated, leading to a state of chronic neuroinflammation.

The pathogenesis of AD suggests a number of therapeutic approaches, but none has proved effective at stopping or reversing disease progression.[77] Given deficiencies in central cholinergic activity, a mainstay of medical therapy of AD is use of anticholinesterases such as tacrine and donepezil.[88] Widely used, these drugs have a favorable but mild effect on neuropsychiatric and functional outcomes, particularly in the early stages of the disease.[89] These drugs also have a variety of side effects, including reversible hepatotoxicity, gastrointestinal symptoms, (nausea, vomiting, diarrhea, dyspepsia, abdominal pain), and dermatitis and the potential for interactions with hepatically metabolized drugs such as cimetidine and warfarin.[77]

Administration of tacrine has been reported to prolong the action of succinylcholine but may cause resistance to nondepolarizing muscle relaxants.[77,90] Donepezil has similar efficacy but fewer side effects and is associated with fewer drug interactions.[77] A newer pharmacologic approach to treatment is memantine, a mild partial N-methyl-D-aspartate receptor antagonist that blocks glutamatergic transmission.[77] Like the anticholinesterases, memantine produces some improvement in cognition and global dementia, but it is marginal.[88]

Approaches to alter the progression of AD are numerous and include use of agents such as antioxidants (e.g., vitamin E), estrogens, and anti-inflammatory agents.[77] The last deserve special attention because they have been studied fairly extensively, albeit with conflicting results. Multiple epidemiologic studies have demonstrated an association between use of non-aspirin nonsteroidal anti-inflammatory drugs and decreased risk for development of AD, but results of randomized controlled studies have been conflicting. For example, two studies published in 2008 suggest that long-term use of ibuprofen, but not celecoxib or naproxen, reduces the risk for development of AD.[91,92] Some of the confusion may relate to the age of the study cohort and duration of treatment as well as to the fact that some nonsteroidal anti-inflammatory drugs have cyclooxygenase-independent effects on Aβ processing but others do not.[93] Therefore, any benefit of such agents may be unrelated to their anti-inflammatory actions and may be greater when treatment begins before age 65 years.[93]

Perhaps the most direct and promising approaches to modifying the course of AD are those that reduce Aβ accumulation or increase its clearance. Drugs that inhibit the formation of Aβ by blocking the proteolytic enzymes β- and γ-secretase, which cleave the large amyloid precursor protein (APP) to generate Aβ, are being studied in early human trials.[94] Likewise, operating under the assumption that Aβ is the main neurotoxic factor in development of AD, trials are under way with vaccines intended to eliminate existing Aβ deposits in the brain.[95] An early clinical trial with one such vaccine was aborted owing to development of encephalitis, but the results were encouraging enough that newer, less immunogenic vaccines are being tested. Whether these more sophisticated and targeted molecular approaches to AD prevention and treatment are successful remains to be seen, but there is hope that AD will soon yield to medical management.

Perioperative care of the patient with Alzheimer's disease is challenging. First, the anticholinesterases used to treat AD may interfere with metabolism of drugs such as succinylcholine and remifentanil, which are degraded by plasma anticholinesterases.[96] Second, because preexisting cognitive impairment predisposes to delirium, the patient with AD is at high risk for postoperative confusion.[56,97,98] There is, however, no reason to think that the precipitating causes of delirium in the demented patient differ from those in the normal patient, although the threshold of a demented patient for development of a cognitive disturbance is presumably lower. Thus, one should assiduously avoid precipitators of delirium, such as cerebral hypoxia and hypoperfusion, endocrine or ionic imbalances, postoperative pain, sepsis, bowel or bladder distention, and use of medications prone to trigger delirium, such as high-dose steroids, neuroleptics, benzodiazepines, ketamine, tertiary anticholinergics, opioids, histamine H_2 blockers, and droperidol.[56]

Whether general anesthesia worsens preexisting dementia is not clear. Studies that demonstrate persistent postoperative cognitive dysfunction, including specific deficits in memory and executive function, in elderly surgical patients have excluded patients with mild cognitive impairment or AD.[99,100] Thus, although it is reasonable to infer that a demented patient might be at greater risk for additional cognitive decline perioperatively than a cognitively intact person, this idea is unproven. Moreover, because poor baseline cognitive performance makes further decline difficult to detect with standard testing, it may be unprovable.[101] Data from the laboratory, however, are cause for concern.[102] Evidence in animals and cultured cells indicates that commonly used general anesthetic agents and some perioperative events enhance molecular events associated with AD.[103] Thus, hyperventilation and the volatile anesthetic agents increase Aβ levels, and hypothermia produces profound but reversible phosphorylation of τ protein.[79,104-106] The clinical significance of these laboratory findings is unclear. The few retrospective epidemiologic studies on the topic provide no convincing evidence for an association between anesthetic exposure and the subsequent risk for development of AD, but the risk ratio was higher in the patients exposed, suggesting that a larger study is needed.[85,86,107,108] In any case, the patient with AD who has amnesia and severe cortical atrophy and synaptic loss will be exquisitely sensitive to the central nervous system depressant effects of general anesthetic agents. This sensitivity implies that lower dosages are necessary and that emergence from general anesthesia may be slow.

DEMYELINATING DISEASES

Guillain-Barré Syndrome (Acute Idiopathic Polyneuritis)

Guillain-Barré syndrome (GBS) is the most common demyelinating paralytic disease in western countries, with an incidence of 1 per 100,000 in patients younger than 30 years and about 4 per 100,000 in patients older than 70 years.[109] Prevailing theories define it as a postinfectious autoimmune disease; it usually develops after a prodromal bacterial or viral illness (with *Campylobacter jejuni*, cytomegalovirus, Epstein-Barr virus, or human immunodeficiency virus).[109] Most cases result from antibody-mediated segmental demyelination of peripheral nerves and varying degrees of secondary axonal degeneration, but the most severe forms involve antibody-mediated primary axonal degeneration.[109]

The clinical course of GBS is characterized by an acute (days) or subacute (weeks), progressive, ascending, symmetrical paralysis usually beginning in the lower limbs and progressing to the upper limbs, trunk, and cranial nerves.[109] There is significant variability in the clinical course of the disease. Typically, the disease progresses for 1 to 3 weeks, plateaus for several weeks, and then slowly recedes. Dysautonomia, paresthesias, numbness, and pain without objective sensory loss are common findings.[109] All brainstem functions, including pupillary responses, corneal reflexes, and vestibulo-ocular reflexes, may be lost such that the condition mimics brainstem death.[110,111] Outcome is variable; 70% of patients have complete functional recovery at 1 year but 20% are left with severe motor sequelae.[109] Even most patients with complete functional recovery have persistent weakness or numbness that does not affect daily life. The mortality rate is 5% to 15%.[109] Risk factors for an unfavorable outcome, defined as less than a 20% probability of walking 6 months after diagnosis, include advanced age, rapid onset and progression of the disease, and a requirement for ventilatory support.[109] The diagnosis is usually made on clinical grounds and verified by cerebrospinal fluid analysis.[109]

A number of therapies have been used to alter the course of this disease but none is curative. Based on the assumption that GBS is an immune-mediated disease, high-dose steroids have been employed, but their efficacy is not substantiated by controlled studies.[109] On the basis of the same theory, plasma exchange and high-dose intravenous immunoglobulins have been evaluated as therapy for GBS. In prospective randomized studies, they are equally effective in producing functional improvement and are often used early in the disease to both shorten the duration and decrease the risk of respiratory failure.[109] Because such therapies are not curative, symptomatic and supportive care is often required. Mechanical ventilation and hemodynamic support may be necessary owing to respiratory failure and autonomic insufficiency, respectively.[112] Severe pain is common in GBS and may manifest prior to onset of weakness. Unfortunately, pain associated with GBS is often difficult to control, being resistant to narcotics and nonsteroidal and steroidal anti-inflammatory agents.[112,113] Both carbamazepine and gabapentin decrease fentanyl consumption during the acute phase in patients admitted to the intensive care unit, however, and pain scores are lower among patients with GBS who are treated with gabapentin.[114] Chronic pain is also common and is often managed with tricyclic antidepressants, tramadol, gabapentin, carbamazepine, or mexiletine.[112]

Anesthetizing the patient who has GBS presents challenges related to abnormal responses to muscle relaxants, dysautonomia, pulmonary insufficiency, and cranial nerve dysfunction. First, because muscle denervation is prominent, patients recovering from GBS are at risk for a hyperkalemic response to succinylcholine.[115,116] The response to nondepolarizing muscle relaxants is also variable. Resistance to neuromuscular block may appear early, whereas sensitivity to blockade occurs later and has persisted for up to 4 years following the initial illness.[117]

Autonomic dysfunction occurs in two thirds of patients with GBS and affects both the sympathetic and parasympathetic nervous systems.[118] This dysautonomia is due to both under-activity and over-activity of the sympathetic and parasympathetic nervous systems; indeed, some patients are hypertensive and have elevated plasma catecholamine levels especially during the acute phases of the disease. This dysfunction can lead to a range of autonomic abnormalities, including sweating, gastrointestinal dysfunction, hypotension, hypertension, abnormal hemodynamic responses to drugs, abnormal thermoregulation, arrhythmias, and even death.[118] Hence, the ability of the patient to compensate for the vasodilative effects of regional or general anesthesia may be compromised, potentially leading to severe hemodynamic instability and even circulatory collapse. There may also be exaggerated responses to vasoactive agents, so vasodilators should be used with extreme caution. Similarly, antiarrhythmics should be used with caution because they may have unexpected pro-arrhythmic effects in patients with GBS, in whom the heart is relatively denervated.[118]

Ventilatory impairment is a principal characteristic of the disease. Diaphragmatic, intercostal, and accessory muscle weakness produces a restrictive pulmonary defect, and respiratory failure manifests initially as weakness of forced exhalation and an impaired cough.[112] Rapid shallow breathing pattern, asymmetrical movement of the chest and abdomen during inspiration, and use of accessory respiratory muscles suggest impending respiratory failure. Decreased minute ventilation and hypercarbia lead to rapidly progressive ventilatory failure despite intact carbon dioxide responsiveness and ventilatory drive.[112] Vital capacity is a good predictor of the need for mechanical ventilation.[112] When the vital capacity value drops below 15 mL/kg, mechanical ventilation is often required because further deterioration is likely as the disease progresses. However, these criteria may be altered in the anesthetized patient. To the extent that volatile anesthetics have intrinsic muscle relaxant properties and high spinal or epidural anesthesia impairs intercostal muscle function, preoperative status may not predict postoperative respiratory function. Thus, patients with GBS who have adequate ventilatory function preoperatively may need ventilatory support postoperatively.

Finally, cranial nerve dysfunction results in inability to handle secretions and a predisposition to aspiration pneumonitis and positional airway obstruction.[112] Accordingly, aspiration prophylaxis should be considered perioperatively, although it is unlikely to mitigate aspiration risk in patients with GBS. In fact, one indication for early tracheostomy is that bulbar muscle weakness, and aspiration risk, may persist long after ventilatory function returns to normal.

Multiple Sclerosis

Multiple sclerosis (MS) is an acquired disease of the central nervous system characterized by demyelinating plaques within the brain and spinal cord.[119] The precise etiology is unknown, but autoimmune, viral, and inflammatory mechanisms, combined with genetic susceptibility, have been implicated.[119,120] The incidence varies by geographic latitude, being lowest near the equator (1:100,000) and increasing as one moves toward the poles.[121] In the United States and Canada, the incidence varies between 6 and 80 per 100,000, with urban dwellers and members of higher socioeconomic groups at greatest risk.

Symptoms generally develop between the ages of 20 and 40 years, with clinical manifestations reflecting the site of central nervous system demyelination.[122] A predilection for periventricular white matter, optic nerves, pons, medulla, and spinal cord leads to the common clinical manifestations. These include optic neuritis, decreased visual acuity, diplopia, nystagmus, weakness, impotence, paresthesias, spasticity, ataxia, bladder dysfunction, and autonomic insufficiency. This disease is marked by periods of unpredictable exacerbation and remission. Typically, symptoms develop over a few days, remain stable for a few weeks, and then improve. Improvements are most likely due to a correction in nerve conduction physiology and not remyelination. Ultimately, therefore, remission is incomplete, and severe disability can result. There are no specific diagnostic tests for MS, so the diagnosis is based on clinical findings supported by laboratory and radiologic tests. Evidence for the diagnosis includes neurologic abnormalities that are separated both in time and place, plaques seen on head or spinal cord MRI or computed tomography, delayed conduction on visual, somatosensory, or auditory evoked potentials, and elevations of cerebrospinal fluid levels of immunoglobulin G and myelin basic protein.[122] Death is usually the result of respiratory muscle paralysis and infection.[123]

There is no definitive therapy for multiple sclerosis.[122] Treatment is directed toward amelioration of acute exacerbations, prevention of relapses, and relief of symptoms.[124] Immunomodulation with adrenocorticotropic hormone, corticosteroids, glatiramer acetate, interferon, azathioprine, methotrexate, or cyclophosphamide enhances recovery from acute episodes, reduces the number of relapses in some patients, and prolongs progression of the disease.[124]

Perioperative issues generally relate to disease severity and progression, associated disorders, preoperative drug therapy, and complications of therapeutic regimens. Because of the waxing and waning clinical course of the disease and the fact that perioperative exacerbation can occur, it is important to document the location and severity of neurologic deficits preoperatively. Autonomic insufficiency, as indicated by a history of impotence, bladder and bowel dysfunction, sweating, and cardiovascular disturbances, is also important because of the possibility of perioperative hemodynamic instability and inability to compensate for the vasodilative effects of general, spinal, or epidural anesthesia.[118] Interestingly, catecholamine values may be either elevated (chronic progressive multiple sclerosis) or reduced (relapsing-remitting multiple sclerosis) in patients with the disease. Whether sensitivity to vasopressors is altered remains unknown, but because 20% to 50% of patients with multiple sclerosis have evidence of autonomic insufficiency, the potential for altered responses should be anticipated.[118,125] Spasticity, contractures, and limitation of movement become problems as the disease progresses, making surgical positioning difficult and occasionally complicating airway management. Cranial nerve involvement and respiratory muscle weakness are also common in MS. In particular, patients should be questioned about a history of upper airway incompetence, inability to clear secretions, and aspiration. Clinical assessment is usually adequate for evaluating the severity of respiratory muscle weakness in patients with MS, but pulmonary function tests may be indicated in some cases.[126]

One important consideration for patients with MS in the operating room or intensive care unit is that they are exquisitely sensitive to hyperthermia.[124,127] Small increases in body temperature can cause profound deterioration in neurologic function and make subclinical lesions clinically apparent. Therefore, active warming devices should be used cautiously during the perioperative period, and even mild hyperthermia should be treated aggressively.

A controversial and poorly investigated allegation is that surgery, anesthesia, or particular anesthetic agents can exacerbate MS.[128] The greatest controversy concerns traditional reluctance to use spinal or epidural anesthesia in a patient with MS.[129,130] This reluctance is based, in part, on potentially greater permeability of the blood-brain barrier to local anesthetics and a demyelination-induced predisposition of the spinal cord to local anesthetic toxicity.[131] One speculation is that epidural is more appropriate than spinal anesthesia because the former produces a lower cerebrospinal fluid concentration of local anesthetic.[132] There are, however, no large, controlled studies to resolve the issue, and there are case reports of both neurologic complications and uncomplicated use of spinal and epidural anesthesia.[132-134] Moreover, although MS is considered to target the central nervous system, one case report suggests that peripheral nerve blocks may produce peripheral nerve injury in patients with MS.[135]

There are also some minor issues related to drug effects that must be considered. First, the patient undergoing long-term therapy with steroids or adrenocorticotropic hormone requires supplemental steroids during the perioperative period. Responses to muscle relaxants may be altered. Succinylcholine-induced hyperkalemia is a risk in the patient with severe neurologic disability and muscle atrophy, but succinylcholine has been used safely in patients in remission or with mild neurologic symptoms. Data concerning the response to nondepolarizing muscle relaxants is limited. Proliferation of extrajunctional cholinergic receptors and resistance to atracurium are reported in patients with MS but, because the disease can be associated with myasthenia gravis, increased sensitivity can also occur.[136,137]

Nitrous Oxide–Induced Myeloneuropathy

In addition to its analgesic-anesthetic properties, nitrous oxide inactivates vitamin B_{12} (cobalamin) and methionine synthase.[138-140] Consequently, use of this drug can lead to the development of subacute combined degeneration (SCD), a myeloneuropathy originally described in patients with vitamin B_{12} deficiency. Vitamin B_{12} and the enzyme methionine synthase are essential for the production of methionine, an amino acid precursor required for maintenance of the myelin sheath. Nitrous oxide inactivates vitamin B_{12} by oxidizing the cobalt in cobalamin, thereby inhibiting the activity of methionine synthase.[138-140]

Subacute combined degeneration after inhalation of nitrous oxide was first described in healthy chronic abusers of the drug,[141,142] but it has also been documented following a single, otherwise uncomplicated period of anesthesia in patients with vitamin B_{12} deficiency.[143] In this context, the condition is sometimes termed "anesthesia paresthetica"[144] but remains pathophysiologically identical to SCD. Vitamin B_{12} deficiency is common in elders and in patients with pernicious anemia, tropical sprue, malnutrition, chronic gastritis, human immunodeficiency virus infection, gastrectomy, or surgical resection of the terminal ileum.[145] Both serum vitamin B_{12} concentration and brain methionine synthase activity typically decrease significantly after a single exposure to nitrous oxide but recover within 48 to 72 hours.[146] The presumption is that repeated, frequent administration of nitrous oxide, or even a single administration to a patient with a vitamin B_{12} deficiency because of a coexisting disease state, is required for the subsequent development of nitrous oxide–induced SCD.[143]

The patient in whom SCD develops after undergoing nitrous oxide exposure is usually normal upon emergence from anesthesia and in the immediate perioperative period but experiences symptoms of the illness weeks to months later.[143,147] Symptoms include paresthesias (pins-and-needles sensations in the hands and legs), impotence, bladder and bowel dysfunction, weakness and spasticity leading to paraplegia, ataxia, personality changes, and progressive intellectual impairment.[143,148] Lhermitte's sign, a characteristic electric shock sensation down the back and into the legs upon flexion of the neck, may also be present.[143,148] Decreased proprioceptive, vibratory, and touch sensations in a stocking and glove distribution, muscle weakness, decreased deep tendon reflexes, and abnormalities on electrophysiologic testing are often identified.[141,148,149] These neurologic findings are the result of progressive demyelination in the posterior columns of the spinal cord; variable degeneration of the lateral and anterior columns of the spinal cord, brain, and optic and peripheral nerves may also occur. Demyelination, which typically begins in the lower cervical or upper thoracic cord, is detectable on MRI and, as demonstrated by enhancement after administration of gadolinium, is associated with breakdown of the blood-brain barrier.[143,150,151]

The most effective treatment of SCD is prevention through preoperative recognition of B_{12} deficiency in at-risk patients.[152] If the disease develops, however, the key is early recognition, because treatment is straightforward and simple: Vitamin B_{12} or cyanocobalamin injections stop progression of the disease. Provided that treatment is begun promptly, complete resolution of symptoms can be expected.[143] Thus, nitrous oxide–induced SCD is unique among the neurologic diseases in this chapter, in that it is caused by an anesthetic agent and can be treated effectively.

REFERENCES

1. Walker FO: Huntington's disease, *Lancet* 369:218–228, 2007.
2. Rodrigo MR: Huntington's chorea: Midazolam, a suitable induction agent? *Br J Anaesth* 59:388–389, 1987.
3. MacPherson P, Harper I, MacDonald I: Propofol and remifentanil total intravenous anesthesia for a patient with Huntington disease, *J Clin Anesth* 16:537–538, 2004.
4. Esen A, Karaaslan P, Can Akgun R, Arslan G: Successful spinal anesthesia in a patient with Huntington's chorea, *Anesth Analg* 103:512–513, 2006.
5. Whittaker M: Plasma cholinesterase variants and the anaesthetist, *Anaesthesia* 35:174–197, 1980.
6. Gualandi W, Bonfanti G: [A case of prolonged apnea in Huntington's chorea], *Acta Anaesthesiol* 19(Suppl 6):235–238, 1968.
7. Costarino A, Gross JB: Patients with Huntington's chorea may respond normally to succinylcholine, *Anesthesiology* 63:570, 1985.
8. Nagele P, Hammerle AF: Sevoflurane and mivacurium in a patient with Huntington's chorea, *Br J Anaesth* 85:320–321, 2000.
9. Kaufman MA, Erb T: Propofol for patients with Huntington's chorea? *Anaesthesia* 45:889–890, 1990.
10. Fernandez IG, Sanchez MP, Ugalde AJ, Hernandez CM: Spinal anaesthesia in a patient with Huntington's chorea, *Anaesthesia* 52:391, 1997.
11. Logroscino G, Traynor BJ, Hardiman O, et al: Descriptive epidemiology of amyotrophic lateral sclerosis: New evidence and unsolved issues, *J Neurol Neurosurg Psychiatry* 79:6–11, 2008.
12. Radunovic A, Mitsumoto H, Leigh PN: Clinical care of patients with amyotrophic lateral sclerosis, *Lancet Neurol* 6:913–925, 2007.
13. Mitchell JD, Borasio GD: Amyotrophic lateral sclerosis, *Lancet* 369:2031–2041, 2007.
14. Cooperman LH: Succinylcholine-induced hyperkalemia in neuromuscular disease, *JAMA* 213:1867–1871, 1970.
15. Azar I: The response of patients with neuromuscular disorders to muscle relaxants: A review, *Anesthesiology* 61:173–187, 1984.
16. Jackson CE, Bryan WW: Amyotrophic lateral sclerosis, *Semin Neurol* 18:27–39, 1998.
17. Hara K, Sakura S, Saito Y, et al: Epidural anesthesia and pulmonary function in a patient with amyotrophic lateral sclerosis, *Anesth Analg* 83:878–879, 1996.
18. Kochi T, Oka T, Mizuguchi T: Epidural anesthesia for patients with amyotrophic lateral sclerosis, *Anesth Analg* 68:410–412, 1989.
19. Jacka MJ, Sanderson F: Amyotrophic lateral sclerosis presenting during pregnancy, *Anesth Analg* 86:542–543, 1998.
20. Moser B, Lirk P, Lechner M, Gottardis M: General anaesthesia in a patient with motor neuron disease, *Eur J Anaesthesiol* 21:921–923, 2004.
21. Boitano LJ, Jordan T, Benditt JO: Noninvasive ventilation allows gastrostomy tube placement in patients with advanced ALS, *Neurology* 56:413–414, 2001.
22. Hebl JR, Horlocker TT, Schroeder DR: Neuraxial anesthesia and analgesia in patients with preexisting central nervous system disorders, *Anesth Analg* 103:223–228, 2006.
23. Marras C, Lang A: Invited article: Changing concepts in Parkinson disease: Moving beyond the decade of the brain, *Neurology* 70:1996–2003, 2008.
24. Zorzon M, Capus L, Pellegrino A, et al: Familial and environmental risk factors in Parkinson's disease: A case-control study in north-east Italy, *Acta Neurol Scand* 105:77–82, 2002.
25. Galvan A, Wichmann T: Pathophysiology of parkinsonism, *Clin Neurophysiol* 119:1459–1474, 2008.
26. Nutt JG, Wooten GF: Clinical practice: Diagnosis and initial management of Parkinson's disease, *N Engl J Med* 353:1021–1027, 2005.
27. Hely MA, Morris JG, Reid WG, Trafficante R: Sydney Multicenter Study of Parkinson's disease: Non–L-dopa-responsive problems dominate at 15 years, *Mov Disord* 20:190–199, 2005.
28. Ferreri F, Agbokou C, Gauthier S: Recognition and management of neuropsychiatric complications in Parkinson's disease, *CMAJ* 175:1545–1552, 2006.
29. Poewe W: Non-motor symptoms in Parkinson's disease, *Eur J Neurol* 15(Suppl 1):14–20, 2008.
30. Aarsland D, Andersen K, Larsen JP, et al: Prevalence and characteristics of dementia in Parkinson disease: An 8-year prospective study, *Arch Neurol* 60:387–392, 2003.
31. Rao SS, Hofmann LA, Shakil A: Parkinson's disease: Diagnosis and treatment, *Am Fam Physician* 74:2046–2054, 2006.
32. Lees AJ: Comparison of therapeutic effects and mortality data of levodopa and levodopa combined with selegiline in patients with early, mild Parkinson's disease. Parkinson's Disease Research Group of the United Kingdom, *BMJ* 311:1602–1607, 1995.

33. Kleiner-Fisman G, Fisman DN, Sime E, et al: Long-term follow up of bilateral deep brain stimulation of the subthalamic nucleus in patients with advanced Parkinson disease, *J Neurosurg* 99:489–495, 2003.

34. Mendez I, Vinuela A, Astradsson A, et al: Dopamine neurons implanted into people with Parkinson's disease survive without pathology for 14 years, *Nat Med* 14:507–509, 2008.

35. McKay R, Kittappa R: Will stem cell biology generate new therapies for Parkinson's disease? *Neuron* 58:659–661, 2008.

36. Nutt JG: Pharmacokinetics and pharmacodynamics of levodopa, *Mov Disord* 23(Suppl 3):S580–S584, 2008.

37. Stotz M, Thummler D, Schurch M, et al: Fulminant neuroleptic malignant syndrome after perioperative withdrawal of antiparkinsonian medication, *Br J Anaesth* 93:868–871, 2004.

38. Young CC, Kaufman BS: Neuroleptic malignant syndrome postoperative onset due to levodopa withdrawal, *J Clin Anesth* 7:652–656, 1995.

39. Nyholm D, Lennernas H: Irregular gastrointestinal drug absorption in Parkinson's disease, *Expert Opin Drug Metab Toxicol* 4:193–203, 2008.

40. Nyholm D, Lewander T, Johansson A, et al: Enteral levodopa/carbidopa infusion in advanced Parkinson disease: Long-term exposure, *Clin Neuropharmacol* 31:63–73, 2008.

41. Pal PK, Sathyaprabha TN, Tuhina P, Thennarasu K: Pattern of subclinical pulmonary dysfunctions in Parkinson's disease and the effect of levodopa, *Mov Disord* 22:420–424, 2007.

42. Vincken WG, Gauthier SG, Dollfuss RE, et al: Involvement of upper-airway muscles in extrapyramidal disorders: A cause of airflow limitation, *N Engl J Med* 311:438–442, 1984.

43. De Letter M, Santens P, De Bodt M, et al: The effect of levodopa on respiration and word intelligibility in people with advanced Parkinson's disease, *Clin Neurol Neurosurg* 109:495–500, 2007.

44. Vincken WG, Darauay CM, Cosio MG: Reversibility of upper airway obstruction after levodopa therapy in Parkinson's disease, *Chest* 96:210–212, 1989.

45. Easdown LJ, Tessler MJ, Minuk J: Upper airway involvement in Parkinson's disease resulting in postoperative respiratory failure, *Can J Anaesth* 42:344–347, 1995.

46. Gdynia HJ, Kassubek J, Sperfeld AD: Laryngospasm in neurological diseases, *Neurocrit Care* 4:163–167, 2006.

47. Backus WW, Ward RR, Vitkun SA, et al: Postextubation laryngeal spasm in an unanesthetized patient with Parkinson's disease, *J Clin Anesth* 3:314–316, 1991.

48. Liu EH, Choy J, Dhara SS: Persistent perioperative laryngospasm in a patient with Parkinson's disease, *Can J Anaesth* 45:495, 1998.

49. Sapir S, Ramig L, Fox C: Speech and swallowing disorders in Parkinson disease, *Curr Opin Otolaryngol Head Neck Surg* 16:205–210, 2008.

50. Miller N, Noble E, Jones D, Burn D: Hard to swallow: Dysphagia in Parkinson's disease, *Age Ageing* 35:614–618, 2006.

51. Jost WH: Gastrointestinal motility problems in patients with Parkinson's disease: Effects of antiparkinsonian treatment and guidelines for management, *Drugs Aging* 10:249–258, 1997.

52. Walter BL: Cardiovascular autonomic dysfunction in patients with movement disorders, *Cleve Clin J Med* 75(Suppl 2):S54–S58, 2008.

53. Oka H, Yoshioka M, Onouchi K, et al: Characteristics of orthostatic hypotension in Parkinson's disease, *Brain* 130:2425–2432, 2007.

54. Senard JM, Valet P, Durrieu G, et al: Adrenergic supersensitivity in parkinsonians with orthostatic hypotension, *Eur J Clin Invest* 20:613–619, 1990.

55. Poewe W, Gauthier S, Aarsland D, et al: Diagnosis and management of Parkinson's disease dementia, *Int J Clin Pract* 62:1581–1587, 2008.

56. Inouye SK: Delirium in older persons, *N Engl J Med* 354:1157–1165, 2006.

57. Voon V, Hassan K, Zurowski M, et al: Prospective prevalence of pathologic gambling and medication association in Parkinson disease, *Neurology* 66:1750–1752, 2006.

58. Salord F, Keita H, Lecharny JB, et al: Halothane and isoflurane differentially affect the regulation of dopamine and gamma-aminobutyric acid release mediated by presynaptic acetylcholine receptors in the rat striatum, *Anesthesiology* 86:632–641, 1997.

59. Mantz J, Varlet C, Lecharny JB, et al: Effects of volatile anesthetics, thiopental, and ketamine on spontaneous and depolarization-evoked dopamine release from striatal synaptosomes in the rat, *Anesthesiology* 80:352–363, 1994.

60. Lefaucheur JP, Gurruchaga JM, Pollin B, et al: Outcome of bilateral subthalamic nucleus stimulation in the treatment of Parkinson's disease: Correlation with intra-operative multi-unit recordings but not with the type of anaesthesia, *Eur Neurol* 60:186–199, 2008.

61. Deogaonkar A, Deogaonkar M, Lee JY, et al: Propofol-induced dyskinesias controlled with dexmedetomidine during deep brain stimulation surgery, *Anesthesiology* 104:1337–1339, 2006.

62. Khatib R, Ebrahim Z, Rezai A, et al: Perioperative events during deep brain stimulation: The experience at Cleveland Clinic, *J Neurosurg Anesthesiol* 20:36–40, 2008.

63. Rozet I, Muangman S, Vavilala MS, et al: Clinical experience with dexmedetomidine for implantation of deep brain stimulators in Parkinson's disease, *Anesth Analg* 103:1224–1228, 2006.

64. Hetherington A, Rosenblatt RM: Ketamine and paralysis agitans, *Anesthesiology* 52:527, 1980.

65. Wiklund RA, Ngai SH: Rigidity and pulmonary edema after Innovar in a patient on levodopa therapy: Report of a case, *Anesthesiology* 35:545–547, 1971.

66. Rivera VM, Keichian AH, Oliver RE: Persistent parkinsonism following neuroleptanalgesia, *Anesthesiology* 42:635–637, 1975.

67. Zoldan J, Friedberg G, Livneh M, Melamed E: Psychosis in advanced Parkinson's disease: Treatment with ondansetron, a 5-HT$_3$ receptor antagonist, *Neurology* 45:1305–1308, 1995.

68. Mets B: Acute dystonia after alfentanil in untreated Parkinson's disease, *Anesth Analg* 72:557–558, 1991.

69. Samadi P, Bedard PJ, Rouillard C: Opioids and motor complications in Parkinson's disease, *Trends Pharmacol Sci* 27:512–517, 2006.

70. Zornberg GL, Bodkin JA, Cohen BM: Severe adverse interaction between pethidine and selegiline, *Lancet* 337:246, 1991.

71. Gravlee GP: Succinylcholine-induced hyperkalemia in a patient with Parkinson's disease, *Anesth Analg* 59:444–446, 1980.

72. Black S, Muzzi DA, Nishimura RA, Cucchiara RF: Preoperative and intraoperative echocardiography to detect right-to-left shunt in patients undergoing neurosurgical procedures in the sitting position, *Anesthesiology* 72:436–438, 1990.

73. Muzzi DA, Black S, Cucchiara RF: The lack of effect of succinylcholine on serum potassium in patients with Parkinson's disease, *Anesthesiology* 71:322, 1989.

74. Davies RG: Deep brain stimulators and anaesthesia, *Br J Anaesth* 95:424, 2005.

75. Minville V, Chassery C, Benhaoua A, et al: Nerve stimulator–guided brachial plexus block in a patient with severe Parkinson's disease and bilateral deep brain stimulators, *Anesth Analg* 102:1296, 2006.

76. Holsinger T, Deveau J, Boustani M, Williams JW Jr: Does this patient have dementia? *JAMA* 297:2391–2404, 2007.

77. Cummings JL: Alzheimer's disease, *N Engl J Med* 351:56–67, 2004.

78. Cummings JL, Cole G: Alzheimer disease, *JAMA* 287:2335–2338, 2002.

79. Xie Z, Tanzi RE: Alzheimer's disease and post-operative cognitive dysfunction, *Exp Gerontol* 41:346–359, 2006.

80. Blennow K, Zetterberg H: Pinpointing plaques with PIB, *Nat Med* 12:753–754, 2006:discussion 754.

81. Masters CL, Cappai R, Barnham KJ, Villemagne VL: Molecular mechanisms for Alzheimer's disease: Implications for neuroimaging and therapeutics, *J Neurochem* 97:1700–1725, 2006.

82. Rowe CC, Ng S, Ackermann U, et al: Imaging beta-amyloid burden in aging and dementia, *Neurology* 68:1718–1725, 2007.

83. Petersen RC: Mild cognitive impairment as a diagnostic entity, *J Intern Med* 256:183–194, 2004.

84. Bertram L, Tanzi RE: Thirty years of Alzheimer's disease genetics: The implications of systematic meta-analyses, *Nat Rev Neurosci* 9:768–778, 2008.

85. Bohnen NI, Warner MA, Kokmen E, et al: Alzheimer's disease and cumulative exposure to anesthesia: A case-control study, *J Am Geriatr Soc* 42:198–201, 1994.

86. Bohnen N, Warner MA, Kokmen E, Kurland LT: Early and midlife exposure to anesthesia and age of onset of Alzheimer's disease, *Int J Neurosci* 77:181–185, 1994.

87. Walsh DM, Selkoe DJ: Deciphering the molecular basis of memory failure in Alzheimer's disease, *Neuron* 44:181–193, 2004.

88. Raina P, Santaguida P, Ismaila A, et al: Effectiveness of cholinesterase inhibitors and memantine for treating dementia: Evidence review for a clinical practice guideline, *Ann Intern Med* 148:379–397, 2008.

89. Trinh NH, Hoblyn J, Mohanty S, Yaffe K: Efficacy of cholinesterase inhibitors in the treatment of neuropsychiatric symptoms and functional impairment in Alzheimer disease: A meta-analysis, *JAMA* 289:210–216, 2003.

90. Davies-Lepie SR: Tacrine may prolong the effect of succinylcholine, *Anesthesiology* 81:524, 1994.

91. Martin BK, Szekely C, Brandt J, et al: Cognitive function over time in the Alzheimer's Disease Anti-inflammatory Prevention Trial (ADAPT): Results of a randomized, controlled trial of naproxen and celecoxib, *Arch Neurol* 65:896–905, 2008.

92. Vlad SC, Miller DR, Kowall NW, Felson DT: Protective effects of NSAIDs on the development of Alzheimer disease, *Neurology* 70:1672–1677, 2008.

93. Scharf JM, Daffner KR: NSAIDs in the prevention of dementia: A cache-22? *Neurology* 69:235–236, 2007.

94. Wilcock GK, Black SE, Hendrix SB, et al: Efficacy and safety of tarenflurbil in mild to moderate Alzheimer's disease: A randomised phase II trial, *Lancet Neurol* 7:483–493, 2008.

95. Holtzman DM: Alzheimer's disease: Moving towards a vaccine, *Nature* 454:418–420, 2008.

96. Crowe S, Collins L: Suxamethonium and donepezil: A cause of prolonged paralysis, *Anesthesiology* 98:574–575, 2003.

97. Rudolph JL, Jones RN, Rasmussen LS, et al: Independent vascular and cognitive risk factors for postoperative delirium, *Am J Med* 120:807–813, 2007.

98. Rudolph JL, Marcantonio ER, Culley DJ, et al: Delirium is associated with early postoperative cognitive dysfunction, *Anaesthesia* 63:941–947, 2008.

99. Monk TG, Weldon BC, Garvan CW, et al: Predictors of cognitive dysfunction after major noncardiac surgery, *Anesthesiology* 108:18–30, 2008.

100. Moller JT, Cluitmans P, Rasmussen LS, et al: Long-term postoperative cognitive dysfunction in the elderly ISPOCD1 study: ISPOCD investigators. International Study of Post-Operative Cognitive Dysfunction, *Lancet* 351:857–861, 1998.

101. Silverstein JH, Steinmetz J, Reichenberg A, et al: Postoperative cognitive dysfunction in patients with preoperative cognitive impairment: Which domains are most vulnerable? *Anesthesiology* 106:431–435, 2007.

102. Kuehn BM: Anesthesia-Alzheimer disease link probed, *JAMA* 297:1760, 2007.

103. Culley DJ, Xie Z, Crosby G: General anesthetic-induced neurotoxicity: An emerging problem for the young and old? *Curr Opin Anaesthesiol* 20:408–413, 2007.

104. Xie Z, Dong Y, Maeda U, et al: The common inhalation anesthetic isoflurane induces apoptosis and increases amyloid beta protein levels, *Anesthesiology* 104:988–994, 2006.

105. Planel E, Richter KE, Nolan CE, et al: Anesthesia leads to tau hyperphosphorylation through inhibition of phosphatase activity by hypothermia, *J Neurosci* 27:3090–3097, 2007.

106. Xie Z, Moir RD, Romano DM, et al: Hypocapnia induces caspase-3 activation and increases Abeta production, *Neurodegener Dis* 1:29–37, 2004.

107. Gasparini M, Vanacore N, Schiaffini C, et al: A case-control study on Alzheimer's disease and exposure to anesthesia, *Neurol Sci* 23:11–14, 2002.

108. Lee TA, Wolozin B, Weiss KB, Bednar MM: Assessment of the emergence of Alzheimer's disease following coronary artery bypass graft surgery or percutaneous transluminal coronary angioplasty, *J Alzheimers Dis* 7:319–324, 2005.

109. Hughes RA, Cornblath DR: Guillain-Barré syndrome, *Lancet* 366:1653–1666, 2005.

110. Stojkovic T, Verdin M, Hurtevent JF, et al: Guillain-Barré syndrome resembling brainstem death in a patient with brain injury, *J Neurol* 248:430–432, 2001.

111. Coad NR, Byrne AJ: Guillain-Barré syndrome mimicking brainstem death, *Anaesthesia* 45:456–457, 1990.

112. Hughes RA, Wijdicks EF, Benson E, et al: Supportive care for patients with Guillain-Barré syndrome, *Arch Neurol* 62:1194–1198, 2005.

113. Ruts L, van Koningsveld R, Jacobs BC, van Doorn PA: Determination of pain and response to methylprednisolone in Guillain-Barré syndrome, *J Neurol* 254:1318–1322, 2007.

114. Pandey CK, Raza M, Tripathi M, et al: The comparative evaluation of gabapentin and carbamazepine for pain management in Guillain-Barré syndrome patients in the intensive care unit, *Anesth Analg* 101:220–225, 2005.

115. Reilly M, Hutchinson M: Suxamethonium is contraindicated in the Guillain-Barré syndrome, *J Neurol Neurosurg Psychiatry* 54:1018–1019, 1991.

116. Feldman JM: Cardiac arrest after succinylcholine administration in a pregnant patient recovered from Guillain-Barré syndrome, *Anesthesiology* 72:942–944, 1990.

117. Fiacchino F, Gemma M, Bricchi M, et al: Hypo- and hypersensitivity to vecuronium in a patient with Guillain-Barré syndrome, *Anesth Analg* 78:187–189, 1994.

118. Flachenecker P: Autonomic dysfunction in Guillain-Barré syndrome and multiple sclerosis, *J Neurol* 254(Suppl 2):II96–II101, 2007.

119. Frohman EM, Racke MK, Raine CS: Multiple sclerosis—the plaque and its pathogenesis, *N Engl J Med* 354:942–955, 2006.

120. Olsson T, Hillert J: The genetics of multiple sclerosis and its experimental models, *Curr Opin Neurol* 21:255–260, 2008.

121. Alonso A, Hernan MA: Temporal trends in the incidence of multiple sclerosis: A systematic review, *Neurology* 71:129–135, 2008.

122. Myhr KM: Diagnosis and treatment of multiple sclerosis, *Acta Neurol Scand Suppl* 188:12–21, 2008.

123. Hirst C, Swingler R, Compston DA, et al: Survival and cause of death in multiple sclerosis: A prospective population-based study, *J Neurol Neurosurg Psychiatry* 79:1016–1021, 2008.

124. Noseworthy JH, Lucchinetti C, Rodriguez M, Weinshenker BG: Multiple sclerosis, *N Engl J Med* 343:938–952, 2000.

125. Labuz-Roszak B, Pierzchala K: Difficulties in the diagnosis of autonomic dysfunction in multiple sclerosis, *Clin Auton Res* 17:375–377, 2007.

126. Smeltzer SC, Skurnick JH, Troiano R, et al: Respiratory function in multiple sclerosis: Utility of clinical assessment of respiratory muscle function, *Chest* 101:479–484, 1992.

127. Guthrie TC, Nelson DA: Influence of temperature changes on multiple sclerosis: Critical review of mechanisms and research potential, *J Neurol Sci* 129:1–8, 1995.

128. Watt JW: Anaesthesia for chronic spinal cord lesions and multiple sclerosis, *Anaesthesia* 53:825–826, 1998.

129. Perlas A, Chan VW: Neuraxial anesthesia and multiple sclerosis, *Can J Anaesth* 52:454–458, 2005.

130. Vercauteren M, Heytens L: Anaesthetic considerations for patients with a pre-existing neurological deficit: Are neuraxial techniques safe? *Acta Anaesthesiol Scand* 51:831–838, 2007.

131. McFarland HF: The lesion in multiple sclerosis: Clinical, pathological, and magnetic resonance imaging considerations, *J Neurol Neurosurg Psychiatry* 6(Suppl 1):S26–S30, 1998.

132. Bader AM, Hunt CO, Datta S, et al: Anesthesia for the obstetric patient with multiple sclerosis, *J Clin Anesth* 1:21–24, 1988.

133. Bamford C, Sibley W, Laguna J: Anesthesia in multiple sclerosis, *Can J Neurol Sci* 5:41–44, 1978.

134. Crawford JS: Epidural analgesia for patients with chronic neurological disease, *Anesth Analg* 62:621–622, 1983.

135. Koff MD, Cohen JA, McIntyre JJ, et al: Severe brachial plexopathy after an ultrasound-guided single-injection nerve block for total shoulder arthroplasty in a patient with multiple sclerosis, *Anesthesiology* 108:325–328, 2008.

136. Brett RS, Schmidt JH, Gage JS, et al: Measurement of acetylcholine receptor concentration in skeletal muscle from a patient with multiple sclerosis and resistance to atracurium, *Anesthesiology* 66:837–839, 1987.

137. Somer H, Muller K, Kinnunen E: Myasthenia gravis associated with multiple sclerosis: Epidemiological survey and immunological findings, *J Neurol Sci* 89:37–48, 1989.

138. Drummond JT, Matthews RG: Nitrous oxide degradation by cobalamin-dependent methionine synthase: Characterization of the reactants and products in the inactivation reaction, *Biochemistry* 33:3732–3741, 1994.

139. Nunn JF: Clinical aspects of the interaction between nitrous oxide and vitamin B_{12}, *Br J Anaesth* 59:3–13, 1987.

140. Chanarin I: The effects of nitrous oxide on cobalamins, folates, and on related events, *Crit Rev Toxicol* 10:179–213, 1982.

141. Layzer RB: Myeloneuropathy after prolonged exposure to nitrous oxide, *Lancet* 2(8102):1227–1230, 1978.

142. Nevins MA: Neuropathy after nitrous oxide abuse, *JAMA* 244:2264, 1980.

143. Singer MA, Lazaridis C, Nations SP, Wolfe GI: Reversible nitrous oxide-induced myeloneuropathy with pernicious anemia: Case report and literature review, *Muscle Nerve* 37:125–129, 2008.

144. Kinsella LJ, Green R: 'Anesthesia paresthetica': Nitrous oxide–induced cobalamin deficiency, *Neurology* 45:1608–1610, 1995.

145. Nilsson-Ehle H: Age-related changes in cobalamin (vitamin B_{12}) handling: Implications for therapy, *Drugs Aging* 12:277–292, 1998.

146. Culley DJ, Raghavan SV, Waly M, et al: Nitrous oxide decreases cortical methionine synthase transiently but produces lasting memory impairment in aged rats, *Anesth Analg* 105:83–88, 2007.

147. Hadzic A, Glab K, Sanborn KV, Thys DM: Severe neurologic deficit after nitrous oxide anesthesia, *Anesthesiology* 83:863–866, 1995.

148. Heyer EJ, Simpson DM, Bodis-Wollner I, Diamond SP: Nitrous oxide: Clinical and electrophysiologic investigation of neurologic complications, *Neurology* 36:1618–1622, 1986.

149. Lin CY, Guo WY, Chen SP, et al: Neurotoxicity of nitrous oxide: Multimodal evoked potentials in an abuser, *Clin Toxicol (Phila)* 45:67–71, 2007.

150. Ilniczky S, Jelencsik I, Kenez J, Szirmai I: MR findings in subacute combined degeneration of the spinal cord caused by nitrous oxide anaesthesia—two cases, *Eur J Neurol* 9:101–104, 2002.

151. Beltramello A, Puppini G, Cerini R, et al: Subacute combined degeneration of the spinal cord after nitrous oxide anaesthesia: Role of magnetic resonance imaging, *J Neurol Neurosurg Psychiatry* 64:563–564, 1998.

152. Holloway KL, Alberico AM: Postoperative myeloneuropathy: A preventable complication in patients with B_{12} deficiency, *J Neurosurg* 72:732–736, 1990.

399

Chapter 22

POSTOPERATIVE AND INTENSIVE CARE INCLUDING HEAD INJURY AND MULTISYSTEM SEQUELAE

Helen R. Stutz • Jean Charchaflieh

Neurologic critical care follows standard critical care practice, with special emphasis on the treatment and prevention of secondary brain injury, through systemic and neurologic monitoring and rapid intervention as needed. Sequelae of traumatic brain injury (TBI) can result from the primary or secondary injury. The lesion sustained at the time of impact, described as the *primary injury,* results from the high-energy acceleration or deceleration of the brain within the cranium. The *secondary injury* consists of a more complex ischemic process induced by alterations in cerebral blood flow (CBF), inflammation, hypermetabolism, and tissue necrosis. Treatment of TBI focuses primarily on prevention and treatment of secondary injury. Independent predictors of poor outcome include hypotension, hypoxia, hypoglycemia, hyperthermia, hypocapnia, and intracranial hypertension.[1] Sequelae of head injury often correlate with the severity of head injury. The Glasgow Coma Scale (GCS) is a commonly used tool for quantifying the severity of head injury. The GCS score ranges from 3 to 15. Scores of 9 through15 indicate mild to moderate head injury, and a score of 8 or less indicates severe injury. Multisystem sequelae of severe head injury include airway obstruction, respiratory dysfunction, cardiovascular dysfunction, fat embolism syndrome, neuromuscular dysfunction, hematologic abnormalities, metabolic abnormalities, electrolyte imbalances, gastrointestinal abnormalities, immunologic abnormalities, endocrine abnormalities, infectious complications, secondary brain injury, and cerebral hyperperfusion syndrome (CHS).

AIRWAY OBSTRUCTION

Asphyxia due to upper airway obstruction is a major cause of death in patients with TBI. Head-injured patients may suffer airway obstruction in the field or during insufficient bag-mask resuscitation because of facial trauma. Maxillary and mandibular fractures, often associated with TBI, may cause displacement of bone fragments and tissues into the pharynx. Basilar skull fractures may cause cranial nerve deficits that compromise the gag reflex and the motor and sensory functions of the airway. Gastric contents may be aspirated into the lungs. Injury to cranial nerves IX, X, and XII may compromise the patient's ability to maintain a patent protected airway owing to difficulty with swallowing and clearing secretions. Tracheal intubation should be performed if the integrity of protective upper airway reflexes is impaired. Endotracheal intubation is the preferred method for securing a patent and protected artificial airway. Cervical spine displacement should be avoided during laryngoscopy and intubation. Cricothyrotomy and tracheostomy may be necessary to secure an airway adequately.

In addition, edema of the mucosa of the upper airway may occur after prolonged surgery. Airway edema is more significant in children owing to the small diameter of their airways. When airway edema is suspected, tracheal extubation should be performed only after absence of airway edema is ascertained by deflating the cuff of the endotracheal tube and confirming the patient's ability to breathe around the tube (leak test). If the patient has difficulty breathing during this maneuver, the trachea should be kept intubated and the patient should be kept sedated until there is evidence edema has resolved. Inhaled racemic epinephrine (0.5 mL of 2% solution in 3 mL saline) may decrease localized mucosal edema and relieve upper airway obstruction. If airway obstruction becomes evident after extubation an artificial airway should be reestablished with the use of endotracheal intubation, the insertion of a laryngeal mask airway (LMA), or even cricothyrotomy if needed.

RESPIRATORY DYSFUNCTION

Respiratory dysfunction may be due to direct lung trauma, pneumonia, alteration in respiratory control, acute respiratory distress syndrome (ARDS), neurogenic pulmonary edema (NPE), or pulmonary embolism (PE).

Direct Lung Trauma

Direct lung trauma may occur in conjunction with rib fractures, pulmonary contusion, hemothorax, pneumothorax, and flail chest. All may produce significant respiratory failure and hypoxemia. Treatment consists of surgical repair, chest tube placement, supplemental oxygen, and mechanical ventilation as needed.

Pneumonia

Nosocomial pneumonia is the second most common complication in patients with TBI,[2] electrolyte imbalances being the most common. Airway colonization with bacteria occurs within 5 days after endotracheal intubation.[3] Risk factors include nasotracheal or orotracheal tubes, nasogastric or orogastric tubes, microaspiration from the pharynx into the lower

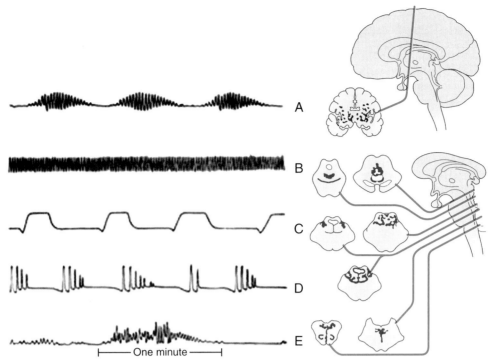

Figure 22–1 Abnormal respiratory patterns associated with pathologic brain lesions. **A,** Cheyne-Stokes respiration. **B,** Central neurogenic hyperventilation. **C,** Apneustic breathing. **D,** Cluster breathing. **E,** Ataxic breathing. *(Adapted from Plum F, Posner JB: Diagnosis of Stupor and Coma, 3rd ed. New York, Oxford University Press, 1980.)*

airway, gastroesophageal reflux, decreased levels of consciousness, lower esophageal sphincter relaxation, prolonged gastric emptying, and increased gastric pH. Early-onset pneumonia is associated with increased morbidity and mortality, higher number of days of mechanical ventilation, and longer stays in the intensive care unit (ICU) and hospital. Risk factors include intubation in the field, GCS score 5 or less, swallowing impairment, and aspiration.

Treatment of pneumonia consists of supportive respiratory therapy plus antibiotics. Broad-spectrum antibiotic therapy is initiated until results of cultures and sensitivity testing are obtained from blood and sputum samples. For hospital-acquired pneumonia, a combination of a β-lactam/β-lactamase inhibitor such as piperacillin-tazobactam plus a macrolide such as azithromycin is used. Coverage against *Pseudomonas* or other resistant gram-negative species may by be provided with the addition of an aminoglycoside or a fluoroquinolone. Vancomycin or linezolid may be added in the presence of an increased risk for methicillin-resistant *Staphylococcus aureus* infection, such as coma, diabetes mellitus, or renal failure. Duration of antimicrobial therapy is until the resolution of pneumonia and is longer (14-21 days) for gram-negative hospital-acquired pneumonia. Radiographic resolution of infiltrates may take 6 weeks or longer and cannot be the sole basis of the duration of therapy.

Alteration in Respiratory Control

Control of respiration is regulated by the apneustic and pneumotaxic centers in the pons, via the reticular formation of the medulla oblongata and then via the ventrolateral portions of the spinothalamic tract. The medulla oblongata modulates the cycle of inspiration and expiration in response to chemical and mechanical stimuli. Changes in arterial P_{CO_2} and CSF pH trigger the chemoreceptors in the medulla to modify breathing patterns. Injury to the brain may disrupt respiratory regulation, leading to hypoxia, hypoventilation, or apnea. Ventilation-perfusion mismatch may occur from decreased consciousness, aspiration, apnea, or pulmonary edema. Ventilation-perfusion mismatch appears to correlate with the severity of TBI as reflected by GCS scores.[4] Abnormal respiratory patterns are commonly seen immediately after brain injury, but they may also develop at a later stage. In mild to moderate brain injury, hyperventilation is the most common respiratory abnormality. In severe brain injury, hypoventilation or apnea may be present. Several types of respiratory patterns have been described in patients with central nervous system (CNS) injury (Fig. 22-1); they are described here.

Cheyne-Stokes Pattern

Cheyne-Stokes respiration refers to periods of hyperpnea alternating with apnea in a smooth crescendo-decrescendo pattern. It is encountered in patients with bilateral damage to the cortex and forebrain. Normally the frontal lobe controls respiratory patterns. In Cheyne-Stokes respiration, there is an excessive reliance upon blood CO_2 levels to trigger brainstem respiratory centers. In a patient with a unilateral mass lesion, onset of Cheyne-Stokes breathing may reveal impending herniation. Another type of faster, short-cycle breathing similar to CheyneStokes respiration is seen in patients with rising intracranial pressure (ICP), posterior fossa lesions, or lower pontine lesions. Patients take one or two waxing breaths followed by three or four rapid breaths, followed by one or two waning breaths.

Ataxic Pattern

Ataxic breathing refers to irregular breathing in both rate and rhythm. It occurs with lesions in the dorsomedial medulla and may be accompanied by hypersensitivity to respiratory depressants. It is considered preterminal.

Apneustic Pattern

Apneustic breathing refers to long, gasping inspiration with insufficient expiration, indicating injury to the pons.

Apneic Pattern

The *apneic pattern* describes the complete absence of breathing, reflecting significant damage to the medulla. It is encountered in acceleration-deceleration injures, which may cause loss of consciousness and apnea, in which the length of apnea is proportional to the degree of trauma.

Cluster Pattern

Cluster breathing refers to episodes of breathing with irregular frequency and amplitude followed by apneic episodes of variable duration. This pattern is typically associated with upper medulla and lower pons lesions. It has also been described in cerebellar hemorrhage, brainstem hemorrhage, Shy-Drager syndrome, anoxic encephalopathy, and subarachnoid hemorrhage (SAH) with severe vasospasm.

Hyperventilation Pattern

Midbrain and upper pontine lesions (usually central tegmentum of the pons) may cause a central neurogenic hyperventilation syndrome with a persistent respiratory rate of 40 to 70 breaths per minute with respiratory alkalosis. Hyperventilation is not considered neurogenic if Po_2 is less than 80 mm Hg or Pco_2 is greater than 40 mm Hg. It can also be seen in the early stages of hepatic coma.

Acute Respiratory Distress Syndrome and Hypoxemia

ARDS may develop as a result of TBI or associated trauma, pulmonary contusions, blood transfusions, and aspiration pneumonia.[5] Hypoxemia may occur because of TBI or associated ARDS, fluid overload, disseminated intravascular coagulation (DIC), fat embolism, and thoracic trauma. Severity and treatment of hypoxemia correspond to the location and severity of brain injury. In mild to moderate brain injury, ICP and ventilatory response may remain intact, and the resulting hypoxemia may be treated with noninvasive supplemental oxygen. The ventilatory response may be affected in severe brain injury, causing both increased $Paco_2$ and severe hypoxemia requiring intubation and mechanical ventilation. Oxygen inhalation therapy is used to prevent or correct tissue hypoxia ($Pao_2 < 60$ mm Hg, or $Sao_2 < 90\%$). All patients with TBI are given supplemental oxygen, because an Sao_2 value less than 90% and systolic blood pressure lower than 12 kPa (90 mm Hg) have been shown to be the most detrimental factors in causing secondary brain injury.

Mechanical ventilation may be necessary. Assist control ventilation is associated with the least work of breathing. However it may be associated with high airway pressures, which may decrease venous return and cardiac output, and with respiratory alkalosis, which may cause a left shift in the oxyhemoglobin curve, arrhythmias, and a decrease in the seizure threshold. Pressure control ventilation is most suitable in patients with reduced lung compliance, in whom it provides lower peak inspiratory pressure as well variable gas flow, which allows better gas distribution and the use of lower tidal volumes. Synchronized intermittent mandatory ventilation enables better synchronization between the ventilator and the patient by allowing patient-initiated breaths to trigger the

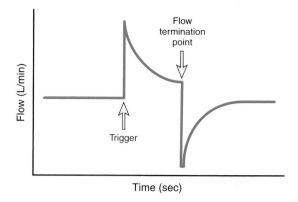

Figure 22–2 Morphology of the pressure support waveform. *(Adapted from Sarkar S, Donn SM: In support of pressure support. Clin Perinatol 2007;34:117-128.)*

machine while also delivering machine-initiated breaths. Pressure support ventilation provides inspiratory pressure assistance during spontaneous breathing; it is a flow-triggered and flow-cycled approach that places greater emphasis on patient control of the ventilator (Fig. 22-2). It is usually used together with synchronized intermittent mandatory ventilation, mainly as a weaning strategy. Positive end-expiratory pressure (PEEP) aids in the redistribution of intra-alveolar water into the interstitial space and improvement of the alveolar recruitment. Transmission of intrathoracic pressure (PEEP) to the intracranial compartment is limited by the presence of valves in the thoracic veins and by the overall decrease in lung compliance due to the use of PEEP and the lung injury itself. It has been shown that in patients with low respiratory system compliance, PEEP had no significant effect on cerebral and systemic hemodynamics. Continuous positive airway pressure is generally used for weaning trials in an intubated patient.

Newer and "smarter" modes of ventilation include pressure-regulated volume control and volume-assured pressure support ventilation. In pressure-regulated volume control ventilation, the machine delivers several breaths to measure several parameters of pressure and compliance and then adjusts the pressure to deliver a selected tidal volume. In volume-assured pressure support ventilation, there are two gas flow sources; the first gives a constant flow pattern, and the second delivers a rapid flow that is set to a pressure limit via pressure support control and is terminated once a preset tidal volume is reached. Both sources of gas flow are activated simultaneously when a breath is triggered. In airway pressure release ventilation, the majority of the respiratory cycle is spent in a high-level continuous positive airway pressure that is terminated only very briefly to allow carbon dioxide to be removed. Airway pressure release ventilation is commonly used in patients with decreased lung compliance in whom volume control ventilation requires unacceptably high airway pressures to ventilate and pressure control ventilation is not adequate to clear carbon dioxide.

Neurogenic Pulmonary Edema

NPE is a rapidly progressing form of pulmonary edema that occurs after CNS insult such as acute cerebral or spinal cord trauma, SAH, intracerebral hemorrhage (ICH), intracranial surgery, meningitis, tumors, venous air embolism, multiple sclerosis, and Guillain-Barré syndrome. NPE is reported to occur in up to 20% of patients with severe head injury, particularly those with hypothalamic lesions.[6] Local ischemic insults in brain "trigger" zones such as the posterior hypothalamus and ventral or dorsal medulla are believed to trigger massive sympathetic activation.[7] α-Adrenergic activation and release of vasoconstrictors such as norepinephrine, neuropeptide Y,[8] endothelin-1, and nitric oxide lead to inflammatory and hemodynamic changes.[9] The intense pulmonary and systemic vasoconstriction leads to increases in pulmonary capillary permeability, venous return, and intrapulmonary shunting. When capillary transmural pressures exceed 40 mm Hg, the pulmonary capillary endothelium and basement membranes are injured, with eventual damage to the epithelium, allowing leakage of proteins and erythrocytes into alveolar spaces.[10] Increased pulmonary capillary permeability is enhanced by inflammatory mediators, such as tumor necrosis factor-α and interleukins (ILs) 1B and 6, which are released into the circulation upon disruption of the blood-brain barrier (BBB) and may be related to the level of cellular cerebral death.[11] Decreases in the Pao_2/Fio_2 ratio to less than 300 have been shown to occur when ICP is elevated and cerebral perfusion pressure (CPP) is decreased. The extent of ventilation-perfusion mismatch correlates with the severity of TBI and with prognosis. It has been suggested that use of catecholamine to maintain CPP may have a pro-inflammatory effect.[12]

Cardiac manifestations of NPE include increased left ventricular workload, decreased contractility, arrhythmias, and arrest. Symptoms of NPE usually appear shortly after CNS injury. Patients present with acute pulmonary edema without signs of left ventricular failure, tachypnea, tachycardia, basal crackles, and respiratory failure. Chest radiographs demonstrate bilateral infiltrates. Electrocardiography, echocardiography, and transesophageal echocardiography findings as well as CVP values are typically within normal limits or may indicate decreased left ventricular function and arrhythmias. An early, transient increase in pulmonary capillary wedge pressure is observed until capillary injury occurs, after which pulmonary artery pressures are within normal range. Brain natriuretic peptide levels are nondiagnostic and are more likely related to catecholamine secretion.[13]

Control of ICP is the first step in the treatment of pulmonary edema. Surgical evacuation of a hematoma or placement of a CSF drain may be necessary to decrease ICP and inhibit the triggering of NPE. Mechanical ventilation may be indicated for the treatment of both TBI and NPE. Moderate PEEP levels (<15 cm H_2O) are recommended to improve oxygenation while avoiding fluctuations in CBF and ICP. Hypercapnia is discouraged because of its potential to raise ICP. Mannitol and hypertonic saline may be useful in decreasing cerebral and pulmonary edema. Goals of cardiac therapy include reducing preload and afterload and increasing cardiac contractility. They are best achieved with the use of α-blockers and avoidance of β-blockers. Diuretics can be used as long as mean arterial pressure (MAP) and CPP are maintained. Appropriate pressor therapy includes dobutamine, which does not alter cerebral oxygenation, and norepinephrine and epinephrine, which do not appear to worsen NPE.[14]

Pulmonary Embolism and Deep Vein Thrombosis

The risk of PE and deep vein thrombosis is increased in brain injury as well as in spinal cord injury (paraplegia), pelvic and lower extremity fractures, multiple trauma, immobilization, and advanced age. Prophylaxis against both of these conditions is recommended for patients with TBI; however, these patients are at significant risk for development of intracranial bleeding after the initial injury or after craniotomy. Therefore, sequential pneumatic compression devices are more suitable than pharmacologic anticoagulation prophylaxis against deep vein thrombosis.

CARDIOVASCULAR DYSFUNCTION

CNS injury causes dysregulation of blood pressure, cardiac output, vasomotor tone, and heart rate. The cardiovascular system response to CNS injury consists of tachycardia, hypertension, and increased cardiac output, which are stimulated by the hypermetabolic state of TBI. However, with severe ICH, bradycardia may occur from increased vagal tone (Cushing's triad). In general, most cases of TBI are associated with increases in both sympathetic nervous system activity and release of catecholamines (epinephrine, norepinephrine, dopamine). Studies have demonstrated that catecholamines are elevated in proportion to the severity of brain injury and are correlated with outcome.[15] Consequences of such catecholamine release include hypertension, myocardial ischemia, and cardiac arrhythmias. Autopsy in patients with severe TBI shows signs of myocardial damage, which is likely due to excess catecholamine release mainly from the hypothalamus.[16] Cardiotoxic effects of catecholamines include myocardial necrosis and fibrosis similar to that found with myocardial infarction, along with elevations in cardiac enzymes.

Patients typically display a biphasic hemodynamic response consisting of an initial tachycardia and increased vascular resistance followed by a vagally mediated bradycardia, decreased vascular resistance, and hypotension. It has been demonstrated that TBI alters cardiovascular reflex responses to acute hemorrhage.[17] Using a murine lateral fluid percussion (LFP) brain injury model, in which mice were subsequently subjected to blood withdrawal approaching 40%, McMahon and colleagues[17] found that acute TBI altered the biphasic cardiovascular response to hemorrhage, with the effect enhanced as the severity of TBI increased. Moderate TBI significantly attenuated the phase two (depressor) response to blood loss, in which MAP and heart rate were maintained at higher values for a longer period with 50% mortality rates (compared to zero mortality in the control group). Presumably, elevations in heart rate and MAP not only lead to increased blood loss but, in the setting of vasomotor paralysis and impaired autoregulation, also result in increased cerebral edema and ICP. Moderate TBI also caused significantly longer apneic periods in the test group than did mild TBI in the test group or hemorrhage without TBI in the control group.[17]

Electrocardiographic Changes

Risk factors of cardiac arrhythmia in patients with TBI include autonomic nervous system dysfunction (dysautonomia), hypoxia, and electrolyte abnormalities.[18] The extent of autonomic dysfunction correlates with the severity of neurologic injury. Dysautonomia leads to an uncoupling of the normal relationship between heart rate and sympathetic regulation that may last for 3 months after injury.[19,20] Arrhythmias are prevalent in TBI. One study demonstrated prolonged QTc intervals in 90% of patients and various nonspecific ST segment and T-wave changes in 53% of patients.[21] The most common arrhythmias are supraventricular tachycardia (SVT), sinus tachycardia, increased P-wave amplitude, and prolonged QT intervals. Heart block is rare.

Electrocardiographic changes occur in 35% to 95% of patients with SAH, usually within the first 48 hours, and may be associated with elevation of cardiac enzymes. ECG changes in SAH include QTc prolongation, ST-T segment abnormalities, shortened PR intervals, inverted T waves, and peaked P waves. Other arrhythmias are premature atrial contractions (PACs), atrial fibrillation, premature ventricular contractions (PVCs), SVT, ventricular tachycardia, torsades de pointes, and heart block. In patients with subdural hematoma, the presence of electrocardiographic changes has been associated with a higher mortality rate.

In children with severe TBI, particularly those with ICH, electrocardiographic changes include prolonged QTc intervals and increased QTc dispersion. In these settings, fatal arrhythmias have been reported in young patients with no preexisting heart disease. Treatment consists of treating the underlying cause, decreasing ICP, supportive therapy for respiration and circulation plus atropine for increased vagal tone (bradycardia), and sympathetic blockade for tachycardia.

Hypertension

Hypertension is the most common cardiovascular complication of TBI, particularly when there is injury to the hypothalamus or the medulla, which are the primary regulators of autonomic activity via catecholamine release. The triggering of catecholamine release could be increased ICP or regional ischemia. However, hypertension may exist without increased catecholamine release. The effects of hypertension on the brain may be worsened during TBI because of impairment of cerebral autoregulation and capillary endothelium. Impaired arterioles fail to constrict in response to hypertension, leading to increases in cerebral blood flow, volume, and pressure and higher risk of cerebral edema. Also, impaired arterioles may fail to dilate in response to hypotension, leading to decreased cerebral perfusion. Patients with chronic hypertension are at increased risk of hypoperfusion owing to rightward shift of the autoregulation curve.

Although the optimal CPP value is not well defined, the Traumatic Brain Injury Foundation recommends keeping CPP higher than 70 mm Hg.[22] In general, systemic hypertension is treated when systolic blood pressure exceeds 200 mm Hg. The most common antihypertensive agents used in TBI are β-blockers because they treat not only hypertension but also complications of excessive catecholamine release such as tachyarrhythmias, myocardial ischemia, and immune suppression.[23,24] Esmolol is an ultra–short-acting (half-life 9 min) β_1-adrenergic blocker that is suitable for use as a continuous intravenous infusion (500 μg/kg over 1 min, then 50-200 μg/kg/min). The β_1-adrenergic blocker metoprolol has a longer half-life than esmolol and is commonly used in the setting of myocardial ischemia and acute myocardial infarction (5 mg IV every 5-15 min to a total of 15 mg). Labetalol, an α_1- and β-adrenergic blocker, with an α_1/β blocking ratio of 1:7. It has rapid onset but long (5 hr) duration of action (initial dose 10-20 mg, then 40-80 mg/10 min to a total dose of 300 mg, then 2 mg/min infusion). It is commonly used in neurosurgical patients because it does not increase ICP. All β-blockers carry the risk of bronchospasm or exacerbation of heart failure in a decompensated patient.

Vasodilators are generally avoided in neurosurgical patients because they may cause cerebrovascular dilation, resulting in increased CBF, increased ICP, and cerebral edema. Short-acting vasodilators such as sodium nitroprusside (SNP; 0.25-10 μg/kg/min) and, to a lesser extent, nitroglycerin (0.25-5 μg/kg/min) are excellent in achieving acute titration of blood pressure. SNP is a rapid-onset, short-acting drug that causes vascular dilation (arteriolar more than venous) through the release of endothelial nitric oxide. It is particularly useful in cases of severe hypertension or when other drugs fail to control blood pressure adequately. It is best used in conjunction with esmolol, which enhances its antihypertensive effects while counteracting its reflex tachycardia effects. SNP dosage is titrated down slowly to avoid rebound hypertension due to the activation of the renin-angiotensin system. Duration of use should be limited to less than 24 to 48 hours to decrease the risk of tachyphylaxis and cyanide toxicity. The latter interferes with cytochrome oxidase, resulting in cellular hypoxia, metabolic acidosis, and increased mixed venous oxygen content. Treatment consists of stopping the SNP infusion and administration of an antidote such as amyl nitrite (inhalation), sodium nitrite (3%, 10 mL), sodium thiosulfate (25%, 50 mL) or hydroxycobalamin (5 g IV). Nitroglycerin causes more venous than arteriolar dilation, leading to decreased venous return and cardiac output, and may raise ICP, particularly in patients with reduced intracranial compliance. It may cause hypoxemia by increasing ventilation-perfusion mismatch due to inhibition of hypoxic regional vasoconstriction in the lungs. It causes minimal or no reflex tachycardia. Hydralazine is a direct, arteriolar, smooth muscle dilator that decreases systemic vascular resistance and blood pressure and may result in reflex tachycardia and increased ICP.

Treatment of increased ICP by evacuation of hematoma or drainage of CSF significantly facilitates treatment of hypertension and achievement of adequate CPP. Assessing the adequacy of CPP in meeting the metabolic needs of the brain is facilitated by the measuring jugular venous oxygen saturation ($Sjvo_2$) or brain tissue oxygen partial pressure ($Pbto_2$). $Sjvo_2$ measurement has been used in TBI and other clinical settings to guide blood pressure management, hyperventilation techniques, fluid therapy, and detection of arteriovenous fistulas. $Sjvo_2$ catheters contain a photosensor and fiberoptic bundles that use either two or three wavelengths of light to determine the percentage of oxygenated hemoglobin (Hb) in jugular venous bulb blood. The catheter is usually placed in the right jugular bulb because most patients (70%) have right-sided dominant venous drainage. Therefore, placement on the dominant side (right) is useful if global oxygenation values are needed, but placement on the ipsilateral side of brain injury is more useful to detect focal changes in $Sjvo_2$. Normal $Sjvo_2$ values are 50% to 75%. Values lower than 50% for more than 5 minutes are considered indicative of abnormal brain metabolism, and those lower than 20% appear to indicate irreversible ischemic injury to the brain. Similarly, values higher than 90% indicate lack of oxygen use by the brain, such as is seen in cases of coma and brain death. Whereas $Sjvo_2$ measures global cerebral oxygenation, $Pbto_2$ measures regional cerebral oxygenation. $Pbto_2$ may be a better monitor of brain oxygenation in TBI, in which regional differences in CBF are likely. Brain oxygenation sensors measure $Pbto_2$ with electromagnetic or fiberoptic technology, and they also monitor temperature. A $Pbto_2$ measurement device is inserted through a craniotomy or through a bolt with fixation. Normal values for $Pbto_2$ are 20 to 40 mm Hg, and critical values are 8 to 10 mm Hg.

Systemic Hypotension (Hypoperfusion)

Support of blood pressure is critical because the injured brain is sensitive to even transient episodes of hypotension, which is an independent predictor of morbidity and mortality in TBI and is common (30%) among patients with TBI.[25] An isotonic crystalloid seems to be the preferred fluid for volume resuscitation because the Saline versus Albumin Fluid Evaluation (SAFE) study found higher mortality rates in patients with TBI who were resuscitated with 4% albumin.[26] This finding was later confirmed by a post hoc analysis performed by the same investigators. Acute anemia and blood loss should be corrected with transfusion of red blood cells (RBCs) to provide Hb for oxygen delivery. The Transfusion Requirements in Critical Care (TRICC) trial showed that in critically ill patients, a restrictive transfusion strategy (transfusing if the Hb is <7 g/dL to keep Hb between 7 and 9 g/dL) is at least as effective as and possibly superior to a liberal transfusion strategy (transfusing if the Hb is <10 g/dL to keep Hb between 10 and 12 g/dL).[27] Whether these findings are applicable to patients with TBI remains to be established.

If hypotension persists despite adequate fluid replacement, then vasopressors or a combination of vasopressors and inotropes is used to raise the CPP to more than 70 mm Hg. Phenylephrine (0.5-2 μg/kg/min) and vasopressin (0.04 unit/min) are pure vasopressors. Norepinephrine (0.1-1 μg/kg/min) is predominantly a vasopressor but also has inotropic effects. Epinephrine (0.1-1μg/kg/min) has more inotropic than vasopressor effects. Although dopamine has mainly dopaminergic (splanchnic vasodilation) effects at doses of 2 to 3 μg/kg/min, it has β-adrenergic (inotropic) effects at doses of 5 to 10 μg/kg/min and mainly α-adrenergic (vasopressor) effects at doses of 10 to 15 μg/kg/min, with significant overlap and individual variations. Low-dose (1-3 μg/kg/min) dopamine infusion has been shown to be of no benefit in the treatment or prevention of renal dysfunction in critically ill patients.

FAT EMBOLISM SYNDROME

Fat embolism syndrome (FES) can complicate TBI. The syndrome consists of the triad cerebral dysfunction, fever, and hypoxemia in the setting of injury to a marrow-containing bone. During such injury, bone intramedullary pressure may become higher than the venous pressure, and fat globules are forced into the vein and then travel to the heart and lungs. The fat globules then embolize in the lung vasculature.[28]

FES is most commonly seen following bone injury but has been also observed in acute pancreatitis, diabetes mellitus, and sickle cell disease. Fat, platelet, and fibrin collections plug cerebral arterioles, leading to ischemia and distal hemorrhage. Similar lesions exist in the liver, kidney, heart, and lung. Additional lesions are pneumonitis, pulmonary edema, and disseminated intravascular coagulation (DIC). Symptoms appear 24 to 48 hours after the initiating injury. Changes in mental status are most commonly seen, with symptoms progressing from restlessness to confusion and then coma. Respiratory failure generally occurs after mental status changes. Chest radiograph reveals diffuse bilateral infiltrates compatible with ARDS. Another finding is petechiae over the neck, chest, and axillae. Retinal fat is observed, and fat is found in clotted blood samples. When FES occurs perioperatively, patients may fail to regain consciousness after general anesthesia.

Therapy for FES consists of support of respiratory and cardiovascular function in the form of supplemental oxygen, mechanical ventilation, and vasopressors. High-dose corticosteroids have been used, although no evidence supports their use. Some case reports describe the successful use of percutaneous cardiopulmonary support to treat an intraoperative case of FES.[29,30] In one case, the patient was stabilized within 10 minutes of initiation of this therapy.[31]

NEUROMUSCULAR DYSFUNCTION

Diaphragmatic paralysis following head trauma has been reported, although it is more commonly seen in patients with stroke (contralateral phrenic nerve paralysis). CNS injury can lead to damage of the central generator of respiratory pattern, resulting in diaphragmatic paralysis. Causes include upper cervical cord injuries, brainstem ischemia and hemorrhage, encephalitis, and neurosurgical complications. About 40% of patients with complete tetraplegia require lifetime mechanical ventilation.[32] Diaphragmatic paralysis may cause difficulty in weaning patients from the ventilator because of poor inspiratory effort and decreased cough reflex. Neuromuscular electrophysiologic studies may help predict respiratory recovery. Traditionally, testing of electromyographic responses has been used. Transcranial magnetic stimulation has now been shown to be a more reliable predictor of recovery of respiratory function. This modality elicits bilateral phrenic nerve stimulation through cervical magnetic stimulation. In one study, transcranial magnetic stimulation was shown to have 100% specificity and 90% sensitivity in predicting recovery of spontaneous ventilatory activity.[33]

HEMATOLOGIC ABNORMALITIES

Anemia

Anemia may be present in patients with TBI as a result of cerebral or extracerebral hemorrhage, either of which may be compounded by preexisting disease. Anemia decreases oxygen-carrying capacity in the blood because Hb carries more than 90% of the oxygen in the blood, which is evident from the blood oxygen content (CaO_2) equation, as follows:

$$CaO_2 = 1.34 \times Hb \times SaO_2 + 0.0031 \times PaO_2$$

Decreased oxygen content in the blood (CaO_2) decreases oxygen delivery (DO_2), which is the product of oxygen content in the blood and cardiac output. Organs with high oxygen requirements, such as the brain and the heart, are most sensitive to the effects of anemia. The heart may be most affected because of a combination of (1) high oxygen requirements (myocardial O_2 consumption [MVO_2] >7.6 mL/min/100 g), in comparison with the total body average (3.5 mL/min/kg), and (2) high oxygen extraction ratio (OER, 65%), in comparison with the total body average (25%).

Treatment of acute anemia consists of replacement of RBCs plus supportive therapy in the form of intravenous fluids, vasopressor therapy, supplemental oxygen, ventilatory support, and sedation. The threshold as well as the target of transfusion of RBCs is not well defined from clinical evidence. As described in the discussion of systemic hypotension, the Transfusion Requirements in Critical Care (TRICC) trial showed that a restrictive transfusion strategy (transfusing when the Hb is <7 g/dL to keep Hb between 7 and 9 g/dL) is at least as effective as and possibly superior to a liberal transfusion strategy (transfusing when the Hb is <10 g/dL to keep Hb between 10 and 12 g/dL).[26] Furthermore, when intravascular volume and other supportive therapies are provided, Hb levels of 5 g/dL seem to be well tolerated. There is no evidence that these findings are applicable to patients with TBI, nor that an Hb level of 10 g/dL is ideal in these patients. The use of intra-Pbto$_2$ or Sjvo$_2$ monitoring may aid in determining the adequacy of oxygen delivery to the brain to meet metabolic requirements. Transfusion of RBCs may be associated with multiple complications, such as hemolytic transfusion reaction, allergic and anaphylactic reactions, transfusion-related acute lung injury, post-transfusion purpura, transfusion-associated graft-versus-host disease, transfusion-related immune modulation (suppression), fever, infection, and hyperbilirubinemia.

Disseminated Intravascular Coagulation

Many patients with head injury have clotting abnormalities, including DIC. Low-grade DIC is seen in 8.4% of patients with primary ICH and is associated with increased morbidity and mortality.[34] The brain is rich in tissue thromboplastin, which is a main activator of DIC. Excessive coagulation that causes DIC may be triggered through different pathways. It can be triggered by endothelial cell injury, which activates the intrinsic pathway; by tissue injury, which activates the extrinsic pathway; or by RBC and platelet injury, which causes the release of procoagulant phospholipids.[35] The development of DIC involves the following four main mechanisms: increased thrombin generation, suppression of anticoagulant pathways, impaired fibrinolysis, and inflammatory activation. Upon cell injury, monocytes and endothelial cells release tissue thromboplastin, and the coagulation cascade is activated. With excessive coagulation, the anticoagulant and fibrinolytic systems are overwhelmed, leading to diffuse microvascular thrombi, which leads to decreased blood supply to various organs. The risk of bleeding is greater because both coagulation factors and platelets are consumed in thrombosis. The fibrinolytic system is activated by the conversion of plasminogen to plasmin, which acts to break down fibrin clots. Plasminogen is consumed and fibrin degradation products (FDPs) accumulate, further raising the risk of bleeding by inhibiting fibrin clot formation and impairing platelet function.

Diagnosis of DIC is based on the presence of a disorder known to be associated with DIC and abnormal results of global coagulation tests, including low platelet count, elevations of fibrin-related markers (e.g., FDPs), increased prothrombin time (PT), and decreased fibrinogen level. These coagulation results are scored on the basis of values and if criteria are met, the diagnosis of DIC is made.[36] Treatment consists of treating the underlying disorder and correcting the resulting coagulopathy and anemia. Coagulopathy is treated with replacement of consumed coagulation products in the form of fresh frozen plasma (FFP), platelets, and cryoprecipitate. Cryoprecipitate is indicated if fibrinogen levels are lower than 100 mg/dL. The goal of treatment is to achieve a fibrinogen level above 100 mg/dL, a platelet count of more than 50,000/mm^3, and an activated partial thromboplastin time close to normal values.

Anemia is treated with transfusion of packed RBCs. Administration of heparin for DIC is controversial, and evidence supporting its use is limited. The use of heparin is based on the finding of clinical evidence of excessive thrombosis. However, it is given at doses lower than those used to treat thrombosis (5-10 units/kg/hr with or without a loading dose). Aminocaproic acid and aprotinin have been used to treat thrombosis associated with DIC. Failure rates have been high, however. Other experimental treatments are antithrombin III concentrate, protein C and protein S concentrates, and direct thrombin inhibitors. The results of clinical trials for these agents have been inconclusive.

METABOLIC ABNORMALITIES

Trauma triggers the neural and endocrine stress response, resulting in increased sympathetic outflow, decreased glucose uptake, and increased insulin resistance, lipolysis, and proteolysis. Manifestations of hypermetabolism and catabolism include increased resting energy expenditure (REE) and muscle breakdown and atrophy. Patients with isolated TBI demonstrate a 140% increase in REE, and there is an inverse relationship between the GCS score and REE.[37,38] Additional factors in increased catabolism include corticosteroid use, enteral feeds administered in bolus form, and expression of cytokines (tumor necrosis factor, IL-1, IL-6), catecholamines, cortisol, and glucagon. With hypercatabolism, glucose use by the brain and blood cells increases. Initially glycogenolysis is used; once glycogen stores are depleted, gluconeogenesis becomes the primary source of glucose production, with the use of amino acids from skeletal muscle breakdown. Protein requirements are further increased by greater synthesis of numerous acute-phase proteins, such as fibrinogen, C-reactive protein, albumin, prealbumin, and α_1-acid glycoprotein. A positive nitrogen balance may be difficult to achieve, and severe protein-calorie malnutrition may occur.

ELECTROLYTE IMBALANCES

Fluid and electrolyte imbalance is the most common complication of TBI. Mechanisms of this imbalance include brain injury, diuretics (mannitol), hypovolemia, myoglobinuria, and renal failure.

Hyponatremia

Hyponatremia is common and is mainly due to the syndrome of inappropriate of antidiuretic hormone secretion (SIADH) or the cerebral salt-wasting syndrome (CSWS). The hypothalamic ADH regulates water balance and osmolality in the body. Hypothalamic baroreceptors are sensitive to minor (1%) increases in serum osmolarity and react by increasing the release of ADH. At serum osmolality greater than 280 mOsm/L, ADH is secreted linearly with increases in osmolarity.[39] The secreted ADH binds to receptors on renal collecting tubules and acts to increase free water absorption. Greater secretion of ADH is common in stress and particularly TBI. SIADH occurs when there is continued release of ADH despite low serum sodium levels and hypervolemia. Laboratory findings in SIADH include serum osmolality less than 280 mOsm/L, serum sodium value less than 135 mEq/L, high urine osmolality, and urinary sodium concentration less than 25 mEq/L. Therapy for SIADH consists of fluid restriction (1-1.5 L/day), furosemide, demeclocycline, and hypertonic

(3%) sodium (HS). The last, reserved for patients whose serum sodium levels are lower than 120 mEq/L, is aimed at achieving an increase in serum sodium at a rate less than 0.5 mEq/L/hr to avoid pontine demyelination syndrome.

CSWS causes profound natriuresis that is stimulated by increased levels of atrial natriuretic factor (ANP), brain natriuretic peptide (BNP), and C-type natriuretic peptide (CNP). These peptides suppress aldosterone synthesis and lead to natriuresis, diuresis, and vasodilatation. Hyponatremia in CSWS results from increased renal excretion of sodium (150-200 mEq/L/day), which is followed by excretion of water, with resultant hypovolemia (unlike the hypervolemia of SIADH). The treatment for CSWS consists of sodium and volume repletion. Hypertonic (3%) NaCl may be used to increase serum sodium levels at a rate less than 0.5 mEq/L/hr.

It is important to distinguish between SIADH and CSWS, because their respective therapies vary greatly. Fluid restriction and diuresis in a patient with CSWS can be fatal because of the possibility of severe hypovolemia and cerebral infarction. Indications for the use of hypertonic (3%) NaCl in the treatment of hyponatremia include serum sodium less than 120 mEq/L, seizures, and cerebral edema. Hypertonic (3%) NaCl is given slowly (100 mL/hr), with frequent monitoring of serum sodium levels to avoid correction at rates above 0.5 mEq/L/hr. Rapid correction of hyponatremia has been associated with central pontine myelinolysis (CPM). The risk of CPM is increased with chronic (>48 hr) hyponatremia. The main risk that hyponatremia and hypo-osmolality pose to the brain is that of cerebral edema, which leads to life-threatening rises in ICP when the increase in intracranial volume exceeds 10%. Compensatory mechanisms consist of CSF displacement from the intracranial to the extracranial compartment and the release of idiogenic osmoles from the intracellular to the extracellular space. These idiogenic osmoles include potassium, glutamate, taurine, and glutamine.

Hypernatremia

Hypernatremia may occur in TBI as a result of inadequate intake of water, high-calorie enteral feeding leading to diarrhea, diabetes insipidus (DI), mannitol, phenytoin, correction of hyperglycemia, and increased total body sodium content resulting from prolonged volume depletion that stimulates aldosterone secretion and causes renal retention of sodium. Chronic hypernatremia is better tolerated than acute hypernatremia. Acute hypernatremia may cause water shift from cerebral tissues and cellular dehydration. Symptoms include lethargy, muscle tremor, rigidity, hyperreflexia, seizures and coma.

DI may be neurogenic (decreased ADH release from the pituitary) or nephrogenic (decreased sensitivity of renal collecting tubules to ADH). Neurogenic DI, which is more common with basilar skull fractures and increased ICP, may indicate impending brain death. Clinical manifestations of DI include increased urinary output (200-300 mL/hr), decreased urinary specific gravity (<1.005), decreased urine osmolality to less than serum osmolality, hypernatremia, and dehydration. Treatment consists of correction of hypovolemia, hypernatremia, and hormonal deficiency. Hypovolemia is corrected with IV fluids at a rate that achieves a 1:1 ratio with urine output. Hypernatremia is corrected with enteral water or parenteral (5% dextrose in water [D_5W]) solution. The use of D_5W is avoided in the neurosurgical patient in order to avoid hyperglycemia, which may worsen neurologic outcome of ischemic

brain injury. Total body water deficit is calculated according to the following formula:

$$H_2O \text{ deficit} = \frac{\text{serum } Na^+ - 140}{140 \times 0.6 \times \text{body wt (kg)}}$$

The goal of free water replacement is to correct serum sodium by a rate no faster than 0.5 mEq/L/h or 12 mEq/L/24h. The goal is to decrease serum sodium to less than 160 mEq/L and serum osmolarity to less than 320 mEq/L.

Hormonal replacement is reserved for cases of severe DI or to avoid administering large volumes of free water. Desmopressin is a synthetic analogue of vasopressin (ADH) that lacks pressor activity and causes free water absorption at the distal tubules and collecting system of the kidneys. It can be administered IV or subcutaneously at 0.3 mcg/kg/day, divided and given twice daily. The oral dose is 0.05 to 1.2 mg/day divided and given twice or three times daily. The intranasal dose is 10-40 mcg one or two times a day. Vasopressin is the pituitary hormone that possesses both pressor and antidiuretic properties. It is used clinically mainly as a vasopressor (0.04 unit/min, IV). However it can be used for the treatment of DI associated with hypotension.

Hypomagnesaemia, Hypokalemia, and Hypocalcaemia

Patients with severe head injury are at high risk for development of hypomagnesaemia, hypokalemia, and hypocalcaemia. These electrolyte abnormalities have been linked to cardiac arrhythmias associated with prolongation of the QT interval. Treatment consists of replacing the electrolyte deficits and correcting the underlying cause. Hypokalemia is most often caused by extracellular shift of potassium due to alkalosis that results from spontaneous or mechanical hyperventilation. In addition, actual potassium loss may occur through the use of corticosteroids or diuretics.

GASTROINTESTINAL ABNORMALITIES AND NUTRITION

Stress Ulcer

Patients with TBI are at increased risk for stress gastritis and ulceration, the risk factors for which include TBI itself, critical illness, and steroid use. Prophylaxis against stress gastritis and ulceration in the form of proton pump inhibitors (PPIs) such as esomeprazole (40 mg IV daily) or H_2-antagonists such as famotidine (40 mg IV daily) is recommended for all critically ill patients with TBI.

Nutrition

Nutrition is an important aspect of the care of the critically ill patient with TBI. TBI is associated with hypermetabolism, hypercatabolism, hyperglycemia, and nitrogen wasting. Patients with TBI are at risk for malnutrition, immunocompromise, and poor healing if their nutritional, specifically protein, requirements are not met. Nutrition should be provided to patients with TBI as soon as the acute issues of stabilization and treatment are addressed. Appropriate nutritional support has been shown to improve patient outcomes.[40] Recommendations based on level II evidence suggest that patients should be fed to attain full caloric replacement by day 7 after injury.[41]

Enteral nutrition is the preferred route of nutrition because it is associated with less risk of hyperglycemia and septic complications than total parenteral nutrition (TPN).[42] TBI is associated with decreased gastric emptying and increased reflux.[43] Increased ICP and low GCS scores at admission are associated with higher rates of gastric atony, ileus, and stress-related gastritis. Early (<36 hr from TBI) enteral nutrition is associated with shorter ICU stays and fewer infectious complications than late (>36 hr from TBI) enteral nutrition.[44] Tighter control of serum glucose levels without reduction of nutritional support may improve the prognosis in TBI. Aspiration of enteral feeds occurs in up to 45% of patients with TBI and is not reduced by jejunal placement of feeding tubes. Precautions include checking gastric residual content after 4 hours of stopping feeding, elevating the head of the bed to at least 30 degrees, and observing for abdominal distention. Metoclopramide (10 mg IV every 8 hr) may improve gastric motility and decreases reflux. Jejunal placement of feeding tubes may overcome the problem of gastric atony and ileus but does not necessarily decreases the risk of aspiration.

If enteral nutrition is not tolerated or not feasible, TPN is used. Benefits of TPN include a lesser degree of negative nitrogen balance, which may improve survival by avoiding protein malnutrition and the associated immunosuppression. Complications of TPN include fluid overload, cerebral edema, hyperglycemia, electrolyte imbalance, and catheter-related complications such as sepsis. About 75% of the total calorie requirements are provided in the form of glucose or dextrose to avoid the use of amino acids as a source of energy. The electrolyte content of TPN is adjusted daily on the basis of the patient's electrolyte levels. Insulin is provided either as part of the TPN solution or, preferably, as a separate infusion to keep blood glucose levels between 110 and 150 mg/dL. TPN provided via a large central vein allows higher (70% dextrose) concentration of the TPN solution. Peripheral parenteral nutrition (PPN) places a limit on the concentration of the solution (30% dextrose) and results in administration of larger fluid volumes. Peripherally inserted central catheters (PICC lines) allow the use of the higher concentrations (70%) of TPN solutions.

Caloric requirements in TBI vary from 25 to 50 kcal/kg/day. Caloric requirements are calculated with use of indirect calorimetry or one of the standard formulas, such as the Harris-Benedict formula. This formula calculates REE as follows:

$$REE \text{ in a male} = 66.473 + 13.7516(\text{weight}) + 5.0033(\text{height}) - 6.755(\text{age})$$

$$REE \text{ in a female} = 65.595 + 9.563(\text{weight}) + 1.8496(\text{height}) - 4.6756(\text{age})$$

The REE is then multiplied by a stress factor. The stress factor for TBI is 1.4 when no steroids are used and 1.4 to 2 when steroids are used.

Indirect calorimetry may be more accurate in assessing caloric requirements than the Harris-Benedict formula. It compares O_2 consumption and CO_2 production relative to the oxidation of carbohydrates, fat, and protein to determine REE. This calculation is accomplished through a metabolic bedside cart that uses the Weir calculation—kcal/min = 3.9

(O_2 consumption) + 1.1 (CO_2 production)—to obtain the value of kilocalories per minute and multiplies this number by 1440 min/day. It is recommended that indirect calorimetry be performed several times per week and that caloric intake be adjusted accordingly.

Total calories are calculated on the basis that fat provides 9 kcal/g, and glucose and protein provide 4 kcal/g each. However, protein is provided mainly to meet nitrogen requirements and not as a calorie source. Nitrogen requirements are calculated on the basis of excreted nitrogen in the urine, urine urea nitrogen (UUN), plus an additional 4 g for other estimated losses. Nitrogen requirements are multiplied by 6.25 to calculate the amount of protein to be provided to achieve a positive nitrogen balance of 0 to 4. Because of the increased protein catabolism in TBI, the goal of achieving a positive nitrogen balance may not be attained until several days after TBI, and patients may require twice as much protein (2 g/kg/day) as in a standard diet (0.8 kg/kg/day). One study demonstrated that a positive nitrogen balance could be obtained earlier with the use of insulin-like growth factor-1 (IGF-1) and growth hormone therapy.[39] Patients with moderate to severe TBI were treated with IGF-1 infusion and subcutaneous growth hormone within 72 hours of injury. Within the treatment group, a positive nitrogen balance was achieved within the first 24 hours following therapy.[39] Prealbumin, a serum protein with a half-life of 2 to 3 days, and urine urea nitrogen (UUN) levels are measured to assess nitrogen balance and guide protein supplementation.

IMMUNOLOGIC ABNORMALITIES

TBI is associated with immunosuppression that correlates in magnitude with the severity of TBI. Manifestations of immunosuppression include increased levels of IL-4, IL-6, IL-10, and prostaglandin E_2 (PGE_2); impaired function of T-cell lymphocytes; and decreased expression of major histocompatibility class (MHC) II molecules by monocytes. This immunosuppression is induced by both humoral and hormonal mechanisms. The humoral mechanism is mediated through decreased expression of cell surface antigens, such as CD4+, RTIA+, Thy-1+, and ICO-111+ lymphocytes.[45] The hormonal mechanism is mediated through stimulation of β_2-adrenergic receptors, which increases expression of the immunoinhibitory cytokine IL-10, in response to increases in ICP and catecholamine release. β_2-Adrenergic antagonists have been shown to block this effect.[46] In addition, induction of proinflammatory cytokines such as IL-1α, IL-1β, and tumor necrosis factor-α may contribute to delayed tissue damage similar to that seen during infection. This effect is mediated through the CNS, endocrine, and paracrine/autocrine signaling mechanisms. In contrast, increased expression of the IL-1 receptor-antagonist (IL-1RA) has neuroprotective effects, through blocking of the binding of IL-1 to its signaling receptor.[47] The immunomodulatory heat shock protein (HSP) 60 stimulates inflammatory cytokines and chemokines and is associated with both proinflammatory and anti-inflammatory effects. It is expressed during stressful situations such as infection, cancer, glucose deprivation, and temperature change. Patients with TBI who were subjected to mild hypothermia had decreased expression of HSP 60 from polymorphonuclear leukocytes (PMNLs) and had a higher risk of infectious complications.[48]

ENDOCRINE ABNORMALITIES

Hyperglycemia and Hypoglycemia

Maintaining euglycemia is vital after TBI and neurosurgery. Both hyperglycemia and hypoglycemia can exacerbate neurologic injury. Hyperglycemia during neuronal injury such as ischemic stroke, cerebral hemorrhage, or cerebral trauma is associated with increased morbidity and mortality.[49,50] During severe TBI, hyperglycemia (serum glucose >170 mg/dL) is associated with a lower rate of survival.[51] Hyperglycemia and the infusion of glucose-containing fluids have been shown to worsen neurologic outcome of cerebral ischemia and stroke mainly because during focal ischemia, glucose is converted to lactate, which exacerbates secondary neuronal injury.[52-54] Intensive insulin therapy in patients with TBI and in patients with non-neurologic critical illnesses is associated with decreases in occurrence of polyneuropathy of critical illness, in days of ventilator dependency, in ICP, and in incidence of seizures, as well as better long-term rehabilitation.[55] In addition to providing strict glucose control, insulin may have neuroprotective effects because it shares significant homology with nerve growth factor (NGF), which facilitates neuronal repair.

On the other hand, hypoglycemia is associated with worse outcome during SAH, ICH, TBI, and cerebral infarction. The brain may suffer an "energy crisis" when brain glucose levels are less than 0.7 mmol/L (mg/dL) or the lactate-to-pyruvate ratio is less than 40. In one study, the risk of brain energy crisis was 23% more likely with each 1 mmol/L decrease in systemic glucose concentration and 10% more likely with each 1 unit/L increase in insulin infusion, despite adjustment for ICP and GCS score. Among patients receiving neurointensive care, episodes of low brain glucose levels and high levels of metabolic distress markers are associated with greater mortality and poorer outcome among survivors. A reasonable balanced goal of glycemic control among patients with TBI may be to maintain serum glucose between 5.5 and 8.25 mmol/l (100-150 mg/dL).

Syndrome of Inappropriate Antidiuretic Hormone Secretion

As previously described, increased ADH secretion following TBI may result in SIADH, which causes water retention with continued sodium excretion, leading to hyponatremia. The mechanism of continued sodium excretion is not well understood but may be due to suppression of proximal tubular reabsorption of sodium in response to an expanded extracellular volume.[56] Laboratory findings in SIADH include decreased serum osmolality and increased urine osmolality. Symptoms of water intoxication include nausea, vomiting, headache, mood lability, confusion, seizures, and coma. SIADH is also seen in patients with SAH, brain tumor, brain abscess, meningitis, and encephalitis. Treatment of SIADH involves water restriction to achieve a negative water balance, loop diuretics, and the infusion of hypertonic saline. In mild cases, water restriction alone may be adequate. However, a high urine osmolarity may not allow adequate water excretion. Therefore, in moderate cases, loop diuretics are used to decrease urine osmolarity, because they impair renal concentrating ability. In more severe cases (serum sodium levels <120 mEq/L), hypertonic saline is used as a slow infusion (2 mL/kg/hr), which compensates for the diuretic-induced natriuresis. Serum sodium, urine osmolality, and urine specific gravity should be measured at regular intervals (4-6 hr) to guide therapy. Hyponatremia should be corrected faster than 0.5 mEq/L/hr or 12 mEq/L/day to minimize the risk of pontine demyelination syndrome, which may lead to seizures, behavioral changes, movement disorders, and coma.

Hypopituitarism

Hypopituitarism secondary to TBI may be partial or complete and immediate or delayed.[57] Within 1 to 2 years of TBI, 28% to 57% of patients have one or more anterior pituitary hormone deficiencies. Isolated growth hormone deficiency is the most common (20%),[58] followed by adrenocorticotropic hormone (ACTH) deficiency (10%).[59] TBI-induced hypopituitarism may be due to infarction, which could be caused by compression from increased ICP, hypoxia, or skull fracture. During the early period of TBI, levels of serum cortisol and ACTH release both increase, with some correlation with the severity of injury.[60,61] However, within 1 week to 2 months after injury, adrenal failure may be encountered in cases of moderate to severe TBI, resulting in significant decrease in cortisol levels.[62]

Therefore, all patients in whom secondary hypoadrenalism due to decreased ACTH is suspected should receive corticosteroid coverage until testing indicates an intact pituitary-adrenal axis. An occult ACTH and cortisol deficiency may become acutely apparent during acute stress and may manifest as hyponatremia and hypovolemic shock. Less acute deficiency may manifest as mild to moderate hypotension, fatigue, lethargy, weight loss, abdominal pain, hypoglycemia, frequent hunger, headaches, and light-headedness. During acute TBI, about 50% of patients have low triiodothyronine (T_3) syndrome (euthyroid sick syndrome [ESS]), which consists of a low level of free T_3 with normal levels of free thyroxine (T_4) and thyroid-stimulating hormone. At 12 months after injury, about 6% of patients have TSH deficiency.[63] Thyroid hormone replacement therapy is not administered to treat low T_3 syndrome, which occurs because of impairment of conversion of T_4 to T_3 due to inhibition of type I deiodinase, which is inhibited during stress or illness. Although animal studies have supported the use of liothyronine in low T_3 syndrome (in dogs undergoing cardiac bypass),[64] human trials of T_3 replacement (levothyroxine or liothyronine) in patients with the disorder have failed to show benefit.

Decreased secretion of pituitary ADH leads to DI. Treatment of DI consists of treatment of the underlying cause (trauma, elevated ICP), replacement of water deficits, correction of electrolyte imbalance, and pharmacologic therapy. Free water is given at volumes that match urine output until the polyuria is resolved. Enterally, up to 1 to 2 L/hr of free water can be given via a gastric tube. Alternatively, D_5W can be given IV at infusion rates that are adjusted to match urine output. Enteral free water is preferred in order to avoid the possible hyperglycemia that may result from D_5W infusions. Free water deficits can be estimated by using the following formula:

$$H_2O \text{ deficit} = \frac{\text{serum Na}^+ - 140}{140 \times 0.6 \times \text{body wt (kg)}}$$

Serum electrolyte levels should be monitored every 4 hours until hypernatremia is resolved. Blood glucose should be monitored frequently and treated with IV insulin, because hyperglycemia may cause additional osmotic diuresis. Pharmacologic treatment of central (neurogenic) DI consists of hormonal replacement, in the form of desmopressin or vasopressin. Desmopressin (DDAVP) may be administered intravenously, subcutaneously, or as a nasal spray. Its effects last 8 to 20 hours. It is given as an initial dose of 10 to 20 μg, with repeated dosing every 30 to 60 minutes (up to 60 μg), until urine output is decreased to less than 100 mL/hr. This initial dose is repeated when urine output increases again to 200 mL/hr. Excessive doses of desmopressin can cause oliguria, hyponatremia, and water intoxication. Vasopressin, which possesses antidiuretic, vasoconstrictive, and oxytocic effects, may also be used. Its effects last 4 to 6 hours, necessitating frequent dosing. Vasopressin therapy is used less commonly than desmopressin because of the former's potentially serious side effects such as hypertension, myocardial infarction, mesenteric infarction, peripheral ischemia, allergic reactions, and abscesses at injection sites.

Hypopituitarism is associated with a twofold increase in mortality due to cardiovascular, respiratory, or cerebrovascular disease.[65] Affected patients are advised to remain under the care of an endocrinologist and to have their cardiovascular risks assessed regularly.

INFECTIOUS COMPLICATIONS

Sepsis is the most common cause of late mortality in TBI. Risk factors include prolonged ventilatory support, massive transfusion, and nutritional insufficiency. Urinary tract infections (UTIs) are the most common nosocomial infections, followed by pneumonia. Risk factors for UTI include indwelling urinary catheters, prolonged antibiotic use, urinary stasis, unsealed collection ports, and elevated serum creatinine concentration. Treatment consists of appropriate selective antibiotic therapy and removal of the infected catheters.

Respiratory tract infections are generally separated into early- and late-onset infections. Early-onset infections tend to be caused by antibiotic-sensitive organisms, and late-onset infections are often caused by antibiotic-resistant organisms. The resistant organisms either are selected through previous antibiotic treatment or are hospital-acquired species. Nosocomial infections are associated with increased mortality.[66]

Intravenous catheter–related infections are the cause of bacteremia in less than 1% of ICU patients.[67] The incidence of meningitis in TBI is about 13%. Risk factors include dural tears with CSF leakage, CSF rhinorrhea or otorrhea, ICP monitoring for longer than 72 hours, ICP catheter manipulation, and antibiotic flushes of ICP catheters. Penetrating brain injuries increase the risk of brain abscess and empyema, particularly subdural empyemas, which are most common in frontal and compressed skull fractures (up to 66% mortality rate).

Fever seems to be an independent predictor of poor outcome in TBI.[68] Systemic temperatures higher than 38.5° C should be treated, but lower temperature treatment thresholds should be used in patients with increased ICP.

SECONDARY BRAIN INJURY

Prevention of secondary brain injury is continued in the postoperative period. Studies have shown that patients who sustain secondary brain injury have less favorable outcomes.[69,70]

Hypotension, hypoxia, hyperthermia, hyperglycemia, hypoglycemia, increased ICP, and any aggravating factors, such as pain, nausea, vomiting, seizures, hypertension, hypercarbia, and impaired cerebral venous drainage, should all be prevented and treated. Conscious, mechanically ventilated patients are sedated with a short-acting agent, such as propofol or dexmedetomidine, to allow intermittent neurologic assessment. Pain due to the operative procedure or the primary or associated injury is relieved with an opioid such as morphine or fentanyl. Nausea and vomiting are treated with stomach suctioning, provided that no basilar skull fractures are present, and with pharmacologic agents such as ondansetron. Seizure prophylaxis after head trauma is somewhat controversial. Phenytoin may be given for 2 weeks after head injury if there have been no seizures, or longer if there has been seizure activity.

Sedation and Analgesia

Sedation and analgesia in post-TBI and postoperative patients presents a unique challenge. Sedation and analgesia are necessary because both pain and agitation increase ICP. In addition, inadequate analgesia may lead to agitation, hypertension, and vomiting, which may raise the risk of intracranial bleeding or other neurologic complications. On the other hand, narcotic analgesics may cause respiratory depression and hypercapnia, leading to cerebral vasodilation and increased ICP. Similarly, oversedation may mask neurologic deficits and interfere with proper neurologic examination. There is evidence that pain after neurosurgical procedures is more severe than expected, which may result in undertreatment by the perioperative team.[71] Pain experienced by patients after craniotomy seems to be of somatic origin, most likely involving the scalp, pericranial muscles, and soft tissue, and from manipulation of the dura mater.[72] Although pain may often be treated as a secondary concern, uncontrolled pain has systemic effects that may directly affect patient outcome (Box 22-1).

In general, short-acting agents are preferred because they allow interruption for neurologic examination. To avoid peaks and troughs with the use of short-acting agents, administration by continuous intravenous infusion is preferred. Commonly used drugs include propofol, midazolam, fentanyl, remifentanil, and dexmedetomidine. The last is a highly selective α_2-adrenergic agonist. It allows patients to be comfortably sedated yet easily arousable for serial neurologic examinations. It is also used intraoperatively for awake craniotomy and preoperatively for sedation of patients with aneurysmal SAH. The administration of dexmedetomidine toward the end of major inpatient surgical procedures has been associated with opioid-sparing effects, reducing morphine requirements by as much as 60%.[73]

Opioids are commonly used for postoperative analgesia. However, in neurosurgical patients, their use increases the risk of respiratory depression, with a higher risk of neurologic complications. Patient-controlled analgesia (PCA) has been used to control pain effectively in patients who have undergone craniotomy. Morphine is the most commonly used opioid. Side effects of opioid use include nausea, vomiting, decreased gastrointestinal motility, constipation, pruritus, and respiratory depression. These side effects may lengthen both recovery time and length of hospital stay.

Nonsteroidal anti-inflammatory drugs are excellent alternatives to opioids in providing analgesia for most postoperative patients. However, they are associated with platelet

---

BOX 22–1	*Systemic Organ Responses to Pain*
Respiratory	Increased skeletal muscle tension
	Decreased total lung compliance
Endocrine	Increases in adrenocorticotropic hormone, cortisol, glucagon, epinephrine, aldosterone, antidiuretic hormone, catecholamines, and angiotensin II
	Decreases in insulin and testosterone
Cardiovascular	Increased myocardial work (mediated by catecholamines, angiotensin II)
Immunologic	Lymphopenia
	Depression of reticuloendothelial system
	Leukocytosis
	Reduced killer T-cell cytotoxicity
Hematologic	Increased platelet adhesiveness
	Diminished fibrinolysis
	Activation of coagulation cascade
Gastrointestinal	Increased sphincter tone
	Decreased smooth muscle tone
Genitourinary	Increased sphincter tone
	Decreased smooth muscle tone

Adapted from: Ortiz-Cardona J, Bendo AA: Perioperative pain management in the neurosurgical patient. Anesthesiol Clin 2007;25:655-674.

---

dysfunction and they might increase the bleeding time. This can lead to a higher risk of post-operative bleeding, particularly after hematoma evacuation, aneurysm repair, and resection of arterial venous malformations (AVM). The use of *N*-methyl-D-aspartate receptor antagonists such as ketamine in patients who have undergone craniotomy should be avoided, given the resulting increase in ICP seen with their use in both human and animal studies.[74,75] Ketamine also causes increases in both CBF and cerebral metabolic rate. Scalp blocks have been used successfully to provide transitional analgesia, similar to that of intravenous morphine, in the immediate postoperative period after remifentanil-based anesthesia.[76] Scalp blocks decrease pain and pain medication requests and increase the time between the end of the procedure and the first request for postoperative analgesics.[77] Although commonly practiced, infiltration of the wound incision site has not been shown to be effective in improving post-craniotomy pain scores.

Control of Intracranial Pressure

The brain, blood, and CSF contents within the cranium constitute a nearly incompressible system, with some capacitance afforded by blood vessels and vertebral spaces. Once capacitance has been maximized, ICP rises dramatically with small increases in intracranial volume. Normally ICP is 10 mm Hg or less, and changes in ICP are generally tolerated over a CPP range of 50 to 150 mm Hg. But as CPP is reduced, vasodilatation and increased ICP occur at a logarithmic rate.[78] Increased ICP may be due to greater cerebral blood volume (CBV) or brain edema. Increased ICP leads to decreased CBF, which leads to a compensatory increase in MAP and a compensatory decrease in cerebrovascular resistance, which is maximal at CPP values of about 50 mm Hg. Although an increase in cerebral vasodilation is a compensatory mechanism to increase CBF, it does reduce CBV, which may further raise ICP, perpetuating a vicious circle of increased ICP and decreased perfusion. Therefore it is essential to break this circle by treating any increase in ICP once the compensatory mechanisms have been maximized.

In TBI, increased ICP may be caused by an increase in volume of any of the cranial compartment intravascular blood, intracellular water, or CSF. In addition, extravascular blood, depressed skull fractures, and foreign bodies may further raise ICP. Decreased cerebral venous drainage may cause diastolic decreases in CPP or interrupted perfusion leading to anaerobic metabolism and lactate production, which leads to cerebral edema and to further increases in ICP.

With end-stage cerebral edema, ICP may exceed CPP, leading to cessation of blood flow to the brain and eventual brain death. Indeed, studies of ICP monitoring in the 1960s showed the appearance of "plateau waves" when ICP levels reached systemic blood pressure levels; these waves were associated with decreased neuronal function. Subsequent studies revealed that plateau waves occurred when MAP decreased to 70 to 80 mm Hg and resolved with either an increase in MAP or a decrease in ICP with hyperventilation, which decreased CBF and CBV. This observation led to the common practice of hyperventilation as a means of reducing ICP and improving CPP, but this practice was proved in later studies to be associated with greater risk of cerebral ischemia and is no longer recommended as routine practice in TBI. Similarly, the utility of ICP monitoring and ICP-guided intensive care of TBI has come under question.[79] One study showed that ICP monitoring was associated with increased risk of prolonged mechanical ventilation and other complications and that it limited the benefits from therapeutic interventions, including medications, hyperventilation, and keeping CPP above 70 mm Hg. This finding may prompt a larger randomized clinical trial to assess the role of ICP monitoring in the management of TBI.

Until the results of such a trial are known, ICP monitoring should be performed according to the guidelines for surgical and neurointensive therapy published by the Brain Trauma Foundation and other professional organizations. These guidelines recommend ICP monitoring for patients with severe TBI and some patients with moderate TBI according to coexisting conditions. An ICP reading higher than 20 mm Hg is considered an indication for ICP-reducing therapy and for maintaining an MAP of 80 to 100 mm Hg. In general, intraparenchymal and intraventricular ICP monitoring devices are considered more accurate and preferable to subdural, subarachnoid, or epidural monitors. Imaging signs of increased ICP include cerebral edema (particularly progressive), midline shift, and cisternal compression. These signs may exist without confirmation by an ICP monitor. Patients with imaging signs of increased ICP should be monitored and treated aggressively in an ICU setting for a period of 10 to 14 days or until resolution of neurologic symptoms and imaging abnormalities.

The aim of treating increased ICP is to ensure adequate CPP, because CPP = MAP – ICP. The definitive treatment of increased ICP is to eliminate or minimize the primary cause of increased ICP. In addition, measures aimed at reducing the volume of one of the three normal components of the cranium (blood, CSF, and cellular water) are performed. Intravascular cerebral blood volume may be reduced by reducing CBV, improving venous drainage, or both. Acute reductions in CBF and CBV can be achieved almost immediately with hyperventilation, which decreases $PaCO_2$ causing vasoconstriction. Risks of this systemic vasoconstriction include cerebral and myocardial ischemia. The efficacy of a hyperventilation-induced decrease in ICP is most prominent during the first 12 to 24 hours of hyperventilation.[80]

Reducing the cerebral metabolic rate may be a safer way of achieving a "coupled" decrease in CBF and CBV. Decreases in cerebral metabolic rate may be achieved with physiologic or pharmacologic measures. Drugs that have been shown to decrease cerebral metabolic rate include barbiturates, benzodiazepines, etomidate, propofol, opioids, and lidocaine. Reports of seizure activity and worsening of ischemic and traumatic brain injury in animals exposed to high doses of opioids have not been substantiated in humans.[81,82] Instead opioid-induced analgesia has been shown to prevent pain- and catecholamine-induced spikes in ICP, and opioid analgesics are used for analgesia and enhancement of sedation in patients with TBI. Osmotic diuretics such as mannitol are used to reduce ICP by shifting water from the intracellular and interstitial spaces into the intravascular space and then into the renal excretory system. This osmotic shift of intracellular water is induced through the presence of an intact semipermeable vascular membrane, the BBB. With a damaged BBB, hyperosmolar agents may shift water from the vascular space into the cellular and interstitial compartments, thus increasing ICP. A rebound increase in cerebral edema and ICP may occur once mannitol has been discontinued, owing to the formation and accumulation of idiogenic osmoles in the brain. Idiogenic osmoles consist mainly of taurine and other amino acids and are formed in the brain secondary to long-standing hyperosmolality. Once formed, osmoles are removed at a rate that could be slower than the rate of normalizing extracellular osmolality, possibly leading to an osmotic intracellular shift of water. Maintaining intravascular osmolality or hyperosmolality is essential in avoiding this complication.

Hypertonic saline (HS) achieves shifting of water into the intravascular space as mannitol does, but without the associated diuresis. Also like mannitol, HS requires the presence of a semipermeable membrane to exert its water-shifting effect. With an intact BBB, HS can achieve a rapid (maximum effect at 20 min) and significant (40%) decrease in ICP.[83] The efficacy of HS in reducing ICP has been shown in ischemic stroke, ICH, SAH, TBI, and postoperative cerebral edema.[84] Because of its lack of diuretic effect, HS may increase CBF while decreasing ICP, which may be an advantage in cases of hypotension or decreased CBF.[85] In the presence of an intact BBB, HS has been shown to be more effective than mannitol in controlling ICP[86,87] and to be effective when other medical therapies had failed.[88,89] Assessing the integrity of the BBB may be facilitated by serum assay of the SB-100 protein, which is an astrocyte-specific an astrocyte-specific protein that leaks into the vascular space when BBB integrity is compromised. Astrocytic foot processes cover approximately 90% of the basement membrane of cerebral capillaries and form the BBB, which prevents movement of most water-soluble molecules that are more than 500 Da from the vascular space into the extravascular space. The accuracy of the SB-100 protein test in predicting the integrity of the BBB compares favorably to that of the gold standard, Q_A, which is the ratio of CSF albumin to serum albumin ($Q_A = [albumin_{CSF}]/[albumin_{serum}]$).

CSF drainage may decrease ICP by decreasing SCF volume. This is usually achieved by placement of a cerebral ventricular catheter, which can be used both to monitor ICP as well as drain CSF. The rate and volume of SCF drainage are controlled to avoid bleeding, ventricular collapse, and brain herniation due to rapid or excessive SCF drain. Surgical intervention may provide the most definitive therapy of increased ICP by removing blood clots or other mass-forming tissues. Acute change in neurologic status or level of consciousness may warrant surgical intervention in addition to other therapeutic measures aimed at decreasing ICP and improving CPP. Evacuation of acute epidural or cerebellar hematoma has been shown to improve outcome in TBI with raised ICP, but no such improvement has been shown consistently in ICH or subdural hematoma.[90]

Acute change in neurologic status or level of consciousness may warrant surgical intervention in addition to other therapeutic measures aimed at decreasing ICP and improving CPP. In cases of increased ICP that is refractory to medical treatment and is not associated with mass lesion, decompressive craniectomy may prevent transtentorial herniation, breaks the self-propagating cycle of increasing ICH and cerebral edema, and improves overall CPP. It may be performed as a hemicraniectomy when there is unilateral focal injury or as a bifrontal craniectomy when there is frontal injury or diffuse injury. Hemicraniectomy consists of removing large bone flaps from portions of the frontal, parietal, temporal, and occipital cranium to expose the middle cerebral fossa and open the dura. Bifrontal craniectomy consists of removing bilateral portions of the frontal bone following placement of bilateral bur holes in the posterior sagittal sinus, the root of the zygoma, and in the temporal region. The craniectomy is then extended posteriorly to the parietal bones several centimeters past the coronal sutures, and the sagittal sinus is then exposed and divided anteriorly to improve CSF and blood flow.

Brain Oxygenation Monitoring

Brain oxygenation monitoring has been used to guide management of ICP, MAP, and FiO$_2$. Systemic hypoxemia (PaO$_2$<50-60 mm Hg) is associated with systemic, including cerebral, vasodilation, which is a compensatory mechanism to increase oxygen delivery (DO$_2$) to body tissues, including the brain. Tissue hypoxia (PbtO$_2$<20 mm Hg) is definitely detrimental to cell function and survival.[91] On the other hand, high FiO$_2$ (>0.6) may lead to the generation of free radicals, which may cause cellular and mitochondrial injury, leading to decreased neuronal recovery.[92]

CEREBRAL HYPERPERFUSION SYNDROME

CHS is a hyperemic state characterized by cerebral edema, swelling, and/or hemorrhage that develops after the restoration of CBF to chronically hypoperfused areas. The ensuing cerebral swelling and hemorrhage cause neurologic dysfunction. It is most commonly seen after repair of AVM, carotid endarterectomy (CEA) or carotid artery stenting (CAS).

Cerebral Hyperperfusion Syndrome after Repair of Arteriovenous Malformation

CHS may occur in areas surrounding large AVMs that have chronic diversion of blood flow to them. These hyperperfused areas lose their ability to autoregulate blood flow and are usually maximally vasodilated. Following embolization or surgical repair of the AVM, the large amount of blood flow flowing through the previously hypoperfused AVM is now shunted back to these maximally dilated vessels, leading to cerebral hyperemia, edema, hemorrhage, or a combination.

Risk factors are preoperative ischemic symptoms of AVM and angiographic evidence of high or inverse flow in a large, deep, border-zone AVM. Preventive measures include strict control of blood flow through the AVM, deliberate hypotension, pretreatment with barbiturates, clamping of the cervical carotid artery, and staged embolization or surgical repair of the feeding vessels to allow the surrounding tissues to regain their autoregulatory function. Treatment is targeted toward the presenting symptoms and the underlying physiology; it may involve mechanical hyperventilation, osmotic diuresis, blood pressure control, and barbiturate coma.

Cerebral Hyperperfusion Syndrome after Carotid Endarterectomy

CHS is a rather rare (1.4%) complication of CEA.[93] It is likely due to failure of autoregulation of cerebral blood flow in cerebral arterioles that are maximally dilated preoperatively because of chronic hypoperfusion and that fail to constrict postoperatively when normal perfusion pressure is restored.[94] This hyperperfusion can lead to cerebral edema or hemorrhage with headache, seizures, decreased level of consciousness, and focal neurologic deficit. The overall incidence of intracranial hemorrhage among patients undergoing CEA ranges from 0.6% to 4.4%, but among patients with CHS it may be as high as 44%.[95] Onset of cerebral edema and intracranial hemorrhage after CEA or CAS ranges from immediately postprocedurally to 17 days postoperatively, with an average of 3 to 7 days.[96] Risk factors include severely (>90%) stenotic carotid artery, a history of hypertension and neurologic deficit, transcranial Doppler ultrasonography (TCD) peak flow velocities or pulsatility indices greater than 100%, intraoperative systemic blood pressure higher than 140 mm Hg, and poor collateral flow.[97,98] Prevention consists of careful intraoperative and postoperative control of blood pressure.

Mild elevation of blood pressure need not be treated in the postoperative period, whereas moderate to severe hypertension should be reduced. It is recommended to keep systemic blood pressure lower than 140 mm Hg in the first 48 hours after CEA or CAS.[99] Titratable, short-acting agents such as SNP and esmolol are preferable in this setting. The β-blocking effects of esmolol offset the sympathetic hyperactivity from SNP. Nitroglycerin is often used because it causes a less precipitous drop in blood pressure than SNP. Alternative agents are labetalol and nicardipine infusions. Intraoperative airway management using a laryngeal mask airway instead of an endotracheal tube has been suggested as a means of decreasing blood pressure lability during surgery.[100] Differential diagnosis of acute neurologic deficits after CEA or CAS should include CHS, intraparenchymal hemorrhage, cerebral edema, and ischemic stroke.

REFERENCES

1. Seppelt I: Intracranial hypertension after traumatic brain injury, *Indian J Crit Care Med* 8:120–126, 2004.
2. Helling T, Evans L, Fowler DL, et al: Infectious complications in patients with severe head injury, *J Trauma* 28:1575–1577, 1988.
3. Cardoso TC, Lopes LM, Carneiro AH: A case-control study on risk factors for early-onset respiratory tract infection in patients admitted in ICU, *BMC Pulm Med* 7:12, 2007.
4. DemLing R, Riessen R: Pulmonary dysfunction after cerebral injury, *Crit Care Med* 18:768–774, 1990.
5. Jia X, Malhotra A, Saeed M, et al: Risk factors for ARDS in patients receiving mechanical ventilation for > 48 h, *Chest* 133:853–861, 2008.
6. Baumann A, Audibert G, McDonnell J, Mertes PM: Neurogenic pulmonary edema, *Acta Anaesthesiol Scand* 51:447–455, 2007.
7. Inobe JJ, Mori T, Ueyama H, et al: Neurogenic pulmonary edema induced by primary medullary hemorrhage: A case report, *J Neurol Sci* 172:73–76, 2000.
8. Mertes PM, Beck B, Jaboin Y, et al: Microdialysis in the estimation of interstitial myocardial neuropeptide Y release, *Regul Pept* 49:81–90, 1993.
9. Lu YC, Liu S, Gong QZ, et al: Inhibition of nitric oxide synthase potentiates hypertension and increases mortality in traumatically brain-injured rats, *Mol Chem Neuropathol* 30:125–137, 1997.
10. Hachenberg T, Rettig R: Stress failure of the blood-gas barrier, *Curr Opin Anaesthesiol* 11:37–44, 1998.
11. Fisher AJ, Donnelly SC, Hirani N, et al: Elevated levels of interleukin-8 in donor lungs is associated with early graft failure after lung transplantation, *Am J Respir Crit Care Med* 16:259–265, 2001.
12. Grande PO, Asgeirsson B, Nordstrom CH: Volume-targeted therapy of increased intracranial pressure: The Lund concept unifies surgical and non-surgical treatments, *Acta Anaesthesiol Scand* 46:929–941, 2002.
13. Meaudre E, Polycarpe A, Pernod G, et al: Contribution of the brain natriuretic peptide in neurogenic pulmonary oedema following subarachnoid haemorrhage, *Ann Fr Anesth Reanim* 23:1076–1079, 2004.
14. Deehan SC, Grant IS: Haemodynamic changes in neurogenic pulmonary oedema: effect of dobutamine, *Intensive Care Med* 22:672–676, 1996.
15. Ríos-Romenets S, Castaño-Monsalve B, Bernabeu-Guitart M: Pharmacotherapy of the cognitive sequelae secondary to traumatic brain injury, *Rev Neurol* 45:563–570, 2007.
16. Neil-Dwyer G, Cruickshank JM, Doshi R: The stress response in subarachnoid haemorrhage and head injury, *Acta Neurochir Suppl (Wien)* 47:102–110, 1990.
17. McMahon CG, Kenny R, Bennett K, Kirkman E: Modification of acute cardiovascular homeostatic responses to hemorrhage following mild to moderate traumatic brain injury, *Crit Care Med* 36:216–224, 2008.
18. Ozdemir D, Ozdemir N, Unal N, Tektas S: QTc dispersion in children with severe head trauma, *Pediatr Emerg Care* 21:658–661, 2005.
19. Baguley IJ, Heriseanu RE, Felmingham KL, Cameron ID: Dysautonomia and heart rate variability following severe traumatic brain injury, *Brain Inj* 20:437–444, 2006.
20. Keren O, Yupatov S, Radai MM, et al: Heart rate variability (HRV) of patients with traumatic brain injury (TBI) during the post-insult subacute period, *Brain Inj* 19:605–611, 2005.
21. Hackenberry LE, Miner ME, Rea GL, et al: Biochemical evidence of myocardial injury after severe head trauma, *Crit Care Med* 10:641–644, 1982.
22. The Brain Trauma Foundation. The American Association of Neurological Surgeons. The Joint Section on Neurotrauma and Critical Care. Guidelines for cerebral perfusion pressure. *J Neurotrauma.* 2000 Jun-Jul;17(6-7):507-11.
23. Neil-Dwyer G, Cruickshank J, Stratton C: Beta-blockers, plasma total creatine kinase and creatine kinase myocardial isoenzyme, and the prognosis of subarachnoid hemorrhage, *Surg Neurol* 25:163–168, 1986.
24. Neil-Dwyer G, Walter P, Cruickshank JM, et al: Effect of propranolol and phentolamine on myocardial necrosis after subarachnoid hemorrhage, *Br Med J* 2:990–992, 1978.
25. Chesnut RM, Marshall LF, Klauber MR, et al: The role of secondary brain injury in determining outcome from severe head injury, *J Trauma* 34:216–222, 1993.
26. Finfer S, Bellomo R, Boyce N, et al: SAFE Study Investigators: A comparison of albumin and saline for fluid resuscitation in the intensive care unit, *N Engl J Med* 350:2247–2256, 2004.
27. Hébert PC, Wells G, Blajchman MA, et al: A multicenter, randomized, controlled clinical trial of transfusion requirements in critical care. Transfusion Requirements in Critical Care Investigators, Canadian Critical Care Trials Group [erratum in: N Engl J Med 1999;340:1056], *N Engl J Med* 340:409–417, 1999.
28. Kao SJ, Yeh DY, Chen HI: Clinical and pathological features of fat embolism with acute respiratory distress syndrome, *Clin Sci (Lond)* 113(6):Sep 85–279, 2007.
29. Igarashi M, Kita A, Nishikawa K, Nakayama M, Tsunoda K, Namiki A: Use of percutaneous cardiopulmonary support in catastrophic massive pulmonary fat embolism, *Br J Anaesth* 96:213–215, 2006.
30. Niwa T, Kawase M, Hasegawa S, Hasegawa R, Osanai H, Sakurai H: A case of fulminant fat embolism syndrome rescued by percutaneous cardiopulmonary support, *J Jpn Soc Intensive Care Med* 13:445–49, 2006.

31. Arai F, Kita T, Nakai T, et al: histopathologic features of fat embolism in fulminant fat embolism syndrome, *Anesthesiology* 107:509–511, 2007.

32. DeVivo MJ, Go BK, Jackson AB: Overview of the national spinal cord injury statistical center database, *J Spinal Cord Med* 25:335–338, 2002.

33. Duguet A, Demoule A, Gonzalez J, et al: Predicting the recovery of ventilatory activity in central respiratory paralysis, *Neurology* 67:288–292, 2006.

34. Rajajee V, Brown DM, Tuhrim S: Coagulation abnormalities following primary intracerebral hemorrhage, *J Stroke Cerebrovasc Dis* 13:47–51, 2004.

35. Levi M: Disseminated intravascular coagulation, *Crit Care Med* 35:2191–2195, 2007.

36. Gando S, Iba T, Eguchi Y, Ohtomo Y, Okamoto K, Koseki K, Mayumi T, Murata A, Ikeda T, Ishikura H, Ueyama M, Ogura H, Kushimoto S, Saitoh D, Endo S, Shimazaki S; Japanese Association for Acute Medicine Disseminated Intravascular Coagulation (JAAM DIC) Study Group. A multicenter, prospective validation of disseminated intravascular coagulation diagnostic criteria for critically ill patients: comparing current criteria. *Crit Care Med* 2006 Mar; 34(3):625–31.

37. Robertson CS, Clifton GL, Grossman RG: Oxygen utilization and cardiovascular function in head-injured patients, *Neurosurgery* 15:307–314, 1984.

38. Weekes E, Elia M: Observations on the patterns of 24-hour energy expenditure changes in body composition and gastric emptying in head-injured patients receiving nasogastric tube feeding, *JPEN J Parenter Enteral Nutr* 20:31–37, 1996.

39. Robertson GL, Shelton RL, Athar S: The osmoregulation of vasopressin, *Kidney Int* 10:25–37, 1976.

40. Hatton J, Kryscio R, Ryan M, et al: Systemic metabolic effects of combined insulin-like growth factor-I and growth hormone therapy in patients who have sustained acute traumatic brain injury, *J Neurosurg* 6:843–852, 2006.

41. Brain Trauma Foundation; American Association of Neurological Surgeons; Congress of Neurological Surgeons; Joint Section on Neurotrauma and Critical Care, AANS/CNS, Bratton SL, Chestnut RM, Ghajar J, et al: Guidelines for the management of severe traumatic brain injury: XII: Nutrition, *J Neurotrauma* 24(Suppl 1):S77–S82, 2007.

42. Heyland DK, Dhaliwal R, et al: Canadian Critical Care Clinical Practice Guidelines Committee: Canadian clinical practice guidelines for nutrition support in mechanically ventilated, critically ill adult patients, *JPEN J Parenter Enteral Nutr* 27:355–373, 2003.

43. Jackson MD, Davidoff G: Gastroparesis following traumatic brain injury and response to metoclopramide therapy, *Arch Phys Med Rehabil* 70:535–553, 1989.

44. Grahm TW, Zadrozny DB, Harrington T: The benefits of early jejunal hyperalimentation in the head-injured patient, *Neurosurgery* 25:729–735, 1989.

45. Sholkina MN, Lebedev MY, Babaev AA, et al: Effect of brain injury on immunophenotype of peripheral blood lymphocytes in rats, *Russ J Immunol* 7:365–470, 2002.

46. Woiciechowsky C, Volk HD: Increased intracranial pressure induces a rapid systemic interleukin-10 release through activation of the sympathetic nervous system, *Acta Neurochir Suppl* 95:373–376, 2005.

47. Tehranian R, Andell-Jonsson S, Beni SM, et al: Improved recovery and delayed cytokine induction after closed head injury in mice with central overexpression of the secreted isoform of the interleukin-1 receptor antagonist, *J Neurotrauma* 19:939–951, 2002.

48. Hashiguchi N, Shiozaki T, Ogura H, Tanaka H, Koh T, Noborio M, Fugita K, Akimau P, Kuwagata Y, Shimazu T, Sugimoto H: Mild hypothermia reduces expression of heat shock protein 60 in leukocytes from severely head-injured patients. *J Trauma* 2003 Dec; 55(6):1054–60.

49. Bhalla A, Tilling K, Kolominsky-Rabas P, et al: Variation in the management of acute physiological parameters after ischaemic stroke: A European perspective, *Eur J Neurol* 10:25–33, 2003.

50. Walia S, Sutcliffe AJ: The relationship between blood glucose, mean arterial pressure and outcome after severe head injury: An observational study, *Injury* 33:339–344, 2002.

51. Jeremitsky E, Omert LA, Dunham CM, et al: The impact of hyperglycemia on patients with severe brain injury, *J Trauma* 58:47–50, 2005.

52. Baird TA, Parsons MW, Phanh T, et al: Persistent poststroke hyperglycemia is independently associated with infarct expansion and worse clinical outcome, *Stroke* 34:2208–2214, 2003.

53. Bruno A, Levine SR, Frankel MR, et al: NINDS rt-PA Stroke Study Group: Admission glucose level and clinical outcomes in the NINDS rt-PA Stroke Trial, *Neurology* 59:669–674, 2002.

54. Rovlias A, Kotsou S: The influence of hyperglycemia on neurological outcome in patients with severe head injury, *Neurosurgery* 46:335–342, 2000.

55. Van den Berghe G, Wilmer A, Hermans G, et al: Intensive insulin therapy in the medical ICU, *N Engl J Med* 354:449–461, 2006.

56. Mattson DL: Importance of the renal medullary circulation in the control of sodium excretion and blood pressure, *J Physiol Regul Integr Comp Physiol* 284:R13–R27, 2003.

57. Leal-Cerro A, Flores JM, Rincon M, et al: Prevalence of hypopituitarism and growth hormone deficiency in adults long-term after severe traumatic brain injury, *Clin Endocrinol (Oxf)* 62:525–532, 2005.

58. Tanriverdi F, Senyurek H, Unluhizarci K, et al: High risk of hypopituitarism after traumatic brain injury: A prospective investigation of anterior pituitary function in the acute phase and 12 months after trauma, *J Clin Endocrinol Metab* 91:2105–2111, 2006.

59. Agha A, Rogers B, Sherlock M, et al: Anterior pituitary dysfunction in survivors of traumatic brain injury, *J Clin Endocrinol Metab* 89:4929–4936, 2004.

60. Barton RN, Stoner HB, Watson SM: Relationships among plasma cortisol, adrenocorticotrophin, and severity of injury in recently injured patients, *J Trauma* 27:384–892, 1987.

61. Feibel J, Kelly M, Lee L, Woolf P: Loss of adrenocortical suppression after acute brain injury: Role of increased intracranial pressure and brain stem function, *J Clin Endocrinol Metab* 57:1245–1250, 1983.

62. Dimopoulou I, Tsagarakis S, Douka E, et al: The low-dose corticotropin stimulation test in acute traumatic and non-traumatic brain injury: Incidence of hypo-responsiveness and relationship to outcome, *Intensive Care Med* 30:1216–1219, 2004.

63. Tsagarakis S, Tzanela M, Dimopoulou I: Diabetes insipidus, secondary hypoadrenalism and hypothyroidism after traumatic brain injury: Clinical implications, *Pituitary* 8:251–254, 2005.

64. Novitzky D, Matthews N, Shawley D: Triiodothyronine replacement on the recovery of stunned myocardium in dogs, *Ann Thorac Surg* 51:10–17, 1991.

65. Toogood AA, Stewart PM: Hypopituitarism: Clinical features, diagnosis, and management, *Endocrinol Metab Clin N Am* 37:235–261, 2008:x.

66. Girou E, Brun-Buisson C, Taillé S, et al: Secular trends in nosocomial infections and mortality associated with noninvasive ventilation in patients with exacerbation of COPD and pulmonary edema, *JAMA* 290:2985–2991, 2003.

67. Hugonnet S, Sax H, Eggimann P, Chevrolet JC, Pittet D: Nosocomial bloodstream infection and clinical sepsis. *Emerg Infect Dis* 2004 Jan; 10(1):76–81.

68. Jones PA, Andrews PJ, Midgley S, et al: Measuring the burden of secondary insults in head-injured patients during intensive care, *J Neurosurg Anesthesiol* 6:4–14, 1994.

69. Pietropaoli JA, Rogers FB, Shackford SR, et al: The deleterious effects of intraoperative hypotension on outcome in patients with severe head injuries, *J Trauma* 33:403–407, 1992.

70. Sarrafzadeh AS, Peltonen EE, Kaisers U, et al: Secondary insults in severe head injury—do multiply injured patients do worse? *Crit Care Med* 29:1116–1123, 2001.

71. Rahimi SY, Vender JR, Macomson SD, et al: Postoperative pain management after craniotomy: Evaluation and cost analysis, *Neurosurgery* 59:852–857, 2006.

72. De Benedittis G, Lorenzetti A, Migliore M, et al: Postoperative pain in neurosurgery: A pilot study in brain surgery, *Neurosurgery* 38:466–469, 1996.

73. Arain SR, Ruehlow RM, Uhrich TD, Ebert TJ: The efficacy of dexmedetomidine versus morphine for postoperative analgesia after major inpatient surgery, *Anesth Analg* 98:153–158, 2004.

74. Belopavlovic M, Buchthal A: Modification of ketamine-induced intracranial hypertension in neurosurgical patients by pretreatment with midazolam, *Acta Anaesthesiol Scand* 26:458–462, 1982.

75. Crosby G, Crane AM, Sokoloff L: Local changes in cerebral glucose utilization during ketamine anesthesia, *Anesthesiology* 56:437–443, 1982.

76. Ayoub C, Girard F, Boudreault D, et al: A comparison between scalp nerve block and morphine for transitional analgesia after remifentanil-based anesthesia in neurosurgery, *Anesth Analg* 103:1237–1240, 2006.

77. Bala I, Gupta B, Bhardwaj N, et al: Effect of scalp block on postoperative pain relief in craniotomy patients, *Anaesth Intensive Care* 34:224–227, 2006.

78. Kofke WA, Stiefel M: Monitoring and intraoperative management of elevated intracranial pressure and decompressive craniectomy, *Anesthesiol Clin* 25:579–603, 2007.

79. Cremer OL, van Dijk GW, van Wensen E, Brekelmans GJ, Moons KG, Leenen LP, Kalkman CJ: Effect of intracranial pressure monitoring and targeted intensive care on functional outcome after severe head injury. *Crit Care Med* 2005 Oct; 33(10):2207–13.

80. Muizelaar JP, Marmarou A, Ward JD, et al: Adverse effects of prolonged hyperventilation in patients with severe head injury: A randomized clinical trial, *J Neurosurg* 75:731–739, 1991.

81. Kofke WA, Attaallah AF, Kuwabara H, et al: The neuropathologic effects in rats and neurometabolic effects in humans of large-dose remifentanil, *Anesth Analg* 94:1229–1236, 2002.

82. Kofke WA, Garman RH, Garman R, Rose ME: Opioid neurotoxicity: Fentanyl-induced exacerbation of cerebral ischemia in rats, *Brain Res* 818:326–334, 1999.

83. Lescot T, Degos V, Zouaoui A, et al: Opposed effects of hypertonic saline on contusions and noncontused brain tissue in patients with severe traumatic brain injury, *Crit Care Med* 34:3029–3033, 2006.

84. Qureshi AI, Suarez JI, Bhardwaj A, et al: Use of hypertonic (3%) saline/acetate infusion in the treatment of cerebral edema: Effect on intracranial pressure and lateral displacement of the brain, *Crit Care Med* 26:440–446, 1998.

85. Tseng MY, Al-Rawi PG, Pickard JD, et al: Effect of hypertonic saline on cerebral blood flow in poor-grade patients with subarachnoid hemorrhage, *Stroke* 34:1389–1396, 2003.

86. Schwarz S, Schwab S, Bertram M, et al: Effects of hypertonic saline hydroxyethyl starch solution and mannitol in patients with increased intracranial pressure after stroke, *Stroke* 29:1550–1555, 1998.

87. Vialet R, Albanèse J, Thomachot L, et al: Isovolume hypertonic solutes (sodium chloride or mannitol) in the treatment of refractory posttraumatic intracranial hypertension: 2 mL/kg 7.5% saline is more effective than 2 mL/kg 20% mannitol, *Crit Care Med* 31:1683–1687, 2003.

88. Horn P, Münch E, Vajkoczy P, et al: Hypertonic saline solution for control of elevated intracranial pressure in patients with exhausted response to mannitol and barbiturates, *Neurol Res* 21:758–764, 1999.

89. Suarez JI, Qureshi AI, Bhardwaj A, et al: Treatment of refractory intracranial hypertension with 23.4% saline, *Crit Care Med* 26:1118–1122, 1998.

90. Manno EM, Atkinson JL, Fulgham JR, Wijdicks EF: Emerging medical and surgical management strategies in the evaluation and treatment of intracerebral hemorrhage, *Mayo Clin Proc* 80:420–433, 2005.

91. van den Brink WA, van Santbrink H, Steyerberg EW, et al: Brain oxygen tension in severe head injury, *Neurosurgery* 46:868–876, 2000.

92. Fiskum G, Rosenthal RE, Vereczki V, et al: Protection against ischemic brain injury by inhibition of mitochondrial oxidative stress, *J Bioenerg Biomembr* 36:347–352, 2004.

93. Ogasawara K, Sakai N, Kuroiwa T, et al: Japanese Society for Treatment at Neck in Cerebrovascular Disease Study Group: Intracranial hemorrhage associated with cerebral hyperperfusion syndrome following carotid endarterectomy and carotid artery stenting: Retrospective review of 4494 patients, *J Neurosurg* 107:1130–1136, 2007.

94. Schroeder T, Sillesen H, Engell HC: Hemodynamic effect of carotid endarterectomy, *Stroke* 18:204–209, 1987.

95. Morrish W, Grahovac S, Douen A, et al: Intracranial hemorrhage after stenting and angioplasty of extracranial carotid stenosis, *AJNR Am J Neuroradiol* 21:1911–1916, 2000.

96. Sundt TM Jr: The ischemic tolerance of neural tissue and the need for monitoring and selective shunting during carotid endarterectomy, *Stroke* 14:93–98, 1983.

97. Abou-Chebl A, Reginelli J, Bajzer CT, Yadav JS: Intensive treatment of hypertension decreases the risk of hyperperfusion and intracerebral hemorrhage following carotid artery stenting, *Catheter Cardiovasc Interv* 69:690–696, 2007.

98. Torgovnick J, Sethi N, Arsura E: Cerebral hyperperfusion syndrome occurring three weeks after carotid endarterectomy, *Rev Bras Cir Cardiovasc* 22:116–118, 2007.

99. Cheung AT, Hobson RW 2nd: Hypertension in vascular surgery: Aortic dissection and carotid revascularization, *Ann Emerg Med* 51(Suppl) S28–S33, 2008.

100. Marietta DR, Lunn JK, Ruby EI, Hill GE: Cardiovascular stability during carotid endarterectomy: Endotracheal intubation versus laryngeal mask airway, *J Clin Anesth* 10:54–57, 1998.

Chapter 23

ANESTHESIA FOR NEUROSURGERY IN THE PREGNANT PATIENT

David J. Wlody • Lela Weems

Neurologic disorders requiring surgical intervention during pregnancy are surprisingly common, and most anesthesiologists eventually encounter a pregnant woman with such a disorder. The anesthetic management of these patients can be complicated by the significant maternal physiologic changes that occur during pregnancy. These changes may require alterations in anesthetic management that would be considered inappropriate for a nonpregnant patient with the same neurosurgical condition.

Additionally, although maternal considerations must remain our primary concern, it is important to recognize that interventions that benefit the mother might have the potential for harming the fetus. Thus, the major challenge in providing anesthesia for neurosurgery performed during pregnancy is to provide an appropriate balance between competing, or even contradictory, clinical goals.

In this chapter we discuss the anesthetic management of pregnant women undergoing resection of intracranial neoplasms, aneurysm clipping, and resection of arteriovenous malformations (AVMs). There is also a brief discussion of the management of spontaneous spinal epidural hematoma. Finally, we consider the small but growing experience in the use of interventional neuroradiology techniques for the management of neurovascular disease in pregnancy. Because the anesthetic management of these procedures is discussed elsewhere in this book, this chapter deals primarily with the ways the anesthetic management is altered by pregnancy.

MATERNAL PHYSIOLOGIC ALTERATIONS DURING PREGNANCY

Pregnancy is associated with changes in structure and function in nearly every organ system. The following discussion deals with those changes that are most pertinent to the anesthetic management of women undergoing surgery, particularly intracranial neurosurgery.

Nervous System

Inhalation Anesthetic Requirements

The minimum alveolar concentration (MAC) for inhalation anesthetics is decreased by approximately 30% during pregnancy, a change that occurs as early as the first trimester.[1,2] This change has been postulated to be a result of higher levels of circulating endorphins.[3] Alternatively, an increase in the concentration of progesterone, a hormone with known sedative effects, might account for the diminished anesthetic requirement.[4] As a result of the pregnant patient's greater sensitivity to inhalation anesthetics, inspired anesthetic concentrations that would be appropriate in nonpregnant patients can lead to severe cardiopulmonary depression during pregnancy.

Local Anesthetic Requirements

Local anesthetic requirements for neuraxial anesthesia are decreased by 30% to 40% during pregnancy. This reduction is in part due to the decreased volume of cerebrospinal fluid (CSF) in the lumbar subarachnoid space secondary to engorgement of the epidural veins.[5] The decrease in local anesthetic requirements predates the onset of significant epidural venous engorgement, however. In vitro preparations of vagus nerves obtained from pregnant rabbits show increased sensitivity to local anesthetic–induced blockade of nerve conduction.[6] When nerves obtained from nonpregnant rabbits are bathed in a progesterone-containing solution, however, this greater sensitivity is not seen.[7] It is therefore suggested that long-term but not short-term exposure to progesterone leads to changes in the neuronal membrane Na^+ channel that increase its sensitivity to local anesthetics.

Respiratory System

Upper Airway Mucosal Edema

The accumulation of extracellular fluid produces soft tissue edema during pregnancy, particularly in the upper airway, where marked mucosal friability can develop. Nasotracheal intubation and the insertion of nasogastric tubes should be avoided unless absolutely necessary because of the risk of significant epistaxis. Laryngeal edema can also reduce the size of the glottic aperture, leading to difficult intubation; this problem can be significantly enhanced in preeclampsia. A 6.0-mm endotracheal tube is therefore appropriate for most pregnant patients.

Functional Residual Capacity

Functional residual capacity (FRC) decreases by as much as 20% by the end of the third trimester, whereas closing capacity remains unchanged.[8] The FRC drops further in the supine position, a situation in which closing capacity commonly exceeds FRC. This decrease leads to closure of small airways, increased shunt fraction, and a greater potential for arterial desaturation. Additionally, because FRC represents the store of oxygen available during a period of apnea, decreases in FRC can be expected to lead to the more rapid development of hypoxemia when a patient becomes apneic, as occurs during the induction of anesthesia. Because oxygen consumption rises by as much as 60% during pregnancy,[9] significant desaturation can occur even when intubation is performed expeditiously. This process was demonstrated in a computer model of pregnancy in which apnea was simulated after 99% denitrogenation. Desaturation to 90% occurred in approximately 5 minutes in the pregnant model, versus 7.5 minutes in the nonpregnant model.[10] Thus, at least 2 minutes of preoxygenation and denitrogenation with a tightly fitting face mask is mandatory before the induction of general anesthesia during pregnancy.[11]

Ventilation

Significant increases in minute ventilation occur as early as the end of the first trimester. At term, minute ventilation increases by 45%, owing to an increase in tidal volume; respiratory rate is essentially unchanged.[12] It is postulated that this increase occurs due to a progesterone-induced increase in the ventilatory response to carbon dioxide (CO_2); there also appears to be an effect due to pregnancy-induced changes in wakefulness.[13] Because the increase in ventilation exceeds the increase in CO_2 production, the normal arterial partial pressure of CO_2 (Pa_{CO_2}) diminishes to approximately 32 mm Hg. The greater renal excretion of bicarbonate partially compensates for the hypocarbia, so that pH rises only slightly, to approximately 7.42 to 7.44.

Cardiovascular System

Blood Volume

Blood volume increases by 45% during pregnancy,[14] with the majority of this increase occurring by the end of the second trimester. Because plasma volume increases to a greater extent than red blood cell mass, a dilutional anemia commonly occurs. Normal hematocrit at term ranges from 30% to 35% and is often lower in women not receiving supplemental iron.

Cardiac Output

Significant increases in cardiac output (CO) occur as early as the first trimester. Capeless and Clapp[15] demonstrated a 22% rise in CO by 8 weeks' gestation, which represents 57% of the total change seen at 24 weeks.[15] Cardiac output rises steadily throughout the second trimester. After 24 weeks, CO remains stable or increases slightly. Older studies demonstrating a decrease in CO in the third trimester reflect measurements made in the supine position with consequent aortocaval compression. At term, cardiac output is approximately 50% above pre-pregnancy baseline.[16]

Cardiac output can increase by an additional 60% during labor.[17] Part of this increase is caused by the pain and apprehension associated with contractions, an increase that can be blunted with the provision of adequate analgesia. There is a further rise in CO, unaffected by analgesia, from the autotransfusion of 300 to 500 mL of blood from the uterus into the central circulation with each contraction. Finally, CO increases further in the immediate postpartum period, by as much as 80% above pre-labor values, because of autotransfusion from the rapidly involuting uterus as well as the augmentation of preload secondary to alleviation of the aortocaval compression.

Aortocaval Compression

When a woman assumes the supine position after 20 weeks' gestation, the enlarged uterus can compress the inferior vena cava against the vertebral column. Collateral flow through the epidural venous plexus and paravertebral vessels can partially compensate for decreased caval blood flow, but the net return of blood to the heart can be significantly decreased, leading to reduced CO. This result has the potential for decreasing uterine blood flow (UBF) to a level that can impair uteroplacental oxygen delivery. Supine positioning may also produce aortic compression. If this occurs, upper extremity blood pressure might be normal but distal aortic pressure and thus uterine artery perfusion pressure will be significantly decreased. Because both regional and general anesthetics reduce venous return, the effects of aortocaval compression will be magnified in the anesthetized patient. Therefore, the supine position must be avoided in pregnant patients undergoing anesthesia after the mid-second trimester. Tilting the operating table 30 degrees to the left or placing a roll under the patient's right hip will prevent significant aortocaval compression.

Gastrointestinal System

Gastric Acid Production

Ectopic gastrin is produced by the placenta. However, plasma gastrin levels appear to be unchanged during pregnancy, and there appears to be no significant difference in either the volume or the acidity of gastric secretions in pregnancy.[18,19]

Gastric Emptying

Contrary to common belief, gastric emptying is not significantly altered during pregnancy.[20] With the onset of painful contractions, however, gastric emptying is slowed. Systemic opioids administered during labor will have a similar effect.

Gastroesophageal Sphincter

The enlarging uterus causes elevation and rotation of the stomach, which interfere with the pinchcock mechanism of the gastroesophageal sphincter. This change increases the likelihood of gastroesophageal reflux.

Pregnancy and Aspiration Pneumonia

The changes described make it more likely that a pregnant patient will regurgitate and aspirate during anesthesia. The time frame for the development of these changes is unclear, but most anesthesiologists begin to use "full stomach" precautions between the end of the first trimester and the mid-second trimester, by which time uterine growth is such that alterations of gastroesophageal structure and function are likely to occur. Pregnant patients should therefore receive aspiration prophylaxis with either a nonparticulate antacid or a combination of a histamine H_2 blocking drug and metoclopramide. Anesthetic induction is influenced by the presence of a full stomach but, as described later, techniques designed to minimize the risk of aspiration might not be ideal for the patient who has an intracranial lesion.

Renal and Hepatic Systems

Aldosterone levels rise during pregnancy, with concomitant increases in total body sodium and water.[21] These changes can increase edema in an intracranial neoplasm and lead either to worsening signs and symptoms or to the onset of symptoms from a previously unrecognized mass lesion. Renal blood flow and glomerular filtration rate increase by approximately 60% at term, paralleling the increase in CO. Thus, blood urea nitrogen (BUN) and serum creatinine values are usually one half to

417

two thirds those seen in nonpregnant women.[22] What would be considered normal or only mildly elevated BUN and creatinine values in nonpregnant women should be a cause for concern during pregnancy.

Slight increases in serum levels of alanine aminotransferase (ALT), aspartate transaminase (AST), and lactate dehydrogenase (LDH) are not uncommon during normal pregnancy.[23] Plasma cholinesterase levels are decreased, but prolonged neuromuscular blockade does not occur in normal parturients receiving succinylcholine.[24]

Epidural Vascular Changes

Epidural Venous Pressure

A generalized increase in intra-abdominal pressure as well as direct compression of the inferior vena cava leads to a rise in epidural venous pressure. It has been suggested that elevated epidural venous pressure, in association with the hemodynamic changes of pregnancy, may predispose to rupture of a preexisting pathology of the venous wall. Epidural veins contain no valves; therefore, abrupt pressure changes, such as produced by coughing, sneezing, or a forceful Valsalva maneuver during the second stage of labor, could be transmitted directly to the epidural veins, causing rupture.[25]

Epidural Arterial Vessels

The epidural arterial vessels may undergo degenerative changes during pregnancy secondary to elevations of progesterone and estrogen.[26] The arterial vessels of pregnant women have been shown to demonstrate numerous histologic changes, including fragmentation of the reticulin fibers, diminished acid mucopolysaccharide concentration, and hypertrophy and hyperplasia of smooth muscle cells.[25] These structural changes, in combination with the hemodynamic changes of pregnancy, may predispose to rupture of an epidural artery and subsequent hematoma formation.

EFFECTS OF ANESTHETIC INTERVENTIONS ON UTERINE BLOOD FLOW

At term, normal UBF is approximately 700 mL/min, which is approximately 10% of total maternal blood flow.[27] The magnitude of UBF is determined by the following equation:

$$UBF = (UAP - UVP)/UVR$$

where *UAP* is uterine arterial pressure, *UVP* is the uterine venous pressure, and *UVR* is the uterine vascular resistance. Alterations in any of these parameters influence UBF and, therefore, the delivery of oxygen and nutrients to the fetus.

Factors that *decrease uterine arterial pressure* include hypovolemia, sympathetic blockade due to neuraxial anesthesia, aortocaval compression, anesthetic overdose, vasodilators, and excessive positive pressure ventilation. Factors that *increase uterine venous pressure* include vena caval compression, uterine contractions, uterine hypertonus, oxytocin overstimulation, and α-adrenergic stimulation, through adrenergically mediated increases in uterine tone. Factors that *increase uterine vascular resistance* include endogenous catecholamines, untreated pain or noxious stimulation (laryngoscopy and intubation, skin incision), preeclampsia, chronic hypertension, and exogenous vasoconstrictors.

Ephedrine has been considered the drug of choice for treating maternal hypotension, largely on the basis of animal studies showing decreases in UBF despite increased maternal blood pressure after the administration of high doses of pure α-adrenergic agonists.[28] This finding has been interpreted to indicate that uterine vascular resistance is increased to a greater extent than maternal blood pressure when these agents are used. However, later studies using low doses of phenylephrine (50-100 µg) show no evidence of any deleterious effect on fetal well-being.[29,30] Furthermore, there is a growing body of evidence that fetal well-being is in fact *improved* when phenylephrine is used to treat maternal hypotension.[31,32] The reasons for this improvement are unclear, but it has been proposed that transplacental passage of ephedrine leads to increases in fetal metabolism, resulting in a perhaps clinically insignificant, but nevertheless measurable fetal metabolic acidosis when compared to phenylephrine.

UTEROPLACENTAL DRUG TRANSFER AND TERATOGENESIS

A detailed consideration of the various mechanisms (active transport, facilitated diffusion, pinocytosis) by which substances are transported across the placenta is beyond the scope of this chapter.[33] This discussion concentrates on *passive diffusion,* the mechanism by which most anesthetic drugs administered to the mother reach the fetus. This process does not require the expenditure of energy. Transfer can occur either directly through the lipid membrane or through protein channels that traverse the lipid bilayer.

Determinants of Passive Diffusion

Concentration gradient is the primary determinant of the rate of transfer of drugs across the placenta. As an example, the initial rate of transfer of an inhalation anesthetic is quite rapid. As the partial pressure of the drug increases in the fetus, the rate of transfer decreases. Substances that have a low molecular weight cross the placenta more readily than those that have a higher molecular weight. Drugs with high lipid solubility readily traverse the placenta. Ionization limits placental transfer. Membrane thickness can be increased in certain pathologic states, including chronic hypertension and diabetes. The effects of these conditions on drug transfer are of less concern than the resultant limitation of the transport of oxygen and nutrients, which can lead to intrauterine growth restriction or, in severe cases, fetal demise.

Specific Drugs

The inhalation anesthetics cross the placenta freely owing to their low molecular weight and high lipid solubility. The longer the period of fetal exposure to the drug (induction-to-delivery interval), the more likely the newborn is to be depressed.

The induction drugs, thiopental, etomidate, and propofol are highly lipophilic and un-ionized at physiologic pH. Placental transfer is quite rapid. Because most of the blood returning to the fetus from the umbilical vein passes through the fetal liver, extensive first-pass metabolism occurs and neonatal depression after an induction dose of these drugs is uncommon. Some studies suggest that newborn depression is more common with propofol than with thiopental.[34]

Both depolarizing and nondepolarizing muscle relaxants are highly ionized at physiologic pH. Placental transfer is minimal.

The opioids freely traverse the placenta because of their high lipid solubility and low molecular weight.

The muscle relaxant reversal drugs neostigmine and edrophonium are highly ionized and demonstrate minimal placental transfer.

The anticholinergic drugs atropine and scopolamine freely pass the placenta. Glycopyrrolate is highly ionized and thus crosses the placenta to a minimal degree.

The commonly used anticoagulants heparin and warfarin have remarkably different placental transfer characteristics. Heparin, a highly ionized polysaccharide molecule, does not reach the fetus. Warfarin, which is uncharged and has a molecular weight of only 330, readily passes across the placenta. Because warfarin can cause birth defects, its use is contraindicated during the period of organogenesis (see later).

Of the antihypertensive drugs, all of the β-blocking drugs that have been studied cross the placenta. Labetalol, which is both effective for the mother and safe for the fetus, is the drug of choice for treatment of maternal hypertension.[35] High-dose infusions of esmolol have been reported to cause persistent fetal bradycardia lasting up to 30 minutes after the termination of the infusion.[36] The effect of a single dose is not known, but there are numerous case reports of its safe use as a bolus during anesthetic induction. Sodium nitroprusside (SNP) freely passes the placenta, a characteristic that has implications for fetal toxicity (see later).

Anesthesia during Pregnancy and the Risk of Birth Defects

Principles of Teratology

It is an established principle that any substance, if administered in large enough quantities for a prolonged period of time during critical periods of gestation, can produce fetal injury ranging from growth restriction to major structural anomalies to death. Thus, it should be a goal of anesthesiologists caring for pregnant women to minimize the exposure of their fetuses to potentially toxic substances. Nevertheless, our fears regarding the potential for injury should be tempered by the following considerations:

- Most anesthetics are administered for such a brief period that the potential for toxicity is minimal.
- There is no convincing *human* evidence that any of the commonly used anesthetics is dangerous to the fetus.
- Maternal hypotension and hypoxemia pose a much greater risk to the fetus than any of the anesthetic drugs.
- Maternal well-being must be our paramount concern. If avoiding a potentially teratogenic drug leads to a poor maternal outcome or maternal death, fetal outcome will be equally compromised.

Evaluation of Teratogenic Potential

Because of the ethical and logistical difficulties inherent in large-scale prospective studies of the teratogenic effects of anesthetics in humans, we must rely on more indirect evidence to evaluate the teratogenic potential of these drugs. The principal investigative tools used are small animal studies, retrospective studies of the offspring of women who received anesthesia during pregnancy, and, in the case of inhalation anesthetics, studies of operating room personnel who were exposed to low-level waste anesthetic gases during pregnancy. In the discussion of specific drugs that follows, reference is made to the studies supporting or opposing their teratogenic potential.

Specific Anesthetic Drugs

Animal studies of the potent inhalation anesthetics have demonstrated conflicting results.[37-40] Their reproductive effects appear to be dose-related. These effects are more likely to be from the physiologic disturbances (hypothermia, hypoventilation, poor feeding) produced by the anesthetic state rather than the anesthetic drug itself. When animals are exposed to inspired concentrations of inhalational anesthetics that do not impair feeding behavior or level of consciousness, reproductive effects are minimal.[41]

Nitrous oxide has clearly been shown to increase the incidence of structural abnormalities and fetal loss in rats; the timing of exposure appears to determine the extent of the effect.[42,43] This effect was initially thought to be the result of inhibition of the enzyme methionine synthetase and subsequent decreases in the levels of methionine and tetrahydrofolate.[44] The mechanism has been called into question, however, because maximal inhibition of methionine synthetase activity occurs at levels of anesthetic exposure that do not have teratogenic effects. Later evidence suggests that the fetal effects of nitrous oxide are from α-adrenergic stimulation and subsequent decreases in UBF.[45] These effects can be reversed by the simultaneous administration of a potent inhalation drug. Studies of operating room personnel exposed to trace levels of nitrous oxide and of women receiving nitrous oxide anesthesia have not shown any teratogenic effect. The reader is referred to the detailed reviews by Burm[46] and Weimann[47] of the reproductive toxicology of nitrous oxide.

Muscle relaxants do not have any teratogenic effect at clinically appropriate doses. Opioids have not been shown to be teratogenic in either human or animal studies.

Several retrospective human studies have suggested that long-term benzodiazepine therapy during pregnancy increases the incidence of cleft lip and cleft palate.[48,49] These studies have been faulted for failure to control for concomitant exposure to other potentially teratogenic substances. There is little evidence to suggest that a single dose of a benzodiazepine during pregnancy poses any risk to the fetus.[50-52]

There is no human evidence suggesting that clinically useful local anesthetics are teratogenic. Chronic cocaine abuse has been linked to birth defects.

Warfarin therapy during pregnancy has been correlated with ophthalmologic, skeletal, and central nervous system abnormalities, presumably from microhemorrhages during organogenesis. Because heparin does not cross the placenta, it is the drug of choice in women requiring anticoagulation during pregnancy.

EPIDEMIOLOGY OF INTRACRANIAL DISEASE IN PREGNANCY AND THE EFFECT OF PREGNANCY ON INTRACRANIAL DISEASE

Subarachnoid Hemorrhage: Aneurysm and Arteriovenous Malformation

There are numerous causes for subarachnoid hemorrhage (SAH) during pregnancy, including hypertensive intracerebral hemorrhage, vasculitis, and bacterial endocarditis, but by far the most common are aneurysmal rupture and bleeding from an AVM. The overall incidence of SAH during pregnancy is approximately 1 in 10,000,[53] which is similar to the incidence in the general population. The 2003-2005 Confidential Enquiry into Maternal Deaths in the United Kingdom indicates that approximately 4% of total maternal deaths, and 7% of indirect (i.e., nonobstetric) deaths, were secondary to SAH.[54]

In 1990, Dias and Sekhar[55] published a review of 154 published cases of SAH during pregnancy. The ratio of aneurysms to AVMs was approximately 3:1. There was no link between increasing parity and the incidence of hemorrhage. For both AVMs and aneurysms, there was a rising incidence of hemorrhage with advancing gestational age, which may be due to increases in cardiac output or, possibly, from hormonal influences on vascular integrity. Interestingly, few of the women bled during labor and delivery, a finding consistent with the observation that more than 90% of all hemorrhages in nonpregnant patients occur at rest. Thirty-four percent of the patients whose rupture occurred during labor and delivery had hypertension, proteinuria, or both, suggesting that the differentiation between SAH and preeclampsia may be difficult on clinical grounds alone.

Neoplastic Lesions

The incidence of intracranial neoplasms does not appear to be appreciably different in pregnant and nonpregnant women. However, as mentioned previously, some tumors appear to grow more rapidly or become symptomatic during pregnancy. The reason may be an increase either in peritumoral edema secondary to increased sodium and water retention, or increased blood volume in vascular tumors such as meningiomas.

There is considerable evidence that hormonal influences affect the growth of brain tumors, particularly meningiomas. As early as 1958, a relationship among the menstrual cycle, pregnancy, and symptomatology of meningioma was identified.[56] The incidence of meningioma is higher in women than in men but decreases significantly after menopause, particularly when surgically induced by oophorectomy.[57] Progesterone receptors have been identified in meningiomas[58]; in vitro growth of human astrocytoma cell lines is enhanced by progesterone.[59] Therefore, accelerated tumor growth during pregnancy is likely due, at least in part, to hormonal stimulation.

MANAGEMENT OF ANESTHESIA FOR CRANIOTOMY DURING PREGNANCY

Timing of Surgery in Relation to Delivery

General Concerns

Whenever craniotomy during pregnancy is contemplated, the physicians caring for the pregnant woman must decide whether the pregnancy will be allowed to proceed to term or whether simultaneous operative delivery will occur. The choice is determined by the gestational age of the fetus, with 32 weeks commonly used as the cutoff. Before this time, pregnancy is allowed to continue; after 32 weeks, cesarean delivery is performed and is followed by immediate craniotomy. This is not because viability begins at 32 weeks, but rather because at this time the risks of preterm delivery are believed to become

less than the risks to the fetus of such maternal therapies as controlled hypotension, osmotic diuresis, and mechanical hyperventilation.

Aneurysm Clipping

Dias and Sekhar[55] demonstrated a significantly higher rate of survival for both mother and fetus when aneurysm clipping was performed after SAH in comparison with nonsurgical management.[55] Therefore, in patients with good clinical grade after SAH, aneurysm clipping should be performed as soon as possible to prevent rebleeding. Clipping of unruptured contralateral aneurysms can be delayed until the postpartum period.

Arteriovenous Malformation Resection

The risk of AVM rupture is greatly increased if a patient has come to clinical attention with a hemorrhagic event.[60,61] Resection of unruptured AVMs can be delayed until after delivery with no apparent increase in maternal mortality, especially for patients at lowest risk of spontaneous rupture.[62] Conversely, resection of ruptured AVMs is more controversial. Improved maternal outcome with early operation has been demonstrated, but this difference did not reach statistical significance.[55] The question of early operation for ruptured AVM during pregnancy remains unanswered at this time. The risk of rupture is probably determined primarily by the underlying risk of the lesion, not the pregnancy. An informed decision must weigh the risk of exposing the mother to neurosurgical intervention against the natural history risk of rupture due to characteristics of the lesion or its presentation.

Neoplasm Resection

Resection of a histologically benign neoplasm such as a meningioma can be delayed until after delivery, but only if frequent follow-up and careful monitoring for neurologic deterioration can be ensured. Surgery for presumed malignant tumors and for those masses producing worsening neurologic deficits—for example, pituitary adenoma with worsening visual field defect—should be performed regardless of gestational age.

Anesthetic Management

Sedative *premedication* may be appropriate in extremely anxious patients, but the risk of hypoventilation, hypercarbia, and subsequent increases in intracranial pressure (ICP) should be considered and guarded against. It might be more appropriate to defer the administration of sedative medications until the patient arrives in the preoperative holding area, where careful observation can be maintained. Because pregnant patients must be considered to be at increased risk of regurgitation and aspiration of gastric contents, medications to decrease the acidity and the volume of the gastric contents should be administered. These include a nonparticulate antacid such as Bicitra 30 mL, metoclopramide 10 mg, and an H_2 blocking drug such as ranitidine 150 mg.

Anesthesia *induction* in the pregnant patient who has an intracranial lesion provides the clearest example of the need to reconcile competing clinical goals. A rapid-sequence induction designed to prevent aspiration does little to prevent the hemodynamic response to intubation that can be catastrophic for the patient who has an intracranial aneurysm or increased ICP. At the same time, a slow "neuro-induction" with thiopental, an opioid, a nondepolarizing muscle relaxant, and mask ventilation does little to reduce the risk of aspiration. This technique can also be expected to lead to neonatal depression if cesarean section is performed as part of a combined procedure. The decision to proceed with or modify a standard rapid-sequence induction without ventilation must weigh the risk of aspiration against the patient's level of increased intracranial pressure and ability to tolerate a period of hypercarbia.

One acceptable technique for anesthetic induction is described in Box 23-1; other approaches that accomplish the stated goals are equally acceptable. As described previously, aspiration prophylaxis is mandatory. Cricoid pressure should be maintained from the point at which consciousness is lost until intubation is confirmed by capnography. If cesarean delivery is performed as part of a combined procedure, the physician caring for the newborn should be made aware of the likelihood of neonatal depression and the need to provide ventilatory support.

The use of fetal heart rate (FHR) monitoring during non-obstetric surgery remains controversial. A 2003 Committee Opinion of the American College of Obstetricians and Gynecologists (ACOG) stated, "there are no data to allow us to make specific recommendations" about the use of fetal monitoring during nonobstetric surgery.[63] Furthermore, decreases in short- and long-term FHR variability, as well as a decreased baseline FHR, are commonly seen even in the healthy, uncompromised fetus whose mother is receiving general anesthesia. Because the evidence base in support of fetal monitoring is primarily anecdotal,[64] the decision to use such monitoring should be individualized. It is probably unrealistic to expect that an emergency cesarean section could be performed expeditiously during craniotomy because of an ominous FHR value; rather, FHR monitoring may be useful because significant changes should lead to a rapid search for potentially reversible causes of decreased uteroplacental perfusion, such as hypotension and hypoxemia.

Anesthesia *maintenance* is not appreciably different in pregnant and nonpregnant women undergoing craniotomy (Box 23-2). As is the case during induction of anesthesia, every effort should be made to maintain hemodynamic stability as well as to avoid increases in cerebral blood volume that could interfere with surgical exposure. As stated previously, potentially teratogenic drugs should be avoided, but the commonly used anesthetics do not appear to fall into this category.

BOX 23–1 *Anesthetic Induction for Craniotomy in a Pregnant Patient*

Thiopental 5-7 mg/kg
Fentanyl 3-5 µg/kg
Lidocaine 75 mg
Rocuronium 0.9-1.2 mg/kg
Mask ventilation with cricoid pressure, 100% O_2

BOX 23–2 *Anesthetic Maintenance for Craniotomy in a Pregnant Patient*

Fentanyl 1-2 µg/kg/hr
Isoflurane 0.5-1%/nitrous oxide
Nondepolarizing muscle relaxant
Thiopental 5-6 mg/kg/hr for "tight brain"

Adjuvants to Surgery

Osmotic diuresis with mannitol is commonly used to decrease brain bulk and facilitate exposure during craniotomy. Because mannitol has been demonstrated in both animal and human studies to produce fetal dehydration,[65,66] some have advised against its use during pregnancy. However, the doses given in these early studies were considerably higher than those currently in clinical use. There is no evidence that mannitol 0.25 to 0.5 g/kg has any significant adverse effect on fetal fluid balance.[67] Furosemide may be an alternative to mannitol.[68]

Maternal hyperventilation can facilitate surgical exposure by decreasing cerebral blood volume. Severe hypocarbia may impair fetal oxygen delivery, however, by shifting the maternal oxygen-hemoglobin dissociation curve to the left. Hyperventilation can also decrease maternal cardiac output by raising intrathoracic pressure. Modest hyperventilation to a Pa_{CO_2} value of 25 to 30 mm Hg should provide adequate surgical conditions without significantly compromising the fetus.[68]

Controlled hypotension has been largely supplanted by the use of temporary clip occlusion of proximal vessels. There may be situations, however, in which the former technique becomes necessary. Because UBF varies directly with perfusion pressure, severe hypotension can lead to fetal asphyxia. Blood pressure should therefore be lowered only to that level deemed necessary for maternal well-being, and for as brief a period as possible. FHR monitoring might alert the anesthesiologist to the development of fetal hypoxia and lead to the restoration of blood pressure if the need for hypotension is not critical at that time.

There is an additional concern when sodium nitroprusside is used as the hypotensive agent. Because of the limited ability of the fetal liver to metabolize cyanide, it is possible for fetal intoxication to occur in the absence of any signs of maternal toxicity.[69] Although there are several case reports of the safe use of sodium nitroprusside during pregnancy,[70,71] the duration of administration should be limited to a period deemed essential to maternal well-being. The total dose of sodium nitroprusside can also be limited through the administration of adjuvants such as a β-blocking drugs and inhalation anesthetics.

Although intraoperative hypothermia to 33° C has not been shown to improve neurologic outcome after craniotomy for SAH,[72] mild permissive hypothermia is still used by a number of practitioners. This level of hypothermia has no significant fetal effects. More profound levels of hypothermia, however, can cause fetal arrhythmias and should be avoided.

Emergence from Anesthesia

Before the removal of the endotracheal tube, the pregnant patient should be fully awake and her airway reflexes intact to minimize the risk of aspiration. Bringing the patient to alertness will also facilitate early neurologic evaluation and eliminate the need for emergency radiologic evaluation of the persistently obtunded patient. At the same time, however, every effort should be made to prevent coughing and straining on the endotracheal tube, which may cause catastrophic intracranial hemorrhage. Prevention may be facilitated through the administration of lidocaine 75 to 100 mg and fentanyl 25 to 50 µg at the end of the operation. Because placement of the head dressing is associated with movement that produces airway stimulation and "bucking" of the patient on the endotracheal tube, it is appropriate to maintain neuromuscular blockade until the dressing has been secured. These guidelines do not apply to patients who were obtunded preoperatively or who had a significantly complicated intraoperative course with bleeding, brain swelling, or ischemia. Such patients should remain intubated until their neurologic status can be evaluated.

SPONTANEOUS SPINAL EPIDURAL HEMATOMA

Spontaneous spinal epidural hematoma (SSEH) is a rare cause of spinal cord compression. The lesions are usually associated with congenital or acquired bleeding disorders, hemorrhagic tumors, spinal AVMs, or increased intrathoracic pressure. In a review published in 2003, Kreppel and associates[73] identified 613 cases reported in the literature since 1682. As of 2005, there were 6 reported cases during pregnancy.[74] In these 6 cases, the women had profound neurologic deficits, were managed surgically, and exhibited significant neurologic improvement after surgery. Pregnancy was carried to term in 3 cases, and emergency cesarean section was performed before evacuation of the spinal epidural hematoma in 3 cases.

When an SSEH occurs in the thoracic or lumbar region, the initial presentation consists of lower extremity radicular pain as well as bladder and bowel dysfunction. Motor and sensory deficits are usually progressive within hours of presentation. The definitive diagnosis is made radiologically, with magnetic resonance imaging appearing to be the preferred modality during pregnancy. For patients who have profound and progressive neurologic deficits, the treatment of choice is immediate surgical evacuation of the hematoma. Lawton and coworkers[75] concluded that neurologic outcome was significantly improved in patients who underwent decompression within 12 hours of the onset of symptoms. Although Duffill and colleagues[76] reported the successful nonoperative management of SSEH,[76] *there are no case reports of pregnant patients who were managed conservatively.*

Cywinski and associates[25] address the possibility of conservative management of the pregnant patient with SSEH. They suggest that the hemodynamic changes seen during vaginal delivery might precipitate expansion of the hematoma. Further, they suggest that cesarean section during conservative management of SSEH would be inappropriate, because of the inability to monitor the patient's neurologic status.[25]

Timing of delivery in relation to SSEH surgery depends on gestational age. If the fetus is deemed viable (>25 weeks' gestation) at the time SSEH is diagnosed, cesarean section may be performed before neurosurgical evacuation of the hematoma to facilitate optimal neurologic outcome for the patient. If the fetus is determined to be nonviable (≤24 weeks' gestation), neurosurgical intervention should be undertaken as soon as possible to improve neurologic outcome, with implementation of specific considerations for surgery in the pregnant patient.[25]

Anesthetic Management of Surgical Evacuation

The concerns and techniques outlined for anesthetic management of intracranial lesions should be followed for evacuation of SSEH with or without cesarean section, including the recommendations for sedative premedication, anesthetic induction and maintenance, FHR monitoring, and emergence.

Anesthetic maintenance is not appreciably different from that for patients undergoing operation for intracranial lesions,

except for the need to maintain the mean arterial blood pressure in the high normal range (70 to 85 mm Hg in normotensive patients) to ensure adequate perfusion of the spinal cord.

Positioning considerations are extremely important in the pregnant patient before thoracic or lumbar laminectomy for hematoma evacuation. Aortocaval compression must be avoided to prevent significant reductions in maternal cardiac output, systemic blood pressure, and uteroplacental perfusion in patients for whom prior cesarean section is not performed. Physiologic studies reveal better relief of uterine compression of the large maternal vessels in the prone position than in the sitting or lateral position, with the lateral position actually being associated with a higher incidence of aortocaval compression.[77,78]

Jea and colleagues[74] described the use of the four-post Wilson frame for surgery in a patient with SSEH; two posts were placed just below the clavicles on the chest and the other posts centered on the anterosuperior iliac spines to support the pelvis.[74] In this position, the abdomen hung free of compression between the four posts, preventing compression of the abdominal aorta and vena cava. Positioning the patient on a Jackson table would similarly reduce aortocaval compression.

Emergence is managed as for pregnant patients undergoing surgery for intracranial lesions. Additional precautions must be taken to assess the patient's readiness for extubation after being in the prone position for surgery because of possible edema of the airway. A leak test should be performed when the patient is fully awake before the endotracheal tube is removed.

INTERVENTIONAL NEURORADIOLOGY IN PREGNANCY

With improvements in techniques and equipment, coiling of both ruptured and unruptured intracranial aneurysms increasingly provides an alternative to surgical clipping, with reduced incidence of vasospasm and procedural complications and a similar incidence of obstructive hydrocephalus, albeit a smaller rate of successful aneurysmal obliteration.[79] There are several case reports of the successful use of endovascular techniques during pregnancy.[80,81] Concerns have been raised regarding fetal radiation exposure during coiling procedures, but if appropriate shielding is used, the level of uterine radiation exposure is comparable to that from normal background radiation.[82] Because rapid manipulation of blood pressure may be necessary, for instance if the aneurysm ruptures, intra-arterial blood pressure monitoring is indicated. General endotracheal anesthesia is generally used during these procedures; the techniques used to blunt the sympathetic response to laryngoscopy and intubation during craniotomy should be used in this setting as well.[83] Finally, although emergency cesarean section in response to a nonreassuring FHR value is unlikely to be an option in most neuroradiology suites that are distant from the operating room, FHR monitoring may provide some guidance regarding the range of blood pressure that provides adequate uteroplacental perfusion and oxygen delivery.

REFERENCES

1. Chan MT, Mainland P, Gin T: Minimum alveolar concentration of halothane and enflurane are decreased in early pregnancy, *Anesthesiology* 85:782–786, 1996.

2. Gin T, Chan MT: Decreased minimum alveolar concentration of isoflurane in pregnant humans, *Anesthesiology* 81:829–832, 1994.

3. Gintzler AR, Liu NJ: The maternal spinal cord: Biochemical and physiological correlates of steroid-activated antinociceptive processes, *Prog Brain Res* 133:83–97, 2001.

4. Dattas S, Migliozzi RP, Flanagan HL, Krieger NR: Chronically administered progesterone decreases halothane requirements in rabbits, *Anesth Analg* 68:46–50, 1989.

5. Igarashi T, Hirabayashi Y, Shimuzu R, et al: The fiberscopic findings of the epidural space in pregnant women, *Anesthesiology* 92:1631–1636, 2000.

6. Flanagan HL, Datta S, Lambert DH, et al: Effect of pregnancy on bupivacaine-induced conduction blockade in the isolated rabbit vagus nerve, *Anesth Analg* 66:123–126, 1987.

7. Bader AM, Datta S, Moller RA, Covino BG: Acute progesterone treatment has no effect on bupivacaine-induced conduction blockade in the isolated rabbit vagus nerve, *Anesth Analg* 71:545–548, 1990.

8. McAuliffe F, Kametas N, Costello J, et al: Respiratory function in singleton and twin pregnancy, *BJOG* 109:765–769, 2002.

9. Spätling L, Fallenstein F, Huch A, et al: The variability of cardiopulmonary adaptation to pregnancy at rest and during exercise, *Br J Obstet Gynaecol* 99(Suppl 8):1–40, 1992.

10. McClelland SH, Bogod DG, Hardman JG: Apnoea in pregnancy: An investigation using physiological modeling, *Anaesthesia* 63:264–269, 2008.

11. McClelland SH, Bogod DG, Hardman JG: Pre-oxygenation in pregnancy: An investigation using physiological modeling, *Anaesthesia* 63:259–263, 2008.

12. Alaily AB, Carrol KB: Pulmonary ventilation in pregnancy, *Br J Obstet Gynaecol* 85:518–524, 1978.

13. Jensen D, Duffin J, Lam Y- M: Physiological mechanisms of hyperventilation during pregnancy, *Respir Physiol Neurobiol* 161:76–86, 2008.

14. Ueland K: Maternal cardiovascular dynamics: VII: Intrapartum blood volume changes, *Am J Obstet Gynecol* 126:671–677, 1976.

15. Capeless EL, Clapp JF: Cardiovascular changes in early phase of pregnancy, *Am J Obstet Gynecol* 161:1449–1453, 1989.

16. Clark SL, Cotton DB, Lee W, et al: Central hemodynamic assessment of normal term pregnancy, *Am J Obstet Gynecol* 161:1439–1442, 1989.

17. Robson SC, Dunlop W, Boys RJ, Hunter S: Cardiac output during labor, *Br Med J* 295:1169–1172, 1987:(Clin Res Ed).

18. Van Thiel DH, Gavaler JS, Joshi SN, et al: Heartburn of pregnancy, *Gastroenterology* 72:666–668, 1977.

19. O'Sullivan GM, Bullingham RE: The assessment of gastric acidity and antacid effect in pregnant women by a non-invasive radiotelemetry technique, *Br J Obstet Gynaecol* 91:973–978, 1984.

20. Wong CA, McCarthy RJ, Fitzgerald PC, et al: Gastric emptying of water in obese pregnant women at term, *Anesth Analg* 105:751–755, 2007.

21. Escher G, Mohaupt M: Role of aldosterone availability in preeclampsia, *Mol Aspects Med* 28:245–254, 2007.

22. Sims EAH, Krantz KE: Serial studies of renal function during pregnancy and the puerperium in normal women, *J Clin Invest* 37:1764–1774, 1958.

23. Bacq Y, Zarka O, Bréchot JF, et al: Liver function tests in normal pregnancy: A prospective study of 103 pregnant women and 103 matched controls, *Hepatology* 23:1030–1034, 1996.

24. Leighton BL, Cheek TG, Gross JB, et al: Succinylcholine pharmacodynamics in peripartum patients, *Anesthesiology* 64:202–205, 1986.

25. Cywinski JB, Parker BM, Lozada LJ: Spontaneous spinal epidural hematoma in a pregnant patient, *J Clin Anesth* 16:371–375, 2003.

26. Nolte JE, Rutherford RB, Nawaz S, et al: Arterial dissections associated with pregnancy, *J Vasc Surg* 21:515–520, 1995.

27. Weiner CP, Eisenach JC: Uteroplacental blood flow. In Chestnut DH, editor: *Obstetric Anesthesia, Principles and Practice*, ed 3, Philadelphia, 2004, Elsevier Mosby, pp 37–48.

28. Ralston DH, Shnider SM, DeLorimier AA: Effects of equipotent ephedrine, metaraminol, mephentermine, and methoxamine on uterine blood flow in the pregnant ewe, *Anesthesiology* 40:354–370, 1974.

29. Ramanathan S, Grant GJ: Vasopressor therapy for hypotension due to epidural anesthesia for cesarean section, *Acta Anesthesiol Scand* 32:559–565, 1988.

30. Moran DH, Perillo M, LaPorta RF, et al: Phenylephrine in the prevention of hypotension following spinal anesthesia for cesarean delivery, *J Clin Anesth* 3:301–305, 1991.

31. Ngan Kee WD, Khaw KS: Vasopressors in obstetrics: What should we be using? *Curr Opin Anaesthesiol* 19:238–243, 2006.

32. Lee A, Ngan Kee WD: Gin T: A quantitative, systematic review of randomized controlled trials of ephedrine versus phenylephrine for the management of hypotension during spinal anesthesia for cesarean delivery, *Anesth Analg* 94:920–926, 2002.

33. Zakowski MI, Herman NL: The placenta: Anatomy, physiology, and transfer of drugs. In Chestnut DH, editor: *Obstetric Anesthesia, Principles and Practice*, ed 3, Philadelphia, 2004, Elsevier Mosby, pp 49–65.

34. Celleno D, Capogna G, Tomassetti M, et al: Neurobehavioral effects of propofol on the neonate following elective cesarean section, *Br J Anaesth* 62:649–654, 1989.

35. Ghanem FA, Movahed A: Use of antihypertensive drugs during pregnancy and lactation, *Cardiovasc Ther* 26:38–49, 2008.

36. Eisenach JC, Castro MI: Maternally administered esmolol produces fetal beta-adrenergic blockade and hypoxemia in sheep, *Anesthesiology* 71:718–722, 1989.

37. Basford A, Fink BR: Teratogenicity of halothane in the rat, *Anesthesiology* 29:1167–1173, 1968.

38. Pope WDB, Halsey MJ, Lansdown ABG, et al: Fetotoxicity in rats following chronic exposure to halothane, nitrous oxide, or methoxyflurane, *Anesthesiology* 48:11–16, 1978.

39. Mazze RI: Fertility, reproduction, and postnatal survival in mice chronically exposed to isoflurane, *Anesthesiology* 63:663–667, 1985.

40. Mazze RI, Wilson AI, Rice SA, et al: Fetal development in mice exposed to isoflurane, *Teratology* 32:339–345, 1985.

41. Mazze RI, Fujinaga M, Rice SA, et al: Reproductive and teratogenic effects of nitrous oxide, halothane, isoflurane, and enflurane in Sprague-Dawley rats, *Anesthesiology* 64:339–344, 1986.

42. Fink BR, Shepard TH, Blandau RJ: Teratogenic activity of nitrous oxide, *Nature* 214:146–148, 1967.

43. Mazze RI, Wilson AI, Rice SA, Baden JM: Reproduction and fetal development in rats exposed to nitrous oxide, *Teratology* 30:259–265, 1984.

44. Fujinaga M, Baden JM: Methionine prevents nitrous oxide-induced teratogenicity in rat embryos grown in culture, *Anesthesiology* 81:184–189, 1994.

45. Fujinaga M: Teratogenicity of nitrous oxide, *Best Pract Res Clin Anaesthesiol* 15:363–375, 2001.

46. Burm AG: Occupational hazards of inhalational anesthetics, *Best Pract Res Clin Anaesthesiol* 17:147–161, 2003.

47. Weimann J: Toxicity of nitrous oxide, *Best Pract Res Clin Anaesthesiol* 17:47–61, 2003.

48. Saxén I: Associations between oral clefts and drugs taken during pregnancy, *Int J Epidemiol* 4:37–44, 1975.

49. Safra MJ, Oakley GP Jr: Association between cleft lip with or without cleft palate and prenatal exposure to diazepam, *Lancet* 306:478–480, 1975.

50. McElhatton PR: The effects of benzodiazepine use during pregnancy and lactation, *Reprod Toxicol* 8:461–475, 1994.

51. Rosenberg L, Mitchell AA, Parsells JL, et al: Lack of relation of oral clefts to diazepam use during pregnancy, *N Engl J Med* 309:1282–1285, 1983.

52. Ornoy A, Arnon J, Shectman S, et al: Is benzodiazepine use during pregnancy really teratogenic? *Reprod Toxicol* 12:511–515, 1998.

53. Selo-Ojeme DO, Marshman LAG, Ikomi A: Aneurysmal subarachnoid hemorrhage in pregnancy, *Eur J Obstet Gynecol Reprod Biol* 116:131–143, 2004.

54. Lewis G: *The Confidential Enquiry into Maternal and Child Health (CEMACH). Saving Mothers' Lives: Reviewing maternal deaths to make motherhood safer, 2003-2005. The Seventh Report on Confidential Enquiries into Maternal Deaths in the United Kingdom.* London, 2007, CEMACH.

55. Dias MS, Sekhar LN: Intracranial hemorrhage from aneurysms and arteriovenous malformations during pregnancy and the puerperium. *Neurosurgery* 71990;:855–865.

56. Bickerstaff ER, Small JM, Guest IA: The relapsing course of certain meningiomas in relation to pregnancy and menstruation, *J Neurol Neurosurg Psychiatry* 21:89–91, 1958.

57. Schlehofer B, Blettner M, Becker N, et al: Association between brain tumors and menopausal status, *J Natl Cancer Inst* 84:1346–1349, 1992.

58. Cahill DW, Bashirelahi N, Solomon LW, et al: Estrogen and progesterone receptors in meningiomas, *J Neurosurg* 60:983–985, 1984.

59. Gonzalez-Aguero G, Gutierrez AA, Gonzalez-Espinosa D, et al: Progesterone effects on cell growth of U373 and D54 human astrocytoma cell lines, *Endocrine* 32:129–135, 2007.

60. Kim H, Sidney S, McCulloch CE, et al: Racial/ethnic differences in longitudinal risk of intracranial hemorrhage in brain arteriovenous malformation patients, *Stroke* 38:2430–2437, 2007.

61. Mast H, Young WL, Koennecke H-C, et al: Risk of spontaneous haemorrhage after diagnosis of cerebral arteriovenous malformation, *Lancet* 350:1065–1068, 1997.

62. Stapf C, Mast H, Sciacca RR, et al: Predictors of hemorrhage in patients with untreated brain arteriovenous malformations, *Neurology* 66:1350–1355, 2006.

63. ACOG Committee on Obstetric Practice: ACOG Committee Opinion Number 284, August 2003: Nonobstetric surgery in pregnancy, *Obstet Gynecol* 102:431, 2003.

64. Macarthur A: Craniotomy for suprasellar meningioma during pregnancy: Role of fetal monitoring, *Can J Anesth* 51:535–538, 2004.

65. Bruns PD, Linder RO, Drose VE, Battaglia F: The placental transfer of water from fetus to mother following the intravenous infusion of hypertonic mannitol to the maternal rabbit, *Am J Obstet Gynecol* 86:160–167, 1963.

66. Battaglia F, Prystowsky H, Smisson C, et al: Fetal blood studies: XIII: The effect of the administration of fluids intravenously to mothers upon the concentrations of water and electrolytes in plasma of human fetuses, *Pediatrics* 25:2–10, 1960.

67. Bharti N, Kashyap L, Mohan VK: Anesthetic management of a parturient with cerebellopontine-angle meningioma, *Int J Obstet Anesth* 11:219–221, 2002.

68. Wang LP, Paech MJ: Neuroanesthesia for the pregnant woman, *Anesth Analg* 107:193–200, 2008.

69. Naulty J, Cefalo RC, Lewis PE: Fetal toxicity of nitroprusside in the pregnant ewe, *Am J Obstet Gynecol* 139:708–711, 1981.

70. Willoughby JS: Sodium nitroprusside, pregnancy, and multiple intracranial aneurysms, *Anaesth Intensive Care* 12:351–357, 1984.

71. Conklin KA, Herr G, Fung D: Anaesthesia for caesarean section and cerebral aneurysm clipping, *Can Anaesth Soc J* 31:451–454, 1984.

72. Todd MM, Hindman BJ, Clarke WR, Torner JC: Mild intraoperative hypothermia during surgery for intracranial aneurysm, *N Engl J Med* 352:135–145, 2005.

73. Kreppel D, Antoniadis G, Seeling W: Spinal hematoma: A literature survey with meta-analysis of 613 patients, *Neurosurg Rev* 26:1–49, 2003.

74. Jea A, Moza K, Levi AD, Vanni S: Spontaneous spinal epidural hematoma during pregnancy: Case report and literature review, *Neurosurgery* 56:E1156, 2005.

75. Lawton MT, Porter RW, Heiserman JE, et al: Surgical management of spinal epidural hematoma: Relationship between surgical timing and neurological outcome, *J Neurosurg* 83:1–7, 1996.

76. Duffill J, Sparrow OC, Millar J, et al: Can spontaneous spinal epidural hematoma be managed safely without operation: A report of four cases, *J Neurol Neurosurg Psychiatry* 69:816–819, 2000.

77. Andrews PJ, Ackermann WE, Juneja MM: Aortocaval compression in the sitting and lateral decubitus positions during extradural catheter placement in the parturient, *Can J Anaesth* 40:320–324, 1993.

78. Nakai Y, Mine M, Nishio J, et al: Effects of maternal prone position on the umbilical arterial flow, *Acta Obstet Gynecol Scand* 77:967–969, 1998.

79. Taha MM, Nakahara I, Higashi T, et al: Endovascular embolization vs. surgical clipping in treatment of cerebral aneurysms: Morbidity and mortality with short-term outcome, *Surg Neurol* 662006;:277–284.

80. Piotin M, de Souza Filho CBA, Kothimbakam R: Moret J: Endovascular treatment of acutely ruptured intracranial aneurysms in pregnancy, *Am J Obstet Gynecol* 185:1261–1262, 2001.

81. Meyers PM, Halbach VV, Malek AM, et al: Endovascular treatment of cerebral artery aneurysms during pregnancy: Report of three cases, *AJNR Am J Neuroradiol* 21:1306–1311, 2000.

82. Marshman LAG, Aspoas AR, Rai MS, Chawda SJ: The implications of ISAT and ISUIA for the management of cerebral aneurysms during pregnancy, *Neurosurg Rev* 30:177–180, 2007.

83. Allen G, Farling P, McAtamney D: Anesthetic management of the pregnant patient for endovascular coiling of an unruptured intracranial aneurysm, *Neurocrit Care* 4:18–20, 2006.

Chapter 24

ETHICAL CONSIDERATIONS IN THE CARE OF PATIENTS WITH NEUROSURGICAL DISEASE

Jonathan D. Moreno • Angelique M. Reitsma • Connie Zuckerman • Alex John London

Research advances and heightened clinical capabilities have enabled those who care for patients with neurosurgical disease to make great strides toward restoring the health and well-being of such patients and reducing their morbidity and mortality. Yet for every new technologic advance and clinical application, new issues have also arisen for caregivers, such as (1) the appropriate selection of patients for application of new technologies and enrollment in clinical trials, (2) the involvement of patients and families in balancing the risks of new treatments against their possible benefits, and (3) how to make decisions for patients who may not be able to participate in the decision-making process yet for whom significant decisions must be made concerning the kind of care to be delivered.

Such questions demand that clinicians look beyond their clinical training and subspecialty expertise when facing the genuine ethical dilemmas that are now an integral part of the clinical setting. Determining the moral status of one's actions can be a troubling and sometimes arduous process for even the most enlightened of clinicians. Because such moral issues permeate clinical practice and because their resolution often requires serious and extended deliberation, clinicians should become familiar with the systems of "clinical ethics" and research ethics that have emerged over the last 35 years. Such familiarity will enable clinicians to deal more effectively with these difficult issues by applying philosophical reasoning and ethical analysis to the problems they encounter in the course of research and clinical practice.

Heightened sensitivity to ethical concerns in the clinical setting has also been accompanied by increased awareness of and concern for the role of the legal system in clinical practice. As medical and surgical care has become ever more sophisticated and developments in the legal process have both educated patients and encouraged them to assert themselves in the provider-patient relationship, physicians have naturally become more sensitive to the legal status of their actions. A clinical ethics framework that incorporates a perspective of legal concerns as it also tries to determine the appropriateness of an action may lie well beyond narrow legal definitions applicable in a particular situation. Although it is incumbent on the clinician to be aware of the legal backdrop for clinical practice, many ethical dilemmas move beyond mere legal technicalities, requiring the clinician to evaluate concurrent and, at times, conflicting duties, rights, and values that are an inevitable part of the provider-patient relationship. In this chapter, we address the ethical issues that confront caregivers of the neurosurgical patient population.

AN INTRODUCTION TO THE HISTORY AND THEORY OF MEDICAL ETHICS

We begin with an overview of the historic development of medical ethics. The account concentrates mainly on the Western secular tradition that begins with followers of Hippocrates and emerges in a fundamentally altered form in the current framework of clinical ethics. We then describe the essential features of the current framework.

Origins of Contemporary Medical Ethics

Western medical ethics is believed to have originated with the Hippocratic cult (about 450 to 300 BC), a group of early physicians who are thought to have been heavily influenced by the Pythagorean thinkers. Rather than ascribing disease to be solely the province of supernatural or deistic causes, this group was one of the first systemized efforts to impart a *naturalistic* approach to the study and practice of medicine. In addition to their accomplishments in mathematics, the Pythagoreans developed a moral philosophy that emphasized respect for life. This outlook would account, for example, for the apparent strictures on abortion and euthanasia that are features of a prominent version of the Hippocratic Oath. For different reasons, the oath also prohibits surgery, which was not regarded as a proper part of physicians' activities. The attitudes held by the Hippocratic physicians apparently were not widely held among other physician cults of the ancient world.[1]

The Hippocratic tradition urges physicians to "do no harm" and to use their skills for the welfare of the individual patient. For many years these principles were thought to justify medical paternalism because they seemed to generate duties mainly to minimize physical harm and to improve the patient's physical well-being. Given that the physician possessed specialized knowledge of the physical structures and causal processes of the patient's body, the physician and not the patient was considered most qualified to determine a patient's health care goals and the means to achieving them. On the basis of this reading of the Hippocratic Oath, patients were not thought qualified to shape the course of their individual care because of their general lack of scientific insight into the nature and workings of their own physical condition.

The last 40 years or so have witnessed a trenchant and often passionate critique of the idea that a patient's best interests are limited to or exhausted by his or her physical well-being. Because a patient's best interests must be determined in light of his or her values and life goals and because the value a patient places on physical well-being depends on how it fits within this larger framework of values and projects, the competent and well-informed patient is generally recognized as the best judge of appropriate health care goals. Few would deny the accuracy of the Hippocratic conception of medicine as a science whose goal is the health and physical welfare of the patient nor challenge the claim that physicians must always look after the best interests of their patients. However, the fact that a competent patient lacks specialized medical knowledge is generally recognized to be less important than the fact that each patient is the most qualified judge of the relative value of his or her physical well-being in relation to his or her larger life goals and projects. For this reason, patient self-determination, as well as its culmination in the doctrine of informed consent, represents the bedrock of contemporary clinical ethics.

As medical science has progressed and physicians have developed the ability to alter the course of a person's life with the use of an array of medical technology, patients have taken a greater interest in determining the way their lives should be shaped.[2] The early seeds of patient self-determination and the doctrine of informed consent began developing as early as the latter part of the 19th century. This period and the early part of the 20th century saw many legal cases involving surgical patients whose consent to excision of tissues had not been obtained.[3] Under prevailing legal theories, these actions were at first considered torts, such as battery or "unconsented touching."[4] As medical and judicial systems evolved, they were then gradually brought under a negligence theory.[4] This change strengthened the growing expectation that informing a patient of the reason for the procedure and obtaining consent for it were proper parts of the physician-patient relationship.[5] In theory, at least, obtaining the patient's informed consent became an essential aspect of the developing standard of care. However, honoring this legal requirement in clinical reality awaited the increased attention to ethical issues that emerged in the late 1960s.

Although we focus here on clinical ethics, no survey of the history of medical ethics can omit society's reaction to the abuses of human beings perpetrated by physicians and scientists in the concentration camps of Nazi Germany. The revelations at Nuremberg led to the promulgation in Helsinki and Geneva of international standards for the protection of research subjects.[6] Unfortunately, these efforts did not prevent blatantly unethical practices in the context of subsequent research by American investigators.[7] As a result, strict statutory protections were established to ensure the informed consent of research participants, including protocol review by institutional committees.[8,9] Public recognition of research abuses led to heightened scrutiny of the physician-patient relationship in the clinical setting and greater support for the concept of informed consent.

Technologic advances once again profoundly influenced the direction of medical ethics, beginning in the later 1960s with the arrival of practical artificial respiratory equipment and, in the early 1970s, with the development of materials that facilitated artificial hydration and nutrition. These advances—combined with social and political changes, including the civil rights movement—culminated in the celebrated legal case of Karen Ann Quinlan in 1976.[10] In the Quinlan decision, the New Jersey Supreme Court established that the right to refuse medical treatment was fundamental and could be exercised on behalf of an incompetent patient by informed surrogates who were knowledgeable about the patient's previous values and

lifestyle.[10] The family was found to be in the best position to represent the wishes of their close relative.[10]

In summary, the history of Western medical ethics has featured a transition from the "beneficence" orientation (doing good for the patient) of premodern medicine to the view that the patient must ultimately decide what his or her best interests are after going through a process of informed consent. Both morally and legally, patient self-determination has become the gold standard of modern biomedical ethics. In the next section, we review the prevailing philosophical principles and theories that are often used to further assess ethical problems in modern medicine.

Prevailing Theories and Principles

The term *medical ethics*, as it is used in contemporary society, is somewhat ambiguous. It may refer to those rules of conduct established by the formal bodies of the medical profession in the course of regulating itself, such as the prohibition of the sexual exploitation of one's patients, or it may refer to novel ethical dilemmas that actually confront health care workers and have no obvious solution in terms of traditional values and ethical codes, such as the removal of life support systems from irreversibly comatose patients.

Two philosophical approaches dominate the literature. Tracing its roots to the German philosopher Immanuel Kant (1724-1804), the Kantian tradition holds that people have a fundamental right to be treated as ends in themselves and not merely as a means to some other end. The basis of the Kantian view is that each person has the capacity to take on projects and to give a distinctive shape to his or her own life. This capacity must be respected in each individual because the value of all other things is derived from the exercise of this capacity. Patient self-determination and informed consent are therefore the preeminent Kantian values for clinical ethics, because without them we cannot freely set the ends for ourselves that give all other things their moral worth. As such, they represent necessary conditions for treating a patient as an end in himself or herself.

Utilitarianism traces its roots back to the English philosophers Jeremy Bentham (1748-1832) and John Stuart Mill (1806-1873).[11] Utilitarianism is a form of consequentialism, which holds that actions or policies are right in proportion to the extent to which they promote the aggregate happiness or well-being. Whereas the Kantian can claim that physicians have special duties to their patients, which derive from the need to respect their patients as ends in themselves, the utilitarian must argue that any duties physicians owe to their patients are rooted in the fact that fulfilling those duties maximizes overall happiness.

Although the principle of autonomy is commonly regarded as the first principle of contemporary medical ethics, those with a more utilitarian slant believe that it is conceptually balanced by the principle of beneficence, the obligation to do good for the patient.[12] Beneficence is closely associated with the traditional Hippocratic obligation to at least not harm the patient, or the principle of nonmaleficence.[12] Arguments that establish the moral basis of beneficence and nonmaleficence are available both to Kantian and utilitarian theories. The main difference between these theories therefore lies not in the principles they recognize but in the way they justify those principles and the way they order them in relation to one another.

The Provider-Patient Relationship

Self-Determination

Strictly speaking, *autonomy* refers to the potential for the individual to be self-determining. Self-determination is, in this line of thinking, regarded as a good thing in itself and also as a means to an end. It is the expression of an individual's personality. Self-determination is thought to be the best means of identifying an individual's best interest, a determination that involves the incorporation of that person's values into a decision. This concept suggests that each individual is in the best position to assess aspects of decision making in the context of his or her own value system. In the clinical setting, self-determination is exercised through the informed consent process, which allows the patient ultimately to determine the most individually appropriate health care choice on the basis of his or her own values and preferences.[13]

Because self-determination is regarded as good, certain individuals may be obligated to foster another's self-determination, if they have a certain type of relationship with that individual. An example is a parent who has a unique opportunity to help the developing child realize his or her individuality by helping to prepare the child to make his or her own choices. Choices are not thought to be truly the result of self-determination until they are considered judgments that encompass the person's reflective deliberation. It is implicit that these judgments would then also be authentic and reliable representations of that person's character and values.

The promotion of a patient's self-determination is a major responsibility, and many conditions could prevent its realization in the clinical setting.[14] One of these is the sense of vulnerability that can accompany illness. Physicians and other health care providers are in a powerful position, either to exploit this sense of vulnerability or to reduce it and instead promote a feeling that the patient has some measure of control over the situation. Ensuring the patient's control would be a first important step in promoting the patient's self-determination. A second important step would be to help the patient identify his or her own authentic preferences among the diagnostic or treatment options available.

Confidentiality

Confidentiality is one of the pillars of the Hippocratic tradition,[15] and it is a fundamental concept that still forms an essential aspect of the physician-patient relationship.[4] Although its strong theoretical basis is maintained, however, it is a concept under continuous assault in the clinical setting. Computerized databases containing sensitive information, team coverage of patient needs, and the demands of third-party insurers have all converged to threaten this fundamental aspect of the bond between patient and provider.[16]

At its core, the concept of confidentiality means that all information that the patient shares with the provider during the course of being treated should remain private and confidential; it should not be revealed to those outside the patient-provider relationship. The trusting bond and fiduciary nature of the relationship should allow the patient to feel comfortable when revealing to the provider all information necessary to ensure a comprehensive understanding of the patient's circumstances and a correct diagnosis of the patient's condition, thereby fostering an individually appropriate caregiver response. In turn, as a means to encouraging the patient to be forthcoming, the provider ensures that no one else will come to know this highly personal and perhaps embarrassing information. Currently, "intrusions" are permitted into this relationship. Examples are multiple caregivers who learn of the patient's circumstances in acute care settings and the insurance company that learns of the patient's condition to determine whether reimbursement is warranted. Nonetheless, the notion that those who do not need to know these intimate details of the patient's condition will not know is still an essential factor in the bond that ties the patient to the provider.

The costs of not guaranteeing confidentiality or breaching it when previously assured are significant both for the individual patient and for society. Patients who believe they cannot trust their providers and are therefore less than candid in their descriptions are likely to suffer the consequences of an incomplete assessment or even a misdiagnosis of their condition. They lose out on what their physicians may have to offer.[17] Also, providers who breach their duty to keep information confidential fail in their ultimate obligation to act beneficently toward their patients and to do them no harm.[17] Moreover, society as a whole is not served well when individuals in need of medical care feel inhibited or are unwilling to seek that care.

Our legal system has recognized the fundamental requirement of confidentiality between doctor and patient.[4] Under most circumstances, information that passes between doctor and patient during the course of care is "privileged," that is, inaccessible in a court of law; a judge or jury will be unable to learn of it.[4] This special exclusion of possibly relevant information further ensures that patients do not feel inhibited when conversing with providers. Despite the essential drive in our court systems to bring out all possibly pertinent information in an individual case, society has nonetheless recognized that our interests as a whole are better served when patients and providers can feel assured that their discussions are private and confidential.

To further safeguard and protect an individual's health information in an era of technologic sophistication, Congress enacted the Health Insurance Portability and Accountability Act (HIPAA) in 2003.[18] The Privacy Rule of HIPAA limits the ability of health plans, hospitals, physicians, and other covered entities to use and share a patient's personal medical information through oral or written communication, computer transmission, and other communication methods. Many have criticized the burden and cost of the implementation of HIPAA and have expressed concern about its impact on research and clinical care,[19] although few would question the challenges to privacy and confidentiality that exist in modern health care environments.

Nonetheless, in certain circumstances, other societal interests are believed to outweigh the interests served by confidentiality. For example, in the midst of certain public health epidemics, in which the obligation to protect the health of society may conflict with the desire to maintain individual confidentiality, a societal consensus is morally and legally justifiable to breach individual confidentiality under certain limited conditions.[4] One example involves laws requiring the reporting of certain diagnoses to health departments[4] and perhaps the tracing of contacts who may have been exposed to an individual's illness. Another example concerns the need to protect the public from harm. Under the state's "police power" (a constitutional concept), physicians have the obligation to report certain medical conditions, such as gunshot wounds.[20] A third example occurs with respect to the state's obligation to protect its most vulnerable members, also known as the state's *parens patriae* power, which obliges health care providers to routinely breach confidentiality and report instances of known or suspected child abuse.[4] Although the circumstances permitting the breach of confidentiality are limited, they clearly represent instances in which other significant societal interests make such a breach justifiable and even desirable, despite the potential harm that may befall an individual patient.

The Informed Consent Process

As stated earlier, the informed consent process permits the expression of individual self-determination in the clinical setting. From a legal perspective, this means that providers are obligated to disclose to patients all information that will allow them to arrive at an informed decision about their choices, including such information as the patient's diagnosis and prognosis, a description of the proposed intervention and its risks and benefits to the patient, and the existence of alternative interventions, along with their risks and benefits.[21] In some jurisdictions, there is the requirement that information "material" to that individual patient be disclosed.[21-24] This requirement might oblige the provider to disclose certain details that he or she might not normally discuss under routine circumstances. Overall, it is essential that the physician provide information to the patient, so that the patient can consider the options and select the choice that promotes the patient's best interests as the patient assesses them.

Philosophically, autonomy and its promotion both undergird the legal doctrine of informed consent and exert greater demands than the doctrine does.[13] Indeed, one seminal philosophical account of the legal doctrine of informed consent process exhibits a more detailed conceptual scheme than is found in the law (Box 24-1) as we will discuss below.[12]

Competence

The possession of sufficient capacity to either consent to or refuse a proposed intervention is obviously a "threshold" requirement in the informed consent process[13]; that is, only those patients capable of making health care choices reflective of personal values have the ability to give informed consent and to be considered self-determining. Patients whose decisional capacity is impaired or lost are generally considered unable to integrate factual information with personal preferences and are thus viewed as in need of assistance with choices or even protection from harmful choices, through the use of either a surrogate decision maker or some other method of deciding on care.[13] Therefore consideration of how the "capacity to decide" is to be determined in the clinical setting is essential.

Strictly speaking, the word *competence* denotes a legal concept,[21] meaning that only a court of law can determine whether to suspend the legal presumption of competency, which generally attaches to all who reach the age of 18 years. The legal presumption of competency enables adults to involve themselves in all fundamental activities of citizenship, including the ability to vote, to contract with another, to write a will, and to get married. It is an empowering concept, covering a range of activities in which the individual is presumed capable of participating. A judicial declaration of incompetency is generally intended to apply globally, that is, to formally disempower the individual in most, if not all, major aspects of controlling his or her life.[21]

The routine assessment of competence in the clinical setting usually has little connection with the sort of global assessment that informs a judicial determination. Rather, competence in this setting is generally judged in the context of whether the patient is capable of either consenting to or refusing a particular proposed intervention.[25] The determination is usually made by an attending physician, sometimes with the assistance of a professional from another discipline, such as a psychiatrist.[4]

Competence to decide about medical treatment may call on various abilities, depending on the demands of the task at hand.[25,26] Yet some general abilities are required in the process of becoming involved in treatment decisions. These include the ability to understand or appreciate the nature of various alternatives and their consequences and the ability to communicate a preference.[27] In reaching a personal preference, one must also be capable of reasoning and deliberation, the latter term signaling that this is a process in which the decision maker's own values are gradually brought to bear on the question.[13] Accordingly, the competent decision maker's values will be more or less stable and consistent over time; they will be values that the decision maker recognizes as his or her own.

Information

The patient with decisional authority (or the properly identified surrogate decision maker) is entitled to all the information available about his or her condition that would be relevant to making a decision about treatment. This information includes not only known or estimated risks and benefits of proposed therapies and their alternatives but also the implications of having no treatment at all.[28] The free flow of information to the patient, however sensitively it may need to be conveyed, is obviously vital for a valid consent process. Likewise, for the provider to suggest an individually appropriate treatment course for that patient, the patient must be encouraged to communicate openly with the provider.[13]

Full information is one of the legal pillars of informed consent, the other being the free and uncoerced consent itself.[13] Exceptions to such disclosure do exist, namely, the "therapeutic privilege," which permits the physician to withhold information from the patient or to seek consent from an appropriate surrogate when provision of such information would be so detrimental that the result would be counter-therapeutic and would bring about harm.[21] Concern is often expressed about doing harm to the patient, particularly by physicians in fields in which terminal illness is common, about the "inhumanity" of telling the patient the unvarnished truth.[29] However, distinguishing between the inherently unwelcome nature of bad medical news and information that might actually induce negative physical consequences in the patient is important. The majority of patients who have been surveyed desire to have information given, even if it foretells their coming demise.[30] In fact, the real need for the therapeutic privilege is rare if it is employed for its actual intent, rather than for the purpose of affording the physician the opportunity to avoid a difficult discussion. Although it is appropriate that information be imparted in a sensitive manner, imparted it should be, nonetheless.

At such times it might be tempting to speak first with, for example, the patient's adult child to enlist his or her support before an encounter with an older patient. For several reasons, this temptation should be avoided. First, certain classes of patients, such as those who are elderly, are too easily stereotyped as unable to manage emotionally powerful information, even though they may be quite functional in other areas of their lives and lacking any psychiatric history relevant to this issue. Second, the information is, after all, confidential information. Because it is of more concern to the patient than to anyone else, he or she has the right to hear it first. Third, the misguided attempt to enlist the adult child's help could backfire in several ways. The grown child may not be prepared for the loss of a parent, may not enjoy the patient's confidence, or may even have a personal agenda that is in conflict with or opposed to the best interests of the patient. There is no barrier to asking the patient whether it would be desirable for the physician to have a conversation with a particular relative, whether privately or with the patient, so that all three can cooperate in planning for the patient's future. In the final analysis, however, the confidentiality of the patient must be respected.

Understanding

A somewhat different objection to the idea of the patient's rendering informed consent is the argument that some medical decisions are so complex that the lay patient cannot be expected to understand their components, thus calling into question the entire foundation of the informed consent concept. Clearly a medical school education should not be a prerequisite for a workable consent process; fortunately, it is not required. Some patients will benefit from a technical presentation of their situation, but such a presentation is not necessarily required for the consent process to be valid. Information should be conveyed to patients so that they clearly understand how the proposed or available options will affect their lives; patients should be able to clearly articulate and understand the risks and benefits of these options as they concretely pertain to their lifestyles and preferences. Such an informing process is inevitably more satisfactory for both patient and provider when the informer knows the patient personally and understands the values that infuse the patient's life.[13] This is a difficult relationship to achieve, particularly for specialists who only briefly come to know the patient in the context of a specific acute situation. Nonetheless, a certain level of intimacy with the patient is essential to truly adhere to the principles that underlie the informed consent process and to help ensure that the patient truly understands the information of critical relevance to his or her personal decision.[21]

Clinically, certain factors are inherent in both the patient's condition and the environment of care that may lessen or even prevent the patient from understanding the information conveyed, no matter how precisely or sensitively it has been imparted. For example, a provider may be unsure whether a patient in an intensive care unit who has been sedated for pain relief can understand sufficiently to engage in informed consent. In addition, the distracting machinery of the environment or the disrupted schedule to which patients must conform also work against full comprehension and understanding on the patient's part. The provider's duty is to do everything possible to lessen or remove impediments that prevent the patient from fully participating in an informed consent process. Such actions might include temporarily moving a patient to more private or serene quarters to carry on a conversation or perhaps lessening a dosage of pain medication so that, although less comfortable, the patient may nonetheless better comprehend and consider the choices that lie before him or her. As well, the physician should be satisfied that there is no metabolic basis (such as a toxic reaction to new medication) to contribute to the patient's lack of understanding.

Consent

Consent refers to the voluntary and uncoerced agreement of the patient. Consent is a more active process than mere assent or dissent. Ideally, it implies deliberation and perhaps also reflection based on one's own values. Obstacles to truly reflective consent in the hospital include such previously cited factors as the physical conditions commonly associated with treatment for acute illness and the disorientation imparted by impersonal hospital routines and protocols. For example, mechanical restraints may be used for legitimate or illegitimate purposes, but they compromise the sense of control and voluntariness that enables a person to make well-considered choices.

Other sorts of constraints on the patient may be more subtle but no less undermining. Examples range from pressures associated with familial dynamics to concern with the financial consequences of one alternative in comparison with another. In extreme circumstances, the physician may be justified in assuming an active role as patient advocate in attempting to determine whether a stated choice is truly what the patient would want for himself or herself or whether it is reflective of certain pressures inflicted on the patient.

Authorization

An action is authorized when the individual with the appropriate authority gives approval. In accordance with the previous discussion, this individual is either the patient or some appropriately appointed representative of the patient. In certain circumstances, such as when an incompetent patient requires emergency care, the requirement for authorization is usually suspended because the immediate needs of the patient are thought to be so critical that time cannot be expended in locating someone other than the patient to provide authorization.[4] In true emergency situations, when a patient's background is unknown (i.e., providers are not aware of any previously expressed wish on the patient's part to decline the type of care about to be provided) and care must be provided immediately to avoid irreparable harm to the patient, the requirement for authorization is generally waived.[4] In such cases, the legal presumption is that (1) reasonable persons would consent to such necessary care, (2) there is no reason to believe this patient would refuse the proposed care, and (3) the time needed to locate an appropriate surrogate might otherwise jeopardize the patient's condition. Such a suspension of consent is temporary, however, because if the patient should subsequently regain capacity or an appropriate surrogate later becomes identified, then, of necessity, authorization would have to be obtained for any future interventions.

In a system preoccupied with documentation and record keeping, the signed consent form presumably giving authorization tends to substitute for the consent process itself.[21] Of course, a form that purports to represent an actual event (that of informing the patient), but does not, is neither ethically nor legally valid. Similarly, verbal consent without a form signed by the patient or surrogate may be valid, although documentation of one kind or another is usually advisable (though sometimes not possible).[31] Of overall importance is the dialogue that supports the documentation and that the consent form theoretically reflects.

Decision Making for Incapacitated Patients

The Importance of Prior Discussions

A common remark about the medical profession in the modern world is that some of the physician's traditional "art" has succumbed to a preoccupation with applied science. Patients are often examined more in terms of their discrete diseases requiring investigation and intervention than as suffering individuals who face the dilemmas and perhaps deterioration brought on by medical crises. Whether or not this criticism is fair or historically accurate, many dilemmas arising out of confusing treatment circumstances could be ameliorated if the wishes of the patient were expressed and discussed with the physician before the patient's loss of capacity.[32]

Given that many people in our health care system do not have regular contact with a physician before the onset of serious illness, the opportunity for such ongoing discussions are not available to everyone.[33] In addition, because few physicians are specially trained to undertake such intimate and personal discussions and because such discussions often require a significant amount of (unreimbursed) time, modern conditions for providing care are often not hospitable to fostering this kind of dialogue.[33]

Still, conversations with patients either by primary care physicians or by specialists who have ongoing relationships with the patient provide excellent occasions for the practice of what is known as "preventive ethics." Properly conducted and documented, such conversations can provide critical guidance even if they do not determine the nature of treatment for a patient who is no longer cogent. The point of such information gathering is not merely to relieve the professional of legal liability. Rather, when physicians discuss preferences in advance, they are acting in a respectful manner that the majority of patients appreciate. These discussions permit the patient to maintain control and to be self-determining, despite any future loss of capacity that may render the patient nonautonomous.[34]

Advance Directives and Proxy Appointments

Because patients' prospective treatment wishes often involve matters of withholding or withdrawing life-sustaining treatment and because of the potential for legal involvement when such treatment decisions are made, attempts should be made to document these advance discussions. Such documentation is more likely to provide clarity in the midst of uncertainty or memory lapses and may also provide the type of legal evidence that may be necessary before life-sustaining care can be withheld or withdrawn.[32,35]

Making sure that the medical record reflects the details of discussions between providers and patients is wise, and specific mechanisms exist in most communities to highlight the nature of these advance planning discussions. Depending on the legal jurisdiction, patients and physicians have the opportunity to document such preferences via several methods. (Readers should consult their local medical society for the precise arrangements legally available in their own jurisdictions.)

The two most commonly accepted methods for such advance planning documentation are the living will[36] and the durable power of attorney for health care, also known as the health care proxy.[32] Both mechanisms are used only if the patient loses the capacity to participate in the decision-making process. A *living will* is a document that patients execute before their loss of decisional capacity. The document serves to record for caregivers and loved ones what the patient's preferences are about future treatment options, in terms of either desired treatment or the treatment the patient would wish to be withheld or withdrawn.[28] Both afford the patient and provider ample opportunity to specify particular wishes and preferences, although the benefits of each method differ. Depending on patient circumstance, one method may be preferable to the other. Typically, such documents detail the types of interventions that patients wish to avoid as the ends of their lives approach. Many states have specified the precise form and content that such documents must follow to be legally binding; other states are generally more concerned with the clarity and the substance contained in the document.[28]

In general, when executing a living will, the patient should be as explicit as possible, using precise language that is not susceptible to differing interpretations or misunderstanding. For example, language discussing "heroic" or "extraordinary" care might have different meanings to different interpreters. If a patient is specifically concerned about such potentially intrusive interventions as mechanical ventilation or artificial nutrition and hydration, then the patient should state this concern precisely.[28] Patients are also advised to specify the precise physical circumstances under which they would want to trigger such withholding or withdrawal.[28] For example, they should make clear whether they desire that permanent loss of consciousness or unremitting pain be present before treatment is withheld or withdrawn. The average lay person would of necessity need the input of a medical provider, both in terms of deciphering what future options may face the patient and determining the benefits and burdens of each option.

Even the most precise and specific living will may not cover every possible option that may confront the incapacitated patient; in addition, certain decisions may not be discernible from the contents of the document.[36] Written documents are also helpful only if they are available (as opposed to being locked away in a drawer) and actually enforced. Therefore many individuals choose to accompany or even replace their living wills with a durable power of attorney for health care or health care proxy.[31] Such a mechanism allows the patient (known as the principal) to legally empower another individual to make whatever treatment decisions the patient would have made had the patient had capacity.[33] Such a mechanism ensures that a healthy advocate will be legally available to assert the patient's prior wishes and also permits flexibility and interpretation should a situation arise that the patient had not previously addressed.[33]

Surrogate Decision Making: Who Decides and on What Basis?

Surrogates or agents specifically appointed by the patient in advance usually have the moral and legal authority to substitute for the patient if the patient becomes incapacitated.[33] Depending on the jurisdiction, legally binding mechanisms can be used before the loss of capacity. In some circumstances, court appointment of a surrogate may be necessary.[4] In some jurisdictions, the fact of biological or spousal connection may be sufficient to both morally and legally empower the surrogate, regardless of a lack of a previously executed document or the lack of court involvement.[4] Once an appropriate surrogate is identified, that person has the responsibility to determine the best course of action for the now incapacitated patient. Just as for the patient, it is essential for the surrogate to go through an "informed consent" process with the patient's providers to ascertain all of the clinically relevant details necessary to understanding the patient's circumstances.[21] However, such decisions clearly extend beyond the realm of medicine and usually involve value judgments that the patient brings to the process.

When a surrogate substitutes for the patient, the ideal method of making a decision is to consider and account for those values that defined the patient while capable, infused that patient's actions, and determined the patient's lifestyle.[33] The ideal requirement is that the surrogate render a "substituted judgment" on the patient's behalf, making the same sort of choice the patient would have made had he or she had the capacity to participate.[33] This is no easy task, although the existence of a well-documented advance directive usually provides the surrogate with the type of information necessary to render such a judgment. In some circumstances, the surrogate may have to interpret or surmise what the patient would have wanted, on the basis of the surrogate's knowledge of the patient as a person and how the patient lived his or her life.[33] In some jurisdictions, such surrogate "interpretations" may not be legally acceptable, depending on the nature of the surrogate appointment and the clarity of the patient's previously expressed wishes.[33]

If such a substituted judgment is not possible, either because the surrogate has insufficient knowledge of the patient as a person or because whatever knowledge is available sheds little light on the current choice at hand, the surrogate would then be morally obligated to make the choice that promotes the patient's "best interests."[12] This judgment is meant to incorporate considerations of a more "objective" nature, such as the patient's prognosis, the patient's pain and suffering,[37] and the patient's present and projected quality of life relative to the life the patient previously experienced, rather than a derogatory evaluation of personal worth in comparison with other members of society.[28] In most circumstances, particularly those involving decisions to withhold or withdraw life-sustaining treatment, surrogates work with providers to determine the patient's best interests in light of what can be done for the patient's current situation, the patient's underlying health and prognosis, and the burdens the patient may experience as a result of any measurable benefits to be achieved.[27] However, in certain jurisdictions, the legality of such judgments may be challenged, and a concern about bias or prejudice always exists when discussions about "quality of life" emerge.[12]

Particularly when discussion of the patient's best interests focuses on treatments that might be "futile" and in no way beneficial to the patient, there is the potential for tremendous discord because the precise meaning of the concept of "futility" may change, depending on the specific orientation of the decision maker.[38] For example, clinicians may view a course of treatment as "futile" if it does nothing to address the underlying condition that forms the subtext of the patient's current situation.[39] Yet others may regard "futility" as only apparent if no measurable benefit of any sort can be derived from a particular intervention.

Treatment Decisions Requiring Special Attention

"Do Not Resuscitate" Orders

Decisions as to whether to attempt resuscitative measures if a patient experiences a cardiac or pulmonary arrest should theoretically be no different from other patient treatment choices. Ideally, a provider would discuss the possible options and their risks and benefits with the patient in advance of any intervention, so that a decision to initiate cardiopulmonary resuscitation (CPR) would reflect the patient's desire that the provider intervene in such circumstances.

However, the reality and mythology that have developed around acute care decisions to resuscitate or to not resuscitate a patient have, for several reasons, brought this particular treatment situation into a different category. Cardiopulmonary resuscitation protocols for the restoration of oxygenation and circulation have been remarkably successful, in terms of both their standardization (by the National Research Council in 1966) and their public acceptance: By 1977, more than 12 million people had been trained in cardiopulmonary resuscitation.[40] Second, because the use of cardiopulmonary resuscitation is often brought on by emergency circumstances, there may be no prior discussion of patient preference upon which to draw and often no knowledge of the patient at all. Third, decisions not to resuscitate require consent not to intervene, which is contradictory to the normal situation of consent to intervene in a particular circumstance. "Do not resuscitate" (DNR) orders require a conscious and, perhaps courageous, effort on the part of a team to recognize before a catastrophic event the inevitability of its occurrence and the likely outcome of intervention. Such forethought must happen in a climate that does little to foster discussion of death and does much to encourage the escalated use of sophisticated acute care technology merely because of its existence, rather than because of its likely benefit.[51]

In one state (New York), legislation exists to actually define the legal parameters of DNR orders,[42] but in most jurisdictions, the use of such orders must, of necessity, become more familiar and comfortable a process for those who often confront patients in the midst of an arrest. As with any other treatment decision, the ethically preferable process for making the DNR decision would be to undergo an informed consent process with the patient or, if the patient is incapacitated, with an appropriate surrogate. In the course of such a discussion, the provider's duty would be to disclose the likelihood and definition of "success" for a person in this particular patient's circumstances and would, as well, require a thorough discussion of all possible aspects of the intervention, including the possibility of connection to a ventilator or injury resulting from the aggressive nature of some resuscitation attempts.[37] Although many patients unexpectedly have an arrest, other patients are likely to fall into a category of arrest "suspects"; their clinical condition would dictate that a discussion of DNR orders, among other possible treatment interventions, would be mandatory as soon in their hospitalization as possible.[36] The goal is to solicit patient input and foster self-determination before the patient loses the capacity to participate in the decision-making process.[41]

Ideally, advance discussions of DNR orders would come in the context of a more general discussion of future treatment options for the particular patient's condition. However, it is possible that permission will be given to place a DNR order in the patient's chart, yet the patient or the surrogate will nonetheless insist on other types of aggressive care that may seem inconsistent with the decision to consent to a DNR order. Such inconsistency may be due to a lack of mutual agreement or understanding about the goals of the treatment process; it may also be the result of a reasoned decision on the part of the patient or surrogate that some interventions are worth certain risk but others are not.[37]

For example, a patient may be willing to undergo the toxic side effects of aggressive, experimental chemotherapy or the bruising recovery that may follow significant surgery yet be unwilling to risk the possibility of winding up dependent on a ventilator as a result of a resuscitation attempt. From the patient's or surrogate's perspective, such choices may not appear inconsistent, although providers would be wise to have the patient or surrogate vocally express reasons for the specific treatment choices made, to ensure full understanding and comprehension by both the patient and the provider.

Of particular concern and difficulty are surgical candidates with preexisting DNR orders in place. Such patients typically have underlying chronic or terminal illnesses that provide the basis for the patient's previous decision to consent to a standing DNR order. However, there may be circumstances in which such patients nonetheless become candidates for surgical intervention, perhaps for palliative purposes or for reasons unconnected to their underlying disease process. In such cases, the decision as to whether the DNR order will remain in place during the surgical intervention should be thoroughly discussed by the patient, surrogate (if involved), surgeon, and anesthesiologist, if possible. It is of critical importance for patients or their surrogates to realize the distinct nature and characteristics of cardiac arrest during the perioperative period. In particular, the facts that cardiac arrest during that period is often directly linked to either the surgical or anesthetic intervention and that resuscitative interventions during such arrests have a very high success rate must be made clear to a patient who seeks surgery for certain, specific objectives. For many providers, the concept of a DNR order during surgery seems incompatible with professional and moral obligations to a patient during the surgical procedure. The often direct linkage between the caregiver's actions and the patient's arrest creates an inescapable obligation for many providers to intervene in the case of arrest.

An evolving approach to this difficult dilemma involves the protocol of "required reconsideration" whenever a patient with a DNR order in place becomes a candidate for surgery.[43,44] Such an approach demands active reconsideration of the DNR decision before the surgical intervention. Such discussion must necessarily involve the patient and the patient's surrogate, if appropriate, and should carefully review the distinct quality of perioperative arrest as well as the goals of the patient for the surgical intervention. In most cases, an accommodation can be worked out whereby a temporary suspension of the DNR order is agreed on, with specific parameters set for its re-institution, either depending on the cause of the perioperative arrest or because of circumstances that arise after the patient's recovery from the surgical intervention. Such a protocol should reflect the patient's values and wishes to the extent possible. If an acceptable agreement cannot be worked out, the involved physicians may either have the option to proceed with the surgery, with a carefully delineated DNR order in place, or choose to decline to intervene, with the obligation to assist the patient in accessing other providers who may be willing to perform the operation despite the constraint of the existing DNR order.

Ultimately, when considering the applicability of a DNR order for a particular patient, one must remember that although the decision not to resuscitate might logically be accompanied by other choices about reducing the aggressiveness of care, this does not necessarily have to be so. A patient may logically, ethically, and legally desire intensive care intervention yet be unwilling to be resuscitated should an arrest occur. Each type of intervention should be considered in its own distinct context, and the merits of any particular intervention should be judged; an appropriate surrogate must decide on behalf of the patient, on the basis of an evaluation of what promotes the best interests of the patient.[13]

The "Never" Competent

Decision making for patients who never possessed capacity is similar to the process described for those who are congenitally retarded or severely impaired or for other reasons never had the opportunity or ability to develop a system of values and preferences that could be used to direct the course of care despite the lack of capacity. Thus "substituted judgment" cannot be rendered on their behalf because they never possessed the original judgment.[13] Rather, the needs and course of care for those never competent must be based on an objective determination of their specific circumstances. This decision should be based on an examination of the patient's diagnosis and prognosis as well as the benefits and burdens associated with the various care options. The assessment of benefits and burdens includes considerations of pain, suffering, palliation, extension of life, and other determinable measures. In all cases, these considerations are limited to benefits and burdens imposed on the individual patient. To the extent that this involves an assessment of the patient's "quality of life," this assessment is limited to determining whether the benefits of continued care for the individual patient outweigh the burdens of care experienced by that patient. This does not involve an assessment of the patient's quality of life in comparison to what might be achievable by others.[38]

As surrogates, parents cannot call on their child's background or lifestyle to form a "substituted judgment." The natural course of surrogate decision making is one that relies on evaluation of the child's best interests, and in such determinations, the parents are generally afforded significant latitude to discern the nature and course of their child's care.[32] When parents' decisions clearly contrast with promoting their child's health and medical well-being, others may be empowered to challenge the choice made by the parents.[4] For these reasons, should parental conduct appear concretely neglectful—or even abusive—of a child's needs, grounds might be found to disempower the parents and allow others to decide on the child's behalf. Principled choices of parents that they could assert for themselves, such as prioritizing religious faith above risk of death, are considered unacceptable when applied to the children of such individuals.[4] Therefore parents who subscribe to the Jehovah's Witness faith may refuse lifesaving blood transfusions for themselves but not on their child's behalf. Parental empowerment does not include the ability to risk death for a child who has not yet attained the capacity to choose such a course for himself or herself.[4]

Children who are on the cusp of capacity (i.e., those approaching the murky line that separates adolescence from adulthood) may in certain circumstances be considered to possess sufficient judgment to participate in the decision making process.[4] Even if their consent is technically not required, from a moral perspective their concerns and desires should warrant serious attention and play a significant, if not determinative, part in the deliberation process.[32]

Critical Care and End-of-Life Decision Making: Special Concerns

The circumstances that surround critical care and end-of-life decision making are often made more controversial and problematic for both patients and providers because of uncertainty about the moral and legal permissibility of certain actions or decisions. This is particularly true when death is a likely or even intended consequence of a choice. In addition, many philosophically based terms are sometimes interjected into discussions without universal clarity or certainty about their intended meanings. For example, comparisons such as *ordinary* versus *extraordinary* or *withholding* versus *withdrawing* sometimes conjure up misguided notions about what is or is not acceptable in the course of delivering patient care.[45] The unnecessary inclusion of confusing terms often clouds the underlying reasons and justifications for choices made either by or on behalf of a patient.

For patients who possess decisional capacity, the choice of whether to initiate, withhold, or withdraw care is one solely within the orbit of the patient's value system, even if the likely or intended consequence of the patient's choice is significant harm or even death.[45] Despite the discomfort that many providers have with this concept, it is one in accord with the moral and legal frameworks supporting patient autonomy.[46] Thus a patient can decline the option of life-prolonging surgery, can ask that mechanical ventilation be withheld if respiratory distress occurs, and can even ask for the withdrawal or cessation of such life-prolonging measures as dialysis, artificial nutrition, and hydration (in most jurisdictions), as long as the patient possesses the capacity and information to assess the benefits and burdens of such choices.[38,46] However, in some jurisdictions, such choices may nonetheless require a legal process to carry out the request.[4] This step may stem more from concern about injecting safeguards into such decision processes rather than any move away from fundamental moral or common law support for such patient decisions. Moreover, in most jurisdictions, such patient requests would be accorded respect even if they were transmitted through an appropriately executed living will or appointed surrogate once the patient loses decisional capacity.

Questions of whether there is any moral or legal difference between withholding and withdrawing care, whether the care involved is of an "ordinary" versus "extraordinary" nature, or whether it is acceptable to omit an action that may lead to the patient's death but not to purposefully act in such a way that may bring about death raise concerns about word origins and their current meaning and significance in the context of care. Many of these terms—although perhaps drawing some useful distinctions in their earlier, theologic origins or perhaps pointing to areas that warrant additional attention—in and of themselves do not determine the morality or legality of the choice carried out.[37] For example, a provider who makes the distinction that "extraordinary" care may be withheld or withdrawn, yet "ordinary" care must be initiated or continued tells us little about the precise nature of the care or its effect on the patient at issue.[28,46]

Although in simpler times distinguishing what was ordinary from what was not perhaps seemed easier, the sophistication of the machinery or commonness of its application in today's sophisticated acute care environment creates situations in which an appropriate intervention for one patient may not be acceptable or even beneficial to another similarly situated patient. In such determinations, the importance is not in what the care is labeled but rather how it affects that patient and fits into the patient's perspective in terms of benefits versus burdens.[37] One patient may believe the receipt of artificial nutrition via a gastrostomy tube is desirable and acceptable, whereas another may view it as extraordinarily burdensome and inconsistent with his or her view of what best suits his or her interests. Such different meanings between patients only underscores how physicians and patients may view choices differently. A provider should not presume that a patient regards a certain course of care in a way similar to how the provider regards it.

Similarly, attempts to explain omissions or withholdings as being morally or legally permissible and actions or withdrawals as impermissible only confuse and distort the reasons and justifications that will make such choices either permissible or not. Merely because a provider decides not to initiate a process does not necessarily relieve that provider of responsibility if the outcome was one intended or foreseen.[28] This is particularly so in the context of patient-provider relationships, in which the provider owes duties to the patient and in which decisions not to act may be as influential and responsible for patient outcomes as any concrete activity that the provider undertakes. For example, a decision to withdraw artificial ventilation from a patient, which may or may not bring about the patient's death, is not necessarily any less permissible or unacceptable than the choice to omit or withhold its use in the first place. Some people may believe a distinction exists between an act that is believed to cause the death of the patient and one that merely holds back a possibility from an already dying patient, but from a moral and legal point of view, arguments used to withhold treatment should be equally justifiable and binding as decisions to withdraw or cease.[38] Judicial decisions that have addressed this matter concur that no logical distinction exists.[38]

A decision not to initiate care can be viewed just as "causative" in terms of patient outcome as any act of withdrawing, if the outcome was one that was foreseen and could have been avoided if a different choice was made. In such circumstances the important point is not so much whether one is acting or omitting or withholding or withdrawing, but rather why one is undertaking that course and whether it can be justified in terms of the patient's preference or the best interests of the patient as determined by an appropriate surrogate.[32] Moreover, many commentators have clarified that decisions not to initiate care, because of fear that once started a treatment cannot later be stopped, may actually harm certain patient populations.[28] Some patients might benefit from a trial of therapy, even if later on the therapy may no longer serve the patient's interests and should be withdrawn in the name of beneficence, nonmaleficence, or patient autonomy. Not to have tried an intervention for fear of not being able to stop it lacks logic and defies the nature of providing medical care, which often means that certain risks are undertaken for certain potential benefits. One must always remember the provider's duty to relieve pain and suffering and not to cause harm to the patient.[28]

Nonetheless, certain actions on the part of providers and requests on the part of patients trigger additional scrutiny and other societal interests that may take priority over a pure vision of patient autonomy or provider beneficence. For example, societal interests in the sanctity of life and concern for the prevention of suicide are generally used to deny support for patient requests for suicide assistance[38,47] or for provider services to purposefully administer a medication or another intervention for the purpose of causing the patient's death (what is sometimes known as "active euthanasia").[38,47] Although much sympathy is generated for the plight of desperately ill patients seeking relief from their terminal conditions and often grand jury investigations of such matters fail to indict involved parties,[28] most states maintain strict theoretical sanctions and legal prohibitions on provider involvement in such cases.

In two decisions the U.S. Supreme Court reiterated the traditional American condemnation of suicide and upheld the value of the individual human life by unanimously striking down two lower court decisions that had found a constitutional right to die with the aid of a doctor. Although the Court ruled that the constitution does not guarantee Americans such a right, it left the individual states with the power to determine the legality of physician-assisted death.[47,48] In October of 1997, the state of Oregon enacted the Death with Dignity Act into law, becoming the first state to legalize and regulate physician-assisted death. The state's first legal physician-assisted death took place on March 24, 1998. In 2006, the Supreme Court specifically addressed a challenge to this Oregon law in the case of Gonzales v Oregon.[49] Ruling that the United States Attorney General could not enforce the Controlled Substances Act against Oregon physicians who prescribed drugs for assisted suicide in the terminally ill, in accord with the Oregon law, the Court affirmed the ability of a state to pass legislation permitting physician-assisted death under defined circumstances.

As these events in Oregon attest, we may be witnessing a shift in societal consensus about how to prioritize values when fundamental questions about the meaning of life and death are the issue. The debate concerns the precise role of the physician and the nature of physician-patient relationship in an era of such sophisticated and often partially successful care that it is sometimes difficult to discern whether, on the whole, an intervention would benefit or burden a patient. Some argue that supporting physician involvement in the intended death of a patient destroys the essential role of the provider as healer and would create an air of uncertainty that would ultimately damage the trust that exists between patient and provider.[27] Others believe that one essential role of the modern physician is relief of suffering, and the possibility of such physician involvement might encourage otherwise desperate patients to try one more round of therapy or intervention, comforted by the knowledge that failure would not lead to unremitting pain or unendurable misery.[27] As the effects of Oregon's Death with Dignity Act become clear and as more states move to enact legislation, the debate over these issues will intensify.

Although the Supreme Court found no constitutional right to physician-assisted death, the Court seemed to recognize the existence of a legitimate conflict between the needs of some terminally ill individuals and the larger interests of society. In fact, some have argued that although patients cannot legally ask physicians to end their suffering by invoking a constitutional right to assistance in dying, patients may very well have a constitutional right to palliative care.[50]

However, all judicial decisions that have examined cases of the withholding or withdrawal of patient care have distinguished such circumstances from cases of active euthanasia or other forms of killing or suicide.[28] No physician who has participated in treatment decisions to withhold or withdraw care has ever been found criminally liable and responsible for the patient's death.[28] Cases of assisted suicide and euthanasia have been distinguished on the basis of the nature of the patient's prognosis and clinical circumstances. Patients who refuse care

or ask for its withdrawal and who will then die from their underlying conditions are not considered to be committing suicide, nor are providers who respect such decisions considered to be assisting suicide or killing the patients.[48]

One final distinction deserves examination: the administration of pain relief with the knowledge, though perhaps not the intent, that such medication may ultimately shorten the patient's life or even cause the patient's death. Under the theologic doctrine of "double effect," such action is usually explained and justified by referring to the primary effect and intent of the action, that of relieving pain, while recognizing the possibility or even likelihood that another effect, that of the patient's shortened life or even death, is a possible result of the action.[12] The action is considered permissible because the intent was to relieve suffering, not to cause death.

Theoretically, in current legal climates, the knowledge that an outcome is possible—though not necessarily intended—might still lead to liability on the part of the provider.[45] However, we know of no successful litigation against a provider for administering pain relief to a patient with significant need, even if the outcome of the relief also meant an earlier death for the patient. Justification for such actions are usually, in current climates, based on either the patient's choice to risk death to achieve pain relief (or a similar decision by an authorized surrogate) or on the widely recognized additional role of the provider to relieve pain when possible. Such provider actions are generally distinguished in legal forums from more common examples of "active euthanasia."[36] In fact, many commentators have suggested that it would be unusually cruel and harmful to a patient to respect the patient's wish that care be withdrawn or withheld, yet not provide him or her with pain medication to ease the transition to death.[37]

Artificial Nutrition and Hydration

The use of artificial means to nourish and hydrate patients who are unable to take in food on their own has generated significant debate concerning definitions of "medical care" versus "comfort care."[36] For many caregivers, the question raised is whether there are any limits to patient self-determination or provider obligations in the context of the physician-patient relationship. Many believe that withholding or withdrawing "medical care" in accord with patients' self-determination is permissible, whereas the provision of artificial nutrition and hydration represents the intrinsic "caring" nature of human interaction and therefore must always be provided as a fundamental demonstration of humanity and compassion.[51]

All courts of law that have addressed this question, including the U.S. Supreme Court, have equated the use of artificial nutrition and hydration with the use of other medical technologies and "high-tech" progenies, such as mechanical ventilation and dialysis. They have thus permitted its withholding or withdrawal in accord with the interests of patient self-determination. In the political arena, some legislatures have even made exceptions to their living will or health care proxy legislation to make allowance for such a distinction[4] and, in some circumstances, to refuse to grant permission for patients or surrogates to have such care withheld or withdrawn.[4] Given the sometimes passionate nature of the debate and the pluralistic nature of our society, a compromise has been reached in many instances that recognizes the right of individuals to determine the course of their care, particularly when providers feel unable to abide by such patients' requests. This accommodation usually calls on either individual or institutional providers to disclose to patients and families, before the onset of a relationship, the perspective of the provider about this type of care.[32]

Dilemmas in Team Decision Making: The Role of the Anesthesiologist

Dilemmas in the clinical setting may emerge not only from interaction with patients and families but also in the relationships that are forged under a system of team coverage of patient care needs. Particularly for the neurosurgical patient—whose problems may span the disciplines of neurology, surgery, and anesthesiology, among others—the collection of providers who join to meet the specific needs of an individual patient may generate interdisciplinary disputes, rivalry, or even antagonisms, which may subtly, or perhaps not so subtly, affect patient care. In this regard, the role of the consultant anesthesiologist is briefly examined as just one example.

A cardinal rule of the Hippocratic tradition, which emphasized the appropriateness of calling in consultants, was that physicians were never to disagree with their colleagues in front of the patient.[15] In our own time, the notion of a "united front" before the laity has perhaps a greater command over medicine than in other professions, so that even when physicians are in substantial disagreement over the appropriate course, they rarely present their disagreement to the patient. Considering that the patient whose condition is serious enough to warrant consultation is often in an emotionally vulnerable position, this policy might not seem to be an unwise one.

However, modern legal analysis and case law support the independent authority and responsibility of the anesthesiologist as separate and distinct from other members of the health care team. Although the anesthesiologist may have little or no participation in the initial decision to intervene surgically, he or she has separate responsibility to review the patient's condition and to obtain an independent informed consent directly from the patient or the patient's surrogate for the use of anesthetics. In effect, the anesthesiologist must review the feasibility of anesthetic intervention for the particular patient and separately determine whether the surgery should proceed on the basis of this review. The actions or determinations of the anesthesiologist are no longer viewed as subordinate to those of the surgeon. The anesthesiologist has an independent duty to the patient, separate and apart from that of the surgeon or any other member of the health care team. Such duty carries through the entire perioperative period, until such time as the anesthesiologist discharges the patient from his or her care.

Ethical Issues in Innovative Neurosurgery: Role of the Anesthesiologist

The anesthesiologist's specific duties toward the surgical patient, as discussed in the previous paragraph on team decision making, also extend toward patients undergoing experimental or innovative procedures. Such innovations may occur within or outside of formal clinical studies, as we explain here. Perhaps even more pressing than during standard operations, the anesthesiologist may function as an important consultant to the neurosurgeon (and perhaps, sometimes, as an advocate for the patient) by helping the neurosurgeon appropriately identify those procedures that are in fact experimental enough to warrant additional scrutiny and review. The additional review and patient protections required for experimental surgery may not always be apparent to the neurosurgeon, because they traditionally have not always been recognized by the surgical profession

in general. Prior research has shown that surgeons generally do not readily identify those innovations that are in fact experimental or that amount to research with human subjects; they do not often submit their innovative procedures to rigorous testing in the form of (controlled) clinical trials nor their innovative surgical techniques to their institutional review boards (IRBs) for prior review and monitoring.[52,53]

Every day, US surgeons modify existing operations, attempting to improve their techniques and outcomes. Sometimes this modification occurs on an individual patient basis; sometimes a group of patients undergoes an innovative procedure. Sometimes a group of patients serves as a prospective or historical control. Innovative operations find their way into the professional journals and conferences as case reports, case series, or case-control studies, and a very small percentage as prospective clinical trials. But many, perhaps most of them, have one thing in common: They were performed under the heading of therapy, not of research. Whether they started out as spontaneous technique modifications necessary for a particular patient situation or as informal studies with or without protocols, most of these studies were done without prior IRB review and without specific research consent from patients.[54] In some instances, such review and consent would have been appropriate and necessary, but uncertainties and disagreements exist among surgeons as to what constitutes routine variations on surgical techniques that require no prior approval and what are new or innovative techniques warranting IRB review and patients' specific informed consent for an experimental procedure or a research study.[53,55] This area is where the neurosurgical anesthesiologist can become an important ally of both patients and science, by helping surgeons correctly identify those innovations that would better be performed under the heading of research. It is therefore of paramount importance that anesthesiologists be familiar with the definitions and regulations for human subject research and with the workings of the local IRB.

Necessary knowledge to make judgments about research and innovative practice can be found in documents from both federal agencies and professional societies. The oversight of research, innovation, and standard health care involves multiple jurisdictions: The separate states; federal agencies involved with regulation, funding, or reimbursement; professional societies; and health maintenance organizations (themselves operating under state and/or federal rules) may all be involved. Increasingly, the courts may play a significant role.

At the federal level, there are the regulations of the U.S. Department of Health and Human Services (DHHS) and its Office of Human Research Protections (OHRP; formerly Office for Protection of Research Risks [OPRR]). DHHS has issued a Code of Federal Regulations Title 45 Part 46, on "Protection of Human Subjects."[9] "45 CFR 46," or the Common Rule, so called because it has been adopted by all but 17 state agencies, provides formal definitions of *research* and *human subject* of such research. Subpart A of 45 CFR 46, or the Federal Policy for the Protection of Human Subjects, sets out definitions and general regulations for performing research with human subjects. *Research* is defined as any systematic investigation designed to develop and contribute to generalizable knowledge. *Human subject* is defined as a living individual about whom an investigator obtains either (1) data through interaction or intervention (e.g., surgery) or (2) identifiable private information. The other subparts of the document specify what additional guidelines are to be followed in case of vulnerable populations.

The Common Rule applies to all research involving humans that is conducted, supported, or otherwise subject to regulation by any federal department or agency. In other words, any institution that receives federal funding falls under and must abide by the Common Rule. This makes the DHHS ultimately responsible over *all* human subject research that is directly or indirectly funded by federal money. DHHS thus technically has jurisdiction over all surgical clinical research as well, as long as it is conducted in health care institutions that receive federal money. DHHS's definitions of research and human subject are applicable in surgery as much as they are in non-interventional specialties. However, the problem lies in the fact that not all surgical research activities are *defined* as such and thereby escape the overview of local IRBs and, ultimately, of the Office of Human Research Protections and DHHS. Part of the reason is that surgeons do not always *recognize* their efforts to improve surgical technique as research (which sometimes is appropriate, sometimes not) and another part is that surgeons are not always adequately aware of the fact that DHHS definitions sometimes *do* apply to their innovative activities. The lack of awareness is most probably due to inadequate familiarity with the Common Rule and its definitions and regulations.[52,53]

The U.S. Food and Drug Administration (FDA) gained regulatory powers to ensure the safety and effectiveness of new medical devices and medications. The law stipulates that all medical devices manufactured after 1976 are subject to an approval process and then subjected to regulatory controls according to their level of patient risk. However, unless an innovative surgical technique involves such an investigational device or an experimental drug, the FDA has no responsibility or jurisdiction over surgical research.[56]

Local agents under the DHHS Common Rule that do have formal jurisdiction are institutional review boards (IRBs). The IRB, also known as the research ethics committee, has been the local protection mechanism for human research subjects since the latter part of the 20th century. IRBs have the authority and responsibility for approving or disapproving proposals to conduct research involving human subjects.

Voluntary guidelines have been issued by surgical societies such as the American College of Surgeons (ACS). The Committee on Emerging Surgical Technologies (CESTE) of the ACS has issued statements specifically addressing the ethical and responsible implementation of new surgical techniques and innovations.[57]

These self-imposed guidelines for emerging surgical technologies and their application to the care of patients were formulated in 1994 and 1995. In part, they read as follows:

1. The development of a new technology must be accompanied by a scientific assessment of safety, efficacy, and need....
2. Diffusion into clinical practice requires appropriate education of surgeons and evaluation of their use of the new technology....
3. Widespread application of new technologies must be continuously assessed and compared with alternative therapies to ensure appropriateness and cost-effectiveness through outcome studies.

The introduction of new technology to surgeons and the public must be done ethically in accordance with the *Statement on Principles of the American College of Surgeons.*

These principles require prior and continued IRB (or equivalent) review of the protocol, full description of the procedure, and informed consent of the patient. However,

current guidelines remain open to individual interpretation and are not restrictive in character. Other than issuing a reprimand or expelling an unruly surgeon from the Fellowship, the ACS does not have responsibility or legal jurisdiction over the practices of its Fellows, let alone over U.S. surgeons who are not members of the ACS. As such, the Statement on Emerging Surgical Technologies is not legally binding. Other surgical organizations, such as the Society of University Surgeons (SUS), have also attempted to address the challenge of surgical innovations by offering guidance.[58]

Until definitive guidelines or laws regulating innovative and experimental surgery have become established, it is up to individual neurosurgeons, aided by their team, including neuro-anesthesiologists, to determine which procedures should be introduced as innovative practice and which should be submitted to more formal scrutiny, such as IRB review and other oversight mechanisms.

Ethical Issues Concerning Managed Care

Finally, as financial considerations become an increasingly prolific feature of the health care landscape, providers and patients alike must be aware of the important ethical dilemmas that can arise from interactions with third-party payers. Although this section focuses on the problems that can arise in the context of managed care, similar problems can also arise within the context of more traditional insurance programs.

Since at least the advent of the Hippocratic tradition, providers have had the moral duty to distribute care equitably among the patients within their practice and to ensure that financial means does not determine access to health care services. Therefore each patient is entitled to skillful, knowledgeable, and diligent care, regardless of insurance status. The provider's fiduciary commitment to the patient's best interests, as that patient understands them, is not a function of the patient's financial resources. Although a patient's membership in a particular managed care organization (MCO) might set limits on the resources to which the patient is entitled in certain circumstances, this limitation should not affect the provider's duty to make the most skillful and effective use of the resources that are available.

Similarly, providers have the moral obligation to ensure the equitable use of health care resources, including technologic and pharmacologic modalities and the use of subspecialty referrals. The traditional fee-for-service system provides physicians with incentives to overuse many of these resources. In response to the skyrocketing health care costs that have resulted from this system of health care allocation, however, MCOs arose with the explicit aim of reining in escalating health care costs. To do so, many MCOs use a variety of financial incentives to encourage providers to adopt more medically and financially prudent patterns of using resources. However, this development means that third-party payers are now giving providers incentives to underuse many of these same resources.

The equitable use of health care resources requires that patients on traditional indemnity plans should not receive referrals or modalities of treatment that are not medically indicated and that patients covered by MCOs should not be denied access to treatment options or subspecialty care that is genuinely medically indicated. In both cases, the provider has a duty to make the most effective use of existing health care resources, avoiding both wastefulness and inadequacy.

Finally, there are often important ways a patient's membership in an MCO may limit or affect access to certain treatment options, by constraining the process by which such access is made available, denying access to certain options altogether, or simply limiting the amount of resources patients can themselves command. The general agreement is that the patient's right to self-determination and the doctrine of informed consent require providers to inform patients of relevant ways their membership in an MCO constrains or limits their health care options.[45,59]

SUMMARY

Full and comprehensive care of the neurosurgical patient requires a thorough understanding of the ethical principles that guide the treatment decision-making process. Caregivers must be sensitive to the right of patients to be self-determining and to participate in the treatment decision-making process to the extent possible. Although decisional incapacity may render a patient unable to participate, the involvement of informed surrogates and the use of advance directives help ensure that treatment decisions are in accord with the patient's wishes and values, even if the patient can no longer participate in those decisions. It is essential to plan proactively for decisional incapacity through the use of advance planning mechanisms.

Particular problems may arise in connection with neurosurgical intervention, such as when DNR orders are in place or with the use of other life-sustaining measures. Clinicians must be cognizant of the autonomous rights of patients, yet patients and surrogates must also be informed of the unique and special characteristics of neurosurgical interventions, which may give rise to a reexamination of the reasons to withhold or withdraw life-sustaining treatments. Providers have a particular obligation to communicate such issues to patients. Anesthesiologists have separate and distinct obligations to the patient, including the obligations to interact directly with the patient, review the patient's readiness for anesthetic intervention, and monitor and oversee the patient's condition during the entire perioperative process in connection with the use of anesthetics. In addition to the reference list for this chapter, readers are encouraged to explore the additional resources listed in Box 24-2.

BOX 24–2 *Additional Readings*

Angell M: The case of Helga Wanglie: A new kind of right to die case. N Engl J Med 1991;325:511.

Cruzan v Director, 110 US 2841 (1990).

Gostin L: Life and death choices after Cruzan. Law Med Health Care 1991;19:9-12.

Gostin L, Weir RF: Life and death choices after Cruzan: Case law and standards of professional conduct. Milbank Q 1991;69:143-173.

In re Helga Wanglie, No. PX-91-283, 4th Judicial District Ct, Hennepin County, Minn (July 1, 1991).

Jonsen A: Watching the doctor. N Engl J Med 1983;308:1531-1535.

Kant E: Foundations of the Metaphysics of Morals. Beck LW, trans. Indianapolis, IN, Bobbs-Merrill, 1959.

REFERENCES

1. Carrick P: *Medical Ethics in Antiquity*, Dordrecht, 1985, D Reidel.
2. Starr P: *The Social Transformation of American Medicine*, New York, 1982, Basic Books.
3. Schloendorff v Society of New York Hospital, 211 NY 125,105 NE 92 (1914).
4. MacDonald M, Meyer K, Essig B: *Health care law*, New York, 1991, Matthew Bender.
5. Salgo v Leland Stanford Jr, University Board of Trustees, 154 Cal App 2d 560, 317 P2d 170 (1st Dist.) (1957).
6. Declaration of Geneva. *World Med Assoc Bull* 1:109–110, 1949.
7. Beecher HK: Ethics and clinical research, *N Eng J Med* 274:1354–1360, 1966.
8. The National Commission for the Protection of Human Subjects of Biomedical and Behavioral Research: *The Belmont Report: Ethical Principles and Guidelines for the Protection of Human Subjects of Research (DHEW Publication No [OS] 78-0012, Appendix I, DHEW Publication No [OS] 78-0013, Appendix 11, DHEW Publication No [OS] 78-0014)*, Washington, DC, 1978, US Government Printing Office.
9. United States Department of Health and Human Services: Protection of Human Subjects. Title 45, Code of Federal Regulations §46 (revised as of March 8, 1983).
10. In re Quinlan, 70 NJ 10, 355 A.2d 647, rev'd 137 NJ Super. 227, 348 A.2d 801 (1975), cert. denied, 429 US 922(1976).
11. Mill JS: *On Liberty*, London, 1863, JW Parker.
12. Beauchamp T, Childress J, *Principles of Biomedical Ethics*, ed 4, New York, 1994, Oxford University Press.
13. President's Commission for the Study of Ethical Problems in Medicine and Biomedical and Behavioral Research: Making Health Care Decisions, Washington, 1982, US Government Printing Office, vol. 1.
14. Katz J: Informed consent: A fairy tale? Law's vision, *U Pitt Law Rev* 39:137–174, 1977.
15. Hippocrates: *Oeuvres Completes d'Hippocrate. Littre, trans*, Paris, 1939-1961, Javal et Bourdeaux.
16. Siegler M: Confidentiality in medicine: A decrepit concept, *N Engl J Med* 307:1518–1521, 1982.
17. US Dept of Health and Human Services: Health Information Privacy. Available at www.hhs.gov/ocr/hipaa
18. Wilson JF: Health Insurance Portability and Accountability Act Privacy Rule causes ongoing concerns among clinicians and researchers, *Ann Intern Med* 145:313–316, 2006.
19. Brody BA, Englehardt HT: Bioethics: *Readings and Cases*. Englewood Cliffs, NJ, Prentice-Hall, 1987.
20. Whalen v Roe, 429 US 589 (1977).
21. Appelbaum P, Lidz C, Meisel A: Informed Consent, *Legal Theory and Clinical Practice*, New York, 1987, Oxford University Press.
22. Canterbury v Spence, 464 F2d 772 (DC Cir 1972), cert denied, 409 US 1064 (1972).
23. Cobbs v Grant, 8 Cal 3d 229, 502 P2d 1, 104 Cal Rptr 505 (1972).
24. Wilkinson v Vesey, I 10 RI 606, 295 A2d 676 (1972).
25. Buchanan A, Brock DW: Deciding for Others, *The Ethics of Surrogate Decision Making*, New York, 1989, Cambridge University Press.
26. Drane J: The many faces of competency, *Hastings Cent Rep* 15:17–21, 1985.
27. Pelligrino E: Doctors must not kill, *J Clin Ethics* 3:98, 1992.
28. Meisel A: *The Right to Die*, New York, 1989, John Wiley & Sons.
29. Novack DH, Plumer R, Smith RL: Changes in physicians' attitudes toward telling the cancer patient, *JAMA* 241:897, 1979.
30. Harris L: Associates: Views of informed consent and decision-making: Parallel surveys of physicians and the public, *President's Commission for the Study of Ethical Problems in Medicine and Biomedical and Behavioral Research*, vol 2, Washington, DC, 1982, US Government Printing Office, Appendices (Empirical Studies of Informed Consent).
31. Annas G: *The Rights of Patients*, ed 2, Totowa, NJ, 1992, Humana Press.
32. The New York State Task Force on Life and the Law: When Others Must Choose, *Deciding for Patients without Capacity*, Albany, NY, 1992, The New York State Task Force on Life and the Law.
33. New York State Task Force on Life and the Law: Life-Sustaining Treatment, *Making Decisions and Appointing a Health Care Agent*, Albany, NY, 1987, The New York State Task Force on Life and the Law.
34. Brody H: The physician/patient relationship. In Veatch R, editor: *Medical Ethics*, Boston, 1989, Jones & Bartlett, pp 65–91.
35. Cantor N: *Advance Directives and the Pursuit of Death with Dignity*, Bloomington, IN, 1993, Indiana University Press.
36. Dubler NN, Nimmons D: *Ethics on Call*, New York, 1992, Harmony Books.

37. President's Commission for the Study of Ethical Problems in Medicine and Biomedical and Behavioral Research: *Deciding to Forgo Life-Sustaining Treatment*, Washington, DC US, 1983, Government Printing Office.

38. The Hastings Center: *Guidelines on the Termination of Life-Sustaining Treatment and the Care of the Dying*, Bloomington, IN, 1987, Indiana University Press.

39. Schneiderman LJ, Jecker NS, Jonsen AR: Medical futility: Its meaning and ethical implications, *Ann Intern Med* 2:949–954, 1990.

40. Donegan JH: New concepts in cardiopulmonary resuscitation, *Anesth Analg* 60:100, 1981.

41. Sulmasy D, Geller G, Faden R, et al: The quality of mercy: Caring for patients with "do not resuscitate" orders, *JAMA* 267:682–686, 1992.

42. New York State Public Health Law, Article 29-B (McKinney Suppl 1992).

43. Cohen CB, Cohen PJ: Do-not-resuscitate orders in the operating room, *N Engl J Med* 325:1879–1882, 1991.

44. Truog RD, Rockoff MA: DNR in the OR: Further questions, *J Clin Anesth* 4:177–180, 1992.

45. Orentlicher D: Health care reform and the patient-physician relationship, *Health Matrix: J Law-Med* 5:141–180, 1995.

46. Beauchamp TL, Veatch RM: *Ethical Issues in Death and Dying*, ed 2, Upper Saddle River, NJ, 1996, Prentice-Hall.

47. Vacco v Quill, I 17 S.Ct. 2293 (1997).

48. Washington v Glucksberg, 117 SCt 2258 (1997).

49. Gonzales v Oregon, 546 US 243 (2006).

50. Burt RA: The Supreme Court speaks: Not assisted suicide but a constitutional right to palliative care, *N Eng J Med* 337:1234–1235, 1997.

51. Lynn J, Childress JF: Must patients always be given food and water? *Hastings Cent Rep* 13:17–21, 1983.

52. Reitsma AM, Moreno JD: Ethical regulations for innovative surgery: The last frontier? *J Am Coll Surg* 194:792–801, 2002.

53. Reitsma AM, Moreno JD: Ethics of innovative surgery: US surgeons' definitions, knowledge, and attitudes, *J Am Coll Surg* 40:103–110, 2005.

54. Margo CE: When is surgery research? Towards an operational definition of human research, *J Med Ethics* 27:40–43, 2001.

55. Angelos P, Lafreniere R, Murphy T, Rose W: Ethical issues in surgical treatment and research, *Curr Probl Surg* 40:345–448, 2003.

56. US Food and Drug Administration. CFR 21, Parts 50 and 56, additional FDA regulations: parts 312 (Investigational New Drug Application), 812 (Investigational Device Exemptions) and 860 (Medical Device Class Procedures). Available at www.fda.gov.

57. American College of Surgeons. Statements on Issues to be considered before new surgical technology is applied to the care of patients. *Bull Am Coll Surg* 1995;80:46–47.

58. American College of Surgeons: Statements on Principles. Available at www.facs.org/fellows-info/statements/stonprin.html

59. Biffl WL, Spain DA, Reitsma AM, et al: Society of University Surgeons Surgical Innovations Project Team: Responsible development and application of surgical innovations: A position statement of the Society of University Surgeons, *J Am Coll Surg* 206:1204–1209, 2008.

60. Morreim EH: *Balancing Act: The New Medical Ethics of Medicine's New Economics*, Washington, DC, 1995, Georgetown University Press.

Chapter 25

FUTURE ADVANCES IN NEUROANESTHESIA

W. Andrew Kofke

Numerous clinical situations remain as problematic issues that continue to vex neuroanesthesiologists and neurointensivists as they work to optimize outcomes for their patients. Nascent research ongoing at this time may provide a window to the future approaches to these problems. In this chapter I review many of these new research areas and speculate as to how they may eventually translate to clinical care of neurosurgical patients in the operating room and neurointensive care unit. Areas to be reviewed are genomics, stem cells, neuroprotection, intracranial pressure (ICP) management, technology, and pharmacology.

GENOMICS

Each cell has to produce proteins in order to function. The specific protein structure is determined by the sequence of base pairs on the organism's DNA combined with post-translational modifications. One estimate is that there are some 35,000 to 40,000 genes with about 6000 proteins active at any given time. However, actual protein composition varies according to the needs (and regulation) of the moment, such that it is thought that as many as 100,000 proteins can be transcribed by a cell.[1] Thus the actual genetic structure of an individual has an important role in the development of and response to disease and the response to therapy.

The field of genomics is significantly complex.[2] Notably the word *gene* has a multitude of definitions,[3] reflecting the wide variety of approaches to the field. The field includes work with single-nucleotide polymorphisms (SNPs), transcript messenger RNA (mRNA) studies, short interfering RNA (siRNA) epigenetics, and copy number variants. SNPs are naturally occurring variation in the specific DNA nucleotides that code for specific proteins resulting in naturally occurring variations in proteins with associated variations in function. After a gene has been transcribed into mRNA, further regulation with potential for variation arises such that there can be heritable changes in a gene's expression or translation without a change in DNA sequence, described in epigenetics[2] work. This concept is more specifically described in siRNA epigenetics studies, wherein a transcribed mRNA is bound by a complementary siRNA, thus interfering with (or regulating) the translation of the DNA nucleotide sequence into a protein. These observations have spawned an area of genetics research examining the possible uses of these interfering RNAs as future research or therapeutic tools.[4]

To date, SNPs are the variant type of choice for association studies in common diseases and complex traits.[5] Many case-control and association studies have produced valuable information on age-related macular degeneration, diabetes, obesity, cardiovascular diseases, prostate cancer, and breast cancer.[5] However, SNPs are not the only source of polymorphism of the human genome. Another abundant source of polymorphism, the copy number variants, involves deletions, insertions, duplications, and complex rearrangements of genomic regions. Such polymorphisms can result in deletion of specific genes, as occurs with rhesus blood type, or with higher numbers of copies of genes, as has been demonstrated with α-hemoglobin. Indeed, up to 10% of the variation in the human genome has been attributed to copy number variation (also called copy number polymorphism).[5]

Notably, the number of combinations and permutations of these causes of variation seem endless. Thus biostatistical issues with sample size, repeated measures, sample independence, association versus causation, and such become essential considerations in experimental design and the ability to draw conclusions from the data. One practical result of these constraints with SNP and other studies is that the most robust conclusions can be derived only from variants that have a high enough frequency to reasonably allow inferences to be drawn. It is my opinion that association studies drawn from genome-wide and other, similar sorts of screening studies require prospective focused testing to confirm the suggestions drawn from such large studies.

These and other current advances in causes of genomic variation foretell a day when an individual patient's genome will be part of his or her history and physical examination. This information will be used to allow the anesthesiologist to optimize specific anesthetic effects, such as hyperemia or neuroexcitation in specific brain areas, define likely anesthetic tolerance and thus appropriate dosing, foretell susceptibility to ischemic and other types of brain damage, and apply general medical therapies to a person's specific genomic signature.[6,7] Moreover, this information will undoubtedly lead to efforts to alter an individual's genotype, genomic regulation, or phenotype, either with respect to diseases anesthesiologists see in the operation or with respect to specific responses to anesthetic interventions. A series of annual reviews has underscored these issues, along with a more thorough overview of advances in the genetics of stroke and cerebrovascular disease.[7-9]

Specific Anesthetic Effects of Genetic Factors

Blood Flow and Metabolism

A 2007 study is the first to detail a neurophysiologic effect of an anesthetic drug based on an SNP. Kofke and associates[10] determined the cerebral blood flow (CBF) response to increasing doses of remifentanil in human volunteers, determining an element of limbic system activation. However, subjects with an apolipoprotein (ApoE$_4$) genotype had a different pattern of limbic system response from those who did not possess this SNP. If similar analogous effects of anesthetics are found with other SNPs, we can expect the development of an SNP-determined selection of anesthetics based on an agent's likelihood to produce some side effects, such as cerebral hyperemia, ictal activation or suppression, and variable neuroprotection.

In a nonneurologic context, early studies in rodents indicate that changes in chromosome composition affect cardiovascular responses to propofol.[11] Countless other physiologic responses to anesthetics will also undoubtedly be determined, with each patient's genome studied for anticipated interactions between genome and the reaction to an anesthetic or other perioperative drug.

Minimum Alveolar Concentration

Red-haired patients are known to require more anesthesia than others.[12] This feature represents probably the first observation of a heritable condition's effect on minimum alveolar concentration (MAC), although the specific SNP or set of SNPs or other causes of genetic variation that produce red hair is not known. Early studies in nematodes have isolated specific genes that affect the sensitivity to anesthetics.[13,14] Moreover, specific genetic alterations in mice are being found to affect anesthetic sensitivity to such disparate anesthetics as pentobarbital, ketamine, and nitrous oxide.[15] One might suggest that this field is not that important, because future management paradigms will most likely entail individual titration. Nonetheless, this type of information will likely relate also to pain tolerance[16] and anticipated needs for postoperative pain control regimens and, possibly, to susceptibility to addiction or delirium.

Pharmacokinetics

Genetic influences on pharmacokinetics have become reasonably well known for a handful of antihypertensive drugs as they relate to genetic effects on metabolism (e.g., hydralazine).[17] Certainly genetic factors are known for such entities as pseudocholinesterase deficiency,[18] the interaction of thiopental with porphyria,[19] and the genetics of malignant hyperthermia.[20] Cytochrome P-450 is important in the metabolism of many drugs, including anesthetics. These genomic variations have been reported to affect the metabolism of midazolam,[21] with the clinical relevance made manifest by a report that genomic differences between cytochromes contributed to death from nonmedical fentanyl ingestion.[22] Multiple other effects of genetic variation on anesthetic metabolism and side effects have been reviewed.[23] It is clear that more information will become available with respect to SNPs, arrays of SNPs, and other causes of genetic variation and their impact on anesthetic metabolism.[20]

Ischemic Tolerance

One group has reported that up to 10% or more of genes undergo alteration in expression after brain ischemia.[24,25,26,27] In humans, alterations in expression of genes responsible for the inflammatory response have similarly been reported after stroke.[28,29] Many other investigators report higher risks of stroke to be associated with different genotypes. Thus, the effect of one's genomic inheritance on predisposition to stroke and *susceptibility to its sequelae* may be an important piece of information. However, the preponderance of such research *in humans* deals with genomic contribution to *risk* of stroke and not with direct genomic contribution to tolerance of, or *vulnerability* to, brain ischemia.

These risk-oriented studies are nonetheless important areas of research. However, their findings are confounded by the natural heterogeneity of clinical stroke and provide no information on the possible genomic contributors in humans to congenitally determined ischemic tolerance or vulnerability.

Three lines of genetic research have introduced the notion of gene-based ischemic tolerance as a therapeutic target. In the first line, altering the genetic makeup of animals subsequent to cerebral ischemia has been shown to alter the animals' ischemic tolerance.[30-33] In the second line of work, researchers have demonstrated that environmental factors introduced in advance of a severe ischemic insult can induce genes to produce proteins that provide tolerance to subsequent ischemia. The prototypical paradigm is one in which ischemia or another insult induces up-regulation of heat shock proteins, which are important contributors to subsequent tolerance to a greater ischemic stress.[34] Other genes have also been suggested as contributing to ischemic preconditioning.[35,36] Indeed, some authorities are now suggesting induction of ischemic tolerance as the basis for recovery in an ischemic penumbra.[37] In the third line of research, Kofke and associates[38] have observed that genomic factors apparently contribute to greater release of biomarkers of brain damage during cardiac surgery.

Cerebral ischemia clearly has a significant effect on transcription and translation of important genes, perhaps in relation to organismal survival and evolution.[24,25,39,40] The phenomenon of ischemic tolerance has been known for many years. Although it is incompletely understood, a basis in altered genetic regulation seems likely,[24,25,40] with the most attractive corollary that *such information will lead to gene-based therapeutics.*[39,40] Gidday and colleagues[41] observed that the extent of cerebral infarction in a neonatal rat model was substantially attenuated if animals were pretreated with small doses of hypoxia. This work was further developed and supported with similar observations in other ischemic models. Later work has suggested convincingly that elaboration of heat shock proteins has an important role in ischemic tolerance.[34] Other candidate contributing genes have also been suggested. HIF-1 (hypoxia inducible factor-1) is one such alternative inducible protective protein.[35] Also described in this context are erythropoietin,[36] glial cell line–derived neurotrophic factor,[42] and tumor growth factor-β_1.[43] One report provides convincing evidence that a significant component of hypoxia inducible factor is, in fact, induced expression of erythropoietin.[44]

The pre-ischemic stress does not necessarily have to be a hypoxic-ischemic stress, because fever and acidosis[45] (among other stressors) also induce subsequent ischemic tolerance mediated by induction of a protective protein. Similarly, ischemic tolerance can be pharmacologically induced by pretreatment with estrogen (Bcl-2),[46] cobalt chloride (HIF-1),[35] desferrioxamine (HIF-1),[35] or isoflurane anesthesia.[47] In contrast, ischemia, despite the induction of a plethora of putative protective genes, also induces the *BRCA-1* gene–associated protein BARD-1 that mediates apoptosis,[48] which is thought to be deleterious. Genetic manipulation of mice has been used to demonstrate how genetic factors can alter endogenous vulnerability to an ischemic insult.[31-33,29,49,50] Bernaudin and coworkers[51] identified several genes that appear to be regulated by hypoxia, leading these investigators to suggest these genes could have a role in genetic predisposition to ischemic tolerance.[51] Genetic makeup and gene expression clearly contribute to a person's vulnerability to brain ischemia.

Hundreds of nucleotide polymorphisms are under active investigation of their contribution to stroke and other cardiovascular diseases (for further information, see the website Gene Canvas, at http://genecanvas.idf.inserm.fr/). Such studies in humans generally deal with the role of a gene in *risk* of stroke. Many genes have been suggested, on the basis of animal work such as that already described, to have

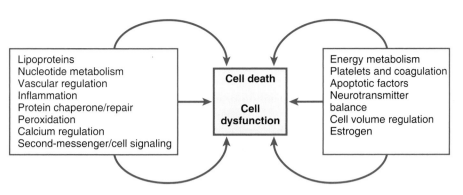

important roles in determination of tolerance to ischemia. However, of the apparent myriad of potentially important genes, only a relative handful has been studied. Nonetheless, one can surmise, from knowledge about the pathophysiology of cerebral ischemia, that evaluation of pathogenetically grouped genes would be a rational approach to screening for SNPs and other causes of genetic variation with potential therapeutic value. From such an approach one could develop "ischemic axes" with corresponding variants in structure and regulation of genes, gene number, transcription, and translation, as depicted in Figure 25-1. This knowledge could be used to develop new neuroprotective therapies or, for an individual patient, to tailor optimal neuroprotective therapy. Finding such clinically relevant effects for a given patient's or patient group's genetic variables will then lead to more intense scrutiny of the protein eventually translated that is transcribed by a given gene. Such information will then lead to rational selection of genes for possible gene delivery or, perhaps, for development of drugs that mimic the effect of favorable proteins or inhibit the effects of unfavorable proteins. Examples of the validity of this approach are now appearing.

At the 2007 American Society of Anesthesiologists meeting, two exemplary abstracts were presented on the neuroprotective efficacy of ApoE–mimetic peptide.[52,53] These abstracts follow several years of work by many investigators showing the relevance of ApoE polymorphisms to neurologic outcomes. Thus it should be clear that unlike most gene association studies used to predict a given patient's risk on the basis of his or her genomic profile, knowledge of SNP associations with ischemic tolerance will likely result in new genome-based gene, proteomic, or other categories of neuroprotective therapies.

Risk of Comorbidities

Gene association studies of stroke are just one example of the role of genomics in defining a given medical risk. Such studies are burgeoning regarding a host of medical conditions. Some studies have shown statistical associations between specific SNPs and specific postoperative complications[54]; examples are renal failure,[55,56] post-transplantation kidney infection,[57] total hip arthroplasty failure,[58,59] allograft dysfunction,[60] pain intensity and analgesic requirements,[61-67] vasopressor requirements,[68] myocardial infarction,[69] inflammatory response,[70] thromboembolism,[71,72] stroke,[73] and vascular graft patency.[74,75] These studies will undoubtedly contribute to risk assessment in individual patients and lead to new therapeutic strategies designed to minimize perioperative complications. Many of the studies deal with cardiac

surgery, but few can[73] be found at this time in the context of neurosurgery.

Application of Therapies to Specific Genomic Signature

As of this writing, characterization of the entire genomes of at least three humans has been accomplished.[76] This accomplishment, combined with previously noted findings, indicates a future that will encompass patients arriving for surgery with their entire genomes on record. Such information should then allow designation of risks and rectification of genomic deficits with drugs specifically tailored to a given patient's genomic endowment.

Stem Cells

Stem cells seem certain to be an important future therapeutic tool[77,78] that will have important implications for neuroanesthesiologists. Neuroanesthesiologists are likely to encounter patients in whom neural stem cells are placed as part of an operative procedure or in whom stem cells were placed earlier, with variable extent of post-implantation differentiation. Given the data suggesting specific neurotoxicity of some anesthetics in the developing brain,[79] it becomes reasonable to suggest that anesthetics used in the context of stem cell placement could significantly affect the success of the procedure. Moreover, the physiologic milieu of the implantation may also be important. One well-known example is the effect of hyperoxia on immature retinal cells.[80] Blood pressure, P_{CO_2}, temperature, and other aspects of anesthetic administration may have similar important effects. Future research will be needed to resolve these issues.

NEUROPROTECTION

Neuroprotection has long been and should continue to be a central focus of neuroanesthesia and neurocritical care. As of this writing, very few neuroprotectant strategies have sustained scrutiny in clinical trials. Significant laboratory work forms much of the basis of neuroanesthesia practice. Much of such work is based on the notion that a physiologic or anesthetic decision must be made and that, in the absence of satisfactory human data, the laboratory data are used to justify a decision.[81] This current situation should eventually be rectified. Some encouraging approaches are currently being evaluated. They probably represent only a small fraction of what will eventually become a part of an evidence-based approach to neuroprotection during neurosurgical procedures.

Hypothermia

Definition of Patient Subsets Suitable for Hypothermia

Hypothermia currently has evidence-based support for its use after global brain ischemia.[82,83] The multi-institutional study in traumatic brain injury performed by Clifton and associates[84] indicated that a patient with traumatic brain injury who arrives at the hospital in a hypothermic state should not be rewarmed, although a protective effect of de novo induction of hypothermia could not be demonstrated. This study was thought to have problems with consistency of critical care practices[85] and must be redone. The Intraoperative Hypothermia for Aneurysm Surgery Trial (IHAST), involving more than 1000 patients undergoing aneurysm surgery, showed no efficacy from the global practice of inducing moderate hypothermia in all patients undergoing cerebral aneurysm surgery.[86] These findings still leave open the question of the potential efficacy of hypothermia for a specific patient with active severe intraoperative focal temporary brain ischemia, without dealing statistically with all of the patients who did not need the hypothermia. The overwhelming evidence of the efficacy of hypothermia in animal studies suggests a need to focus the clinical studies to better identify the clinical patient subsets in which the maneuver will be found efficacious.[87]

New Methods to Induce Hypothermia

As with most neuroprotective therapies, the efficiency and efficacy of the induction of hypothermia seems an important factor. Thus some research is ongoing that suggests important advances in the means by which hypothermia can be induced and maintained.

ICE CRYSTALS

Cold fluids have long been used to decrease temperature,[88] but the approach involved problems with the volume of fluid needed to effect the desired endpoints. Studies on the use of an ice slurry given intravenously[89] may result in an improved method to induce hypothermia quickly, safely, and in a controlled manner. Work is needed to ensure that the infused ice crystals have no sharp edges and thus will have no potential for endothelial trauma.

HEAT EXCHANGE TECHNIQUES

Newer devices available for inducing hypothermia use either surface cooling[90] or intravascular cooling.[91] Future versions of such devices will certainly have servocontrol systems to enable the physicians to program or prescribe the desired central temperature as well as software to ensure maintenance of an unchanging level of hypothermia. A current conundrum in temperature reduction therapy is shivering, which can have adverse systemic effects and prevent achievement of the normothermic or hypothermic therapeutic endpoints.[92,93] It is likely that better understanding of this process will yield a reliable and safe pharmacologic approach to prevent shivering.

HIBERNATION

Hibernating animals routinely tolerate physiologic insults that are known to be deleterious in the nonhibernating state. These animals can induce profound decreases in temperature, can adjust immune function, and have enhanced antioxidant defenses. They are capable, in a regulated manner, to decrease metabolic rate to as low as 2% of normal.[94] This knowledge has led to the notion that whatever neuroprotective mechanisms are operating in hibernating animals may have potential for translation to neuroprotection in humans.[95] A variety of neurally controlled biochemical processes that underlie hibernation have been reported.[94] Neural regulatory mechanisms include hibernation protein complex and a variety of neurotransmitter systems, hydrogen sulfide[94,96,97] and neural circuits.[94,97] Molecular mechanisms of the organismic tolerance of this condition include a switch to lipid-based biofuel, inactivation of pyruvate dehydrogenase, altered structure and concentration of thyroid hormones, altered neuronal morphology,[97] delta opioids,[98,99] and altered pH regulation.[100-102] Moreover, because the heart ordinarily develops lethal arrhythmias at hibernating temperatures, a variety of gene-regulated processes have been postulated to allow continued cardiac contraction.[97] Evaluation of the genomes of hibernating animals is ongoing, with the hope that identification of similarities to the human genome will lead to therapies to activate these otherwise latent genes to better allow humans to tolerate ischemia or hypoxia without neural or other organ injury.[97] These notions form the basis for ongoing research to develop suspended animation methods, with the overt intent of copying hibernation biochemistry and physiology[95,96,103,104] and then translating them to attenuate problems in human neuroprotection.

Infrared Laser Therapy

Recent work suggests that infrared light can be used to penetrate the skull to improve tissue energetics, notwithstanding an anaerobic condition. Data are very preliminary at this time, but laboratory studies are encouraging. Shining low-level infrared light at a specific wavelength improves production of adenosine triphosphate in neuronal culture[105] and improves neurologic outcome in animal stroke models,[106-108] and there are encouraging results from preliminary studies in humans with stroke.[109] If these promising early results are borne out in future studies, infrared laser therapy would certainly become an element of neuroanesthesia management. One can envision the intraoperative use of transcranial or transcortical low-level laser light any time there is an ischemic process or perhaps to attenuate retractor injury.

Spinal Cord Injury

Many avenues are being explored with many indications that spinal cord injury may be amenable to protection in the acute stage and restoration over the long term. Current research suggests the following as approaches likely to be translated eventually to clinical care.

Acute Protection

Promising studies of acute protection include the use of pharmacologic therapies,[110] surgical decompression,[110,111] and hypothermia. Early laboratory studies demonstrated the therapeutic potential of surgically applied hypothermia for several hours in the acute management of spinal cord injury, with dramatic attenuation of paraplegia, as demonstrated by Albin and colleagues.[112-114]

Stem Cell Therapy

The possible use of stem cell therapy in spinal cord injury is based on the use of embryonic stem cells or progenitor cells from other sources, such as bone marrow, to promote regeneration of cells and remyelination.[115-118] Animal studies support the feasibility of this approach, showing the capability of embryonic stem cells to develop into glial cells and into neural cells that make synaptic contacts.[115] In addition to these sources, the nervous system itself may also be a source of endogenous stem cells.[115]

Neurotrophin Therapy

A variety of approaches using neurotrophin therapy[110] are currently being explored, including cytokine blockade,[119] implantation of trophin-producing cells,[118,120] viral gene transfer,[121] and implantation of stem cell progenitors of glial cells.[122]

Activity-Based Restorative Therapy

Animal studies indicate that the paradigm of Brus-Ramer and colleagues[123] and others[110,124] offers promising opportunities to restore motor function through the use of activity-dependent processes to strengthen the connectivity between "top-down" and "bottom-up" pathways. This notion has been further elaborated with early studies evaluating nanotechnology to produce focused electrical stimulation while monitoring consequent neurochemical processes deriving from such stimulation.[125] Clinical implementation of this approach is in the early stages of study and implementation,[115,126] using functional electrical stimulation (FES). The encouraging results indicate the capability of this approach, perhaps combined with stem cell therapy, to promote neural proliferation in the sub-injury areas of the cord.[115] Notably, baclofen therapy seems to inhibit such regeneration.[115] A functional translation of this approach is the FES bicycle, used for years to promote return of function.[115] The best known example of this sustained, determined approach to achieve some recovery after a severe spinal cord injury is the case of actor Christopher Reeve, who improved by two American Spinal Injury Associates grades over 5 to 8 years after his spinal cord injury.[115]

Overall, for spinal cord injury, once considered a hopeless injury, there is now ongoing research suggesting that a probable multimodality battery of therapies may eventually be available.

Multimodality Therapy

Establishing the efficacy of new neuroprotective therapies in neurocritical care and stroke has proved to be an exercise in futility.[127] More than 475 completed clinical trials are listed on the Internet Stroke Trials Registry,[128] with few apparent reproducible results of any demonstrable efficacy in the acute context. However, these many "negative" studies belie the supportive basic laboratory studies that justified the time and enormous expense for such translational clinical trials. I will provide a rationale to show that such results, in retrospect, are altogether predictable and provide an explanatory model for such reproducible futility in a complex biologic system. Many of the points discussed are supported in an editorial by Grotta.[127] It is my expectation that these issues will eventually lead to a commonplace approach to the use of multimodal therapies for neuroprotection. As Donnan,[129] in the 2007 Feinberg Lecture suggests, "We have reached a stage at which research in this area should stop altogether or radical new approaches adopted." The new approaches may include a reevaluation of prospective randomized studies as the only path to new knowledge.

Imagine a factory that makes widgets. A number of processes are important for the quality of the final widget as it

proceeds: conveyor speed (x_1), presence of raw materials and power (x_2), quality of bolts (x_3), quality of steel (x_4), and type of metal used for circuits (x_5). A weighting factor can be applied to each variable (w_i) leading to the following general equation describing the final widget quality (Q):

$$Q = w_1x_1 + w_2x_2 + w_3x_3 + w_4x_4 + w_5x_5$$

Each variable x can be precisely known with very small variation, so any change in any of the variables will produce a reproducible and predictable change in the widget quality.

In a biological system characterized by severity of a pathophysiologically complex injury (S), a similar equation can be derived with important pathophysiologic factors (x_i) and weighting factors (w_i) as follows:

$$S = w_1x_1 + w_2x_2 + w_3x_3 + w_4x_4...$$

Notably different from widget production, however, is that a large number of disparate and potentially interacting factors are known to contribute to S, with also an unknown number of as yet unknown factors with correspondingly unknown weighting factors and variability, partially represented in Figure 25-1. Moreover, each pathophysiologic factor has to be described over a biologically diverse population, such that each factor has an associated central tendency and large normal or non-normal distribution about that mean. Also, the weighting factors and pathophysiologic factors vary as a function of time after the onset of the insult. Thus the importance of CBF is very high early on, but late in the course it becomes a less important contributor to final outcome (e.g., thrombolysis works well if performed promptly but is fruitless if performed a day later).

Additionally, in the context of clinical medicine, there are also associated system factors (H_i), such as nursing ratio, nursing experience, availability of drugs and technology, and efficiency of rapid response teams. A further element of H_i is the variable penetrance of evidence-based, accepted protocols, such as hypothermia after cardiac arrest. All of these local system factors are variables that are also important to the severity of injury, such that the equation can be written as follows:

$$S = \Sigma w_ix_i + \Sigma w_iH_i$$

Given the preceding characterization of the multiple, highly variable biologic and system factors that enter into a given outcome, it should come as no surprise that clinical studies directed at improving only one of the numerous complex factors tend to show no effect, especially if they are multi-institutional in design (increasing variation in H factors), unless it is truly a breakthrough phenomena (large W factor, such as early thrombolysis in ischemic stroke) or the therapy exerts a multifaceted effect (e.g., hypothermia). This situation then leads to the notion that (1) the current, widely accepted methods of advancing clinical knowledge for complex problems is generally a fruitless waste of public resources that produces *innovation paralysis* on the part of institutions, third party payers, clinicians, pharmaceutical companies, and investigators and (2) an alternative method is needed that is based on a multifactorial approach. Rogalewski and associates[130] have reviewed and endorsed this concept, but they failed to suggest a rational means for building the multimodal approach other than trying everything at once, which is perhaps another prescription for trouble. A rational method is needed. It is my expectation that such a method may entail a hybridization of quality improvement methods and standard research techniques to create a new model of incremental addition of therapies with ongoing evaluation of effects. More details on this speculation can be found at http://mkeamy.typepad.com/anesthesiacaucus/2008/01/incrementally-a.html.

Management of Intracranial Pressure

Traditional methods of managing intracranial hypertension are primarily phenomenologic; that is, the ICP is elevated and therapy is implemented to decrease it. If warranted, investigation may be implemented to evaluate for hydrocephalus or masses. However, vascular factors contributing to intracranial hypertension typically receive scant attention for their contribution to an ICP problem. These vascular factors include systemic hypertension, cerebral venous hypertension, and hyperemia. Grande and coworkers[131] have emphasized the role of systemic hypertension in exacerbating hydrostatic brain edema, leading to venous outflow obstruction that in turn further exacerbates hydrostatic edema, and so on, in a positive feedback cycle. Piechnik and associates[132] provide a mathematical model that underscores this issue, in which, although triggered by systemic hypertension, high ICP is propagated by cerebral venous hypertension. Early experimental support for this approach is provided by Hayreh and colleagues[133] and Nemoto and coworkers.[134]

Another little-appreciated factor is the role of hyperemia in the genesis of hydrostatic edema. Observations after arteriovenous malformation resection and carotid endarterectomy suggest a role for hyperemia in contributing to a normal perfusion pressure breakthrough syndrome. Moreover, static observations of multiple patients at different points on the path from normal to hepatic encephalopathy provides strong circumstantial support for the notion that hyperemia precedes brain edema and intracranial hypertension.[135,136]

It seems likely that once appropriate monitors have been developed to provide reliable information regarding cerebral venous pressure and volume and CBF, manipulation of these physiologic variables will become part of the standard paradigm in the treatment of intracranial hypertension.

TECHNOLOGY

Monitoring

Neuromonitoring has long been an area of active research and clinical contributions in anesthesia. Such a tradition is to be expected into the future. However, this area is full of challenges regarding validation of new monitors as accurately reflecting the desired parameter and, moreover, showing that making such measurements matters. Crosby and Todd,[137] in an editorial on ICP measurement, quote Pickering's remark "Not everything that counts can be counted, and not everything that can be counted, counts."

Continuous regional blood flow and metabolic rate monitoring, long a holy grail of neuromonitoring, should eventually be realized as a clinical reality. Currently attractive noninvasive methods tend to be based on near infrared spectroscopy (NIRS), and other, invasive techniques may also be useful.

Near Infrared Spectroscopy–Based Techniques

NIRS-based methods have been explored as a means to discern quantitative continuous bedside information about regional CBF (rCBF) and metabolism. Regional CBF methods that are in early stages of development entail use of an injected chromophore, such as indocyanine green (ICG), or diffuse correlation spectroscopy (DCS). Indeed, these techniques offer the potential that noninvasive techniques will provide important bedside information about cerebrovascular physiology.

Since being first described by Jobsis[138] in 1977 and hailed as the "monitor of the future"[139] in 1983, NIRS has been developed as a noninvasive monitor of cerebral chromophores, such as oxyhemoglobin, deoxyhemoglobin, and cytochrome aa$_3$. This is made possible by the fact that infrared light penetrates into tissue much deeper than visible light.[140,141] Researchers have been reporting the use of NIRS to facilitate continuous bedside rCBF monitoring. The NIRS-based methods DCS, diffuse reflectance spectroscopy (DRS), and ICG–blood flow index (BFI) monitoring hold significant promise as bedside monitors of rCBF and cerebral metabolic rate (CMRo$_2$). DCS and DRS are in earlier stages of development but offer the potential for a truly continuous rCBF and CMRo$_2$ monitor whereas the ICG-BFI method will not provide continuous rCBF monitoring. Nonetheless the capability to perform up to 50 such ICG-BFI studies in one day can allow it to approach continuous monitoring in its capability. These methods are discussed in more detail here.

INDOCYANINE GREEN–BLOOD FLOW INDEX MONITORING

NIRS also allows detection of other infrared chromophores, such as ICG, which has several attributes that make it an ideal tracer to monitor rCBF. ICG has an infrared absorption peak at 805 nm[142] and, after intravenous injection, is limited to the intravascular compartment.[143] These properties make the use of ICG as a marker of tissue blood flow feasible. It is nontoxic,[144] and serious adverse reactions to it are rare.[144-147] Notably, ICG is rapidly removed from the circulation by the liver, followed by biliary excretion[148] with a circulation half-time of 3.3 minutes.[143,149] These kinetic properties make ICG suitable for repetitive measurements even with short between-study intervals without accumulation of dye.[149] With a maximal likely daily dosage of 5 mg/kg based on animal studies[150] and a study dose of 0.1 mg/kg, up to 50 rCBF determinations can be made daily. Thus, although ICG-BFI monitoring is not true moment-to-moment monitoring, being able to evaluate BFI as a proportionate indicator of rCBF every 30 minutes as one manipulates and optimizes physiology or pharmacology at the bedside according to rCBF values is nonetheless a very attractive notion.

The BFI is based on fluorescein flowmetry for measurement of relative blood flow changes in the intestine using intravital fluorescence microscopy.[151] This method entails the use of the ratio of the maximum fluorescence and the rise time of the fluorescence curve. Keubler and associates[152] adapted the mathematical basis for fluorescein flowmetry to the first circulatory passage of an ICG bolus through the brain (Fig. 25-2).

Several approaches to the use of ICG NIRS for rCBF determination or estimation have been reported. The reports can be roughly categorized as feasibility studies, animal validation studies, and human validation studies.

Feasibility Studies. Roberts and colleagues[153] described the use of ICG NIRS in children during hypothermic cardiopulmonary bypass. After making some assumptions regarding

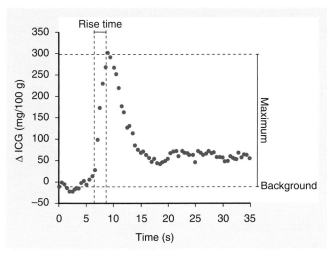

Figure 25–2 Calculation of blood flow index (BFI) from indocyanine green (ICG) kinetics monitored in an intact porcine head by near-infrared spectroscopy.

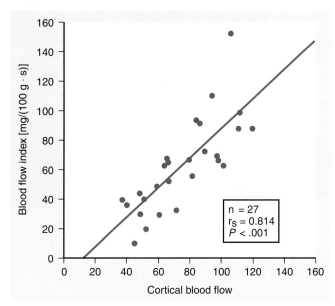

Figure 25–3 Correlation of blood flow index assessed by near-infrared spectroscopy in intact porcine head and cortical blood flow (CBF) in cortical gray matter as measured simultaneously by radioactive microspheres. r_s, Spearman's coefficient of correlation; n = 27 measurements in 8 animals.[150]

the Fick equation, they derived rCBF values, although they did not compare them with any other standard techniques. They concluded that NIRS CBF is a feasible technique warranting further study. In 12 human volunteers, Gora and coworkers[154] evaluated the BFI derived from the brain washout curves and, using the Fick equation and dye-densitometer evaluation of arterial ICG concentration, demonstrated the possibility of using both measures in humans. The coefficient of variation was 10% to 12%. Although they did not compare their results with any other standard rCBF methods, they concluded that the technique is feasible and promising as a bedside monitor of absolute rCBF or of rCBF trends. Kuebler and associates[152] evaluated for extracerebral contamination in a porcine model, comparing BFI from NIRS ICG with quantitative rCBF as assessed by radioactive microspheres. They used a Hamamatsu NIRS system with optodes placed in an anterior-posterior configuration for a transmission (rather than reflectance) NIRS mode. Their data showed an excellent correlation of the NIRS ICG method with rCBF and a very poor correlation with galeal blood flow, although Bland-Altman analysis showed rather wide limits of agreement.

At least part of the significant variability in NIRS rCBF estimates is the result of the noninvasive nature of NIRS and the fact that measurements must be made through an unknown volume of extracerebral blood, which has different flow and phase (timing) characteristics from those of brain blood flow.[155] Leung and colleagues[156] developed a computer simulation using a two-layer analytical model of light transport in tissue proposed by Kienle and associates.[157] Modeled optical data were converted into tissue ICG concentrations through the use of either a single-detector modified Beer-Lambert law method or a two-detector spatially resolved method. CBF values were estimated by the deconvolution method using the arterial input function and the previously described blood flow index techniques.[152] The single-detector technique suffered from significant underestimation of CBF, which was attributed to the lower flow in the extracerebral layer, but the spatially resolved technique improved both accuracy and robustness, especially when used as a relative measure of change.[156]

Validation Studies in Animals. Several animal studies comparing NIRS ICG CBF measurement with other CBF methods have been performed. DeVisscher and colleagues,[158]

in rats, and Kuebler and associates,[152] in pigs, compared NIRS ICG-BFI with CBF measurement using microspheres. The porcine study found an excellent correlation between the two methods, with a near doubling of CBF across the experimental conditions (Fig. 25-3).[152] Springett and coworkers[159] measured arterial ICG concentration with a peripherally placed densitometer and combined this with NIRS ICG evaluation to determine rCBF under a variety of $Paco_2$ conditions, reporting excellent precision in terms of reproducibility, with the absolute numbers for CBF in agreement with previously published values.

Validation Studies in Humans. Keller and associates[160] used NIRS ICG, deriving the ratio of cerebral blood volume to mean transit time, to calculate the rCBF in human volunteers. CBF was altered through CPAP breathing, with studies performed in separate sessions over 3 days. The NIRS ICG rCBF data were compared with data acquired under similar conditions, but not concurrently, with bolus contrast perfusion magnetic resonance imaging (MRI). These investigators found good correlation. However this validation suffers from the following weaknesses: a true CBF measure was not used as the gold standard, the range of CBF values tested was low, and the measures were not made concurrently.

Terborg and colleagues[161] evaluated the capability of NIRS BFI to assess low flows in patients with middle cerebral artery infarctions, performing interhemispheric comparisons of patients with controls. They did not measure blood flow with another method and thus assumed a low-flow condition in the infarcted areas. Nonetheless, receiver operating characteristic analysis of their data indicated excellent sensitivity and specificity of the method in detecting a low-flow state.

DIFFUSE CORRELATION SPECTROSCOPY AND DIFFUSE REFLECTANCE SPECTROSCOPY

DCS for continuous evaluation of rCBF[162] and DRS for continuous evaluation of $CMRo_2$ and oxygen extraction fraction (OEF) are new methods using infrared light to provide real-time continuous information on changes in rCBF and regional $CMRo_2$ and quantitative information on OEF. Promising studies have been reported on the use of these methods in subprimate animal models (Fig. 25-4).

Diffuse Correlation Spectroscopy. Near-infrared photons diffuse through thick living tissues.[163] When diffusing photons scatter from moving blood cells, they experience phase shifts that cause the intensity of detected light on the tissue surface to fluctuate in time. These fluctuations are more rapid for faster-moving blood cells. Therefore, one can derive information about tissue blood flow far below the tissue surface from measurements of temporal fluctuations impressed on diffusing light. Further details of the DCS method can be found elsewhere.[162,164-167]

Diffuse Reflectance Spectroscopy. It is well known that the near-infrared photon fluence rate, a measure of particle flux obeys a diffusion equation in highly scattering media such as tissue. In DRS, light measurements employ intensity-modulated light sources (i.e., the frequency domain technique). The amplitude of the input source is sinusoidally modulated, producing a diffusive wave within the medium. These disturbances are called *diffuse photon density waves or* simply *diffusive waves.* When everything works, a best estimate of the absorption and scattering coefficients at one or more optical wavelengths is obtained that can be derived from contributions from different tissue chromophores. Oxyhemoglobin and deoxyhemoglobin concentrations along with water concentration are the most significant tissue absorbers in the near infrared (NIR). Their combination gives total hemoglobin concentration, which can be referred to as blood volume and blood oxygen saturation or Sto_2, both of which are useful physiologic parameters. Combined with DCS calculation of CBF, these measurements lead to a real-time bedside assessment of $CMRo_2$ and OEF.[168,169] Publications from the University of Pennsylvania Physics and Astronomy Department related to these issues with a detailed theoretical treatment can be found at http://www.lrsm.upenn.edu/pmi/nonflash-ver/publicationNF.html.

In early experiments, University of Pennsylvania investigators compared DCS measurements of flow variation with other standards. Direct comparisons were made to Doppler ultrasound,[170,171] to laser Doppler flowmetry,[172] to arterial spin-labeled MRI,[173-175] and to reports in the literature.[162,172,177-180] Moreover, this group carried out extensive studies in phantoms, wherein the medium's viscosity and the flow speed of scatterers are varied.[162,172,181] Overall, these validation studies have shown that DCS measurements of blood flow variations are in good agreement with theoretical expectation and with other measurement techniques. In rodents this method has been demonstrated to detect hyperemia due to hypercapnea[160,177] and ischemia due to middle cerebral artery occlusion[174] and cardiac arrest[177] with appropriate changes in OEF and $CMRo_2$ (see Fig. 25-4). Human validation studies are needed.

OTHER METHODS

Smith and colleagues[182] have reported an alternative approach, also using NIRS, to measure OEF at the bedside. Two other groups, using the Fick principle, suggested measuring CBF by monitoring changes in oxygenated hemoglobin in response to changes in Fio_2 as a tracer.[183,184] This technique was found to correlate with xenon rCBF measurements in neonates.[185,186] However, subsequent studies in animals and in adults showed an unacceptably high coefficient of variation, and the method did not correlate with other established methods.[155,187] Moreover, there were concerns that altering Fio_2 could be deleterious in brain-injured patients.[184]

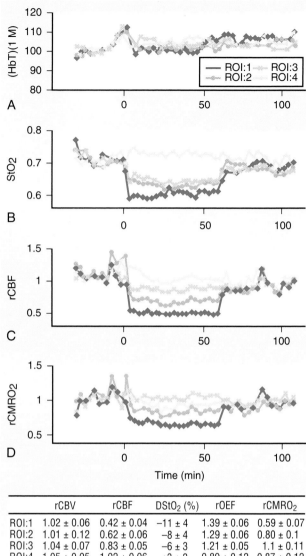

	rCBV	rCBF	DStO2 (%)	rOEF	rCMRO2
ROI:1	1.02 ± 0.06	0.42 ± 0.04	−11 ± 4	1.39 ± 0.06	0.59 ± 0.07
ROI:2	1.01 ± 0.12	0.62 ± 0.06	−8 ± 4	1.29 ± 0.06	0.80 ± 0.1
ROI:3	1.04 ± 0.07	0.83 ± 0.05	−6 ± 3	1.21 ± 0.05	1.1 ± 0.11
ROI:4	1.05 ± 0.05	1.02 ± 0.06	+3 ± 2	0.89 ± 0.12	0.87 ± 0.12

* All values are mean ± SD (n = 5). rCBV, rCBF, rOEF and $rCMRO_2$ are relative to respective baseline values before occlusion. $DStO_2$ is (%) change from baseline.

Figure 25–4 Diffuse correlation spectroscopy and diffuse reflectance spectroscopy results with temporary focal ischemia in rats.[174] *Top panel* shows the time traces of HbT (A), Sto_2 (B), regional cerebral blood flow (rCBF) (C), and regional cerebral metabolic rate ($rCMRo_2$) (D) in four regions of interest (ROIs). Both Sto_2 and rCBF are most reduced in the ischemic ROI-1 and are reduced to lesser degrees in both peri-ischemic regions. Although $rCMRo_2$ is reduced in the ischemic ROI-1 (see table) and in peri-ischemic ROI-2, the changes in rCBF and Sto_2 are balanced in ROI-3. The cerebral blood volume is nominally constant throughout all four ROIs. *Bottom table* shows summary data for all five rats. Regions of interest within the images were defined relative to bregma for ROI-1, an ischemic region; ROI-2, a peri-ischemic region toward midline; ROI-3, a posterior peri-ischemic region; and ROI-4, a contralateral control region.

Reliable Measurement of Depth of Hypnosis and Analgesia

Bispectral index and patient state index (PSI) monitors have undergone extensive evaluation as monitors of depth of hypnosis, with reasonable evidence for a role in some neurosurgical settings.[188] However, this depth of anesthesia monitoring approach provides little insight into adequacy of analgesia. Early work in this area suggests that depth of

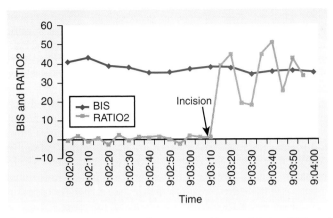

Figure 25–5 Comparison of concurrent bispectral index (BIS) and electromyelography (EMG) ratio monitoring in a human during surgery. Pain induced by surgical incision is not associated with a change in BIS, and the EMG ratio detects the lack of analgesia with appropriate response to administration of analgesic drugs. *From Bennett HL, Patel L Farida N, Beddell S, Bobbin M, et al: Separation of the hypnotic component of anesthesia and facial EMG responses to surgical stimulation. Anesthesiology 2007;107:A730.*

analgesia monitoring will also eventually be developed and validated (Fig. 25-5).[189] Studies performed on facial electromyography, palmar conductance,[190,191] and pupillometry[192] have yielded reasonable results, suggesting that such monitoring should be clinically feasible for future applications. The availability of values indicating depth of hypnosis, analgesia, and neuromuscular blockade, along with cardiovascular monitoring, will then enable the neuroanesthesiologist to precisely titrate the anesthetic drug as a "magic bullet" directed to that element of the anesthetic state most in need of attention.

Continuous Blood Levels of Intravenous Anesthetics

Currently, no clinically available technology provides continuous direct measurement of blood levels of anesthetics. One approach has been to use a pharmacodynamic measure, such as the bispectral index, to derive the blood level that works, even if the exact level is not known, and then to titrate anesthetic dosage in comparison with its effect rather than with a blood level.

Nonetheless, reports now indicate that sensitive exhaled gas monitoring can measure end-tidal concentrations of propofol. Indications are that such a monitor provides a reliable measure of blood concentration.[193] No comparable technology has been reported for other intravenous anesthetic drugs. One might speculate that a hypnotic, paralytic, or analgesic drug of the future might be designed with a chromophore in its structure that would allow its detection and thus continuous monitoring by transcutaneous spectroscopy. One finger for the pulse oximeter, one for the analgesic monitor, one for the hypnotic ....

Brain Tissue Oxygen Level and Chemistry

Brain tissue Po_2 ($Pbto_2$) monitoring has been receiving significant attention. There is ample retrospective evidence to associate a low $Pbto_2$ value with poor outcome,[194] and certainly it makes physiologic sense. Nonetheless, there is a chance that $Pbto_2$ monitoring, akin to the story with ICP monitoring, could become so widely accepted without high-quality evidence that it will become difficult to properly design a study. Certainly one should expect that this monitoring will eventually find a place in titration of the physiologic contributors to

brain $Pbto_2$ to thus ensure that it be neither too high, as that might be deleterious,[195] nor too low.

Exhaled Gas Monitoring

Previously the province of nonportable gas chromatography–mass spectrometry types of equipment, improved sensor and computing technology has led to the capability to place a highly sensitive array of chemical sensors in exhalation tubing of a patient to make significant physiologic inferences.[196] Currently published examples suggest an ability to detect bacterial pneumonia[197] and sinusitis,[198] asthma,[199] aerodigestive tract tumor cells,[200] lung cancer,[201] and tuberculosis.[202] The technology has been reported able to detect lipid peroxidation in food.[203] Given that lipid peroxidation[204-207] or perhaps release of other volatile organic compounds occurs with ischemia, it becomes plausible to suggest that this technology will have a place in screening for immediate evidence of ongoing cerebral (or other organ) ischemia in neuroanesthesia and neurocritical care.

Feedback Loops: The Anesthesia Robot

Multiple physiologic parameters can be measured with digital output that is amenable to feedback loops. Technology is now available or in development that is demonstrating the feasibility of this concept for parameters such as neuromuscular blockade, depth of hypnosis monitors, facial electromyography (analgesia), and blood pressure. Given that the administration of an anesthetic entails provision of hypnosis, analgesia, immobility, and sympathetic reflex control, all of which can be monitored, this then presents the notion of the anesthesiologist's *explicitly prescribing an effect* of a drug rather than a dose as the primary goal in the administration of anesthesia. Moreover, for the neuroanesthesiologist, brain-oriented parameters such a brain Po_2, tissue lactate or glutamate, CBF, and other measures may also be amenable to such an approach. In addition, the notion of providing[208,209] and measuring amnesia is also an attractive possibility, although amnesia monitors at this time remain undescribed (other than as an after-the-fact inquiry).

Putting all of these concepts together produces the concept of an anesthesia robot. After all the physical elements of an anesthetic and surgery are initially set up, the anesthesiologist will prescribe the desired physiologic and anesthetic endpoints, and the computer-robot will ensure adherence to these goals from minute to minute or perhaps even second to second to ensure the most optimal homeostatic system possible. In a manner conceptually akin to a voltage clamp, changes in the rate at which the robot administers therapeutics will provide an additional alarm perhaps before the usual alarm criteria arise.

Blood Substitutes

Two categories of blood substitutes have shown encouraging results that may translate to the future neurosurgery operating room or neurointensive care unit, perfluorocarbons and stroma-free hemoglobin.[210]

Perfluorocarbons (PFCs) were the first-generation blood substitute. They have a linear oxygen dissociation relationship such that high Fio_2 is needed and discharge of oxygen into the capillaries may not be as desired. Multiple trials have been done over the years but without a safety and efficacy profile that has enabled approval from the U.S. Food and Drug Administration. Fluosol-DA was approved but subsequently withdrawn. Other PFC products are Perftoran (Synthetic

Blood International, Costa Mesa, CA; also developed and in use in Russia), Oxycyte (Synthetic Blood International; entering phase II trials), and Oxyfluor (HemaGen/perfluoro-carbon, St Louis, MO; discontinued because of safety issues).

Stroma-free hemoglobin has many theoretical advantages, but numerous disadvantages have proved so far to be insurmountable. The molecule has substantially higher affinity for oxygen, so there is difficulty with its release of O_2 to tissue, it produces problematic hypertension likely related to nitric oxide binding, and there have been problems with renal dysfunction. Nonetheless, research is continuing and may eventually produce chemically modified hemoglobin that will be safe and efficacious.

For the neuroanesthesiologist, these products may have special advantages due to their not being limited to perfusion of areas that allow passage of erythrocytes. They thus may find a unique role for situations with microcirculatory compromise.

Magnetic Resonance Imaging in the Operating Room

MRI is undergoing evaluation as an aid during neurosurgery. The primary impetus is that this modality may help to provide more complete tumor resection and can be used to reevaluate stereotactic coordinates intraoperatively because brain anatomy may be altered during the course of a procedure.[211] This use of MRI introduces a variety of logistical challenges that can substantially increase the time in the operating room.[212] Nonetheless, the introduction of this technology may translate into a modality that provides information of value to both neurosurgeon and anesthesiologist, including biochemical information such as levels of high-energy phosphates, lactate, N-acetylphosphate, and other chemicals. In addition, rCBF and metabolic rate information may also become available during neurosurgical procedures through MRI methodology.

PHARMACOLOGY

"Fast On, Fast Off" Anesthesia

Work has been ongoing for decades in an effort to elucidate mechanisms of anesthesia. Implicit in such work has been the assumption that induction of and emergence from anesthesia are equal and opposite biologic processes. However, Kelz and associates[213] now suggest that the neural substrates that underlie induction and emergence are different. In their work they describe the role of the endogenous orexin system in emergence from, but not entry into, the anesthetized state. This finding suggests that future pharmacologic work in this area may lead to methods to manipulate the process of emergence from anesthesia such that, rather than awaiting dissipation of or antagonizing the induction anesthetic drugs, the anesthesiologist may perform specific manipulation of the neural substrates of emergence from anesthesia in order to achieve faster, more reliable emergence from anesthesia after neurosurgical procedures.

Nonneurotoxic Agents

Postoperative cognitive dysfunction is an object of increasing scrutiny, because it has a fairly robust incidence in elderly patients after noncardiac surgery, ranging from 10% to 15%.[214-216]

Although the precise mechanism of this phenomenon remains to be elucidated, there are ample data to suggest that specific neurotoxic effects of anesthetics could be important factors. Eckenhoff and coworkers[217] reported the amyloidogenic properties of halothane and isoflurane, and Bianchi and colleagues[218] have described behavioral changes after isoflurane but not sevoflurane anesthesia. Moreover, Wei and associates[219] have reported that intracellular calcium homeostasis may be an important factor: Sevoflurane does not induce an increase in intracellular calcium and there is no apoptosis, whereas isoflurane induces release of calcium from intracellular stores with associated apoptosis. In immature brains, some anesthetics appear to induce unplanned apoptosis with delayed cognitive deficits (see earlier discussion in this chapter for possible impact on stem cell function).[79] Nitrous oxide has dose-dependent and paradoxical protective and neurotoxic effects.[220] Finally, opioids used in moderate to high doses produce hypermetabolism and histologically verifiable brain damage.[221-225]

All of these observations and others strongly implicate at least a partial role for many anesthetics in the pathogenesis of postoperative cognitive dysfunction. Moreover, a provocative set of studies by Bohnen and colleagues[226,227] suggest a possible role of cumulative lifetime anesthetic (and surgical) experience in the genesis of Alzheimer's disease, with a relevant study by Kofke and associates[12] suggesting a differential pattern of brain blood flow with remifentanil as a function of a subject's $ApoE_4$ status. The $ApoE_4$ allele of the ApoE SNP relates to a person's likelihood to later experience Alzheimer's disease.[228,229]

As answers begin to accumulate as to factors that contribute to anesthetic neurotoxicity and postoperative cognitive dysfunction, it is to be expected that anesthetic paradigms will be developed that will not have such deleterious side effects.

SUMMARY

In this chapter I have reviewed current research in areas relevant to neuroanesthesia and neurocritical care. Some clinical problem areas have been suggested as important objects of research with a distillation of nascent work that can be reasonably anticipated to translate to clinical care. If these speculations are borne out, the neuroanesthesia operating room of the future will indeed look a good deal different from and better than the one of today.

REFERENCES

1. National Institute on Alcohol Abuse and Alcoholism: Concepts and Terms in Genetic Research—A Primer. 2005 Available at http://pubs.niaaa.nih.gov/publications/arh26-3/165-171.htm.
2. National Institute of General Medical Sciences: The New Genetics: Glossary. Available at http://publications.nigms.nih.gov/thenewgenetics/glossary.html.
3. Chitty M: Gene definitions and taxonomy for pharmaceuticals. Available at http://www.genomicglossaries.com/content/gene_def.asp.
4. Reynolds A, Leake D, Boese Q, et al: Rational siRNA design for RNA interference, Nat Biotech 22:326–330, 2004.
5. Beckmann JS, Estivill X, Antonarakis SE: Copy number variants and genetic traits: Closer to the resolution of phenotypic to genotypic variability, Nat Rev Genetics 8:639–646, 2007.
6. Allen PD: Anesthesia and the human genome project: the quest for accurate prediction of drug responses, Anesthesiology 102:494–495, 2005.
7. Dichgans M, Hegele RA: Update on the genetics of stroke and cerebrovascular disease 2006, Stroke 38:216–218, 2007.

8. Hegele RA, Dichgans M: Update on the genetics of stroke and cerebrovascular disease 2007, *Stroke* 39:252–254, 2008.

9. Alberts MJ, Tournier-Lasserve E: Update on the genetics of stroke and cerebrovascular disease 2004, *Stroke* 36:179–181, 2005.

10. Kofke WA, Blissitt PA, Rao H, et al: Remifentanil-induced cerebral blood flow effects in normal humans: Dose and ApoE genotype, *Anesth Analg* 105:167–175, 2007.

11. Stekiel TA, Weber CA, Contney SJ, Bosnjak ZJ: Differences in cardiovascular sensitivity to propofol in a chromosome substitution rat model, *Croat Med J* 48:312–318, 2007.

12. Liem EB, Lin CM, Suleman MI, et al: Anesthetic requirement is increased in redheads, *Anesthesiology* 101:279–283, 2004.

13. Rajaram S, Sedensky MM, Morgan PG: Unc-1: A stromatin homologue controls sensitivity to volatile anesthetics in *Caenorhabditis elegans*, *Proc Natl Acad Sci U S A* 95:8761–8766, 1998.

14. Kayser EB, Morgan PG, Sedensky MM: GAS-1: A mitochondrial protein controls sensitivity to volatile anesthetics in the nematode *Caenorhabditis elegans*, *Anesthesiology* 90:545–554, 1999.

15. Sato Y, Seo N, Kobayashi E: Genetic background differences between FVB and C57BL/6 mice affect hypnotic susceptibility to pentobarbital, ketamine and nitrous oxide, but not isoflurane, *Acta Anaesthesiol Scand* 50:553–556, 2006.

16. Liem EB, Joiner TV, Tsueda K, Sessler DI: Increased sensitivity to thermal pain and reduced subcutaneous lidocaine efficacy in redheads, *Anesthesiology* 102:509–514, 2005.

17. Ludden TM, McNay JL Jr, Shepherd AM, Lin MS: Variability of plasma hydralazine concentrations in male hypertensive patients, *Arthritis Rheum* 24:987–993, 1981.

18. Hanel HK, Viby-Mogensen J, de Muckadell OB: Serum cholinesterase variants in the Danish population, *Acta Anaesthesiol Scand* 22:505–507, 1978.

19. Dundee JW, McCleery WN, McLoughlin G: The hazard of thiopental anaesthesia in porphyria, *Anesth Analg* 41:567–574, 1962.

20. Galley HF, Mahdy A, Lowes DA: Pharmacogenetics and anesthesiologists, *Pharmacogenomics* 6:849–856, 2005.

21. He P, Court MH, Greenblatt DJ, von Moltke LL: Factors influencing midazolam hydroxylation activity in human liver microsomes, *Drug Metab Dispos* 34:207–1198, 2006.

22. Jin M, Gock SB, Jannetto PJ, Jentzen JM, Wong SH: Pharmacogenomics as molecular autopsy for forensic toxicology: Genotyping cytochrome P450 3A4*1B and 3A5*3 for 25 fentanyl cases, *J Anal Toxicol* 29:590–598, 2005.

23. Palmer SN, Giesecke NM, Body SC, et al: Pharmacogenetics of anesthetic and analgesic agents, *Anesthesiology* 102:663–671, 2005.

24. Tang Y, Lu A, Aronow BJ, et al: Genomic responses of the brain to ischemic stroke, intracerebral hemorrhage, kainate seizures, hypoglycemia, and hypoxia, *Eur J Neurosci* 15:1937–1952, 2002.

25. Schwarz D, Morris TL, Ford OH 3rd, et al: Identification of differentially expressed genes induced by transient ischemic stroke, *Mol Brain Res* 101:12–22, 2002.

26. Tang Y, Xu H, Du X, Lit L, Walker W, Lu A, Ran R, Gregg JP, Reilly M, Pancioli A, Khoury JC, Sauerbeck LR, Carrozzella JA, Spilker J, Clark J, Wagner KR, Jauch EC, Chang DJ, Verro P, Broderick JP, Sharp FR: Gene expression in blood changes rapidly in neutrophils and monocytes after ischemic stroke in humans: a microarray study, *J Cereb Blood Flow Metab* 26:1089–1102, 2006.

27. Sharp FR, Xu H, Lit L, Walker W, Pinter J, Apperson M, Verro P: Genomic profiles of stroke in blood, *Stroke* 38:691–693, 2007.

28. Tang Y, Xu H, Du X, et al: Gene expression in blood changes rapidly in neutrophils and monocytes after ischemic stroke in humans: A microarray study, *J Cereb Blood Flow Metab* 26:1089–1102, 2006.

29. Sharp FR, Xu H, Lit L, et al: Genomic profiles of stroke in blood, *Stroke* 38(Suppl):691–693, 2007.

30. Kitagawa K, Matsumoto M, Kuwabara K, et al: Delayed, but marked, expression of apolipoprotein E is involved in tissue clearance after cerebral infarction, *J Cereb Blood Flow Metab* 21:1199–1207, 2001.

31. Panahian N, Yoshiura M, Maines M: Overexpression of heme oxygenase-1 is neuroprotective in a model of permanent middle cerebral artery occlusion in transgenic mice, *J Neurochem* 72:1187–1203, 1999.

32. Lukkarinen J, Kauppinen RA, Gröhn OH, et al: Neuroprotective role of ornithine decarboxylase activation in transient focal cerebral ischaemia: A study using ornithine decarboxylase-overexpressing transgenic rats, *Eur J Neurosci* 10:2046–2055, 1998.

33. Weisbrot-Lefkowitz M, Reuhl K, Perry B, et al: Overexpression of human glutathione peroxidase protects transgenic mice against focal cerebral ischemia/reperfusion damage, *Mol Brain Res* 53:333–338, 1998.

34. Rajdev S, Hara K, Kokubo Y, et al: Mice overexpressing rat heat shock protein 70 are protected against cerebral infarction, *Ann Neurol* 47:782–791, 2000.

35. Sharp F, Bergeron M, Bernaudin M: Hypoxia-inducible factor in brain, *Adv Exper Med Biol* 502:273–291, 2001.

36. Siren A, Ehrenreich A: Erythropoietin—a novel concept for neuroprotection, *Eur Arch Psych Clin Neurosci* 251:179–184, 2001.

37. Schaller B, Bahr M, Buchfelder M: Pathophysiology of brain ischemia: penumbra, gene expression, and future therapeutic options, *Eur Neurol* 54:179–180, 2005.

38. Kofke W, Konitzer P, Meng QC, et al: The effect of apolipoprotein E genotype on NSE and S-100 levels after cardiac and vascular surgery, *Anesth Analg* 99:1323–1325, 2004.

39. Yenari M, Dumas TC, Sapolsky RM, Steinberg GK: Gene therapy for treatment of cerebral ischemia using defective herpes simplex viral vectors, *Neurol Res* 23:543–552, 2001.

40. Koistinaho J, Hökfelt T: Altered gene expression in brain ischemia, *NeuroReport* 81997:i–viii.

41. Gidday J, Fitzgibbons JC, Shah AR, Park TS: Neuroprotection from ischemic brain injury by hypoxic preconditioning in the neonatal rat, *Neurosci Lett* 168:221–224, 1994.

42. Arvidsson A, Kokaia Z, Airaksinen MS, et al: Stroke induces widespread changes of gene expression for glial cell line-derived neurotrophic factor family receptors in the adult rat brain, *Neuroscience* 106:27–41, 2001.

43. Krupinski J, Kumar P, Kumar S, Kaluza J: Increased expression of TGF-beta 1 in brain tissue after ischemic stroke in humans, *Stroke* 27:852–857, 1996.

44. Prass K, Scharff A, Ruscher K, et al: Hypoxia-induced stroke tolerance in the mouse is mediated by erythropoietin, *Stroke* 34:1981–1986, 2003.

45. Narasimhan P, Swanson RA, Sagar SM, Sharp FR: Astrocyte survival and HSP70 heat shock protein induction following heat shock and acidosis, *Glia* 17:147–159, 1996.

46. Alkayed N, Goto S, Sugo N, et al: Estrogen and Bcl-2: Gene induction and effect of transgene in experimental stroke, *J Neurosci* 21:7543–7550, 2001.

47. Blanck T, Haile M, Xu F, et al: Isoflurane pretreatment ameliorates postischemic neurologic dysfunction and preserves hippocampal Ca^{2+}/calmodulin-dependent protein kinase in a canine cardiac arrest model, *Anesthesiology* 93:1285–1293, 2000.

48. Irminger-Finger I, Leung WC, Li J, et al: Identification of BARD1 as mediator between proapoptotic stress and p53-dependent apoptosis, *Mol Cell* 8:1255–1266, 2001.

49. Siushansian R, Bechberger JF, Cechetto DF, et al: Connexin43 null mutation increases infarct size after stroke, *J Comp Neurol* 440:387–394, 2001.

50. Bruce A, Boling W, Kindy MS, et al: Altered neuronal and microglial responses to excitotoxic and ischemic brain injury in mice lacking TNF receptors, *Nat Med* 2:788–794, 1996.

51. Bernaudin M, Tang Y, Reilly M, et al: Brain genomic response following hypoxia and re-oxygenation in the neonatal rat: Identification of genes that might contribute to hypoxia-induced ischemic tolerance, *J Biol Chem* 277:39728–39738, 2002.

52. Wang H, Sheng H, Vitek MP, et al: An apoE-mimetic peptide improves outcome after transient focal ischemia in mice (A1432). In Abstracts of the Annual Meeting of the American Society of Anesthesiologists. Available at www.asaabstracts.com/strands/asaabstracts/abstract.htm;jsessionid=5014B6559219E13AAAA18EA3576CC207?year=2007&index=10&absnum=2149

53. Sheng H, Li J, Vitek MP, et al: Persistent administration of ApoE peptide improves neurological deficit in mouse spinal cord injury (A1434). In Abstracts of the Annual Meeting of the American Society of Anesthesiologists. Available at: http://www.asaabstracts.com/strands/asaabstracts/abstract.htm;jsessionid=AAD238218DB88421CC91C4C09C802D24?year=2007&index=10&absnum=1336

54. Ausman JI: Perioperative genomics, *Surg Neurol* 65:422, 2006.

55. Isbir SC, Tekeli A, Ergen A, et al: Genetic polymorphisms contribute to acute kidney injury after coronary artery bypass grafting, *Heart Surg Forum* 10:E439–E444, 2007.

56. Grigoryev DN, Liu M, Cheadle C, et al: Genomic profiling of kidney ischemia-reperfusion reveals expression of specific alloimmunity-associated genes: Linking "immune" and "nonimmune" injury events, *Transplant Proc* 38:3333–3336, 2006.

57. Rodrigo E, Sánchez-Velasco P, Ruiz JC, et al: Cytokine polymorphisms and risk of infection after kidney transplantation, *Transplant Proc* 39:2219–2221, 2007.

58. Malik MH, Jury F, Bayat A, et al: Genetic susceptibility to total hip arthroplasty failure: A preliminary study on the influence of matrix metalloproteinase 1, interleukin 6 polymorphisms and vitamin D receptor, *Ann Rheum Dis* 66:1116–1120, 2007.

59. Kolundzic R, Orli D, Trkulja V, et al: Single nucleotide polymorphisms in the interleukin-6 gene promoter, tumor necrosis factor-alpha gene promoter, and transforming growth factor-beta1 gene signal sequence as predictors of time to onset of aseptic loosening after total hip arthroplasty: Preliminary study, *J Orthop Sci* 11:592–600, 2006.

60. de Alvarenga MP, Pavarino-Bertelli EC, Abbud-Filho M, et al: Combination of angiotensin-converting enzyme and methylenetetrahydrofolate reductase gene polymorphisms as determinant risk factors for chronic allograft dysfunction, *Transplant Proc* 39:78–80, 2007.

61. Sery O, Hrazdilová O, Didden W, et al: The association of monoamine oxidase B functional polymorphism with postoperative pain intensity, *Neuro Endocrinol Lett* 27:333–337, 2006.

62. Janicki PK, Schuler G, Francis D, et al: A genetic association study of the functional A118G polymorphism of the human mu-opioid receptor gene in patients with acute and chronic pain, *Anesth Analg* 103:1011–1017, 2006.

63. Kim H, Lee H, Rowan J, et al: Genetic polymorphisms in monoamine neurotransmitter systems show only weak association with acute postsurgical pain in humans, *Mol Pain* 2:24, 2006.

64. Chou WY, Yang LC, Lu HF, et al: Association of mu-opioid receptor gene polymorphism (A118G) with variations in morphine consumption for analgesia after total knee arthroplasty, *Acta Anaesthesiol Scand* 50:787–792, 2006.

65. Chou WY, Wang CH, Liu PH, et al: Human opioid receptor A118G polymorphism affects intravenous patient-controlled analgesia morphine consumption after total abdominal hysterectomy (see comment), *Anesthesiology* 105:334–337, 2006.

66. Bessler H, Shavit Y, Mayburd E, et al: Postoperative pain, morphine consumption, and genetic polymorphism of IL-1beta and IL-1 receptor antagonist, *Neurosci Lett* 404:154–158, 2006.

67. Lee YS, Kim H, Wu TX, et al: Genetically mediated interindividual variation in analgesic responses to cyclooxygenase inhibitory drugs (see comment), *Clin Pharmacol Ther* 79:407–418, 2006.

68. Ryan R, Thornton J, Duggan E, et al: Gene polymorphism and requirement for vasopressor infusion after cardiac surgery, *Ann Thorac Surg* 82:895–901, 2006.

69. Podgoreanu MV, White WD, Morris RW, et al: Perioperative Genetics and Safety Outcomes Study (PEGASUS) Investigative Team: Inflammatory gene polymorphisms and risk of postoperative myocardial infarction after cardiac surgery, *Circulation* 114(Suppl):I275–I281, 2006.

70. Bittar MN, Carey JA, Barnard JB, et al: Tumor necrosis factor alpha influences the inflammatory response after coronary surgery (see comment), *Ann Thorac Surg* 81:132–137, 2006.

71. Miriuka SG, Langman LJ, Evrovski J, et al: Thromboembolism in heart transplantation: Role of prothrombin G20210A and factor V, *Leiden. Transplantation* 80:590–594, 2005.

72. Ozbek N, Ataç FB, Yildirim SV, et al: Analysis of prothrombotic mutations and polymorphisms in children who developed thrombosis in the perioperative period of congenital cardiac surgery, *Cardiol Young* 15:19–25, 2005.

73. Grocott HP, White WD, Morris RW, et al: Perioperative Genetics and Safety Outcomes Study (PEGASUS) Investigative Team: Genetic polymorphisms and the risk of stroke after cardiac surgery, *Stroke* 36:1854–1858, 2005.

74. Unno N, Nakamura T, Mitsuoka H, et al: Single nucleotide polymorphism (G994→T) in the plasma platelet-activating factor-acetylhydrolase gene is associated with graft patency of femoropopliteal bypass, *Surgery* 132:66–71, 2002.

75. Walter DH, Schächinger V, Elsner M, et al: Statin therapy is associated with reduced restenosis rates after coronary stent implantation in carriers of the Pl(A2)allele of the platelet glycoprotein IIIa gene (see comment), *Eur Heart J* 22:587–595, 2001.

76. Chi KR: The year of sequencing, *Nat Methods* 5:11–14, 2008.

77. Csete M: Cellular transplantation, *Anesthesiol Clin N Am* 22:887–901, 2004.

78. Rosser AE, Zietlow R, Dunnett SB: Stem cell transplantation for neurodegenerative diseases, *Curr Opin Neurol* 20:688–692, 2007.

79. Jevtovic-Todorovic V, Hartman RE, Izumi Y, et al: Early exposure to common anesthetic agents causes widespread neurodegeneration in the developing rat brain and persistent learning deficits, *J Neurosci* 23:876–882, 2003.

80. Cunningham S, Fleck BW, Elton RA, McIntosh N: Transcutaneous oxygen levels in retinopathy of prematurity, *Lancet* 346(8988):1464–1465, 1995.

81. Kofke WA: Making clinical decisions based on animal research data, *Pro J Neurosurg Anesthesiol* 8:68–72, 1996.

82. Hypothermia after Cardiac Arrest Study Group: Mild therapeutic hypothermia to improve the neurologic outcome after cardiac arrest, *N Engl J Med* 346:549–556, 2002.

83. Bernard S, Gray TW, Buist MD, et al: Treatment of comatose survivors of out-of-hospital cardiac arrest with induced hypothermia, *N Engl J Med* 346:557–563, 2002.

84. Clifton G, Allen S, Barrodale P, et al: A phase II study of moderate hypothermia in severe brain injury, *J Neurotrauma* 10:263–271, 1993.

85. Clifton G, Choi SC, Miller ER, et al: Intercenter variance in clinical trials of head trauma—experience of the National Acute Brain Injury Study: Hypothermia, *J Neurosurg* 95:751–755, 2001.

86. Todd M, Hindman BJ, Clarke WR, Torner JC: Intraoperative Hypothermia for Aneurysm Surgery Trial (IHAST) Investigators: Mild intraoperative hypothermia during surgery for intracranial aneurysm, *N Engl J Med* 352:135–145, 2005.

87. Marion D: Moderate hypothermia in severe head injuries: The present and the future, *Curr Opin Crit Care* 8:111–114, 2002.

88. Baumgardner JE, Baranov D, Smith DS, Zager EL: The effectiveness of rapidly infused intravenous fluids for inducing moderate hypothermia in neurosurgical patients, *Anesth Analg* 89:163–169, 1999.

89. Vanden Hoek TL, Kasza KE, Beiser DG, et al: Induced hypothermia by central venous infusion: Saline ice slurry versus chilled saline, *Crit Care Med* 32(Suppl):S425–S431, 2004.

90. Mayer SA, Kowalski RG, Presciutti M, et al: Clinical trial of a novel surface cooling system for fever control in neurocritical care patients (see comment), *Crit Care Med* 32:2508–2515, 2004.

91. Diringer MN: Neurocritical Care Fever Reduction Trial Group: Treatment of fever in the neurologic intensive care unit with a catheter-based heat exchange system, *Crit Care Med* 32:559–564, 2004.

92. De Witte J, Sessler DI: Perioperative shivering: physiology and pharmacology, *Anesthesiology* 96:467–484, 2002.

93. Mahmood MA, Zweifler RM: Progress in shivering control, *J Neurol Sci* 261:47–54, 2007.

94. Drew KL, Buck CL, Barnes BM, et al: Central nervous system regulation of mammalian hibernation: Implications for metabolic suppression and ischemia tolerance, *J Neurochem* 102:1713–1726, 2007.

95. Bellamy R, Safar P, Tisherman SA, et al: Suspended animation for delayed resuscitation, *Crit Care Med* 24(Suppl):S24–S47, 1996.

96. Volpato GP, Searles R, Yu B, et al: Inhaled hydrogen sulfide: A rapidly reversible inhibitor of cardiac and metabolic function in the mouse, *Anesthesiology* 108:659–668, 2008.

97. Andrews MT: Advances in molecular biology of hibernation in mammals, *Bioessays* 29:431–440, 2007.

98. Borlongan CV, Wang Y, Su TP: Delta opioid peptide (D-Ala 2, D-Leu 5) enkephalin: Linking hibernation and neuroprotection, *Front Biosci* 9:3392–3398, 2004.

99. Su T: Delta opioid peptide (D-Ala, D-Leu) enkephalin promotes cell survival, *J Biomed Sci* 7:195–199, 2000.

100. Swain JA: Hypothermia and blood pH: A review, *Arch Inter Med* 148:1643–1646, 1988.

101. Rahn H: Why are pH of 7.4 and P_{CO_2} of 40 normal values for man? *Bull Eur Physiopathol Resp* 12:5–13, 1976.

102. Rahn H, Garey WF: Arterial CO2, O2, pH, and HCO3− values of ectotherms living in the Amazon, *Am J Physiol* 225:735–738, 1973.

103. Wu X, Drabek T, Kochanek PM, et al: Induction of profound hypothermia for emergency preservation and resuscitation allows intact survival after cardiac arrest resulting from prolonged lethal hemorrhage and trauma in dogs, *Circulation* 113:1974–1982, 2006.

104. Tisherman SA: Hypothermia and injury, *Curr Opin Crit Care* 10:512–519, 2004.

105. Oron U, Ilic S, De Taboada L, Streeter J: Ga-As (808 nm) laser irradiation enhances ATP production in human neuronal cells in culture, *Photomed Laser Surg* 25:180–182, 2007.

106. Oron A, Oron U, Chen J, et al: Low-level laser therapy applied transcranially to rats after induction of stroke significantly reduces long-term neurological deficits, *Stroke* 37:2620–2624, 2006.

107. Detaboada L, Ilic S, Leichliter-Martha S, et al: Transcranial application of low-energy laser irradiation improves neurological deficits in rats following acute stroke, *Lasers Surg Med* 38:70–73, 2006.

108. Lapchak PA, Wei J, Zivin JA: Transcranial infrared laser therapy improves clinical rating scores after embolic strokes in rabbits, *Stroke* 35:1985–1988, 2004.

109. Lampl Y, Zivin JA, Fisher M, et al: Infrared laser therapy for ischemic stroke: A new treatment strategy. Results of the NeuroThera Effectiveness and Safety Trial-1 (NEST-1), *Stroke* 38:1843–1849, 2007.

110. Rossignol S, Schwab M, Schwartz M, Fehlings MG: Spinal cord injury: Time to move? *J Neurosci* 27:11782–11792, 2007.

111. Baptiste DC, Fehlings MG: Update on the treatment of spinal cord injury, *Prog Brain Res* 161:217–233, 2007.

112. Albin MS, White RJ, Acosta-Rua G, Yashon D: Study of functional recovery produced by delayed localized cooling after spinal cord injury in primates, *J Neurosurg* 29:113–120, 1968.

113. Albin MS, White RJ, Locke GS, et al: Localized spinal cord hypothermia—anesthetic effects and application to spinal cord injury, *Anesth Analg* 46:8–16, 1967.

114. Albin MS, White RJ, Locke GE, Kretchmer HE: Spinal cord hypothermia by localized perfusion cooling, *Nature* 210(5040):1059–1060, 1966.

115. McDonald JW: Repairing the damaged spinal cord: From stem cells to activity-based restoration therapies, *Clin Neurosurg* 51:207–227, 2004.

116. McDonald JW, Howard MJ: Repairing the damaged spinal cord: A summary of our early success with embryonic stem cell transplantation and remyelination, *Prog Brain Res* 137:299–309, 2002.

117. Coutts M, Keirstead HS: Stem cells for the treatment of spinal cord injury, *Exp Neurol* 209:368–377, 2008.

118. Yoshihara T, Ohta M, Itokazu Y, et al: Neuroprotective effect of bone marrow–derived mononuclear cells promoting functional recovery from spinal cord injury, *J Neurotrauma* 24:1026–1036, 2007.

119. Genovese T, Mazzon E, Crisafulli C, et al: TNF-alpha blockage in a mouse model of SCI: Evidence for improved outcome, *Shock* 29:32–41, 2008.

120. Zhang X, Zeng Y, Zhang W, et al: Co-transplantation of neural stem cells and NT-3-overexpressing Schwann cells in transected spinal cord, *J Neurotrauma* 24:1863–1877, 2007.

121. Koda M, Kamada T, Hashimoto M, et al: Adenovirus vector-mediated ex vivo gene transfer of brain-derived neurotrophic factor to bone marrow stromal cells promotes axonal regeneration after transplantation in completely transected adult rat spinal cord, *Eur Spine J* 16:2206–2214, 2007.

122. Biernaskie J, Sparling JS, Liu J, et al: Skin-derived precursors generate myelinating Schwann cells that promote remyelination and functional recovery after contusion spinal cord injury, *J Neurosci* 27:9545–9559, 2007.

123. Brus-Ramer M, Carmel JB, Chakrabarty S, Martin JH: Electrical stimulation of spared corticospinal axons augments connections with ipsilateral spinal motor circuits after injury, *J Neurosci* 27(50):13793–13801, 2007.

124. Frigon A, Yakovenko S, Gritsenko V, et al: Strengthening corticospinal connections with chronic electrical stimulation after injury (comment), *J Neurosci* 28:3262–3263, 2008.

125. Andrews RJ: Neuroprotection at the nanolevel—part II: Nanodevices for neuromodulation: Deep brain stimulation and spinal cord injury, *Ann N Y Acad Sci* 1122:185–196, 2007.

126. McDonald JW, Becker D, Holekamp TF, et al: Repair of the injured spinal cord and the potential of embryonic stem cell transplantation, *J Neurotrauma* 21:383–393, 2004.

127. Grotta J: Neuroprotection is unlikely to be effective in humans using current trial designs (see comment), *Stroke* 33:306–307, 2002.

128. Stroke Trials Registry: The Internet Stroke Center. Available at: http://www.strokecenter.org/trials/.

129. Donnan GA: The 2007 Feinberg lecture: A new road map for neuroprotection, *Stroke* 39:242, 2008.

130. Rogalewski A, Schneider A, Ringelstein EB, Schäbitz WR: Toward a multimodal neuroprotective treatment of stroke, *Stroke* 37:1129–1136, 2006.

131. Grande P, Asgeirsson B, Nordstrom C: Volume-targeted therapy of increased intracranial pressure: The Lund concept unifies surgical and non-surgical treatments, *Acta Anaesth Scand* 46:929–941, 2002.

132. Piechnik SK, et al: Cerebral venous blood outflow: A theoretical model based on laboratory simulation, *Neurosurgery* 49:1214–1222, 2001: discussion 1222–1223.

133. Hayreh SS, Edwards J: Ophthalmic arterial and venous pressures: Effects of acute intracranial hypertension, *Br J Ophthalmol* 55:649–663, 1971.

134. Nemoto EM: Dynamics of cerebral venous and intracranial pressures (see comment), *Acta Neurochir Suppl* 96:435–437, 2006.

135. Aggarwal S, Kramer D, Yonas H, et al: Cerebral hemodynamic and metabolic changes in fulminant hepatic failure: A retrospective study, *Hepatology* 19:80, 1994.

136. Aggarwal S, Obrist W, Yonas H, et al: Cerebral hemodynamic and metabolic profiles in fulminant hepatic failure: Relationship to outcome, *Liver Transpl* 11:1353–1360, 2005.

137. Crosby G, Todd MM: On neuroanesthesia, intracranial pressure, and a dead horse, *J Neurosurg Anesthesiol* 2:143–144, 1990.

138. Jobsis FF: Noninvasive, infrared monitoring of cerebral and myocardial oxygen sufficiency and circulatory parameters, *Science* 198(4323):1264–1267, 1977.

139. Fox EJ: The monitor of the future? *Anaesthesia* 38:433, 1983.

140. Hongo K, Kobayashi S, Okudera H, et al: Noninvasive cerebral optical spectroscopy: Depth-resolved measurements of cerebral haemodynamics using indocyanine green, *Neurol Res* 17:89–93, 1995.

141. Cui W, Kumar C, Chance B: Experimental study of migration depth for the photons measured at sample surface. In *Proceedings of Time-Resolved Spectroscopy and Imaging of Tissues*, Los Angeles, 1991, The International Society for Optical Engineering.

142. Landsman ML, Kwant G, Mook GA, Zijlstra WG: Light-absorbing properties, stability, and spectral stabilization of indocyanine green, *J Appl Physiol* 40:575–583, 1976.

143. Cherrick GR, Stein SW, Leevy CM, Davidson CS: Indocyanine green: Observations on its physical properties, plasma decay, and hepatic extraction, *J Clin Invest* 39:592–600, 1960.

144. Fox IJ, Wood EH: Indocyanine green: Physical and physiologic properties, *Mayo Clin Proc* 35:732–744, 1960.

145. Garski TR, Staller BJ, Hepner G, et al: Adverse reactions after administration of indocyanine green, *JAMA* 240:635, 1978.

146. Speich R, Saesseli B, Hoffmann U, et al: Anaphylactoid reactions after indocyanine-green administration, *Ann Intern Med* 109:345–346, 1988.

147. Benya R, Quintana J, Brundage B: Adverse reactions to indocyanine green: A case report and a review of the literature, *Cathet Cardiovasc Diagn* 17:231–233, 1989.

148. Wheeler HO, Cranston WI, Meltzer JI: Hepatic uptake and biliary excretion of indocyanine green in the dog, *Proc Soc Exp Biol Med* 99:11–14, 1958.

149. Haller M, Akbulut C, Brechtelsbauer H, et al: Determination of plasma volume with indocyanine green in man, *Life Sci* 53:1597–1604, 1993.

150. http://www.drugs.com/pdr/indocyanine-green.html

151. Perbeck L, Lund F, Svensson L, Thulin L: Fluorescein flowmetry: A method for measuring relative capillary blood flow in the intestine, *Clin Physiol* 5:281–292, 1985.

152. Kuebler WM, Sckell A, Habler O, et al: Noninvasive measurement of regional cerebral blood flow by near-infrared spectroscopy and indocyanine green, *J Cereb Blood Flow Metab* 18:445–456, 1998.

153. Roberts I, Fallon P, Kirkham FJ, et al: Estimation of cerebral blood flow with near infrared spectroscopy and indocyanine green, *Lancet* 342(8884):1425, 1993.

154. Gora F, Shinde S, Elwell CE, et al: Noninvasive measurement of cerebral blood flow in adults using near-infrared spectroscopy and indocyanine green: A pilot study, *J Neurosurg Anesthesiol* 14:218–222, 2002.

155. Newton CR, Wilson DA, Gunnoe E, et al: Measurement of cerebral blood flow in dogs with near infrared spectroscopy in the reflectance mode is invalid, *J Cereb Blood Flow Metab* 17:695–703, 1997.

156. Leung TS, Tachtsidis I, Tisdall M, et al: Theoretical investigation of measuring cerebral blood flow in the adult human head using bolus indocyanine green injection and near-infrared spectroscopy, *Appl Opt* 46:1604–1614, 2007.

157. Kienle A, Patterson MS, Dögnitz N, et al: Noninvasive determination of the optical properties of two-layered turbid media, *Appl Opt* 37:779–791, 1998.

158. De Visscher G, Leunens V, Borgers M, et al: NIRS mediated CBF assessment: Validating the indocyanine green bolus transit detection by comparison with coloured microsphere flowmetry, *Adv Exp Med Biol* 540:37–45, 2003.

159. Springett R, Sakata Y, Delpy DT: Precise measurement of cerebral blood flow in newborn piglets from the bolus passage of indocyanine green, *Phys Med Biol* 46:2209–2225, 2001.

160. Keller E, Nadler A, Alkadhi H, et al: Noninvasive measurement of regional cerebral blood flow and regional cerebral blood volume by near-infrared spectroscopy and indocyanine green dye dilution, *Neuroimage* 20:828–839, 2003.

161. Terborg C, Bramer S, Harscher S, et al: Bedside assessment of cerebral perfusion reductions in patients with acute ischaemic stroke by near-infrared spectroscopy and indocyanine green, *J Neurol Neurosurg Psychiatry* 75:38–42, 2004.

162. Cheung C, Culver JP, Takahashi K, et al: In vivo cerebrovascular measurement combining diffuse near-infrared absorption and correlation spectroscopies, *Phys Med Biol* 46:2053–2065, 2001.

163. Yodh A, Chance B: Spectroscopy and imaging with diffusing light, *Physics Today* 48:34–40, 1995.

164. Boas D, Yodh A: Spatially varying dynamical properties of turbid media probed with diffusing temporal light correlation, *J Opt Soc Am* 14:192–215, 1997.

165. Boas DA, Campbell LE, Yodh AG: Scattering and imaging with diffusing temporal field correlations, *Phys Rev Lett* 75:1855–1858, 1995.

166. Maret G, Wolf PE: Multiple light scattering from disordered media: The effect of brownian motion of scatterers. *Z Phys B:, Condens Matter* 65:409–413, 1987.

167. Pine DJ, Weitz DA, Chaikin PM, Herbolzheimer E: Diffusing wave spectroscopy, *Phys Rev Lett* 60:1134–1137, 1988.

168. Corlu A, Durduran T, Choe R, et al: Uniqueness and wavelength optimization in continuous-wave multispectral diffuse optical tomography, *Opt Lett* 28:2339–2341, 2003.

169. Corlu A, Choe R, Durduran T, et al: Diffuse optical tomography with spectral constraints and wavelength optimization, *Appl Opt* 44:2082–2093, 2005.

170. Yu G, Durduran T, Zhou C, et al: Noninvasive monitoring of murine tumor blood flow during and after photodynamic therapy provides early assessment of therapeutic efficacy, *Clin Cancer Res* 11:52–3543, 2005.

171. Menon C, Polin GM, Prabakaran I, et al: An integrated approach to measuring tumor oxygen status using human melanoma xenografts as a model, *Cancer Res* 63:7232–7240, 2003.

172. Durduran T: *Non-invasive measurements of tissue hemodynamics with hybrid diffuse optical methods* [PhD thesis], Philadelphia, 2004, University of Pennsylvania.

173. Durduran T, Yu G, Burnett MG, et al: Diffuse optical measurement of blood flow, blood oxygenation, and metabolism in a human brain during sensorimotor cortex activation, *Opt Lett* 29:1766–1768, 2004.

174. Durduran T, Zhou C, Yu G, et al: Preoperative measurement of CO2 reactivity and cerebral autoregulation in neonates with severe congenital heart defects, San Jose, CA, 2007, Presented at SPIE Photonics West.

175. Yu G, Floyd TF, Durduran T, et al: Validation of diffuse correlation spectroscopy for muscle blood flow with concurrent arterial spin labeled perfusion MRI, *Opt Expr* 15:1064–1075, 2007.

176. Culver JP: Diffuse optical tomography of cerebral blood flow, oxygenation, and metabolism in rat during focal ischemia, *J Cereb Blood Flow Metab* 23:911–924, 2003.

177. Li J, Dietsche G, Iftime D, et al: Noninvasive detection of functional brain activity with near-infrared diffusing-wave spectroscopy, *J Biomed Opt* 10:44002, 2005.

178. Durduran T, Choe R, Yu G, et al: Diffuse optical measurement of blood flow in breast tumors, *Opt Lett* 30:2915–2917, 2005.

179. Culver JP, Durduran T, Furuya D, et al: Diffuse optical measurement of hemoglobin and cerebral blood flow in rat brain during hypercapnia, hypoxia and cardiac arrest, *Adv Exp Med Biol* 510:293–297, 2003.

180. Jaillon F, Li J, Dietsche G, et al: Activity of the human visual cortex measured noninvasively by diffusing-wave spectroscopy, *Opt Expr* 15:6643–6650, 2007.

181. Boas D: *Diffuse photon probes of structural and dynamical properties of turbid media: theory and biomedical applications in physics* [PhD thesis], Philadelphia, 1996, University of Pennsylvania.

182. Smith M, Leung T, Tisdall M, et al: Measurement of cerebral oxygen extraction fraction using near infrared spectroscopy in healthy adult volunteers, *J Neurosurg Anesthesiol* 19:324, 2007.

183. Edwards AD, Wyatt JS, Richardson C, et al: Cotside measurement of cerebral blood flow in ill newborn infants by near infrared spectroscopy, *Lancet* 2(8614):770–771, 1988.

184. Elwell CE, Cope M, Edwards AD, et al: Quantification of adult cerebral hemodynamics by near-infrared spectroscopy, *J Appl Physiol* 77:2753–2760, 1994.

185. Bucher HU, Edwards AD, Lipp AE, Duc G: Comparison between near infrared spectroscopy and ^{133}xenon clearance for estimation of cerebral blood flow in critically ill preterm infants, *Pediatr Res* 33:56–60, 1993.

186. Skov L, Pryds O, Greisen G: Estimating cerebral blood flow in newborn infants: Comparison of near infrared spectroscopy and ^{133}Xe clearance, *Pediatr Res* 30:570–573, 1991.

187. Elwell CE, Cope M, Edwards AD, et al: Measurement of cerebral blood flow in adult humans using near infrared spectroscopy—methodology and possible errors, *Adv Exp Med Biol* 317:235–245, 1992.

188. Punjasawadwong Y, Boonjeungmonkol N, Phongchiewboon A: Bispectral index for improving anaesthetic delivery and postoperative recovery, *Cochrane Database Syst Rev* (4)2007:CD003843.

189. Bennett HL, Patel L, Farida N, Beddell S, Bobbin M, et al: Separation of the hypnotic component of anesthesia and facial EMG responses to surgical stimulation, *Anesthesiology* 107:A730, 2007.

190. Gjerstad AC, Storm H, Hagen R, et al: Comparison of skin conductance with entropy during intubation, tetanic stimulation and emergence from general anaesthesia, *Acta Anaesthesiol Scand* 51:8–15, 2007.

191. Storm H, Shafiei M, Myre K, Raeder J: Palmar skin conductance compared to a developed stress score and to noxious and awakening stimuli on patients in anaesthesia, *Acta Anaesthesiol Scand* 49:798–803, 2005.

192. Larson MD, Kurz A, Sessler DI, et al: Alfentanil blocks reflex pupillary dilation in response to noxious stimulation but does not diminish the light reflex, *Anesthesiology* 87:55–849, 1997.

193. Takita A, Masui K, Kazama T: On-line monitoring of end-tidal propofol concentration in anesthetized patients (see comment), *Anesthesiology* 106:659–664, 2007.

194. Stiefel M, Spiotta A, Gracias VH, et al: Reduced mortality rate in patients with severe traumatic brain injury treated with brain tissue oxygen monitoring, *J Neurosurg* 103:805–811, 2005.

195. Fiskum G, Rosenthal RE, Vereczki V, et al: Protection against ischemic brain injury by inhibition of mitochondrial oxidative stress, *J Bioenerg Biomembr* 36:347–352, 2004.

196. Thaler ER, Hanson CW: Medical applications of electronic nose technology, *Expert Rev Med Devices* 2:559–566, 2005.

197. Hockstein NG, Thaler ER, Lin Y, et al: Correlation of pneumonia score with electronic nose signature: A prospective study, *Ann Otol Rhinol Laryngol* 114:504–508, 2005.

198. Thaler ER, et al: Use of an electronic nose to diagnose bacterial sinusitis, *Am J Rhinol* 20:170–172, 2006.

199. Dragonieri S, Schot R, Mertens BJ, et al: An electronic nose in the discrimination of patients with asthma and controls, *J Allergy Clin Immunol* 120:856–862, 2007.

200. Gendron KB, Hockstein NG, Thaler ER, et al: In vitro discrimination of tumor cell lines with an electronic nose, *Otolaryngol Head Neck Surg* 137:269–273, 2007.

201. Electronic nose shows promise for detecting early-stage lung cancer, *Disease Man Advis* 11:71–72, 2005.

202. Fend R, Kolk AH, Bessant C, et al: Prospects for clinical application of electronic-nose technology to early detection of *Mycobacterium tuberculosis* in culture and sputum, *J Clin Microbiol* 44:2039–2045, 2006.

203. Olsen E, Vogt G, Veberg A, et al: Analysis of the early stages of lipid oxidation in freeze-stored pork back fat and mechanically recovered poultry meat, *J Agric Food Chem* 53:338–348, 2005.

204. Behn C, Araneda OF, Llanos AJ, et al: Hypoxia-related lipid peroxidation: Evidences, implications and approaches, *Resp Physiol Neurobiol* 158:143–150, 2007.

205. Adibhatla RM, Hatcher JF: Phospholipase A2, reactive oxygen species, and lipid peroxidation in cerebral ischemia, *Free Rad Biol Med* 40:376–387, 2006.

206. Warner DS, Sheng H: Batinić-Haberle I: Oxidants, antioxidants and the ischemic brain, *J Exp Biol* 207:3221–3231, 2004.

207. Salvemini D, Cuzzocrea S: Superoxide, superoxide dismutase and ischemic injury, *Curr Opin Invest Drugs* 3:886–895, 2002.

208. Sonner JM, Li J, Eger EI 2nd: Desflurane and the nonimmobilizer 1,2-dichlorohexafluorocyclobutane suppress learning by a mechanism independent of the level of unconditioned stimulation, *Anesth Analg* 87:200–205, 1998.

209. Pastalkova E, Serrano P, Pinkhasova D, et al: Storage of spatial information by the maintenance mechanism of LTP, *Science* 313:1141–1144, 2006.

210. Grethlein S, Rajan A, Bartz RR, Pryzbelski R, Coursin D, Williams EC, et al: Blood substitutes. eMedicine 2007 February 24, 2008. Available at: http://www.emedicine.com/med/topic3198.htm.

211. Yrjana SK, Tuominen J, Koivukangas J: Intraoperative magnetic resonance imaging in neurosurgery, *Acta Radiol* 48:540–549, 2007.

212. Archer DP, McTaggart Cowan RA, Falkenstein RJ: Sutherland GR: Intraoperative mobile magnetic resonance imaging for craniotomy lengthens the procedure but does not increase morbidity, *Can J Anaesth* 49:420–426, 2002.

213. Kelz MB, Sun Y, Chen J, et al: An essential role for orexins in emergence from general anesthesia, *Proc Natl Acad Sci U S A* 105:1309–1314, 2008.

214. Johnson T, Monk T, Rasmussen LS, et al: ISPOCD2 Investigators: Postoperative cognitive dysfunction in middle-aged patients, *Anesthesiology* 96:1351–1357, 2002.

215. Moller J, Cluitmans P, Rasmussen LS, et al: Long-term postoperative cognitive dysfunction in the elderly: I SPOCD1 study. ISPOCD investigators. Internation Study of Post-Operative Cognitive Dysfunction, *Lancet* 351:857–861, 1998.

216. Abildstrom H, Christiansen M, Siersma VD, et al: Apolipoprotein E genotype and cognitive dysfunction after noncardiac surgery, *Anesthesiology* 101:855–861, 2004.

217. Eckenhoff R, Johansson JS, Wei H, et al: Inhaled anesthetic enhancement of amyloid-beta oligomerization and cytotoxicity, *Anesthesiology* 101:703–709, 2004.

218. Bianchi SL, Tran T, Liu C, et al: Brain and behavior changes in 12-month-old Tg2576 and nontransgenic mice exposed to anesthetics, *Neurobiol Aging* 29:1002–1010, 2008.

219. Wei H, Kang B, Wei W, et al: Isoflurane and sevoflurane affect cell survival and BCL-2/BAX ratio differently, *Brain Res* 1037:139–147, 2005.

220. Jevtovic-Todorovic V, Todorović SM, Mennerick S, et al: Nitrous oxide (laughing gas) is an NMDA antagonist, neuroprotectant and neurotoxin, *Nat Med* 4:460–463, 1998.

221. Kofke W, Attaallah AF, Kuwabara H, et al: The neuropathologic effects in rats and neurometabolic effects in humans of high-dose remifentanil, *Anesth Analg* 94:1229–1236, 2002.

222. Kofke W, Garman RH, Janosky J, Rose ME: Opioid neurotoxicity: Neuropathologic effects of different fentanyl congeners and effects of hexamethonium-induced normotension, *Anesth Analg* 83:141–146, 1996.

223. Kofke W, Garman RH, Stiller RL, et al: Opioid neurotoxicity: Fentanyl dose response effects in rats, *Anesth Analg* 83:1298–1306, 1996.
224. KofkeW, Garman RH, Tom WC, et al: Alfentanil-induced hypermetabolism, seizure, and neuropathology in rats, *Anesth Analg* 75:953–964, 1992.
225. Sinz E, Kofke W, Garman R: Phenytoin, midazolam, and naloxone protect against fentanyl-induced brain damage in rats, *Anesth Analg* 91:1443–1449, 2000.
226. Bohnen N, Warner MA, Kokmen E, et al: Alzheimer's disease and cumulative exposure to anesthesia: A case-control study, *J Am Geriatr Soc* 42:198–201, 1994.
227. Bohnen N, Warner MA, Kokmen E, Kurland LT: Early and midlife exposure to anesthesia and age of onset of Alzheimer's disease, *Int J Neurosci* 77:181–185, 1994.
228. Corder E, Saunders AM, Strittmatter WJ, et al: Gene dose of apolipoprotein E type 4 allele and the risk of Alzheimer's disease in late onset families, *Science* 261:921–923, 1993.
229. Roses A, Saunders A: ApoE, Alzheimer's disease, and recovery from brain stress, *Ann N Y Acad Sci* 826:200–212, 1997.

Page numbers followed by f indicates figures; t, tables; b, boxes.

455

464